OXFORD MEDICAL PUBLICATIONS

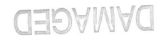

Paediatric exercise science and medicine

Paediatric exercise science and medicine

Edited by

Neil Armstrong

Professor of Paediatric Physiology and Director of the Children's Health and Exercise Research Centre,
School of Postgraduate Medicine and Health Sciences, University of Exeter, UK

and

Willem van Mechelen

Professor of Social Medicine, Department of Social Medicine and Institute for Research in Extramural Medicine,
Vrije Universiteit, Amsterdam, The Netherlands

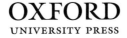

OXFORD
UNIVERSITY PRESS

OXFORD
UNIVERSITY PRESS

Great Clarendon Street, Oxford OX2 6DP

Oxford University Press is a department of the University of Oxford.
It furthers the University's objective of excellence in research, scholarship,
and education by publishing worldwide in

Oxford New York

Athens Auckland Bangkok Bogotá Buenos Aires Calcutta
Cape Town Chennai Dar es Salaam Delhi Florence Hong Kong Istanbul
Karachi Kuala Lumpur Madrid Melbourne Mexico City Mumbai
Nairobi Paris São Paulo Singapore Taipei Tokyo Toronto Warsaw

with associated companies in
Berlin Ibadan

Oxford is a registered trade mark of Oxford University Press
in the UK and in certain other countries

Published in the United States
by Oxford University Press, Inc., New York

British Library Cataloguing in Publication Data
Data available

Library of Congress Cataloging in Publication Data

1 3 5 7 9 10 8 6 4 2

ISBN 0 19 262977 8

Typeset by Newgen Imaging Systems (P) Ltd., Chennai, India

Printed in Great Britain on acid-free paper by
Butler and Tanner Ltd, Frome, Somerset

Contents

Preface

Sports and exercise medicine has evolved over the last 60 years into a major specialism in medicine and over the last decade there has been a dramatic increase in published research focusing on the exercising child and adolescent. This emerging, discipline of paediatric exercise science and medicine is comprehensively addressed in this book. The contributors are internationally recognized leaders in the field and their chapters are extensively referenced to allow the reader to pursue areas of interest in more depth.

Children and adolescents are not mini-adults and measurement techniques developed with adults are often not appropriate for use with young people. Children are growing and maturing at their own rate and their physiological responses to physical activity are difficult to interpret as they progress through childhood and adolescence into adult life. The initial sections of the book address these issues. Part I is devoted to the assessment and interpretation of exercise data and Part II examines the development of exercise performance in relation to growth and maturation.

The beneficial effects of appropriate physical activity during adult life are well-documented but the potential of physical activity to confer health benefits during childhood and adolescence has not been explored fully. Part III reviews the extant literature and discusses the role of physical activity in the promotion of young people's health and well-being and Part IV focuses on physical activity for children and adolescents with chronic health conditions.

Intensive training and participation in sports competitions may start at a young age and even prepubertal children may be engaged in several hours per week of strenuous exercise. Injury is an inevitable risk of exercise and sport regardless of age and Part V considers the aetiology and prevention of injuries during youth sport in addition to the diagnosis and management of common sports injuries during childhood and adolescence.

Paediatric Exercise Science and Medicine provides a state of the art, reference work which is designed to support and challenge those involved in developmental exercise science and medicine. Throughout the text emphasis is placed upon critical analysis of the research literature and potential areas for future research are identified. If the book stimulates further interest in the study of the exercising child and adolescent and encourages exercise scientists and paediatricians to initate research programmes in paediatric exercise science and medicine it will have served its purpose.

Exeter and Amsterdam   Neil Armstrong
January 2000   Willem Van Mechelen

Contributors

Neil Armstrong, Professor of Paediatric Physiology, Director, Children's Health and Exercise Research Centre and Head, Department of Exercise and Sport Sciences, School of Postgraduate Medicine and Health Sciences, University of Exeter, Exeter, EX1 2LU, UK.

Frank J. G. Backx, Netherlands Olympic Committee and Netherlands Sports Confederation, Department of Sports and Health, P O Box 302, 6800 AH Arnhem, The Netherlands.

Gerald Barber, VP Cardiovascular Management, Applied Clinical Communications, IV Gatehall Drive, Parsippany, NJ 07054, USA.

Adam D. G. Baxter-Jones, Lecturer, Department of Child Health, University of Aberdeen Medical School, Foresterhill, Aberdeen, AB25 2ZD, UK.

Gaston Beunen, Professor of Kinesiology and Chairman, Centre for Physical Development Research, Faculty of Physical Education and Physiotherapy, Katholieke Universiteit Leuven, Tervuursevest 101, 3001 Heverlee (Leuven), Belgium.

Cameron J. R. Blimkie, Professor and Foundation Chair, Children's Hospital Institute of Sports Medicine, The New Children's Hospital, Sydney, P O Box 3515, Parramatta, NSW 2124 Australia and the Australian Catholic University, P O Box 968, North Sydney, NSW 2059, Australia.

Colin Boreham, Professor of Sports Science, Department of Sports Studies, Ulster University, Jordanstown, BT37 0QB, Northern Ireland, UK.

Wolfgang Bruns, Senior House Officer, Department of Orthopaedic Surgery, University of Aberdeen Medical School, Polwarth Building, Foresterhill, Aberdeen, AB25 2ZD, UK.

Nuala M. Bryne, School of Human Movement Studies, Queensland University of Technology, Victoria Park Road, Kelvin Grove, Queensland 4059, Australia.

Keith D. Buchanan, Professor, Wellcome Research Laboratories, Department of Medicine, Mulhouse, Grosvenor Road, Belfast BT12 6JB, Northern Ireland, UK.

Robert C. Cantu, Chief, Neurosurgery Service and Director, Service Sports Medicine, Emerson Hospital, Concord, MA 01742, USA.

Albrecht L. Claessens, Professor of Kinesiology, Faculty of Physical Education and Physiotherapy, Katholieke Universiteit Leuven, Tervuursevest 101, 3001 Heverlee (Leuven), Belgium.

Roger Eston, Reader in Human Physiology, School of Sport, Health and Physical Education Sciences, University of Wales, Bangor, LL57 2EN, UK.

Bareket Falk, Director, Department of Physiology, Ribstein Centre for Sports Medicine and Research, Wingate Institute, Netanya 42902, Israel.

Marc Gewillig, Professor of Paediatric Cardiology, University Hospital, Gasthuisberg Herestraat 49, 3000, Leuven, Belgium.

Maarike Harro, Docent of Health Promotion, Department of Public Health, Faculty of Medicine, University of Tartu, Ylikooli 18, Tartu EE 50090, Estonia.

Helge Hebestreit, Privat dozent, Universitäts-Kinderklinik Würzburg, Josef-Schneidestr. 2, 97080 Würzburg, Germany.

Andrew P. Hills, Associate Professor, School of Human Movement Studies, Queensland University of Technology, Victoria Park Road, Kelvin Grove, Queensland 4059, Australia.

David A. Jones, Professor of Sport and Exercise Sciences, School of Sport and Exercise Sciences, University of Birmingham, Birmingham, BT15 2TT, UK.

Han C. G. Kemper, Professor of Health Sciences, Institute for Research in Extramural Medicine, Faculty of Medicine, Vrije Universiteit, van der Boechorstraat 7, 1081 BT Amsterdam, The Netherlands.

Mininder S. Kocher, Fellow, Department of Orthopedic Surgery, Boston Children's Hospital, Instructor of Orthopedic Surgery, Harvard Medical School, Boston, MA 02115, USA.

Gerjo Kok, Professor of Applied Psychology, Faculty of Psychology, Maastricht University, P O Box 616, 6200 MD Maastricht, The Netherlands.

Susi Kriemler, Klinik für Kinder und Jugendliche, Stadtspital Triemli, Birmensdorferstr 497, 8063 Zurich, Switzerland.

Kevin Lamb, Senior Lecturer, Department of Physical Education and Sports Science, Chester College, Parkgate Road, Chester, CH1 4BJ, UK.

Sarah Levin, Research Assistant Professor, Department of Exercise Science, School of Public Health, University of South Carolina, Columbia, SC 29208, USA.

David Macauley, Director, Children's Hospital Institute of Sports Medicine, The New Children's Hospital, Sydney, P O Box 3515, Parramatta, NSW 2124, Australia.

Nicola Maffulli, Clinical Senior Lecturer and Consultant Orthopaedic Surgeon, Department of Orthopaedic Surgery, University of Aberdeen Medical School, Polwarth Building, Foresterhill, Aberdeen, AB25 2ZD, UK.

Per Mahler, Médécin Adjoint, Service de Santé de la Jeunesse, 11 Rue des Glacis-de-Rive, 1211 Geneve 3, Switzerland.

Anthony D. Mahon, Associate Professor, Human Performance Laboratory, Ball State University, Muncie, IN, 47306, USA.

Robert M. Malina, Director, Institute for the Study of Youth Sports, 213 IM Sports Circle, Professor of Kinesiology and Adjunct Professor of Anthropology, Michigan State University, East Lancing, MI 48824-1049, USA.

Ree Meertens, Associate Professor, Department of Health Education and Promotion, Maastricht University, P O Box 616, 6200 MD, Maastricht, The Netherlands.

Lyle J. Micheli, Division of Sports Medicine, Boston Children's Hospital and Associate Clinical Professor of Orthopedic Surgery, Harvard Medical School, 300 Longwood Ave, Boston, MA 02115, USA.

Don W. Morgan, Associate Professor, 237E HHP Building, Department of Exercise and Sport Science, University of North Carolina at Greensboro, P O Box 26169 Greensboro, NC 27402-6169, USA.

Nancy G. Murray, Center for Health Promotion Research and Development, School of Public Health, University of Texas—Houston Health Science Center, 1200 Herman Pressler, W-904, Houston, TX 77030, USA.

J. Alberto Neder, Honorary Research Fellow, Department of Physiology, St George's Hospital Medical School, University of London, London, SW17 0RE, UK.

Patricia A. Nixon, Associate Professor, Department of Health and Exercise Science, Wake Forest University, Winston-Salem, North Carolina, 27109, USA.

Russell R. Pate, Professor of Exercise Science and Chair, Department of Exercise Science, School of Public Health, University of South Carolina, Columbia, SC 29208, USA.

Tony Reybrouck, Professor of Physiology and Cardiac Rehabilitation, Gasthuisberg University Hospital, Herestraat 49, 3000 Leuven, Belgium.

Chris Riddoch, Senior Lecturer, Department of Exercise and Health Science, Graduate Dean, Faculty of Social Sciences, University of Bristol, 8 Woodland Road, Bristol, BS8 1TN, UK.

Susan Rochat-Griffith, Centre de Médecine d'Exercise, Service de Santé de la Jeunesse. 11 Rue des Glacis-de-Rive, 1211 Geneve 3, Switzerland.

Carlos Rodriguez, Centre de Médecine d'Exercise, Service de Santé de la Jeunesse. 11 Rue des Glacis-de-Rive, 1211 Geneve 3, Switzerland.

Joan M. Round, Senior Research Fellow, School of Sport and Exercise Sciences, University of Birmingham, Birmingham, B15 2TT, UK.

Thomas W. Rowland, Professor of Pediatrics and Director of Pediatric Cardiology, Baystate Medical Center, Springfield, MA 01199, USA.

Anthony Sargeant, Research Professor, Neuromuscular Biology Research Group, Department of Sport and Exercise Science, Manchester Metropolitan University, UK; and the Institute for Fundamental and Clinical Human Movement Sciences of the Vrije University, Amsterdam and the University of Nijmegen, The Netherlands.

Herman Schaalma, Assistant Professor, Department of Health Education and Promotion, Maastricht University, P O Box 616, 6200 MD, Maastricht, The Netherlands.

Jost Schnyder, Director, Centre de Médecine d'Exercise, Service de Santé de la Jeunesse. 11 Rue des Glacis-de-Rive, 1211 Geneve 3, Switzerland.

David A. Sugden, Professor of Special Needs in Education and Pro Vice Chancellor, University of Leeds, Leeds, LS2 9JT, UK.

Wendell C. Taylor, Associate Professor, Center for Health Promotion Research and Development, School of Public Health, University of Texas—Houston Health Science Center, 1200 Herman Pressler, W-904, Houston, TX 77030, USA.

Susan R. Tortolero, Center for Health Promotion Research and Development, School of Public Health, University of Texas—Houston Health Science Center, 1200 Herman Pressler, W-904, Houston, TX 77030, USA.

Stewart G. Trost, Research Assistant Professor, Department of Exercise Science, School of Public Health, University of South Carolina, Columbia, SC 29208, USA.

Jos W. R. Twisk, Senior Researcher, Department of Social Medicine and Institute for Research in Extramural Medicine, Faculty of Medicine, Vrije Universiteit, van der Boechorststraat 7, 1081 BT Amsterdam, The Netherlands.

Willem van Mechelen, Professor of Social Medicine, Department of Social Medicine and Institute for Research in Extramural Medicine, Faculty of Medicine, Vrije Universiteit, van der Boechorststraat 7, 1081 BT Amsterdam, The Netherlands.

Evert A. L. M. Verhagen, Researcher, Department of Social Medicine and Institute for Research in Extramural Medicine, Faculty of Medicine, Vrije Universiteit, van der Boechorststraat 7, 1081 BT Amsterdam, The Netherlands.

James Watkins, Senior Lecturer, Scottish School of Sport Studies, University of Strathclyde, Glasgow, G13 1PP, UK.

Joanne R. Welsman, Senior Research Fellow and Deputy Director, Children's Health and Exercise Research Centre, School of Postgraduate Medicine and Health Sciences, University of Exeter, Exeter, EX1 2LU, UK.

Brian J. Whipp, Professor of Physiology, Department of Physiology, St George's Hospital Medical School, University of London, London, SW17 0RE, UK.

Helen C. Wright, Associate Professor, School of Physical Education, Nanyang Technological University, 469 Bukit Timah Road, Singapore 259756.

Merrilee N. Zetaruk, Director of Pediatric Sports and Dance Medicine, Winnipeg Children's Hospital, Assistant Professor of Pediatrics, University of Manitoba, 840 Sherbrook Street, Winnipeg, R3A 1S1, Canada.

PART I

Assessment in Paediatric Exercise Science

1.1 Interpreting exercise performance data in relation to body size

Joanne R. Welsman and Neil Armstrong

Introduction

The appropriate normalization of exercise performance data for differences in body size underpins the elucidation of the growth and maturation of physiological function. Therefore, scaling is an issue of fundamental importance for all paediatric exercise scientists. The selection and application of a scaling method appropriate for the data and research question being addressed is at least as important as ensuring that the methodology used to collect the data is valid, reliable and appropriate for use with young people. Several scaling methods are available and some methods can be applied in different ways. Unfortunately, taken as a whole, the extant literature presents a confusing picture as to which of these techniques is preferable, how they should be applied, and the meaning of the results obtained. The aim of this chapter is to clarify these issues through a description of the techniques available for analysing both cross-sectional and longitudinal data-sets, highlighting their statistical and theoretical derivations. Where appropriate, brief examples are included to illustrate how the application of appropriate scaling has produced new insights into the interpretation of growth- and maturity-related exercise performance previously obscured by traditional scaling methods.

It is important to emphasize from the outset that all methods described below are valid and useful in certain applications; but equally, all techniques are constrained by underlying statistical assumptions which, if ignored, may invalidate findings or confuse interpretations based upon them. The technique of choice will depend upon the research question being addressed or context within which it is being applied. Confusions will arise not only when an inappropriate technique is applied, but also when a more suitable method is applied incorrectly or indiscriminately.

Ratio scaling

Conventional scaling consists of constructing the simple ratio Y/X where Y is the size-dependent exercise performance measure and X is the body size variable, usually body mass, for example peak oxygen uptake (peak $\dot{V}O_2$) expressed as $ml\,kg^{-1}\,min^{-1}$. Stature, body surface area or lean body mass are also, if less commonly, used as denominators but the accuracy with which the latter two measures can be obtained in children and adolescents raises questions as to their validity as dependent variables.[1]

This ratio will produce appropriately size-adjusted values only when the data conform to the mathematical expression of a simple linear model,

$$Y = bX + \epsilon$$

This equation describes a straight line which passes through the origin (zero), where b is the linear coefficient (the slope of the line describing the bivariate relationship) and ϵ is the additive, or constant, error term.

It has long been recognized that, where the aim of scaling is to remove the influence of body size, i.e. to create a size-free variable, the simple per body mass ratio is frequently deficient in achieving this goal.[2–4]

Albrecht et al.[4] list three criteria by which the effectiveness of the per body mass ratio to produce a size-free performance variable can be judged. Of these, perhaps the simplest and most revealing is the statistical criterion which requires a product–moment correlation coefficient between Y/X and X which is not significantly different from zero. However, significant negative correlations (ranging from $r = -0.35$ to -0.41) have been observed between mass-adjusted peak $\dot{V}O_2$ and body mass in adults.[5–7] The data summarized in Fig. 1.1.1, representing 212 12-year-olds, confirm the inability of the simple ratio to remove the influence of body mass from peak $\dot{V}O_2$ in young people, with significant negative coefficients of $r = -0.48$ and $r = -0.64$ obtained for boys and girls, respectively. The practical implication of this tendency to 'overscale'[6] is to artefactually penalize heavier individuals whilst advantaging those of light body mass.[8] This can lead to statistical difficulties when ratio standards are incorporated into subsequent correlation or regression analyses leading to potentially spurious results.[5,9]

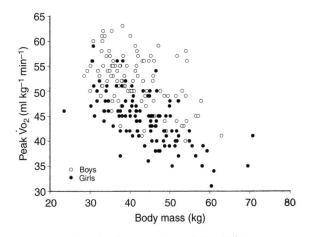

Fig. 1.1.1 The relationship between ratio-scaled peak $\dot{V}O_2$ ($ml\,kg^{-1}\,min^{-1}$) and body mass in 12-year-olds (Armstrong and Welsman, unpublished).

Despite long-standing concerns with their validity, much of our current understanding of developmental exercise science is based upon data interpreted via ratio standards and they continue to be widely used in studies with young people. However, 'continued usage does not confer validity when the application is inappropriate'[10] and unless it can be demonstrated that a data-set truly conforms to a simple linear model (as for example has been shown for sprint running performance in adults[6]) and the computed ratio is uncorrelated with the body size variable, an alternative method should be considered.

Linear regression scaling (regression standards)

In recognition of the limitations of ratio standards several authors[3,5] have proposed a scaling method based upon a least squares linear regression model which incorporates an intercept term,

$$Y = a + bX + \epsilon$$

Here a is the intercept, i.e. the point at which the regression line joins the Y axis, b is the slope of the line and ϵ is the error term (residual), which, as with the simple ratio model, is assumed to be constant (additive) throughout the range of X.

This scaling technique may be used to construct 'regression-adjusted scores' or 'regression standards', i.e. where the individual's residual error (predicted minus observed score) is added to the group's arithmetic mean score.[4,5] Katch and Katch[5] demonstrated, within the same data set, a significant correlation of $r = -0.460$ ($p < 0.05$) between body mass and $\dot{V}O_2$ max expressed in $ml\,kg^{-1}\,min^{-1}$ (i.e. the ratio standard) reduced to non-significance ($r = -0.002$, $p > 0.05$) for the regression adjusted scores, these latter values therefore representing a size-free variable.

An alternative approach suitable for group comparisons is to use analysis of covariance (a statistical technique which combines linear regression and analysis of variance) to compare the slopes and intercepts of regression lines generated for different subject groups.[6,11–13] Where the slopes are shown to be parallel (a requirement of the analysis) differences in the intercept and computed adjusted means reflect differences of magnitude between groups. Using this technique to model peak $\dot{V}O_2$ in 10 and 15 year old boys, Williams et al.[11] demonstrated no significant difference in the ratio standards (values of 49 and 50 $ml\,kg^{-1}\,min^{-1}$, respectively). However, as illustrated in Fig. 1.1.2, the analysis of covariance demonstrated a significant difference between the groups with higher values for the older boys. Similarly, Eston et al.[14] demonstrated how differences between young boys and men in ratio-scaled submaximal running economy ($\dot{V}O_2$ in $ml\,kg^{-1}\,min^{-1}$) disappeared when linear regression modelling was used to interpret the data.

The improved statistical fit provided by linear adjustment scaling, demonstrated by a reduction in residual sum of squares compared with the simple ratio method,[6] has given rise to the recommendation that this should be the scaling technique of choice.[12] However, authors have cautioned that this is not appropriate given the limitations of the technique:[15] although it may be more appropriate to model data with an intercept term rather than forcing the relationship through the origin (as is the case for simple ratio scaling), the incongruity of a model which, through the finding of a positive intercept term, implies a physiological response for zero body size has long been noted.[16] Furthermore, statistical assumptions underlying the use of linear

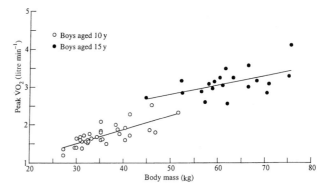

Fig. 1.1.2   The linear relationship between peak $\dot{V}O_2$ and body mass in 10 and 15 year old boys. Redrawn from Williams et al.[11] with permission.

regression techniques require the residuals to have constant variance with a mean of zero. Residuals should also be mutually independent, independent of the body size variable and, in order to carry out parametric tests of significance, these residuals should be normally distributed.[17–19] Unfortunately, these conditions are rarely met by body-size related performance variables in which the data are frequently skewed with heteroscedastic (multiplicative) residuals.[20–22]

Allometric (log-linear) scaling and power function ratios

Where the relationship between the body size and performance variable is proportional but not necessarily linear, a scaling technique based upon the allometric or power function model[23] may be appropriate,

$$Y = aX^b\epsilon$$

This equation describes a curvilinear relationship in which the value of the b exponent describes the curvature of the line and the influence of the body size variable upon the performance measure. Where the dependent variable (X) increases at a slower rate than the independent variable (Y), the b exponent will be less than one, for example mammalian metabolic rate[24] scales to $mass^{0.75}$. Conversely, a mass exponent greater than 1.0 indicates that the dependent variable is increasing faster than the independent variable—as is the case for the mammalian skeleton[24] which is proportional to $mass^{1.08}$. A slope exponent of 1.0 indicates direct proportionality in which the relationship is not curvilinear but described by the straight line of the simple linear model (ratio standard) described above.

The multiplicative error termed assumed by the allometric/log-linear model is an important feature of this scaling technique as it accommodates the heteroscedasticity frequently observed in size-related performance measures.[6,21] Log-linearization of data will also correct skewness and, although the effect of outliers and their possible exclusion should always be carefully considered, their effect will be minimized in allometric scaling.[18,25]

Parameters a and b of the allometric relationship are usually solved by applying standard least-squares regression (LSR) to logarithmically transformed data, the linear form of the allometric equation being,

$$\log Y = \log a + b \log X \log \epsilon$$

This is appropriate providing, as previously mentioned, the log of the error term is independent and has a normal distribution with constant variance.[19,26]

Frequently in the biological sciences[4,27] and recently in the longitudinal interpretation of paediatric exercise performance[28] reduced major axis regression (RMAR) or major axis regression (MAR) of logarithmically transformed data have been used to solve for the terms to be used in allometrically adjusted ratios. Albrecht et al.[4] caution against this procedure where the intended purpose is to derive a size-adjusted variable which is uncorrelated with body size. Unless data are collinear (i.e. $r = 1.0$), using parameters derived from RMAR rather than LSR will introduce systematic bias causing the adjusted variables to remain correlated with X, with the magnitude of this residual correlation increasing as the correlation between $\log X$ and $\log Y$ decreases.

Logarithmic transformation of data also facilitates intergroup comparisons using analysis of covariance as described for the linear model above. The derived values of parameter a (its antilog corresponding to the constant multiplier a of the allometric equation) describe differences in magnitude of the Y variable between groups which can be demonstrated to share a common b exponent, i.e. the slopes of the regression lines are not significantly different between groups. Thus, although its significance is often overlooked in preference for solving for the b exponent (see discussion below), the key to understanding differences in size-related performance between, for example, different sex or maturity groups often lies within the parameter a.[6,21,29,30] Although this analysis is, in itself, sufficient to examine group differences, where an appropriately constructed size-free ratio is required for subsequent correlational or regression analyses the derived slope statistic may be used to compute power function ratios by dividing the Y variable by body size raised to the value of b identified (i.e. Y/X^b). The resultant ratios should retain no residual correlation with size although, as for the simple ratio standard, the distributional properties of the allometrically adjusted ratios may be altered.[4]

Echoing concerns expressed in the comparative biology literature,[4,18] several authors have noted the importance of modelling physiological data-sets with regard for the assumptions underlying least-squares linear regression[19,31] and cautioned against indiscriminate application of allometric scaling techniques. As mentioned above, it is essential to examine whether residual errors display homoscedasticity (constant error variance) following log transformation, for example by checking for lack of correlation between the residuals and log body mass[19,21,31] and the assumption of normally distributed errors should be statistically verified.[19,31] However, even where these criteria are fulfilled there may be circumstances where allometric modelling yields a power function ratio which does not represent a dimensionless variable, i.e. the derived ratio is not independent of body size. Batterham and George[31] demonstrated in adult maximal muscle power data that, although the allometrically derived ratio Y/mass^b was not significantly correlated with body mass, visual inspection of the data suggested a quadratic curvature indicative of poor initial model specification and residual mass-dependence. In this data-set the incorporation of a second-order polynomial term (mass^2) into the allometric equation was necessary to appropriately describe the power–mass relationship in this subject sample.

Solving for the b exponent and theoretical alternatives to $b = 1.0$

It has been stated that 'the objective of allometric scaling is to solve for the exponent of the scaling variable'.[7] Indeed there are numerous examples in both the adult and paediatric exercise science literature where allometric scaling is used solely to identify the mass exponent which describes the relationship between exercise performance (usually peak $\dot{V}O_2$) and body size variables in various subject groups.[28,32–35] Intrinsic to many of these studies has been the aim of supporting or refuting one of the theoretically justified exponents (discussed below) in order to provide a universal alternative to the commonly accepted value of $b = 1.0$, i.e. the ratio standard.

This approach is understandable given that the roots of allometric scaling lie in the biological sciences where allometry, more specifically the b exponent, is frequently used to interpret interspecific structure–function relationships in animals ranging vastly in both body size and shape.[24,36] However, it is important to realize that this is only one facet of allometric scaling which, in application to human developmental exercise science (i.e. intraspecific allometry), is of limited utility and underestimates the true potential of allometric scaling to elucidate key issues regarding sex, maturational and age effects upon exercise performance.

To illustrate this point consider the results from our laboratory in which allometric scaling was applied to the interpretation of peak $\dot{V}O_2$ data derived from subjects ranging in maturational age. An initial analysis[37] identified separate b exponents for prepubertal, pubertal and adult males and females yielding values ranging from 0.647 to 0.917. Subsequently, log-linear analysis of covariance demonstrated that these exponents were not significantly different and that the relationship between body mass and aerobic power in all groups could be adequately described by a common mass exponent of 0.798.[21] Significant differences were apparent, however, in the adjusted means derived from the intercept (parameter a) terms demonstrating significant increases in peak $\dot{V}O_2$ across male groups (contrasting to the non-significant change indicated by the ratio standard) whilst in females, peak $\dot{V}O_2$ increased significantly from prepuberty to puberty in females with no decline evident into adulthood as suggested by traditional scaling techniques. Thus, the former analysis which simply solved separate mass exponents for the six groups provided limited meaningful information—different mass exponents preclude comparisons amongst groups as a different denominator would be used in the derived power function ratios for each sex and maturity group. In contrast, appropriate allometric (log-linear) scaling demonstrated, firstly through identification of a common exponent of 0.80, that the ratio standard would not enable valid comparisons among groups independent of body mass and, secondly, through comparison of the derived constant multipliers (or log-linear intercept terms), patterns of change in aerobic fitness which were masked by conventional ratio scaling. Thus appropriate allometric scaling provided important insights into the growth and maturation of peak $\dot{V}O_2$ which have subsequently been confirmed,[30] whereas ostensibly the same scaling technique applied differently simply provided descriptive data of little interpretative value.

Similarly, in one of the earliest studies to interpret aerobic power using allometric techniques, McMiken[32] reanalyzed data from classic studies of trained[38–40] and untrained[40] subjects and concluded that observed differences in mass exponents differentiated the trained ($b = 1.0$) from the untrained subjects ($b = 0.88$). However, this analysis ignored the possibility that the difference in fitness among groups was simply one of magnitude, i.e. reflected by differences in the intercept, with trained and untrained groups sharing a common b exponent.

Appropriate normalization of exercise performance data is fundamental to understanding aspects of developmental exercise performance free from the confounding influence of body size. Thus, where comparisons in exercise performance amongst groups are made using allometric scaling an important first step is to examine, e.g. using log-linear analysis of covariance, whether the groups can be described by a common slope (b exponent) with the magnitude of intergroup differences then described by differences in the constant multiplier. Data should only be modelled allowing separate exponents when this is demonstrated to be statistically justifiable.[6]

Dimensionality theory

Despite the continued and almost universal application of the ratio standard to partition body size effects from exercise performance, it has long been recognized, even within the paediatric exercise science literature,[32,33] that there are scaling exponents for exercise performance measures such as peak $\dot{V}O_2$ derived from theoretical principles which may represent plausible alternatives.

Assuming geometric similarity (isometry) amongst individuals, i.e. that proportions of body components are constant regardless of size, all linear measurements of the body such as stature, breadths and skinfolds etc. have the dimension L; all areas, including body surface area and muscle cross-sectional area, have the dimension L^2; and body mass and volumes (e.g. of lungs and heart etc.) the dimension L^3. From Newton's second law, time has the dimension L in physiological systems. Thus, peak $\dot{V}O_2$ measured as a volume per unit time should be proportional to $L^3 - L = L^2$. In other words, in order to dissociate peak $\dot{V}O_2$ from body size, values should be expressed as ml min^{-1} m^{-2}. Alternatively, as stature^2 is analogous to mass raised to the 2/3 power in geometrically similar bodies, an alternative, equivalent denominator for peak $\dot{V}O_2$ would be mass$^{0.67}$.[41] It is important to note that others have suggested that this is theoretically simplistic,[42] and have demonstrated that simple dimensionality theory does not necessarily predict a mass exponent of 2/3.

Other authors have advocated a scaling exponent of mass raised to the power 3/4 (analogous to stature$^{2.25}$) based upon empirical observations[43,44] that metabolic rate in many species of homeotherms does not appear to conform to the expected surface law, mass$^{0.67}$, but rather increases proportional to mass$^{0.75}$. To provide a rationale for this apparent departure from theoretical predictions, McMahon[45] proposed a model of elastic similarity based upon engineering principles whereby biological proportions and metabolic rates are limited by the elastic properties of the animal, properties which ensure that bending and buckling forces during locomotion do not impair the structural integrity of the limbs and joints. However, the concept of elastic similarity has been questioned[46] and the exponent of 3/4 explained as a statistical artefact caused by fitting a single allometric model to data obtained from a number of different species,[47] which, when analyzed separately, have intraspecific slopes of $b = 0.67$.[24] Other authors maintain that there is no biologically meaningful explanation for the 3/4 power[48] or question the validity of extrapolating an exponent for resting oxygen consumption to describe maximal oxygen uptake,[33] but, nevertheless, both theoretical values have been and continue to be, explored as possibilities of representing a universal alternative to 1.0 for the expression of size-independent peak $\dot{V}O_2$.

Empirical findings

Several studies modelling adult peak $\dot{V}O_2$ data have identified mass exponents close to or equal to 0.67,[6,49,50] which have been interpreted as providing support for more general application of the 2/3 power suggested by geometric similarity and empirical intraspecific allometry. Other authors modelling a broader age range (up to 79 years) have provided data to support the preferential application of the 3/4 power when mass is included as the sole covariate, but demonstrated that this reduces to a value not significantly different from 0.67 when other known covariates are partitioned out.[26]

Empirical data from studies with young people present an inconsistent picture. Review articles summarizing mass exponents for peak $\dot{V}O_2$ identified in cross-sectional studies with young people[51,52] report values which, although typically less than the 1.0 of the ratio standard, range from 0.37 to 1.07 with virtually no two studies yielding the same values. Given this variability in results it is not surprising that some authors have commented that there is no sound reason to abandon general application of the simple ratio standard.[53–55]

What reasons can be offered in explanation for the diversity of exponents reported? One possibility is that the assumption of isometry is untenable during growth and maturation. Although, overall, geometric similarity appears to be a reasonable supposition in children and adults at least from the age of seven years,[56] differential rates of individual growth during puberty may distort the proportional relationship. However, it has been suggested that as children follow a common rhythm of growth, deviations from geometric similarity during growth should themselves be systematic.[57] The range of reported exponents suggests that this is not the case.

Much of the variation in reported mass exponents is likely to be explained by differences in factors such as sample size and heterogeneity. It has been suggested that meaningful exponents will only be observed in large subject groups encompassing a wide range of body size,[58] but homogeneity with respect to other confounding covariates may also be important.[26] In adults, Heil[26] has suggested that an exponent of 0.67 will be identified in groups homogeneous for covariates such as stature, training status and body composition, whereas a value of 0.75 may be a more appropriate descriptor for heterogeneous subject groups.

Such factors are likely to influence mass exponents identified in young people. For example, we reported a mass exponent of 0.65 in a sample of 164 prepubertal children,[29] but this value was reduced to 0.52 in another sample of only 32 prepubescents.[59] Similarly, exponents close to 1.0 have tended to derive from studies where a large age range (and hence body size and maturational age range) is represented.[60–62] In these cases, the mass exponent may be inflated if other confounding variables are not concurrently covaried out. For example, it has been postulated[63] that the theoretical 0.75 exponent is an artefact caused by failing to account for the disproportionate increase in muscle mass which accompanies increasing body size.[64,65] Nevill[63] demonstrated in heterogeneous subject groups how extension of the allometric equation to include stature as an additional covariate reduced the mass exponent to values closer to the theoretically anticipated 0.67. A similar reduction in the mass exponent from 0.80 to 0.71 has been demonstrated in the comparison of peak $\dot{V}O_2$ in prepubertal, pubertal and adult subjects following the incorporation of stature as an additional covariate in the allometric analysis.[21]

Although Nevill's hypothesis has been dismissed as statistical artefact resulting from collinearity between stature and mass in a least-squares regression analysis,[66] studies with adults[26] and young people[21,67] have confirmed a significant, independent contribution of stature to peak $\dot{V}O_2$. Although the significance of the stature exponent remains contentious, perhaps, for example acting as a surrogate for lung function[68] or skinfold thicknesses,[69] these studies do demonstrate the flexibility of the allometric approach and the need to incorporate several covariates into an analysis. The independent effect of mass on the performance variable will be observed only once other covariates, which may include age, stature, skinfold thickness and lung function have been investigated and statistically accounted for.

It is important to emphasize that lack of concordance between empirically derived values and theoretical exponents when scaling peak aerobic performance, no more invalidates allometry as an effective tool for elucidating group differences in a variety of size-dependent exercise performance measures, than does continued usage of ratio standards confer validity upon their use as a scaling technique. As illustrated above, the *b* exponent obtained is often of secondary importance in comparative studies and is evidently sample-specific and influenced by other known covariates.

Scaling for body size differences in longitudinal data-sets

Ontogenetic allometry

The interpretation of size-dependent performance measures in longitudinal data-sets represents a formidable challenge to the paediatric exercise scientist. As discussed above, there is considerable evidence to suggest that the simple ratio approach will fail to produce a size-free variable and thus is unlikely to provide a satisfactory picture of developmental trends. An analysis based upon allometric interpretation is likely to be more revealing. Various approaches to partitioning body size effects from longitudinal data-sets based upon allometric principles have been applied to studies of peak aerobic fitness in young people and these will serve to illustrate their relative merits and disadvantages.

Several studies have adopted an ontogenetic allometric approach,[36] ontogenetic allometry referring to the examination of differential growth rates within the individual growth process. This technique involves the computation of a body size exponent for each subject from the slope of the log-linear regression line describing the individual's longitudinal data-set.[28,57,62,70] These individual exponents can be subsequently averaged to describe, for example, sex[70] or maturity groups.[28]

The range of mean ontogenetic exponents observed in these studies is broadly comparable to that demonstrated in cross-sectional studies. In several of these studies, a stated aim has been to compare the empirically derived mean exponents against the theoretically predicted values (0.67 and 0.74) in order to recommend a universal exponent. However, a common feature of these studies has been an extremely broad interindividual range in mass exponents: Rowland et al.[70] reported values ranging from $b = 0.18$ to 1.74 in 20 children measured annually for five years from the mean age of 9.2 y. This led the authors to comment that

the variability of exponents in this study…suggests that it is unlikely that a single exponent will be identified that accurately normalizes $\dot{V}O_2$ max in the childhood population (Ref. 70, p. 271).

Thus, the application of a theoretical value of 0.67 to assess longitudinal tracking of aerobic fitness[71] is not recommended as, although likely to provide more plausible results than the ratio standard, it is unlikely to provide an exact sample-specific exponent.

One limitation of this approach is its focus upon deriving exponents for individuals or discrete groups. Thus this method has limited utility for the examination of key questions such as identification and quantification of the interactive effect of sex, maturity and body size upon the development of aerobic power,[30,37] although the finding of significantly different mass exponents for boys and girls,[70] albeit in a very small sample, is intriguing and warrants further examination in more representative data-sets. Furthermore, from a statistical viewpoint this approach is inefficient as statistics from the individual analyses (the slope and intercept parameters) can only be partially accommodated in a subsequent between-group analysis.[67]

Multilevel modelling

Multilevel modelling[72] is essentially an extension of multiple regression which is appropriate for analyzing hierarchically structured or nested data. In longitudinal (repeated measures) data this hierarchy can be viewed as occurring at two levels; level 1 being the repeated measurement occasions which are grouped or nested within the level 2 unit—in this case the individual subject.

Multilevel modelling is preferable to conventional analytical approaches for longitudinal data as, in addition to describing the population mean response, random variation around this mean at both levels is recognized and statistically described. For example at level 2, individuals have their own growth rates which are allowed to vary randomly around the underlying mean group response. At level 1, each individual's observed measurements may vary around their own underlying growth trajectory, particularly where the testing occasions are not equally spaced. Furthermore, unlike traditional methods based upon repeated measures analysis of variance which require a complete longitudinal data-set, this method is able to handle unbalanced data, for example where one or more measurement occasions has been missed. Similarly, as individual growth trajectories can be modelled, differing intervals between measurement occasions can be accommodated. The procedure is statistically efficient and easily adaptable to a multivariate approach, allowing the effects and relative importance of a variety of explanatory variables or combinations of explanatory variables to be investigated and quantified.[73]

As with the scaling of cross-sectional data, the same problems and issues regarding the use of an additive linear (polynomial)[74] versus a multiplicative allometric approach[67] apply when using multilevel regression modelling, with the latter demonstrated to be theoretically and statistically superior for longitudinal analyses.[67] The use of multilevel modelling to interpret developmental changes in aerobic fitness is discussed in Chapter 2.8 and elsewhere.[69] The technique has also provided valuable insights into longitudinal changes in young people's submaximal $\dot{V}O_2$,[75] short term power output,[76] and strength.[67]

Summary

Appropriate scaling underpins our interpretation of developmental exercise science and there is now considerable evidence to refute the validity of the ratio standard as the automatic response to the need to remove body size effects from physiological function. Scaling techniques based upon least-squares linear regression have statistical advantages, but as size-related exercise performance data-sets are often skewed with heteroscedastic errors, logarithmic transformation of data prior to analysis is recommended and will allow identification of allometric parameters.

The appropriate application of allometric principles to the interpretation of size-dependent exercise performance in young people has already provided insights previously masked by conventional ratio scaling. However, allometric body size exponents are highly sample specific, reflecting differences in sample size, composition, age, and where other covariates have been accounted for. This lack of generalizability has been supported in longitudinal studies where ontogenetic body size exponents have shown extreme interindividual variation. Multilevel regression modelling techniques using a multiplicative, allometric approach are increasingly being used, and enable a sensitive and detailed interpretation of longitudinal exercise data. However, as eloquently summarized by Ross *et al.* (See Ref. 57, p. 137).

> The use of allometry as an analytic stratagem helps bring a quantitative orderliness to the complexity of the assessment of human structure and function. It does not explain individual differences, it serves to identify them.

The real challenge to the paediatric research scientist, then, is to elucidate the physiological and metabolic processes underlying these differences.

References

1. Rowland, T. W. *Developmental exercise physiology.* Human Kinetics Publishers, Champaign, Il, 1996.
2. DuBois, P. H. On the statistics of ratios. *American Journal of Psychology* 1948; **3**: 309–15.
3. Tanner, J. M. Fallacy of per-weight and per-surface area standards and their relation to spurious correlation. *Journal of Applied Physiology* 1949; **2**: 1–15.
4. Albrecht, G. H., Gelvin, B. R. and Hartman, S. E. Ratios as a size adjustment in morphometrics. *American Journal of Physical Anthropology* 1993; **91**: 441–68.
5. Katch, V. L. and Katch, F. I. Use of weight-adjusted oxygen uptake scores that avoid spurious correlation. *Research Quarterly* 1974; **45**: 447–51.
6. Nevill, A., Ramsbottom, R. and Williams, C. Scaling physiological measurements for individuals of different body size. *European Journal of Applied Physiology* 1992; **65**: 110–7.
7. Davies, M. J., Dalsky, G. P. and Vanderburgh, P. M. Allometric scaling of $\dot{V}O_2$ max and lean body mass in older men. *Journal of Ageing and Physical Activity* 1995; **3**: 324–31.
8. Winter, E. M. Scaling: Partitioning out differences in size. *Pediatric Exercise Science* 1992; **4**: 296–301.
9. Katch, V. L. Use of the oxygen/body weight ratio in correlational analyses: Spurious correlations and statistical considerations. *Medicine and Science in Sports* 1973; **5**: 252–7.
10. Cotes, J. E. and Reed, J. W. Ratios and regressions in body size and function: A commentary. *Journal of Applied Physiology* 1995; **78**: 2328–9.
11. Williams, J. R., Armstrong, N., Winter, E. M. and Crichton, N. Changes in peak oxygen uptake with age and sexual maturation in boys: Physiological fact or statistical anomaly? In. *Children and exercise XVI.* (ed. J. Coudert and E Van Praagh). Masson, Paris, 1992; 35–7.
12. Toth, M. J., Goran, M. I., Ades, P. A., Howard, D. B. and Poehlman, E. T. Examination of data normalization procedures for expressing peak $\dot{V}O_2$ data. *Journal of Applied Physiology* 1993; **75**: 2288–92.
13. Nindl, B. C., Mahar, M. T., Harman, E. and Patton, J. F. Lower and upper body anaerobic performance in male and female adolescent athletes. *Medicine and Science in Sports and Exercise* 1995; **27**: 235–41.
14. Eston, R. G., Robson, S. and Winter, E. A comparison of oxygen uptake during running in children and adults. In. *Kinanthropometry IV* (ed. W. Duquet and J. Day). E. and F. N. Spon, London, 1993; 236–41.
15. Cooper, D. M. and Berman, N. Ratios and regressions in body size and function: A commentary. *Journal of Applied Physiology* 1995; **77**: 2015–7.
16. Kleiber, M. Physiological meaning of regression equations. *Journal of Applied Physiology* 1950; **2**: 417–23.
17. Manaster, B. J. and Manaster, S. Techniques for estimating allometric equations. *Journal of Morphology* 1975; **147**: 299–308.
18. Smith, R. J. Allometric scaling in comparative biology: Problems of concept and method. *American Journal of Physiology* 1984; **246**: R152–60.
19. Nevill, A. M. and Holder, R. L. Scaling, normalizing and per ratio standards: An allometric modelling approach. *Journal of Applied Physiology* 1995; **79**: 1027–31.
20. Nevill, A. M. and Holder R. L. Modelling maximum oxygen uptake—a case-study in non-linear regression model formulation and comparison. *Applied Statistics* 1994; **43**: 653–66.
21. Welsman, J., Armstrong, N., Kirby, B. J., Nevill, A. M. and Winter, E. Scaling peak oxygen uptake for differences in body size. *Medicine and Science in Sports and Exercise* 1996; **28**: 259–65.
22. Nevill, A. M. The appropriate use of scaling techniques in exercise physiology. *Pediatric Exercise Science* 1997; **9**: 295–8.
23. Huxley, J. *Problems of relative growth.* Methuen, London, 1932.
24. Schmidt-Nielsen, K. *Scaling: Why is animal size so important?* Cambridge University Press, Cambridge, 1984.
25. Jolicoeur, P. and Heusner, A. A. The allometry equation in the analysis of the standard oxygen consumption and body weight of the white rat. *Biometrics* 1971; **27**: 841–55.
26. Heil, D. P. Body mass scaling of peak oxygen uptake in 20- to 79-yr-old adults. *Medicine and Science in Sports and Exercise* 1998; **29**: 1602–8.
27. Corruccini, R. S. Multivariate morphometric data transformations. *Journal of Human Evolution* 1986; **15**: 139–41.
28. Beunen, G. P., Rogers, D. M., Woynarowska, B. and Malina, R. M. Longitudinal study of ontogenetic allometry of oxygen uptake in boys and girls grouped by maturity status. *Annals of Human Biology* 1997; **24**: 33–43.
29. Armstrong, N., Kirby, B., McManus, A. and Welsman, J. Aerobic fitness of pre-pubescent children. *Annals of Human Biology* 1995; **22**: 427–41.
30. Armstrong, N., Welsman, J. R. and Kirby, B. J. Peak $\dot{V}O_2$ and maturation in 12-yr olds. *Medicine and Science in Sports and Exercise* 1998; **30**: 165–9.
31. Batterham, A. M., Tolfrey, K. and George, K. P. Nevill's explanation of Kleiber's 0.75 mass exponent: An artefact of collinearity problems in least squares model? *Journal of Applied Physiology* 1997; **82**: 693–7.
32. McMiken, D. F. Maximum aerobic power and physical dimensions of children. *Annals of Human Biology* 1976; **3**: 141–7.
33. Bailey, D. A., Ross, W. D., Mirwald, R. L. and Weese, C. Size dissociation of maximal aerobic power during growth in boys. *Medicine Sport* 1978; **11**: 140–51.
34. Rogers, D. M., Olson, B. and Wilmore, J. H. Scaling for the $\dot{V}O_2$-to-body size relationship among children and adults. *Journal of Applied Physiology* 1995; **79**: 958–67.
35. Rogers, D. M., Turley, K. R., Kujawa K. I., Harper, K. M. and Wilmore, J. H. Allometric scaling factors for oxygen uptake during exercise in children. *Pediatric Exercise Science* 1995; **7**: 12–25.
36. Gould, S. J. Allometry and size in ontogeny and phylogeny. *Biological Reviews* 1966; **41**: 587–640.
37. Armstrong, N. and Welsman, J. Assessment and interpretation of aerobic function in children and adolescents. *Exercise and Sport Sciences Reviews* 1994; **22**: 435–76.
38. Astrand, P. O., Engstrom, L., Eriksson, B. O., Karlberg, P., Nylander, I., Saltin, B. and Thoren, C. Girl swimmers. *Acta Paediatrica* 1963; **47**: 3–75.
39. Daniels, J. T. and Oldridge, N. Oxygen consumption and growth of young boys during running training. *Medicine and Science in Sports* 1971; **3**: 161–5.

40. Klissouras, V. Heritability of adaptive variation. *Journal of Applied Physiology* 1971; **31**: 338–44.

41. Astrand, P. O. and Rodahl, K. *Textbook of work physiology.* McGraw-Hill, New York, 1986.

42. Butler, J. P., Feldman, H. A. and Fredberg, J. F. Dimensional analysis does not determine a mass exponent for metabolic scaling. *American Journal of Physiology* 1987; **253**: R195–9.

43. Brody S., Proctor R. C. and Ashworth U. S. Basal metabolism, endogenous nitrogen, creatine and neutral sulphur excretions as functions of body weight. *University of Missouri Agriculture Experiment Station Research Bulletin* 1934; **220**: 1–40.

44. Kleiber, M. Body size and metabolism. *Hilgardia* 1932; **6**: 315–53.

45. McMahon, T. Size and shape in biology. *Science* 1973; **174**; 1201–4.

46. Cooper, D. M. Development of the oxygen transport system in normal children. In. *Advances in paediatric sports sciences vol. 3* (ed. O. Bar-Or). Human Kinetics Publishers, Champaign, Il, 1989; 67–100.

47. Heusner, A. A. Energy metabolism and body size. Is the 0.75 mass exponent of Kleiber's equation a statistical artefact? *Respiration Physiology* 1982; **48**: 1–12.

48. Heusner, A. A. What does the power function reveal about structure and function in animals of different size? *Annual Reviews in Physiology* 1987; **49**: 121–33.

49. Bergh, U., Sjodin, B., Forsberg, A. and Svedenhag, J. The relationship between body mass and oxygen uptake during running in humans. *Medicine and Science in Sports and Exercise* 1991; **23**: 205–11.

50. Nevill, A. M., Lakomy, H. K. A. and Lakomy, J. Rowing ergometer performance and maximum oxygen uptake of the 1992 Cambridge University boat crews. *Journal of Sports Sciences* 1992; **10**: 574.

51. Rowland, T. W. The development of aerobic fitness in children. In *Children and exercise XIX, promoting health and well-being* (ed. N. Armstrong, B. J. Kirby and J. R. Welsman). E and FN Spon, London, 1997; 179–90.

52. Welsman, J. R. Interpreting young people's exercise performance: Sizing up the problem. In *Children and exercise XIX, promoting health and well-being* (ed. N. Armstrong, B. J. Kirby and J. R. Welsman). E and FN Spon, London, 1997; 191–203.

53. Shephard, R. J. *Physical activity and growth.* Year Book Medical Publishers, Chicago, 1982.

54. Bar-Or O. *Paediatric sports medicine for the practitioner.* Springer-Verlag, New York, 1983.

55. Shephard, R. J. *Aerobic fitness and health.* Human Kinetics Publishers, Champaign, Il, 1994.

56. Asmussen, E. and Heeboll-Nielsen K. A. A dimensional analysis of physical performance and growth in boys. *Journal of Applied Physiology,* 1955; **7**: 593–603.

57. Ross, W. D., Bailey, D. A., Mirwald, R. L., Faulkner, R. A., Rasmussen, R., Kerr, D. A. and Stini, W. A. Allometric relationship of estimated muscle mass and maximal oxygen uptake in boys studied longitudinally age 8 to 16 years. In *Children and exercise, paediatric work physiology XV.* (ed. R. Frenkl and I. Szmodis). National Institute for Health Promotion, Budapest, 1991; 135–42.

58. Calder, W. A. III Scaling energetics of homeothermic vertebrates: An operational allometry. *Annual Reviews in Physiology* 1987; **49**: 107–20.

59. Welsman, J. R., Armstrong, N., Kirby, B. J., Winsley, R. J., Parsons, G. and Sharpe P. Exercise performance and MRI determined muscle volume in children. *European Journal of Applied Physiology* 1997; **76**: 92–7.

60. Cooper, D. M, Weiler-Ravell, D., Whipp, B. J. and Wasserman, K. Aerobic parameters of exercise as a function of body size during growth. *Journal of Applied Physiology,* 1984; **56**: 628–34.

61. Paterson, D. H., McLellan, T. M., Stella, R. S. and Cunningham, D. A. Longitudinal study of ventilation threshold and maximal O_2 uptake in athletic boys. *Journal of Applied Physiology* 1987; **62**: 2051–7.

62. Sjodin, B. and Svedenhag, J. Oxygen uptake during running as related to body mass in circumpubertal boys: A longitudinal study. *European Journal of Applied Physiology* 1992; **65**: 150–7.

63. Nevill, A. The need to scale for differences in body size and mass: An explanation of Kleiber's 0.75 mass exponent. *Journal of Applied Physiology* 1994; **77**: 2870–3.

64. Alexander, R. M., Jayes, A. S., Maloiy, G. M. O. and Wathuta, E. M. Allometry of the leg muscles of mammals. *Journal of Zoology,* London, 1981; **194**: 539–52.

65. Nevill, A. M. Evidence of an increasing proportion of leg muscle mass to body mass in male adolescents and its implication for performance. *Journal of Sports Science* 1994; **12**: 163–4.

66. Batterham, A. M. and George, K. P. Allometric modelling does not determine a dimensionless power function ratio for maximal muscular function. *Journal of Applied Physiology* 1997; **83**: 2158–66.

67. Nevill, A. M., Holder, R. L., Baxter-Jones, A., Round, J. M. and Jones, D. A. Modelling developmental changes in strength and aerobic power in children. *Journal of Applied Physiology* 1998; 963–70.

68. Nevill, A. M., Holder, R. L. and McConnell, A. K. Lung function in human beings. Its relationship to maximal oxygen uptake and lifestyle. *Journal of Physiology* 1998; **506**: 115P.

69. Armstrong, N., Welsman, J. R., Nevilll, A. M. and Kirby, B. J. Modeling growth and maturation changes in peak oxygen uptake in 11–13-year olds. *Journal of Applied Physiology,* 1999; **87**: 2230–6.

70. Rowland, T., Vanderburgh, P. and Cunningham, L. Body size and the growth of maximal aerobic power in children: A longitudinal analysis. *Paediatric Exercise Science* 1997; **9**: 262–74.

71. Janz, K. F. and Mahoney, L. T. Three-year follow-up of changes in aerobic fitness during puberty: The Muscatine study. *Research Quarterly for Exercise and Sport* 1997; **68**: 1–9.

72. Goldstein, H., Rasbash, J., Plewis, I., Draper, D., Browne, W., Yang, M., Woodhouse, G. and Healy, M. *A user's guide to MlwiN.* University of London, Institute of Education, London, 1998.

73. Duncan, C., Jones, K. and Moon, G. Health-related behaviour in context: A multilevel modelling approach. *Social Science and Medicine* 1996; **42**: 817–30.

74. Baxter-Jones, A., Goldstein, H. and Helms, P. The development of aerobic power in young athletes. *Journal of Applied Physiology* 1993; **75**: 1160–7.

75. Welsman, J. R. and Armstrong, N. Longitudinal changes in submaximal oxygen uptake in 11–13 year olds. *Journal of Sports Sciences* 2000; **18**: 183–9.

76. Armstrong, N., Welsman, J. R. Kirby, B. J. and Williams, C. A. Longitudinal changes in young people's short term power output. *Medicine and Science in Sports and Exercise* (in press).

1.2 Anthropometry, physique, body composition and maturity

Albrecht L. Claessens, Gaston Beunen and Robert M. Malina

Introduction

Anthropometry is an embracing term for a series of systematized techniques that quantify the external dimensions of the human body. It is often viewed as the traditional and perhaps basic tool of physical anthropology,[1,2] but also has a long tradition of use in physical education and the physical activity and sports sciences.[2,3]

The importance and applicability of anthropometry, and related techniques (somatotype, body composition), and biological maturity to sports medicine and sports sciences in general, and to the paediatric exercise sciences in particular, is well documented and established.[4–6] In addition to providing a basis for understanding and explaining the impact of sports training and physical activity on growth and maturation,[7–11] the assessment of morphological and maturational traits is also of relevance in the context of talent identification and development.[12–15]

The purposes of this chapter are:

(1) to describe a series of anthropometric dimensions and several ratios that have relevance to the paediatric sport sciences;

(2) to briefly discuss somatotype methodology as a means of estimating physique;

(3) to review methodological aspects and techniques of body composition assessment; and

(4) to provide an overview of methods for assessing maturity status of children and adolescents.

Anthropometry in assessing size and proportional characteristics

Choice of measurements and standardized procedures

Choice of measurements

Anthropometry is a method and should be treated as such, a means to an end and not an end in itself (Ref. 2, p. 206).

The number of measurements that can be taken on an individual is almost limitless. Thus, a key issue in the use of anthropometry is the selection and choice of measurements. This depends on the purpose of the study and on the specific questions under consideration. Measurements should be *selected* to provide specific information within the context of the study design. Thus, no single battery of measurements will meet the needs of every study.[16] According to Cameron[17] the choice of measurements for any particular situation depends on five criteria: relevance, accuracy and reliability, equipment, convenience, and cost. *Relevance* refers to the choice of measurements which will test most accurately the research hypothesis. Only measurements which can be taken with a high degree of *accuracy and reliability* should be selected. A measurement is of limited utility if it cannot be obtained accurately and reliably. Appropriate *equipment*, if correctly handled and regularly checked and calibrated, is vital and will help reduce errors. Other factors being equal, the *convenience* of one particular measurement may give it preference over another; this is labelled as '*accessibility and subject participation*'.[18] The final criterion is the *cost*, which is a major factor in many studies and which may lead to the use of cheaper versions of recommended instruments. A related factor is time investment. It is thus recommended that only those measurements which are absolutely essential in the context of the purposes of the study be taken. It makes no sense to take an extensive battery of measurements simply because one has the opportunity to measure.[2,16–18]

Standardized procedures

Anthropometric dimensions should be taken in a '*standardized*' manner, according to well-described and agreed upon procedures. Although there are several '*standardized*' protocols in the literature,[11,17,19,20] it is well known that similarly labelled techniques and perhaps measurement sites, are not always identical. A series of anthropometric dimensions relevant to the paediatric exercise sciences is subsequently described. The procedures for taking the measurements are based in part on those used in the Leuven Growth Studies of Belgian Boys[21] and Flemish Girls,[22] which principally followed the procedures described by Cameron.[17] For some of the descriptions reference is made to the *Anthropometric standardisation reference manual* edited by Lohman, Roche and Martorell.[19]

Measuring body size

Overall body size

Body mass and stature, are the two 'base-line' measurements or indicators of an 'overall' estimate of body size, and have been incorporated into almost every measuring protocol. *Body mass* should be measured on an accurately calibrated balance and recorded to the nearest 0.1 kg. Ideally, the subject should be nude (but this is usually impractical), or with minimal clothing and without shoes. If this is not possible, the subject should be weighed in clothing of known weight, so that a correction can be made. *Stature* (standing height) can be measured in several ways:

(1) free standing;
(2) standing against a wall or fixed stadiometer (with or without stretch); and
(3) in a recumbent position (for subjects who are unable to stand upright, such as small children, the elderly and handicapped).

The method described here is standing against a fixed stadiometer, without stretch, but the subject is instructed 'to stand as erect as possible'. The subject without shoes, stands upright against the stadiometer so that the heels, buttocks and scapulae are in contact with the backboard, and the feet are together. The head should be positioned in the Frankfort plane, and the headboard of the instrument should be moved down to make contact, with a small pressure, to compress the hair onto the vertex of the skull. Stature is recorded to the last completed unit (mm) and expressed in m or cm.

It is important to note that mass and stature are affected by *diurnal variation*, i.e. variation in a dimension during the course of a day. This is of special interest for short-term longitudinal studies, in which observed 'changes' may not reflect 'real' changes, but are simply a reflection of the time of the day at which the measurements were taken. On average, the individual is lightest in the morning and then body mass increases gradually during the course of the day. Mass is also affected by diet and physical activity, and daily changes in body mass, which may reach about 1 kg, are most likely to be due to variations in the amount of body water or gastrointestinal contents.[2,23] In menstruating girls, variation in the phase of the menstrual cycle also affects diurnal variation in body mass.[2,24]

Stature is also affected by the time of the day at which it is measured. It is greatest in the morning and decreases gradually during the day. This 'shrinking' is limited to the vertebral column (and thus to sitting height), and is related to the compression of the intervertebral cartilages. Depending on measurement technique, diurnal change in stature varies from about 10 to 20 mm.[2,25–27] These figures should not be ignored since, on average, the diurnal variation in stature is greater than measurement error.[26] The diurnal change in stature may also be influenced by vigorous high impact physical activity.

Segment lengths

Although many segment lengths can be measured (directly or indirectly as projected lengths—for an overview see references 11 and 19), two measurements, sitting height and leg length, are often used in paediatric exercise, and more specifically in growth studies. *Sitting height* is measured with an anthropometer (or with a Sitting Height Table). It is the distance from the sitting surface to the top of the head. The subject is sitting on a bench or table, and is positioned so that the head is in the Frankfort plane, the shoulders relaxed, the back straight, the legs are at right angles into the knees. The subject is instructed to sit as straight (erect) as possible. *Leg length* (or subischial length) is estimated as the difference between stature and sitting height. Note, there is no method of measuring true leg length.

Skeletal breadths

Breadth (width) measurements are taken across specific bone marks. They provide an indication of skeletal robustness. The apparatus can be the upper end of an anthropometer, a spreading caliper, a sliding caliper or a Vernier caliper. The more commonly taken breadth dimensions are biacromial and bicristal breadths on the trunk, and humerus and femur breadths on the extremities. The two latter breadth dimensions are used in the Heath–Carter technique for estimating the mesomorphy component of somatotype (see below). *Biacromial breadth* is the distance between the tips of the acromial processes. It is measured from the rear of the subject accurate to 1 mm. The position of the lateral tips of the acromial processes is slightly different in each subject; it is recommended that landmarks are carefully marked before applying the instrument. When the subject stands with relaxed shoulders, the technician applies the anthropometer points to the lateral tips of the processes. The points of the instrument must be pressed firmly so that the thickness of tissues that cover them is minimized. The measurement is read to the nearest mm, and expressed in cm. *Bicristal breadth* is the distance between the most lateral points of the iliac crests. The subject stands with the front to the measurer, in a relaxed position, with the arms somewhat away to ensure a clear view of the iliac crests. The anthropometer is held horizontally and the blades are applied to the most lateral points of the iliac crests. To obtain this 'bony' measurement, the blades must be pressed firmly against the crests so that the soft tissues are compressed and minimized. The measurement is read to the nearest mm, and expressed in cm.

Biepicondylar breadth is the distance between the most lateral points of the epicondyles of the humerus. Either a broad-blade or a small sliding spreading caliper, accurate to 1 mm, is used. The subject stands relaxed facing the measurer with the arm raised to the horizontal and the elbow flexed to 90 degrees. The caliper is applied to the medial and lateral epicondyles of the humerus with some pressure to compress the soft tissue. *Bicondylar breadth* is the distance between the two most lateral points of the condyles of the femur and is best measured with a small spreading caliper. The subject stands facing the technician with the (left or right) foot on a small bench so that there is a right angle in the knee. Alternatively, the subject is sitting on a chair or table with the legs flexed 90 degrees at the knees and the feet on the floor. The caliper is applied to the medial and lateral condyles of the femur with sufficient pressure to compress the soft tissue.

Circumferences

Circumference measurements are ordinarily taken on the limbs and trunk. Commonly used circumferences are upper arm, both relaxed and flexed, forearm, calf and thigh circumferences. Limb circumferences are mostly used as indicators of relative muscularity. The flexed upper arm and calf girths are used in calculating mesomorphy in the Heath–Carter Anthropometric Protocol (see below). Two trunk girths, waist and hip circumferences, are often taken as indicators of relative subcutaneous fat distribution.

A flexible, non-stretchable tape, accurate to 1 mm, is required. The tape is applied at the appropriate site, and should be at a right angle to the long axis of the body part measured. Contact with the skin should be continuous along the tape but without compressing the underlying soft tissues. For measuring *upper arm circumference relaxed* (cm), the subject stands relaxed with his/her side to the technician the arm hanging freely at the side and the palm facing the thigh. The tape is passed around the arm at the level of the midpoint of the upper arm. This landmark is the point on the lateral side of the upper arm midway between the lateral border of the acromial process and the tip of the olecranon process when the arm is flexed at 90 degrees. The measurement is performed with the arm relaxed and hanging beside the body. For measuring *upper arm circumference flexed* (sometimes referred to as *biceps circumference*) (cm) the subject stands upright and contracts m. biceps brachii as much as possible. The tape is passed around the arm so that it touches the skin surrounding the maximum circumference. *Forearm circumference* (cm) is measured at a point immediately distal to the elbow joint. The subject stands relaxed, facing the technician, with the arm slightly upward and the hand supinated. The tape is passed around the arm at the maximum horizontal or at the greatest bulge of the muscles of the forearm.

Calf circumference (cm) is measured with the subject in a standing position (preferable on a small bench) with the feet slightly apart and body mass distributed equally on both feet. The tape is positioned horizontally around the calf (perpendicular to its long axis) and moved up and down to locate the maximum circumference. If a calf skinfold will be measured later, this level should be marked on the medial side of the calf. *Thigh circumference* can be measured on three different levels: proximal, mid-thigh and distal.[19] *Proximal thigh circumference* is measured just below the gluteal fold and perpendicular to its long axis. The subject stands erect with the feet slightly apart and the body mass evenly distributed between both legs. For practical reasons, the subject is standing on a small bench, so that the measurer can be close to eye level with the upper thigh. *Mid-thigh circumference* is measured at the level midway between the centre of the inguinal crease and the proximal border of the patella. This level is marked while the subject is seated (and will also serve as the landmark for measuring the front thigh skinfold). The circumference is taken with the subject standing and body mass evenly distributed between the legs. For *distal thigh circumference*, the tape is placed around the thigh just proximal to the femoral epicondyles, while the subject stands in an erect position, preferably on a bench.

Waist circumference is most often measured at the level of the natural waist, i.e. at the narrowest part of the torso. This level is approximately one-half the distance between the costal border and iliac crest. The subject stands erect with the abdomen relaxed, and the arms hanging slightly away from the body. *Hip circumference* (sometimes called *buttocks circumference*) is taken at the level of maximum protrusion of the buttocks. The subject stands erect, with the body mass distributed equally on both feet. In most cases, hip circumference is taken with the subject wearing light clothing. In this case, pressure may need to be applied to compress the clothing.

Skinfolds thicknesses

Skinfold thicknesses (in short *skinfolds*) are thicknesses of double folds of skin plus subcutaneous adipose tissue at specific sites on the body. The utility of skinfold thicknesses is twofold: (i) they provide a relatively simple and non-invasive method of estimating general fatness; and (ii) they characterize in a certain way the distribution of subcutaneous adipose tissue over the whole body (relative fat patterning). The following general description is independent of the type of the caliper used and is based on the assumption that the measurer is right-handed. After the site is located, and in some cases marked, the thumb and index finger of the left hand are used to raise a skinfold about 1 cm above to the site at which the skinfold is to be measured. The fold is grasped firmly and held throughout the measurement. The caliper is then applied at the site for approximately 3 s.

Skinfold thicknesses are measured to the nearest 0.1 mm, and expressed in mm.

The skinfold sites often used in paediatric exercise and sport sciences are the triceps, biceps, subscapular, suprailiac, front thigh and medial calf. The *triceps skinfold* is measured at the marked level midway between the acromial and the olecranon processes (this is the same level as for upper arm circumference relaxed) over the posterior surface of m. triceps brachii. The subject stands with the back to the measurer, and the skinfold is picked up about 1 cm above the marked midpoint. The *biceps skinfold* is measured on the anterior aspect of the arm, over the m. biceps brachii at the same midpoint level as described for the triceps skinfold. The subject stands facing the measurer, the arm hanging relaxed with the palm facing forward. The site of the *subscapular skinfold* is located immediately below the inferior angle of the scapula. The subject stands with the back to the measurer with the shoulders relaxed, and the arms hanging loosely at the sides. The skinfold is picked up at an angle laterally and downward, following the natural cleavage line of the skin. The *suprailiac skinfold* is measured approximately 1 cm above the iliac crest in the midaxillary line.

The skinfold used in estimating endomorphy in the Heath–Carter anthropometric method is measured over the anterior superior iliac spine. It is presently called the 'suprasilane skinfold' (see below). The *front thigh skinfold* is located in the midline of the anterior aspect of the thigh, midway between the inguinal crease and the proximal border of the patella. The subject is seated on a bench for locating the measuring point. The thickness of a vertical fold is measured on the thigh while the subject is standing and body mass is shifted to the non-measured leg; the measured leg is relaxed with the knee slightly flexed and the foot flat on the floor. The *medial calf skinfold* is measured as a vertical fold at the level of maximum calf circumference on the medial aspect of the calf with the subject sitting on a bench and the knee at a right angle.

Measuring proportions

Anthropometric measurements provide specific information about *absolute* dimensions of the human body. They can also be related to each other and expressed as indices or ratios, in order to assess body proportions. Although in theory any two measurements can be related to each other, the following indices are commonly used in the paediatric sport science setting: mass-for-stature; sitting height to stature; bicristal diameter to biacromial diameter; (3 × biacromial diameter) — bicristal diameter; and the waist to hip ratio.[2,24]

The *mass-for-stature ratios* express the subject's body mass relative to his/her stature. They are often used in the context of under- or overweight and obesity. The most commonly used mass-for-stature ratio at present is the Quetelet index or *body mass index* (BMI), mass (in kg) divided by stature^2 (in m²). Another 'mass/stature' relationship is the so-called reciprocal ponderal index or *somatotype ponderal index*, in which *stature (cm) is divided by the cube root of mass (kg)*. It is used in estimating ectomorphy in somatotype assessment protocols (see below).

The *sitting height/stature* ratio provides an estimate of head, neck and trunk length relative to stature, or conversely, relative leg length. It is calculated as: *sitting height (cm) × 100/stature (cm)*.

A very widely used ratio in the paediatric exercise sciences, especially in surveys of young athletes, is the bicristal/biacromial ratio, expressing the breadth of the hips relative to that of the shoulders. This relationship is considered in the context of *androgyny* of physique, i.e. the degree of masculinity in the female or the degree of femininity in the male.[28–30] To estimate the degree of androgyny, two indices are at hand. The ratio *bicristal diameter × 100/biacromial diameter*;[28] and the androgyny index[30] calculated as: (*3 × biacromial diameter*) − *bicristal diameter*.

The ratio of *waist-to-hip circumferences* provides an index of relative fat distribution, i.e. waist circumference is an indicator of adipose tissue in the waist and abdominal region, while hip circumference is an indicator of adipose tissue over the hips and buttocks. This ratio, however, has limited utility as an indicator of relative fat distribution in children and youth.[31]

Estimating physique by somatotyping

General concepts

Somatotyping is a method for describing the human physique as it refers to an individual's body form as a whole, the configuration of the entire body rather than of specific features. The concept of *somatotype* was introduced by William Sheldon and coworkers,[32] and is perhaps the most commonly used conceptual approach to physique today. An individual's somatotype is a composite of the contributions of three *more or less independent* components: endomorphy, mesomorphy and ectomorphy. These three components are always recorded in this order, each describing the value of a particular component of physique. *Endomorphy,* the first component, describes the relative degree of fatness of the body, regardless of where the fat tissue is distributed. It also characterizes a predominance of digestive organs, softness and roundness of the body, and relative volume of the abdominal trunk and distal tapering of the limbs. The second component, *mesomorphy,* is characterized by the predominance of muscle, bone and connective tissue. It also describes corresponding physical aspects such as the 'robustness' of the body, and the relative volume of the thoracic trunk. *Ectomorphy,* the third component, is characterized by linearity, slenderness and fragility of build, with poor muscular development, and a predominance of surface area over body mass.

Sheldon's method is basically photoscopic or anthroposcopic, based on the visual observation and evaluation of the configuration of the body as 'Gestalt'. In this concept, an evaluation is made of the shape of the body as a whole; size is not a factor. Each component is assessed individually on a seven-point scale from a standardized somatotype photograph (front, side and back views), with one representing the least expression and seven representing the fullest expression. The three ratings together comprise the somatotype; they should be treated as a unit and not individually. Based on this system, the three extreme somatotypes are 7–1–1 (extreme endomorph), 1–7–1 (extreme mesomorph), and 1–1–7 (extreme ectomorph). Sheldon initially viewed the *somatotype* as an estimate of the 'genotype'.[32,33] This provoked a stream of criticism, which has led to modification of the method for estimating somatotype, although not the concept of somatotype. The modifications proposed by Parnell[34] and by Heath and Carter[35] incorporate anthropometry to determine each component. Further, many individuals recognized that the somatotype was not fixed and that it could be modified, e.g. by extreme diet and/or training. Parnell as well as Heath and Carter viewed the somatotype as a *phenotype*, based on body measurements at a given point in time.

The method of Heath and Carter appears to be applied world-wide, most probably because of its practical applicability, especially in the sports sciences with a focus on the study of the somatotype of elite athletes, both youth and adult.[36] In the late 1950s, Sheldon developed a new somatotype method, called the *Trunk Index,* in an attempt to eliminate some of the subjectivity of the original method and to account for variation with age.[37] However, this Trunk Index method is difficult to apply, especially in children, and is not used very often.

The Heath–Carter somatotype method

The complete Heath–Carter method actually combines photoscopic and anthropometric procedures.[36,38] In practice, however, the technique is used primarily in its anthropometric form for the reasons that anthropometry is more objective and, more importantly, obtaining standardized somatotype photographs (in front, side and back views) is quite difficult and costly.[24] The anthropometric Heath–Carter somatotype is calculated from a set of ten dimensions: body mass, stature, four skinfolds, two bone breadths and two limb girths. The first component, endomorphy, is derived from the sum of three skinfolds: the triceps, subscapular and suprailiac, adjusted for stature. The second component, mesomorphy, is derived from biepicondylar (humerus) and bicondylar (femur) breadths, flexed-arm and calf circumferences corrected for the triceps and medial calf skinfolds, respectively, and stature. These four limb measurements are adjusted for stature. The third component, ectomorphy, is based on the somatotype ponderal index. The ten dimensions were described in the preceding section.

To estimate the Heath–Carter anthropometric somatotype, two methods are available:

(1) the traditional approach which uses the Heath–Carter Somatotype Rating Form, and

(2) specific equations for each component.

The *step-by-step* procedures for the estimation of the anthropometric Heath–Carter somatotype by means of the *Rating Form* are described in Carter and Heath[36] (p. 371) and Duquet and Carter[38] (p. 40). The algorithms for calculating the Heath–Carter anthropometric somatotype are given in Table 1.2.1.

Specific attention must be given when the Heath–Carter method is applied to children. The rating forms for anthropometric somatotypes, as originally designed by Heath and Carter,[35] provide mesomorphy and ectomorphy scales adjusted for stature, but no similar adjustments for endomorphy and the sum of three skinfolds. However, on the assumption that skinfolds diminish during growth in proportion to an increase in stature, it was suggested that the sum of three skinfolds be multiplied by 170.18/stature (cm) before rating endomorphy in children.[36,39]

It is of interest to observe that endomorphy and mesomorphy as described in the Heath–Carter somatotype method are related to specific body composition concepts. Endomorphy is defined as relative fatness (or leanness), whereas mesomorphy is described as relative musculoskeletal development adjusted for stature, expressing the relative amount of fat-free mass in the body. However, results of several studies[40–45] do not support these notions, especially for children and young adults. Although moderate correlations are observed between endomorphy and percentage body fat, there are rather low correlations between mesomorphy and the fat-free mass, questioning the validity of

Table 1.2.1 Formulae for the calculation of the anthropometric Heath–Carter somatotype

---

Endomorphy = $-0.7182 + 0.1451(X) - 0.00068(X^2) + 0.0000014(X^3)$

where X is the sum of the triceps, subscapular and suprailiac skinfolds, in mm (for application to children, X is multiplied by 170.18/height (cm) to yield height-corrected endomorphy).

Mesomorphy = 0.858 (**humerus breadth, cm**) + 0.601 (**femur breadth, cm**) + 0.188 (**corrected arm girth, cm**) + 0.161 (**corrected calf girth, cm**) − 0.131(**height, cm**) + 4.5

where corrected arm girth is flexed arm girth (cm) minus the triceps skinfold (cm), and corrected calf girth is calf girth (cm) minus the medial calf skinfold (cm).

Ectomorphy = $0.732(HWR) - 28.58$ (if $HWR > 40.74$)

= $0.463(HWR) - 17.615$ (if $39.65 < HWR \leqslant 40.74$)

= 0.5 (if $HWR \leqslant 39.65$)

where **HWR** is height (cm) divided by the cube root of weight (kg).

Adapted from Duquet and Carter,[38] and Malina[2].

referring to mesomorphy as fat-free mass in the context of body composition (see below). Furthermore, it should be realized that the dimensions for estimating mesomorphy are based on limb measurements with the exclusion of trunk dimensions, and that the three somatotype components are by no means independent, i.e. they are moderately to highly interrelated and these interrelations change with gender and age.[46,47]

The definition of somatotype and procedures for estimating somatotype with the Heath–Carter method are not identical to those as described by Sheldon, although the same terms are used. In the original 'Sheldonian' concept, somatotype refers only to the individual's *body shape* and not to body composition. Although both methods use the term *somatotype*, it has a different meaning in each.[2,24,46,47]

For statistical analysis of somatotype data, it must be recognized that the somatotype is a 'Gestalt' and that it must be treated as a unit. However, in most studies relating somatotype to other aspects of sports and paediatric exercise sciences, or health aspects, each component is commonly treated as an independent variable. For a summary of the most appropriate statistical methods to analyse somatotype data, reference is given to Cressie et al.[48]

Body composition assessment: Methodological aspects and techniques

Introduction

A variety of methods are available for estimating body composition in children and adolescents, including densitometry, hydrometry, body potassium, neutron activation analysis, creatinine excretion and anthropometry.[49–53] More recent, new and sophisticated technologies, such as infrared interactance, magnetic resonance imaging, computerized tomography scanning, dual-energy X-ray absorptiometry and bioelectrical impedance analysis (BIA), have been developed[51,54] and applied to children and adolescents. Although all of the innovative methods have been utilized for estimating body composition

of children and adolescents, they are largely limited to the clinical or laboratory setting with some exceptions. This chapter gives specific emphasis to densitometry or the hydrostatic weighing technique, and to body composition methods which can be applied in field testing, specifically anthropometry and BIA.

Densitometry: The hydrostatic weighing technique

Although, the use of densitometry as a criterion method to validate new methods of body composition assessment in children and adolescents is limited and questionable,[49–52,55] this method will be briefly discussed because a considerable amount of past and present paediatric research is based on densitometry, and most field techniques are validated and calibrated against this method. Readers who are interested in a full description of this method are referred to Going[56] and Pollock et al.[53]

Body density is the ratio of body mass to body volume. Total body volume is normally measured by the hydrostatic weighing technique corrected for pulmonary residual volume and the amount of gas in the gastrointestinal tract. The residual volume, or the air remaining in the lungs after full expiration, is measured independently. For the amount of gastrointestinal gas, a constant of 100 ml is usually used. The hydrostatic weighing technique utilizes Archimedes' principle that a body immersed in a fluid is acted upon by a buoyancy force that is evidenced by a loss of mass equal to the mass of the displaced fluid.[53] Body density is subsequently transformed into its fat and fat-free components.

Density of the whole body can be represented in four components, including fat mass and the fat-free mass which consists of water, mineral and residual components, mostly protein.[51] Although this four-component chemical model is conceptually the most valid approach, in practice, the two-component model as proposed by Brozek et al.[57] and Siri[58], consisting of a fat component with density d_f and a fat-free component (including muscle, bone and other non-fatty tissues) with density d_{ffm}, is more commonly used in research and clinical settings.[49–52] However, this model is not without problems, especially related to the paediatric population. This system assumes that the composition of fat and FFM is constant for all individuals, with density values of 0.900 and 1.100 g ml^{-1}, respectively. Based on the dissection data of 25 cadavers, it has been demonstrated that there is a considerable variation among subjects in density of bone and muscle,[59] and any difference between the assumed value and the true value of fat-free density will result in an error in prediction of per cent body fat.[52] The standard deviation of the density of FFM in adults is about 0.016 g ml^{-1},[60] and although this is seemingly a small variability, in fact, it leads to large errors in percentage body fat.[52]

Although concerns have been raised,[49–51] the Brozek and Siri formulae have been more or less universally utilized for children and adolescents. However, relative to the adult, a child's FFM proportionally has a greater water and a lower bone mineral fraction. This will lower the fat-free density, with the consequence that the use of both equations results in an overestimation of body fat and an underestimation of the FFM in the paediatric population.[49] Fat-free density, however, varies greatly during the growth period. Estimates range from 1.063 g ml^{-1} and 1.064 g ml^{-1} at birth in boys and girls, respectively, to 1.100 g ml^{-1} at maturity.[49,50] However, it should be noted that these are mean values of groups without mention of variability within the groups.[52] To estimate percentage body fat from total body density accurately in children and adolescents, the density of the FFM representative of the growth and maturation status must thus be known.[51] Paediatric-specific equations have been developed for the estimation of percentage fat from density for 1–16 year old boys and girls by Lohman[50] based on multicomponent estimates of FFM. By this approach it is possible to express water, mineral and protein as fractions of the whole FFM.[51] Several reviews dealing with variability in density of the FFM during growth and maturation are available.[49–51]

Besides the assumption of a constant density of the FFM, there are also some practical problems associated with hydrostatic weighing of the paediatric population.[24,52] In general, this procedure requires considerable subject cooperation, and in fact, very young children cannot be measured with this technique. Its lower age limit is about seven or eight years.[24] At the time of weighing, subjects must empty their lungs as much as possible to residual volume while fully submerged. This may not be possible for young children, with the consequence of a poor reproducibility for the technique. The reproducibility of the measurement was about 0.0006 g ml^{-1} in adults and about 0.0048 g ml^{-1} in children,[61] resulting in errors of 0.3% and 2.5% body fat, respectively. These results reflect the practical problems in estimating body composition by hydrostatic weighing in the paediatric population, especially younger children.

Field methods for estimating body composition

Anthropometry

By far the most common technique for estimating body composition by anthropometry is the use of skinfold thicknesses. A skinfold thickness is a double layer of skin and subcutaneous adipose tissue at selected sites. Calipers with a constant pressure of 10 g mm^{-2} are recommended, although some cheaper plastic calipers are also acceptable for use in the non-research setting.[53] Skinfolds are relatively easy and inexpensive to obtain. Standardization of skinfold sites and techniques were described earlier.

Typically, a sum of several skinfolds is entered into a regression equation to predict either body density (from which percentage body fat can be derived) and/or percentage body fat. Skinfold equations have been developed in several paediatric samples.[61–64] Although the use of skinfolds to predict body fat in children and adolescents is promising, there are some major limitations.[51]

A first limitation concerns the use of total body density, or percentage body fat, as the dependent variable. In most equations, however, the adult model (the Siri or Brozek equations) is used without consideration of the chemical immaturity of children and adolescents.[51]

A second limitation concerns the problem of accuracy of the developed equations (by cross-validation) and, as a consequence, the lack of applicability to other samples (of children and adolescents, or others such as athletic, obese or handicapped youth). For example, the Slaughter et al.[64] skinfold equations, which were thought to be the most accurate for children and adolescents, were recently cross-validated. In a cross-validation study of the Slaughter equations on 122 children and adolescents, ages 8–17 years,[65] the criterion method against which the equations were cross-validated was the Siri age-adjusted body density equations.[50] Only the Slaughter (triceps + subscapular) equation for females was successfully cross-validated. The authors[65] concluded, however, that a

> … combined effort should be directed toward reducing error for all of the Slaughter equations and in eliminating the statistically significant differences between the criterion method and the triceps and calf skinfold equation for females. Further on the significant method by gender interaction indicates a need for further refinement of the triceps and calf skinfold equation in adolescent males. (p. 1076.)

These expectations, however, are not easily addressed. In a sample of 24 boys and 23 girls, both prepubertal and pubertal,[66] it was demonstrated that the Slaughter (triceps + calf [T + C]) and the (triceps + subscapular [T + S]) equations overestimated percentage body fat (%BF) by 0.31% and 0.09%, respectively, compared to %BF determined by the four-component model. Limits of agreement (+ 2SD) were 8.10%BF and 9.88%BF, respectively. The Slaughter T + C equation did not predict well when %BF > 30%, and overpredicted %BF more in boys than in girls. The Slaughter T + S equation tended to underpredict body fat in female subjects and overpredict body fat in males[66] (p. 933). Based on these observations, the authors[66] concluded that the Slaughter equations are not sufficiently accurate for the paediatric population and require further refinement.

A third limitation concerns the relationship of skinfolds to body density. This relationship varies with maturity status, with prepubescent and pubescent boys and girls having significantly different relationships compared to adults.[51] This can be partly explained by variability in the density of FFM during growth, and also by maturity-related variability in the distribution of subcutaneous fat at various sites of the body and by the ratio of internal to external fat stores.[51] In addition to these limitations, and even if the individual being measured conforms to the description of those in the original samples (e.g. in gender, age, race, general physique, physical activity level, etc.), there is considerable potential for error in prediction, especially in the paediatric population.[52] The standard error of estimation (SEE) in a adult population averages about 3.7% body fat.[67] This means that in approximately two out of three predictions, the true percentage body fat will be within + 3.7% of the estimated value.[52] The SEE in children is somewhat higher, on average, 4.5% body fat,[61] with the consequence of considerable margins of error within individual predictions. To minimize problems associated with converting skinfold values to percentage body fat, the sum of skinfolds by itself can be used as a reflection of total body fat. This is especially useful in relation to national or population-specific norms.[50,52,65,68] However, skinfolds are only an indication of subcutaneous adipose tissue, and to estimate total fatness from a sum of skinfolds means that a constant relationship between the amount of subcutaneous adipose tissue and the amount of adipose tissue stored internally (viscerally) is assumed. Little is known about this relationship in children. Another complication of using a sum of skinfolds in children is that there are large and rapid changes in body size during growth, with the consequence that the same set of skinfold thicknesses in two boys who differ in size will not represent the same amount of adipose tissue, either in absolute or relative terms. This poses a problem in interpreting skinfold thicknesses, especially around the period of peak height velocity at puberty.[52] Notwithstanding these limitations, and until more accurate equations are developed, the sum of skinfolds as a simple and useful indicator of total body fatness is recommended for the paediatric population.[66]

Bioelectrical impedance analysis

Bioelectrical impedance analysis is a relatively new technique for estimating body composition in humans.[69] The fundamental theory and physical principles on which BIA is based are somewhat complicated and beyond the scope of this chapter. In depth information is given in two recent readable reviews.[69,70] BIA is a non-invasive, rapid and easy technique for estimating body composition. The equipment is relatively inexpensive and portable. Hence, BIA has potential for use with individuals across a broad age spectrum and in a variety of settings.[69,71,72] Although BIA has potential as a method for estimating body composition in the paediatric population,[51,70] neither its validity nor precision as a measure of body composition for children and youths is sufficiently established.[51,52,65,72] Cross-validation of two BIA equations for children and adolescents[51,73] against a four-component body composition model in prepubescent and pubescent boys ($n = 24$) and girls ($n = 23$) demonstrated that both BIA equations produced a mean bias in %BF of 0.68% and 2.18%, respectively.[66] The limits of agreement (+ 2 SD), as statistically analysed by the Bland and Altman method,[74] were 11.04%BF and 12.02%BF, respectively. In addition, the bias of both BIA equations was dependent on %BF. Both equations overestimated %BF of lean subjects in males, and underestimated %BF of fatter individuals. The BIA equation of Houtkooper et al.[73] tended to overestimate %BF in pubertal boys and underestimate %BF in pre- and early-pubertal girls. The bias in estimating %BF with the BIA equation of Boileau[51] was dependent on both gender and maturation of the subjects.[65] This lack of agreement for %BF between both BIA equations and the four-component model was rather surprising, because both the Houtkooper et al.[73] and the Boileau[51] BIA equations were originally validated against a four-component body composition model.

The method of estimating body composition from BIA is based on the principle that biological tissues act as conductors or insulators, and the flow of current through the body will follow the path of least resistance.[71] Because bone-free lean tissue has a greater electrolyte and water content, and greater conductivity than adipose and bone tissues,

an estimate of FFM from the magnitude of the body's electrical conductivity can be made. BIA uses an injected current, and impedance (Z) to the flow of the weak electric current is directly related to the length (L) of the conductor and inversely related to its cross-sectional area (A): $Z = \rho(L/A)$, where ρ is the specific resistivity of the body's tissues and is assumed to be constant. Impedance yields a measure of resistivity, and resistance (R) is used with stature (S) in the form of S^2/R as an index of total conductive volume of the body.[71,72]

Some problems, however, arise when the BIA method is applied to the paediatric population. A first problem relates to conductor length and its configuration. Impedance is proportional to the geometry of the conductor, and it is assumed that the human body is shaped like a perfect cylinder with a uniform length and cross-sectional area. Although stature is used as the indicator of conductor length, body shape varies considerably among individuals of the same stature. The impact of the size and shape of the human body as the conductor on the resistance value in adults has been demonstrated.[75–77] However, this principle is even more important in regard to children and adolescents, where the geometry of the conductor changes during growth as size increases and shape alters considerably.[72] Hence, changes in size and proportions during growth have to be taken into account when BIA equations are developed.

A second problem relates to the chemical immaturity of the FFM in children. The resistive index (S^2/R) is the basis of the common BIA method for assessing body composition in adults. However, the equations used mostly in the BIA instruments are derived from studies of adults and thus reflect the relationship between the S^2/R index and FFM found in adults.[52,72] A third problem concerns racial variation. BIA estimates of body composition in the paediatric population are mainly limited to white subjects;[51] racial variation in body composition and proportions may influence BIA.[72] A last problem concerns measurement issues. The accuracy of the BIA method is highly dependent on some controlling factors that may increase the measurement error of this method. One of these factors deals with the standardization of the BIA procedure, especially the placement of the electrodes.[78,79] The positioning of electrodes on children is generally based on conventional landmarks defined on adults. However, given the small size of extremities in young children, placement of electrodes too close together influences measured values of resistance.[72]

Assessing maturational status

Growth and maturation are concepts that are often used together and sometimes considered as synonymous. Growth refers to the increase in size of the whole body or the size attained by specific parts of the body. The changes in size are outcomes of the increase in cell number or hyperplasia, increase in cell size or hypertrophy, or increase in intercellular material or accretion. Growth is a dominant biological activity during the first two decades of life. It starts at conception and continues until the late teens or into the early twenties for some individuals. Maturation refers to the process of becoming fully mature. It gives an indication of the distance that an individual has travelled along the way to the adult state. Maturation refers to the tempo and timing of progress towards the mature biological state and consequently varies with the biological system that is used to assess this state. Chronological age or the time that an individual has lived has limited utility as an indicator of biological maturity. There is considerable variability in physical characteristics among individuals of the same chronological age, especially during the pubertal years.

The processes of growth and maturation are related, and both influence physical performance. Those engaged in teaching physical education or coaching youth are certainly familiar with the following scenario: John is 13.5 years chronological age, with a stature of 171 cm, body mass 60 kg, and arm pull strength 65 kg, while Jim also 13.5 years has a stature of 150 cm, body mass 40 kg, and arm pull strength score is 32 kg. These boys of exactly the same chronological age are often required to compete against each other in a variety of sports, and often on fitness tests[7,80] (see Chapter 2.1). One of the main reasons for this size and strength gap between John and Jim is the difference in biological maturation. John is advanced in biological maturation and has a skeletal age of 15.5 years, whereas Jim is later in biological maturation and has a skeletal age of 11.5 years. The skeletal maturity of both boys, however, falls within the range of normal variation for boys of this age level. It is entirely possible that Jim will catch-up and eventually become taller, heavier and stronger than John as a adult.

This section briefly considers different methods used to estimate the biological maturity status of youth.

A good technique to assess maturity should meet the following conditions:

(1) reflect changes in a biological system;
(2) be to some degree independent of growth;
(3) be applicable from birth to adulthood;
(4) reach the same adult state in all individuals; and
(5) show a continuous increase over the entire process.

The first is obvious; biological maturation should deal with biological systems. The second implies that the system should be related to growth, since there normally is harmony in growth and maturation, but there is need for a system that does not measure growth (size attained or changes in size attained, i.e. growth velocity). What is needed is an indicator with its own scale that marks the progress towards the mature, adult state. Preferably the system should be applicable throughout the whole maturation process, from birth to adulthood. It can be argued that the system should even be applicable from conception to adulthood or, in a life-time perspective, until old age to death. Most systems, however, are limited to the period of birth to adulthood, or to shorter intervals. The fourth criterion is of utmost importance since it reflects the essence of maturation, namely every individual should ultimately reach adulthood and this adult state should be the same for all individuals. Finally, the system of choice should show a continuous increase, i.e. it cannot decrease because by definition maturity is progress towards the mature state.

Since Boas[81] first realized that chronological age is not an adequate timescale for identifying tempo and timing of changes in biological characteristics, and biological milestones, such as age at peak height velocity or age at menarche in girls, are required, considerable efforts have been made to develop adequate techniques to assess biological maturation. Four biological systems have been and are still used:

(1) sexual maturity;
(2) dental maturity;
(3) morphological maturity; and
(4) skeletal maturity.

Sexual maturity

Sexual maturity refers to the changes in secondary sex characteristics that occur during puberty, the period of becoming sexually mature. Sexual maturity is most often assessed using a five-stage scale for pubic hair and genital development in boys, and pubic hair and breast development in girls, together with age at menarche. Menarche is the age at occurrence of the first menstrual flow; it does not signify regular ovulation and regular menstrual cycles. The five-stage scales have been described by Tanner,[82] based upon the work of others. Although often referred to as 'Tanner's stages', this custom is incorrect since these stages were in use long before Tanner described them. Furthermore it is essential to mention which of the secondary sex characteristics are assessed because there is considerable variation within and among individuals in the timing and sequence of the stages. The five stages for breast, pubic hair and genital development should be assigned by visual inspection of the nude subject at clinical examination. Since this procedure is invasive and sensitive to adolescents, self-assessment has been proposed as an alternative. Several studies have reported reasonable validity and reliability of self-assessments. There is still a need for further validation of self-assessment.

Age at menarche can be obtained with three approaches. First, prospective or longitudinal, in which a representative sample of non-menstruating girls (starting at about eight years) are followed and monitored at regular intervals about their first menstrual period. This design leads to reasonable information about the exact time at which individual girls reach menarche. Second, retrospective or recall, in which a representative sample of girls who are menstruating is questioned about the age at which they experienced their first menstrual flow. The data obtained with this method are influenced by memory, and large errors have been reported in recalling the exact dates. However, recall data correspond quite closely to those obtained with the prospective approach, and provide a reasonable estimate for groups.[24] Note, however, the retrospective method is of limited value in samples of young adolescent girls, since a great number of girls have not yet attained menarche thus biasing the group mean. Third, cross-sectional or status quo design, in which a representative sample of girls, 8–17 years, is questioned about whether or not their first menstrual flow has already occurred. The discrete responses, i.e. yes or no, are grouped by age; a probit or logit is fitted through the observed data to estimate the median age for the sample. It does not refer to individuals. The main shortcoming of sexual maturity assessment is the relatively short period during which the system is applicable, i.e. puberty. Further, the stages are discrete categories superimposed on a continuous change in the characteristics. Reference data for the ages at which stages of each secondary characteristic are attained in different populations are available.[24,82–84]

A final word of caution, it is common to group children by stage of pubertal development, independent of chronological age. This overlooks chronological age *per se* as a source of variation in size, physique and performance capacity; e.g. the explosive strength as measured by vertical jump of a 12 year old boy in genital stage four may be quite different from the jumping power of a 16 year old boy in genital stage four.

Morphological maturity

Morphological age refers to the maturational progress in morphological or somatic characteristics. In this respect, height age, i.e. the average age at which a certain stature is attained in a given population, is an inadequate indicator of biological maturation. The main disadvantage of height age as an indicator of biological maturation is that the endpoint is different for each individual. For a small person 160 cm can already signify adult stature, i.e. 100% reached, whereas for a tall basketball player it can signify that only 75% of adult stature is reached. Height age violates the requirement that the endpoint should be the same for all individuals.

The biological milestone, age at peak height velocity, is a good morphological maturity indicator. Age at peak height velocity is the age at which the individual growth curve reaches maximum velocity during the adolescent growth spurt. It occurs, on average, at about 14.0 years in boys, and two years earlier at about 12.0 years in girls.[7,24,83] The drawback of this procedure is that it is only one point in time and that it requires longitudinal data for individuals followed over several years across adolescence.

Another approach to morphological maturity is to calculate the percentage of adult stature attained at a given age. By definition the endpoint is the same for each individual, i.e. reaching one's own adult stature. The problem is to define adult stature for the individual child or adolescent. Several techniques have been developed to predict adult stature. The techniques developed by Bayley,[85] Roche et al.[86] and Tanner et al.[87] are the most accurate and commonly used. The predictors in these methods are actual stature, chronological age, skeletal age and, in some techniques, parental stature and/or age at menarche for girls. Recently, Beunen et al.[88] proposed a method using stature, sitting height, chronological age and two skinfolds as predictors in boys 12 to 15 years of age. This technique has similar accuracy as the technique of Tanner et al.[87] and may be useful when skeletal age cannot be assessed.

Dental maturity

Dental maturity can be estimated from the age of eruption of deciduous or permanent teeth, or from the number of teeth present at a certain age.[89] Eruption is, however, only one event in the calcification process of the teeth and has limited biological meaning. For this reason, Demirjian et al.[90] constructed a scale for the assessment of dental calcification, based on the principles developed by Tanner et al.[87] for the assessment of skeletal maturity. However, dental maturity does not closely correspond to sexual, morphological and skeletal maturity.

Skeletal maturity

Skeletal maturity is the most commonly used indicator of biological maturation. It is widely recognized as the best single biological maturity indicator.[82] At present, three techniques are in use: the atlas technique first introduced by Todd[91] and later published in two revisions by Greulich and Pyle;[92] the bone-specific Tanner–Whitehouse technique first described in the late 1950s and 1960s, and subsequently revised[87] (TWII method); and finally the bone-specific method developed by the group of Roche, one for the knee[93] and one for the hand and wrist.[94] It should be mentioned that other methods have been proposed and used, but from the literature on biological maturation and its applications it is clear that the above mentioned methods are the ones presently in use.

In the development of systems to assess skeletal age, the contribution of Todd is of great significance, since he first introduced the concept of maturity indicators which are characteristic features of the maturity status of ossification centres that are universal and occur in an irreversible, regular order. This concept has resulted in the development of what later was identified as the bone-specific approach in which skeletal maturity status of each ossification centre is assessed and then combined in a skeletal maturity score (Tanner–Whitehouse technique[87]) or in an overall skeletal age (Roche or Fels techniques[94]). The description of specific maturity indicators of individual bones was already included in the atlas technique, but how to use them in the assessment of skeletal age was not clearly explained.

The atlas method consists of a number of X-rays representative of the maturity status at a given age level. This means that, for boys and girls separately, a number of plates of the hand and wrist are published in an atlas. These plates were selected from a large number of radiographs and represent the median appearance of the skeletal maturity status at a given age. Skeletal age for a boy or girl is then rated by comparing the X-ray of the hand and wrist with the plates of the atlas. When using the atlas techniques, the most accurate bone age assessments are obtained when a bone age is assigned for each bone separately and the median age of all bones is taken as the skeletal age of the hand and wrist.

The Tanner–Whitehouse technique[87] is a bone-specific approach in which the bones of the hand and wrist are graded on a scale and then converted to a maturity score for the hand and wrist, for which population specific reference standards are made. For the radius, ulna, metacarpals and phalanges, adult status is characterized by fusion of the epiphysis and diaphysis. For each of these bones, specific stages from initial ossification to union have been defined and described. For all these stages of each bone a maturity scale has been constructed so that the scores on these scales

> … are defined in such a way as to minimise the overall disagreement between the different bones, this disagreement being totalled over a large sample of individuals covering the whole developmental span. (p. 3)

Subsequently the stages of the bones are converted into a weighted score (for example the radius and ulna are given four times more weight than the metacarpals or phalanges of the third and fifth finger) and these weighted scores are added to obtain an overall maturity score of the hand and wrist. For these maturity scores reference standards were constructed for the British and other populations. It should be mentioned that in the TWII method the ossification centres of the second and fourth finger are not estimated since the maturity stages of the phalanges in each row of the fingers (for example, the distal phalanges) are very similar. Furthermore, three different scales are available: one for the 20 bones of the hand and wrist (TWII scale), one for the 13 short and long bones (RUS scale including radius, ulna and short bone), and one for the carpal bones (CARP scale). In practice, the maturity stages are assigned to 20 (TWII scale), 13 (RUS scale) or seven (CARP scale) bones of the hand and wrist following carefully the description of the stages given in Tanner et al.[87] Depending on the scale used the corresponding sex-specific scores are given, then summed and compared to the reference standards of the population. Very often the maturity score is converted into skeletal age, which is the corresponding chronological age at which, on the average, an overall maturity score is reached. In the Belgian population a TWII score of 848 corresponds in boys to a skeletal age of 13.5 years, and this is the same as in the British population. At other age levels, however, there are considerable differences between Belgian and British children.[95]

The Fels method of assessing skeletal maturity of the hand and wrist[94] is based upon maturity indicators that are, as previously mentioned, radiographic features that must occur during the maturation of every child to be useful in the assessment. One hundred and thirty possible maturity indicators were initially tested. Also selected were metric maturity indicators that consisted of ratios between linear measurements of radius, ulna, metacarpals and phalanges. The potential of each maturity indicator was subsequently tested on the basis of its ability to discriminate between children of the same chronological age, and its universal appearance, reliability, validity and completeness. This very thorough selection procedure was first completed for boys and then applied to girls. The resulting Fels method is based upon a final selection of 85 graded maturity indicators for radius, ulna, carpals, metacarpals and phalanges, and 13 metric indicators of measured ratios for radius, ulna, metacarpals and phalanges. Each of these indicators is useful in both boys and girls. Sixty-one of the indicators are simply presence–absence indicators, 17 are three-grade, five are four-grade and two are five-grade indicators. The Fels method is a computer-assisted procedure. The number of indicators to be assessed at an age is large, but most of these indicators are assessed simply, quickly and easily. The system provides not only a skeletal age but also, and importantly, a standard error for that assessment.

Finally it should be mentioned that sexual, morphological and skeletal maturity indicators are highly interrelated but not so that one can predict skeletal maturity from secondary sex characteristics or vice versa.

Summary

If measurements are taken by a well-trained observer, anthropometric analysis of children and adolescents is highly reliable. The key to effective anthropometry, however, lies in understanding the meaning of specific measurements, so that a set can be taken that effectively answers the research question(s) addressed or meets the needs of the desired application(s). Anthropometric measurements should be treated as a means to an end rather than an end in themselves.

Human physique can be described through somatotyping. This chapter has focused on the techniques of Sheldon et al.[32] and Heath–Carter.[36,38] The term somatotyping, however, has different meanings in each of the methods, as in the Sheldon method somatotype refers only to the individual body shape and not to body composition. The Heath–Carter anthropometric somatotype technique is probably the most practically useful method in paediatric exercise science.

Densitometry is widely used to assess body composition but in the paediatric population it has some shortcomings due to the assumption of a constant density of the fat-free mass during growth and maturation. The use of anthropometric prediction equations to estimate body density or percentage body fat also has limitations with children and adolescents. The sum of skinfolds is recommended as a simple and useful indicator of total body fatness, although single skinfolds are also useful as indicators of body fat patterning in young people. The use of BIA as a field method of estimating children's and adolescents' body composition is growing in popularity but more research is required before it can be recommended for use in the paediatric population.

A number of methods for the assessment of maturational status are available and include the use of sexual, dental, morphological and skeletal maturity. In future, more attention needs to be given to the refinement of non-invasive methods for the assessment of maturity status. Self-reporting methods of sexual maturity need to be standardized and validated. The use of predicted adult stature as an indicator of maturity status needs to be explored, and routine measurement of parental statures and incorporation of these dimensions into evaluation of growth, should be promoted within paediatric exercise science.

References

1. **Lasker, G. W.** The place of anthropometry in human biology. In *Anthropometry: The individual and the population* (ed. S. J. Ulijaszek and C. G. N. Mascie-Taylor). Cambridge University Press, Cambridge, 1994; 1–6.
2. **Malina, R. M.** Anthropometry. In *Physiological assessment of human fitness* (ed. P. J. Maud and C. Foster). Human Kinetics Publishers, Champaign, Il, 1995; 205–19.
3. **Malina, R. M.** Anthropometry in physical education and sport sciences. In *History of physical anthropology* (ed. F. Spencer), Vol. 1. A. L. Garland Publishing, New York, 1997; 90–4.
4. **Bar-Or, O.** (ed.) *The child and adolescent athlete.* Blackwell, Oxford, 1996.
5. **Docherty, D.** (ed.) *Measurement in pediatric exercise science.* Human Kinetics Publishers, Champaign, Il, 1996.
6. **Harries, M., Williams, C., Stanish, W. D.** and **Micheli, L. J.** (ed.) *Oxford textbook of sports medicine.* Oxford University Press, New York, 1994.
7. **Beunen, G.** and **Malina, R. M.** Growth and biological maturation: Relevance to athletic performance. In *The child and adolescent athlete* (ed. O. Bar-Or). Blackwell, Oxford, 1996; 3–24.
8. **Hergenroeder, A. C.** and **Klish W. J.** Body composition in adolescent athletes. *Pediatric Clinics of North America* 1990; **37**: 1057–83.
9. **Malina, R. M.** Physical growth and biological maturation of young athletes. *Exercise and Sport Sciences Reviews* 1994; **22**: 389–433.
10. **Malina, R. M.** and **Beunen, G.** Monitoring of growth and maturation. In *The child and adolescent athlete* (ed. O. Bar-Or). Blackwell, Oxford, 1996; 647–72.
11. **Ross, W. D.** Anthropometry in assessing physique status and monitoring change. In *The child and adolescent athlete* (ed. O. Bar-Or). Blackwell, Oxford, 1996; 538–72.
12. **Bloomfield, J.** Talent identification and profiling. In *Textbook of science and medicine in sport* (ed. J. Bloomfield, P. A. Fricker and K. D. Fitch). Blackwell Scientific Publication, Melbourne, 1992; 187–98.
13. **Komadel, L.** The identification of performance potential. In *The olympic book of sports medicine* (ed. A. Dirix, H. G. Knuttgen and K. Tittel). Blackwell Scientific Publications, Oxford, 1988; 275–85.
14. **Malina, R. M.** and **Beunen, G.** Matching of opponents in youth sports. In *The child and adolescent athlete.* (ed. O. Bar-Or). Blackwell, Oxford, 1996; 202–13.
15. **Matsudo, V. K. R.** Prediction of future athletic excellence. In *The child and adolescent athlete* (ed. O. Bar-Or). Blackwell, Oxford, 1996; 92–109.
16. **Malina, R. M.** Physical anthropology. In: *Anthropometric standardisation reference manual* (ed. T. G. Lohman, A. F. Roche and R. Martorell). Human Kinetics Publishers, Champaign, Il, 1988; 99–102.
17. **Cameron, N.** *The measurement of human growth.* Croom Helm, London, 1984.
18. **Micozzi, M. S.** Applications of anthropometry to epidemiologic studies of nutrition and cancer. *American Journal of Human Biology* 1990; **2**: 727–39.
19. **Lohman, T. G., Roche, A. F.** and **Martorell, R.** (ed.) *Anthropometric standardisation reference manual.* Human Kinetics Publishers, Champaign, Il, 1988.
20. **Norton, K.** and **Olds, T.** (ed.) *Antropometrica.* University of New South Wales Press, Sydney, 1996.
21. **Renson, R., Beunen, G., Van Gerven, D., Simons, J.** and **Ostyn, M.** Description of motor ability tests and anthropometric measurements. In *Somatic and motor development of Belgian secondary schoolboys*

(ed. M. Ostyn, J. Simons, G. Beunen, R. Renson and D. Van Gerven). Leuven University Press, Leuven. 1980.

22. **Claessens, A. L. M., Vanden Eynde, B., Renson, R.** and **Van Gerven, D.** The description of tests and measurements. In *Growth and fitness of Flemish girls. The Leuven growth study* (ed. J. Simons, G. P. Beunen, R. Renson, A. L. M. Claessens, B. Vanreusel and J. A. V. Lefevre). Human Kinetics Publishers, Champaign, Il, 1990; 21–39.

23. **Jones, P. R. M.** and **Norgan, N. G.** Anthropometry and the assessment of body composition. In *Oxford textbook of sports medicine* (M. Harries, C. Williams, W. D. Stanish and L. J. Micheli). Oxford University Press, New York: 1994; 149–60.

24. **Malina, R. M.** and **Bouchard, C.** *Growth, maturation, and physical activity.* Human Kinetics Publishers, Champaign, Il, 1991.

25. **Kobayashi, M.** and **Togo, M.** Twice-daily measurements of stature and body weight in two children and one adult. *American Journal of Human Biology* 1993; 5: 193–201.

26. **Lampl, M.** Further observations on diurnal variation in standing height. *Annals of Human Biology* 1992; 19: 87–90.

27. **Whitehouse, R. H., Tanner, J. M.** and **Healy, M. J. R.** Diurnal variation in stature and sitting height in 12–14-year-old boys. *Annals of Human Biology* 1974; 1: 103–6.

28. **Bayley, N.** and **Bayer, L. M.** The assessment of somatic androgyny. *American Journal of Physical Anthropology* 1946; 4: 433–61.

29. **Malina, R. M.** and **Merrett, D. M. S.** Androgyny of physique of women athletes: comparisons by sport and over time. In *Essays on auxology presented to James Mourilyan Tanner by former colleagues and fellows* (ed. R. Hauspie, G. Lindgren and F. Falkner). Castlemead Publications, London, 1995; 355–63.

30. **Tanner, J. M.** Current advances in the study of physique. Photogrammetric anthropometry and an androgyny scale. *Lancet* 1951; **March 10**: 574–9.

31. **Mueller, W. H.** and **Malina, R. M.** Relative reliability of circumferences and skinfolds as measures of body fat distribution. *American Journal of Physical Anthropology* 1987; 72: 437–9.

32. **Sheldon, W. H., Stevens, S. S.** and **Tucker, W. B.** *The varieties of human physique. An introduction to constitutional psychology.* Hafner, Darien, Connecticut, 1940.

33. **Sheldon, W. H., Dupertuis, C. W.** and **McDermott, E.** *Atlas of men. A guide for somatotyping the adult male at all ages.* Hafner, Darien, Connecticut, 1954.

34. **Parnell, W. H.** *Behaviour and physique. An introduction to practical and applied somatometry.* Greenwood, Westport, Connecticut, 1958.

35. **Heath, B. H.** and **Carter, J. E. L.** A modified somatotype method. *American Journal of Physical Anthropology* 1967; 27: 57–74.

36. **Carter, J. E. L.** and **Heath, B. H.** *Somatotyping. Development and applications.* Cambridge University Press, Cambridge, 1990.

37. **Sheldon, W. H., Lewis, N. D. C.** and **Tenney, A. M.** Psychotic patterns and physical constitution. In *Schizophrenia. Current concepts and research* (ed. D. V. Siva Sanker). PJD Publications, Hicksville, New York, 1969; 839–911.

38. **Duquet, W.** and **Carter, J. E. L.** Somatotyping. In *Kinanthropometry and exercise physiology laboratory manual* (ed. R. Eston and T. Reilly). E. and F. N. Spon, London, 1996; 35–50.

39. **Hebbelinck, M., Duquet W.** and **Ross, W. D.** A practical outline for the Heath–Carter somatotyping method applied to children. In *Pediatric work physiology. Proceedings of the fourth international symposium* (ed. O. Bar-Or). Wingate Institute, Israel, 1973; 71–84.

40. **Lohman, T. G., Slaughter, M. H., Selinger, A.** and **Boileau, R. A.** Relationship of body composition to somatotype in college men. *Annals of Human Biology* 1978; 5: 147–57.

41. **Slaughter, M. H.** and **Lohman, T. G.** Relationship of body composition to somatotype. *American Journal of Physical Anthropology* 1976; 44: 237–44.

42. **Slaughter, M. H.** and **Lohman, T. G.** Relationship of body composition to somatotype in boys ages 7 to 12 years. *Research Quarterly* 1977; 48: 750–8.

43. **Slaughter, M. H., Lohman, T. G.** and **Boileau R. A.** Relationship of Heath and Carter's second component to lean body mass and height in college women. *Research Quarterly* 1977; 48: 759–68.

44. **Song, J. K.** *Somatotye and body composition in males followed longitudinally from 17 to 35 years of age* (Doctoral dissertation). Faculty of Physical Education and Physiotherapy, Leuven, 1995.

45. **Wilmore, J. H.** Validation of the first and second components of the Heath–Carter modified somatotype method. *American Journal of Physical Anthropology* 1970; 32: 369–72.

46. **Claessens, A., Beunen, G.** and **Simons, J.** Anthropometric principal components and somatotype in boys followed individually from 13 to 18 years of age. *Humanbiologia Budapestinensis* 1985; 16: 23–36.

47. **Claessens, A., Beunen, G.** and **Simons, J.** Stability of anthroposcopic and anthropometric estimates of physique in Belgian boys followed longitudinally from 13 to 18 years of age. *Annals of Human Biology* 1986; 13: 235–44.

48. **Cressie, N. A. C., Withers, A. T.** and **Craig, N. P.** The statistical analysis of somatotype data. *Yearbook of Physical Anthropology* 1986; 29: 197–208.

49. **Lohman, T. G.** Applicability of body composition techniques and constants for children and youth. *Exercise and Sport Sciences Reviews* 1986; 14: 325–57.

50. **Lohman, T. G.** Assessment of body composition in children. *Pediatric Exercise Science* 1989; 1: 19–30.

51. **Boileau, R. A.** Body composition assessment in children and youths. In *The child and adolescent athlete.* (ed. O. Bar-Or). Blackwell, Oxford, 1996; 523–37.

52. **Martin, A. D., Ward R.** Body composition. In *Measurement in pediatric exercise science* (ed. D. Docherty). Human Kinetics Publishers, Champaign, Il, 1996; 87–128.

53. **Pollock, M. L., Garzarella L.** and **Graves J. E.** The measurement of body composition. In *Physiological assessment of human fitness* (ed. P. J. Maud and C. Foster). Human Kinetics Publishers, Champaign, Il, 1995; 167–204.

54. **Roche, A. F., Heymsfield, S. B.** and **Lohman, T. G.** (ed.) *Human body composition.* Human Kinetics Publishers, Champaign, Il, 1996.

55. **Klish, W. J.** The 'Gold Standard'. In *Body composition measurements in infants and children* (ed. W. J. Klish and N. Kretchmer). Report of the Ninety-Eighth Ross Conference on Pediatric Research. Ross Laboratories, Columbus, Ohio, 1989; 4–7.

56. **Going, S. B.** Densitometry. In *Human body composition* (ed. A. F. Roche, S. B. Heymsfield and T. G. Lohman). Human Kinetics Publishers, Champaign, Il, 1996; 3–23.

57. **Brozek, J., Grande, F., Anderson, J. T.** and **Keys, A.** Densitometric analysis of body composition, revision of some quantitative assumptions. *Annals New York Academy of Science* 1963; 110: 113–40.

58. **Siri, W. E.** Body composition from fluid spaces and density: Analysis of methods. In *Techniques for measuring body composition* (ed. J. Brozek and A. Henschel). National Academy of Sciences, Washington, DC, 1961; 223–44.

59. **Clarys, J. P., Martin, A. D.** and **Drinkwater, D. T.** Gross tissue weights in human cadaver dissection. *Human Biology* 1984; 56: 459–73.

60. **Martin, A. D.** and **Drinkwater, D. T.** Variability in the measures of body fat, assumptions or technique ? *Sports Medicine* 1991; 11: 277–88.

61. **Deurenberg, P., Pieters, J. J. L.** and **Hautvast, J. G. A. J.** The assessment of the body fat percentage by skinfold thickness measurements in childhood and young adolescence. *British Journal of Nutrition* 1990; 63: 293–303.

62. **Boileau, R. A., Wilmore, J. H., Lohman, T. G., Slaughter, M. H.** and **Riner, W. F.**. Estimation of body density from skinfold thickness, body circumferences and skeletal widths in boys age 8 to 11 years: Comparison of two samples. *Human Biology* 1981; 53: 575–92.

63. **Slaughter, M. H., Lohman, T. G., Boileau, R. A., Stillman, R. J., Van Loan, M.** and **Horswill, C. A.,** *et al.* Influence of maturation on relationship of skinfolds to body density: A cross-sectional study. *Human Biology* 1984; 56: 681–9.

64. **Slaughter, M. H., Lohman, T. G., Boileau, R. A., Horswill, C. A., Stillman, R. J.** and **Van Loan, M. D.,** *et al.* Skinfold equations for estimation of body fatness in children and youth. *Human Biology* 1988; 60: 709–23.

65. **Janz, K. F., Nielsen, D. H., Cassady, S. L., Cook, J. S., Wu Y-T.** and **Hansen, J. R.** Cross-validation of the Slaughter skinfold equations for children and adolescents. *Medicine and Science in Sports and Exercise* 1993; 25: 1070–6.

66. **Roemmich, J. N., Clark, P. A., Weltman, A.** and **Rogol, A. D.** Alterations in growth and body composition during puberty. I. Comparing multicompartment body composition models. *Journal of Applied Physiology* 1997; **83**: 927–35.

67. **Lohman, T. G.** Skinfolds and body density and their relation to body composition: A review. *Human Biology* 1981; **53**: 181–225.

68. **Lohman, T. G.** *Advances in body composition assessment.* Human Kinetics Publishers, Champaign, Il, 1992.

69. **Chumlea, Wm. C.** and **Guo, S. S.** Bioelectrical impedance: A history, research issues, and recent consensus. In *Emerging technologies for nutrition research* (ed. S. J. Carlson-Newberry and R. B. Costello). National Academy Press, Washington, DC, 1997; 169–92.

70. **Baumgartner, R. N.** Electrical impedance and total body electrical conductivity. In *Human body composition* (ed. A. F. Roche, S. B. Heymsfield and T. G. Lohman). Human Kinetics Publishers, Champaign, Il, 1996; 79–107.

71. **Heyward, V. H.** and **Stolarczyk, L. M.** *Applied body composition assessment.* Human Kinetics Publishers, Champaign, Il, 1996.

72. **Malina, R. M.** Application of bioelectric impedance analysis to children and adolescents. In *Body composition measurements in infants and children* (ed. W. J. Klish and N. Kretchmer). Report of the Ninety-Eighth Ross Conference on Pediatric Research. Ross Laboratories, Columbus, Ohio, 1989; 14–21.

73. **Houtkooper, L. B., Going, S. B., Lohman, T. G., Roche, A. F.** and **Van Loan, M.** Bioelectrical impedance estimation of fat-free body mass in children and youth: A cross-validation study. *Journal of Applied Physiology* 1992; **72**: 366–73.

74. **Bland, J. M.** and **Altman, D. G.** Statistical methods for assessing agreement between two methods of clinical measurements. *Lancet* 1986; **February 8**: 307–10.

75. **Baumgartner, R. N., Chumlea W. M.** and **Roche, A. F.** Associations between bioelectric impedance and anthropometric variables. *Human Biology* 1987; **59**: 235–44.

76. **Claessens, A. L., Van Langendonck, L., Lefevre, J., Thomis, M.** and **Beunen, G.** Body shape as a relevant parameter in estimating body composition by bioelectrical impedance analysis. *Journal of Sports Sciences* 1999; **17**: 552–3.

77. **Van Langendonck, L., Claessens, A. L., Philippaerts, R., Lefevre, J., Thomis, M.** and **Beunen, G.** Associations between bioelectrical impedance and anthropometric variables. *Paper presented at the 3rd Annual Congress of the European College of Sports Science*, Manchester, July 15–18, 1998.

78. Bioelectrical impedance analysis in body composition measurement; National Institutes of Health Technology Assessment Conference Statement 1994, Dec. 12–14. *American Journal of Clinical Nutrition* 1996; **64**: 524S–32S.

79. **Deurenberg, P.** International Consensus Conference on impedance in body composition. *Age and Nutrition* 1994; **5**: 142–5.

80. **Beunen, G.** Physical growth, maturation and performance. In *Kinanthropometry and exercise physiology laboratory manual* (ed. R. Eston and T. Reilly). E. and F. N. Spon, London, 1996; 51–71.

81. **Boas, F.** The growth of children. *Science* 1892; **19/20**: 257–7; 281–2; 351–2.

82. **Tanner, J. M.** *Growth at adolescence.* Blackwell Scientific Publications, Oxford, 1962.

83. **Tanner, J. M.** *Foetus into man. Physical growth from conception to maturity.* Harvard University Press, Cambridge, MA, 1989.

84. **Eveleth, P. B., Tanner, J. M.** *Worldwide variation in human growth.* Cambridge University Press, Cambridge, 1990.

85. **Bayley, N.** Tables for predicting adult height from skeletal age and present height. *Journal of Pediatrics* 1946; **28**: 49–64.

86. **Roche, A. F., Wainer H., Thissen, D.** Predicting adult stature for individuals. *Monographs in Pediatrics* 1975; **3**: 1–114.

87. **Tanner, J. M., Whitehouse, R. H., Cameron, N., Marshall, W. A., Healy, M. J. R.** and **Goldstein, H.** *Assessment of skeletal maturity and prediction of adult height (TW2 method).* Academic Press, London, 1983.

88. **Beunen, G. P., Malina, R. M., Lefevre, J., Classens, A. L., Renson, R.** and **Simons, J.** Prediction of adult stature and noninvasive assessment of biological maturation. *Medicine and Science in Sports and Exercise* 1997; **29**: 225–30.

89. **Demirjian, A.** Dentition. In *Human growth. Postnatal growth* (ed. F. Falkner and J. M. Tanner), Vol. 2. Plenum Press, New York, 1978; 413–44.

90. **Demirjian, A., Goldstein, H.** and **Tanner, J. M.** A new system for dental age assessment. *Human Biology* 1973; **45**: 211–27.

91. **Todd, J. W.** *Atlas of skeletal maturation: Part 1. Hand.* Mosby, London, 1937.

92. **Greulich, W. W.** and **Pyle, I.** *Radiographic atlas of skeletal development of the hand and wrist.* Standford University Press, Standford, 1950, 1959.

93. **Roche, A. F., Wainer, H.** and **Thissen, D.** *Skeletal maturity: Knee joint as a biological indicator.* Plenum Press, New York, 1975.

94. **Roche, A. F., Chumlea, W. C.** and **Thissen, D.** *Assessing the skeletal maturity of the hand-wrist: Fels method.* Thomas, Springfield, 1988.

95. **Beunen G., Lefevre, J., Ostyn, M., Renson, R., Simons, J.** and **Van Gerven, D.** Skeletal maturity in Belgian youths assessed by the Tanner–Whitehouse method (TW2). *Annals of Human Biology* 1990; **17**: 355–76.

1.3 Muscle strength

Cameron J. R. Blimkie and David Macauley

Introduction

This chapter focuses on laboratory-based strength assessment techniques and considerations for the paediatric population. The theoretical and practical considerations underlying strength assessment in adults,[1,2] and children and adolescents[3,4] have been previously and thoroughly reviewed. This chapter will supplement, but not replicate, the material covered in these references. The topic of strength development and its correlates or determinants during childhood are beyond the scope of this chapter. These issues have been thoroughly reviewed elsewhere,[5–8] (see Chapter 2.4 in this volume). The reader is encouraged to refer to these previous works for a more complete understanding of the general issues pertaining to strength development and assessment in children.

Strength is a construct which is generally understood to represent the ability of muscles to exert force either for the purpose of resisting or moving external loads (including the body) or to propel objects (again including one's own body) against gravity. In youth sport, strength is recognized as a variable, but nonetheless important, determinant of performance success in many activities, especially during the adolescent years. Strength may exert its influence on sports performance in a permissive manner, e.g. by increasing joint stability and thereby minimizing risk of musculoskeletal injury, or it may have a more direct influence by providing the increased force required to differentiate successful from less successful performances in sports where strength is a factor. Strength is but one of numerous traits, however, which may influence success in sports. The relationship between strength and other fitness components including anaerobic power, aerobic power and speed, and their relative importance in determining success in sport remain to be satisfactorily determined in the paediatric population.

Strength is also an important health-related fitness component, which, for example, may influence the timing of, and success of re-entry into sport after injury, or one's physical independence, e.g. ability to move about freely without assistance, particularly in children with chronic paediatric diseases. Strength may also be an enabling factor which facilitates the development of persistent physical activity habits in youth and the establishment of positive attitudes toward exercise, which may carry over into adulthood. Again, the importance of strength, in relation to health status during childhood and adolescence, and in later adult life has not been extensively addressed. Given its potential importance in the realm of sport, rehabilitation medicine and health, not surprisingly, strength assessment is a relevant and important issue for the paediatric population.

There are numerous rationales for strength assessment in the paediatric population, and many of these are exemplified in current practices of strength testing by various groups working with children. Strength testing may be used to describe developmental patterns of muscle function for the purpose of establishing normative values, against which to compare muscle function of children with various paediatric diseases. Standardized strength testing may be used to examine secular trends among different cohorts of children, trends which may be predictive of future population health risk or which may influence the direction of public policy in the areas of health and fitness planning and programming. Since muscle is a major storage cite for body protein, strength testing may provide a useful and non-invasive means of assessing the adequacy of skeletal muscle function and protein nutritional status in at-risk paediatric populations. Clinically, strength assessment may be used to describe functional profiles of specific neuro-muscular diseases, to determine the level of residual function following injury or surgical intervention, and to assess the effectiveness of various rehabilitation procedures. In sport, strength assessment may be used to determine the relative importance of strength for performance success, and subsequently to assist in the process of talent identification, providing a better match between the strength profiles of young athletes and the strength requirements of specific sports or positions within sports. Strength assessment may also be used to identify specific areas of muscle weakness in athletes which are then targeted for remedial training. Lastly, strength assessment may be used in paediatric research to examine any number of issues, such as the effectiveness of resistance training on strength development and sports performance, or the functional adaptation of muscle to various other controlled interventions such as weight loss and re-feeding.

Terminology

From a scientific perspective, strength is a specific construct which refers to the ability of muscle (single or group) to produce measurable force, torque or moment, about a single joint or multiple joints, under a defined set of controlled conditions. For the purpose of this chapter, a slightly modified version of the definition of strength provided by Knuttgen and Kraemer[9] will be used: strength is defined as 'the maximal force, torque or moment developed by a muscle or muscle groups during one maximal voluntary or evoked action of unlimited duration, at a specified velocity of movement'. This definition captures the essence of traditional approaches to strength assessment which incorporates maximal voluntary efforts, but also includes the assessment of strength under conditions of involuntary or electrically stimulated conditions; the latter is a less common, but nevertheless viable, additional condition for assessment of muscle function in humans, including children. For the purposes of this chapter, strength assessment will be considered for both voluntary and electrically stimulated conditions.

In most laboratories, muscle strength is usually expressed in units of force, torque and moment, terms which similarly refer to the measurable tension generated by muscle in its activated state. In certain situations, particularly with athletic populations, strength is still measured in the units of the external load, e.g. pounds (lb) or kilograms (kg), which are lifted in the execution of a weight lifting manoeuvre. These units adequately reflect the muscle forces required and applied to overcome external loads and are legitimate expressions of strength in this context. For most other purposes, however, and for the sake of international standardization, strength results should be expressed in units defined by The Système Internationale d'Unités (SI System): force in Newtons (N), torque in Newton meters (N m) and moment in Newton meters (N m)[2]. Some of the earlier literature reported strength in foot pounds (ft lb), which, for purposes of comparison, can be converted to N m simply by multiplying by 1.355 818.

The term force typically refers to the level of active tension generated by isolated muscle preparations *in vitro*, or to *in vivo* measurements of muscle tension where force is measured directly at the site of load application, e.g. dynamometer pad, rather than distally to the point of application, such as the central axis of rotation of a dynamometer. In isolated muscle preparations, the measured tension is largely determined by the underlying morphological (size), physiological (muscle fibre type distribution, size, length and activation) and biochemical (enzyme profiles) characteristics of the muscle, without regard to biomechanical influences, such as the angle of muscle insertion on joint articulations, which can influence external forces measured *in vivo* in humans. By contrast, *in vivo* measurements of strength in humans, measured at the site of load application, are also influenced by factors extrinsic to the muscle *per se*, such as muscle angle of insertion.

The terms force and torque are often used interchangeably in the strength assessment literature, although in the strictest sense, torque represents the product of both intrinsic (muscle) and extrinsic (anatomical, biomechanical and mechanical) factors on muscle strength expression. Torque is an expression of the effective measurable tension, which will vary as a function of the intrinsic muscle characteristics as above, the distance of the point of muscle insertion on the skeletal lever from the axis of rotation of the involved joint, and the angle of insertion of the active muscle's tendon on the skeletal lever.

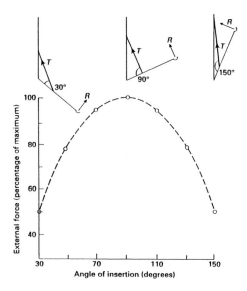

Fig. 1.3.1 The effect of angle of muscle insertion on the external torque produced by a muscle during a concentric shortening action. *T* is the direction of muscle contraction (shortening) and *R* is the external load or resistance. Adapted from Lakomy.[10]

This relationship is presented schematically in Fig. 1.3.1 and is described by the equation: Torque $(Tq) = Td\sin\Phi$; where T is the intrinsically generated constant force or tension of the active muscle transmitted via the tendon to the bone, d is the distance from the point of tendon insertion on the bone to the axis of joint rotation, and Φ is the angle of tendon insertion on the bone.[10]

Static strength measured at discrete joint angles with the joint position fixed and the dynamometer axis of rotation proximal to the point of application of the resistance, e.g. during isometric testing using an isokinetic dynamometer, is typically expressed in terms of torque. If tension is measured directly at the source of application of the resistance, such as with hand grip dynamometry or manometry, or with custom built-dynamometers, then strength is more appropriately expressed as force.

Lastly, activated muscles may also cause continuous dynamic angular rotation of skeletal segments around joint axes: strength measured under these conditions is expressed more commonly as torque or joint moments. As with static torque measurements, the measured tension at any point throughout the range of motion is also dependent on the parameters T, d, and $\sin\Phi$. *In vivo*, statically determined torques and dynamically determined moments are also influenced by extrinsic mechanical factors, such as the length of the moment arm, the distance between the point of attachment of the limb segment to the testing device and the joint axis of rotation—not to be confused with the anatomical factor d, the distance from the point of tendon insertion on the bone to the axis of joint rotation. While it is important conceptually to understand how muscle morphology and physiology, muscle–tendon anatomy, joint biomechanics and the mechanics of dynamometry relate to the terminology used to describe muscle strength in children, it is even more important to understand and account for the potential influence of these myriad factors in the interpretation of strength assessment in the paediatric population. The significance of each of these factors in the interpretation of strength assessment in children will be addressed in a later section.

It is evident from above, that both static and dynamic muscle strength, regardless of the terminology by which strength is expressed are influenced not only by the intrinsic physiological characteristics of the active muscle, but also by joint specific musculo-skeletal anatomical and biomechanical factors. Whereas the distance between the muscle insertion and joint axis of rotation remains constant within individuals during any particular strength assessment manoeuvre, in many joint actions (such as elbow flexion), the angle of muscle insertion will change with varying limb position within its range of motion, resulting in variable measurable torques at different joint positions. Additionally, differences in the distance of muscle insertion from the axis of joint rotation among individuals of varying size, e.g. short and tall children of the same age, will influence external torque measurements and must be considered when assessing and comparing 'muscle function' *per se*, independent of biomechanical influences among heterogeneously sized children.

It is important to understand how the various intrinsic and extrinsic factors described above can influence the outcome and interpretation of strength assessment results. For example, the reproducibility of repeated strength measurements (torques or moments) for a given individual, made under varying conditions of moment arm length would be poor, if correction was not made for the differences in moment arm length between testing sessions. Likewise, higher measured torques or moments in a tall child compared to a shorter child of the same age and with comparable muscle cross-sectional area, might be attributed falsely to a greater intrinsic force producing capacity of the taller boy's muscle, when in fact the difference might be wholly accounted for by the biomechanical advantage afforded the taller boy by the greater distance of tendon insertion from the joint axis of rotation—assuming that the tendon insertion distance from the axis of rotation varies in proportion to the length of the skeletal segment being acted upon. Numerous other factors including age, gender, maturity, level of physical activity and training status can also influence the expression of strength,[6,8] and like biomechanical influences must be considered carefully in the interpretation of strength assessment data from children.

Skeletal muscle active states

For all practical purposes, whether strength is being measured under voluntary or involuntary conditions, muscle activation results in one of three different muscle action types: concentric, isometric or eccentric actions. A schematic representation of these different types of muscle actions is presented in Fig. 1.3.2. It is important to understand the differences between these different types of muscle actions, because their differences dictate in large part, which is the most relevant type of action to incorporate during strength testing.

In a concentric action, the distance between the origin and insertion of the muscle becomes shorter (the muscle length shortens), and the generated muscle tension is greater than the opposing resistance. These types of actions result in dynamic limb or trunk movement of variable or constant external velocity. Concentric actions of variable velocity are more common in activities of daily living and sports than the more rarely occurring constant velocity or isokinetic actions; however, the latter are easily achievable now with sophisticated dynamometry, and are rapidly becoming the norm rather than the exception in strength testing in rehabilitation medicine, fitness testing and exercise science research.

Confusion has arisen in the past regarding the proper usage of the terms concentric and isotonic muscle actions. The term isotonic typically was used to describe dynamic muscle actions which were common manoeuvres in various sports, e.g. knee extension in kicking a soccer ball, or elbow flexion in single arm biceps curl strength training

exercise. As the roots of the term suggest, isotonic actions imply that a constant (iso) force (tonic) is applied throughout the range of motion of a manoeuvre. While the external resistance or load may remain constant in these situations (mass of the soccer ball or dumb-bell), the intrinsic muscle tension is not constant during these actions and will vary as a function of muscle length (external joint angles) and contraction speed (external angular velocities), as described by the force–velocity–length relationship.[2,10] Truly isotonic muscle actions rarely occur in human performance and continued use of this term to describe 'muscle action type' in the strength assessment literature should be discouraged.[9] The term isotonic, has nevertheless become solidly entrenched in the exercise science literature, and because of its familiarity may still be utilized legitimately to describe strength assessment techniques which incorporate constant external loading, e.g. a weightlifting task, where the limb velocity and intrinsic muscle tension will vary as a function of joint angle during the manoeuvre. The term isoinertial has recently been used to replace and describe traditional isokinetic strength tests.[1] This term provides a more accurate description of the mechanics of these types of manoeuvres, but perhaps with the expense of further terminological confusion.

A word of caution also about concentric isokinetic actions. The term implies that the movement velocity (kinetic) is constant (iso) throughout the range of movement. Although isokinetic movements are performed at a constant pre-set angular velocity selected by the test administrator, the proportion of the movement which is actually performed under truly isokinetic conditions is variable and dependent upon the chosen angular velocity and the range of motion of the exercise.[3] Generally, the higher the pre-set angular velocity and the smaller the range of motion of the exercise, the smaller the isokinetic portion of the exercise (Fig. 1.3.3). Muscle moments reported from the non-isokinetic portion of a strength testing manoeuvre misrepresent the true isokinetic capability of the muscle and are problematic to the valid interpretation of strength results. This effect may be even more problematic in testing situations involving children with muscle weakness, where movements are comprised solely of limb acceleration and deceleration without a plateau phase to the strength curve, or in situations where the joint range of motion is limited due to injury or

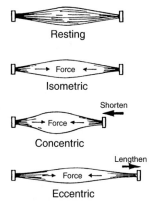

Fig. 1.3.2 The three basic types of muscle actions: isometric (no change in length with fixed attachments), concentric (force generation brings the bony attachments closer together), and eccentric (muscle is forcibly lengthened because external force is pulling the bony attachments further apart while the muscle is attempting to shorten). Adapted from Knuttgen and Kraemer.[9]

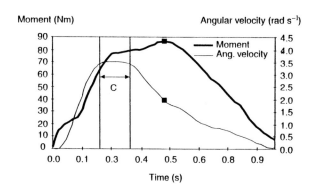

Fig. 1.3.3 Moment and angular velocity data during a knee extension test at a pre-set angular velocity of 3.15 rad s[-1]. Notice the shorter constant-velocity phase and the longer acceleration and deceleration periods. The maximum moment indicated by the square is clearly outside the isokinetic phase, and was recorded when angular velocity of the joint was decreasing and was approximately 2.0 rad s[-1]. Adapted from Baltzopoulos and Kellis.[3]

chronic disease, e.g. arthritis. In these situations, recorded moments from the non-isokinetic phase of the movement should be corrected,[11] or perhaps an alternative muscle action, e.g. isometric, would provide a more valid measure of the strength capability of the muscle in these situations.

Eccentric muscle actions represent a second type of dynamic muscle activity. In eccentric muscle actions, the intrinsic muscle tension is less than the externally applied load or resistance, the muscle lengthens and the distance between limbs or the joint angular displacement increases. Eccentric muscle actions are quite common in activities of daily living, e.g. walking down stairs, and in sports performance, e.g. dipping action at the knee in preparation for jumping in volleyball, but compared to isometric and concentric muscle actions have not been used as extensively in strength assessment, especially in the paediatric population.

In isometric muscle actions, the intrinsic muscle tension matches the external resistance, and although the muscle is in an active state, there is no visible or measurable change in the external length of the muscle, and therefore no resultant movement. Isometric actions occur frequently in sport to stabilize joints, e.g. during the neck bridging manoeuvre in free-style wrestling, and the drive swing in golf, as well as in activities of daily living, e.g. trunk stabilization when lifting groceries or sneezing. Since there is no apparent joint movement, isometric muscle actions result in static muscle activity.

It should be evident that each of these three specific muscle actions will provide measures of strength which reflect muscle activation under specific testing conditions of variable muscle length (lengthened or shortened), joint position, and/or movement velocity. Comparison of the strength-producing capacity of muscle during concentric, isometric and eccentric actions, across the continuum of variable muscle lengths, joint positions and shortening/lengthening velocities, has been extensively investigated *in vitro* (isolated muscle preparations) and *in vivo* in adults, and described by the classic muscle length–joint angle–tension[12] and force–velocity relationships.[9,12,13] These relationships are depicted schematically in Fig. 1.3.4.

In short, at a given joint angle or muscle length, isometric static strength is typically greater than concentric strength measured at the same joint angle during a dynamic shortening action, but is perhaps slightly less or not different *in vivo* from eccentric strength measured at the same joint angle during a dynamic lengthening action. During dynamic concentric muscle action, strength typically decreases with increasing joint angular velocity, whereas it may increase only slightly initially or not change with increasing dynamic eccentric muscle action, throughout a muscle's range of motion. During static isometric muscle action, peak strength occurs at an optimal muscle length or joint angle, which varies for different muscles or muscle groups; strength is typically (for most muscle groups) lower on either side of this optimal length and decreases progressively with increased shortening or lengthening beyond this point (Fig. 1.3.5). These classic relationships have been established mostly for adults, although limited studies in children suggest that the length–tension and force–velocity relationships generally also hold true for isometric, concentric and eccentric muscle actions in the paediatric population.[14–18]

These relationships have a significant influence on strength outcome, and the accuracy of the interpretation of strength assessment results is highly dependent upon a full appreciation of the interaction between these relationships. The validity of strength comparisons among different children, within the same child at different times, or between children and adults requires first and foremost that similar muscle actions be contrasted, and that comparisons are made either at

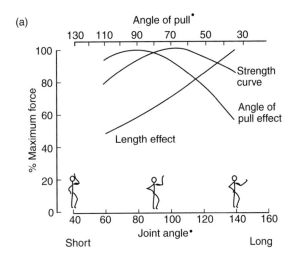

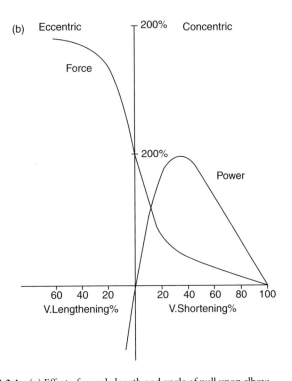

Fig. 1.3.4 (a) Effect of muscle length and angle of pull upon elbow flexion strength. The length–tension effect and the angle of pull effect interact to produce the strength curve for elbow flexion. The length effect acts to increase muscle tension from the shortest to longest muscle lengths, through the range of movement depicted. The longest length corresponds to an elbow joint angle (bottom horizontal axis) of 140°. In contrast, the optimum angle of pull (90°—top horizontal axis) occurs at a joint angle of 80°. Thus the peak of the resultant strength curve, expressed as a percentage of maximum force, would be expected to occur somewhere between joint angles of 80° and 140°; in this example it occurs at a joint angle of about 100°. Adapted from Sale and Norman.[12] (b) Schematic representation of the effect of velocity of contraction, expressed as a percentage of the maximum velocity, on force production (force–velocity relationship) in relation to isometric (0 velocity at the mid-point of the horizontal axis), concentric (shortening) velocity to right of the centre axis, and eccentric (lengthening) velocity to the left of the centre axis. Adapted from Sale and Norman.[12]

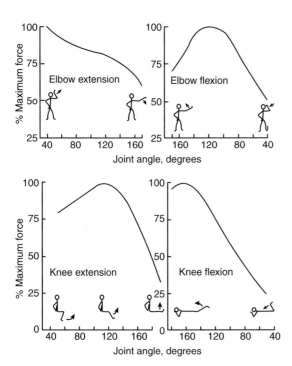

Fig. 1.3.5 Schematic representation of strength curves for selected muscle groups and exercise tests through given ranges of movement. Notice that the shape of the strength curves varies in the different movements. Adapted from Sale and Norman.[12]

the same joint angle or muscle length for isometric actions, or identical angular velocities or limb movement speeds for dynamic concentric or eccentric muscle actions. Other factors besides these, which will be addressed later in the chapter, will particularly influence the validity and reliability of strength assessment results in children, but these are by far the most salient issues to consider in assuring the validity of strength assessment procedures in children and adults.

Determinants of a strength assessment method

In keeping with the principle of specificity,[2,19] the strength assessment method should include the specific prime movers involved in the action of interest; isolate the type of muscle action which is most characteristic of its involvement in sport, training or rehabilitation; and include exercises which mimic the activity movement pattern of interest as closely as possible in terms of range of joint angle involvement and velocity or speed of limb movement. Selection of the most appropriate testing method depends first and foremost on identifying and isolating as closely as possible, the specific muscle or muscle groups to be tested. A decision must then be made about the relevancy of the different types of muscle actions in relation to the specific purpose of the test. Decisions regarding the joint angle of testing, the testing velocity and the degree of replication of the movement pattern are then made, while trying to satisfy both the requirements of the specificity principle and individual constraints imposed by the peculiarities of various sports, injuries, rehabilitative exercises or current medical status. Practical issues such as the availability of size-appropriate or disability-modified equipment, will also influence the testing method to be selected. As a general principle, the more specific the strength

testing method, the more valid the strength assessment results. At the very least, the selected method should satisfy the principle of muscle or muscle group specificity; muscle action type is perhaps not as important to mimic since there is a moderate to strong positive correlation[20] between the three muscle action types (at least in adults), and although not ideal, strength results from one type of muscle action may serve as a surrogate for another type.

The validity of strength assessment results and particularly the interpretation of these results is also strongly influenced by the reliability or reproducibility of the test measurement. Reliability, which reflects the amount of variability in repeated measurements made at different intervals (short term or long term), is determined primarily by biological variation and experimental sources of error. Biological variability reflects the consistency with which an individual can perform a given task, and this is dependent primarily on intrinsic biological, physiological and psychological factors. The main purpose of strength assessment is to isolate and detect biological sources of variation in strength performance, free of experimental sources of error. Experimental error is inevitable in any testing situation, but it should be kept to a minimum. Standard testing procedures for minimizing experimental error, with special considerations for children, which apply to strength testing for all muscle action types, will be provided later in the chapter. These will improve the reliability of the strength assessment results and provide greater sensitivity to detect biological sources of variation in the child's ability to exert maximal muscle force.

The decision to incorporate a specific mode of muscle action or a specific type of test in strength assessment will depend in part on the level of required precision, and the reliability of the selected strength measurement. If extremely precise measurements are required to detect subtle changes in strength, e.g. short-term changes in twitch torque due to nutritional intervention, then the greater the importance of the reliability of the measurement. Reliability tolerances, although always important, are perhaps less critical, the larger the expected or anticipated difference in strength performance.

Strength assessment techniques
Isometric strength assessment

In the laboratory, isometric strength is usually assessed by cable tensiometry, dedicated isometric dynamometers, e.g. hand grip dynamometer, or by custom designed dynamometers consisting of a testing frame which is configured with a force transducer or strain gauge. The former provides greater versatility in terms of the number of muscle groups that can be tested, whereas the two latter approaches are usually a bit more constricting and limit testing to only a select number of muscles or muscle groups. Examples of custom made dynamometers used to test isometric elbow flexion and ankle plantar flexion strength in children are depicted in Fig. 1.3.6.[21,22] Because custom designed dynamometers usually provide a greater degree of muscle or muscle group isolation and stability, these are often the dynamometers of choice when assessing muscle function using electrical stimulation protocols. Additionally, most commercially available isokinetic dynamometers can also be used to test isometric muscle strength, simply by pre-setting the joint angular velocity control at $0 \, \text{rad s}^{-1}$ or $0 \, \text{degrees s}^{-1}$ ($1.0 \, \text{rad s}^{-1} = 57.307 \, \text{degrees s}^{-1}$).

Since muscle strength varies as a function of muscle length or joint angle, a complete assessment of the muscle's isometric force producing

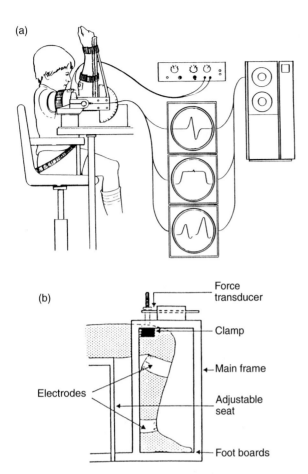

Fig. 1.3.6   (a) Schematic representation of the experimental procedures for determination of voluntary strength, motor unit activation and contractile properties of the elbow flexor muscle group in children. Adapted from Blimkie *et al.*[21] (b) Schematic representation of the dynamometer and experimental set-up for measuring maximal voluntary and electrically evoked ankle plantar flexor forces in children. Adapted from Davies.[22]

capacity requires multiple tests at various joint angles throughout the range of motion of interest. Repetitive testing of this nature is time consuming and fatiguing to both the subject and the test administrator. Multiple joint angle isometric testing protocols can also be very tedious, contributing to boredom and poor subject motivation. This may be of greater concern when testing children, who generally have shorter attention spans than adults, or children with chronic diseases which may predispose to early onset central (anaemias) or peripheral muscle (mitochondrial myopathies) fatigue. Nevertheless, isometric strength testing can be accomplished relatively inexpensively if cable tensiometry or dedicated isometric dynamometers, e.g. hand grip or back lift dynamometers are used, and cable tensiometry has the additional advantage of being more readily modifiable than commercially available isokinetic dynamometers for the extreme variations in body size experienced in paediatric exercise testing. An additional advantage of isometric strength testing, especially in a clinical setting, is that it can be used to measure strength safely, without risk of aggravation, within the residual functional range of an injured or pathological joint.

There is no agreed upon standard protocol for assessing isometric strength in children, or for that matter, adults. When performing isometric testing, adequate time must be provided to permit the development of peak force. In adults this is usually achieved within 5 s from the initiation of the test. Likewise in children, voluntary peak isometric strength is usually achieved within 2 to 5 s of a given trial.[22–28] A minimum of 30 s is usually given between consecutive trials and subjects typically perform between two to five trials for a specific muscle group. The highest of all trials' results, or the average of the most consistent results, when more than one trial is performed, may be used as the criterion measure of isometric strength.[27,29,30]

If only one joint angle is to be assessed which represents the isometric peak force producing capacity of the muscle, then the test administrator must establish *a priori*, on the basis of the length–tension relationship, the optimal joint angle at which to perform the test. It is important to remember that the optimal joint angle varies across muscle groups. The isometric length–tension relationship has not been thoroughly described for all major muscle groups in children, and neither should this relationship be assumed to be constant across different developmental stages, disease conditions, or identical to adults. Ideally, if testing is to be done at only a single joint angle, the selection should be based on individually determined muscle-specific length–tension relationships, akin to the procedure used to determine optimal braking force for assessment of peak anaerobic power from the force–velocity and force–power relationships during leg cycling[31] (and see Chapter 1.4). In practice, however, and to reduce assessment time, isometric tests are usually carried out at one or several predetermined joint angles which are constant for all subjects. The pre-selected joint angle may be optimal for some, but certainly not for all, and testing expediency is gained at the price of compromised validity. Additionally, the optimal joint angle might change with developmentally associated increases in muscle size and limb segment lengths, and these changes may compromise the validity of isometric strength comparisons (at both the individual and group levels) made at a constant joint angle, across different stages of development.

Although there are no supporting comparative data, habituation time to achieve consistent peak voluntary isometric force measures within the proscribed 5 s window may be greater in very young children compared to adolescents or adults. It may also be influenced by the level of prior testing or practice experience and the size of the muscle tested. In the author's experience, younger children (under eight years of age) are unfamiliar with the concept of rapid, almost instantaneous force development, and the idea of force maintenance or plateau once the peak force is achieved. Consequently, there is a tendency for a slower rise phase to the peak and then oscillation between peak and suboptimal force production during the hold phase of the testing protocol. Consequently, longer habituation may be required for younger children first exposed to isometric strength testing. This process can be shortened by providing the child with visual feedback on an oscilloscope or computer screen, and as with adults, by offering verbal coaching to exert greater effort. Similarly, children seem to find it more difficult to elicit and consistently reproduce maximal voluntary isometric effort with larger than with smaller muscle groups, e.g. knee extension versus elbow flexion, and when the required action is unfamiliar, e.g. maximal sustained dorsi flexion; slightly longer periods of habituation and more practice trials may also be required to improve the efficiency of isometric testing under these latter conditions.

The reliability of isometric strength measurements has not been examined extensively in children. Test–retest variations in the range of 3.7% to 11.0% have been reported for several muscle groups in samples ranging from 10–18 years of age,[30,32,33] whereas slightly poorer reproducibility (15%) has been reported for a younger population (4–13 years of age) of both sexes, using myometry.[34] Test–retest correlations for isometric hand grip and leg strength in boys between 7 and 12 years of age were moderately high, ranging between 0.86 to 0.90 and reliability was slightly higher for simultaneous double ($r = 0.90$), compared to single right ($r = 0.86$) and left ($r = 0.88$) leg strength measures.[35] High reliability has also been reported for isometric strength measures in boys with Muscular Dystrophy.[36] The variability reported in children lies within the range for adults, with a tendency towards the higher end of the range.[37] Clearly, more information is required regarding the effects of age, gender, disease, dynamometer type, muscle group and exercise complexity (e.g. single joint versus multiple joint, unilateral versus bilateral) on the reliability of isometric strength measurements in the paediatric population.

Isokinetic concentric strength assessment

Today, isokinetic concentric muscle testing is more the norm, than the exception, in many research laboratories, orthopaedic clinics and rehabilitation centres throughout the world. Although not yet used as extensively as with adults, isokinetic concentric strength testing is also being used more commonly with children. There are numerous commercially available dynamometers which provide an array of strength testing modalites, of which isokinetic concentric mode testing is one. The technical specifications and capabilities of these systems have been thoroughly reviewed elsewhere.[2,13]

Isokinetic assessment has several advantages over isometric testing. Most activities of daily living or actions in sport involve phases of dynamic concentric muscle action, and in this sense isokinetic testing may provide more specificity in terms of muscle action type than isometric or static testing. With isokinetic testing the peak functional capacity of most major prime mover muscles can be assessed throughout their entire functional range of motion, in a single effort without the need for repositioning; this improves the efficiency of strength assessment, which may be especially important when assessing children. Perhaps most important, however, is the inherent safety of isokinetic actions, afforded by the mechanism of accommodating resistance. This, in addition to the pre-set velocity control, are the two primary features which distinguish isokinetic strength testing from most other modes. Accommodating resistance is a particularly important feature with naive subjects such as children, or in testing situations involving injured muscles, since the resistance mechanism will disengage when overexertion might otherwise initiate or cause a reoccurrence of injury.

Isokinetic testing is not without its limitations, however. Human activities of daily living or actions in sport are rarely if ever executed in an isokinetic mode, and often the joint angular velocity of movements of interest in youth sports, e.g. pitching in baseball, far exceed the velocity capabilities of most commercially available dynamometers. Additionally, reliable isokinetic measurements are possible only through the three cardinal planes of movement for the body, and most activities of humans are not constrained in such a manner. These limitations detract somewhat from the specificity principle, but no more so than any of the other strength testing methods or modalities. Most commercially available isokinetic dynamometers have been designed for adults, necessitating equipment and procedural modifications when testing children.[4] Inconsistent equipment and procedural modifications within and between testing centres will have a negative impact on the reliability and reproducibility of isokinetic strength

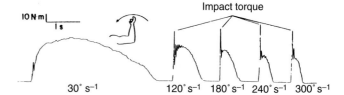

Fig. 1.3.7 Schematic representation of impact torque recordings during an isokinetic concentric elbow flexion exercise test at various joint angular velocities on a Cybex dynamometer. Note the predominance of the impact torque at the higher joint angular velocities, e.g. from 120 degrees s^{-1} and above. Adapted from Sale.[2]

measures and compromise the validity of isokinetic strength comparisons. Additionally, printed data reports from most of these isokinetic dynamometers will uncritically report the peak torque detected within the range of movement of the test, whether it occurs within or beyond the true isokinetic phase of a test manoeuvre. Particularly at high testing velocities, and perhaps more so for children with relative muscle weakness, the highest peak torque will be caused by the impact artefact,[2] which is not a true measure of the isokinetic force producing capacity of the muscle (Fig. 1.3.7). These data would not provide a valid measure of isokinetic torque and should not be accepted as representative of the maximal voluntary isokinetic torque producing capacity of the muscle.

Notwithstanding these largely mechanical considerations, perhaps the other most important potential limitation of isokinetic testing for children is the novelty of the accommodating resistance action. Whereas the concept and feel of providing maximal voluntary effort against a resisting force throughout the full range of joint motion is foreign to children and adults alike, it is perhaps more difficult for children to grasp the idea and adapt to this type of action than adults. Either because of their immature motor control or simply the sheer novelty of the action, children seem to find it more difficult than adults to alternate continuously between reciprocal isokinetic concentric flexion and extension actions. Unfamiliarity with these testing modes and protocols may require either longer periods of habituation, or separate testing of the agonist and antagonist muscles in a reciprocal pair for younger children. The requirement for sometimes different testing protocols in children, depending on age and level of motor development, confounds the interpretation of test results. Strength results obtained under the two conditions (continuous reciprocal versus separate agonist and antagonist) may not be directly comparable, since the physiological conditions (e.g. regional blood flow, muscle temperature, muscle pre-stretch, co-contraction and inhibition) under which force is measured probably vary considerably between testing protocols.

As for isometric strength testing, there are no officially accepted testing protocols for concentric isokinetic strength testing for children. Testing guidelines and protocols are provided for each of the major muscle groups by most of the isokinetic manufacturers, but little if any consideration is ever given to potential modifications to these procedures which might enhance the validity and reliability of isokinetic strength measurements in children. Since the primary purpose of isokinetic strength testing is to elicit maximal force production throughout the full range of joint motion, adequate warm up is essential to minimize risk of injury. There are no physiological reasons for providing a longer warm-up for children than for adults, but given the novelty of the isokinetic action a greater number of submaximal warm-up trials might be warranted to help facilitate habituation. Typically, children are provided a minimum of two and sometimes as many as eight sub-maximal trials at a given pre-set velocity, followed by two or three maximal efforts, a recovery period of at least 30 s and then the criterion test which may consist of a minimum of two and usually a maximum of six all-out efforts using either a continuous or interrupted protocol.[16,18,30,38,39] An alternative during the warm-up phase is to ask the subject to gradually increase the effort over the course of the practice trials so that maximal effort is achieved only during the last or penultimate effort. Discounting the impact (Fig. 1.3.7) or overshoot torque,[2,40] the highest peak torque of all trials,[16,27,30,41,42] or the average peak torque of several trials,[38,39] at given angular velocities has been used as the criterion measure of isokinetic concentric strength in children. Generally, during multiple velocity isokinetic testing, warm-up and criterion trials progress from lower to higher test velocities[38,41–43] as recommended by most manufacturers of commercial isokinetic dynamometers. Others[18,27,30] have randomized isokinetic testing velocity to eliminate ordering effects. This latter approach has proven safe with children, provided an adequate generalized and muscle-specific warm-up is given which incorporates all the pre-selected test velocities. Information regarding the effects of test protocol variability on the reliability and reproducibility of isokinetic concentric strength test results in children is sadly lacking. Standardization of isokinetic concentric test protocols for children is required.

The reliability and reproducibility of isokinetic concentric strength measures has not been investigated extensively in children. The mean score deviations in maximal isokinetic concentric strength of eight muscle groups (angular velocity unspecified) in 7–15 year old boys and girls was 5.3% to 5.8% for within-trial results and 7.9% to 9.8% for trials conducted seven to ten days apart.[44] Isokinetic concentric hip flexion and extension peak torques were moderately reliable ($0.63 < r < 0.84$) at angular velocities of 30 and 90 degrees s^{-1} in boys 6–10 years of age, whereas hip abduction and adduction measures were less reliable ($0.49 < r < 0.59$) at the same angular velocities, when retested one to two weeks apart.[38] More recently, isokinetic knee extension and flexion peak torques at an angular velocity of 100 degrees s^{-1} were shown to be highly reliable ($0.85 < r < 0.95$) and quite reproducible (8% and 12% coefficients of variation, respectively) in young boys, 6–8 years of age.[39] Similar results (coefficients of variation between 5% and 11%) have been reported for the reproducibility of between-trial (same day) isokinetic elbow flexion and knee extension strength measures in 10 year old boys;[6] the reproducibility worsened, however, when measurements were made on separate days (10.8% to 16.2% coefficients of variation).

Reliability can also be influenced by the number of testers performing the isokinetic strength assessment. It stands to reason that the greater the number of testers used, the poorer the procedural standardization and the lower the reliability of the test results. Although not examined extensively, the between-tester mean score deviations in one study[44] for shoulder and hip flexion and abduction, and knee and elbow flexion and extension ranged between 8.7% and 10.0%. The mean peak torques did not differ significantly when the assessment was done by different testers, but the magnitude of the differences were generally greater than those obtained with repeat testing by a single tester. These observations suggest that isokinetic concentric strength results may be more reliable when administered by a single rather than by multiple testers.

Reliability of isokinetic concentric strength measurements may also be influenced by limb dominance. Regrettably, there is little clear direction offered by the literature as to which limb might provide the most reproducible and reliable results. Several studies have reported no difference in bilateral isokinetic concentric strength results,[17,39,43,45–47] suggesting good reproducibility regardless of limb dominance. Others, however, have reported significant and substantial differences between dominant and non-dominant limbs, implying poor reproducibility.[42,48,49] There are no data to our knowledge which compare the reliability coefficients of repeated isokinetic concentric test results of dominant and non-dominant limbs. Correlations for isokinetic concentric peak torque between dominant and non-dominant limbs for knee and elbow flexion and extension are moderately high and range between $r = 0.65$ and $r = 0.94$ in 6–8 year old boys,[39,43] whereas at least in one study[43] the correlations for shoulder flexion and extension strength were considerably lower ($r = 0.37$ to 0.76). These bilateral limb comparisons provide no information about the reliability of strength measures in the dominant and non-dominant limbs, but rather suggest that there is considerable individual variability in the ability to produce peak isokinetic torque between limbs. On a practical basis and to ensure optimal testing reliability, these observations suggest that measurements should be made consistently on the same limb.

Lastly, isokinetic concentric test reliability may also be influenced by dynamometer type. Although each of the commercially available isokinetic dynamometers measures isokinetic peak torque, the absolute torques may vary considerably for essentially the same muscle action, across different dynamometers. One study[50] of adolescent male high school athletes reported no difference in peak torques at 60 degrees s^{-1} for knee flexion or extension among three different brand name dynamometers at a relatively slow angular velocity (60 degrees s^{-1}), but statistically significant and substantial differences at higher testing velocities of 180 and 300 degrees s^{-1}. Differences in isokinetic concentric peak torques across dynamometer types have also been reported for adults.[50,51] Although there are no comparable data on children, observations in adults suggest that differences in peak torque might also occur across different models of the same commercial dynamometer.[52] These observations suggest that the reliability of isokinetic peak torque assessments in children will be enhanced if measurements are made consistently with the same type and model of commercial dynamometer.

Isokinetic eccentric strength assessment

The advantages and disadvantages of isokinetic concentric dynamometry as described above, generally also apply to isokinetic eccentric dynamometry. In contrast to concentric strength testing, however, isokinetic eccentric strength testing is a relatively under-utilized testing modality in children. This, despite the availability of the eccentric testing mode on most newer models of commercially available isokinetic dynamometers.[2,13]

The paucity of information on eccentric muscle function in children may stem in part from the unsubstantiated concern that eccentric testing with its high peak torque producing capacity might predispose children to higher risk of muscle injury. This issue needs to be investigated more thoroughly, for there is no *a priori* reason to expect greater muscle injury with controlled isokinetic eccentric, compared to the other forms of testing, provided children are adequately instructed in the manoeuvre and given sufficient warm-up, familiarization and recovery between trials. Perhaps the more important reason for the under-utilization of this testing mode, however, is the novelty and complexity of performing isolated eccentric muscle actions for children.

Children apparently find it more difficult to comprehend the nature of the manoeuvre and to exert the level of motor coordination required for smooth and consistent executions of eccentric muscle testing[3,4] compared to adults. Whether it is due to limited attention span, lack of understanding or immature motor control, these limitations will necessitate greater patience and more thorough explanations by the tester, and longer periods of familiarization for the subjects. Learning may be facilitated by providing simple, thorough and non-technical instructions,[3] relating the required action to actions that the child may be familiar with from sport or activities of daily living, and by providing actual demonstrations of the testing manoeuvre.

There are no accepted standardized protocols for eccentric muscle testing for children. In the few studies that have utilized this testing mode in children, the testing procedures and protocols have not been described thoroughly or differentiated from the concentric testing mode,[14,16,17] and the tests have been restricted to the elbow flexor[16] and knee extensor[14,17,18] muscle groups. The testing sequences used to date involve initiation of the manoeuvre with an isokinetic concentric action, followed by the eccentric action. In three of these studies it is unclear whether the eccentric actions were tested immediately following concentric manoeuvres or if they were assessed individually.[14,16,18] In the other study, the eccentric action followed immediately after and as a continuation of the concentric action.[17] In the studies conducted to date, strength was assessed at the same joint angular velocities as during concentric testing (i.e. 0.21 to 3.14 rad s^{-1} or 12 to 180 degrees s^{-1}) and the mean of two or three trials was used as the criterion measure. With the exception of the study by Mohtadi et al.,[17] information regarding warm-up procedures, instructions and familiarization are sadly lacking.

Given the complexity and novelty of eccentric muscle actions, it may be advisable to perform concentric and eccentric muscle testing separately.[4] Testing of these actions separately removes the possible effect of potentiation from prior loading, on subsequent muscle actions, as would occur in the more common continuous combined concentric–eccentric testing protocols. Concentric–eccentric muscle strength ratios derived from the continuous and separate protocols are therefore not comparable across these different testing conditions. Additionally, there is only one report to our knowledge of the reproducibility of eccentric muscle strength in children, and none of its reliability. In a small sample of 10–12 year old boys, there were no significant test–retest (within a two week period) differences in eccentric knee extension torques, and the coefficients of variation were 4.0% and 9.9% for the non-dominant and dominant legs, respectively.[17] Clearly, the utility of eccentric strength testing in children cannot be established until issues of reliability and reproducibility are clarified and age-appropriate protocols are established and standardized. The agonist concentric–antagonist eccentric muscle action is common in many every day and sport activities, and the concentric-agonist to eccentric-antagonist peak strength ratio may be a useful index of functional muscle status in children.[3] The utility of this ratio, however, will depend on the yet to be established reliability and reproducibility of the peak eccentric strength component in children.

Isotonic strength testing

Isotonic or isoinertial testing has been used extensively in the past with adults, and especially with athlete groups to measure peak strength. These tests are often considered as field- rather than laboratory-based tests, even though they have been, and legitimately can be considered as a component of a thorough laboratory strength assessment battery. Isotonic testing is typically conducted using free weights (dumb-bells or barbells), weight-stack machines and many commercially available isokinetic dynamometers.[2,13] Isotonic testing incorporates dynamic muscle actions which, depending on exercise sequencing, may activate the stretch–shortening cycle and more closely mimic actions in sport than isometric actions. Moreover, isotonic testing can incorporate multiple joint manoeuvres which may more closely mimic sport actions while perhaps also eliciting greater co-contraction of agonist muscles, thereby providing greater joint stability and protection against injury than other testing modes. Limitations of the isotonic testing mode, however, include the variability in joint angular velocity throughout the range of motion of a manoeuvre and the inability to control contributions from other ancillary muscle groups: these factors limit the validity of strength comparisons across muscles within individuals and for similar muscles amongst individuals. Additionally, the actions executed in most isolated isotonic strength manoeuvres do not resemble very closely, in pattern or speed, typical actions in sport or daily living. Lastly, maximal isotonic strength testing, especially for multi-joint exercises, e.g. squat press, involve substantial skill and experience to be executed properly and safely.

Isotonic strength testing has been used less extensively in children than in adults, perhaps because of the putative increased risk of injury with this mode of testing compared to isometric and isokinetic modes. The one repetition maximum (1RM) lift, expressed in lb, kg or N of weight lifted, has been the traditional method of determining peak isotonic strength in adults. This is the maximum external load or resistance that an individual can lift just once with proper technique throughout the entire range of motion of an action. In this sense the 1RM qualifies as a true measure of maximal voluntary strength as defined earlier in the chapter. Because of the high skill requirement, and the potential for injury, the 1RM test is generally not recommended for pre-pubertal children.[53,54] The concern over the 1RM stems largely from injuries associated with training for, or execution of, maximal lifts in junior competitive weightlifting competitions.[55] There is no evidence that 1RM strength testing of fairly simple exercises such as the bench press, double leg press or arm curl, done in the laboratory, with modified weight stack machines and with proper adherence to lifting technique exposes a child to higher risk of injury than isometric or isokinetic testing.

The 1RM approach has been used only sparingly, however, to assess maximal voluntary isotonic strength in prepubescent children[27,30,56] and adolescent girls.[57] With the exception of the study by Ozum et al.,[56] testing in these studies was always conducted on commercially available or custom-made weight stack machines. Free weights in the form of dumb-bells were used in the study by Ozum et al.[56] Typically, with these protocols, children are given proper technical instruction in the execution of each exercise, the exercise is usually demonstrated by the tester, and then the subject attempts several repetitions of each lift, at minimal load, while receiving feedback. Novice subjects are usually given one session of habituation to the various isotonic exercises and the criterion 1RM test is usually performed the next day or within a couple of days. During the criterion test, subjects are given a warm-up consisting of three to eight repetitions of the specific exercise at low to moderate load. The 1RM load is searched for by performing a graduated series of single repetitions of increasing load separated by 30 to 60 s of recovery, beginning with the warm-up load. Each increment in loading should be perceptively more difficult and the 1RM load should be reached between six to eight trials. Once the 1RM load is identified, the subject can be given a few moments rest and the 1RM load can be attempted again. This will confirm whether the true 1RM maximum load has been achieved.

There are no published data on the reliability and reproducibility of the 1RM approach in children. In one of the authors' (CJB) own experiences, 1RM bench press, double leg press and arm (biceps) curl were found to be highly reliable (test–retest correlation of $r > 0.90$) and reproducible (coefficient of variation of less than 8%) in children nine years of age and older (unpublished observations). Improved accuracy of the 1RM load assessment can be achieved by modifying the weight machine such that smaller weight increments than those provided by the manufacturer can be added to the stack, without exceeding the subject's 1RM peak. It is the authors' opinion that relatively simple 1RM isotonic strength tests, such as the bench press, double leg press and arm curl exercises, can be performed safely and effectively in the laboratory with children nine years of age or older on weight stack type machines, provided subjects are properly instructed in the technique, given adequate familiarization, and the testing protocol includes adequate warm-up and incremental loading to maximum. If testing is not done on equipment especially designed for children, then special care is required to ensure that technical adjustments and the testing set-up permit biomechanically correct and safe execution of the exercises. Attempts at 1RM testing in the field, under less controlled conditions and using free weights and multi-joint manoeuvres may predispose the child to a higher risk of injury and should not be attempted with young children.

Several variations of multiple repetition submaximum load protocols, e.g. 5RM, 6RM and 10RM lifts have also been used to test isotonic strength in children.[58–60] These are generally claimed as safer alternatives to the 1RM procedure. These protocols are similar to the 1RM in that they all require an initial series of trials with different loads to search for the target load that will lead to exhaustion at a predetermined number of repetitions. For example, the criterion strength measure for a 5RM test will be the load or resistance which brings the child to failure at five repetitions, e.g. can lift the load only five times. This target load is usually identified within three to four sets or trials. Once the target load is determined, subjects should be given a rest period and then the criterion test load should be attempted again to verify that the true repetition maximum load has been identified. These multiple repetition submaximum protocols have been used to test isotonic strength for the squat, bench or chest press, overhead press, leg extension, leg curl and arm curl exercises using free weights[60] and child-sized dynamic constant resistance machines.[58,59] These protocols provide highly reliable measures of isotonic strength in children between 8 and 13 years of age with test–retest reliability coefficients ranging from 0.88 to 0.99.[58–60] There are no available published data on the reproducibility of these measures in children.

While seeming as an attractive alternative to the 1RM protocol, the multiple submaximum repetition protocols do not satisfy our earlier definition of maximal voluntary strength. While there is little doubt that these protocols measure at least in part, the functional strength of the child, they also measure the endurance capacity of the muscle or muscle group being tested; the greater the number of repetitions in the protocol, the more the test becomes a measure of muscle endurance rather than strength. Additionally, although being lauded as safer than the 1RM protocols, there is no published information comparing the safety of the multiple submaximum versus 1RM protocols, or of the isotonic approaches generally, with isometric or isokinetic testing

approaches. Lastly, many of the commercially available isokinetic dynamometers also have isotonic testing capability.[2,13] There are, however, no published reports to our knowledge of maximal isotonic strength measures in children obtained on isokinetic dynamometers. Clearly, more work needs to be done in this area to establish the relationship between 1RM and multiple repetition submaximum isotonic strength measures, between isotonic strength measurements and peak isometric and isokinetic strength, and the relative risk of injury associated with these different strength testing approaches in children.

Electrically evoked muscle strength

The preceding sections have discussed various approaches that have been used to measure maximal voluntary strength in children. The validity of these approaches rests entirely on the assumption that the child is firstly, capable of, and secondly, willing to exert maximal effort during testing. Test results are dependent on the degree to which instructions are understood, the skill level in executing the manoeuvre, the degree of cooperation and motivation of the child during the test, and whether there is any underlying pathology which might directly or indirectly influence the force producing capacity of the muscle. These conditions may vary within an individual over time, among individuals within a given population, and between different populations, e.g. younger versus older children, normal healthy children versus young athletes, and healthy children compared with children with various chronic paediatric diseases. These factors directly influence the validity, reliability and reproducibility of strength results and ultimately their utility in research and clinical practice.

Various electrical stimulation protocols have been used in experimental studies and clinical practice to assess evoked (involuntary) measures of muscle force production in healthy children[22,23,25–28,61] and children with various paediatric diseases.[21,28,34,62] The advantage of evoked protocols is that strength measurements are independent of most of the factors mentioned above which can influence the validity, reliability and reproducibility of maximal voluntary strength measures. Perhaps most importantly, they are independent of skill and volition. Evoked protocols have been applied successfully to measure twitch torque or tetanic force production for the extensor hallucis brevis,[63] adductor pollicis,[26,61] elbow flexors,[21,28,62] plantar flexors,[23,62] dorsi flexors,[23] triceps surae[22,25] and knee extensor[24,26–28,62] muscle groups in children as young as four years old,[26] but more typically from nine years of age and older.

Ironically, there are no published data to our knowledge of the reliability and reproducibility of evoked twitch or tetanic strength measures in children. Unpublished observations (Blimkie *et al.*, unpublished results), however, indicate that evoked twitch torque measures for the elbow flexor and knee extensor muscle groups are just as reproducible as isometric and isokinetic strength measures in ten year olds (coefficients of variation between 5.5 and 8.7%). The relationship between twitch torque and maximal voluntary isometric strength has not been extensively examined in children. Twitch torque of the triceps surae increases in concordance with maximal voluntary isometric strength in boys and girls between 9 and 21 years of age,[22,25] and twitch torque and maximal voluntary strength are highly correlated ($r = 0.81$) in children and adolescents for the plantar flexors,[23] but only moderately correlated for the dorsi flexors ($r = 0.65$ to 0.67).

For evoked twitch protocols, the muscle group of interest is secured in a custom-made dynamometer which is configured with a sufficiently sensitive force transducer or strain gauge to record the resultant electrically stimulated isometric force. Since this procedure is basically measuring isometric force production, the measurable resultant force will be influenced not only by the intrinsic force producing capacity of the muscle, but also by the length of the muscle or joint angle position.[64] The optimal muscle length or joint angle will vary for different muscle groups and among individuals, and should not be presumed to be identical for children and adults. As for maximal voluntary isometric strength assessment, the joint angle and muscle length for optimal peak twitch torque determinations should be established on an individual and muscle-specific basis. This will provide the most valid measure of the peak twitch torque capacity of the muscle under investigation. If this procedure is not followed, then at the very least, measurements should be made consistently at the same muscle length or joint angle for all subjects.

Evoked protocols involve either percutaneous electrical stimulation applied directly over the motor end point of the muscle as is the case for the elbow flexors, or over a portion of the muscle belly in the case of larger muscle groups, such as the quadriceps, plantar flexors or triceps surae. Twitches can also be induced by direct stimulation of the main nerve serving the muscle group such as the femoral nerve for the quadriceps, the ulnar nerve for the adductor pollicis and the tibial nerve for the tibialis anterior muscle. Whereas full muscle activation can only be assured during direct nervous stimulation of the muscle, there appears to be a fairly strong relationship between force production patterns of the percutaneous and directly stimulated quadriceps muscle,[28] suggesting that at least for this muscle group, the percutaneously evoked twitch measure is an acceptable surrogate of the true intrinsic force producing capacity of the muscle. Absolute twitch torques will differ, however, between techniques, and valid comparisons of twitch torques can only be made when measurements are obtained using the same technique.

Evoked twitch protocols typically involve the application of unidirectional square wave pulses of varying duration (depending on muscle size) and increasing voltage delivered via a stimulator through surface electrodes until maximal activation of the muscle is achieved. Maximal muscle activation is achieved when there is no further increase in twitch force production or when there is a plateau in the muscle electrical activity as measured by electromyography. To ensure that the peak twitch response has been obtained, the stimulation voltage is increased above that which elicited the peak twitch torque: if full activation is achieved the supramaximal stimulation will not elicit any further increase in twitch torque. Twitch torques can be substantially potentiated by prior voluntary muscle contractions[28,64] so these protocols are usually performed prior to tests of maximal or even submaximal voluntary effort, or after a recovery period of known sufficient duration to normalize the twitch response to its pre-potentiated state (Fig. 1.3.8).

The technical preparation involved with these protocols, and the novelty of the evoked muscle isometric actions may cause apprehension and fear in some children and negatively influence compliance to the protocol. These tests are not suitable for all children and the tester must be sensitive to the situation and the feelings of the child. The child's comfort, welfare and wishes should be upheld at all costs. Nevertheless, these protocols have been used successfully in several laboratories throughout the world with children of various ages, but mostly from nine years of age and above. Twitch protocols are a valid and feasible means of assessing intrinsic muscle strength in children, but perhaps these techniques are most applicable for strength assessment in the clinical and research areas. More work is required to establish the reliability and reproducibility of twitch strength measurements for different muscle groups and

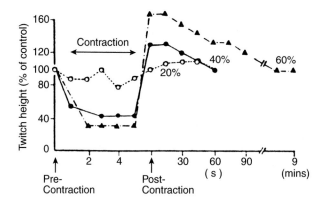

Fig. 1.3.8 Effect of prior muscle contraction on recorded twitch force production expressed as a percentage of the pre-contraction twitch height. Note that the twitch force (% height) decreases during the 5-s contraction in two subjects compared to the control in the open circles, but is augmented or potentiated immediately post-contraction in subjects who performed prior exercise. Adapted from Rutherford *et al.*[28]

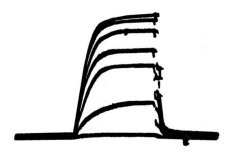

Fig. 1.3.9 Representation of tetanic force of the triceps surae muscle group with a stimulus frequency of 50 Hz and increasing voltage. Adapted from Davies.[22]

with different stimulation procedures, and their relationship to maximal voluntary strength measured by isokinetic and isotonic techniques.

Electrically evoked tetanic protocols have been used less extensively in children than the evoked twitch protocols. Tetanic force is measured using the same dynamometers and testing set-up as for the twitch protocols. With these protocols, a series of stimulation trials of variable duration, increasing stimulation frequency (5 to 50 Hz), and sometimes increasing voltage, separated by a brief period of recovery between trials is applied until there is a plateau in tetanic tension. The peak torque is taken as the criterion measure of tetanic tension (Fig. 1.3.9). Tetanic force has been measured and reported for the elbow flexors,[28] adductor pollicis,[34,61] quadriceps[28,34] and triceps surae[22,25] muscle groups. For the triceps surae muscle group[22,25] the maximal voluntary isometric force always exceeded the peak tetanic force at the highest stimulation frequency of 50 Hz by about 15%. This difference could be due to either the additional contribution of synergistic muscles to the maximal voluntary force output or to suboptimal tetanic stimulation at 50 Hz.

There is little information regarding the relationship between maximal voluntary isometric strength and tetanic torque in children. For the triceps surae, tetanic force increases in concordance with maximal voluntary strength between 9 and 21 years of age in both sexes and tetanic force at 50 Hz was highly positively correlated ($r = 0.83$) with maximal voluntary isometric force.[22,25] Similar concordance has also been observed between increases in tetanic force of the adductor pollicis and hand grip strength in both sexes between 9 and 15 years of age.[61] There is no information to our knowledge of the reliability and reproducibility of tetanic force measurements in children. Although tetanic protocols may provide the most valid index of intrinsic muscle or muscle groups' isometric force producing capacity, forces produced under these conditions cannot be considered representative of maximal strength capability under voluntary effort or for more complex isokinetic and isotonic manoeuvres.

Whereas most children can tolerate twitch protocols, the level of compliance for tetanic protocols is substantially poorer. Only 25 out of 53 children successfully completed the 50 Hz tetanic stimulation of the triceps surae.[25] Fewer than 50% of the nine year olds but 69% of adolescent girls and 79% of adolescent boys completed the 50 Hz tetanic protocol for the adductor pollicis.[61] Tetanic protocols at high stimulation frequencies are noxious and discomforting to many children. Children seem to have slightly greater tolerance of the tetanic protocol at lower stimulation frequencies (10 versus 50 Hz) and the correlation ($r = 0.79$) between tetanic forces at 10 Hz and 50 Hz is quite good,[22] suggesting that perhaps lower frequency stimulation protocols might be used instead of higher frequency protocols to improve compliance. The noxious nature of tetanic stimulation protocols raises an interesting question of ethics regarding the use of this technique in young children. The reliability and reproducibility of tetanic force measurements in children need to be established and these protocols should be reserved for research purposes and clinical applications in children with suspected or diagnosed neuromuscular disease.

Evoked isometric twitch torque measurements have also been used in combination with maximal voluntary isometric testing to determine level of motor unit activation during volitional effort in children.[21,23,24,27,28,62] This procedure (the interpolated twitch technique) does not strictly measure maximal strength, but rather provides an estimate of the degree of activation of a muscle or muscle group at various levels of volitional effort. It is a useful technique to confirm level of motivation during the execution of a manoeuvre in otherwise healthy individuals, or the degree of inhibition associated with pathology or injury. A more detailed description of this procedure is provided by Belanger and McComas[23] and Rutherford et al.[28]

Interpretative considerations

Normalization of strength results

Isometric, isokinetic and isotonic strength measures are all influenced to various degrees by intrinsic (muscle size and composition) and extrinsic (biomechanical and mechanical) factors which vary among individuals of a given age and within individuals over time, especially in growing children. These factors influence absolute force or torque measures and confound interpretations of strength results.

If strength comparisons are made between children of similar age and generally similar body composition, but different sizes, and the muscle in question is a large muscle important in weight-bearing and locomotion, then perhaps normalizing the strength score by body mass provides the most convenient and still valid basis of comparison. This may, however, underestimate the true force producing capacity of children with abnormal body composition, e.g. obese children, and this may bias the interpretation of their test results.

Normalizing by body mass, however, is more problematic when strength comparisons are made across different age and maturity groups or between genders following puberty, since the ratio of muscle mass to body mass is not constant and varies with age and gender during childhood (see Chapter 1.1). If, however, strength is considered for one of the smaller muscles, particularly of the upper body, then perhaps normalizing by the muscle size or estimated cross-sectional area (from anthropometry or medical imaging) is a more appropriate means of controlling for size differences.

Since force output is also influenced by biomechanical factors such as moment arm lengths or mechanical advantage, these factors should also be considered in the normalization of strength scores. In a practical sense it is difficult to measure precisely, the distance of insertion of tendons from the axis of rotation about a joint, but if one assumes that these distances will vary in proportion to stature or segment length, then crude adjustments on this basis can be made which will minimize the potential biomechanical advantage of taller compared to shorter children. This is perhaps a more important factor to consider when comparing strength results across different age groups and at different stages of growth and development.

Mechanical considerations

Considerable size differences exist between children of similar age, and individual children change dramatically in size during the course of childhood. This variability in growth, if not accounted for, may impose mechanical constraints on the interpretation of strength test results. The external position of the mechanical load or resistance in relation to limb segment length can have a significant effect on measurable torques or forces in isometric and isokinetic strength testing, and confound data interpretation. Standard positioning of external loads in relation to limb segment length (specific proportion of limb length) under these testing conditions should be adhered to when testing children of similar age but different size, and perhaps more importantly when testing the same child at different stages of growth and development. Failure to account for this potential mechanical influence will lead to erroneous and biased interpretations of strength results.

Contralateral limb comparisons

In certain situations, and perhaps more so in clinical practice and rehabilitative medicine, strength of an injured muscle or limb is compared to that of the uninjured contralateral side. Acutely, this is a legitimate means of assessing the severity of injury. However, if there is a substantial lapse in time between reassessments, and if the contralateral limb has increased its functional load to compensate for reduced function in the injured limb, then contralateral strength results may provide an inflated reference for the recovering limb. In this case, the strength of the contralateral limb at the time of injury would perhaps provide a more suitable baseline against which to assess degree of recovery in the injured limb.

Additionally, when testing young athletes, and for the sake of testing efficiency, a decision must be made whether to test the dominant or non-dominant limb. The literature on the effects of limb dominance on voluntary strength is at best equivocal. In sports where there is clearly a limb preference, and if only one limb is to be tested, then clearly the dominant limb for that activity should be selected. This may be a more important consideration in post- than pre-pubertal children where a combination of increased training intensity and more mature neuro-endocrinological development may facilitate greater differentiation between dominant and non-dominant limbs. Whether to test dominant or non-dominant limbs or both will depend on the purpose of the test; regardless of purpose, however, consistency in limb selection should be adhered to when performing strength testing of children.

Test instructions

Like size, there is considerable variability in intelligence, attention span and motivation among children of the same age and within children as they mature. The first priority in strength testing children is to ensure safety. This is achieved by thorough instruction in the techniques to be used and by the adequacy of familiarization and warm-up procedures. The younger the child, the greater the need for simplicity in instructions, and generally the longer the familiarization procedure. This will depend also on the complexity of the movement required during testing and the child's familiarity with the movement pattern from life experience. Learning occurs fairly rapidly for simple manoeuvres, such as isometric elbow flexion testing, but may take a bit longer for novel activities such as isokinetic concentric testing and even longer for eccentric testing or weightlifting exercises, especially for children. Motivation is a key factor to reliable testing and may be even more important for a young child who is unaccustomed to providing maximal effort on demand. To enhance reliability, standardized motivational procedures should be used consistently within and across different strength testing procedures and muscle action types.

Summary

Strength testing serves numerous meaningful functions in the paediatric population. There is a substantial literature base on isometric strength testing of children but surprisingly little about isokinetic and isotonic strength testing. The reliability and reproducibility of various testing modes, especially isokinetic and isotonic testing, and their relative safety for children of different ages needs to be further elaborated. Additionally, more research is required to define the relationship between strength as assessed by these different testing modalities and its relationship to health, injury prevention and sports performance at different ages and for both sexes during childhood.

References

1. **Abernethy, P., Wilson, G.** and **Logan P.** Strength and power assessment. Issues, Controversies and Challenges. *Sports Medicine* 1995; **19**: 401–17.
2. **Sale D. G.** Testing strength and power. In *Physiological testing of the high-performance athlete*, 2nd edn. (ed. J. D. MacDougall, H. A. Wenger and H. J. Green). Human Kinetics Publishers, Champaign, Il, 1991; 21–106.
3. **Baltzopoulos, V.,** and **Kellis, E.** Isokinetic strength during childhood and adolescence. In *Pediatric anaerobic performance* (ed. E. Van Praagh). Human Kinetics Publishers, Champaign, Il, 1998; 225–40.
4. **Gaul, C. A.** Muscular strength and endurance. In *Measurement in pediatric exercise science* (ed. D. Docherty). Human Kinetics Publishers, Champaign, Il, 1996; 225–58.
5. **Beunen, G.** Muscular strength development in children and adolescents. In *Exercise and fitness—benefits and risks* (ed. K. Froberg, O. Lammert, H. St. Hansen and C. J. R. Blimkie). Odense University Press, Odense, DK, 1997; 193–207.
6. **Blimkie, C. J. R.** Age-and-sex-associated variation in strength during childhood: Anthropmetric, morphologic, neurologic, biomechanical, endocrinolgic, genetic, and physical activity correlates. In *Perspectives in exercise science and sports medicine. Vol 2. Youth, exercise and sport* (ed. C. V. Gisolf and D. R. Lamb). Benchmark Press, Indianapolis, 1989; 99–163.
7. **Blimkie, C. J. R.,** and **Sale, D. G.** Strength development and trainability during childhood. In *Pediatric anaerobic performance* (ed. E. Van Praagh). Human Kinetics Publishers, Champaign, Il, 1998; 193–224.
8. **Froberg, K.,** and **Lammert, O.** Development of muscle strength during childhood. In *The child and adolescent athlete. The encyclopedia of sports medicine* (ed. O. Bar-Or), Vol IV. Blackwell Scientific, London, 1996; 25–41.
9. **Knuttgen, H. G.,** and **Kraemer, W. J.** Terminology and measurement in exercise performance. *Journal of Applied Sport Science Research* 1987; **1**: 1–10.
10. **Lakomy, H. K. A.** Strength. In *Oxford textbook of sports medicine* (ed. M. Harries, C. Williams, W. D. Stanish and L. J. Micheli. Oxford University Press, Oxford, 1994; 112–7.
11. **Baltzopoulos, V.** Muscular and tibiofemoral joint forces during isokinetic knee extension. *Clinical Biomechanics* 1995; **10**: 208–14.
12. **Sale, D. G.,** and **Norman, R. W.** Testing strength and power. In *Physiological testing of the elite athlete* (ed. J. D. MacDougall, H. A. Wenger and H. J. Green), 1st edn. Mutual Press, Ottawa, 1982; 7–37.
13. **Perrin, D. H.** *Isokinetic exercise and assessment.* Human Kinetics Publishers, Champaign, Il, 1993.
14. **Abe, T., Kawakami, Y., Ikegawa S., Kanehisa H.,** and **Fukunaga, T.** Isometric and isokinetic knee joint performance in Japanese ski racers. *Journal of Sports Medicine and Physical Fitness* 1992; **32**; 353–7.
15. **Calmers P., Borne, I. V. D., Nellen, M., Domenach, M., Minaire, P.** and **Drost M.** A pilot study of knee isokinetic strength in young, highly trained, females gymnasts. *Isokinetic Exercise Science* 1995; **5**; 69–74.
16. **Kawakami, Y., Kanehisa, H., Ikegawa, S.** and **Fukunaga, T.** Concentric and eccentric muscle strength before, during and after fatigue in 13 year-old boys. *European Journal of Applied Physiology* 1993; **67**; 121–4.
17. **Mohtadi, N. G. H., Kiefer, G. N., Tedford, K.** and **Watters, S.** Concentric and eccentric quadriceps torque in pre-adolescent males. *Canadian Journal of Sport Sciences* 1990; **15**: 240–3.
18. **Seger, J. Y.** and **Thorstensson, A.** Muscle strength and myoelectric activity in prepubertal and adult males and females. *European Journal of Applied Physiology* 1994; **69**: 81–7.
19. **Hakkinen, K., Komi, P. V.** and **Kauhanen, H.** Electromyographic and force production characteristics of leg extensor muscles of elite weight lifters during isometric, concentric and various stretch-shortening cycle exercises. *International Journal of Sports Medicine* 1986; **7**: 144–51.
20. **Knapick, J. J., Wright, J. E., Mawdsley, R. H.** and **Braun, J. M.** Isokinetic, isometric and isotonic strength relationships. *Archives of Physical Medicine and Rehabilitation* 1983; **64**: 77–80.
21. **Blimkie, C. J. R., Ebbesen, B., MacDougall, D., Bar-Or, O.** and **Sale D.** Voluntary and electrically evoked strength characteristics of obese and nonobese preadolescent boys. *Human Biology* 1989; **61**: 515–32.
22. **Davies, C. T. M.** Strength and mechanical properties of muscle in children and young adults. *Scandinavian Journal of Sports Science* 1985; **7**: 11–5.
23. **Belanger, A. Y.** and **McComas, A. J.** Contractile properties of human skeletal muscle in childhood and adolescence. *European Journal of Applied Physiology* 1989; **58**: 563–7.
24. **Blimkie, C. J. R., Sale, D.** and **Bar-Or O.** Voluntary strength, evoked twitch contractile properties and motor unit activation of the knee extensors in obese and non-obese adolescent males. *European Journal of Applied Physiology* 1990; **61**: 313–8.
25. **Davies, C. T. M., White M. J.** and **Young, K.** Muscle function in children. *European Journal of Applied Physiology* 1983; **52**: 111–4.
26. **Hosking, G. P., Young, A., Dubowitz, V.** and **Edwards, R. H. T.** Tests of skeletal muscle function in children. *Archives of Disease in Childhood* 1978; **53**: 224–9.
27. **Ramsay, J. A., Blimkie, C. J. R., Smith, K., Garner, S., MacDougall, D.** and **Sale D.** Strength training effects in prepubescent boys. *Medicine and Science in Sports and Exercise* 1990; **22**: 605–14.
28. **Rutherford, O. M., Jones, D. A.** and **Newham, D. J.** Clinical and experimental application of the percutaneous twitch superimposition technique for the study of human muscle activation. *Journal of Neurology, Neurosurgery, and Psychiatry* 1986; **49**: 1288–91.
29. **Anderson, L. B.** and **Henckel, P.** Maximal voluntary isometric strength in Danish adolescents 16–19 years of age. *European Journal of Applied Physiology* 1987; **56**: 83–9.

30. **Blimkie, C. J. R., Ramsay, J., Sale, D. G., MacDougall, J. D., Smith, K.** and **Garner, S.** Effects of 10 weeks of resistance training on strength development in prepubertal boys. In *Children and exercise XIII. International series on sport sciences* (ed. S. Oseid and K. H. Carlson). Human Kinetics Publishers, Champaign, Il, 1989; 183–97.

31. **Van Praagh, E.** and **Franca, N. M.** Measuring maximal short-term power output during growth. In: *Pediatric anaerobic performance* (ed. E. Van Praagh). Human Kinetics Publishers, Champaign, Il, 1998; 155–89.

32. **Asmussen, E.** Growth in muscular strength and power. In *Physical activity human growth and development* (ed. G. L. Rarick). Academic Press, New York, 1973; 60–79.

33. **Edwards, R. H. T., Chapman, S. J., Newham, D. J.** and **Jones, D. A.** Practical analysis of variability of muscle function measurements in Duchenne Muscular Dystrophy. *Muscle and Nerve* 1987; **10**: 6–14.

34. **Hosking, G. P., Bhat, U. S., Dubowitz, V.** and **Edwards, R. H. T.** Measurement of muscle strength and performance in children with normal and diseased muscles. *Archives of Diseases in Childhood* 1976; **51**: 957–63.

35. **Teeple, J. B., Lohman, T. G., Misner, J. E., Boileau, R. A.** and **Massey, B. H.** Contribution of physical development and muscular strength to the motor performance capacity of 7–12 year old boys. *British Journal of Sports Medicine* 1975; **9**: 122–9.

36. **Scott, O. M., Hyde, S. A., Goddard, C.** and **Dubowitz, V.** Quantitation of muscle function in children: A prospective study in Duchene muscular dystrophy. *Muscle and Nerve* 1982; **5**: 291–301.

37. **Tornvall, G.** Assessment of physical capabilities with special reference to the evaluation of maximal working capacity. *Acta Physiologica Scandinavica* 1963; **58**: 1–101.

38. **Burnett, C. N., Betts, E. F.** and **King, W. M.** Reliability of isokinetic measurements of hip muscle torque in young boys. *Physical Therapy* 1990; **70**: 244–9.

39. **Merlini, L., Dell'Accio, D.** and **Granata, C.** Reliability of dynamic strength knee muscle testing in children. *Journal of Orthopaedic and Sports Physical Therapy* 1995; **22**: 73–6.

40. **Baltzopoulos, V.** and **Brodie, D. A.** Isokinetic dynamometry. Applications and limitations. *Sports Medicine* 1989; **13**: 101–16.

41. **Gilliam, T. B., Villanacci, J. F., Freedson, P. S.** and **Sady, S. P.** Isokinetic torque in boys and girls ages 7–13: Effect of age, height and weight. *Research Quarterly* 1979; **50**: 599–609.

42. **Henderson, R. C., Howes, C. L., Erickson, K. L., Heere, L. M.** and **DeMasi, R. A.** Knee flexor-extensor strength in children. *Journal of Orthopaedic and Sports Physical Therapy* 1993; **18**: 559–63.

43. **Weltman, A., Tippett, S., Janney, C., Strand, K., Rians, C., Cahill, R.** and **Katch, F.** I. Measurement of isokinetic strength in prepubertal males. *Journal of Orthopaedic and Sports Physical Therapy* 1988; **9**: 345–63.

44. **Molnar, G. E., Alexander, J.** and **Gutfeld, H.** Reliability of quantitative strength measurements in children. *Archives of Physical Medicine and Rehabilitation* 1979; **60**: 218–21.

45. **Burnie, J.** Factors affecting selected reciprocal muscle group ratios in preadolescents. *International Journal of Sports Medicine* 1986; **8**: 40–5.

46. **Burnie, J.** and **Brodie, D. A.** Isokinetic measurements in preadolescent males. *International Journal of Sports Medicine* 1986; 7: 205–9.

47. **Capranica, L., Cama, G., Fanton, F., Tessitore, A.** and **Figura, F.** Force and power of preferred and non-preferred leg in young soccer players. *Journal of Sports Medicine and Physical Fitness* 1992; **32**: 358–63.

48. **Sunnegardh, J., Brattbey, L.-E., Nordesjo, L.-O.** and **Nordgren B.** Isometrics and isokinetic muscle strength, anthropometry and physical activity in 8 and 13 years old Swedish children. *European Journal of Applied Physiology* 1988; **58**: 291–7.

49. **Molnar, G. E.** and **Alexander, J.** Quantitative muscle testing in children: A pilot study. *Archives of Physical Medicine and Rehabilitation* 1973; **54**: 224–8.

50. **Wilk, K. E., Johnson, R. D.** and **Levine, B.** A comparison of peak torque values of knee extension and flexor muscle groups using Biodex, Cybex and Kin-Com isokinetic dynamometers. *Physical Therapy* 1987; **67**: 789–90.

51. **Heinrichs, K. I., Perrin, D. H., Weltman, A., Gieck, J. H.** and **Ball, D. W.** Effect of protocol and assessment device on isokinetic peak torque of the quadriceps muscle group. *Isokinetics and Exercise Science* 1995; **5**: 7–13.

52. **Thigpen, L. K., Blanke, D.** and **Lang, P.** The reliability of two different Cybex isokinetic systems. *The Journal of Sports Physical Therapy* 1990; **12**: 157–62.

53. **Freedson, P. S., Ward, A.** and **Rippe, J. M.** Resistance training for youth. In *Advances in sports medicine and fitness* (ed. W. A. Grana, J. A. Lombardo and B. J. Sharkey), Vol. 3. Year Book Medical, Chicago, 1990; 57–63.

54. National Strength and Conditioning Association (NSCA). Position paper on prepubescent strength training. *National Strength and Conditioning Association Journal* 1985; 7: 27–31.

55. **Brown, E. W.** and **Kimbell, R. G.** Medical history associated with adolescent powerlifting. *Pediatrics* 1983; **72**: 636–44.

56. **Ozum, J. C., Mikesky, A. E.** and **Surburg, P. R.** Neuromuscular adaptations following prepubescent strength training. *Medicine and Science in Sports and Exercise* 1994; **26**: 510–4.

57. **Rice, S., Blimkie, C. J. R., Webber, C. E., Levy, D., Martin, J., Parker, D.** and **Gordon, C. L.** Correlates and determinants of bone mineral content and density in healthy adolescent girls. *Canadian Journal of Physiology and Pharmacology* 1993; **71**: 923–30.

58. **Faigenbaum, A. D., Westcott, W. L., Micheli, L. J., Outerbridge, A. R., Long, C. J., LaRosa-Loud, R.** and **Zaichkowsky, L. D.** The effects of strength training and detraining on children. *Journal of Strength and Conditioning Research* 1996; **10**: 109–14.

59. **Faigenbaum, A. D., Zaichkowsky, L. D., Westcott, W. L., Micheli, L. J.** and **Fehlandt, A. F.** The effects of a twice-a-week strength training program on children. *Pediatric Exercise Science* 1993; **5**: 339–46.

60. **Sailors, M.** and **Berg, K.** Comparison of responses to weight training in pubescent boys and men. *Journal of Sports Medicine* 1987; **27**: 30–6.

61. **Backman, E.** and **Henriksson, K. G.** Skeletal muscle characteristics in children 9–15 years old: Force, relaxation rate and contraction time. *Clinical Physiology* 1988; **8**: 521–7.

62. **Hanning, R. M., Blimkie, C. J. R., Bar-Or, O., Lands, L. C., Moss, L. A.** and **Wilson, W. M.** Relationships among nutritional status and skeletal and respiratory muscle function in cystic fibrosis: Does early dietary supplementation make a difference? *American Journal of Clinical Nutrition* 1993; **57**: 580–7.

63. **McComas, A. J., Sica, R. E. P.** and **Petito, F.** Muscle strength in boys of different ages. *Journal of Neurology, Neurosurgery and Psychiatry* 1973; **36**: 171–3.

64. **Bulow, P. M., Norregaard, J., Danneskiold-Samsoe, B.** and **Mehlsen, J.** Twitch interpolation technique in testing of maximal muscle strength: Influence of potentiation, force level, stimulus intensity and preload. *European Journal of Applied Physiology* 1993; **67**: 462–6.

1.4 Anaerobic performance

Neil Armstrong and Joanne R. Welsman

Introduction

Muscle contraction through cross-bridge cycling between the actin and myosin filaments is supported by the energy released during the hydrolysis of adenosine triphosphate (ATP) to adenosine diphosphate (ADP) and inorganic phosphate (Pi), catalysed by the enzyme myosin ATPase.

$$ATP + H_2O \xrightarrow{ATPase} ADP + Pi + energy$$

The intramuscular stores of ATP are limited and for muscle contraction to be sustained ATP must be rapidly resynthesized. At the onset of exercise ATP is regenerated from ADP through an intramuscular reservoir of another high energy phosphate, creatine phosphate (CP), in the presence of the enzyme creatine kinase. This energy pathway is often called anaerobic alactic because it does not require oxygen or generate lactate.

$$CP + ADP \xrightarrow{\text{Creatine kinase}} ATP + C$$

The energy provided by these anaerobic reactions can be released at a very fast rate but, even when ATP is augmented by CP, muscle activity cannot be sustained for more than a few seconds without the assistance of other energy pathways. The first of these to be brought into play is referred to as anaerobic lactic as it produces ATP during the anaerobic degradation of glycogen, via a complex series of enzymatic reactions, to pyruvate which is subsequently reduced to lactate. The capacity of this pathway to produce ATP is significantly greater than the other anaerobic pathway but the maximal rate of ATP resynthesis is only about half that of the anaerobic alactic pathway.

$$Glycogen \rightarrow lactate + ATP$$

The aerobic pathway is the slowest to respond to the demands of exercise and the rate at which ATP can be generated anaerobically greatly exceeds that of the aerobic energy pathway. The aerobic pathway, however, has the ability to use pyruvate, free fatty acids (FFA) and even amino acids as substrates and it has a much greater capacity for energy generation than the anaerobic pathways. Prolonged muscle activity therefore depends upon the ability to deliver oxygen to the muscles.

$$(\text{Pyruvate and FFA and amino acids}) + oxygen \rightarrow CO_2 + H_2O + ATP$$

During exercise energy pathways do not operate in isolation and the relative intensity and duration of the activity dictates which pathways are the predominant providers of ATP. In near-maximal dynamic exercise the anaerobic pathways will provide the majority of energy during the initial stages of the activity but the aerobic pathway will make a gradually increasing contribution as the exercise progresses. This overlapping provision of energy by the aerobic and anaerobic pathways makes it very difficult to determine the rate or capacity of ATP production by a single pathway. Several proposed tests of 'anaerobic performance' include a significant contribution of energy from aerobic sources (e.g.[1,2]).

Phosphorus nuclear magnetic resonance spectroscopy (^{31}PNMR) offers a promising non-invasive technique for quantifying anaerobic energy yield[3] and exploratory work with both children[4] and adolescents[5] has been reported. Research is, however, limited to leg or arm exercise as currently available magnets do not allow assessment of whole-body exercise. An elegant study during short-term dynamic exercise in adults has demonstrated that, using needle biopsy of muscle and venous and arterial catheterization, direct quantitative measurement of anaerobic energy turnover is possible.[6] However, the use of these techniques with children or adolescents is unethical and paediatric exercise scientists must normally rely upon non-invasive methodology.[7,8]

Indirect estimates of children's anaerobic metabolism have been made from determination of the accumulated oxygen deficit (AOD).[9,10] AOD is measured as the difference between the actual oxygen uptake ($\dot{V}O_2$) of a supramaximal exercise bout (i.e. at say, 110% of peak $\dot{V}O_2$) and the oxygen demand predicted by extrapolation from the linear regression of exercise intensity and $\dot{V}O_2$ within a series of submaximal 'steady state' $\dot{V}O_2$ exercise bouts (see reference 11, p 122 for a sample calculation). The security of the premises underlying the technique has been challenged[12,13] and estimates of young people's 'anaerobic capacity'[11] from AOD must be interpreted cautiously.

Further development of technologies such as ^{31}PNMR may provide new insights into young people's anaerobic characteristics but direct measurement of children's and adolescents' anaerobic energy turnover is not presently possible. This chapter will therefore focus on the plethora of tests which have been developed to measure short-term power output.

Assessment of short-term power output

The two components of anaerobic performance of most interest are peak and mean power output. Peak power output is the maximum rate at which energy is transferred to the external system and mean power output is the total work done during the performance test divided by the time taken.[14] Young people's short-term power output has been assessed using jumping, cycling, running and, more recently, isokinetic dynamometry but the validity of these tests is often difficult to assess.

For a test to be valid it must also be reliable, and because of the widespread and inappropriate use of the correlation coefficient as a measure of test–retest reliability[15,16] there is little information on the variation in repeated measurements by the same short-term power output test on the same subject. Even if short-term power output tests have acceptable reliability, it is difficult to confirm their validity as there is no 'gold standard' test against which to compare. Furthermore, as short-term power output is predominantly dependent on energy supply intrinsic to the active muscles, performance test data are specific to the movement pattern used.[17] In other words, we cannot assume that power output in running tests will be similar to power output generated during cycling, as the contribution of the muscles involved may vary markedly between the two activities.[17]

Jump tests

According to Van Praagh[18,19] the first scientific investigation of leg power was carried out by Marey[20] who recorded the simultaneous measurement of force (pneumatic force platform) and displacement during a vertical jump (VJ). Other jumps, such as the standing broad jump, have been proposed as tests of anaerobic power[21] and some investigators[22] have advocated the use of a repeated series of VJs but the simple VJ has proved the most popular of this type of test.

Sargent[23] popularized the VJ as a measure of muscular power and a range of protocols have evolved from his original test. In most protocols subjects are allowed counter-movements (e.g. momentary crouch, forward arm swing) to aid their performance[24] but in others counter-movements are minimized.[25] Typically, subjects are required to jump vertically as high as they can and the highest point reached by the fingers, with the arms extended, is compared with the height reached by the fingers when the subject is standing erect, with arms extended upwards.

VJ performance is highly dependent on protocol and the general lack of standardization across studies confounds inter-study comparisons.[26] Furthermore, with young people growth and development and the resulting increase in neuromuscular activation and motor coordination must be considered. Only about 40% of 9 to 13 year olds perform the VJ with a mature pattern.[27] VJ performance appears to improve linearly with age during childhood, but during adolescence, VJ performances of girls reach a plateau while those for boys show evidence of an adolescent spurt.[28] Nevertheless, Bar-Or[29] has compared VJ scores with peak power (PP) in the Wingate anaerobic test (WAnT) and reported 'fair to good' validity.

The VJ as described by Sargent[23] has the dimension of work not power, and several formulae have been proposed to add velocity to the body mass and vertical height components[30,31] but the validity of these formulae is questionable.[26] Use of a force platform allows the calculation of instantaneous power from the product of instantaneous force exerted by the subject on the force platform and the acceleration of the subject's centre of mass.[32–34] Using this method with ten 11 year old children (six boys and four girls) Davies and Young[35] reported PP in the VJ to be 45% lower than that obtained during the first 5 s of all-out cycling. Interestingly, the same study reported that externally loading the children (from 5% to 30% body mass) resulted in a linear decrease in PP proportional to the added load. This finding indicates that body mass is not less than optimal for maximal PP output in a VJ.

Jumping is, however, an impulsive activity with the height jumped being a function of the product of force and time and not the product of force and velocity (see Chapter 2.2). The VJ has therefore been strongly criticized as a measure of power output[36] and although it remains a popular field test it is rarely used as a laboratory measure of young people's anaerobic performance.

Monoarticular force–velocity tests

Torque during movement across a single joint can be measured using isokinetic dynamometers[37] and as the angular velocity can be pre-set it is possible to calculate power output. This approach enables the characteristics of single muscle groups to be measured under controlled conditions. There are, however, several potential problems associated with the use of commercially available isokinetic dynamometers, not the least of which is the necessity to modify appropriately for children equipment which was designed for use by adults. Isokinetic dynamometer readings are rarely generated under true constant angular velocity,[38] and the difficulty of voluntarily accelerating a limb to optimal velocity for PP output has been noted.[17] Results are often difficult to interpret because of the range of angular velocities at which torque is reported. Van Praagh[18] has commented that the force–velocity relationship is highly specific and the torque–velocity relationship cannot be simply evaluated by an isolated movement at a markedly different velocity. Adult data suggest that the maximal power measured during monoarticular exercises is less than half the maximal power measured during polyarticular exercise.[39] This is partly explained by the additional power produced by other joints which act simultaneously during a polyarticular movement.[26]

Some studies have investigated total work output using monoarticular isokinetic techniques.[41] Bar-Or[29] has described a test involving 25 maximal knee extensions and flexions at an angular velocity of $3.14\ \mathrm{rad\ s^{-1}}$ and he reported, in 48 9–17 year old boys, a correlation between total work of the extensors and total work in the WAnT of $r = 0.94$. With the subjects classified according to maturational status and body mass 'corrected for' (see Chapter 1.1 for a critique) by expressing the work output in ratio with mass (i.e. $\mathrm{J\ kg^{-1}}$) the correlation coefficients were 0.68, 0.80 and 0.21 for pre-, mid- and late-pubescents, respectively.[41]

Monoarticular force velocity data from children are sparse and focus on peak torque rather than power output.[42–47] Coefficients of repeatability[15,16] for peak torque do not appear to have been published but research in our Centre (De Ste Croix and Armstrong, unpublished data) revealed, with 23 ten year old boys tested one week apart, repeatability coefficients varying from 12.4 to 21.8 Nm (mean torque values, 42.7 to 66.3 Nm) for extension and from 12.6 to 21.0 Nm (mean torque values, 33.7 to 48.2 Nm) for flexion, over velocities ranging from 0.52 to $3.14\ \mathrm{rad\ s^{-1}}$. Repeatability was more variable at slower velocities. More research is clearly required before this technique of assessing young people's short-term power output can be recommended.

Cycle tests

At the Fourth International Symposium on Pediatric Work Physiology, Cumming[48] introduced a 30-s friction-braked cycle ergometer test which was further developed under the innovative leadership of Oded Bar-Or at the Wingate Institute in Israel.[49] As the WAnT it has become the most widely used test of anaerobic performance providing measures of PP and MP.[50] Pirnay and his associates[51,52] focused specifically on PP and proposed a cycle test consisting of short maximal sprints (5 to 7 s) against several braking forces on a friction-braked ergometer. The highest recorded power output was assumed to correspond to PP. This protocol has been subsequently modified and, as the force–velocity test (F–V test), it has gained popularity with adults[26,53] and children[54,55] and been adapted for use with isokinetic cycle ergometers.[56,57]

Wingate anaerobic test

The WAnT involves pedalling a cycle ergometer, against a constant braking force, with maximal effort for 30 s, and the majority of data on young people's anaerobic performance have been generated with the WAnT.[7,8] The WAnT can be easily modified for upper body assessment and several studies of children's and adolescents' short-term power output during arm cranking have been published.[58,59] The WAnT has been demonstrated to be highly related to young people's performances in a range of predominantly anaerobic tasks[60] and it has been found to be both feasible and informative when used with children with a neuromuscular disability.[29] High test–retest correlation coefficients have been reported[60] but only one published study has reported coefficients of repeatability.[95] In our Centre, we have observed, in a series of studies with 70 nine and ten year old children, repeatability coefficients[15] in the range 44 to 50 W for PP and 34 to 42 W for MP for WAnT test–retests one week apart (see section on running tests for detailed data on WAnTs repeated over two days).

The WAnT requires a cycle ergometer in which the braking force can be kept constant and a means of monitoring pedal or flywheel revolutions. Most paediatric exercise science laboratories have developed and customized on-line automated data collection systems to retrieve the number of pedal (or flywheel) revolutions and calculate the performance indices, but several versions of appropriate software are commercially available. Monark or Fleisch friction-loaded cycle ergometers are the instruments of choice and the use of toe clips has been demonstrated to improve power output by five to 12% in adults.[61] With small children the cycle crank length may be problematic and if the crank length is inappropriate for the child's leg length the muscle length–tension relationship may adversely affect power output.[62] Bar-Or[63] has observed this effect to be small within the usual range of subject size and he reported that a change in optimal crank length of 5 cm would be expected to alter PP by only 1.24%.

Several laboratories have modified the original Wingate protocol and the lack of standardization across studies makes it difficult to interpret data from different laboratories. The advantages of a pre-test warm-up have been demonstrated[64] and, as changes in muscle temperature change the rate of cross-bridge detachment and therefore the maximal velocity of shortening,[65] it is advisable to carefully standardize the warm-up and build it into the test protocol.[62] With children, a rolling start is generally preferred and the ergometer seat and handlebars need to be adjusted appropriately for each subject. A typical protocol,[66] following a 3 to 4 min standardized warm-up which includes three or four short sprints, would be to commence the WAnT from a rolling start, at 60 rev min^{-1} against minimal resistance (weight basket supported). When a constant pedal rate of 60 rev min^{-1} is achieved, a countdown of '3—2—1—go' is given, the test braking force applied and the on-line data collection system activated. Subjects must remain seated but they are verbally encouraged to pedal maximally throughout the test. Power output is conventionally calculated from the formula:

$$P(W) = \omega T_r$$

Where ω is the angular velocity of the flywheel in rad s^{-1} and T_r is the resistive torque in Nm given by the product of the braking force and the radius of the flywheel.

This method of calculating power output in the WAnT does not take into account the work done in overcoming the inertia of the flywheel or the internal resistance of the cycle ergometer. Using a Monark 814E cycle ergometer, Chia et al.[67] factored in these components and calculated adjusted power output from:

$$P_{adj} = \omega[T_i + T_r] = \omega[I(d\omega/dt) + L_{plus\ 9\%} r]$$

where ω is the angular velocity of the flywheel; T_r is the resistive torque given by the product of $L_{plus\ 9\%}$ and r; $L_{plus\ 9\%}$ is the applied force plus the frictional loss in overcoming the internal force of the ergometer;[52,53] r is the radius of the flywheel; T_i is the inertial torque given by the product of inertia (flywheel inertia[67] plus sprocket and crank inertia[68] and angular acceleration of the flywheel (dω/dt)).

Chia et al.[67] demonstrated that when the corrected method of calculation was applied to the PP of nine year old children, PP occurred earlier in the test and values were about 20% higher in both boys and girls. These findings are in accord with those for adults[14] but to date there are no similar data available from young people despite the simplicity of the technique.

In the traditional WAnT, the Wingate team initially recommended calculating PP over a 5-s time interval and assumed that this was a reflection of alactic anaerobic performance. However, subsequent research in adults demonstrated a dramatic surge in muscle lactate concentration during the first few seconds of the test,[69] and the convention was adopted that PP represented the highest mechanical power generated during a cycling or arm cranking motion without reference to the energy pathways supporting the activity.[29] Experimenters have reported PP over 1, 3 or 5 s time segments and it has been recommended that with the relative ease of computer-driven data collection systems PP over several time periods should be reported to facilitate cross-study comparisons.[67] The total work done over 30 s was originally referred to as 'anaerobic capacity',[70] but as protocols longer than 30 s have yielded more anaerobic work than the WAnT[71] the term MP has been adopted to describe the power output over the 30 s period. A typical WAnT power curve is illustrated in Fig. 1.4.1.

The choice of a 30 s duration for the WAnT was influenced by the work of Cumming[48] and Margaria et al.[72] and by pilot work which indicated that some adult subjects were unable to complete longer all-out cycle tests.[63] The 30-s WAnT is, however, well-tolerated by young people and a recent study[73] demonstrated that children recover following a WAnT much faster than adults. Bar-Or[29] has suggested that if a WAnT needs to be repeated, a rest period for children need not exceed 5 to 10 min, but investigators following this advice should be wary of a possible cumulative temperature effect on cross-bridge cycling.

The 30 s duration of the WAnT guarantees a significant contribution from the aerobic energy pathway which, in children, may be as high as 40%,[67,74] and investigators should be aware that MP is not an exclusively anaerobic variable. Some studies have indicated that during the WAnT children and adolescents attain about 70% of their peak $\dot{V}O_2$.[75,76] Nevertheless, blood lactate levels following a WAnT progressively rise as lactate diffuses from muscle and accumulates in blood. In children, peak blood lactate following a WAnT occurs at 2 to 3 min post-exercise,[54,67,77] which is somewhat earlier than in adults.[78] The interpretation of post-exercise blood lactates is complex and confounded by methodological problems related to sampling sites and assay techniques[79,80] (see Chapter 1.7). The scarcity of longitudinal

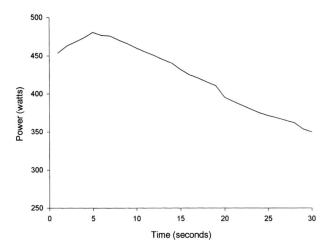

Fig. 1.4.1 Typical Wingate Anaerobic Test power curve.

Table 1.4.1 Blood lactate following a Wingate anaerobic test in children and adolescents

Study	Sex	Age (y)	n	Blood lactate (mmol litre^{-1})
Van Praagh et al.[77]	M	7.4 (0.3)	19	7.0 (3.2)
Falgairette et al.[88]	M	7.7 (0.4)	36	6.2 (2.1)
Falgairette et al.[88]	M	9.3 (0.7)	27	5.1 (1.8)
Armstrong and Welsman (unpublished)	F	9.9 (0.3)	17	5.2 (1.4)
Falgairette et al.[104]	M	11.3 (1.0)	26	8.0 (1.8)
Falgairette et al.[88]	M	11.6 (0.5)	34	7.7 (2.1)
Armstrong et al.[66]	M	12.2 (0.4)	100	6.2 (1.6)
Armstrong et al.[66]	F	12.2 (0.4)	100	6.0 (1.3)
Van Praagh et al.[54]	F	12.8 (0.4)	12	9.0 (1.8)
Van Praagh et al.[54]	M	12.9 (0.5)	15	10.0 (1.6)
Falgairette et al.[88]	M	13.1 (0.4)	29	8.4 (2.1)
Armstrong and Welsman (unpublished)	M	13.2 (0.4)	78	6.2 (1.7)
Armstrong and Welsman (unpublished)	F	13.1 (0.4)	67	6.1 (1.8)
Armstrong and Welsman (unpublished)	M	14.1 (0.3)	16	7.3 (1.3)
Falgairette et al.[88]	M	14.4 (0.4)	18	7.8 (1.6)

Values are mean (standard deviation)

data make it impossible to identify accurately the rate and timing of the progression of children's post-exercise lactates toward the higher values normally found in adults.[7,80] Table 1.4.1 presents typical data on post-WAnT lactates with the blood sampled from either the fingertip or earlobe, 2 to 3 min post-exercise and a whole blood assay used.

Power is the product of force and velocity, and as each combination of braking force and pedal revolutions may produce a different power output, optimal performance on the WAnT is dependent upon the selection of an appropriate braking force for each subject. The prototype of the WAnT[48] used the same braking force for all subjects but subsequent versions of the test have related the braking force to body mass. Bar-Or[60] has published tables of optimal braking forces for both boys and girls according to body mass but there is some evidence to suggest that, at least with 6–12 year olds, PP is independent of braking force on the Monark cycle ergometer, in the range 0.64 N kg^{-1} to 0.78 N kg^{-1}.[81] A braking force of 0.74 N kg^{-1} is commonly used with older children and adolescents.[66,82] However, as the WAnT progresses, fatigue will cause a decrease in pedalling rate, thus affecting the power/velocity ratio, and consequently a further fall in power output in addition to that directly caused by fatigue. In other words, the braking force will not be optimal for both MP and PP. This problem has been addressed with the development of special isokinetic cycle ergometers which maintain velocity at a constant level throughout the test.[57] Few studies with children have been reported and it appears that appropriately sophisticated isokinetic cycle ergometers are not readily available for purchase.[56,83]

The limitations of setting a braking force in relation to body mass when performance is better related to muscle mass are readily apparent.[17,84] Identification of an appropriate braking force is particularly difficult during growth and maturation due to the complex changes in body composition which occur at this time.[7,28] This was clearly illustrated in a recent study[85] which determined the thigh muscle volume of nine year old children using magnetic resonance imaging. A common braking force of 0.74 N kg^{-1} was applied to both boys and girls but further analysis revealed that, despite their similar body mass, the girls were exercising against a braking force which was, on average, 19% higher than that of the boys in relation to their thigh muscle volume. Individual differences varied by 49%. As much of the available data on young people's anaerobic performance are from the WAnT the use of body mass-related braking forces may have clouded our understanding of sex differences and changes in PP and MP in relation to growth and maturation.

Force–velocity test

The F–V test focuses on optimized peak power (OPP) and overcomes the methodological problem, experienced by the WAnT, of selecting the appropriate braking force to elicit PP. The test consists of a series (typically four to eight) of maximal 5 to 8 s sprints by a seated subject, performed against a range of constant braking forces. In contrast to the characteristic curvilinear relationship between force and velocity in the contracting muscle, quasi-linear braking force–velocity and parabolic braking force–power relationships have been widely observed during cycling at pedal rates between 50 and 150 rev min^{-1}.[26,53] These relationships enable the optimal velocity and braking force for OPP to be clearly identified for each subject as illustrated in Fig. 1.4.2. According to Vandewalle et al.,[26] the force (F) and velocity (V) which elicit OPP are about 50% of F_o and V_o, respectively, where F_o corresponds to the extrapolation of F for zero braking force and V_o corresponds to the extrapolation of V for zero velocity. OPP is therefore equal to 25% of the product of F_o and V_o. Winter[53,86] has provided details of the calculation of OPP from the relationship between pedalling rate and braking force and a simple computer program facilitates the process (Fig. 1.4.3).

The F–V test is being increasingly used in studies of young people[54,55,87–89] but the number of sprints employed, the rest period between sprints, the use of a rolling or standing start, the randomization and increments of braking forces applied, and the standardization of warm-ups all need to be addressed before meaningful comparisons can be made between studies. No published studies with young people have taken into account the inertia of the flywheel or the internal resistance of the cycle ergometer and coefficients of repeatability of the test are not available.

The principal disadvantage of the F–V test is the total time required for completion in relation to other anaerobic tests and there is a possibility of lactate stacking over the series of sprints.[55] However, the F–V test deserves further attention because the PP achieved is more likely to reflect the 'true' PP cycling than that measured by the WAnT or other cycling protocols, and the inter-relationship of optimal braking force and optimal velocity during growth and maturation is worthy of study. Some investigators have advocated the use of the F–V test to identify the optimal braking force for the WAnT[29,54] but this is contentious as the optimal braking force for a sprint of about 5 s is unlikely to also be optimal for a 30 s sprint. The F–V test provides a promising model for the investigation of young people's short-term power output in its own right and not just as a prerequisite for another test.

Running tests

A number of running tests have been used to estimate young people's anaerobic performance,[18,19] but the development of a running test which measures short-term power output remained elusive until Margaria *et al.*[90] solved the problem by requiring subjects to run up a flight of stairs. Knowing the height ascended, the time taken and the subject's body mass external power output was calculated. The Margaria Step Test (MST) became the most popular test of anaerobic

performance for two decades and it is still widely used as a measure of young people's short-term power.

In the laboratory, assessment of power output while running on a motorized treadmill is problematic[91] although some investigators have used the time subjects can maintain a set exercise intensity (fixed slope and constant belt velocity) as a measure of young people's anaerobic performance.[1] However, the non-motorized treadmill (NMT) has the potential to provide a running model for the assessment of both adults'[92,93] and children's[94,95] short-term power output.

Margaria step test

In the original MST protocol subjects were invited to sprint up a flight of stairs, two steps of 17.5 cm each at a time, after a 2 m run on the flat. The time taken to climb an even number of stairs was measured with an electronic clock driven by two photoelectric cells. The reason for an even number of steps was to have the subject intercept the beam of light while in the same position and in the same phase of movement. Margaria *et al.*[90] reported that maximal speed was attained in 1.5 to 2 s and then maintained constant for at least 4 to 5 s. It was assumed that all the external work was done in raising the centre of mass of the body and that this rise was the same as the level difference between the steps. Power was then calculated from the formula:

$$\begin{aligned} \text{Power (W)} &= \text{force} \times \text{velocity} \\ &= \text{body weight (N)} \times \text{vertical speed (m s}^{-1}) \\ &= [\text{body mass (kg)} \times 9.81 \text{ m s}^{-1}] \times [h\,(\text{m})/t\,(\text{s})] \end{aligned}$$

where h is the level difference between the steps where the cells are set, t is the time taken, and 9.81 is the acceleration due to gravity.

Margaria *et al.*[90] reported data on 131 subjects of both sexes, aged about 10–70 years. They claimed the data to be very reproducible with repeated tests in the same session giving values that never exceeded $\pm 4\%$ of the average. Pressure-activated switchmats linked to an electronic timer superseded the use of photocells[96] and subsequent modifications of the original protocol have shown that variations in step height, length of run-up and the use of external loading can markedly affect the external power recorded in both adults and children.[96–98]

With the realization that good motor coordination is essential for optimal performance and the likelihood of a considerable learning effect, especially with young children, the popularity of the MST waned. Although the MST has generally been replaced by the WAnT as the principal measure of young people's short-term power output, Margaria's elegant work provided a methodology which stimulated research into anaerobic performance and provided several insights into the topic. For example, the MST generated the first data to suggest that children's anaerobic performance may be inferior to that of adults.[90]

Non-motorized treadmill test

A 30 s maximal sprint on a NMT was proposed by Lakomy and his associates[92,93] as a useful way of investigating human responses to brief periods of high intensity exercise. Van Praagh's research group used the test with trained and untrained 8–13 year olds, but only for periods of less than 10 s. They reported, in abstract form, a correlation of $r = 0.94$ between PP on the NMT and PP during a F–V test.[94,99] PP during the F–V test was significantly higher than 'running power' on the NMT and Van Praagh and Franca[19] reported that, whereas no learning effects were observed during the F–V test, a significant learning effect was observed (test–retest) during running on the NMT. No further details on reliability

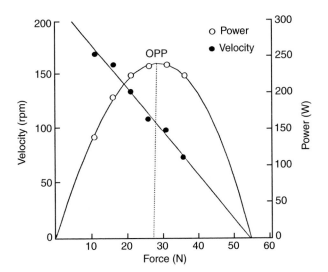

Fig. 1.4.2 The interpolation of optimal peak power for force–velocity and force–power relationships. (Reprinted from Armstrong and Welsman,[7] with permission.)

The relationship between peak pedalling rate in $\mathrm{rev\,min^{-1}}$ (R) and applied braking force (F) in Newtons is of the form:

$$R = a + bF$$

Where a is the intercept and b is the slope.

On Monark ergometers, one revolution of the pedals moves a point on the flywheel a distance of 6 m. Consequently, an expression for power output (P) in Watts can be produced:

$$P = \frac{R}{60} \times 6 \times F$$

$$\therefore P = \frac{a + bF}{60} \times 6 \times F$$

$$\therefore P = \frac{aF}{10} + \frac{bF^2}{10}$$

By differentiating this expression the gradient at any point on the power force curve can be identified:

$$\frac{\mathrm{d}P}{\mathrm{d}F} = a + 2bF$$

At the apex of the curve, the gradient is zero:

$$\therefore O = a + 2bF$$

$$\therefore F = \frac{-a}{2b}$$

Substituting this value of F in the original equation yields the peak value of power output (OPP)

$$\mathrm{OPP} = \frac{a(-a/2b)}{10} + \frac{b(-a/2b)^2}{10} = \frac{-0.025a^2}{b}$$

As b is negative, OPP and the braking force and pedalling rate corresponding to OPP can be identified.

Fig. 1.4.3 Determination of optimized peak power from pedalling rate and applied braking force. (Adapted from Winter et al.[86] and reproduced with Dr Winter's permission.)

were reported and, despite stressing the potential of NMT tests for the measurement of an individual's running power, this group do not appear to have published further research on this topic.

Falk *et al.*[100,101] tested 11–17 year old athletes on an NMT and reported PP over 2.5 s. The young athletes were instructed to sprint 'all-out' for 30 s but as most subjects found this duration of exercise too difficult to complete MP was reported over a 20 s period. The PP and MP scores were compared to WAnT performances of similarly aged but untrained young people. The NMT scores were generally higher but as the WAnT PP and MP were calculated over 5-s and 30-s periods this was not unexpected. The subjects appear to have only experienced the test once and no habituation period was described in the reports. Test–retest reliability was determined with 29 males and females aged 10–31 years who performed the test twice. Nineteen of these subjects performed the test three times. Test–retest coefficients of 0.80 and 0.81 for PP and MP, respectively, were found between the second and third tests but the relationship between the first and second tests was found to be less consistent.[101] The findings of both

Falk and Van Praagh emphasize the importance of a period of habituation prior to performance on an NMT.

Work in our Centre[95,102,103] has refined Lakomy's model and developed a permanent anaerobic test station for children as illustrated in Fig. 1.4.4. A safety frame bolted to the floor with the harness clipped to the child provides a safe environment in which following habituation the children are confident to sprint maximally. The internal resistance of the NMT is standardized through an external motor fixed to the front drum of the NMT which rotates the belt at a constant velocity for 5 min prior to each trial. A strain gauge, fixed to a wall bracket adjustable to the size of the child and an extensible tether, with the other end of the tether attached to a non-elastic belt around the child's waist, provides the horizontal force component. Power output is calculated from the product of the restraining force and the treadmill belt velocity, which is monitored on-line with an electronic sensor.

In the Exeter NMT test (ExNMT)[95] the children are fully habituated to the test during a comprehensive habituation session conducted in the testing week. The recorded test is held on a subsequent day and the subjects warm-up and commence the test from a rolling start with the belt speed at $1.67\,\mathrm{m\,s^{-1}}$. When a constant belt speed is attained a countdown of '3—2—1—go' is given, the computerized on-line system is activated and the child sprints maximally for a period of 30 s.

Sutton *et al.*[95] reported a study in which 19 well-habituated ten year olds completed two ExNMTs and two WAnTs carried out, counterbalanced, over two days. The PP and MP for the ExNMT and WAnT were $212.7 \pm 39.6\,\mathrm{W}$, $150.2 \pm 29.3\,\mathrm{W}$ and $256.8 \pm 88.2\,\mathrm{W}$, $226.1 \pm 77.8\,\mathrm{W}$, respectively. Significantly higher 2 min post-exercise blood lactates were reported following the ExNMT ($7.1 \pm 1.4\,\mathrm{mmol\,litre^{-1}}$ versus $5.2 \pm 1.2\,\mathrm{mmol\,litre^{-1}}$). The correlations between PP and MP on the ExNMT and WAnT were 0.82 and 0.88, respectively. The ExNMT demonstrated repeatability coefficients[15,16] of 26.6 W for PP and 15.3 W for MP. The corresponding values for the WAnT were 44.5 W for PP and 42.1 W for MP. The same authors[95] demonstrated that following habituation the ExNMT was appropriate for eight year olds and reported average PP over two tests of 207.9 W and average MP of 143.6 W. The repeatability coefficients were 28.4 W and 14.1 W for PP and MP, respectively. These are the only studies to date which have reported the test–retest repeatability of a NMT test.

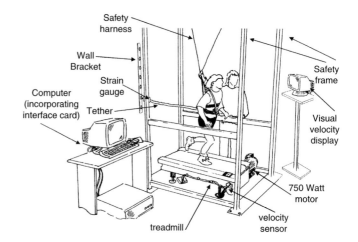

Fig. 1.4.4 The Exeter non-motorized treadmill test. (Reproduced with permission of the Children's Health and Exercise Research Centre, University of Exeter.)

Summary

In young people, although new technologies such as ^{31}PNMR have potential for the future, it is not possible to obtain direct measurements of anaerobic energy turnover during whole-body exercise. The only viable alternative currently available is to measure maximal short-term power output. No performance test will allow accurate determination of the contribution to total anaerobic metabolism of the two anaerobic systems, and the appropriate test to use depends upon the question the experimenter is addressing.

If PP is to be measured then the external force should be optimally matched with the ability of the muscle groups exercised to operate at their optimal velocity. The F–V test is therefore the method of choice, especially as it also provides information on the force and velocity components of power output. Data on young people, however, are sparse and the reliability of the test with this population requires further investigation.

For a more sustained test of power output (i.e. > 10 s) the WAnT is likely to retain its current popularity despite the well-documented problems associated with the selection of an appropriate braking force to determine PP and MP. Isokinetic cycle ergometers which can maintain velocity at a constant level throughout the test may eventually replace the WAnT, but appropriate isokinetic cycle ergometers are not commercially available at a reasonable cost. The ExNMT provides a promising laboratory model for the assessment of short-term power output during running but further research is required before it can be evaluated fully.

References

1. Paterson, D. H. and Cunningham, D.A. Development of anaerobic capacity in early and late maturing boys. In *Children and exercise XI* (ed. R. A. Binkhorst, H. C. G. Kemper and W. H. M. Saris). Human Kinetics Publishers, Champaign, Il, 1985; 119–28.

2. De Bruyn-Prévost P. and Sturbois, X. Physiological responses of girls to aerobic and anaerobic endurance tests. *Journal of Sports Medicine and Physical Fitness* 1984; **24**: 149–54.

3. Cooper, D. M. and Barstow, T. J. Magnetic resonance imaging and spectroscopy in studying exercise in children. *Exercise and Sport Sciences Reviews* 1996; **24**: 475–99.

4. Zanconato, S., Buchthal, S., Barstow, T. J. and Cooper, D. M. 31P-magnetic resonance spectroscopy of leg muscle metabolism during exercise in children and adults. *Journal of Applied Physiology* 1993; **74**: 2214–8.

5. Kuno, S., Takahashi, H., Fujimoto, K., Akima, H., Miyamaru, M., Nemoto, I., Itai, Y. and Katsuta, S. Muscle metabolism during exercise using phosphorus-31 nuclear magnetic resonance spectroscopy in adolescents. *European Journal of Applied Physiology* 1995; **70**: 301–4.

6. Bangsbo, J., Gollnick, P. D., Graham, T. E., Juel, C, Kiens B., Mizuno M. and Saltin, B. Anaerobic energy production and O_2 deficit-debt relationship during exhaustive exercise in man. *Journal of Physiology* 1990; **422**: 539–59.

7. Armstrong, N. and Welsman, J. R. *Young people and physical activity*. Oxford University Press, Oxford, 1997.

8. Rowland, T. W. *Developmental exercise physiology*. Human Kinetics Publishers, Champaign, Il, 1996.

9. Naughton, G. A. and Carlson, J. S. Anaerobic capacity assessment in male and female children with all-out isokinetic cycling exercise. *Australian Journal of Science and Medicine in Sport* 1995; **27**: 83–7.

10. Naughton, G. A., Carlson, J. S., Buttifant, D. C., Selig, S. E., Meldrum, K., McKenna, M. J. and Snow, R. J. Accumulated oxygen deficit measurements during and after high-intensity exercise in trained male and female adolescents. *European Journal of Applied Physiology* 1997; **76**: 525–31.

11. Carlson, J. S. and Naughton, G. A. Assessing accumulated oxygen deficit in children. In *Pediatric anaerobic performance* (ed. E. Van Praagh). Human Kinetics Publishers, Champaign, Il, 1998; 118–36.

12. Bangsbo, J. Oxygen deficit: a measure of the anaerobic energy production during intense exercise. *Canadian Journal of Applied Physiology* 1996; **21**: 350–63.

13. Zoladz, J. A., Rademaker, A. and Sargeant, A. J. Oxygen uptake does not increase linearly with power output at high intensities of exercise in humans. *Journal of Physiology* 1995; **488**: 211–8.

14. Lakomy, H. K. A. Assessment of anaerobic power. In *Oxford textbook of sports medicine* (ed. M. Harries, C. Williams, W. D. Stanish and L. J. Micheli). Oxford University Press, Oxford, 1994; 180–187.

15. Bland, J. M. and Altman, D. G. Statistical methods for assessing agreement between two methods of clinical measurement. *Lancet* 1986; I: 307–10.

16. Bland, J. M. and Altman, D. G. Comparing two methods of clinical measurement: a personal history. *International Journal of Epidemiology* 1995; **24 (Suppl 1)**: S7–S14.

17. Sargeant, A. Short-term muscle power in children and adolescents. In *Advances in pediatric sports sciences* (ed. O. Bar-Or),Vol 3. Human Kinetics Publishers, Champaign Il, 1989; 41–63.

18. Van Praagh, E. Testing of anaerobic performance. In *The encyclopaedia of sports medicine. The child and adolescent athlete* (ed. O. Bar-Or). Blackwell Scientific, London, 1996; 602–16.

19. Van Praagh, E. and Franca, N. M. Measuring maximal short-term power output during growth. In *Pediatric anaerobic performance* (ed. E. Van Praagh). Human Kinetics Publishers, Champaign, Il, 1998: 155–89.

20. Marey, E. J. and Demeny, G. Locomotion humaine: méchanisme du saut (Human locomotion: the jump mechanism). *Compte Rendu Séances Acad Sci* 1885: 489–94.

21. Baumgartner, T. A. and Jackson, A. S. *Measurement for evaluation in physical education and exercise science*. Brown, Dubuque, Ia, 1991.

22. Bosco, C., Luhtanen, P. and Komi, P. V. A simple method for measurement of mechanical power in jumping. *European Journal of Applied Physiology* 1983; **50**: 273–82.

23. Sargent, L. W. The physical test of a man. *American Physical Education Review* 1921; **26**: 188–94.

24. Kirby, R. F. *Kirby's guide for fitness and motor performance tests*. Ben Oak, Cape Girardeau, MO, 1991.

25. Ferretti, G., Gussoni, M., di Prampero P. E. and Ceretelli, P. Effects of exercise on maximal instantaneous muscular power of humans. *Journal of Applied Physiology* 1987; **62**: 2288–94.

26. Vandewalle, H., Pérès, G. and Monad, H. Standard anaerobic exercise tests. *Sports Medicine* 1987; **4**: 268–89.

27. Martin, J. C. and Malina, R. M. Developmental variations in anaerobic performance associated with age and sex. In *Pediatric anaerobic performance* (ed. E. Van Praagh). Human Kinetics Publishers, Champaign, Il, 1998; 45–64.

28. Malina, R. M and Bouchard, C. *Growth, maturation and physical activity*. Human Kinetics Publishers, Champaign, Il, 1991.

29. Bar-Or, O. Anaerobic performance. In *Measurement in pediatric exercise science* (ed. D. Docherty). Human Kinetics Publishers, Champaign, Il, 1996; 161–82.

30. Gray, R. K., Start, K. B. and Glencross, DJ. A test of leg power. *Research Quarterly* 1962; **33**: 44–50.

31. Fox, E. L., Bowers, R. and Foss, M. *The physiological basis for exercise and sport*. Brown and Benchmark, Madison, 1993; 657–8.

32. Davies, C. T. M. Human power output in exercise of short duration in relation to body size and composition. *Ergonomics* 1971; **14**: 245–56.

33. Davies, C. T. M. and Rennie, R. Human power output. *Nature* 1968; **217**: 770.

34. Offenbacher, E. L. Physics and the vertical jump. *American Journal of Physiology* 1970; **38**: 7.

35. **Davies, C. T. M.** and **Young K.** Effects of external loading on short-term power output in children and young male adults. *European Journal of Applied Physiology* 1984; **52**: 351–4.

36. **Adamson, G. T.** and **Whitney, R. J.** Critical appraisal of jumping as a measure of human power. *Medicine and Sport* 1971; **6**: 208–11.

37. **Baltzopoulos, V.** and **Kellis, E.** Isokinetic strength during childhood and adolescence. In *Pediatric anaerobic performance* (ed. E. Van Praagh). Human Kinetics Publishers, Champaign, Il, 1998; 225–40.

38. **Murray, D. A.** and **Harrison, E.** Constant velocity dynamometer: an appraisal using mechanical loading. *Medicine and Science in Sports and Exercise* 1986; **6**: 612–24.

39. **Avis, F. J., Hoving, A** and **Toussaint, H. M.** A dynamometer for the measurement of force, velocity, work and power during an explosive leg extension. *European Journal of Applied Physiology* 1985; **54**: 210–5.

40. **Saavedra, C., Lagassé, P., Bouchard, C.** and **Simoneau, J-A.** Maximal anaerobic performance of the knee extensor muscles during growth. *Medicine and Science in Sports and Exercise* 1991; **23**: 1083–9.

41. **Calvert, R. E., Bar-Or, O., McGillis, L. A** and **Suei, K.** Total work during an isokinetic and Wingate endurance tests in circumpubertal males. *Pediatric Exercise Science* 1993; **5**: 398.

42. **Faro, A., Silva, J., Santos, A., Iglesias, P.** and **Ning, Z.** A study of knee isokinetic strength in preadolescence. In *Children and exercise XIX* (ed. N. Armstrong, B. J. Kirby and J. R. Welsman). E. and F. N. Spon, London, 1997; 313–8.

43. **De Ste Croix, M. B. A., Armstrong, N., Welsman, J. R., Winsley, R. J., Parsons, G.** and **Sharpe, P.** Relationship of muscle strength with muscle volume in young children. In *Children and exercise XIX* (ed. N. Armstrong, B. J. Kirby and J. R. Welsman). E. and F. N. Spon, London, 1997; 319–24.

44. **Weltman, A., Tippett, S., Janney, C., Strand, K., Rians, C., Cahill, B.R.** and **Katch, F. I.** Measurement of isokinetic strength in prepubertal males. *Journal of Orthopaedic and Sports Physical Therapy* 1988; **9**: 345–51.

45. **Gilliam, T. B., Villanacci, J. F.** and **Freedson, P. S.** Isokinetic torque in boys and girls ages 7 to 13: effect of age, height and weight. *Research Quarterly* 1979; **50**: 599–609.

46. **Burnie, J.** and **Brodie, D. A.** Isokinetic measurement in preadolescent males. *International Journal of Sports Medicine* 1986; **7**: 205–9.

47. **Kanecisa, H., Ikagawa, S., Tsunoda, N.** and **Fukunaga, T.** Strength and cross-sectional areas of knee extensor muscles in children. *European Journal of Applied Physiology* 1994; **65**: 402–5.

48. **Cumming, G.R.** Correlation of athletic performance and aerobic power in 12– 17-year-old children with bone age, calf muscle, total body potassium, heart volume and two indices of anaerobic power. In *Pediatric work physiology* (ed. O. Bar-Or). Wingate Institute, Netanya, Israel, 1973; 109–14.

49. **Ayalon, A., Inbar, O.** and **Bar-Or, O.** Relationships between measurements of explosive strength and anaerobic power. In *International series on sports sciences: Vol 1, Biomechanics IV* (ed. R. C. Nelson and C. A. Morehouse). University Park Press, Baltimore, 1974; 527–32.

50. **Inbar, O., Bar-Or, O.** and **Skinner, J. S.** *The Wingate anaerobic test.* Human Kinetics Publishers, Champaign, Il, 1996.

51. **Maréchal, R., Pirnay, F., Creilaard** and **J. M., Petit, J. M.** *Influence de l'age sur la puissance anaerobie (Influence of age on anaerobic power).* Economica, Paris, 1979.

52. **Pirnay, F.** and **Creilaard, J. M.** Mesure de la puissance anaerobic alactique. *Med de Sports* 1979; **53**: 13–6.

53. **Winter, EM.** Cycle ergometry and maximal exercise. *Sports Medicine* 1991; **11**: 351–7.

54. **Van Praagh, E., Fellmann, N., Bedu, M., Falgariette, G.** and **Coudert, J.** Gender difference in the relationship of anaerobic power output to body composition in children. *Pediatric Exercise Science* 1990; **2**: 336–48.

55. **Williams, C.** and **Armstrong, N.** Optimized peak power output of adolescent children during maximal sprint pedalling. In *Children in sport* (ed.F. J. Ring). University Press, Bath, 1995; 40–4.

56. **Sargeant, A. J.** and **Dolan, P.** Optimal velocity of muscle contraction for short-term (anaerobic) power output in children and adults. In *Children*

and exercise XII (ed. J. Rutenfranz, R. Mocellin and F. Klimt). Human Kinetics Publishers, Champaign, Il, 1986; 39–42.

57. **Sargeant, A. J., Hoinville, E.** and **Young, A.** Maximum leg force and power output during short-term dynamic exercise. *Journal of Applied Physiology* 1981; **51**: 1175–82.

58. **Blimkie, C. J. R., Roache, P., Hay, J. T., Bar-Or, O.** Anaerobic power of arms in teenage boys and girls: relationship to lean tissue. *European Journal of Applied Physiology* 1988; **57**: 677–83.

59. **Nindle, B. C., Mahar, M. T., Harman, E. A.** and **Patton, J. F.** Lower and upper body anaerobic performance in male and female adolescent athletes. *Medicine and Science in Sports and Exercise* 1995; **27**: 235–41.

60. **Bar-Or, O.** Noncardiopulmonary pediatric exercise tests. In *Pediatric laboratory exercise testing* (ed. T. W. Rowland). Human Kinetics Publishers, Champaign, Il, 1993; 165–85.

61. **Lavoie, N., Dallaier, J., Brayne, S.** and **Barrett, D.** Anaerobic testing using the Wingate and the Evans-Quinney protocols with and without toe stirrups. *Canadian Journal of Applied Sport Science* 1984; **9**: 1–5.

62. **Sargeant, A. J.** The determinants of anaerobic muscle function during growth. In *Pediatric anaerobic performance* (ed. E. Van Praagh). Human Kinetics Publishers, Champaign, Il, 1998; 97–117.

63. **Bar-Or, O.** The Wingate anaerobic test: An update on methodology, reliability and validity. *Sports Medicine* 1987; **4**: 381–94.

64. **Inbar, O.** and **Bar-Or, O.** The effects of intermittent warm-up on 7- to 9-year-old boys. *European Journal of Applied Physiology* 1975; **34**: 81–9.

65. **Sargeant, A. J.** Effect of muscle temperature on leg extension force and short-term power output in humans. *European Journal of Applied Physiology* 1987; **56**: 693–8.

66. **Armstrong, N., Welsman, J. R.** and **Kirby, B. J.** Performance on the Wingate anaerobic test and maturation. *Pediatric Exercise Science* 1997; **9**: 253–61.

67. **Chia, M., Armstrong, N.** and **Childs, D.** The assessment of children's anaerobic performance using modifications of the Wingate anaerobic test. *Pediatric Exercise Science* 1997; **9**: 80–9.

68. **Monger, L. S., Allchom, A.** and **Doust, J.** An automated bicycle ergometer system for the measurement of Wingate Test indices with allowance for inertial and accelerative influences. *Journal of Sports Science* 1993; **7**: 77–8.

69. **Jacobs, I., Tesch, P. A., Bar-Or, O., Karlsson, J.** and **Dotan, R.** Lactate in human skeletal muscle after 10 and 30 s of supramaximal exercise. *Journal of Applied Physiology* 1983; **55**: 365–7.

70. **Bar-Or, O.** *Pediatric sports medicine for the practitioner.* Springer-Verlag, New York, 1983.

71. **Katch, V., Weltman, A., Martin, R.** and **Gray, L.** Optimal test characteristics for maximal anaerobic work on the bicycle ergometer. *Research Quarterly* 1977; **48**: 319–27.

72. **Margaria, R., Oliva, D., di Prampero P. E.** and **Ceretelli P.** Energy utilization in intermittent exercise of supramaximal intensity. *Journal of Applied Physiology* 1969; **26**: 752–6.

73. **Hebestreit, H., Minura, K-I.** and **Bar-Or, O.** Recovery of muscle power after high intensity short-term exercise: comparing boys to men. *Journal of Applied Physiology* 1994; **74**: 2875–80.

74. **Williams, C. A.** *Anaerobic performance of prepubescent and adolescent children.* Unpublished doctoral dissertation. University of Exeter, United Kingdom, 1995.

75. **Van Praagh, E., Bedu, M., Falgairette, G., Fellmann, N.** and **Coudert, J.** In *Children and exercise: pediatric work physiology XV* (ed. R. Frenkl and I. Szmodis). National Institute for Health Promotion, Budapest, 1991; 281–7.

76. **Chia, M.** *Anaerobic fitness of young people.* Unpublished doctoral dissertation. University of Exeter, United Kingdom, 1998.

77. **Van Praagh, E., Falgairette, G., Bedu, M., Fellmann, N.** and **Coudert, J.** Laboratory and field tests in 7-year-old boys. In *Children and exercise XIII* (ed. S. Oseid and K. H. Carlsen). Human Kinetics Publishers, Champaign, Il, 1989; 11–7.

78. **Creilaard, J. M.** and **Franchimont, P.** La mesure de la capacité anaérobie lactique: mise au point actuelle. *Medicine Sport* 1985; **59**: 150–2.

79. **Williams, J., Armstrong, N.** and **Kirby, B.** The influence of site of sampling and assay medium upon the measurement and interpretation of blood lactate responses to exercise. *Journal of Sports Science* 1992; **10**: 95–107.

80. **Welsman, J.** and **Armstrong, N.** Assessing post-exercise lactates in children and adolescents. In *Pediatric anaerobic performance* (ed. E. Van Praagh). Human Kinetics Publishers, Champaign, Il, 1998; 137–54.

81. **Carlson, J.** and **Naughton, G.** Performance characteristics of children using various braking resistances on the Wingate anaerobic test. *Journal of Sports Medicine and Physical Fitness* 1994; **34**: 362–9.

82. **Falk, B.** and **Bar-Or, O.** Longitudinal changes in peak aerobic and anaerobic mechanical power of circumpubertal boys. *Pediatric Exercise Science* 1993; **5**: 318–31.

83. **Sargeant, A. J., Dolan, P.** and **Thorne, A.** Optimal velocity of muscle contraction for short-term output in children and adults. In *Children and sport* (J. Ilmarinen and I. Valimaki). Springer-Verlag, Berlin, 1984; 93–8.

84. **Sargeant, A. J.** Problems in, and approaches to the measurement of short term power output in children and adolescents. In *Children and exercise XVI, Pediatric work physiology* (ed. J. Coudert and E. Van Praagh). Masson, Paris, 1992; 11–7.

85. **Welsman, J. R., Armstrong, N., Kirby, B. J., Winsley, R. J., Parson, G.** and **Sharpe, P.** Exercise performance and magnetic resonance imaging determined thigh muscle volume in children. *European Journal of Applied Physiology* 1997; **76**: 92–7.

86. **Winter, E. M., Brown, D., Roberts, N. K. A., Brookes, F. B. C.** and **Swaine, I. L.** Optimized and corrected peak power output during friction-braked cycle ergometry. *Journal of Sports Science* 1996; **14**: 513–21.

87. **Duché, P., Falgairette, G., Bedu, M., Fellmann, N., Lac, G., Robert, A.** and **Coudert, J.** Longitudinal approach of bio-energetic profile in boys before and during puberty. In *Pediatric work physiology* (ed. J. Coudert and E. Van Praagh). Masson, Paris, 1992; 43–5.

88. **Falgairette, G., Bedu, M., Fellmann, N., Van Praagh, E.** and **Coudert, J.** Bioenergetic profile in 144 boys aged from 6 to 15 years with special reference to sexual maturation. *European Journal of Applied Physiology* 1991; **62**: 151–6.

89. **Mercier, B., Mercier, J., Ganier, P., La Gallais, D.** and **Préfaut, C.** Maximal anaerobic power: relationship to anthropometric characteristics during growth. *International Journal of Sports Medicine* 1992; **13**: 21–6.

90. **Margaria, R., Aghemo, P.** and **Rovelli, E.** Measurement of muscular power (anaerobic) in man. *Journal of Applied Physiology* 1966; **21**: 1662–4.

91. **Asmussen, E.** and **Bonde-Petersen, F.** Storage of elastic energy in skeletal muscle in man. *Acta Physiol Scand* 1974; **91**: 385–92.

92. **Lakomy, H. K. A.** The use of a non-motorized treadmill for analysing sprint performance. *Ergonomics* 1987; **30**: 627–37.

93. **Cheetham, M. F., Williams, C.** and **Lakomy, H. K. A.** A laboratory running test: metabolic responses of sprint and endurance trained athletes. *British Journal of Sports Medicine* 1985; **19**: 81–4.

94. **Fargeas, M. A., Van Praagh, E., Léger, L., Fellmann, N.** and **Coudert, J.** Comparison of cycling and running power outputs in trained children. *Pediatric Exercise Science* 1993; **5**: 415.

95. **Sutton, N. C., Childs, D. J., Bar-Or, O.** and **Armstrong, N.** A non-motorized treadmill test to assess children's short-term power output. *Pediatric Exercise Science* 2000; **12**: 89–98.

96. **Armstrong, N.** and **Ellard R.** The measurement of alactacid anaerobic power in trained and untrained adolescent boys. *Physical Education Review* 1983; **7**: 73–9.

97. **Davies, C. T. M., Barnes, C.** and **Godfrey, S.** Body composition and maximal exercise performance in children. *Human Biology* 1972; **44**: 195–214.

98. **Caiozzo, V. J.** and **Kyle, C. R.** The effect of external loading upon power output in stair climbing. *European Journal of Applied Physiology* 1980; **51**: 750–4.

99. **Van Praagh, E., Fargeas, M. A., Léger, L., Fellmann, N.** and **Coudert, J.** Short-term power output in children measured on a computerized treadmill ergometer. *Pediatric Exercise Science* 1993; **5**: 482.

100. **Falk, B., Weinstein, Y., Epstein, S., Karni, Y.** and **Yarom, Y.** Measurement of anaerobic power among young athletes using a new treadmill test. *Pediatric Exercise Science* 1993; **5**: 414.

101. **Falk, B., Weinstein, Y., Dotan, R., Abramson, D. A., Mann-Segal, D.** and **Hoffman, J. R.** A treadmill test of sprint running. *Scandinavian Journal of Medicine and Science in Sports* 1996; **6**: 259–64.

102. **Armstrong, N., Williams, J. R., Williams, C.** and **Frost, J.** Methods of assessing children's anaerobic performance. Paper presented to *British Association of Sports Science Conference, Children in Sport.* Bedford, 1987.

103. **Armstrong, N.** and **Welsman, J. R.** Laboratory testing of young athletes. In *Colour atlas and text of sports medicine in childhood and adolescence* (ed. N. Maffulli). Mosby-Wolfe, London, 1995; 109–22.

104. **Falgairette, G., Duché, P., Bedu, M., Fellman, N., Coudert, J.** Bioenergetic characteristics in prepubertal swimmers: comparison with active and non-active boys. *International Journal of Sports Medicine* 1993; **14**: 444–8.

1.5 Pulmonary function

Patricia A. Nixon

Introduction

At rest and during exercise, the lungs serve two major functions: (1) to pump sufficient air to and from the alveoli along the airways or conduits; and (2) to exchange oxygen and carbon dioxide between the alveoli and the capillary blood flow. Together, these functions help to maintain acid–base balance. In healthy children, the lungs are not thought to be limiting to exercise. However, children with pulmonary disorders may exhibit abnormal pulmonary responses which may ultimately contribute to a limitation to exercise.

The focus of this chapter is the assessment and interpretation of pulmonary function during exercise in children, with emphasis on the parameters commonly measured in the paediatric setting. The measurements of resting pulmonary function (i.e. lung volumes and expiratory flow rates) are presented to provide the basic foundation for understanding changes that occur with exercise. Some measurements are more relevant to children with pulmonary disorders, and examples of normal and abnormal responses are provided. In some instances, data on children are lacking, so responses of adults are presented. A more detailed discussion of the physiology and the changes in lung function that occur with growth and development in healthy children is provided in Chapter 2.6. In view of these changes throughout childhood and adolescence, 'normal' values are not provided in this chapter, but can be found in the extensive works of Polgar and Promadhat[1] and Zapletal[2] for resting pulmonary function, and Godfrey[3] for exercise responses.

The assessment of pulmonary function at rest

The assessment of resting pulmonary function via spirometry and the measurement of lung volumes are not routinely done as part of the exercise evaluation of the healthy child. However, this information may be useful for understanding the pulmonary responses to exercise, particularly in the child with a pulmonary disorder. Additional information may be obtained via the less common measurements of lung compliance and respiratory muscle strength which are discussed in Chapter 2.6.

Lung volumes

Static lung volumes and capacities are presented schematically in Fig. 1.5.1.[4] Capacities are defined as the sum of two or more volumes. The spirographic tracing starts with resting breathing providing the tidal volume (V_T), i.e. the volume of air that is breathed in or out during normal respiration. Inspiratory reserve volume (IRV) is the volume of air that can be maximally inspired above V_T. The volume of air that can be maximally expired below V_T is the expiratory reserve volume

(ERV). The volume of air that remains in the lungs after a maximal expiration is the residual volume (RV). The volume of air that is left in the lungs after a normal expiration is functional residual capacity (FRC) and is the sum of RV and ERV. Total lung capacity (TLC) is the volume of air that is in the lungs after a maximal inspiration, and is the sum of IRV, V_T, ERV and RV. The vital capacity (VC) is the maximum amount of air that can be expired from TLC and is the sum of IRV, V_T and ERV. All of these static lung volumes and capacities increase non-linearly with increasing age, body surface and stature, correlating most closely with stature.[2]

Functional residual capacity is generally measured by one of three methods:

(1) the nitrogen washout method;
(2) the inert gas (usually helium) dilution technique; or
(3) plethsymography.[5]

For the first two methods, a known volume and concentration of a tracer gas is inhaled, and the lung volume is calculated based on the concentration of gas in the expired air, assuming complete mixing of the tracer gas in the lungs. These methods underestimate FRC in patients with airway obstruction who have poorly ventilated regions of the lung. The last method, plethysmography, calculates RV and TLC based on the theory of Boyle's law which assumes that in a closed container, such as the plethysmograph or body box, changes in lung volumes can be calculated from changes in pressure under constant temperature.[6] This method is better suited for patients with poorly

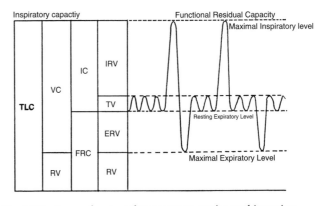

Fig. 1.5.1 Lung volumes as they appear on a spirographic tracing. TLC = total lung capacity, VC = vital capacity, RV = residual volume, IC = inspiratory capacity, FRC = functional residual capacity, IRV = inspiratory reserve volume, TV = tidal volume, ERV = expiratory reserve volume. From Comroe *et al.*[4] (reprinted with permission).

ventilated regions of the lung because it measures virtually all of the gas in the lungs.

Airway patency or flow

Airway patency is assessed by examining expiratory air flow rates and volumes, most commonly in the form of a flow/volume loop, and measured via standard spirometric techniques.[7,8] The components of the flow/volume loop in a healthy child are shown in Fig. 1.5.2. Forced vital capacity (FVC) is the maximal volume of air expired after a maximal inspiration. The maximal or peak expiratory flow rate (PEFR) occurs early in the forced expiratory manoeuvre. The amount of air expired during the first second of a forced maximal manoeuvre is the forced expiratory volume in one second (FEV_1). It provides a measure of large airway function or patency. Smaller airway function or patency is provided by the forced expiratory flow rate between 25 and 75% of FVC (FEF_{25-75}). Smaller airway function is also reflected by the flow rate after 75% of FVC has been exhaled (FEF_{75}). In this example, the maximal inspiratory flow (MIF) loop (the curve below the x-axis) is also shown. The tidal volume loop during normal breathing is also provided for comparison with the maximal manoeuvre. Measures of FVC, PEFR, FEV_1 and MIF are effort-dependent, whereas the measures of smaller airway function or the 'tail' of the expiratory curve are considered to be relatively independent of effort.[2]

The flow/volume loop of a child with obstructive lung disease is presented in Fig. 1.5.3. In obstructive disorders, there is limited airway patency and reduced expiratory flow. As shown, the FVC of the patient is normal, but there is evidence of both larger and smaller airway obstruction, as reflected in reduced FEV_1, FEF_{25-75} and FEF_{75}. In contrast, with restrictive lung disorders, the flow rates are normal, but the amount of air that the lungs contain is decreased, as shown in the

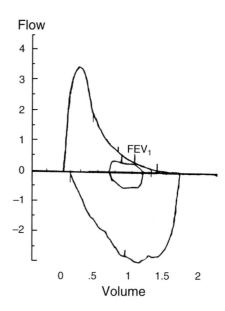

Figure 1.5.3 The flow/volume loop of a child with obstructive lung disease. The FVC is normal, but flow rates are decreased.

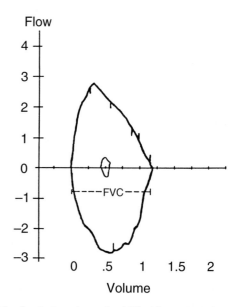

Fig. 1.5.4 The flow/volume loop of a child with restrictive lung disease. The FVC is decreased, but flow rates are normal.

reduced FVC in Fig. 1.5.4. However, it may appear that the child with the restrictive defect also has airway obstruction because the FEV_1 will be reduced compared to normal predictive values, as a consequence of all lung volumes being reduced. For this reason, the ratio of FEV_1/FVC is examined to obtain a more accurate measure of airway patency relative to lung volume. Children tend to have higher FEV_1/FVC (up to 90%) compared with adult values (75 to 85%).[5]

Maximal voluntary ventilation

The resting measure of maximal voluntary ventilation (MVV) is also often performed to provide a measure of the mechanical capacity of the

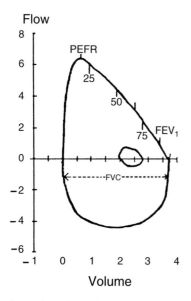

Fig. 1.5.2 The flow/volume loop of a healthy child. Peak expiratory flow rate (PEFR), forced expiratory volume in one second (FEV_1), and forced vital capacity (FVC) are labelled. The 25, 50 and 75 refer to the forced expiratory flow rates at 25, 50 and 75% of FVC. The curve below the x-axis reflects inspiration.

lungs. For this test, the child is instructed to breathe as deeply and quickly as they can for 12 s.[7] The volume of air breathed is then extrapolated to one minute. Some investigators suggest that MVV in children can be estimated from the product of $FEV_1 \times 35$.[3,9]

A variety of spirometers can be used to determine flow rates, FVC and MVV.[6] The majority of spirometers operate either by measuring volume displacement or by directly measuring flow. The volume-displacement spirometers include water-sealed spirometers, dry rolling-seal spirometers, bellows or wedge-bellows spirometers. The volume of air expired or inspired into a closed system mechanically displaces a recording pen on a chart recorder or activates a potentiometer which measures the volume and flow rates. The advantage of these systems is that they provide a mechanical tracing of the flow/volume curve. The disadvantages are that some systems are not very mobile (water-sealed), the closed systems can possibly become contaminated and are cumbersome to clean, and they may not be computerized.[6]

More recently, flow-sensing pneumotachometers, including pressure-differential flow sensors, heated wire flow sensors and turbine flow sensors, have become popular devices for determining minute ventilation. With these pneumotachometers, the flow of gas produces a signal from which flow can be measured and gas volumes integrated. The most common type of flow sensor is the pressure-differential pneumotachometer. Based on Poiseuille's law, gas flow and pressure drop are linearly related, assuming laminar (non-turbulent) flow. The change in air pressure across a resistive element (either capillary tubes or metal screens) is detected and measured by a pressure transducer from which flow and volume can be calculated. The heated-wire pneumotachometer senses the change in temperature in a heated element (thermistor) with changes in gas flow. The gas flow is determined by the amount of current necessary to maintain a pre-set temperature of the thermistor, from which flow and volume can likewise be calculated. Both the pressure-differential and heated-wire pneumotachometers can be affected by debris and moisture collected on the sensing elements. Furthermore, to reduce measurement error, the pneumotachometer should be the appropriate size and calibrated in the expected range of flow rates for the test subject.

The turbine flow sensor consists of a lightweight impeller or vane connected to a series of gears that move with and directly measure the volume of gas flow. The accuracy of the turbine may also be affected by moisture and saliva. In addition, the impeller may be slow to start up at the beginning of each breath and to slow down at the end of each breath, due to inertia, leading to measurement error.[10]

The assessment of pulmonary function during exercise

Minute ventilation

The pulmonary parameter most commonly measured during exercise is minute ventilation ($\dot{V}_E$), i.e. the volume of air exhaled during one minute and expressed as litres per minute (BTPS). Minute ventilation is a required component for the calculation of oxygen uptake ($\dot{V}O_2$) using open-circuit spirometry. In earlier days, expired air was collected in Douglas bags or meteorological balloons, and the volume was measured as the bag was manually emptied into a dry gas meter or a large Tissot type water sealed spirometer. The dry gas meter and the water sealed spirometer could also be connected to the breathing circuit for direct measurements of minute ventilation.

More recently, flow-sensing pneumotachometers, as described previously, have become the most popular devices for determining minute ventilation during exercise. The potential error measurements, due to moisture, inertia etc., become exaggerated with the higher flow rates during exercise. In addition, the density and viscosity of different gases such as 100% oxygen can also affect the pressure–flow relationship. Consequently, calibration should be performed under the same conditions as the testing to avoid measurement error.[11]

During progressive exercise, $\dot{V}_E$ increases linearly with increasing $\dot{V}O_2$ until a point at which the increase in $\dot{V}_E$ is accelerated, probably due to the addition of anaerobic metabolism (see section on ventilatory anaerobic threshold). $\dot{V}_E$ is determined by age, body size, fitness and exercise intensity, and therefore, has wide normal variation which limits its interpretation as a single measure of ventilatory function.

Tidal volume and respiratory rate

The components of $\dot{V}_E$ are tidal volume (V_T) and respiratory rate or the frequency of breathing (f_R). During progressive exercise, the increase in ventilation is met initially by increases in V_T up to about 50% of vital capacity.[12] V_T encroaches on both inspiratory and expiratory reserve volumes, resulting in an end-expiratory lung volume (EELV) that falls below the resting functional residual capacity of the lungs. The lower EELV helps to lessen the work of the diaphragm during inspiration.[13] As exercise becomes more intense, f_R increases to meet the higher ventilatory and metabolic demands.[3] The child with restrictive lung disease has to compensate for limited V_T by increasing f_R to meet the ventilatory demands of exercise. In healthy adults, V_T generally does not exceed 70% of inspiratory capacity (IC), whereas V_T has been shown to approach 100% of IC in adults with restrictive lung disease.[14] Similar results may be anticipated in the child with restrictive lung disease.

Breathing reserve

The ratio of minute ventilation at peak exercise to the resting maximal voluntary ventilation ($\dot{V}_E$/MVV) gives some indication of the proportion of mechanical ventilatory capacity used at peak exercise. The unused portion is considered to be the breathing reserve.[14] In the healthy child, the minute ventilation at peak or maximal exercise is usually well below the MVV obtained at rest ($\dot{V}_E$/MVV = 60 to 70%), indicating sufficient mechanical reserve.[3] In contrast, the peak $\dot{V}_E$ of the child with obstructive lung disease may approach or even exceed the MVV, leaving little or no ventilatory reserve, and suggesting ventilatory limitation to exercise.[15] The fact that $\dot{V}_E$ can exceed MVV may be attributed to bronchodilation during exercise, but may also be due to the problem or limitation of comparing an effort-dependent resting voluntary manoeuvre (MVV) with an 'involuntary' exercise measure. The forced expiratory manoeuvre of MVV in the 'artificial' laboratory setting may cause the airways to collapse somewhat.

Ventilatory equivalent for oxygen

The ventilatory equivalent for oxygen, or the ratio of minute ventilation to oxygen uptake ($\dot{V}_E/\dot{V}O_2$), provides a measure of ventilatory efficiency at various levels of exercise. In general, children exhibit a higher $\dot{V}_E/\dot{V}O_2$ compared to adults, suggesting ventilatory inefficiency in children.[16] Normally, the $\dot{V}_E/\dot{V}O_2$ increases at work rates above the anaerobic threshold (AT). However, in patients who have a mechanical ventilatory limitation or chemoreceptor insensitivity, the $\dot{V}_E/\dot{V}O_2$ may fail to increase above AT.[11]

In children with obstructive lung disease such as cystic fibrosis, $\dot{V}_E/\dot{V}O_2$ may be elevated to compensate for increased dead space (i.e. ventilated regions of the lung where gas exchange does not occur because of limited capillary blood flow).[17]

Ventilatory equivalent for carbon dioxide

The ventilatory equivalent for carbon dioxide, or the ratio of minute ventilation to carbon dioxide production ($\dot{V}_E/\dot{V}CO_2$), provides a non-invasive measure of dead space, subject to influence by arterial carbon dioxide tension (P_aCO_2).[11] Higher than normal values of $\dot{V}_E/\dot{V}CO_2$ are observed in patients with increased dead space ventilation.[11] The plotting of $\dot{V}_E/\dot{V}CO_2$ and $\dot{V}_E/\dot{V}O_2$ against work rate may provide a non-invasive way to obtain information on ventilation/perfusion (V_A/Q) matching (i.e. the matching of ventilated alveoli with perfused capillaries). Elevated ventilatory equivalents for O_2 and CO_2 can reflect either hyperventilation or uneven V_A/Q, depending on the arterial carbon dioxide tension (P_aCO_2).[11] Furthermore, the plotting of $\dot{V}_E/\dot{V}CO_2$ against $\dot{V}_E/\dot{V}O_2$ can be used as one method to determinate ventilatory anaerobic threshold.[18]

Ventilatory anaerobic threshold

The ventilatory anaerobic threshold (VAT) has been described as the point during progressive exercise where $\dot{V}_E$ increases disproportionately with the increase in $\dot{V}O_2$.[18] It is believed that the accelerated increase in $\dot{V}_E$ occurs in response to the excess CO_2 produced by the buffering of lactate, the by-product of anaerobic metabolism. While many studies have shown that the threshold for the accelerated increase in ventilation corresponds to the threshold for increase in lactate,[19–23] controversy exists as to whether this represents a cause-and-effect relationship.[24,25] Despite this controversy, the measurement of VAT may be quite useful in the testing of paediatric populations for several reasons:

(1) the measurement is non-invasive and therefore avoids the discomfort of blood sampling;
(2) it has been shown to correlate with $\dot{V}O_2$ max and endurance performance in adults,[26] and with tests of physical work capacity in children;[27]
(3) it does not require a maximal effort which is sometimes hard to obtain in children;
(4) it has good test–retest reliability;[28,29]
(5) it can be used to prescribe exercise intensity; and
(6) it has been shown to increase with endurance training.[30]

In general, the VAT of children occurs at a higher percentage of $\dot{V}O_2$ max than in adults,[19,31] decreases with age,[32,33] and is lower in girls than boys.[33]

There are several commonly used methods for determining VAT. In general, the VAT is more easily determined using breath-by-breath measurement of gas exchange and ramp or one minute increments in work rate. The VAT is identified as the $\dot{V}O_2$ at which an accelerated

non-linear increase in $\dot{V}_E$ occurs[20] (Fig. 1.5.5). Since the $\dot{V}_E$ is driven by excess CO_2, VAT can also be determined by the point at which the $\dot{V}_E/\dot{V}O_2$ increases while the $\dot{V}_E/\dot{V}CO_2$ does not change.[18,34] Likewise, the VAT has also been identified as the $\dot{V}O_2$ at which end-tidal oxygen tension (P_{ETO_2}) and $\dot{V}_E/\dot{V}O_2$ increase without a commensurate decrease in end-tidal CO_2 tension (P_{ETCO_2}).[11]

In patients whose ability to increase $\dot{V}_E$ sufficiently at higher work rates is impaired due to increased airway resistance or abnormal chemoreceptor sensitivity, VAT may be more clearly detected by examining the relationship between $\dot{V}CO_2$ and $\dot{V}O_2$, or the V-slope method.[35] With this method, VAT is the point at which an accelerated linear increase in $\dot{V}CO_2$ occurs relative to $\dot{V}O_2$ (Fig. 1.5.6). It has also been shown that the slope of $\dot{V}CO_2/\dot{V}O_2$ (the respiratory exchange ratio, RER) versus time increases abruptly at the VAT, and can be used to refine the determination of VAT.[36] Normal VAT values for children range from 58 to 83% of $\dot{V}O_2$ max, and vary according to age, gender and fitness level.[31] As previously mentioned, the measurement of VAT provides information on a child's aerobic fitness, and can be used to prescribe exercise, and follow changes that may occur with growth or training.

The VAT may also provide useful information in some children with chronic diseases, particularly when maximal exercise testing may be deemed too stressful or potentially unsafe. For instance, Reybrouck et al.[37] found the VAT to be more sensitive in detecting subnormal exercise performance in children with congenital heart disease than

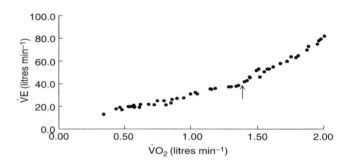

Fig. 1.5.5 The ventilatory anaerobic threshold (indicated by the arrow) occurs at the oxygen uptake ($\dot{V}O_2$) where there is an accelerated increase in minute ventilation ($\dot{V}E$).

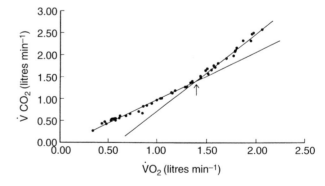

Fig. 1.5.6 Determination of ventilatory anaerobic threshold (indicated by the arrow) using the V-slope method.

other estimates of exercise performance capacity, such as the $\dot{V}O_2$ at a given submaximal heart rate (e.g. $\dot{V}O_2170$). Twice as many children were found to have below normal values ($<95\%$ confidence interval) for VAT compared with below normal values for exercise capacity observed in only 28% of the children for the $\dot{V}O_2170$ test.

In contrast, the VAT may not be detectable in children with increased airway resistance, such as asthma or cystic fibrosis, who may exhibit hyperventilation at very low levels of exercise and are unable to increase ventilation sufficiently at higher work rates.[3] Similarly, the VAT may not be detectable in very sick children with extremely limited exercise capacity such as those with tricuspid atresia, whose VAT may already be surpassed at the onset of exercise.[38]

Measurements of pulmonary gas exchange

Arterial blood gases

Pulmonary gas exchange during exercise is most accurately determined by direct measurement of arterial O_2 and CO_2 tension (P_aO_2 and P_aCO_2). However, arterial sampling can be quite painful and therefore is not warranted in the healthy child, and is often refused by the sick child. Consequently, a number of investigators advocate the use of arterialized ear lobe blood samples as a less invasive alternative to direct arterial blood gas sampling.[39–41] With proper techniques,[38] the validity and reliability of arterialized ear lobe measurements have been supported by many studies,[38–41] while a more recent investigation of a large sample of adults suggests that arterial PO_2 (measured at rest only) may be underestimated by the assessment of arterialized ear lobe blood.[42] However, differences between arterial and ear lobe measures of PCO_2 were negligible in the same study.[42] Despite the potential error with ear lobe measurements, this method is superior to non-invasive indirect estimates of arterial PO_2 and PCO_2, such as pulse oximetry and transcutaneous monitoring.

Transcutaneous PO_2 and PCO_2

Transcutaneous measures of PO_2 and PCO_2 via the attachment of electrodes to the skin are not considered to be accurate indirect indices of arterial PO_2 and PCO_2, and, therefore, should not be used with exercise testing.[43,44]

Oxyhaemoglobin saturation

Similarly, the measurement of oxyhaemoglobin saturation (S_aO_2) via pulse oximetry should not be considered an indirect estimate of P_aO_2. However, pulse oximetry measurements of S_aO_2 are useful in the clinical setting for providing information about oxyhaemoglobin saturation. Pulse oximetry works by detecting differences in light wavelengths absorbed by oxygenated versus desaturated haemoglobin.[44] Measurement error may be introduced by poor finger or ear lobe perfusion, dark skin pigmentation, pierced ear holes, finger nail polish, movement, stray light and increased levels of carboxy- and methaemoglobin. True values of arterial S_aO_2 have been shown to be overestimated as well as underestimated by pulse oximetry with inaccuracy worsening during episodes of hypoxemia ($S_aO_2 < 90\%$).[45–47]

Except for elite athletes who may exhibit oxyhaemoglobin desaturation with very intense exercise,[48] S_aO_2 should be near 100% and not decrease during exercise in healthy children. In patients with cardiac defects and/or pulmonary disease, S_aO_2 may be normal or decreased at rest, and may remain stable or decrease or even increase during exercise.[49]

End-tidal CO_2 tension

The measurement of CO_2 tension in the expired air at the end of expiration (P_{ETCO_2}) should also *not* be used as an indirect estimate of P_aCO_2. However, it provides some information about P_aCO_2 assuming:

(1) CO_2 equilibrium is achieved between end-capillary blood and alveolar gas;
(2) P_{ETCO2} approximates the time-weighted average of the ventilation-weighted alveolar CO_2 tension;
(3) the lung is sufficiently uniform in terms of ventilation to perfusion ratio (V_A/Q).[44]

The difference between P_{ETCO_2} and P_aCO_2 varies with V_T, f_R and CO_2 output, limiting the usefulness of P_{ETCO_2} as an index of P_aCO_2 during exercise, particularly in patients with ventilation/perfusion abnormalities.[50] However, a general pattern of response can be observed during progressive exercise. During progressive exercise, P_{ETCO_2} increases by several mmHg above resting values because of increased CO_2 production and delivery to the lungs, until heavy exercise, when P_{ETCO2} begins to fall as the respiratory rate increases substantially to eliminate excess CO_2 and maintain acid–base balance. (Fig. 1.5.7) In patients with severe obstructive lung disease such as asthma or cystic fibrosis, P_{ETCO_2} *may* continue to increase or fail to decrease despite a levelling off of carbon dioxide production, which *may* suggest hypoventilation or the inability to increase ventilation sufficiently to eliminate excess CO_2 and maintain acid–base balance. It is important to note that children are often apprehensive and may hyperventilate prior to exercise, resulting in a low 'resting' P_{ETCO_2} for comparison with exercise.

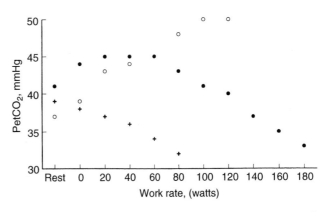

Fig. 1.5.7 The end-tidal carbon dioxide (P_{ETCO_2}) response to progressive exercise in a healthy child ($\bullet$), a child with *severe* obstructive lung disease (O), and a child with a *severe* restrictive lung defect (+). In children with milder obstructive or restrictive defects, the P_{ETCO_2} response pattern will be similar to the healthy child's response.

Dead space

At rest, 25 to 35% of inspired air is wasted ventilation, in the sense that it does not participate in gas exchange, creating physiological dead space. Physiologic dead space includes the conducting airways such as the mouth, nose, trachea, bronchi and bronchioles (anatomic dead space) and the alveoli that are not adequately perfused by blood flow (alveolar dead space). The portion of inspired air that participates in gas exchange is alveolar ventilation (V_A). In the healthy young child, physiologic dead space is about one third of the V_T.[2] For a given level of ventilation, dead space increases and alveolar ventilation decreases if V_T falls and f_R rises.

During exercise, dead space increases as V_T increases but to a lesser extent. As exercise intensity increases, the ratio of dead space to tidal volume (V_D/V_T) falls by about one third reaching values in the range of 0.20 to 0.25 in both children and adults.[51]

Measurement of V_D/V_T requires the measurement of arterial P_aCO_2 for accuracy. Some automated testing systems estimate V_D/V_T from equations that use P_{ETCO2} as a substitute for P_aCO_2.[52] However, this non-invasive method has been shown to overestimate P_aCO_2 and thus V_D/V_T in normal persons,[53] and has been shown to be unreliable and inaccurate in patients with lung disease.[54,55]

For optimal gas exchange, the capillaries supplying the ventilated alveoli must be properly perfused; that is, there must be adequate ventilation to perfusion (V_A/Q) matching. Pulmonary blood flow and the perfusion of the pulmonary capillary bed are determined by cardiac output, pulmonary vascular resistance and pulmonary arterial pressure. When ventilated regions are underperfused, hypoxemia (i.e. a drop in P_aO_2) will occur. Conversely, when perfused regions are underventilated, hypoventilation (i.e. an increase in P_aCO_2) will occur.

Less common measurements

Diffusion capacity

Gas exchange may also be determined by the diffusion of gases across the alveolar–capillary membrane. The diffusion capacity of the lungs is dependent on:

(1) the gas pressure gradient between the alveoli and capillary;
(2) the transit time of the red blood cell;
(3) the solubility of the gases in the liquids and tissues;
(4) the permeability and thickness of the alveolar–capillary membrane; and
(5) the amount and quality of haemoglobin.[2]

The diffusion capacity of the lungs is most easily measured by determining the diffusion of carbon monoxide (DL_{CO}) using the single-breath technique.[5] Zapletal *et al.*[2] found DL_{CO} to increase with increasing stature and TLC and age. However, the ratio of DL_{CO}/TLC decreased with increasing stature and age. Pulmonary diffusion capacity is decreased in patients with anaemia or with thickened alveolar–capillary membranes, such as sarcoidosis, lupus and pulmonary fibrosis.[5]

During exercise, DL_{CO} increases significantly, reaching values nearly three times greater than rest.[56] The increase in DL_{CO} correlates directly with $\dot{V}O_2$, and the slope of $DL_{CO}/\dot{V}O_2$ was found to be twice as high in children as in adults.[57] In healthy children and adults, diffusion capacity does not affect exercise tolerance; however, in patients with

decreased diffusion capacities, it may be predictive of oxyhaemoglobin desaturation during exercise.[58,59]

Flow/volume loops with exercise

It is possible to record flow/volume loops during exercise to provide information about mechanical air flow limitation. As previously mentioned, with light-to-moderately intense exercise, the increase in ventilation is met by increases in V_T up to about 60% of VC. At higher intensities, f_R increases to meet the higher ventilatory and metabolic demands. Even at maximal exercise, the tidal loop does not approach the resting forced expiratory loop in the healthy person (Fig. 1.5.8A). In contrast, the tidal loop of the child with obstructive lung disease encroaches upon or even exceeds the resting maximal expiratory flow/volume loop during exercise, which may be due to airway narrowing after deep inspiration for the maximal forced expiratory manoeuvre, non-uniform lung emptying and thoracic gas compression (Fig. 1.5.8B).[60]

More commonly, measurement of the expiratory flow rates are performed before and after exercise, rather than during, to aid in the diagnosis of airway reactivity to exercise, or exercise-induced asthma (EIA). The standard EIA testing protocol is performed on a motorized treadmill with the exercise intensity increasing rapidly to a level that can be sustained for 6–8 min and that elicits a heart rate equal to 80 to 90% of age-predicted maximum heart rate.[61,62] Forced expiratory flow rates and volumes are measured pre-exercise, and approximately 2, 5, 10 and 15 min post-exercise, and then after the administration of an inhaled bronchodilator. A decrease in FEV_1 of 15% or greater following exercise (expressed as percentage change from pre-exercise values) is considered to be a positive diagnosis of EIA.[62] In the healthy child, the airways dilate during exercise (as a result of sympathetic stimulation). In the child with exercise-induced asthma, while bronchodilitation may occur initially, bronchoconstriction occurs during or, more commonly, after exercise.[3] Figure 1.5.9 shows a decrease in larger airway flow rates following exercise in a child with exercise-induced asthma.

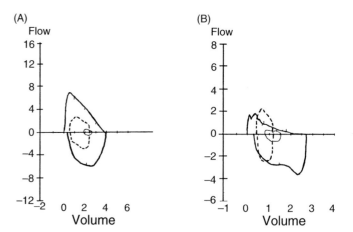

Fig. 1.5.8 Tidal volume loops during exercise (----) superimposed on the resting forced expiratory flow/volume loop (——) in a healthy child (A) and a child with severe obstructive lung disease (B).

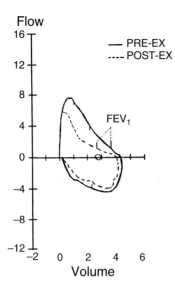

Fig. 1.5.9 Forced expiratory flow/volume loops measured before (—) and after (---) exercise in a child with exercise-induced asthma. Note the lower FEV$_1$ following exercise compared to normal pre-exercise value.

Interpretation of pulmonary exercise testing

For proper interpretation, it is important to choose the appropriate testing protocol. For example, an EIA provocation testing protocol should be followed for the assessment of EIA. Submaximal exercise testing may provide sufficient information when maximal testing is deemed too stressful or unnecessary. Generally, most of the normative data are based on progressive maximal exercise testing, and comparisons to the normative data should be made using the same testing protocol.

The interpretation of exercise test results is ideally based on both numerical data and graphical displays. Different strategies for interpreting test results with emphasis on pulmonary disease are presented by Younes[63], the European Respiratory Society Task Force[43] and Wasserman *et al.*[11] In children, the interpretation of tests is usually limited to non-invasive data and their graphical display. Suggestions for graphical displays include the following *x–y* plots: work rate (or time) on the *x*-axis versus separate plots of $\dot{V}O_2$, heart rate, $\dot{V}_E$, $\dot{V}_E/\dot{V}O_2$ and $\dot{V}_E/\dot{V}CO_2$ combined, and P_{ETCO2} and P_{ETO2} combined on the *y*-axis; $\dot{V}O_2$ on the *x*-axis versus heart rate, $\dot{V}_E$ and $\dot{V}CO_2$ separately; and $\dot{V}_E$ on the *x*-axis versus V_T on the *y*-axis.

For accurate interpretation of the results from a progressive maximal exercise test, it is important to determine if the child gave a maximal effort. A maximal effort may be determined by examining the RER, heart rate, $\dot{V}_E/MVV$ and the subject's effort at peak exercise (see Chapter 1.7). In the healthy child, the peak RER should be greater than 1.05, the peak heart rate should be near age predicted values, the peak $\dot{V}_E/MVV$ should be at least 60%, and the subject should appear to have given a maximal effort. In some cases, the $\dot{V}O_2$ at near-maximal exercise may level off despite further increases in exercise, although this may not always be seen in children or with specific testing protocols, and therefore may not be a useful criterion for determining a maximal effort.

In the child with a health problem, all of the criteria may not be met despite a maximal effort. It is important to realize that one

parameter can appear to be submaximal or abnormal due to the effects of another parameter. For instance, peak heart rate may be reduced because the child has a ventilatory or peripheral limitation to exercise that prevents the cardiovascular system from reaching its maximum capacity. Similarly, the child with a cardiac defect may have a chronotropic limitation to exercise that prevents the ventilatory system from being stressed. Furthermore, the child may terminate exercise because of symptoms, and, as a result, may not meet any of the physiologic criteria for a maximal effort. Consequently, the examiner's subjective assessment of the child's effort plays an important role.

Once it has been determined that the child gave a maximal effort, then the child's physical work capacity and peak oxygen uptake should be compared to normal values specific to the testing protocol. If subnormal, the explanation may lie in one or a combination of the other parameters measured. The other parameters should be examined for abnormalities even if the child's fitness level is normal or above normal.

The submaximal progressive data should also be examined for inappropriate responses or patterns of response. For instance, a high $\dot{V}_E$ for a given $\dot{V}O_2$ or $\dot{V}CO_2$ may reflect ventilatory compensation for increased dead space in a child with obstructive pulmonary disease, or an accelerated increase in $\dot{V}_E$ at a low $\dot{V}O_2$ may indicate a low ventilatory anaerobic threshold in an unfit child.

Finally, the results of the exercise test may not fully explain the child's exercise intolerance. It is possible that peripheral limitations to exercise exist, which are not reflected in the cardiorespiratory data. The child with a chronic disease may also be afraid or unwilling to exercise because of the usually false belief that it is unsafe for him/her to exercise which he/she has learned from the cues of parents, teachers and others.

Summary

The evaluation of pulmonary function at rest and during exercise can provide useful information about the lungs' ability to provide sufficient volume and flow of air, as well as adequate exchange of oxygen and carbon dioxide. In the healthy child, the assessment of pulmonary parameters during exercise can provide information on fitness, and changes that may occur with growth or exercise training. In the child with disease, testing can help to identify abnormal responses which may contribute to exercise intolerance. In turn, this information may be useful for following changes with disease progression, and may ultimately play a role in the clinical care and treatment of the child with a pulmonary disorder.

References

1. **Polgar, G.** and **Promadhat, V.** *Pulmonary function testing in children. Techniques and standards.* W. B. Saunders, Philadelphia, 1971.
2. **Zapletal A., Samanek, M.** and **Paul, T.** *Lung function in children and adolescents.* Karger, Basel, 1987.
3. **Godfrey, S.** *Exercise testing in children.* W. B. Saunders, London, 1974.
4. **Comroe, J. H., Forster, R. E., I. I., Dubois, A. B., Briscoe, W.A.** and **Carlsen E.** *The lung. Clinical physiology and pulmonary function tests.* Year Book Medical Publishers, Chicago, 1962.
5. **Hyatt, R. K., Scanlon, P. D.** and **Nakamura, M.** *Interpretation of pulmonary function tests: A practical guide.* Lippincott-Raven, Philadelphia, 1997.

6. **Ruppel. G. E.** *Manual of pulmonary function testing.* Mosby, St. Louis, 1991.

7. Anonymous. Standardization of spirometry—1987 Update. Statement of the American Thoracic Society. *American Review of Respiratory Disease* 1987; **136**: 1285–98.

8. **Quanjer, Ph. H., Helms, P., Bjure, J.** and **Caultier, C.** Standardization of lung function tests in paediatrics. *European Respiratory Journal* 1989; **2**: 121S–264S.

9. **Fulton, J. E., Pivarnik, J. M., Taylor, W. C., Snider, S. A., Tate, A. L.** and **Rankowski, R. F.** Prediction of maximum voluntary ventilation (MVV) in African-American adolescent girls. *Pediatric Pulmonology* 1995; **20**: 225–33.

10. **Cooper, CB., Harris, ND.** and **Howard, P.** Evaluation of a turbine flow meter (Ventilometer Mark 2) in the measurement of ventilation. *Respiration* 1990; **57**: 243–7.

11. **Wasserman, K., Hansen, J. E., Sue, D. Y.** and **Whipp, B. J.**. *Principles of exercise testing and interpretation.* Lea and Febiger, Philadelphia, 1987.

12. **Jones, N. L., Makrides, L., Hitchcock, C., Chypchar, T.** and **McCartney, N.** Normal standards for an incremental progressive cycle ergometer test. *American Review of Respiratory Disease* 1985; **131**: 700–8.

13. **Henke, K. G., Sharratt, M., Pegelow, D.** and **Dempsey, J. A.** Regulation of end-expiratory lung volume during exercise. *Journal of Applied Physiology* 1988; **64**: 135–46.

14. **Wasserman, K.** and **Whipp, B. J.** Exercise physiology in health and disease. *American Review of Respiratory Disease* 1975; **112**: 219–49.

15. **Nixon, P. A.** Role of exercise in the evaluation and management of pulmonary disease in children and youth. *Medicine and Science in Sports and Exercise* 1996; **28**: 414–20.

16. **Rowland, T. W., Auchinachie, J. A., Keenan, T. J.** and **Green, G. M.** Physiologic responses to treadmill running in adult and prepubertal males. *International Journal of Sports Medicine* 1987; **8**: 292–7.

17. **Cerny, F. J., Pullano, T. P.** and **Cropp, G. J.** Cardiorespiratory adaptations to exercise in cystic fibrosis. *American Review of Respiratory Disease* 1982; **126**: 217–20.

18. **Wasserman, K.** and **McIlroy, M. B.** Detecting the threshold of anaerobic metabolism in cardiac patients during exercise. *American Journal of Cardiology* 1964; **14**: 844–52.

19. **Reybrouck, T. M.** The use of the anaerobic threshold in pediatric exercise testing. In *Advances in pediatric sport sciences* (ed. O. Bar-Or). Human Kinetics Publishers, Champaign, Il, 1989.

20. **Wasserman, K., Whipp, B. J, Koyal, S. N.** and **Beaver, W. L.** Anaerobic threshold and respiratory gas exchange during exercise. *Journal of Applied Physiology* 1973; **35**: 236–43.

21. **Macek, J.** and **Vavra, J.** Anaerobic threshold in children. In *Children and exercise XI.* (ed. R. A. Binkhorst, H. C. G. Kemper and W. H. M. Saris). Human Kinetics Publishers, Champaign, Il, 1985.

22. **Eriksson, B. O.** Physical training, oxygen supply and muscle metabolism in 11–13 year old boys. *Acta Physiologica Scandinavica* 1972; **86**: 1–48.

23. **Eriksson, B. O.** and **Koch, G.** Effects of physical training on haemodynamic response during submaximal and maximal exercise in 11–13 year old boys. *Acta Physiologica Scandinavica* 1973; **87**: 27–39.

24. **Hughes, E., Turner, S. C.** and **Brooks, G. A.** Effects of glycogen depletion and pedalling speed on 'anaerobic threshold.' *Journal of Applied Physiology* 1982; **52**: 1598–1607.

25. **Brooks, G. A.** Anaerobic threshold: review of the concept and directions for future research. *Medicine and Science in Sports and Exercise* 1985; **17**: 22–31.

26. **Davis, J. A.** Anaerobic threshold: review of the concept and directions for future research. *Medicine and Science in Sports and Exercise* 1985; **17**: 6–18.

27. **Reybrouck, T., Weymans, M., Ghesquiere, J., van Gerven, D.** and **Stijns, H.** Ventilatory threshold during treadmill exercise in kindergarten children. *European Journal of Applied Physiology* 1982; **50**: 79–86.

28. **Mahon, A. D.** and **Marsh, M. L.** Reliability of the rating of perceived exertion at ventilatory threshold in children. *International Journal of Sports Medicine* 1992; **13**: 567–71.

29. **Weymans, M.** and **Reybrouck T.** Habitual level of physical activity and cardiorespiratory endurance capacity in children. *European Journal of Applied Physiology* 1989; **58**: 803–7.

30. **Mahon, A. D.** and **Vaccaro, P.** Ventilatory threshold and $\dot{V}O_2$ max changes in children following endurance training. *Medicine and Science in Sports and Exercise* 1989; **21**: 425–31.

31. **Washington, R. L.** Anaerobic threshold in children. *Pediatric Exercise Science* 1989; **1**: 244–56.

32. **Cooper, D. M., Weiler-Ravell, D., Whipp, B. J.** and **Wasserman, K.** Aerobic parameters of exercise as a function of body size during growth in children. *Journal of Applied Physiology* 1984; **56**: 628–34.

33. **Reybrouck, T., Weymans, M., Stijns, H., Knops, J.** and **Van der Hauwaert, L.** Ventilatory anaerobic threshold in healthy children: Age and sex differences. *European Journal of Applied Physiology* 1985; **54**: 278–84.

34. **Wasserman, K.** The anaerobic threshold measurement to evaluate exercise performance. *American Review of Respiratory Disease* 1984; **129**: S35–40.

35. **Sue, D. Y., Wasserman, K., Moricca, R. B.** and **Casaburi, R.** Metabolic acidosis during exercise in patients with chronic obstructive pulmonary disease. Use of the v-slope method for anaerobic threshold determination. *Chest* 1988; **94**: 931–8.

36. **Washington, R. L., Van Gundy, J. C., Cohen, C., Sondheimer, H.** and **Wolfe, R.** Normal aerobic and anaerobic exercise data for North American school-age children. *Journal of Pediatrics* 1988; **112**: 223–33.

37. **Reybrouck, T., Weymans, M., Stijns, H.** and **Van der Hauwaert, L. G.** Ventilatory anaerobic threshold for evaluating exercise performance in children with congenital left-to-right intracardiac shunt. *Pediatric Cardiology* 1986; **7**: 19–24.

38. **Wessel, H. U., Stout, R. L.** and **Paul, M. H.** Exercise in postoperative tricuspid atresia. In *Children and exercise XI.* (ed. R. A. Binkhorst, H. C. G. Kemper and W. H. M. Saris). Human Kinetics Publishers, Champaign, Il, 1985.

39. **Godfrey, S., Wozniak, E. R., Courtney Evans, R. J.** and **Samuels, C. S.** Ear lobe blood samples for blood gas analysis at rest and during exercise. *British Journal of Diseases of the Chest* 1971; **65**: 58–63.

40. **Christoforides, C.** and **Miller, J. M.** Clinical use and limitations of arterialized capillary blood for PO_2 determination. *American Review of Respiratory Disease* 1968; **98**: 653–7.

41. **Spiro, S. G.** and **Dowdeswell, I. R. G.** Arterialized earlobe blood samples for blood gas tensions. *British Journal of Diseases of the Chest* 1976; **70**: 263–8.

42. **Sauty, A., Uldry, C., Debetaz, L. F., Leuenberger, P.** and **Fitting, J. W.** Differences in PO_2 and PCO_2 between arterial and arterialized earlobe samples. *European Respiratory Journal* 1996; **9**: 186–9.

43. European Respiratory Society Task Force. Clinical exercise testing with reference to lung diseases: indications, standardization and interpretation strategies. *European Respiratory Journal* 1997; **10**: 2662–89.

44. **Clark, J. S., Votteri, B., Ariagno, R. L., Cheung, P., Eichhorn, J. H., Fallat, R. J., Lee, S. E., Newth, C. J. L., Rotman, H.** and **Sue, D. Y.** Non-invasive assessment of blood gases. *American Review of Respiratory Disease* 1992; **145**: 220–32.

45. **Hansen, J. E.** and **Casaburi, R.**, Validity of ear oximetry in clinical exercise testing. *Chest* 1987; **91**: 333–7.

46. **Orenstein, D. M., Curtis, S. E., Nixon, P. A.** and **Hartigan, E. R.** Accuracy of three pulse oximeters during exercise and hypoxemia in patients with cystic fibrosis. *Chest* 1993; **104**: 1187–90.

47. **Chapman, K., D'Urzo, A.** and **Rebuck, A.** The accuracy and response characteristics of a simplified ear oximeter. *Chest* 1983; **83**: 860–4.

48. **Williams, J. H., Powers, S. K.** and **Stuart, M. K.** Hemoglobin desaturation in highly trained athletes during heavy exercise. *Medicine and Science in Sports and Exercise* 1986; **18**: 168–73.

49. **Nixon, P. A.** and **Orenstein, D. M.** Exercise testing in children. *Pediatric Pulmonology* 1988; **5**: 107–22.

50. **Jones, H. L., McHardy, G. J. R., Naimark, A.** and **Campbell, E. J. M.** Physiological dead space and alveolar–arterial gas pressure differences during exercise. *Clinical Science* 1966; **31**: 19–29.

51. **Shephard, R. J.** and **Bar-Or, O.** Alveolar ventilation in near maximum exercise. Data on pre-adolescent children and young adults. *Medicine and Science in Sports* 1970; **2**: 83–92.

52. Jones, N. L. *Clinical exercise testing.* W. B. Saunders, Philadelphia, 1988.

53. Robbins, P. A., Conway, J., Cunningham, D. A., Khamnei, S. and Paterson D. J. A comparison of indirect methods for continuous estimation of arterial PCO_2 in men. *Journal of Applied Physiology* 1990; 68: 1727–31.

54. Lewis, D. A., Sietsema, K. E., Casaburi, R. amd Sue, D. Y. Inaccuracy of non-invasive estimates of V_D/V_T in clinical exercise testing. *American Review of Respiratory Diseases* 1993; 147: A185.

55. Yamanaka, M. K. and Sue, D. Y. Comparison of arterial-end-tidal PCO_2 difference and dead space/tidal volume ratio in respiratory failure. *Chest* 1987; 92: 832–5.

56. Andersen, S. D. and Godfrey, S. Transfer factor for CO_2 during exercise in children. *Thorax* 1971; 26: 51–4.

57. Shephard, R. J., Allen, C., Bar-Or, O., Davies, C. T. M., Degre, S., Hedman, R.. and Ishi, K. The working capacity of Toronto school children. Part II. *Canadian Medical Association Journal* 1969; 100: 705–14.

58. Lebecque, P., Lapierre, J. G., Lamarre, A. and Coates, A. L. Diffusion capacity and oxygen desaturation effects on exercise in patients with cystic fibrosis. *Chest* 1987; 91: 693–7.

59. Owens, G. R., Rogers, R. M., Pennock, B. E. and Levin, D. The diffusing capacity as a predictor of arterial oxygen desaturation during exercise in patients with chronic obstructive pulmonary disease. *New England Journal of Medicine* 1984; 310: 1218–21.

60. Gallagher, C. G. Exercise and chronic obstructive pulmonary disease. *Medical Clinics of North America* 1990; 74: 619–41.

61. Cropp, G. J. A. The exercise bronchoprovocation test: Standardization of procedures and evaluation of response. *Journal of Allergy and Clinical Immunology* 1979; 64: 627–33.

62. NHLBI Expert Panel Report. Guidelines for the diagnosis and management of asthma. *Journal of Allergy and Clinical Immunology* 1991; 88: 425–534.

63. Younes, M. Interpretation of clinical exercise testing in respiratory disease. *Clinics in Chest Medicine* 1984; 5: 189–206.

1.6 Cardiovascular function

Gerald Barber

Introduction

This chapter will review the assessment of cardiovascular function at rest and during exercise. It will concentrate on the cardiac parameters typically measured during a paediatric exercise test. Since the cardiovascular system is an important component of a child's exercise response, abnormalities in one or more of these parameters can significantly affect global measurements, such as exercise time, power and anaerobic threshold. These global parameters are discussed elsewhere in this volume

A detailed discussion of various cardiovascular diseases and their treatments is not attempted and the discussion of specific cardiovascular diseases will be limited to examples demonstrating the use and value of the parameters discussed in this chapter. Normative data are addressed in Chapter 2.7.

Cardiovascular parameters

Heart rate

Heart rate is one of the simplest and most frequently used parameters in assessing the cardiac response to exercise.

Maximum exercise heart rate is frequently used to assess a subject's relative exercise intensity by comparing it with that subject's predicted maximum heart rate. While this is a valuable technique in normal individuals, there are several potential problems when it is used in individuals with cardiac disease.

First, the relationship between heart rate and exercise intensity is dependent on normal sinus rhythm. Even if the individual is in sinus rhythm at the start of the exercise test, the test itself may stimulate a tachyarrhythmia more than the effort-dependent sinus rate. While this can frequently be detected by simultaneous electrocardiography, some atrial tachyarrhythmias originate near the sinus node and, in electrocardiographic appearance, mimic normal sinus rhythm.

Second, even if the subject remains in sinus rhythm, this rhythm may be elevated or depressed by many factors other than exercise intensity, such as drugs, anxiety and temperature.

Finally, the individual subject's maximum heart rate may be much less than the predicted maximum heart rate based on population studies. Population data are obtained from normal subjects. Exercise tests are frequently used to assess subjects with known or suspected heart disease, one component of which may be chronotropic incompetence. Even the simple surgical closure of an atrial septal defect can produce chronotropic incompetence.[1] Furthermore, this abnormality is not limited to known cardiac patients. During exercise, cured oncology patients also demonstrate chronotropic incompetence.[2]

Blood pressure

Blood pressure is important in assessing cardiac work and vascular resistance. In order to eject blood from the heart, the left ventricle (LV) must generate a pressure equal to or greater than central aortic pressure. Thus, blood pressure is directly related to the systolic work of the heart. Blood pressure is typically measured in a peripheral artery at the level of the heart. During systole, this pressure is assumed to be equal to LV pressure. It should be noted that even in the absence of left ventricular outflow tract obstruction, this assumption is not entirely true. Vascular patterns are not the same throughout the peripheral arteries and there are varying effects of vascular compliance and pressure wave reflection on the measured blood pressure.

Electrocardiogram

Besides providing an accurate heart rate assessment, electrocardiography has three primary functions in the assessment of cardiovascular function during paediatric exercise testing. Similar to adult exercise studies, electrocardiography is used to assess the adequacy of myocardial perfusion. However, the prevalence of significant coronary artery lesions is much less and the prevalence of significant conduction abnormalities, such as bundle branch block or pre-excitation, is much greater in the paediatric than adult population. For these reasons, exercise electrocardiography is a much less useful technique in paediatric compared to adult exercise studies.

One of the main paediatric uses of the exercise electrocardiogram (ECG) is the assessment of rhythm disturbances. Examples of this use include: suppression of premature ventricular contractions during exercise; conversion of junctional or ectopic atrial rhythms to sinus rhythm during exercise; development of relative bradyarrhythmias secondary to the development of heart block during exercise; and development of supraventricular or ventricular tachyarrhythmias during exercise.[3,4]

Finally, the exercise ECG is useful in assessing pacemaker function and response to exercise. This assessment is essential in individuals with a variable 'rate-responsive' pacemaker. It is helpful, however, even in individuals with fixed rate pacemakers, since during exercise the pacemaker may fail to appropriately sense intrinsic cardiac activity, it may sense artefact as cardiac activity and fail to appropriately stimulate the myocardium, or it may appropriately sense and stimulate, but the myocardium may not appropriately respond to the stimulation ('failure to capture').[5]

Cardiac output, stroke volume and systemic vascular resistance

Cardiac output, stroke volume and systemic vascular resistance are major components in assessing the cardiovascular response to exercise.

The role of the cardiovascular system during exercise is to meet the metabolic requirements of the exercising muscles. This is accomplished by increasing blood flow to these muscles to increase oxygen delivery and facilitate the removal of metabolic waste. Several components of the cardiovascular system are involved in this response. Overall, cardiac output is increased. This results from an increase in both heart rate and stroke volume. This increase in stroke volume results from an increase in both preload and inotropic state. The increased preload results from the muscular activity squeezing or pumping the venous capacitance vessels increasing venous return. In addition, the augmented cardiac output is preferentially directed to the exercising muscles by a localized reduction in systemic vascular resistance. This localized reduction in systemic vascular resistance is reflected in the overall systemic vascular resistance. Thus, assessment of these three parameters provides a significant amount of information about the cardiovascular response to exercise.

All of the cardiovascular parameters must respond in concert for a proper cardiovascular response to exercise. For example, a pacemaker may artificially increase heart rate, but if this increase is not accompanied by an increase in venous return and an increase in inotropic state, cardiac output actually falls instead of rising.[6] The cardiovascular parameters are not mutually independent. They must be considered together in assessing the cardiovascular response to exercise.

Assessment techniques at rest and during exercise

Heart rate

While heart rate may be assessed by a variety of techniques, in exercise tests assessing cardiovascular response, it is usually assessed electrocardiographically. Even in this case, there are various electrocardiographic ways of determining heart rate. The heart rate can be manually determined by measuring the time interval between two or more QRS complexes recorded on ECG paper. The heart rate can be calculated by a computer built into the ECG system by measuring the time interval between rapid electrical signal changes assumed to represent QRS complexes. In this case, the ECG computer may determine the heart rate by analysing the signal from one or more ECG leads. The more leads analysed, the greater the accuracy of the heart rate assessment but also the greater the required computing power and cost of the system. In addition, computer ECG systems rarely measure instantaneous heart rate. Instead, they measure the average heart rate over either a preprogrammed time interval or a preprogrammed number of beats. This preprogramming is frequently not subject to user selection or control. The accuracy of computer ECG systems in determining the aetiology of the electrical signal change *vis-à-vis* atrial activity, QRS complex, pacemaker spikes or artefact varies from one manufacturer to another. Thus, a computer-generated ECG heart rate may be too high, if atrial activity, pacemaker spikes or artefact are incorrectly judged to represent QRS complexes, or too low if QRS complexes are incorrectly judged to represent atrial activity, pacemaker spikes or artefact. Whenever a computer-generated heart rate is used in assessing the cardiovascular response to exercise, electrocardiographic tracings at an appropriate paper speed to assess heart rate (25 mm s^{-1} or faster) should be intermittently obtained to cross-check for the computer-generated measurements.

Blood pressure

Intra-arterial and auscultatory sphygmomanometry are the 'gold standards' for blood pressure assessment at rest. There is no gold standard during exercise. During exercise, intra-arterial measurements of blood pressure significantly overestimate systolic pressure due to wave amplification. Auscultatory sphygmomanometry is frequently used, but it can be difficult to accurately auscultate the Korotkoff sounds given the noise level in the typical exercise laboratory and the noise artefact generated by arm motion during exercise. For these reasons, various automated devices have been developed to determine blood pressure during exercise. With increasing experience, development time and computer power, these devices have become more sophisticated and there are now several algorithms used by the various manufacturers.

The oscillometric technique uses changes in pressure in an airbag positioned over the artery of interest. As pressure in the blood pressure cuff is lowered from above systolic to systolic levels, the arterial wall begins to expand with each cardiac contraction. Pressure changes from this expansion are detected by the airbag. These pressure changes increase, reaching their maximal intensity when the cuff pressure is equal to mean arterial pressure. Signal intensity then drops with further reductions in cuff pressure. There is no differentiation in signal when cuff pressure equals diastolic pressure so diastolic pressure is often estimated by one of a variety of algorithms built into the device. While this technique works well at rest, it is easy to see how the small pressure changes in the airbag caused by the sudden expansion of the arterial wall can easily be lost in the artefact of large pressure changes caused by motion and muscle contraction during exercise.

The auscultatory technique is similar in that it detects arterial wall motion. When the cuff pressure is greater than systolic pressure, the intra-arterial pressure is always lower than the cuff pressure and the artery remains collapsed throughout the cardiac cycle. When the cuff pressure is less than diastolic pressure, the intra-arterial pressure is always greater than the cuff pressure and the artery is continuously open throughout the cardiac cycle. When the cuff pressure is between these two pressures, the artery opens and closes, with resultant wall motion, depending on the relative pressures between the inside (the intra-arterial pressure) and outside (the cuff pressure) of the arterial wall. This wall motion produces the Korotkoff sounds. In the auscultatory technique, a microphone placed over the artery of interest is used to detect the sound produced by this wall motion and, thus, systolic and diastolic blood pressures. Similar to the oscillometric technique, the microphone can pick up sound artefacts due to motion and muscle contraction near the microphone. The effect of these artefacts can be reduced by the addition of an ECG gating on QRS signals to aid in the discrimination of signal from artefact. However, the previous comments about the varying ability of ECG computers to accurately discriminate the electrical signal from the QRS complex from other electrical signals and artefacts also apply to ECG gated blood pressure assessments. Nevertheless, of all the various automated blood pressure techniques, during exercise, the auscultatory technique with ECG gating appears to be the most accurate.[7]

Another technique that is frequently used is a combination of standard auscultatory sphygmomanometry with an automated auscultatory device. Since the automated auscultatory device uses a microphone to detect Korotkoff sounds, the output from this microphone can be amplified and sent to a headset where it can be listened to by an individual while simultaneously observing cuff pressure on a mercury manometer. This amplification helps overcome the difficulty in auscultating Korotkoff sounds due to background laboratory noise. This manually detected blood pressure can be used either to test the reasonableness of or in place of the blood pressure generated by the automated device.

Regardless of the technique used to assess blood pressure, the blood pressure cuff size must be appropriate for the size of the extremity in which blood pressure is being measured. The length of the bladder should be sufficient to completely encircle the extremity and the width of the bladder should be sufficient to cover approximately three-quarters of the length of the upper arm or leg.[8]

Electrocardiogram

Exercise electrocardiography is obtained using commercially available computerized systems. Since the software used in these systems is considered proprietary and beyond the control of the user, critical evaluation of the various systems is essential before purchase. Minimal requirements should include: the ability to produce high quality hardcopy printouts of rhythm strips and 12 lead electrocardiograms; continuous real time display or print out of at least three orthogonal non-averaged ECG leads; and, if the real time ECG data are displayed on a monitor screen, a reasonable time delay between the screen and the hardcopy printer, so that hardcopy recordings of abnormalities can be obtained after they are visualized on the screen. Computerized arrhythmia detection and interpretation in children is difficult, even using Holter monitors in which the data are first collected and then subsequently analysed. It is extremely difficult, if not impossible, to perform during the real-time conditions of an exercise test using current computer equipment. Thus, it is helpful if the ECG system is capable of storing all the exercise data for subsequent review and analysis. If this is not the case, then, throughout the exercise test, either a continuous printout of at least three orthogonal non-averaged ECG leads should be obtained or the ECG display screen should be continuously observed with hardcopy recordings of any potential rhythm disturbance.

One crucial area, which is under the control of the laboratory personnel, is the placement of the ECG leads. A modified lead placement is frequently used during exercise testing. Leads placed at the standard positions on the arms and legs yield poor data because of muscle artefact. Furthermore, they present a potential patient hazard due to the ease with which the lead wires can become entangled in the exercise apparatus. Typically, the arm leads are placed on the upper chest and the leg leads on the lower back. The fact that this position results in a mild right-shifting of the axis compared to the standard arm and leg positions must be considered when interpreting exercise ECGs. Exercise produces significant ECG artefact compared to ECGs obtained under supine resting conditions. For this reason, good lead contact with appropriate skin preparation is essential. Various techniques have been used for this skin preparation including lightly abrading the area with a dental drill or alcohol cleansing to remove oils followed by light abrasion with fine sandpaper.

Not only must one be aware of the ECG changes produced by the slightly abnormal lead placement, one must also be aware of ECG changes caused by positional changes of the heart. Standard ECG criteria apply to an ECG taken in the supine position at rest, not in a sitting or standing position while exercising and hyperventilating. Thus, it is essential to obtain several baseline ECGs before exercise. These ECGs should include ECGs obtained under resting conditions in supine, sitting and standing positions and an ECG obtained while hyperventilating.

It is difficult to make accurate measurements from exercise ECGs. Exercise heart rates are two to three times resting rates. This means that the entire cardiac cycle can occur in 300 ms or less. Adequate precision in measuring parts of this cycle is difficult at standard paper recording speeds of 25 mm s^{-1}, that is 40 ms per grid mark on ECG paper. In studying arrhythmias at similar heart rates in the electrophysiologic laboratory, the electrocardiographic tracings are frequently recorded at 100 mm s^{-1} paper speed. Similarly, exercise ECGs should be recorded at paper speeds of at least 50 mm s^{-1}. However, increasing paper speed is not the only consideration. With increasing sympathetic tone, conduction system properties change during exercise. This causes the PR segment of the ECG to shift from a horizontal to a down-sloping line. This shift should be considered in measuring ST depression. Usually ST depression is assessed by connecting consecutive PQ points and then measuring the J point and the ST depression relative to this line. With a down-sloping PR segment, this technique has a high incidence of false positives.[9] Under these circumstances, a line should be drawn from the beginning of the P wave to the beginning of the Q wave. This line should be projected beyond the QRS complex and J point, and the level of the ST segment should be measured relative to this line. Computer generated ST measurements on commercial ECG systems do not use this technique and, therefore, frequently report erroneous values for ST depression in children. Because of the increased heart rate during exercise, the T wave moves closer to the QRS complex. Thus, the point where ST depression would typically be measured is frequently in the midst of the T wave and it is necessary to measure the ST segment at an earlier point in the cardiac cycle. It is important to note the time interval used for this measurement and to be consistent in order to compare values from different stages of a single exercise test or between serial tests.

It is beyond the scope of this chapter to discuss arrhythmia interpretation. Rhythm disturbances should be interpreted according to standard guidelines. If there are any questions about a particular rhythm, a paediatric cardiologist should be consulted.

Cardiac output, stroke volume and systemic vascular resistance

Both cardiac output and stroke volume can be directly measured. Typically, however, one is measured and the other calculated using the relationship:

$$\text{Cardiac output} = \text{Stroke volume} \times \text{Heart rate}$$

Once cardiac output has been determined, systemic vascular resistance can be calculated using the relationship:

$$\text{Systemic vascular resistance} = \frac{\text{Cardiac output}}{\text{MBP} - \text{MRAP}}$$

where MBP represents the mean arterial blood pressure and MRAP represents the mean right atrial pressure. Mean arterial blood pressure is typically calculated as the diastolic blood pressure plus one-third of the difference between the systolic and diastolic pressures. Most exercise tests are non-invasive and the mean right atrial pressure is, therefore, unknown. Typically, it is assumed to be negligible compared to mean arterial pressure and ignored. While this assumption is reasonable in most paediatric studies, its validity should be assessed for the patient being studied.

When cardiac output is the directly measured parameter, it is usually measured non-invasively using one of two rebreathing techniques. Regardless of the technique used, rebreathing techniques measure effective pulmonary blood flow not cardiac output. There is an implicit assumption that cardiac output and effective pulmonary blood flow are essentially equal within the accuracy of the technique. This assumption is invalid and rebreathing techniques cannot be used in children with left-to-right or right-to-left shunts. Furthermore, rebreathing techniques assume that there is no significant impediment to gas flow between the mouth, where gas concentrations are measured, and the vascular system. Significant pulmonary disease, therefore, also invalidates either technique.[10]

The first technique employs the Fick principle (Carbon dioxide (CO_2) rebreathing technique).

$$\text{Cardiac output} = \frac{CO_2 \text{ Production}}{\text{Mixed venous } P_{CO_2} - \text{Arterial } P_{CO_2}}$$

CO_2 production is calculated prior to the rebreathing manoeuvre using data obtained from a flow meter and a CO_2 gas analyser. Arterial CO_2 concentration is either estimated from the end-tidal CO_2 concentration using one of several equations or invasively measured by blood gas determination from a previously inserted arterial line. The individual then rebreaths a gas mixture containing CO_2 at a concentration presumed to be near the mixed venous concentration. If this is correct, the CO_2 concentration in the rebreathing bag will soon reach a plateau with the plateau concentration equal to the mixed venous concentration. If an equilibrium plateau is not reached, various mathematical formulae have been developed to estimate the mixed venous concentration. This technique has the advantage of being simple, cheap and accurate.[11] There are, however, some problems with the technique. Since the mixed venous CO_2 concentration is unknown, it is difficult to ascertain the appropriate CO_2 concentration to place in the rebreathing bag before starting the rebreathing manoeuvre. If the initial bag concentration is not close to the equilibrium concentration, equilibrium will not be reached during the rebreathing manoeuvre. Another problem is the fact that the equation used to estimate arterial from end-tidal CO_2 concentration may not be valid in the subject being tested, if an arterial line is not inserted in order to directly measure arterial CO_2 concentration.[12] Finally, the Fick principle requires steady state conditions. For this reason, it cannot be used to assess cardiac output at peak exercise.

The second technique employs rebreathing a mixture of a soluble and an insoluble gas. In order for this technique to work, the soluble gas must be physiologically inert with a high lung diffusion capacity and low blood solubility. The typical soluble gas used is acetylene but other gases, such as nitrous oxide (N_2O), are equally acceptable. Typically, helium is used as the insoluble gas. The principal purpose of the insoluble gas is to measure the total volume of the rebreathing circuit, i.e. the volume of the rebreathing bag, the respiratory tubing and valves and the subject's lung volume. The insoluble gas also establishes that the rebreathing system is a closed system with no significant gas leak. When this gas mixture is rebreathed, the soluble gas quickly saturates all the blood in contact with functioning alveoli. Subsequent disappearance of this gas is a function of the alveolar–capillary concentration gradient, the solubility of the gas in blood, and the rate of appearance of new blood at the alveolar capillary interface, i.e. the effective pulmonary blood flow. The rate of disappearance of the gas during the rebreathing procedure can be easily determined. Since the gas chosen is not normally present in blood, its concentration entering the lung is zero. Thus, the alveolar–capillary concentration gradient is equal to the alveolar or end-tidal concentration. Finally, the solubility of the gas in blood is a known constant. Thus, cardiac output (effective pulmonary blood flow) is calculable:

$$\text{Cardiac output} = \text{IV} \times \frac{760}{\text{BP} - 47} \times \frac{(SG_{init}/He_{mean})}{(SG/He)_0}$$

$$\times \frac{-\log(\Delta SG/He)}{\Delta \text{Time}_{min}} \times \frac{1}{\text{Solubility}_{SG}}$$

where IV is the initial volume of rebreathing gas, BP is the barometric pressure, SG is the soluble gas concentration, He is the helium concentration, and Solubility_{SG} is the solubility of the soluble gas in blood. The subscripts init, mean and 0 refer to the initial, mean and time zero gas concentrations, respectively. The rebreathing calculation is not started until the gas in the bag has been evenly distributed throughout the lung. This equilibration accounts for the difference between the initial and time zero concentrations. In essence, the second factor converts the bag volume to standard conditions, and the third factor corrects for the increased volume of distribution when the gas in the rebreathing bag is allowed to equilibrate with the gas in the respiratory system. The fourth factor is the decay slope and the fifth factor is the solubility coefficient. Several studies have demonstrated the accuracy of this technique.[10,13–16]

When stroke volume is the directly measured parameter, it is typically determined by either a Doppler or an impedance technique. Using ultrasound equipment, the Doppler principle can be applied to moving blood cells to measure instantaneous velocity of blood flow. When this velocity signal is measured in the ascending aorta and averaged throughout systole, stroke volume can be calculated from the cross-sectional area of the aorta and the average flow signal:

$$\text{SV} = \text{Aortic cross-sectional area} \times \int^t \frac{\Delta f \times c}{2f_0 \times \cos\phi} \times dt$$

where f_0 is the initial frequency, Δf is the Doppler shift, c is the speed of sound in tissue and ϕ_0 is the incident angle between blood flow and sound wave.

There are several potential problems with this technique, especially in its application during exercise. The cross-sectional area of the aorta is not constant. It changes throughout the cardiac cycle and increases slightly during exercise. In order to calculate the instantaneous velocity from the Doppler shift, ϕ is assumed to be zero degrees, eliminating the cosine factor in the above equation. Anatomic considerations may prevent the examiner from ever achieving a ϕ of zero degrees in the ascending aorta. Furthermore, ϕ may change throughout the exercise protocol. The Doppler sampling site may not be the same as the site where the aortic cross-sectional area was measured and the Doppler sampling site also may vary throughout the exercise protocol. Finally, the calculation requires laminar blood flow since a constant velocity is assumed throughout the cross-sectional area of interest. This assumption may be invalid at rest, let alone during exercise in individuals with cardiovascular disease. Further study is needed to assess the validity of this technique during exercise. While Shaw[17] found a good correlation ($r = 0.95$) between calculated cardiac output and workload using this technique, the cardiac outputs consistently underestimated those obtained by other techniques by approximately 20% during exercise. In another study,[18] correlation coefficients between Doppler and thermodilution cardiac outputs ranged from 0.75 to 0.96 with a 'quite variable' accuracy of the Doppler technique from subject to subject. In children who were exercising, Marx[19] found a correlation coefficient of 0.86 and a SEE of 1.4 litre min^{-1} comparing Doppler and CO_2 rebreathing techniques.

The impedance measurement of stroke volume is based on the relationship between transthoracic electrical impedance and thoracic blood volume and the assumption that the change in thoracic blood volume during any systolic period is equal to the stroke volume ejected by the heart during that period:[20]

$$SV = \text{Blood resistivity} \times \left(\frac{I}{Z_0}\right)^2 \times \frac{dZ}{dt} \times \text{Ejection time}$$

where Z is impedance and I interelectrode distance. The subscript 0 refers to baseline or time zero.

Similar to the other techniques, this technique has several potential problems. Thoracic blood volume is dependent on many factors other than cardiac activity. For example, respiratory changes are several-fold cardiac changes in impedance. Exercise causes the positions of the electrodes and internal organs to vary relative to each other. Furthermore, the relationship between electrical impedance and blood volume is not a simple function. It is geometrically dependent. For this reason, various equations have been proposed running the gamut from a cylinder to a truncated cone. Given the intrinsic variability in human physique, along with the potential variability in lead placement on the chest, a single mathematical model with good fit of all the data is probably impossible. Studies to date suggest that the best use of the impedance method may be in assessing trend data during exercise, not in determining absolute stroke volumes or cardiac outputs.[21] The impedance technique does have one major advantage: It is not affected by intracardiac or extracardiac shunts.[22] It may be especially useful in tracking cardiac output trends in patients with intracardiac or extracardiac shunts where a rebreathing technique is impossible.

Interpretation of abnormal data

Interrelationship of parameters

In assessing abnormalities in cardiovascular exercise parameters, one must be aware that these parameters are either directly or indirectly related. The relationships between heart rate, stroke volume and cardiac output and between cardiac output, systemic vascular resistance and blood pressure have already been discussed. Because of these relationships, chronotropic incompetence will affect more than just the peak exercise heart rate. Either, it will also result in a compensatory increase in stroke volume, as is frequently seen in patients with heart block,[23–25] or it will result in a reduction in cardiac output. Furthermore, if it results in a reduction in cardiac output, this reduction will most likely cause an elevation in systemic vascular resistance in order to maintain blood pressure and cerebral perfusion.

In addition, heart rate and ECG are interrelated. The ECG is a reflection of the conduction properties of the heart and these conduction properties are rate dependent. Thus, ECG intervals can only be interpreted in relationship to the underlying heart rate. Similarly, conduction system abnormalities may affect heart rate. If a portion of

the conduction system is unable to respond appropriately to the increasing sympathetic tone of exercise, heart block occurs producing a heart rate below that appropriate for the level of exercise. If the increasing sympathetic tone produces either a supraventricular or a ventricular tachyarrhythmia, then the resultant heart rate will be more than that appropriate for the exercise intensity.

Oxygen consumption and cardiac output are also interrelated. Oxygen consumption is limited by the cardiac output and the capacity for oxygen extraction. The capacity for oxygen extraction is limited by blood oxygen content. Since very little oxygen is dissolved in blood when breathing room air at standard atmospheric pressure, the oxygen content of the blood is a function of haemoglobin concentration. In children older than ten years of age, the maximum capacity for oxygen extraction, i.e. the maximum difference in oxygen content between the system arteries and veins, is approximately 13.5 ml O_2 per 100 ml blood. This value is slightly lower in younger children due to their lower haemoglobin concentrations.[26] Short of blood doping, the only way to increase oxygen consumption is by increasing cardiac output. Anything that interferes with the cardiac output response to exercise will therefore, of necessity, also interfere with peak oxygen consumption. The relationship between oxygen consumption and cardiac output is so strong that it is often expressed as the 'exercise factor,' that is the change in cardiac output divided by the change in oxygen consumption. In general, it takes an approximately 6-litre increase in cardiac output to produce a 1-litre increase in oxygen consumption.[19,27,28]

Potential effects of non-cardiac parameters on cardiac assessment

In addition to the interrelationships between cardiac parameters, the effects of non-cardiac parameters on cardiac parameters must also be considered. The effect of pulmonary abnormalities on the assessment of cardiac output by rebreathing techniques has already been discussed. The addition of carbon monoxide to a soluble–insoluble rebreathing gas mixture can help in recognizing this problem by permitting the determination of lung diffusion capacity. The validity of one of the rebreathing technique assumptions, i.e. normal lung diffusion capacity, can be directly tested and the calculated cardiac output value rejected when this assumption is proven invalid. Since lung disease causing significant maldistribution of the rebreathing gas mixture will also diminish the lung diffusion capacity, this potential technical problem is also addressed by the addition of carbon monoxide. Unfortunately, the usefulness of this technique is limited to determining when underlying pulmonary disease makes it impossible to determine a valid cardiac output using the soluble gas rebreathing technique. Carbon monoxide has not been used in association with the CO_2 rebreathing technique. In these circumstances, one must rely on an assessment of pulmonary function before or after the rebreathing manoeuvre to determine whether a pulmonary abnormality is likely to have affected the calculated cardiac output.

In addition, one must be aware of the indirect effects of the non-cardiac systems on the cardiovascular system. A person performing a maximum exercise test stops exercising when he or she reaches the maximum capabilities of any of the organ systems necessary for exercise. Typically, it is assumed that the cardiovascular system is the limiting organ system. While this is generally true in normal subjects, it may not be true in individuals with diseases involving other organ systems. For example, an individual with cystic fibrosis may stop exercising due to pulmonary constraints long before reaching maximum cardiac capabilities.[29–31] In this case, the reduced values for peak heart rate, blood pressure, or cardiac output should not be interpreted as indications of cardiovascular disease. They are strictly a function of the demands placed on the cardiovascular system by the exercise level achieved.

Typical abnormalities

Survivors of childhood cancer provide a good example of typical cardiovascular abnormalities and the exercise evaluation thereof. There are many reasons for these patients to have limited exercise ability. They are treated with agents that are potentially toxic to multiple organ systems including the neurologic, musculoskeletal, endocrine, respiratory and cardiovascular. In addition, the cardiovascular toxicity is multifactorial since it involves not only the cardiac muscle but also the entire conduction system.

Since there are disease and treatment specific abnormalities, the exact abnormalities and their severity will depend on the specific oncologic disorders present in the population being studied. In the population studied by Barber and Heise,[32] the survivors of childhood cancer had significant reductions in their total exercise time ($80 \pm 24\%$ predicted), peak power ($81 \pm 23\%$ predicted) and peak oxygen consumption ($65 \pm 18\%$ predicted). While they had a restrictive ventilatory pattern at rest and reduced ventilatory parameters during exercise, the analysis of pulmonary function during exercise demonstrated that the reduction in ventilatory parameters during exercise was the result, not the cause, of their exercise limitation (see Chapter 1.5 for an analysis of the assessment of pulmonary function). The ECG evaluation revealed ventricular arrhythmias including short runs of non-sustained ventricular tachycardia but these abnormalities resulted in termination of the exercise test in only 1–2% of the patients (Barber, unpublished data). Peak heart rate was reduced ($92 \pm 7\%$ predicted) as were the cardiac output ($80 \pm 18\%$ predicted) and stroke volume ($88 \pm 22\%$ predicted) responses to exercise. With the reduction in cardiac output, systemic vascular resistance was elevated ($127 \pm 27\%$ predicted) producing essentially normal systolic ($95 \pm 12\%$ predicted) and diastolic ($101 \pm 16\%$ predicted) blood pressures. Thus, the exercise limitation in these patients was a result of a cardiac output limitation. This limitation was a combined result of abnormalities in both pump function (reduced stroke volume) and conduction (chronotropic incompetence).

The importance of a full cardiovascular assessment including the measurement of stroke volume and cardiac output is illustrated by two other studies.

Hogarty et al.[33] performed serial exercise evaluations in survivors of bone marrow transplantation. Similar to Barber and Heise,[32] they found that a limited cardiac output response to exercise was the primary cause of the exercise abnormality. Linear modelling of their data demonstrated that, while peak oxygen consumption increased (4% per year over five years), neither maximum cardiac index nor anaerobic threshold changed. Thus, the improvement in peak oxygen consumption did not result from an improvement in cardiovascular function. Instead, the authors theorized that the improvement in peak oxygen consumption was a compensatory response at the level of the skeletal muscle to the inadequate cardiac response. This is similar to the response seen in adult survivors of large myocardial infarctions.

Silber et al.[34] used the cardiac output response to exercise to evaluate risk factors for developing cardiac dysfunction in survivors of childhood cancer. Using this technique, the authors discovered that female survivors of childhood cancer were 2.9 times more likely than male survivors to have cardiac dysfunction. In addition, the age at treatment was a significant predictor of subsequent cardiac dysfunction. The younger the patient was at the time of treatment, the more likely they are to have an abnormal cardiac output response to exercise. For example, someone treated at age five years was 2.4 times more likely to have an abnormal cardiac output response to exercise than someone treated at age 18 after controlling for both gender and dose effects.

Obstruction to either right[35] or left ventricular outflow[36] can produce an insufficient blood pressure response to exercise, and coarctation of the aorta[37] can produce an excessive blood pressure response to exercise. Obstructions to either right or left ventricular outflow are typically apparent at rest and primarily evaluated by means other than exercise testing. Exercise testing following coarctation of the aorta, however, produces physiologic information about this lesion not apparent at rest. Typically, relief of the obstruction, either surgically or via balloon catheter dilatation, is adequate with elimination of the aortic arch gradient and normalization of the systemic blood pressure at rest. For a variety of reasons, from intrinsic abnormalities of the vascular tissue of the aorta to scar tissue formation at the site of repair, however, the aorta may not respond appropriately to an increased cardiac output during exercise. In a study of patients with a good coarctation repair based on resting haemodynamic measurements, 28% of the patients developed systolic hypertension and a mean 45 ± 13 mmHg aortic arch gradient during exercise.[37] This development of a relative arch obstruction when cardiac output increased above resting baseline was confirmed by isoproterenol infusion in the cardiac catheterization laboratory in those patients with an abnormal exercise test. While an abnormal blood pressure response to exercise may be the easiest abnormality to detect in these patients, the effect of the abnormal aortic arch on exercise is far reaching. Following successful repair of coarctation of the aorta, Johnson et al.[38] discovered that, even though the vasodilatory response to exercise of the femoral artery was increased, the blood flow response was impaired.

Tetralogy of Fallot is an example of a cardiac lesion in which exercise electrocardiography is essential. Exercise related arrhythmias are seen in 20–35% of patients following tetralogy of Fallot repair.[39–41] These arrhythmias range from sinus pauses to varying degrees of heart block to couplets to ventricular tachycardia. In the study of Wessel et al.,[39] rhythm disturbances had a 76% sensitivity and a 72% specificity in detecting patients with an impaired total exercise time (<75% predicted for age). Hannon et al.[41] demonstrated the importance of evaluating all the cardiovascular parameters in this group of patients. In their study, 25% of the patients had an exercise related arrhythmia. However, stroke volume and cardiac output responses were also abnormal in the subset of patients in which these parameters were measured, providing an additional explanation for the observed reduction in total work performed (63% predicted).

In addition to evaluating the exercise ECG for arrhythmias, it is important to assess the intervals and morphology of the various waveforms. Wolfe–Parkinson–White (WPW) syndrome is an example of a cardiac abnormality with both interval and morphologic abnormalities. In WPW, there is an accessory conduction pathway between the atria and the ventricles. This results in pre-excitation of the ventricles, which is reflected on the surface electrocardiogram as a short PR interval and a slow early component of the QRS complex, commonly referred to as a delta wave. Determining the refractory period of the accessory pathway is essential since accessory pathways with short refractory periods can result in sudden death. The rise in heart rate with exercise may exceed the antegrade refractory period of the accessory pathway if the refractory period is long. In this case, the exercise ECG suddenly normalizes with the loss of the delta wave and the lengthening of the PR interval. The heart rate at the point of this sudden normalization determines both the antegrade refractory period of the accessory pathway and the maximum atrial rate that can be conducted through this pathway to the ventricles. Both Bricker et al.[42] and Yamabe et al.[43] have demonstrated that the antegrade refractory period of the accessory pathway measured during exercise testing correlates with that measured during electrophysiologic study. It is important to note, however, that for an exercise test to be diagnostic of a long antegrade refractory period, it is essential that the normalization occurs suddenly. A delta wave is the result of the rapid conduction through the accessory pathway compared to the slower conduction through the AV node. The sympathetic stimulation of exercise accelerates AV nodal conduction. This acceleration results in a lessening of the difference between AV nodal and accessory pathway conduction, causing the delta wave to gradually diminish. This gradual change reflects the conduction properties of the AV node, not the accessory pathway.[44] In addition, exercise can only determine the accessory pathway's antegrade (atria-to-ventricle) refractory period. It cannot determine the retrograde (ventricle-to-atria) refractory period.

While it is essential to examine the exercise ECG for ST depression, as evidence of myocardial ischemia, the assessment of myocardial ischemia by exercise electrocardiography is less accurate in paediatric than in adult subjects. While coronary artery anomalies causing myocardial ischemia are generally rare in children, they are common after Kawasaki disease. In a study by Paridon et al.,[45] perfusion defects were detected by SPECT in 25 of 41 patients after Kawasaki disease. In these patients, exercise ECG had a sensitivity of only 8% compared with SPECT. The specificity, positive predictive and negative predictive values were 86%, 40% and 44%, respectively. Fukuda et al.[46] recently studied 38 patients with Kawasaki disease. Fifteen of these had marked coronary artery stenosis, defined as greater than 75%. SPECT and exercise ECG were compared. In detecting patients with marked coronary artery stenosis, the sensitivity of the exercise ECG was only 33% compared to 80% for SPECT.

Summary

The primary cardiovascular parameters routinely measured during paediatric exercise testing are the ECG, heart rate, blood pressure, cardiac output, stroke volume and systemic vascular resistance. All of these parameters are readily assessable using standard non-invasive techniques. Assessment of these cardiovascular parameters is an essential component in evaluating a subject's exercise limitation. Numerous studies, such as Hogarty et al.[33] and MacLellan-Tobert et al.,[47] have demonstrated the fallibility of estimating these parameters in subjects with cardiac limitations of their exercise response. They should be measured in any paediatric exercise test in which there is the possibility of an abnormal cardiovascular response.

References

1. Perrault, H., Drblik, S. P., Montigny, M., Davignon, A., Lamarre A., Chartrand, C. et al. Comparison of cardiovascular adjustments to exercise in adolescents 8 to 15 years of age after correction of tetralogy of Fallot, ventricular septal defect or atrial septal defect. American Journal of Cardiology 1989; 64: 213–7.

2. Jakacki, R. I, Goldwein, J. W, Larsen, R. L, Barber, G. and Silber, J. H. Cardiac dysfunction following spinal irradiation during childhood. Journal of Clinical Oncology 1993; 11: 1033–8.

3. Alboliras, E. T., Porter, C. J., Ritter, D. G., Danielson, G. K. and Driscoll, D.J. Progressive atrioventricular block during exercise in univentricular heart. Pacing and Clinical Electrophysiology 1986; 9: 821–5.

4. Weigel, T. J., Porter, C. J., Mottram, C. D. and Driscoll, D. J. Detecting arrhythmia by exercise electrocardiography in paediatric patients: assessment of sensitivity and influence on clinical management. Mayo Clinic Proceedings 1991; 66: 379–86.

5. Bricker, J. T., Garson, A., Traweek, M. S., Smith, R. T., Ward, K.A. and Vargo, T. A. et al. The use of exercise testing in children to evaluate abnormalities of pacemaker function not apparent at rest. Pacing and Clinical Electrophysiology 1987; 8: 656–60.

6. Barber G, Di Sessa, T, Child, J. S., Perloff, J. K., Laks, H., George, B. L. et al. Hemodynamic responses to isolated increments in heart rate by atrial pacing after a Fontan procedure. American Heart Journal 1988; 115: 837–41.

7. Griffin, S. E., Roberds, R. A. and Heyward, V. H., Blood pressure measurement during exercise: a review. Medicine and Science in Sports and Exercise 1997; 29: 149–59.

8. Report of the second task force on blood pressure control in children—1987 Pediatrics 1987; 79: 1–25.

9. Thapar, MK., Strong, W. B., Miller, M. D., Leatherbury, L. and Salehbhai, M. Exercise electrocardiography in healthy black children. American Journal of Diseases of Children 1978; 132: 592–5.

10. Kallay, M. C., Hyde, R. W., Smith, R. J., Rothbard, R. L. and Schreiner, B. F. Cardiac output by rebreathing in patients with cardiopulmonary disease. Journal of Applied Physiology 1987; 63: 201–10.

11. Kirby, T. E., The CO_2 rebreathing technique for determination of cardiac output: Part II. Journal of Cardiac Rehabilitation 1985; 5: 132–8.

12. Pianosi, P. and Hochman, J. End-tidal estimates of arterial PCO_2 for cardiac output measurement by CO_2 rebreathing: a study in patients with cystic fibrosis and healthy controls. Pediatric Pulmonology 1996; 22: 154–60.

13. Sackner, M. A., Greeneltch, D., Heiman, M. S., Epstein, S. and Atkins, N. Diffusion capacity, membrane diffusion capacity, capillary blood volume, pulmonary tissue volume and cardiac output measured by a rebreathing technique. American Review of Respiratory Disease 1975; 111: 157–65.

14. Triebwasser, J. H., Johnson, R. L., Burpo, R.P., Campbell, J. C., Reardon, W. C. and Blomquist, G. Non-invasive determination of cardiac output by a modified acetylene helium rebreathing procedure utilizing mass spectrometer measurements. Aviation Space and Environmental Medicine 1977; 48: 203–9.

15. Smyth, R. J., Gledhill, N., Froese, A.B. and Jamnik, V. K., Validation of noninvasive maximal cardiac output measurement. Medicine and Science in Sports and Exercise 1984; 16: 512–5.

16. Nyström, J., Celsing, F., Carlens, P., Ekblom, B. and Ring, P. Evaluation of a modified acetylene rebreathing method for determination of cardiac output. Clinical Physiology 1986; 6: 253–68.

17. Shaw, J. G., Johnson, E. C., Voyles, W. F. and Greene, E. R. Noninvasive Doppler determination of cardiac output during submaximal and peak exercise. Journal of Applied Physiology 1985; 59: 722–31.

18. Christie, J., Sheldahl, L. M., Tristani, F. E., Sagar, K. B., Ptacin, M. J and Wann, S. Determination of stroke volume and cardiac output during exercise: comparison of two-dimensional and Doppler echocardiography, Fick oximetry, and thermodilution. Circulation 1987; 76: 539–47.

19. Marx, G. R., Hicks, R. W. and Allen, H. D. Measurement of cardiac output and exercise factor by pulsed Doppler echocardiography during supine bicycle ergometry in normal young adolescent boys. Journal of the American College of Cardiology 1987; 10: 430–4.

20. Miles D. S. and Gotshall, R. W. Impedance cardiography: noninvasive assessment of human central hemodynamics at rest and during exercise. Exercise and Sport Sciences Reviews 1989; 17: 231–63.

21. **Miles, D. S., Cox, .M. H., Verde, T. J.** and **Gotshall, R. W.** Application of impedance cardiography during exercise. *Biological Physiology* 1993; **36:** 119–29.

22. **Miles, D. S., Gotshall, R. W., Golden, J. C., Tuuri, D. T. Beekman, R.H** and **Dillon, T.** Accuracy of electrical impedance cardiography for measuring cardiac output in children with congenital heart defects. *American Journal of Cardiology* 1988; **61:** 612–6.

23. **Miyazawa, K., Yamaguchi, I., Komatsu, E., Kagaya, S.** and **Oda, J.** Cardiovascular response to exercise in pacemaker implanted patients with fixed heart rate. *Japanese Heart Journal* 1989; **30:** 809–16.

24. **Alexander, T., Friedman, D. B., Levine B. D., Pawelczyk, J. A.** and **Mitchell, J. H** Cardiovascular responses during static exercise. Studies in patients with complete heart block and dual chamber pacemakers. *Circulation* 1994; **89:** 1643–7.

25. **Nobrega, A. L., Williamson, J. W., Garcia, J. A.** and **Mitchell, J. H.** Mechanisms for increasing stroke volume during static exercise with fixed heart rate in humans. *Journal of Applied Physiology* 1997; **83:** 712–7.

26. **Mocellin, R.,** Exercise testing in children with congenital heart disease. *Pediatrician.* 1986; **13:** 18–25.

27. **Astrand, P. O., Cuddy, T. E., Saltin, B.** and **Stenberg, J.** Cardiac output during submaximal and maximal work. *Journal of Applied Physiology* 1964; **19:** 268–74.

28. **Faulkner, J. A., Heigenhauser, G. J.** and **Schork, M. A.,** The cardiac output–oxygen uptake relationship of men during graded bicycle ergometry. *Medicine and Science in Sports* 1977; **9:** 148–54.

29. **Orenstein, D. M., Henke, K. G.** and **Cerny, F. J.** Exercise and cystic fibrosis. *The Physician and Sports Medicine* 1983; **11:** 57–63.

30. **Freeman, W., Stableforth, D. E., Cayton, R. M.** and **Morgan, M. D.** Endurance exercise capacity in adults with cystic fibrosis. *Respiratory Medicine* 1993; **87:** 541–9.

31. **de Jong W., van der Schans, C. P., Mannes, G. P., van Aalderen, W. M., Grevink, R. G.** and **Koeter, G. H.** Relationship between dyspnoea, pulmonary function and exercise capacity in patients with cystic fibrosis. *Respiratory Medicine* 1997; **91:** 41–6.

32. **Barber, G.** and **Heise, C. T.,** Exercise capacity following successful treatment of childhood cancer. In *Children and exercise XIX: Promoting health and well-being* (ed. N. Armstrong, B. Kirby and J. Welsman). E. & F. N. Spon, London, 1997: 472–6.

33. **Hogarty, A. N., Leahey, A., Bunin, N., Hao, H., Naan, A., Arey, A.** and **Aridon, S. M.** Cardiopulmonary performance during exercise after paediatric bone marrow transplantation. In *Children and exercise XIX: Promoting health and well-being* (ed. N. Armstrong, B. Kirby and J. Welsman). E. & F. N. Spon, London, 1997: 465–71.

34. **Silber, J. H., Jakacki, R. I., Larsen, R. L., Goldwein, J. W.** and **Barber, G.** Increased risk of cardiac dysfunction after anthracyclines in girls. *Medical and Pediatric Oncology* 1993; **21:** 477–9.

35. **Barber, G., Danielson, G. K., Puga, F. J., Heise, C. T.** and **Driscoll, D. J.** Pulmonary atresia with ventricular septal defect: preoperative and postoperative responses to exercise. *Journal of the American College of Cardiology* 1986; **7:** 630–8.

36. **James, F. W., Schwartz, D. C ., Kaplan, S.** and **Spilkin, S. P.** Exercise electrocardiogram, blood pressure, and working capacity in young patients with valvular or discrete subvalvular aortic stenosis. *American Journal of Cardiology* 1982; **50:** 769–75.

37. **Weber, H. S., Cyran, S. E., Grzeszczak, M., Myers, J. L., Gleason, M. M.** and **Baylen, B. G.** Discrepancies in aortic growth explain aortic arch gradients during exercise. *Journal of the American College of Cardiology* 1993; **21:** 1002–7.

38. **Johnson, D., Bonnin, P., Perrault, H., Marchand, T., Vobecky, S. J., Fournier, A,** *et al.* Peripheral blood flow responses to exercise after successful correction of coarctation of the aorta. *Journal of the American College of Cardiology* 1995; **26:** 1719–24.

39. **Wessel, H. U, Cunningham, W. J., Paul, M. H., Bastanier, C. K., Muster, A. J.** and **Idriss, F. S.** Exercise performance in tetralogy of Fallot after intracardiac repair. *Journal of Thoracic and Cardiovascular Surgery* 1980; **80:** 582–93.

40. **James, F. W., Kaplan, S., Schwartz, D. C., Chou, T.C., Sandker, M. J.** and **Naylor, V.** Response to exercise in patients after total surgical correction of tetralogy of Fallot. *Circulation* 1976; **54:** 671–9.

41. **Hannon, J. D., Danielson, G. K, Puga, F. J., Heise, C. T.** and **Driscoll, D. J.** Cardiovascular response to exercise after repair of tetralogy of Fallot. *Texas Heart Institute Journal* 1985; **12:** 393–400.

42. **Bricker, J. T., Porter, C. J., Garson, A., Jr., Gillette, P. C., McVey, P, Traweek, M.S.,** *et al.* Exercise testing in children with Wolff–Parkinson–White syndrome. *American Journal of Cardiology* 1985; **55:** 1001–4.

43. **Yamabe, H., Okumura, K.** and **Yasue, H.** Comparison of the effects of exercise and isoproterenol on the antegrade refractory period of the accessory pathway in patients with Wolff–Parkinson–White syndrome. *Japanese Circulation Journal* 1994; **58:** 22–8.

44. **Daubert, C., Ollitrault, J., Descaves, C., Mabo, P., Ritter, P.** and **Gouffault, J.** Failure of the exercise test to predict the anterograde refractory period of the accessory pathway in Wolff Parkinson White syndrome. *Pacing and Clinical Electrophysiology* 1988; **11:** 1130–8.

45. **Paridon, SM, Galioto, F. M., Vincent, J. A., Tomassoni, T. L., Sullivan, N. M.** and **Bricker, J. T.** Exercise capacity and incidence of myocardial perfusion defects after Kawasaki disease in children and adolescents. *Journal of the American College of Cardiology* 1995; **25:** 1420–4.

46. **Fukuda, T., Akagi, T., Ishibashi, M., Inoue, O., Sugimura, T.** and **Kato, H.** Noninvasive evaluation of myocardial ischemia in Kawasaki disease: comparison between dipyridamole stress thallium imaging and exercise stress testing. *American Heart Journal* 1998; **135:** 482–7.

47. **MacLellan-Tobert, S. G., Driscoll, D. J., Mottram, C. D., Mahoney, D. W., Wollan, P. C.** and **Danielson, G. K.** Exercise tolerance in patients with Ebstein's anomaly. *Journal of the American College of Cardiology* 1997; **29:** 1615–22.

1.7 Aerobic fitness

Neil Armstrong and Joanne R. Welsman

Introduction

Muscle contraction is supported by the energy released during the hydrolysis of adenosine triphosphate (ATP). The intramuscular stores of ATP are limited and for muscle contraction to be sustained ATP must be rapidly resynthesized. At the beginning of exercise ATP is resynthesized anaerobically (see Chapter 1.4) but during prolonged muscle activity ATP resynthesis is predominantly supported by aerobic metabolism.[1,2] This process depends upon the pulmonary, cardiovascular and haematological components of oxygen delivery and the oxidative mechanisms of the exercising muscles.

Maximal oxygen uptake ($\dot{V}O_2$ max), 'the highest amount of oxygen the body can consume during work for the aerobic production of ATP'[3] is widely recognized as the best single measure of adults' aerobic fitness.[4,5] $\dot{V}O_2$ max ultimately limits an individual's capacity to perform aerobic exercise, but it is neither the best index of an individual's ability to sustain aerobic exercise at submaximal levels nor the most sensitive means by which to detect improvements in aerobic fitness following training (see Chapter 2.11). Despite its derivation from anaerobic metabolism, measures of blood lactate accumulation during submaximal exercise provide a valuable measure of aerobic fitness[6,7] and can be used to detect improvements in muscle oxidative capacity with training even in the absence of changes in $\dot{V}O_2$ max.[8,9]

In this chapter we will focus on the measurement of aerobic fitness and on the assessment and interpretation of blood lactate responses to exercise. The interpretation of growth-related changes in aerobic fitness is addressed in Chapter 1.1 and developmental aspects of aerobic fitness are discussed in Chapters 2.6 to 2.8.

Maximal or peak oxygen uptake

Early studies of boys' $\dot{V}O_2$ during treadmill running were carried out in the United States by Robinson[10] and Morse et al.,[11] and Åstrand's[12] investigation of physical working capacity in relation to sex and age was the first major study to include girls as subjects. Since these pioneer studies $\dot{V}O_2$ max has become the most researched variable in paediatric exercise science, with 24% of all research papers published during the first ten years of the journal *Pediatric Exercise Science* (1989–98) involving the direct determination of young people's $\dot{V}O_2$ max.

The traditional model assumes that $\dot{V}O_2$ rises with increasing exercise intensity up to a point beyond which no further increase in $\dot{V}O_2$ takes place, even though a well-motivated subject is still able to increase his/her exercise intensity. Exercise beyond the point of levelling of $\dot{V}O_2$ (a $\dot{V}O_2$ plateau) is assumed to be supported exclusively by anaerobic energy sources resulting in an intracellular accumulation of lactate, acidosis and inevitably termination of the exercise. However, both the methodological[13,14] and theoretical[15,16] bases of the $\dot{V}O_2$ plateau concept have been challenged and the validity of the traditional model is a topic of lively debate.[17,18]

Regardless of the theoretical arguments, in practice, an absolute levelling of $\dot{V}O_2$ with increasing exercise intensity seldom occurs and a number of less rigorous criteria to define a $\dot{V}O_2$ plateau have been proposed[19,20] (see Fig. 1.7.1). The most commonly applied criterion with young people is a body mass-related requirement for an increase in $\dot{V}O_2$ of not more than 2.0 ml kg^{-1} min^{-1} for a 5–10% increase in exercise intensity.[21] However, even with a body mass-related criterion only a minority of children and adolescents demonstrate a $\dot{V}O_2$ plateau during an exercise test to exhaustion.[22,23]

Some authors have argued that the failure to elicit a $\dot{V}O_2$ plateau with young subjects may be related to low levels of motivation or low anaerobic capacity,[24,25] but recent data have demonstrated, with large samples of both children and adolescents, that those who plateau do not have higher $\dot{V}O_2$, heart rate or blood lactate values than those not demonstrating a $\dot{V}O_2$ plateau.[26–28] Nevertheless, as the term $\dot{V}O_2$ max conventionally implies the existence of a $\dot{V}O_2$ plateau, it has gradually become more common in paediatric exercise science to define the highest oxygen consumption observed during an exercise test to exhaustion as peak $\dot{V}O_2$.[29,30]

The general principles underlying the determination of young people's peak $\dot{V}O_2$ are fundamentally the same as those which apply to adults but with children and adolescents there are additional considerations which need to be addressed. These include ethics and pre-test preparation, respiratory gas analysis, appropriate ergometers and protocols, and defining a maximal effort. Subsequent sections will address these issues.

Ethics and pre-test preparation

The involvement of young people in non-therapeutic research raises complex issues which have been debated at length elsewhere,[31–34] and detailed discussion is beyond the scope of this chapter. In essence, researchers must consider carefully whether the procedures they wish to employ are ethical with young subjects, and whether the value of the knowledge gained clearly outweighs the risks, either physiological or psychological, to the child or adolescent.

Young people should only act as subjects in non-therapeutic research when the information required could not be gained by research with adults and when the risk to the child is negligible. Negligible risks have been defined as, 'not greater than those ordinarily encountered in daily life or during the performance of routine physical or psychological examinations or tests' (See Ref. 32, p. 14). Procedures suggested to represent negligible risk include, observation of behaviour, non-invasive physiological monitoring, developmental assessments, physical examinations, changes in diet, and obtaining blood and urine

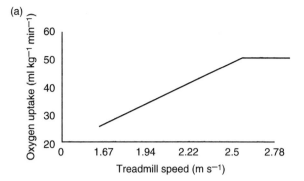

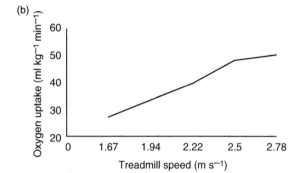

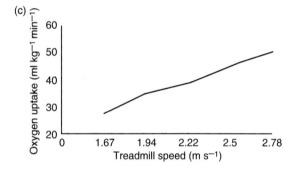

Fig. 1.7.1 Oxygen uptake in relation to exercise intensity (a) A true $\dot{V}O_2$ plateau (b) "$\dot{V}O_2$ plateau" where change in $\dot{V}O_2 \leqslant 2.0$ ml kg^{-1}min^{-1} (c) No plateau in $\dot{V}O_2$ at exhaustion.

samples.[32] The determination of healthy young people's peak $\dot{V}O_2$ clearly falls within these guidelines.

Children's and adolescents' participation in research involving the determination of peak $\dot{V}O_2$ should be through an informed willingness to cooperate rather than coercion. The legal age at which a minor can consent to participate in research projects varies from place to place, but the young person's capacity to provide informed consent depends more upon his/her having sufficient understanding and intelligence to make that decision than chronological age. The responsibility to present the relevant information in a form that the child or adolescent can understand lies with the investigator. It is, however, prudent to ensure that parents or guardians are fully cognisant of all experimental procedures and give their informed consent before proceeding with the research programme.

It is advisable to invite parents and children to attend a pre-project meeting to discuss openly all aspects of the research. The preliminary meeting should be followed up by scheduling a visit to the laboratory by the young subjects so that they can become familiar with the

research team, the equipment and the experimental procedures. At this meeting a pre-test evaluation of each subject may be performed according to recognized procedures.[35–37] If supporting materials, such as purpose-written booklets with background information and space to fill in relevant data (e.g. stature, mass, etc.), are prepared in advance, the testing programme can be designed as an educational experience for the child. The emphasis should, however, be on the young person enjoying the experience despite the need to exercise to exhaustion, which may be alien to many children and adolescents. The experience is enhanced if the laboratory is child-friendly, well-lit, appropriately decorated, spacious, with stable humidity (40 to 60%) and temperature (20 to 22 °C), and staffed with an experienced team who are able to maintain subject interest throughout the visit.

The involvement of local schools is often vital to the success of paediatric exercise science projects and this can be encouraged by giving schools the option of regular input into their curriculum by members of the research team. Although individual subject data must be held in confidence, descriptive data of samples of subjects and interpretative project updates can be fed back to schools periodically, both to enrich their curriculum and to promote long-term partnerships.

Respiratory gas analysis

The determination of $\dot{V}O_2$ is conventionally based on the ability to measure the volume of expired air per unit time ($\dot{V}_E$) and the fraction of oxygen (F_EO_2) and carbon dioxide (F_ECO_2) in the expired air. In addition, the barometric pressure, the gas temperature and the water vapour pressure of the gases are required. Figure 1.7.2 illustrates the calculations necessary to convert the measured variables into $\dot{V}O_2$ which is expressed under standard temperature and pressure, dry (STPD) conditions (i.e. temperature of 0 °C, pressure of 760 mmHg, and completely dry). Measurement error in the determination of $\dot{V}O_2$ has been comprehensively discussed elsewhere[19] and this chapter will focus primarily on issues relevant to children and adolescents.

Young people's $\dot{V}_E$, F_EO_2 and F_ECO_2 are often measured using systems which were designed for use with adults. Facemasks have a tendency to leak and mouthpieces and nose clips are usually preferred with young people although a recent study[38] has supported the use of facemasks and sealants with children as young as 8 y. However, regardless of whether a mouthpiece/noseclip system or a facemask is used they must be matched to the size of the young subject's face. All breathing valves have a dead space and adult-sized valves may therefore cause children to inspire significant volumes of previously expired air during exercise. It has been suggested[39] that a valve dead space of 59 ml may be appropriate for children with body surface area > 1.0 m^2, but that a dead space of 35 ml may be required for smaller subjects. The case to reduce valve dead space must, however, be balanced against the resulting increase in resistance to flow.

Many systems use a mixing chamber which stores gas over a given interval and, with the help of baffles, allows the fractions of O_2 and CO_2 to be mixed before being periodically sampled for measurement of F_EO_2 and F_ECO_2. However, large mixing chambers may cause substantial errors in measurement of gas exchange variables as children have smaller exercise tidal volumes than adults. It has been recommended that mixing chambers should be tailored to the size of the subject,[39] but appropriate dimensions in relation to tidal volume have not been established.

The recent development of rapidly responding flow meters, the ability to measure both inspired and expired ventilation (see Chapter 1.5),

1. Convert volume of expired air at ambient temperature and pressure, saturated (ATPS) to standard temperature and pressure, dry (STPD)

$$\dot{V}_E(STPD) = \dot{V}_E(ATPS) \times \frac{Pb - Patm(H_2O)}{760} \times \frac{273}{273 + Ta}$$

where $\dot{V}_E$ is volume of expired air in litre min^{-1}, Pb is barometric pressure in mmHg, $Patm(H_2O)$ is water vapour pressure in mmHg, and Ta is ambient temperature in $^\circ$C.

2. Calculate volume of inspired air from volume of expired air

$$\dot{V}_I(STPD) = \frac{\dot{V}_E(STPD) \times (1 - F_EO_2 - F_ECO_2)}{0.7904}$$

where $\dot{V}_I$ is volume of inspired air in litre min^{-1}, F_EO_2 is fraction of oxygen in expired air, F_ECO_2 is fraction of carbon dioxide in expired air, and 0.7904 is assumed to be the fraction of inert gases in the inspired air.

3. Calculate oxygen uptake

$$\dot{V}O_2(STPD) = (\dot{V}_I(STPD) \times F_IO_2) - (\dot{V}_E(STPD) \times F_EO_2)$$

where $\dot{V}O_2$ is oxygen uptake in litre min^{-1}, and F_IO_2 is fraction of oxygen in inspired air (often assumed to be 0.2093)

Fig. 1.7.2 Conventional calculation of oxygen uptake from volume of expired air per minute and fraction of oxygen and carbon dioxide in expired air.

and the replacement of the traditional chemical analysis of gas fractions with fast response infrared CO_2 analysers and electrochemical O_2 analysers permit the measurement of gas exchange data on a breath by breath basis. These systems are becoming commonplace in paediatric exercise science laboratories but they are not without their problems. The phasic nature of breathing during exercise makes it difficult to measure ventilation in a rapidly breathing individual, and flow meters need to be validated with flow rates ranging from what is observed for light through maximal exercise.[19,40] Similarly, gas analysers need to be calibrated carefully and a three point calibration incorporating 0%, span and midrange values is necessary for both gas analysers.[19]

Breath by breath data are providing new insights in paediatric exercise science (see Chapter 2.10) but they can also lead to confusion regarding data sampling. It has been demonstrated clearly that the variability in measuring $\dot{V}O_2$ is considerably greater as the sampling interval shortens,[13,14] and this may be a particular problem with children with small peak $\dot{V}O_2$. Myers[40] recommends that in the determination of peak $\dot{V}O_2$ one should resist the temptation to use breath by breath data and configure the system to report test results using 30-s samples printed every 10 s. This smoothes the data but permits adequate resolution for analysis. Regardless of the sample interval chosen, it should be reported as it will influence the $\dot{V}O_2$ observed.

Ergometers

Young people's peak $\dot{V}O_2$ has been determined using a wide range of ergometers[41–43] but, although it may be important to simulate competitive performance when testing young athletes,[36,44,45] the cycle ergometer and the treadmill remain the ergometers of choice in most paediatric exercise science laboratories.

Cycle ergometry provides a portable, relatively cheap, less noisy and more quantifiable mode of exercise than treadmill running and it may induce less anxiety in young subjects.[25,46,47] Limited upper body movement during cycle ergometry facilitates the measurement of ancillary variables such as heart rate, blood pressure and blood lactate. Cycle ergometers may, however, need to be modified for young children[48] who often experience difficulty with the need to maintain a fixed pedal rate when cycling on mechanically braked ergometers.[12] Electronically braked ergometers which adjust resistance to pedalling frequency may alleviate this difficulty to some extent, but the increase in resistance required to maintain exercise intensity following a reduction in pedal rate may in itself cause problems with some youngsters.

Treadmill running engages a larger muscle mass than cycling and the peak $\dot{V}O_2$ obtained is therefore more likely to have been limited by central rather than peripheral factors.[20,21] Peak $\dot{V}O_2$ is typically 8–10% higher during treadmill running than cycle ergometry,[49–51] although some adolescents do achieve higher peak $\dot{V}O_2$ on a cycle ergometer.[44] Correlations between peak $\dot{V}O_2$ determined on a treadmill and a cycle are normally about 0.90.[44,49]

The reported reliability of cycle and treadmill values for peak $\dot{V}O_2$ on repeated testing appears to be similar, with correlation coefficients generally in the range 0.87 to 0.96.[42,49,52,53] However, the use of correlation coefficients to assess the variation in repeated measurements by the same method on the same subject has been criticized as they are a measure of the strength of the relationship between two measures, not of the repeatability in a test–retest model.[54,55] No published study of young people's peak $\dot{V}O_2$ to date has reported the repeatability coefficient[54,55] of either treadmill or cycle ergometer tests.

A major disadvantage of cycle ergometry with children is that a high proportion of the total power output is developed by the quadriceps muscle,[56] and the effort required to push the pedals during the later stages of a progressive test is high in relation to muscle strength.[57] Blood flow through the quadriceps is restricted[58,59] resulting in increased anaerobic metabolism[49,60] and consequent termination of the test through peripheral muscle pain.[61]

Reviews of the extant literature have demonstrated that at 10 to 12 years of age sex differences in peak $\dot{V}O_2$ are generally less when determined on a cycle ergometer than when determined on a treadmill,[28,30] whereas at 16 years of age sex differences are consistent regardless of the ergometer used in the determination of peak $\dot{V}O_2$. This may be a methodological artefact reflecting girls' earlier maturation and the tendency for cycle ergometer tests to be terminated by peripheral rather than central fatigue. The use of cycle ergometers to determine the peak $\dot{V}O_2$ of children may therefore have clouded our understanding of the development of aerobic performance, and the treadmill appears to be the most appropriate mode of exercise in the laboratory determination of healthy young people's peak $\dot{V}O_2$.

Exercise protocols

Peak $\dot{V}O_2$ is a robust variable which has been shown, on a specific ergometer, to be generally independent of exercise protocol.[62–64] In clinical settings standardized exercise protocols with published norms are popular,[34,65,66] but most research laboratories utilize protocols which are suited to the specific aims of the investigation and are appropriate for the age, size and maturity of the subjects.

Progressive exercise tests to exhaustion may be continuous or discontinuous. Continuous tests reduce the total length of the test but the rest period during discontinuous stages facilitates ancillary measurements (e.g. blood sampling), allows the experimenters to encourage and motivate the subject, and compensates for children's shorter attention spans. The duration of each incremental stage may vary according to whether or not near steady-state measures of $\dot{V}O_2$ and blood lactate are required. A near steady-state in $\dot{V}O_2$ can be achieved within 2 min, but it may take up to 3 min for blood lactate to appropriately reflect the exercise intensity.[67,68]

General guidelines for the design of an appropriate exercise test using a treadmill are outlined in Table 1.7.1.

Defining a maximal effort

Exercise tests with children and adolescents are normally terminated when the subject, despite strong verbal encouragement from the experimenters, is unable or unwilling to continue. The experimenters are then left, in the absence of a $\dot{V}O_2$ plateau, with the problem of deciding whether the young subject has delivered a maximal effort. Habituation to the laboratory environment, subjective criteria of intense effort (e.g. facial flushing, sweating, hyperpnoea, unsteady gait), and the paediatric exercise testing experience of the experimenters are vital ingredients in making this decision but supportive physiological indicators are also available.

Heart rate at peak $\dot{V}O_2$

Heart rate rises linearly with exercise intensity and normally starts to level off as peak values are attained. Heart rate therefore provides an indicator of effort but it is dependent on the exercise protocol,[34,62] with heart rate at peak $\dot{V}O_2$ tending to be lower during cycle ergometry than treadmill running.[23,44] Heart rate at peak $\dot{V}O_2$ is also subject to wide individual variations. We have recorded heart rates at peak $\dot{V}O_2$ ranging from 185 to 225 beats min^{-1} in prepubertal children[26,62] and adolescents,[23,70] with mean values of 196 and 201 beats min^{-1} for cycle and treadmill exercise, respectively, and no significant sex difference.

Heart rate is used widely as an indicator of performance with 72% of peak $\dot{V}O_2$ studies published in *Pediatric Exercise Science* (1989–98) utilizing either > 90% or 95% of age-predicted maximum heart rate as a criterion of maximal effort. These criteria may not be rigorous enough to indicate a maximal effort with many young people and as maximal heart rate is fairly stable during childhood and adolescence, the recommendation that target heart rates of 200 beats min^{-1} for treadmill running and 195 beats min^{-1} for cycling[30,34] may be more appropriate, with the additional proviso that heart rate should be levelling off over the final exercise stages.[46]

Respiratory exchange ratio at peak $\dot{V}O_2$

The respiratory exchange ratio (RER) rises during exercise to reflect increased CO_2 production, through buffering lactate as well as substrate utilization, and can therefore indicate intense effort. Seventy six per cent of the peak $\dot{V}O_2$ studies published in *Pediatric Exercise Science* (1989–98) used an RER $\geqslant 1.00$ as a criterion of maximal effort and it

has been advocated as the best criterion of maximal effort.[47] In our laboratory, RERs at peak $\dot{V}O_2$ following a progressive, treadmill protocol have averaged 1.05 in young people[36,70] with no significant sex difference. However, the standard deviation of 0.06 illustrates individual differences and some young subjects can provide an exhaustive effort with an RER at peak $\dot{V}O_2$ of < 1.00.

RER is ergometer dependent and is often higher during cycling than running.[49,65] Furthermore, it is highly dependent on protocol regardless of the ergometer used. For example, following a progressive treadmill protocol the mean RER at peak $\dot{V}O_2$ of 17 nine year old boys was 0.99, but after a continuous 2 min treadmill run at the same speed but up a slope 5% higher than the previous test the mean RER was 1.18, although the mean peak $\dot{V}O_2$ on the two tests was not significantly different.[62] Nevertheless, an RER at peak $\dot{V}O_2 \geqslant 1.00$ following a progressive exercise test is a valuable indicator of a near maximal effort in young people.

Blood lactate at peak $\dot{V}O_2$

High post-exercise blood lactate levels are often used with adults as a subsidiary criterion of peak $\dot{V}O_2$ and some laboratories recommend post-exercise lactates of 6 to 9 mmol litre^{-1} as indicative of maximal effort with children and adolescents.[71,72] There is, however, considerable variability in post-exercise blood lactates of children and adolescents, with levels at peak $\dot{V}O_2$ ranging from less than 4.0 mmol litre^{-1} to over 13.0 mmol litre^{-1} using the same protocol, sampling and assay techniques.[36,73] In the light of the methodological factors discussed later in this chapter and the dependence of lactate on mode of exercise,[49] protocols employed[62] and timing of post-exercise sampling relative to the cessation of the exercise,[74,75] the recommendation of minimum post-exercise blood lactates to validate peak $\dot{V}O_2$ is untenable.

There is no easy solution to the problem of whether in the absence of a $\dot{V}O_2$ plateau the child or adolescent has delivered a maximal effort. However, the view that if, in a progressive exercise test, the subject demonstrates clear subjective symptoms of fatigue, supported by a heart rate which is levelling off at about 200 beats min^{-1} and an RER $\geqslant 1.00$, a maximal effort can be assumed, has recently received strong support.[62,65,76]

Blood lactate

At both rest and exercise lactate is generated in skeletal muscle as a by-product of glycolytic energy generation. Lactate diffuses from muscle into the blood where, both during and post-exercise it can be sampled to provide information regarding, for example, glycolytic stress[78] or aerobic fitness.[79,80]

Although blood lactate is sampled with the aim of obtaining information about muscle lactate production, it is important to emphasize that lactate metabolism during exercise is a dynamic process in which lactate levels measured in blood cannot be assumed to bear a consistent or direct relationship with either rates of muscle lactate production or muscle lactate levels. In skeletal muscle, lactate may be produced in some muscle fibres whilst being simultaneously consumed by adjacent fibres within the same muscle, therefore net lactate output from the muscle does not directly relate to the amount of lactate production.[81] Lactate which diffuses into the blood is removed by several processes, including oxidation in other skeletal muscles and the heart, or used as a gluconeogenic precursor in the liver and kidneys.[82]

Table 1.7.1 Guidelines for designing a treadmill exercise protocol

1. The time of day of the test does not appear to be critical[77] but the test should be conducted at least 2 h after the consumption of solid food.

2. The subject should not have exercised vigorously on the day of testing and should be wearing physical education kit and suitable footwear.

3. The subject should be habituated to the laboratory environment and familiar with treadmill running.

4. Throughout the test the child's safety and well-being are paramount. Contraindication to exercise must be ruled out before the test begins and experimenters should know what indications signal that the test should be terminated.[37]

5. A low intensity exercise warm-up is advisable.

6. The child's age, maturity, and therefore attention span should be considered when designing the protocol. The optimal test duration is about 9 to 12 min of exercise following a warm-up and the exercise periods may be interspersed with standard rest periods (e.g. 1 min).

7. Ancillary measures such as blood sampling are facilitated by discontinuous tests although the length of exercise stage should be at least 3 min for blood lactate to reflect the exercise intensity and at least 2 min for a near steady-state $\dot{V}O_2$.

8. Changes in belt speed or slope should not be excessive and gradients and speeds should be appropriate to the size, age and maturity of the subject.

9. Subjective and objective end-points should be decided prior to the test (e.g. facial flushing, sweating, hyperpnoea, unsteady gait, HR levelling off at about 200 beats min^{-1}, RER $\geqslant$ 1.0).

10. The subject should be allowed to gradually warm-down following the test.

During an incremental exercise test, such as described above for the determination of peak $\dot{V}O_2$, blood lactate typically increases as illustrated in Fig. 1.7.3. The early stages of the test are associated with minimal change in blood lactate with levels perhaps not increasing above resting values (1 to 2 mmol litre^{-1}). As the test progresses a point is reached where blood lactate levels begin to increase rapidly (sometimes called the lactate breakpoint/lactate threshold etc.) with a subsequent steep rise until exhaustion. It cannot be inferred that the first increase above resting levels reflects the onset of muscle lactate production; lactate production is likely to have increased at these low intensities but, as described above, where this is matched by increased removal and metabolism the net result is no observable increase in blood levels.[81]

As shown in Fig. 1.7.3, following appropriate training the entire lactate curve is shifted to the right such that any given exercise intensity is achieved with a lower blood lactate. This response forms the basis of the use of the blood lactate response to exercise as a sensitive and well-established measure of aerobic fitness in adults.[83] Children's blood lactate responses appear to be lower than those of adults during comparable exercise intensities,[84,85] although definitive explanations for these differences remain elusive.[30,46] Similarly, the utility of blood lactate to differentiate aerobic fitness levels in young people remains equivocal,[86] although an appropriate short-term training programme has been shown to elicit similar changes to those illustrated in Fig. 1.7.3 in young girls despite no change in peak $\dot{V}O_2$.[79] Blood lactate responses to exercise are highly influenced by methodological variations such as mode of exercise (cycle ergometer versus treadmill), exercise protocol, site of blood sampling, and blood treatment and assay procedures. Evident in several comprehensive summaries of children's peak and submaximal lactate responses is a lack of interstudy standardization of methodology.[30,46,80,86] These differences must be considered when interpreting young people's blood lactate responses and are likely to have contributed to the controversy surrounding the maturation of children's blood lactate responses.[46]

Methodological considerations

Protocol effects

The concentration of lactate in blood and muscle is influenced by both a time-dependent and an intensity-dependent variation during exercise,[87,88] therefore the duration of each exercise stage during an incremental protocol will influence the observed lactate level, particularly where the exercise intensity exceeds the maximal lactate steady state (see below). The exercise stage should be of sufficient duration to allow adequate diffusion of lactate from muscle to blood.[89,90] If sampled too soon, lactate measured will not accurately reflect intensity of exercise and will influence the determination of fixed blood lactate reference levels.[87,90] With adults, an incremental stage of at least four minutes is recommended but with young people a three minute stage is considered sufficient.[83]

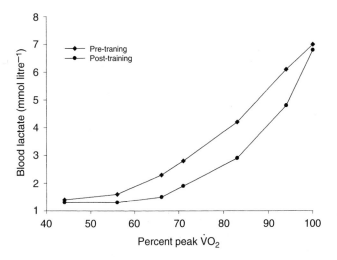

Fig. 1.7.3 Blood lactate responses to exercise.

Site of sampling

Lactate generated in skeletal muscles during leg exercise diffuses into the femoral veins, then rapidly appears in the arterial circulation. Thus blood sampled from the arteries of the arm provides the closest reflection of the extent of lactate diffusion into the systemic circulation.[92,93] The technical and medical hazards associated with arterial blood sampling preclude its use as a routine technique and the procedure is clearly not ethically defensible for research purposes with healthy young people.[94] Fortunately, it has been demonstrated that arterial lactate levels are closely reflected by capillary lactate levels during treadmill exercise[95] providing a good blood flow is maintained at the sampling site. During exercise, following adequate warm-up, this is unlikely to be a problem but at rest or in cold environments external warming of the hand may be required to induce vasodilation. Capillary blood sampling from the fingertip[96] or earlobe[97] is the least invasive and traumatic sampling method, is suited to field situations, and has been extensively used with young people.[30,78] Squeezing the site to obtain an adequate blood sample must be avoided to prevent dilution of the sample by tissue fluid.[98] Similarly, the sampling site should remain clean and dry to prevent contamination by sweat.[99]

To facilitate serial blood sampling, some investigators have drawn venous blood from a catheter inserted into an arm or hand vein. This is not recommended as several studies have shown that, in contrast to arterial blood, femoral lactate levels are not well reflected by venous blood.[100] Furthermore, during cycle ergometry, lactate levels in venous blood have been shown to be significantly lower than in simultaneously sampled arterial or capillary blood,[101] with the discrepancy increasing at higher exercise intensities.[91,102] During steady-state submaximal treadmill exercise arterial–venous lactate differences appear less pronounced, but the trend towards an increasing discrepancy in values between sites remains.[95,103]

Assay methods

Despite its significant impact upon the value of blood lactate obtained, the nature and extent of differences between lactate assay methodologies remain poorly documented and infrequently acknowledged in the interpretation of young people's blood lactate responses during exercise.

Once sampled, blood may undergo a variety of treatments depending upon the analyser, which may require preparation of either serum, plasma, lysed blood or a protein-free preparation (see Table 1.7.2). The modern semi-automatic analyzers used in many paediatric exercise laboratories are based upon an enzymatic electrochemical assay which is usually used to analyze whole blood immediately following sampling. These analysers have many advantages; they are simple to use, do not require large amounts of blood (typically lactate is assayed in 25 µl of blood) and results are available rapidly (usually within 60 to 90 s). Portable versions of several models are available, which facilitates blood lactate measurement in field situations.

Before the availability of this methodology, lactate was often determined using a enzymatic-spectrophotometric assay which required the preparation of a protein-free filtrate (see Table 1.7.2). This is achieved by precipitating the blood proteins by the addition of ice-cold perchloric acid or trichloroacetic acid, centrifuging the sample and assaying lactate in the clear supernatant.

The variation in the results obtained from different assays may be considerable and depends upon two main factors; firstly, whether or not the solids (cells, proteins, cellular debris etc.) have been removed (as in plasma, serum and protein-free preparations) or not (as in whole blood and lysed blood), and secondly whether the sample has been haemolysed to release erythrocyte lactate (as in lysed blood and protein-free preparations). The volume difference accounts for the largest variation in lactate levels observed. In whole blood assays, only the lactate in the plasma fraction is assayed but the sample still contains the solid fraction. Thus lactate levels in whole blood are substantially lower than in preparations from which the solids have been removed. Estimates quantifying the volume difference between protein-free and whole blood lactates vary from 5%[104] to 63.7%,[105] with the difference apparently reducing at high exercise intensities.[105] Lactate values in plasma are approximately 30% higher than in whole blood.[95,101]

The addition of a chemical lysing agent releases intracellular lactate, thus contributing an additional source of lactate to the sample. Therefore, in contrast to a whole blood assay where lactate is measured in the plasma compartment, protein-free and lysed blood assays measure 'total' lactate, that is plasma plus erythrocyte lactate. Individual differences in haematocrit may, therefore, be a confounding factor in lactate levels observed.[101,106] Lactate levels in lysed blood tend to be higher than those in whole blood, with the difference becoming more marked at higher lactate concentrations.[95,105]

The effect of different assay methodologies upon blood lactate levels and the implications of these for performance evaluation can be clearly illustrated using the regression equations generated by Williams et al.[95] If a sample taken during exercise yields a whole blood lactate of 4 mmol litre^{-1}, simply lysing the blood would increase the lactate value to 4.4 mmol litre^{-1} and a value of 5.5 mmol litre^{-1} would be obtained if plasma was assayed.

Table 1.7.2   Blood preparations for lactate assay

Whole blood:	Blood is collected into a capillary tube or cuvette coated with heparin to prevent clotting and is analyzed, usually within minutes, without further treatment.
Plasma:	Blood is collected as above and centrifuged to separate the liquid (plasma) and solid constituents of the blood. Lactate is then measured in the plasma.
Serum:	Blood is allowed to clot and is then centrifuged to separate the clear, straw-coloured serum which is assayed for lactate.
Lysed blood:	Blood is treated with chemicals which break open (lyse) the red blood cells releasing the intracellular lactate. The blood is not separated before assay.
Protein-free preparation:	The blood sample is chemically treated to break down blood proteins and then centrifuged to separate the solids and liquids. The liquid portion is then assayed for lactate

Reprinted from Armstrong and Welsman[46] with permission.

Blood lactate measures for performance assessment

As described above, training-induced improvements in aerobic fitness result in a lower blood lactate response to all levels of submaximal exercise. Therefore, any point on the lactate curve illustrated in Fig. 1.7.3 might be used to detect and monitor intra-individual improvements. However, in order to make comparisons amongst individuals or groups (e.g. by sex or maturity stage), lactate responses are often standardized to some measure of 'lactate threshold'. Most often this term is used to describe the first observable increase in blood lactate above resting levels.[107] This can be determined either from visual inspection of the inflection in blood lactate responses,[108] mathematical interpolation[109–111] or by defining the point of inflection as a 1 mmol litre^{-1} increase over baseline levels.[112] A clear inflection point may not be observable particularly during a discontinuous protocol where peak $\dot{V}O_2$ is attained within relatively few incremental stages (for example, as in the data presented in Fig. 1.7.3, which are typical of a young person's blood lactate responses to incremental exercise). To circumvent this, some authors have recommended the use of a fixed blood lactate reference level and in adults, a value of 4.0 mmol litre^{-1}, originally referred to as the 'onset of blood lactate accumulation',[113,114] has become an accepted assessment standard.[83] One justification for a 4 mmol litre^{-1} criterion was the suggestion that this corresponded to the maximal lactate steady state (MLSS),[87] although subsequent evidence has demonstrated wide inter-individual variation, particularly in athletes.[115,116]

MLSS defines the highest exercise intensity which can be maintained without incurring a progressive increase in blood lactate. As processes of lactate accumulation and elimination are in equilibrium, although elevated above resting levels, exercise can continue for prolonged periods at the MLSS and it represents perhaps the most sensitive and informative measure of aerobic endurance performance.

It is important to re-emphasize that the exercise intensity at which a given threshold or reference level occurs is highly specific to both the exercise protocol and the methods used to determine blood lactate levels. Much of the original work into blood lactate responses which resulted in the general acceptance of a 4 mmol litre^{-1} reference criterion determined lactate in a protein-free preparation. Given that young people respond to any given exercise intensity with lower lactate levels than adults and that the majority of paediatric laboratories assay lactate in whole blood,[30,78] the validity of a 4 mmol litre^{-1} reference level to assess aerobic fitness in children and adolescents may be questioned. In both trained[108,117] and untrained[73,117,118] young people, a whole blood lactate level of 4 mmol litre^{-1} is often not attained until approximately 90% peak $\dot{V}O_2$. In response to this Williams et al.[73] proposed the use of a 2.5 mmol litre^{-1} whole blood criterion, and demonstrated that physiological responses to exercise eliciting this level of blood lactate closely represent those at the maximal lactate steady state in 13 year old boys and girls.[96] In this study, the MLSS, defined as a change in blood lactate $\leqslant 0.5$ mmol litre^{-1} between minutes five and ten of a 10 min continuous exercise bout, occurred at 2.1 and 2.3 mmol litre^{-1} in boys and girls, respectively. The MLSS in young people has not been documented extensively but studies with boys have reported lactate levels at the MLSS ranging from 3.1 to 5.0 mmol litre^{-1}.[97,119–121] These studies used a protein-free assay, therefore the higher values reported are not unexpected. Further sources of interstudy variation in results may include the use of cycle ergometry[120,121] versus treadmill

running,[97,119] and continuous[96,120] versus discontinuous[97,119] exercise stages. The value of lactate obtained has also been shown to vary according to the duration of each exercise stage and the specific criterion used to define the MLSS.[121]

Blood lactate responses to exercise and chronological age

Several studies have investigated children's and adolescents' blood lactate responses to exercise, but a precise description of changes with age and maturation remains elusive largely as a result of inconsistent exercise and blood sampling protocols and small and/or single sex subject samples.

Apparent age-related differences have been noted in several studies of boys. Tanaka and Shindo[122] noted a significant inverse relationship between heart rate at the lactate threshold, expressed as a percentage of peak heart rate, and chronological age in 8–15 year olds. Similarly, Izumi and Ishiko[123] noted that during cycle ergometry, the lactate threshold occurred much closer to peak $\dot{V}O_2$ in teenage boys than in adults (73% versus 63% peak $\dot{V}O_2$). Another comparison of teenage boys with adults[124] also noted higher heart rates at the exercise intensity corresponding to a 4.0 mmol litre^{-1} blood lactate in the younger subjects, although differences became negligible when expressed in relative terms.

In what appears to be the largest single study of both boys and girls, Williams and Armstrong[118] found no significant relationship between age and per cent peak $\dot{V}O_2$ at a blood lactate of 4.0 mmol litre^{-1} in 11 to 16 year olds although this level occurred so close to peak $\dot{V}O_2$ to be of questionable value as a marker of submaximal performance. Interestingly, a significant, although very low, correlation was obtained between age and per cent peak $\dot{V}O_2$ at a lower reference level of 2.5 mmol litre^{-1} in the same boys ($r = -0.226$, $p < 0.05$) and girls ($r = -0.272$, $p < 0.05$). An absence of any age effect has also been noted with respect to the MLSS; Beneke et al.[120] observed no significant relationship between either level of blood lactate or per cent peak $\dot{V}O_2$ at the MLSS determined during cycle ergometry and age in 34 males aged 11 to 20 years. There do not appear to be significant sex differences in performance at fixed submaximal lactate reference levels.[118]

Blood lactate responses to exercise and maturity

Despite early indications that blood lactate responses are related to indices of maturational age,[125] and animal studies suggesting androgenic dependency of muscle glycolytic capacity and consequent lactate production,[126,127] the role of maturity in determining young people's blood lactate responses to exercise remains inconclusive.[30,46]

Studies examining specific relationships between maturity and blood lactate indices of aerobic performance are scarce but consistent in failing to identify an independent maturational effect. For example, we used a regression approach to examine the effects of body size and salivary testosterone upon blood lactate indices including per cent peak $\dot{V}O_2$ at a 2.5 mmol litre^{-1} reference level in 12 to 16 year old boys whose maturation ranged from Tanner stage one to stage five.[128] No significant independent effect of testosterone upon submaximal blood lactate levels was observed.[129] Similarly, no significant differences in the per cent peak $\dot{V}O_2$ at reference levels of 2.5 and 4.0 mmol litre^{-1} were observed in a sample of 119 boys and girls compared by maturity group.[118] Thus it would appear that factors other than hormonal changes with sexual maturation regulate developmental changes in blood lactate responses during exercise.

Summary

$\dot{V}O_2$ max is widely recognized as the best single index of aerobic fitness but only a minority of children and adolescents demonstrate the $\dot{V}O_2$ plateau conventionally associated with $\dot{V}O_2$ max. There is therefore a growing conviction that peak $\dot{V}O_2$ is the appropriate term to use with young people. Peak $\dot{V}O_2$ may be accepted as a maximal index provided appropriate subjective criteria of exhaustion are fulfilled and supported by the achievement of specific heart rate and/or RER values. Prior to a determination of peak $\dot{V}O_2$, ethical issues, pre-test preparation and respiratory gas analysis need to be addressed. The treadmill is the appropriate ergometer for the laboratory determination of healthy young people's peak $\dot{V}O_2$, but the exercise protocol used should be designed with reference to the aims of the study and the age, size and maturity of the subjects. The precise methodology, apparatus and criteria of a maximal effort used in the determination of children's and adolescents' peak $\dot{V}O_2$ should be carefully reported.

Blood lactate responses are highly protocol dependent with most of the variability attributable to differences in site of blood sampling and assay methodology. Exercise lactate measures are not directly comparable between studies unless identical protocols and assay procedures have been followed. Laboratory determined reference markers can only be extrapolated to field conditions if measurement procedures and assay methods remain consistent. Much remains to be elucidated regarding age and maturational influences upon blood lactate responses during exercise, and interpretation will be facilitated by careful intrastudy standardization of methods used, and precise and detailed reporting of these in publication.

References

1. Newsholme, E. A. Fuels used for different athletic events: Quantitative and qualitative analysis. In *Children and exercise XIX* (ed. N. Armstrong, B. J. Kirby and J. R. Welsman). E. and F. N. Spon, London, 1997: 479–93.

2. Newsholme, E. A. and Leech, A. R. *Biochemistry for the medical sciences.* Wiley, Chichester, 1983.

3. Anshel, M. H., Freedson, P., Hamill, J., Haywood, K., Horvat, M. and Plowman, S. A. *Dictionary of the sport and exercise sciences.* Human Kinetics Publishers, Champaign, Il, 1991.

4. Wilmore, J. H. and Costill, D. L. *Physiology of sport and exercise.* Human Kinetics, Champaign, Il, 1994.

5. Astrand, P. O. and Rodahl, K. *Textbook of work physiology.* McGraw-Hill, New York, 1986.

6. Weltman, A., Tippett, S., Janney, C., Strand, K., Rians, C., Cahill, B. R. and Katch, F. I. Measurement of isokinetic strength in prepubertal males. *Journal of Orthopedic and Sports Physical Therapy* 1988; 9: 345–51.

7. Yoshida, T., Chida, M., Khioka, M. and Suda, Y. Blood lactate parameters related to aerobic capacity and endurance performance. *European Journal of Applied Physiology* 1987; 56: 7–11.

8. Henritze, J., Weltman, A., Schurrer, R. L., Barlow, L. Effects of training at and above the lactate threshold on the lactate threshold and maximal oxygen uptake. *European Journal of Applied Physiology* 1985; 54: 84–8.

9. Sjodin, B., Jacobs, I. and Svedenhag, J. Changes in onset of blood lactate accumulation and muscle enzymes after training at OBLA. *European Journal of Applied Physiology* 1982; 49: 45–57.

10. Robinson, S. Experimental studies of physical fitness in relation to age. *Arbeitsphysiologie* 1938; 10: 251–323.

11. Morse, M., Schlutz, F. W. and Cassels, D. E. Relation of age to physiological responses of the older boy to exercise. *Journal of Applied Physiology* 1949; 1: 683–709.

12. Åstrand PO. *Experimental studies of physical working capacity in relation to sex and age.* Munksgaard, Copenhagen, 1952.

13. Myers, J., Walsh, D., Buchanan, N. and Froelicher, V. F. Can maximal cardiopulmonary capacity be recognised by a plateau in oxygen uptake. *Chest* 1989; 96: 1312–6.

14. Myers, J., Walsh, D., Sullivan, M. and Froelicher, V. Effect of sampling on variability and plateau in oxygen uptake. *Journal of Applied Physiology* 1990; 68: 404–10.

15. Noakes, T. D. Implications of exercise testing for prediction of athletic performance: a contemporary perspective. *Medicine and Science in Sports and Exercise* 1988; 20: 319–30.

16. Noakes, T. D. Challenging beliefs: ex Africa semper aliquid novi. *Medicine and Science in Sports and Exercise* 1997; 29: 571–90.

17. Noakes, T. D. Maximal oxygen uptake: 'classical' versus 'contemporary' viewpoints: a rebuttal. *Medicine and Science in Sports and Exercise* 1998; 30: 1381–98.

18. Bassett, D. R. and Howley, E. T. Maximal oxygen uptake: 'classical' versus 'contemporary' viewpoints. *Medicine and Science in Sports and Exercise* 1997; 29: 591–603.

19. Howley, E. T., Bassett, D. R. and Welch, H. G. Criteria for maximal oxygen uptake: review and commentary. *Medicine and Science in Sports and Exercise* 1995; 27: 1292–301.

20. Shephard, R. J. Tests of maximum oxygen intake. A critical review. *Sports Medicine* 1984; 1: 99–124.

21. Shephard, R. J. The working capacity of schoolchildren. In *Frontiers of fitness* (ed. R. J. Shephard). Thomas, Springfield, 1971, pp. 319–45.

22. Armstrong, N., Balding, J., Gentle, P. and Kirby, B. Estimation of coronary risk factors in British schoolchildren: a preliminary report. *British Journal of Sports Medicine* 1990; 24: 61–6.

23. Armstrong, N., Williams, J., Balding, J., Gentle, P. and Kirby, B. The peak oxygen uptake of British children with reference to age, sex and sexual maturity. *European Journal of Applied Physiology* 1991; 62: 369–75.

24. Krahenbuhl, G. S., Skinner, J. S. and Kohrt, W. M. Developmental aspects of maximal aerobic power in children. *Exercise and Sport Sciences Reviews* 1985; 13: 503–38.

25. Rowland, T. W. Aerobic exercise testing protocols. In *Pediatric laboratory exercise testing in children* (ed. T. W. Rowland). Human Kinetics Publishers, Champaign Il, 1993: 19–42.

26. Armstrong, N., Kirby, B. J., McManus, A. M. and Welsman, J. R. Aerobic fitness of pre-pubescent children. *Annals of Human Biology* 1995; 22: 427–41.

27. Armstrong, N. Children and aerobic exercise. In *Sports, exercise and medicine* (ed. J. McCraken and I. Williams). University of Nottingham Press, Nottingham, 1995: 93–116.

28. Armstrong, N. and Welsman, J. The assessment and interpretation of aerobic fitness in children and adolescents: An update. In *Exercise and fitness—benefits and limitations* (ed. K. Froberg, O. Lammert, H. St. Hansen and C. J. R. Blimkie). University Press, Odense, 1997: 173–80.

29. Armstrong, N. and Davies, B. The metabolic and physiological responses of children to exercise and training. *Physical Education Review* 1984; 7: 90–105.

30. Armstrong, N. and Welsman, J. Assessment and interpretation of aerobic fitness in children and adolescents. *Exercise and Sport Sciences Reviews* 1994; 22: 435–76.

31. Nicholson, R. H. *Medical research with children.* Oxford University Press, Oxford, 1986.

32. Working Party on Ethics of Research in Children. Guidelines to aid ethical committees considering research involving children. *British Medical Journal* 1980; 280: 229–31.

33. Working Party on Research in Children. *The ethical conduct of research in children*. Medical Research Council, London, 1991.

34. Rowland, T. W. *Developmental exercise physiology*. Human Kinetics, Champaign, Il, 1996.

35. American College of Sports Medicine. *ACSM's guidelines for exercise testing and prescription*. Williams and Wilkins, Baltimore, 1995.

36. Armstrong, N. and Welsman, J. Laboratory testing of young athletes. In *Color atlas and textbook of sports medicine in childhood and adolescence* (ed. N. Maffulli). Mosby-Wolfe, London, 1995: 109–22.

37. Tomasson, T. L. Conducting the pediatric exercise test. In *Pediatric laboratory exercise testing* (ed. T. W. Rowland). Human Kinetics Publishers, Champaign, Il, 1993: 1–17.

38. Mahon, A. D., Stolen, K. Q. and Gay, J. A. Using a facemask and sealant to measure respiratory gas exchange in children during exercise. *Pediatric Exercise Science* 1998; 10: 347–55.

39. Staats, B. A., Grinton, S. F., Mottram, C. D., Driscoll, D. J. and Beck, K. C. Quality control in exercising testing. *Progress in Pediatric Cardiology* 1993; 2: 11–7.

40. Myers JN. *Essentials of cardiopulmonary exercise testing*. Human Kinetics Publishers, Champaign, Il, 1996.

41. Armstrong, N., Davies, B. and Heal, M. The specificity of energy utilization by trained and untrained adolescent boys. *British Journal of Sports Medicine* 1983; 17: 193–9.

42. Rivera-Brown, A. M. and Frontera, W. R. Achievement of plateau and reliability of $\dot{V}O_2$ max in trained adolescents tested with different ergometers. *Pediatric Exercise Science* 1998; 10: 164–75.

43. Chan, O. L., Duncan, M. T., Sundsten, J. W., Thinakaran, T., Noh, M. N. B. C. and Klissouras, V. The maximum aerobic power of the Temiars. *Medicine and Science in Sports and Exercise* 1976; 8: 235–8.

44. Armstrong, N. and Davies, B. An ergometric analysis of age group swimmers. *British Journal of Sports Medicine* 1981; 15: 20–6.

45. Al-Hazza, H. M., Al-Refaee, S. A., Sulaiman, M. A., Dafterdar, M. Y., Al-Herbish, A. S. and Chukwuemeka, A. C. Cardiorespiratory responses of trained boys to treadmill and arm ergometry: effects of training specificity. *Pediatric Exercise Science* 1998; 10: 264–76.

46. Armstrong, N. and Welsman, J. R. *Young people and physical activity*. Oxford University Press, Oxford, 1997.

47. Léger, L. Aerobic performance. In *Measurement in pediatric exercise science* (ed. D. Docherty). Human Kinetics Publishers, Champaign, Il, 1996: 183–223.

48. Howell, M. L. and MacNab, R. B. J. *The physical work capacity of Canadian children aged 7 to 17*. Canadian Association for Health, Physical Education and Recreation, Toronto Ontario, 1968.

49. Boileau, R. A., Bonen, A., Heyward, V. H. and Massey, B. H. Maximal aerobic capacity on the treadmill and bicycle ergometer of boys 11–14 years of age. *Journal of Sports Medicine and Physical Fitness* 1977; 17: 153–62.

50. Turley, K. R., Rogers, D. M. and Wilmore, J. H. Maximal testing in prepubescent children: treadmill versus cycle ergometry. *Medicine and Science in Sports and Exercise* 1993; 25: S9.

51. Macek, M., Vavra, J. and Novosadova, J. Prolonged exercise in prepubertal boys. I—Cardiovascular and metabolic adjustment. *European Journal of Applied Physiology* 1976; 35: 291–8.

52. Golden, J. C., Janz, K. R., Clarke, W. R. and Mahoney LT. New protocol for submaximal and peak exercise values for children and adolescents: The Muscatine Study. *Pediatric Exercise Science* 1991; 3: 129–40.

53. Baggley, G. and Cumming, G. R. Serial measurement of working and aerobic capacity of Winnipeg schoolchildren during a school year. In *Environmental effects of work performance* (ed. G. R. Cumming, A. W. Taylor and D. Snidal). Canadian Association of Sport Sciences, Canada, 1972: 173–86.

54. Bland, J. M and Altman, D. G. Statistical methods for assessing agreement between two methods of clinical measurement. *Lancet* 1986; i: 307–10.

55. Bland, J. M. and Altman, D. G. Comparing two methods of clinical measurement: a personal history. *International Journal of Epidemiology* 1995; 24 (Suppl 1):S7-S14.

56. Kay, C. and Shephard, R. J. On muscle strength and the threshold of anaerobic work. *Internationale Zeitschrift fur angewandte Physiologie einschliesslich Arbeitsphysiologie* 1969; 27: 311–28.

57. Hoes, M., Binkhorst, R. A., Smeekes-Kuyl, A. and Vissurs, A. C. Measurement of forces exerted on a pedal crank during work on the bicycle ergometer at different loads. *Internationale Zeitschrift fur angewandte Physiologie einschliesslich Arbeitsphysiologie* 1968; 26: 33–42.

58. Katch, F. I., Girandola, F. N. and Katch VL. The relationship of body weight to maximum oxygen uptake and heavy work endurance capacity on the bicycle ergometer. *Medicine and Science in Sports and Exercise* 1971; 3: 101–6.

59. Glassford, R. C., Bayford, G. H. Y., Sedgwick, A. W. and MacNab, R. B. J. Comparison of maximal oxygen uptake values determined by predicted and actual methods. *Journal of Applied Physiology* 1965; 20: 509–13.

60. Skinner, J. S. and McLellan, T. H. The transition from aerobic to anaerobic metabolism. *Research Quarterly* 1980; 51: 234–48.

61. Wirth, A., Trager, E., Scheele, K., Mayer D, Diehm, K., Reisch, K. *et al*. Cardiopulmonary adjustment and metabolic response to maximal and submaximal physical exercise of boys and girls at different stages of maturity. *European Journal of Applied Physiology* 1978; 39: 229–40.

62. Armstrong, N., Welsman, J. and Winsley, R. Is peak $\dot{V}O_2$ a maximal index of children's aerobic fitness? *International Journal of Sports Medicine* 1996; 17: 356–9.

63. Skinner, J. S., Bar-Or, O., Bergsteinova, V., Bell, C. W., Royer, D. and Buskirk, E. R. Comparison of continuous and intermittent tests for determining maximal oxygen intake in children. *Acta Paediatrica Scandinavica* 1971; 217: 24–8.

64. Sheehan, J. M., Rowland, T. W. and Burke, E. J. A comparison of four treadmill protocols for determination of maximal oxygen uptake in 10 to 12 year old boys. *International Journal of Sports Medicine* 1987; 8: 31–4.

65. Rowland, T. W. Does peak $\dot{V}O_2$ reflect $\dot{V}O_2$ max in children? Evidence from supramaximal testing. *Medicine and Science in Sports and Exercise* 1993; 25: 689–93.

66. Freedson, P. S. and Goodman, T. L. Measurement of oxygen consumption. In *Pediatric laboratory exercise testing* (ed. T. W. Rowland). Human Kinetics, Champaign Il, 1993: 91–113.

67. Hale, T., Armstrong, N., Hardman, A., Jakeman, P., Sharp, C. and Winter, E. *The physiological assessment of the elite competitor*. National Coaching Foundation, Leeds, 1989.

68. Williams, J. and Armstrong, N. The maximal lactate steady state and its relationship to performance at fixed blood lactate reference values in children. *Pediatric Exercise Science* 1991; 3: 333–41.

69. Armstrong, N., Balding, J., Gentle, P., Williams, J. and Kirby, B. Peak oxygen uptake and physical activity in 11 to 16 year olds. *Pediatric Exercise Science* 1990; 2: 349–58.

70. Armstrong, N., Welsman, J. R. and Kirby, B. J. Peak oxygen uptake and maturation in 12-year-olds. *Medicine and Science in Sports and Exercise* 1998; 30: 165–9.

71. Cumming, G. R., Hastman, L., McCort, J. and McCullough, S. High serum lactates do occur in children after maximal work. *International Journal of Sports Medicine* 1980; 1: 66–9.

72. Docherty D, Gaul CA. *Critical analysis of available laboratory tests used in evaluating the fitness of children and youth*. Fitness Canada, Ottawa, 1990.

73. Williams, J., Armstrong, N. and Kirby, B. The 4 mM blood lactate level as an index of exercise performance in 11–13 year old children. *Journal of Sports Sciences* 1990; 8: 139–47.

74. Chia, M., Armstrong, N. and Childs, D. The assessment of children's anaerobic performance using modifications of the Wingate anaerobic test. *Pediatric Exercise Science* 1997; 9: 80–9.

75. Shephard, R. J., Allen, C., Bar-Or, O., Davies, C. T. M., Degre, S., Hedman, R., Ishii, K., Kaneko, M., LaCour, J. R., di Prampero, P. E. and Seliger, V. The working capacity of Toronto schoolchildren, I. *Canadian Medical Association Journal* 1969; 100: 560–6, 705–14.

76. Rowland, T. W. and Cunningham, L. N. Oxygen uptake plateau during maximal treadmill exercise in children. *Chest* 1992; 101: 485–9.

77. **Cumming, G. R.** Current levels of fitness. *Canadian Medical Association Journal* 1967; **88**: 351–5.

78. **Welsman, J.** and **Armstrong, N.** Assessing postexercise blood lactates in children and adolescents. In *Pediatric anaerobic performance* (ed. E. Van Praagh). Human Kinetics Publishers, Champaign, Il, 1998: 137–53.

79. **Welsman, J. R., Armstrong, N.** and **Withers, S.** Responses of young girls to two modes of aerobic training. *British Journal of Sports Medicine* 1997; **31**: 139–42.

80. **Pfitzinger, P.** and **Freedson, P.** Blood lactate responses to exercise in children: Part 2. Lactate threshold. *Pediatric Exercise Science* 1997; **9**: 99–307.

81. **Brooks, G. A.** Current concepts in lactate exchange. *Medicine and Science in Sports and Exercise* 1991; **23**: 895–906.

82. **Stainsby, W. N.** and **Brooks, G. A.** Control of lactic acid metabolism in contracting muscles and during exercise. *Exercise and Sports Sciences Reviews* 1990; **18**: 29–63.

83. **Bird, S.** and **Davison, R.** (eds) *Guidelines for the physiological testing of athletes* (3rd Edn). BASES, Leeds, 1997.

84. **Eriksson, B. O.** and **Saltin, B.** Muscle metabolism during exercise in boys aged 11–16 years compared to adults. *Acta Paediatrica Belgica* 1974; **28** (Suppl.): 257–65.

85. **Martinez, L. R.** and **Haymes, E. M.** Substrate utilization during treadmill running in prepubertal girls and women. *Medicine and Science in Sports and Exercise* 1992; **24**: 975–983.

86. **Pfitzinger, P.** and **Freedson, P.** Blood lactate responses to exercise in children: Part 1. Peak lactate concentration. *Pediatric Exercise Science* 1997; **9**: 210–22.

87. **Heck, H., Mader, A., Hess, G., Mucke, S., Muller, R.** and **Hollman, W.** Justification of the 4 mmol litre^{-1} lactate threshold. *International Journal of Sports Medicine* 1985; 6: 117–30.

88. **Campbell, M. E., Hughson, R. L.** and **Green, H. J.** Continuous increase in blood lactate concentration during different ramp exercise protocols. *Journal of Applied Physiology* 1989; **66**: 1104–7.

89. **Karlsson, J.** and **Jacobs, I.** Onset of blood lactate accumulation during muscular exercise as threshold concept. I. Theoretical consideration. *International Journal of Sports Medicine* 1982; **3**: 190–201.

90. **MacDougall, J. D., Wenger, H. A.** and **Green, H. J.** (eds) *Physiological testing of the high-performance athlete* Human Kinetics Publishers, Champaign, Il, 1991.

91. **Yoshida, T.** Effect of exercise duration during incremental exercise on the determination of anaerobic threshold and the onset of blood lactate accumulation. *European Journal of Applied Physiology* 1984; **53**: 196–9.

92. **Newton, J. L.** and **Robinson, S**.The distribution of blood lactate and pyruvate during work and recovery. *Federation Proceedings* 1965; **24**: 590.

93. **Saltin, B., Blomqvist, G., Mitchell, J. H., Johnson, R. L. Jr, Wildenthal, K.** and **Chapman, C.** Response to exercise after bedrest and after training. *Circulation* 1968; 38(Suppl 5): 1–78.

94. **Bar-Or, O.** The growth and development of children's physiologic and perceptional responses to exercise. In *Children and sport* (ed. J. Ilmarinen and I. Valimaki). Springer-Verlag, Berlin, 1984: 3–17.

95. **Williams, J., Armstrong, N.** and **Kirby, B. J.** The influence of the site of sampling and assay medium upon the measurement and interpretation of blood lactate responses to exercise. *Journal of Sports Sciences*, 1992; **10**: 95–107.

96. **Williams, J. R.** and **Armstrong, N.** Relationship of maximal lactate steady state to performance at fixed blood lactate reference values in children. *Pediatric Exercise Science* 1991; **3**: 333–41.

97. **Mocellin, R., Heusgen, M.** and **Gildein, H. P.** Anaerobic threshold and maximal steady-state blood lactate in prepubertal boys. *European Journal of Applied Physiology* 1991; **62**: 56–60.

98. **Tietz, N. W.** *Textbook of clinical chemistry.* W. B. Saunders, Philadelphia, 1986.

99. **Thoden, J. S.** Testing aerobic power. In *Physiological testing of the high-performance athlete* (ed. J. D. MacDougall, H. A. Wenger and H. J. Green). Human Kinetics Publishers, Champaign, Il, 1982: 107–74.

100. **Gisolfi, C.** and **Robinson, S.** Venous blood distribution in the legs during intermittent treadmill work. *Journal of Applied Physiology* 1970; **29**: 368–73.

101. **Foxdal, P., Sjödin, B., Rudstam, H., Östman, C., Östman, B.** and **Hedenstierna, G. C.** Lactate concentration differences in plasma, whole blood, capillary finger blood and erythrocytes during submaximal graded exercise in humans. *European Journal of Applied Physiology* 1990; **61**: 218–22.

102. **Yoshida, T., Suda, Y.** and **Takeuchi, N.** Endurance training regimen based upon arterial blood lactate: Effects on anaerobic threshold. *European Journal of Applied Physiology* 1982; **49**: 223–30.

103. **Busse, M. W., Muller, M.** and **Boning, D.** A method of continuous treadmill testing. *International Journal of Sports Medicine* 1983; (abstract suppl.): 2.

104. **Weil, M. H., Leavy, J. A., Rackow, E. C.** and **Halfman, C. J.** Validation of a semi-automated technique for measuring lactate in whole blood. *Clinical Chemistry* 1986; **32**: 2175–7.

105. **Friedheim, L. C.** and **Town, G. P.** Blood lactate methodologies compared. *Medicine and Science in Sports and Exercise* 1989; 21(Suppl): S21.

106. **Soutter, W. P., Sharp, F.** and **Clark, D. M.** Bedside estimation of whole blood lactate. *British Journal of Anaesthesia* 1978; **50**: 445–50.

107. **Wasserman, K., Whipp, B. J., Koyal, S. N.** and **Beaver, W. L.** Anaerobic threshold and respiratory gas exchange during exercise. *Journal of Applied Physiology* 1973; 35: 236–43.

108. **Maffulli, N., Testa, V., Lancia, A., Capasso, G.** and **Lombardi, S.** Indices of sustained aerobic power in young middle distance runners. *Medicine and Science in Sports and Exercise* 1991; **23**: 1090–6.

109. **Davis, J. A., Caiozzo, V. J., Moore, J. L., Hawksworth, C. A., Prietto, C. A.** and **McMaster, W. C.** Accuracy of the subjective determination of the anaerobic threshold discerned from gas exchange measurements. *International Journal of Sports Medicine* 1983; **4**: 137.

110. **Gladden, L. B., Yates, J. W., Stremel, R. W.** and **Stamford, B. A.** Gas exchange and lactate anaerobic threshold: inter and intraevaluator agreement. *Journal of Applied Physiology* 1985; **58**: 2082–9.

111. **Beaver, W. L., Wasserman, K.** and **Whipp, B. J.** Improved detection of lactate threshold during exercise using a log-log transformation. *Journal of Applied Physiology* 1985; **59**: 1936–40.

112. **Coyle, E. F., Martin, W. H., Ehsani, A. A., Hagberg, J. M., Bloomfield, S. A., Sinacore, D. R.** and **Holloszy, J. O.** Blood lactate threshold in some well-trained ischemic heart disease patients. *Journal of Applied Physiology* 1983; **54**: 18–23.

113. **Sjodin, B., Jacobs, I.** and **Karlsson, J.** Onset of blood lactate accumulation and enzyme activities in m. vastus lateralis in man. *International Journal of Sports Medicine* 1981; **2**: 166–70.

114. **Sjodin, B., Schele, R., Karlsson, J., Linnarsson, D.** and **Wallensten, R.** The physiological background of onset of blood lactate accumulation. In *Exercise and sport biology* (ed. P. Komi). Human Kinetics Publishers, Champaign, Il, 1982: 43–55.

115. **Stegmann, H.** and **Kindermann, W.** Comparison of prolonged exercise tests at the individual anaerobic threshold and the fixed anaerobic threshold of 4 mmol litre^{-1}. *International Journal of Sports Medicine* 1982; **3**: 105–10.

116. **Haverty, M., Kenny, W. L.** and **Hodgson, J. L.** Lactate and gas exchange responses to incremental and steady state running. *British Journal of Sports Medicine* 1988; **2**: 51–4.

117. **Yoshizawa, S., Honda, H., Urushibara, M.** and **Nakamura, N.** Aerobic-anaerobic energy supply and daily physical activity level in young children. In *Children and exercise XIII* (ed. S. Oseid and K-H. Carlsen). Human Kinetics Publishers, Champaign, Il, 1989: 47–56.

118. **Williams, J. R.** and **Armstrong, N.** The influence of age and sexual maturation on children's blood lactate responses to exercise. *Pediatric Exercise Science*, 1991; **3**: 111–20.

119. **Mocellin, R., Heusgen, M.** and **Korsten-Reck, U.** Maximal steady state blood lactate levels in 11-year-old boys. *European Journal of Pediatrics* 1990; **149**: 771–3.

120. **Beneke, R., Heck, H., Schwarz, V.** and **Leithäuser, R.** Maximal lactate steady state during the second decade of age. *Medicine and Science in Sports and Exercise* 1996; **28**: 1474–8.

121. **Beneke, R., Schwarz, V., Leithäuser, R., Hütler, M.** and **von Duvillard, S. P.** Maximal lactate steady state in children. *Pediatric Exercise Science* 1996; **8**: 328–36.

122. **Tanaka, H.** and **Shindo, M.** Running velocity at blood lactate threshold of boys aged 6–15 years compared with untrained and trained young males. *International Journal of Sports Medicine* 1985; **6**: 90–4.

123. **Izumi, I., Ishiko, T.** Lactate threshold in pubescent boys. *Japanese Journal of Physical Education* 1984; **28**: 309–14.

124. **Simon, G., Berg, A., Dickhuth, H. H., Simon-Alt** and **A., Keul, J.** Bestimmung der anaeroben Schwelle in Abhangigkeit von Alter und von der Leistungsfahigkeit. (Determination of the anaerobic threshold depending on age and performance potential). *Deutsche Zeitschrift fur Sportsmedizin* 1981; **32**: 7–14.

125. **Eriksson, B. O., Karlsson, J.** and **Saltin, B.** Muscle metabolites during exercise in pubertal boys. *Acta Paediatrica Scandinavica* 1971; **217** (Suppl.): 154–7.

126. **Dux, L., Dux, E.** and **Guba, F.** Further data on the androgenic dependency of the skeletal musculature: The effect of prepubertal castration on the structural development of the skeletal muscles. *Hormone and Metabolic Research* 1982; **14**: 191–4.

127. **Krotkiewski, M., Kral, J. G.** and **Karlsson, J.** Effects of castration and testosterone substitution on body composition and muscle metabolism in rats. *Acta Physiologica Scandinavica* 1980; **109**: 233–7.

128. **Tanner JM.** *Growth at adolescence* (2nd edn). Blackwell Scientific Publications, Oxford, 1962.

129. **Welsman, J., Armstrong, N.** and **Kirby, B.** Serum testosterone is not related to peak $\dot{V}O_2$ and submaximal blood lactate responses in 12–16 year old males. *Pediatric Exercise Science*, 1994; **6**: 120–7.

1.8   Physical activity
Maarike Harro and Chris Riddoch

Introduction

There is general agreement that children should be regularly active and that a range of physically active pursuits should feature as an important part of children's lifestyles. However, strong evidence to support the physical or psychological health benefits of activity during the childhood period is difficult to locate. Recent reviews[1–3] have concluded that although there is evidence to suggest that physical activity benefits the health of children, the data are in fact very weak (see Chapter 3.1). This is in stark contrast to the voluminous evidence indicating that activity during adulthood is extremely beneficial.[4,5] It is therefore interesting to note that adults, in whom activity levels are low and health links are abundant, commonly express concern about children, in whom activity levels are higher, and where the health links are tenuous.

Nevertheless, the health benefits of activity are so wide-ranging and significant in adults that it would be foolish not to be concerned that children take an appropriate amount of physical activity, as it is quite plausible that childhood activity beneficially affects health. For example, childhood activity may persist into adulthood, modify the evolution of health risk factors, optimize physical and psychological development, and improve quality of life. Such arguments are maybe more relevant at the current time, when children's activity levels are perceived to be declining.[6]

Further data on children's physical activity are required, but physical activity is notoriously difficult to assess. The many problems of assessing activity in adults are further compounded when children are assessed, primarily because the cognitive abilities of children are not as well developed as those of adults, and also because they have more complex and multi-dimensional activity patterns. This chapter will review a range of methods which can be used in field situations, focusing on the issues of precision (validity and reliability), practicality, benefits and limitations, scientific attributes, and their suitability for use with children. The relationship between physical activity and young people's health is addressed in Chapter 3.1.

Dimensions of physical activity

Essentially, physical activity is an infinitely variable and complex behaviour with many dimensions, and this is the root cause of most difficulties. It is not only difficult to choose which dimension to measure, but it is often unclear which dimensions of activity are measured by which instrument. Further, physical activity does not come in handy and easy-to-measure 'packages' (like cigarettes, alcohol or possibly even meals). Physical activity is a variable and unstable behaviour, and there is no single instrument which can capture physical activity in its entirety. Even the most expensive and sophisticated instruments only capture a limited amount of data relating to a narrow range of dimensions of activity. Cost seems to be consistently and inversely related to precision, and the final decision regarding which instrument to choose for a research project is inevitably a trade-off between precision, subject characteristics, cost, time, subject numbers and practicality.

Physical activity is commonly described as having the following main dimensions:

- Duration of sessions
- Intensity—measured as energy expenditure ($kcal\,min^{-1}$ or $kJ\,h^{-1}$), oxygen consumption ($ml\,kg^{-1}\,min^{-1}$) or heart rate ($beats\,min^{-1}$)
- Frequency
- Mode or type

Physical activity can also be thought of, and measured, in terms of the total volume of activity, for example, minutes per day or week, or in terms of its energy expenditure equivalent, kJ per day or week. When assessing activity levels for fitness and performance outcomes, it is necessary to assess frequency, intensity and duration very carefully, whereas when assessing health-related outcomes total volume of activity may be more important, as it is this dimension which is most closely related to health status—at least in adults.

It is possible to transform raw data into other units which are known to be related to health. For example, counts from a motion sensor or heart rate data can be converted to energy expenditure by using algorithms derived from laboratory and field pilot study data. However, it should be remembered that these procedures inevitably require vari-ous assumptions to be made which are often untested and therefore constitute major sources of error. Commonly used units of measurement—each relating to different dimensions of activity— include accumulated time of activity, energy expended through physical activity, amount of physical work performed, 'counts' of directly measured movement, ordinal ratings compared to gender and age peers, or a numerical score derived from responses to a questionnaire.

It can be seen that each dimension of activity is fundamentally different from the others, and for research purposes demands its own assessment technique. As most assessment techniques measure only one or a small number of dimensions, it is very difficult to compare studies or to select a measurement tool for new research.

Range of methods

More than 30 different methods of assessing physical activity can be identified in the scientific literature, but a single, standard technique that can be universally applied does not exist. In general, the easier, cheaper and more practical a method is, the less precise it is. The methods with higher levels of precision require special equipment, which is normally expensive and hence limits its use with large groups of subjects. Table 1.8.1 summarizes the main categories of methods and the dimension(s) of activity which they each assess.

A particular subgroup of methods has been found to be more practical when studying children, and to carry some measure of validity. These are self-report questionnaires and interviews, proxy reports (parent/teacher), diaries, heart rate monitoring, motion sensors, direct observation and the assessment of activity energy expenditure using the 'doubly labelled water' method.

An important distinction should be made between the self-report methods (questionnaire, interview, proxy reports, diary), which are subjective, and the others, which are objective. Subjective methods carry a high probability of measurement error, especially with children, whereas the objective techniques are more precise. It is therefore usual to see the objective instruments used as criterion measures when validating subjective methods. Occasionally, the reverse of this has been done, most notably when a new instrument (e.g. a motion sensor) is manufactured and is in need of validation. It is tempting to validate it against older, tried and trusted methods, e.g. a questionnaire, but it makes no sense to use a method such as a questionnaire with its own limited validity as a criterion measure.

Specific instruments have been comprehensively reviewed elsewhere.[7] We will therefore focus upon the concepts and principles underlying the instruments, their precision and their practicality. In this way we hope to provide the information necessary for researchers to choose a suitable method.

Validity and reliability of methods

Validity and reliability are issues of such importance that an initial discussion of the concept is warranted. Validity refers to the 'accuracy' of an instrument, i.e. whether it measures what you intend it to measure, and reliability refers to 'repeatability', i.e. whether you obtain the same result with repeated tests. An instrument must be reliable in order to be valid, but can demonstrate reliability without actually being valid. In other words, the instrument measures something different to that which was intended, but does so consistently.

Generally, validation studies of instruments to measure physical activity in children tend to be disappointing. Several researchers[8–10] have attributed the lack of strong correlations between different instruments used in validity studies to the possibility that the instruments may assess different dimensions of physical activity. In technical terms, there may be a substantial amount of variance not shared between the two measures of physical activity.[11] It is extremely difficult to assess whether a low validity result is real, or whether an inappropriate choice of criterion measure has been made. If the latter is the case, then both instruments might be measuring in a valid way, but because they are measuring different things, the associations between the two are weak.

During a literature search we identified 90 validity and reliability studies of physical activity measurement techniques conducted with children. A full range of results—from zero correlation to very strong correlations—was apparent. It is not possible here to report the full set of studies, but some general comments are worthy of note. In the following overview, we have concentrated on validity studies which use a criterion method which is at least as accurate as the type of measure under investigation.

Self-report methods correlate very weakly with, for example, heart rate monitoring or motion sensors—typically at $r = 0.2$ to 0.4. Interestingly, reliability scores are much better, typically being $r = 0.3$ to 0.6 but sometimes approaching $r = 0.8$ to 0.9. We might therefore conclude that self-report methods are reasonably reliable, but have limited validity. Results from heart rate studies and motion sensors are comparable, and are much more encouraging. Heart rate monitors correlate typically at $r = 0.4$ to 0.7 with motion sensors, and reliability scores are $r = 0.6$ to 0.9, with the higher scores being obtained over shorter time periods. Motion sensors have received increasing attention over recent years, and it is this area that possibly offers the greatest scope for advancement in this field. Both uniaxial and triaxial instruments correlate typically at $r = 0.5$ to 0.7 with heart rate monitors, and slightly higher than this with observation methods. Triaxial instruments do not perform better than uniaxial instruments and the two correlate highly with each other, at approaching $r = 0.9$. Test–retest scores for motion sensors are variable, and generally lie in the range 0.4 to 0.6. Given that activity behaviour itself can vary between testing occasions, it can be concluded that motion sensors carry a large measure of reliability but see Bland and Altman[12] for a critique of the use of correlation coefficients in this context. Motion sensors correlate well with the doubly labelled water method in field situations, which is extremely encouraging.

Much of the data relating to validity is underpinned, and confounded, by the fact that children, particularly during outside play, engage in a far more diverse range of activities than adults. In particular, children's activity is less 'memorable' because it is normally accumulated via a large number of short sessions which are not normally predetermined. This range of activities is also greater than the more limited activities which can be assessed in a laboratory, where activities are restricted to those which can be performed on an ergometer. This has major implications for validity studies for two reasons. Firstly, children are unable to recall much of their less memorable bursts of activity, and secondly data gathered on a few carefully controlled activities in a laboratory cannot be applied to the more diverse, play-like

Table 1.8.1 Methods of assessing physical activity and related activity dimensions

Method	Dimension(s) of activity*
Doubly labelled water method	EE
Direct calorimetry	EE
Indirect calorimetry	EE
Direct observation/video recording	F,I,T,M
Motion sensors—newer models	F,I,T,P
Heart rate monitoring	F,I,T,P
Motion sensors—older models	EE
Activity diaries	F,I,T,M,P
Interviews	F,I,T,M,P
Self-report questionnaires	F,I,T,M,P
Proxy reports (parent or teacher)	F,I,T,M
Dietary assessment	EE
Job classification	EE

* EE = energy expenditure; F = frequency; I = intensity; T = time; M = mode; P = patterns, settings, etc.

activities of real life. To develop an instrument which can undertake the accurate assessment of the unique, sporadic and variable activities of children, especially younger children, is therefore one of our major current challenges.

When assessing the reliability of instruments, a further set of problems are encountered. The same technique applied one week apart may perform reliably, but the activity itself—especially in field situations—may change, thus rendering the apparent reliability level as inadequate. Thus, test–retest reliability can only be realistically tested in laboratory settings, where standardized bouts of physical activity can be accurately repeated, and the performance of heart rate monitors, movement counters and oxygen analysis equipment can be assessed.

Desirable attributes of instruments

Any instrument which assesses children's habitual physical activity must be considered against a number of factors which are necessary for the activity to be truly representative of a child's activity patterns.

A representative time period for measurement must be selected. For example, if we are investigating habitual levels of activity, the time period of measurement must be long enough to be reasonably representative of a child's behaviour. As a guide, two weekdays plus two weekend days are normally considered sufficient to represent a week, but there are obvious problems when we need to assess longer periods. For example, activity behaviour varies with the seasons—both climatic and sporting.

The instrument must be non-reactive. In other words, the child's normal behaviour must not be altered by either the instrument, or by the knowledge that their activity level is being measured. One obvious attraction of a heart rate monitor for a child is to immediately try to get the heart rate as high as possible, and s/he will perform additional activity in achieving this. In these situations, a period of habituation to the instrument is required, during which all unusual activity behaviour is absorbed.

Further considerations are social acceptability, financial cost and the extent to which the method poses excessive burdens for the participants and/or the staff.[13]

Methods
Questionnaires, interviews, proxy reports and diaries
Self-administered questionnaires and interviews

With self-administered questionnaires children recall their activity over a given period of time. Popular questionnaires use the previous day[14] and also the previous seven days.[14–15] Interviews can also be used, where 'probing' of the child's activities is possible, and sometimes a combination of questionnaire and interview techniques can be used to cross-check responses. However, interviews are time-consuming and therefore expensive in terms of labour, and can only be conducted in relatively small studies. Problems of interpretation between different interviewers introduces a major source of error, and substantial training is therefore required. Whereas it might be expected that interviews are more precise than questionnaires, there is limited evidence to support this contention.

There are many factors which might contribute to measurement error when using self-report methods with children. Questionnaires designed for adults are normally not suitable for children, because children's activity patterns are so different. Adults tend to perform activity in readily identifiable 'sessions', whereas children are 'on the go' all the time—at least within the limitations of a relatively sedentary school day. As children tend to engage in physical activity that is sporadic, both in time and intensity,[16] they find the task of recalling activities extremely difficult. There is evidence to suggest that strenuous activity is recalled more accurately than moderate or mild activity,[17] which might be expected, but it is unfortunate because much of children's activity is sporadic, spontaneous and generally not 'memorable', at least in terms of its frequency, duration and intensity—information which is commonly asked for in questionnaires.

It is difficult to ascertain at what age children become able to provide meaningful data via a questionnaire, because cognitive abilities differ greatly between individual children. However, it is generally considered that children under the age of 12 years cannot recall activities accurately and are unable to quantify the time frame of activity.[18] Wallace et al.[19] have reported that 11 to 13 year old children recalled only 46% of their activities during the previous seven days and 55% to 65% during the last 24 hours, when compared to observation data.

To improve children's recall, it is common to 'cue' them by incorporating a list of common activities or identifiable time periods (for example, a breakdown of the school day). It is helpful for the child if the time frame includes the journey from home to school, physical activity during school recess, organized sports, breaks between the lessons, physical education lessons, and recreational activities performed after school and during weekends.

The language used in interviews and questionnaires must take account of the reading age of the children, and simple but comprehensive instructions must be given. Questionnaires should be assessed for reading age, and a reading age of seven years is normally considered adequate for the majority of children over the age of ten years. The appearance and quality of presentation of the questionnaire is important, and also its length. The use of cartoons and friendly language in the instructions help to maintain interest, and length is important because of the limited attention span of many children. It should be possible for the majority of children to complete a questionnaire within 20 to 30 min. If data are required which describe children's normal activity patterns, then both weekends and weekdays should be included and, ideally, seasons of the year, as activity patterns vary between weekdays and weekends and also by season.

The use of physical activity recall questionnaires is ubiquitous in studies of children, but use in anything but large studies is highly questionable. It is difficult to quantify the measurement error inherent with children's recall of their physical activities, but it is likely that it is of such a magnitude that the validity of the data is questionable whether they are used either for descriptive (activity levels) or analytical (associations with other variables) purposes. In the absence of large numbers and the accompanying high statistical power, questionnaires are likely to give misleading and inaccurate results.

It may be that questionnaire data can—probably on a crude basis—categorize children into ranked activity groups for use in further analyses. We must here differentiate between the twin aims of quantifying the activity (for descriptive purposes) and ranking children (for analytical purposes). It may be that questionnaires can perform the latter, but not the former. In this case it might be said that

the new generation of motion sensors which incorporate extremely sensitive accelerometers. These instruments are very small and are fitted to the child's hip in a small pouch attached via a belt. They monitor body movements directly and objectively, and more recently developed instruments store the data on a minute-by-minute basis for up to three weeks.

The accelerometer monitors movement in a specific plane and stores the data as 'counts'. In the newer models, not only are the number of movements monitored, but also the intensity of the movements. The resulting data are therefore a function of the frequency and intensity of movement. Movements can be registered in a single plane (uniaxial), or in several planes (multiaxial). For the great majority of bodily movements, uniaxial (usually vertical) units are as precise as multiaxial units since movements involving other axes are almost always accompanied by movement in the vertical plane.[39,40] Uniaxial accelerometers are also normally smaller—a significant consideration when working with young children. Although activity in children may involve more non-vertical movements (crawling, climbing) than typical activities performed by adults, multiaxial devices have not been found to be significantly more precise than uniaxial devices in the assessment of physical activity in field situations.

Some models filter out non-human movement (such as the vibration caused by sitting in a moving car), and can be preprogrammed to start recording at a predetermined time in the future. Data are downloaded via an interface to a computer for analysis, and a graphical output can be produced.

Accelerometers have been shown to correlate at $r = 0.86$ with energy expenditure (calculated from oxygen uptake) during carefully assessed laboratory exercise.[41] The acid test for these instruments is whether this level of precision can be reproduced during free-living activities. No published data are yet available, but counts from an accelerometer have been found to correlate at $r = 0.61$ with the volume of physical activity measured by the doubly labelled water method (Ekelund U., personal communication). Further validation work is undoubtedly necessary, but it may be that for assessment of this dimension of activity—most closely related to health status—motion sensors may be the way forward.

Direct observation

Observation of children and the immediate recording of their activities, have been used to study physical activity in both pre-school children (from 20 months) and schoolchildren (to 13 years of age). Children can also be recorded with video cameras, and the records viewed as many times as desired by any number of observers. Substantial observation time in the natural setting is needed to validate instruments and to obtain sufficient data to permit generalization of results to other settings and populations.[42] Observation strategies can be (a) momentary, (b) partial-interval or (c) partial. In momentary observation observed activities are coded and recorded at the end of the observation interval. In partial-interval observation the events are coded if they occur at any time during the observed time period. In partial observation a specific time interval is left for coding/recording. Observational methodology can be improved by the usage of computers or audiocassette to record information.

Observation techniques can yield accurate data and can be undoubtedly useful in small studies. However, multiple observers may be needed in larger studies, and training is necessary to reduce inter-observer variability. Further, it is normally impossible to observe a child for the whole day, and therefore this technique is most useful for assessing activities performed in a specific time period, or setting, for example, a physical education class. In a recent review, Armstrong and Welsman[1] have suggested that further validity work is needed on observational techniques, and also that different observation protocols need to be compared in order to ascertain the most effective procedures.

Doubly labelled water method

The doubly labelled water method (DLW) is now recognized as the reference method of choice—or 'gold standard'—for the assessment of energy expenditure in free living subjects. The method uses stable isotopes of hydrogen and oxygen, ingested as water, and is based on the assumption that oxygen atoms in expired carbon dioxide are in isotopic equilibrium with the oxygen atoms in total body water (TBW). A quantity of water with a known concentration of stable, non-radioactive, naturally occurring isotopes of hydrogen (^{2}H) and oxygen (^{18}O) is ingested and allowed to equilibrate with the TBW. Over time, water lost from the body during normal physiological activity (as urine, sweat and water vapour during respiration) contains the two isotopic labels ^{2}H$_2$O and H$_2$^{18}O in proportion to their concentrations in the TBW. However, the labelled oxygen also leaves the body in expired air as carbon dioxide (C^{18}O$_2$). The principle of the method is to measure the difference in the rate of loss between hydrogen (^{2}H) and oxygen (^{18}O) in urine or saliva.

From the difference in elimination rates of the two isotopes, the production of CO_2 can be calculated.[43] Then, by knowing or estimating the respiratory quotient (RQ), along with the estimated CO_2 production rate, oxygen uptake and energy expenditure can be calculated.[44] In cases where the RQ is unknown, a fixed value of 0.85 can be used, which does not introduce gross errors. Alternatively, an approximation calculated from dietary intake data can be used. Both isotopes are stable, so there is essentially no risk to subjects. The concentration of isotopes ingested has to be greater than occurs in nature, although naturally existing levels need only to be raised minimally because mass spectrometers are ultra-sensitive. This method is normally reserved as a criterion measure against which other methods are validated, because it gives very accurate data on energy expenditure resulting from physical activity. Heart rate monitors and motion sensors are the most likely candidates for validation studies. Because doubly labelled water is very expensive, validation studies are currently sparse.

Summary

It can be seen that the assessment of physical activity is problematical. For the researcher who wishes to measure physical activity in children, Table 1.8.2 gives a summary of how each of the most popular methods compares in terms of some of their key attributes.

It can be seen from Table 1.8.2 that the pattern of validity scores contrast sharply with the patterns of scores for cheapness, ease of administration and feasibility for large studies. Whereas there are many questions researchers need to ask themselves before choosing a method, it may be that the two methods which display an optimum balance of all features are heart rate monitoring and motion sensors. Each of these instruments is non-intrusive, measures a variety of dimensions of activity, can be converted to energy expenditure if necessary, is objective, and has moderate to strong validity coefficients. While these

Table 1.8.2 Summary of attributes of methods used to assess physical activity in children

Method	Valid	Cheap	Objective	Easy to administer	Easy to complete	Measures patterns, modes, and dimensions of activity	Non-reactive	Feasible in large studies	Suitable for ages < 10 y	Suitable for ages > 10 y
Questionnaire	*	***		***	**	***	***	***		***
Interview	**	*		**	**	***	***	**	*	***
Proxy report	*	***		***	**	***	***	**	***	*
Teacher rating	*	***		***	**	*	***	**	***	***
Diary	*	**		*	*	***	*	**		***
Heart rate monitoring	**	*	***	*	**	**	*	*	***	***
Motion sensor	**	*	***	**	**	* (older models) ** (newer models)	*	*	***	***
Observation	**	*	**	*	***	**	**	*	***	***
Doubly labelled water	***	***	***	*	***		**		***	***

methods are relatively expensive, the costs are not so great that they could not be budgeted for within the resources of a large survey, where data collection is spread over, for example, one year. Expensive equipment and materials are used to measure other health-related parameters—e.g. fitness, blood pressure and cholesterol—and it is illogical to under-spend on the measurement of physical activity which is just as strongly related to health. The additional costs are likely to be heavily out-weighed by the considerable gains in measurement precision.

A number of important recommendations can be made, which relate to both choosing a method and the further development of methods:

1. Self report methods should be reserved for very large studies, for example, national surveys. In this situation, their limited validity is compensated for by increased statistical power. For the epidemiologist, a 'marker' of physical activity level can suffice, but the measurement error, and hence misclassification, inherent in these methods mitigates against their use in smaller studies.

2. The increasing sophistication and miniaturization of objective methods (in particular heart rate monitors and motion sensors) makes their use increasingly feasible, practically and financially, in even quite large studies. The great increase in precision of measurement is well worth the additional costs involved. In small studies they are probably mandatory.

3. It is probably impossible to measure every facet of physical activity, and research designs can become very complicated if this is attempted. The burden on the child can increase markedly when questionnaires become over-complicated. Careful consideration should be given to the dimension(s) of activity which is most closely related to the research question, and attention focused on this.

4. Where multiple dimensions of activity need to be assessed, more than one technique can be used. For example, a motion sensor can estimate total activity and also give information about session duration, time of day, intensity and daily patterns. If this were supported by a diary, questionnaire or interview, information on the mode and setting of the activity can also be obtained.

5. Further validation studies are required in relation to how each method performs in terms of the different dimensions of physical activity.

References

1. **Armstrong, N.** and **Welsman, J.**, *Young people and physical activity*. Oxford University Press, Oxford, 1997.

2. **Mutrie, N.** and **Parfitt, G.** Physical activity and its link with mental, social and moral health in young people. In *Young and active? Young people and health-enhancing physical activity—evidence and implications* (ed. S. Biddle, J. Sallis and N. Cavill). Health Education Authority, London, 1998; 49–68.

3. **Riddoch, C. J.** Relationships between physical activity and physical health in young people. In *Young and active?* (ed. S. Biddle, J. Sallis and N. Cavill). Health Education Authority, London, 1998; 17–48.

4. **Powell, K. E., Thompson, P. D., Caspersen, C. J.** and **Kendrick, K. S.** Physical activity and the incidence of coronary heart disease. *Annual Review of Public Health* 1987; **8**: 281–7.

5. **Berlin, J. A.** and **Colditz, A.** A meta-analysis of physical activity in the prevention of coronary heart disease. *American Journal of Epidemiology* 1990; **132**: 612–27.

6. **Durnin, J. V. G. A.** Physical activity levels—past and present. In *Physical activity and health: Symposium of the society for the study of human biology* (ed. N. G. Norgan). Cambridge University Press, Cambridge, 1992; 20–7.

7. **Montoye, H. J., Kemper, H. C. G., Saris, W. H. M.** and **Washburn, R. A.**, *Measuring physical activity and energy expenditure*. Human Kinetics Publishers, Champaign, Il, 1996.

8. **LaPorte, R. E., Montoye, H. J.** and **Caspersen, C. J.** Assessment of physical activity in epidemiological research: problems and prospects. *Public Health Reports* 1985; **100**: 131–46.

9. **Montoye, H. J.** and **Taylor, H. L.** Measurement of physical activity in population studies. *Human Biology* 1984; **56**: 195–216.

10. **Sallis, J. F., Buono, M. J., Roby, J. J., Carlson, D.** and **Nelson, J. A.** The Caltrac accelerometer as a physical activity monitor for school-age children. *Medicine and Science in Sports and Exercise* 1990; **22**: 698–703.

11. **Epstein, L. H., Paluch, R. A., Coleman, K. J., Vito, D.** and **Anderson, K.** Determinants of physical activity in obese children assessed by accelerometer and self-report. *Medicine and Science in Sports and Exercise* 1996; **28**: 1157–64.

12. **Bland, J. M.** and **Altman, D. G.** Comparing two methods of clinical measurement: A personal history. *International Journal of Epidemiology* 1995; **24**(Suppl 1): S7–S14.

13. **Baranowski, T., Bouchard, C., Bar-Or, O., Bricker, T., Heath, G., Kimm, S. Y. S., Malina, R., Obarzanek, E., Pate, R., Strong, W. B., Truman, B.** and **Washington, R.** Assessment, prevalence, and cardiovascular benefits of physical activity and fitness in youth. *Medicine and Science in Sports and Exercise* 1992; **24**: S237–47.

14. **Sallis, J. F., Condon, S. A., Goggin, K. J., Roby, J. J., Kolody, B.** and **Alcaraz, J. E.** The development of self-administered physical activity surveys for 4th grade students. *Research Quarterly for Exercise and Sport* 1993; **64**: 25–31.

15. **Riddoch, C. J., Murphy, N., Nicholls, A., van Wersche, A.** and **Cran, G.**, (eds). *Report of the Northern Ireland health and fitness survey*. The Queen's University of Belfast, Belfast, 1990.

16. **Armstrong, N.** and **Bray, S.** Physical activity patterns defined by continuous heart rate monitoring. *Archives of Disease in Childhood* 1991; **66**: 245–7.

17. **Taylor, C. B., Coffey, T.** and **Berra, K.** Seven-day activity and self-report compared to a direct measure of physical activity. *American Journal of Epidemiology* 1984; **120**: 818–24.

18. **Pate R. R.** Physical activity assessment in children and adolescents. *Critical Reviews in Food Science and Nutrition* 1993; **33**: 321–6.

19. **Wallace, J. P., McKenzie, T. L.** and **Nader, P. R.** Observed versus recalled exercise behaviour: A validation of a seven day exercise recall for boys 11 to 13 years old. *Research Quarterly for Exercise and Sport* 1985; **56**: 161–5.

20. **Strazzullo, P., Cappuccio, F. P., Trevisan, M., De Leo, A., Krogh, V., Giorgione, N.** and **Mancini, M.** Leisure time physical activity and blood pressure in schoolchildren. *American Journal of Epidemiology* 1988; **127**: 726–33.

21. **Sallis, J. F.** Self-report measures of children's physical activity. *Journal of School Health* 1991; **61**: 215–9.

22. **Pate, R. R., Dowda, M.** and **Ross, J. G.** Associations between physical activity and physical fitness in American children. *American Journal of Diseases of Children* 1990; **144**: 1123–9.

23. **Murphy, J. K., Alpert, B. S., Christman, J. V.** and **Willey, E. S.** Physical fitness in children: A survey method based on parental report. *American Journal of Public Health* 1988; **78**: 708–10.

24. **Noland, M., Danner, F., Dewalt, K., McFadden, M.** and **Kotchen, J. M.** The measurement of physical activity in young children. *Research Quarterly for Exercise and Sport* 1990; **61**: 146–53.

25. **Riddoch, C. J., Mahoney, C., Murphy, N., Cran, G.** and **Boreham, C.** Validation of an activity diary to assess children's moderate and vigorous physical activity. In *Children and exercise XVI, paediatric work physiology: methodological, physiological and pathological aspects* (ed. J. Coudert and E. Van Praagh). Masson, Paris, 1992; 115–7.

26. **Durant, R. H., Baranowski, T., Davis, H., Thompson, W. O., Puhl, J., Greaves, K. A.** and **Rhodes, T.** Reliability and variability of heart rate

monitoring in 3-, 4-, or 5-yr-old children. *Medicine and Science in Sports and Exercise* 1992; **24**: 265–71.

27. **Armstrong, N.** Young people's physical activity patterns as assessed by heart rate monitoring. *Journal of Sports Science* 1998; **16**: S9–S16.

28. **Armstrong, N., Balding, J., Gentle, P.** and **Kirby, B.** Patterns of physical activity among 11 to 16 year old British children. *British Medical Journal* 1990; **301**: 203–5.

29. **Riddoch, C. J., Mahoney, C., Murphy, N., Cran, G.** and **Boreham, C.** The physical activity patterns of Northern Irish schoolchildren ages 11–16 years. *Pediatric Exercise Science* 1991; **3**: 300–9.

30. **Livingstone, M. B.** Heart-rate monitoring: The answer for assessing energy expenditure and physical activity in population studies? *British Journal of Nutrition* 1997; **78**: 869–71.

31. **Bergren, G.** and **Christensen, E. H.** Heart rate and body temperature as indices of metabolic rate during work. *Arbeitsphysiologie* 1950; **14**: 255–60.

32. **Riddoch, C. J.** and **Boreham, C. A.** The health-related physical activity of children. *Sports Medicine* 1995; **19**: 86–102.

33. **Bailey, R. C., Olson, J., Pepper, S. L., Porszasz, J., Bartow, T. J** and **Cooper, D. M.** The level and tempo of children's physical activities: An observational study. *Medicine and Science in Sports and Exercise* 1995; **27**: 1033–41.

34. **Sallo, M.** and **Silla, R.** Physical activity with moderate to vigorous intensity in 4 to 10 year old children. *Pediatric Exercise Science* 1997; **9**: 44–54.

35. Department of Health, *Strategy statement on physical activity.* Department of Health, London, 1996.

36. **Pate, R. R., Pratt, M., Blair, S. N., Haskell, W. L., Macera, C. A.** and **Bouchard, C.** *et al.* Physical activity and public health: A recommendation from the centers for disease control and prevention and the American College of Sports Medicine. *Journal of the American Medical Association* 1995; **273**: 402–7.

37. US Department of Health and Human Services, *Physical activity and health: A report of the surgeon general.* Department of Health and Human Services, Centers for Disease Control and Prevention, National Center for Chronic Disease Prevention and Health Promotion, Pittsburgh, PA, 1996.

38. **Saris, W. H. M.** Habitual physical activity in children: methodology and findings in health and disease. *Medicine and Science in Sports and Exercise* 1986; **18**: 253–63.

39. **Janz, K. F.** Validation of the CSA accelerometer for assessing children's physical activity. *Medicine and Science in Sports and Exercise* 1994; **26**: 369–75.

40. **Welk, G. J.** and **Corbin, C. B.** The validity of the Tritrac-R3D activity monitor for the assessment of physical activity in children. *Research Quarterly for Exercise and Sport* 1995; **66**: 202–9.

41. **Trost, S. G., Ward, D. S., Moorehead, S. M., Watson, P. D., Riner, W.** and **Burke, J. R.** Validity of the computer science and applications (CSA) activity monitor in children. *Medicine and Science in Sports and Exercise* 1998; **30**: 629–33.

42. **McKenzie, T. L.** Observational measures of children's physical activity. *Journal of School Health* 1991; **61**: 224–7.

43. **Schoeller, D. A., Ravussin, Schultz, Y., Acheson, K. J., Baertschi, P.** and **Jequier, E.** Energy expenditure by doubly labelled water: validation in humans and proposed calculation. *American Journal of Physiology* 1986; **250**: R823–830.

44. **Stager, J. M., Lindeman, A.** and **Edwards, J.** The use of doubly labelled water in quantifying energy expenditure during prolonged activity. *Sports Medicine* 1995; **19**: 166–72.

1.9   Effort perception

Roger Eston and Kevin L. Lamb

Introduction

Individuals possess a well-developed system for sensing the strain involved in physical effort. Effort perception and perceived exertion are synonymous terms which can be defined as the act of detecting and interpreting the sensations arising from the body during physical exertion.[1] The ability to detect and interpret these sensations has been studied in a wide range of populations in a variety of activities and exercise tasks. The plethora of research activity on perceived exertion in adults in the last 30 years has been the subject of several comprehensive reviews.[2–5] However, research on the efficacy of using perceived exertion in children is still relatively new. This has been the subject of two critical review papers by the authors,[6,7] and some of the information presented here will be drawn from these reviews.

Although there have been over 30 studies of children's perceptions of physical effort, our understanding remains limited. It is only recently that researchers have realized that adult-derived methods and applications of the rating of perceived exertion (RPE) notion are not appropriate for use with children. Most investigators have conducted their research in the same vein as that performed in greater volume on adults, but we believe that the time for progress is now overdue. A lack of consensus currently exists in terms of how data should be gathered and analysed, making interpretations of validity and reliability quite difficult. A rationale is presented here to advocate that future investigations on effort perception in children should consider the ability of children to understand and interpret the scale used. This inevitably means refining existing scales or developing new ones. With regard to the latter, we present ideas and suggestions for future research, with examples of recently developed perceived exertion scales for use with children.

Application and description of traditional RPE scales

A description of the most common methods of assessing perceived exertion and how this information is used to assess and regulate the intensity of exercise follows. A variety of scales have been developed in an attempt to assess perceived exertion. The ubiquitous 15 point alphanumeric RPE Category Scale, developed by Borg in 1970,[8] later revised in 1986[9] (Fig. 1.9.1), and Borg's lesser used Category-Ratio 10 Scale[10] (Fig. 1.9.2) are the most commonly used rating of perceived exertion scales. These scales can be used to assess *overall* feelings of exertion or they can be used to *differentiate* between respiratory–metabolic (central) and peripheral (local) signals of exertion. For example, *differentiated* ratings of perceived exertion may be used to segregate the sensations arising from the upper body and the lower body during cycle ergometry exercise or during rowing, running or stepping.

6	No exertion at all
7	
8	Extremely light
9	Very light
10	
11	Light
12	
13	Somewhat hard
14	
15	Hard (heavy)
16	
17	Very hard
18	
19	Extremely hard
20	Maximal exertion

Fig. 1.9.1   The Borg 6–20 Rating of Perceived Exertion (RPE) Scale. From Borg.[9]

0	Nothing at all
0.5	Extremely weak
1	Very weak
2	Weak (light)
3	Moderate
4	Somewhat Strong
5	Strong (heavy)
6	
7	Very Strong
8	
9	
10	Extremely strong (almost maximal)
•	Maximal

Fig. 1.9.2   The Borg Category-Ratio Rating of Perceived Exertion Scale. From Borg.[10]

It is generally observed that RPE measured during an exercise test increases as exercise intensity increases. Reviews of studies have confirmed the strong positive association between RPE and indices of metabolic demand in adults[1–5,11] and children.[6,7]

In the traditional 15 point and Category-Ratio 10 (CR-10) scales, numbers are anchored to verbal expressions. However, in the CR-10 Scale the numbers have a fixed relationship to one another. For example, an intensity judgement of three would be gauged to be one third that of nine. On this scale there is a point above ten (extremely strong, almost maximal) which may be assigned any number in proportion to ten which describes the proportionate increase in perceived exertion. For example, if the exercise intensity feels 30% harder than ten on the CR-10 Scale, the RPE would be 13. This type of scale has been suggested to reflect the incremental pattern of effort perception in relation to ventilatory drive during exercise, which is discussed later.

Estimation and production of effort

The relationship between RPE and various measures of exercise intensity is most frequently derived from passive *estimation* procedures. In this way, a rating of perceived exertion is given in response to a request from the clinician to indicate how 'hard' the exercise feels. The information is frequently used to compare responses between conditions or after some form of intervention. It may also be used to assist the clinician or coach to prescribe exercise intensities. For example, an exercise intensity (e.g. heart rate, work rate or oxygen uptake), which coincides with a given RPE, may be prescribed by the clinician. Alternatively, the exercise intensity may be adjusted to match a series of pre-specified RPE values. For example, the individual may be requested to *produce* a specific RPE during an exercise bout. Measures of metabolic demand may then be compared at each RPE-derived exercise intensity. Several studies on adults[12–18] and children[19–25] show support for the use of the RPE in this way.

Evidence suggests that the accuracy of RPE in estimation and production procedures is improved with practice, although there are surprisingly few studies which have explored this fundamental concept in adults,[13] and only one (referred to later) which has attempted to address this issue in children. As this is deemed to be an important area of research by the authors, it is appropriate here to consider some of the issues relating to the process of learning. Consideration of the validity and reliability of an RPE scale for children should not ignore age, reading ability, experience and conceptual understanding. The latter is a developmental issue, influenced by the extent of children's experiences of exercise, which was recognized by two of the leading proponents of RPE (Borg[26] and Bar-Or[27]) over 20 years ago.

Surprisingly, however, few investigations on perceived exertion in children have incorporated all of these issues into their design. For a child to perceive effort accurately, and then reliably produce a given intensity at a given RPE, it is logical to assume that learning must occur. Implicit in the process of learning is practice of the skill and the cognitive ability of the child. According to Piaget's stages of development, children around the age of seven to ten years can understand categorization, but find it easier to understand and interpret pictures and symbols rather than words and numbers. Recently, investigators have incorporated various symbols to emulate categories of effort and acute fatigue into paediatric versions of an RPE scale. These developments have also recognized the need for verbal descriptors and terminology which are more pertinent to a child's cognitive development, age and reading ability.

The study of perceived exertion in children: a historical perspective

Oded Bar-Or[27] is credited with being the pioneer of research on perceived exertion in children. In 1975, he presented RPE data on 589 children (aged 7–17 years) at the First International Symposium on Physical Work and Effort, recorded during continuous, incremental cycle ergometry. All six age-groups (7 to 9, 8 to 10, 10 to 11, 11 to 12, 13 to 14, and 16 to 17 years) reported higher RPEs with increases in power output. However, compared with adults, the children tended to report a lower RPE for a given relative exercise intensity.

This research acquired a near-definitive status for the next ten years. With a few exceptions, notably an abstract by Kahle *et al.*[29] which reported an increase in the reproducibility of RPE in healthy girls as they got older, a study by Davies *et al.*[30] which observed that anorexic girls could use RPE to discriminate between differences in exercise intensity and Eston's[31] somewhat prescient discussion paper on the potential for using RPE in the secondary school physical education curriculum, there were no further reports in the academic literature until 1986. In that year, there were at least five simultaneous published reports from Canada, England, Japan and the USA.[32–36] With one exception,[31] researchers focused on the RPE–objective effort (heart rate, work rate) relationship in the laboratory setting and in the passive 'estimation' mode, described above. From 1990, however, pre-specified RPEs were used to compare objective effort measures in children.[19]

The development of child-specific rating scales

Important advances in the study of effort perception in children have occurred in the last decade. Despite recognition that experience of exercise was an important determinant for accurate perception of exercise intensity,[26–28] little regard was given to the creation of a more developmentally appropriate scale using meaningful terminology and symbols until 1989. In that year, Nystad *et al.*[37] published an illustrated RPE scale with all the written descriptors removed. Six stick figures depicted various stages of effort for use with a group of 10–12 year old asthmatic children (Fig. 1.9.3). Despite these attempts to improve the relatively incomprehensible nature of the 6–20 scale, children were still confused by the scale. The investigators concluded that the children lacked physical experience and awareness of different exercise intensities, and therefore could not understand the concept of perceived exertion. A similar idea has been adopted by Mutrie and colleagues at the University of Glasgow, using caricatures at various stages of animation (Fig. 1.9.4). In this scale the original wording used by Borg[8] has been retained, although it can be seen that other vernacular terms, indigenous to the Glasgow area have also been used! At present there are no validity or reliability data on this particular version of the scale.

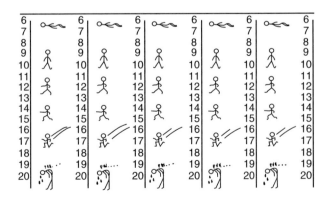

Fig. 1.9.3 Borg RPE Scale with stick figures. From Nystad *et al.*[37]

Other illustrated RPE scales have been applied, including a four point exercising heart scale[38] in a pilot study of 20 boys and girls (aged 9 to 11) during discontinuous cycling (Fig. 1.9.5). This scale utilizes images of a heart exercising on a cycle in progressively increasing states of exertion. Although not shown here, the scale also uses the colour red to reinforce the notion of exertion. The relationship between effort ratings and heart rates (0.62; $p<0.01$) and power output (0.67; $p<0.01$) suggest that this scale, with its limited selection of exertion categories, may be worthy of further investigation.

A significant development in the measurement of children's effort perception occurred in 1994 with the publication of two papers which proposed and validated an alternative child-specific scaling[23] (Fig. 1.9.6). Compared to the Borg Scale, the Children's Effort Rating Table (CERT) has five fewer possible responses, a range of numbers (1–10) more familiar to children (than 6–20) and verbal expressions chosen by children as descriptors of exercise effort. Studies comparing the 6–20 RPE and CERT in children aged 5 to 9 years[39] during stepping and 8 to 11 years[24,25,40] during cycling exercise provided support for the CERT. The potential of CERT attracted positive attention from other investigators interested in paediatric effort perception.[41, 42] The realization that paediatric scales should include some form of illustration has led to a number of pictorial scales, including a pictorial CERT[43] (Fig. 1.9.7).

Robertson[42] advanced the CERT a stage further. As part of a special symposium on effort perception at the European Paediatric Work Physiology Conference in Exeter in 1997, he presented a pilot 1–10 scale called the Omni Scale (Fig. 1.9.8). This has a category format and contains both pictorial and verbal descriptors. Although, currently there are no published data on the validity of this scale, the authors believe that this type of scale provides a significant advancement in procedures for gauging effort perception in children.

Whilst research will assess the efficacy of the Omni Scale, it is pertinent to debate its overall psychophysical structure. It remains to be determined if the gradient depicted in the scale should be linear. It may be justified on the basis of the linear association with physiological variables such as oxygen uptake and heart rate and RPE. However, whilst it is acknowledged that these factors are undoubtedly *associated* with sensations of effort, it is unlikely that they act directly as mediators for the respiratory–metabolic signal of exertion, i.e. they are not *causative*. As Noble and Robertson[1] have acknowledged, the majority of evidence linking heart rate with perceptual signals of exertion is derived from correlational data, but correlational data cannot be used to infer causality. Reviews[11,44] of studies in which heart rate has been experimentally manipulated during exercise indicate that heart rate does not appear to function as a physiological mediator for respiratory–metabolic signals of exertion. However, experimental and clinical evidence strongly supports ventilatory function as a physiological mediator for the respiratory–metabolic signal, particularly at higher relative metabolic rates.[1]

With the exception of the study by Noble[45] on adults, there is a paucity of research on the relationship between category-ratio scale ratings and sensations associated with curvilinear physiological responses such as blood lactate and pulmonary ventilation. Nevertheless, given the indisputable evidence that ventilation is a physiological mediator for respiratory–metabolic signals of exertion, and given that this variable rises in a curvilinear fashion with equal increments in work rate, it would perhaps be more ecologically valid if a symbolic version of a perceived exertion scale for children contained a gradient that is curvilinear in nature, and not linear. We suggest that categorization of perceptual responses could be depicted by a series of four to five linear *stages* of progressively increasing gradients, which

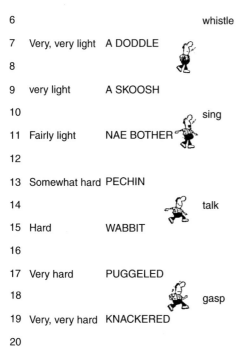

Fig. 1.9.4   University of Glasgow vernacular RPE Scale.

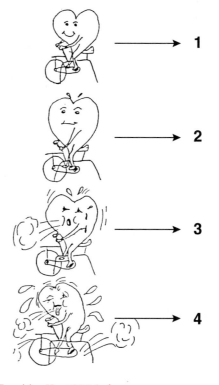

Fig. 1.9.5   Exercising Heart RPE Scale.

1   Very, Very easy
2   Very easy
3   Easy
4   Just feeling a strain
5   Starting to get hard
6   Getting quite hard
7   Hard
8   Very hard
9   Very, Very hard
10   So hard I'm going to stop

Fig. 1.9.6   Children's Effort Rating Table. From Williams et al.[23]

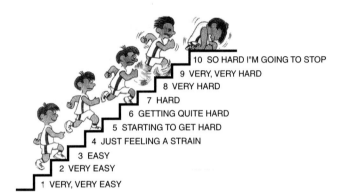

Fig. 1.9.7   Illustrated CERT Scale. From Yelling and Swaine.[43]

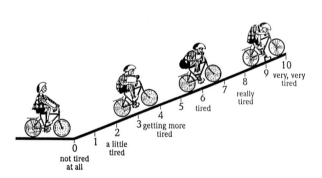

Fig. 1.9.8   Omni Perceived Exertion Scale. From Robertson.[42]

jointly form the basis of a curvilinear response. This removes the difficulty that children may have in assimilating information from a purely curvilinear pattern. We believe that a scale of this nature has face validity. It is readily conceivable that a child will recognize from previous learning and experience that the steeper the hill, the harder it is to ascend. This may also be helpful in the process of 'anchoring' effort perceptions.

The principle of presenting a scale that is readily assimilated by children on the basis of their own experiences and stages of development is very important. Using this principle as a basis for the conceptual framework of an alternative illustrated scale, Fig. 1.9.9 presents a child pulling a cart that is loaded progressively with bricks (Cart and Load Effort Rating, CALER, scale). The number of bricks in the cart is commensurate with numbers on the scale. Wording has been selected from the CERT to accompany some of the categories of effort. A preliminary study,[46] in which 20 boys and girls aged seven to ten years were requested to produce a work rate according to CALER 2, 5 and 8, has demonstrated potential for this type of pictorial scale. We are currently exploring the efficacy of these types of scales, including a stepping scale created by ourselves and Pam Shepherd, in which a backpack carried by a character from the Walt Disney film 'A Bug's Life' is progressively loaded with bricks (Fig. 1.9.10).

Anchoring effort perceptions

Whatever scale is used, it is important to provide the child with an understanding of the range of sensations that correspond to categories of effort within the scale. This is known as 'anchoring'. Whilst this may be partially achieved by reference to previous experience (memory), it is best achieved through directed experience. In this way, the child is exposed to a range of intensities which can be used to set the perceptual anchor points at 'low' and 'high' levels. This can be achieved during habituation to the test or exercise procedures. After an appropriate warm-up at an 'easy' level, the child should be allowed to experience exercise which is perceived as being 'hard' or 'very hard'. To avoid fatigue, a period of time should be allowed to regain full recovery.

Standardizing instructions

It is also important to standardize the instructions before using a perceived exertion scale. For example, the text which depicts the scaling and anchoring instructions accompanying the Omni Scale published in 1997. It should be noted that these instructions are for use in the estimation mode only:

> We would like you to ride on the bicycle for a little while. Every few minutes it will get harder to pedal the bicycle. Please use the numbers on this picture to tell us how your body feels when bicycling.

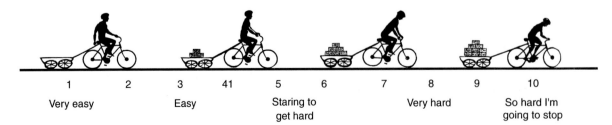

Fig. 1.9.9   Cart and Load RPE Scale. From Eston et al.[46]

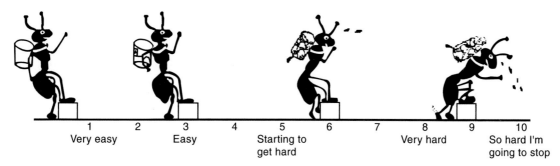

Fig. 1.9.10 Bug and Bag Effort Scale

Please look at the person at the bottom of the hill who is just starting to ride a bicycle (point to left pictorial). If you feel like this person when you are riding you will *not be tired at all*. Give a 0 (zero). Now look at the person who is barely able to ride the bicycle to the top of the hill (point to the right pictorial). If you feel like this person when you are riding you will be *very, very tired*. Give a number 10. If you feel somewhere in between *not at all tired* (0) and *very, very tired* (10), then give a number between 0 and 10.

We will ask you to give a number that tells how your body feels, then a number that tells how your legs feel and then a number that tells how your breathing feels.

Remember, there are no right and wrong numbers. Use both the pictures and words to help select the numbers. Use *any* of the numbers to tell how you feel when riding the bicycle.

Remind subject to point to the number. (Reproduced with the permission of Dr Robertson.)

Validity of effort perception: problems with comparing values from estimation, production, continuous and intermittent procedures

The majority of investigations have typically studied children's perceptions of effort during a passive estimation process. The effort perceptions have then been compared against objective measures of physiological strain, such as heart rate (HR), power output or oxygen uptake, using either intermittent or continuous protocols. Described in more detail by Lamb and Eston,[6] most studies of RPE have used a continuous testing protocol[19,21,27,30,32–34,36,37,47–53] in preference to an intermittent testing protocol.[29,35,54,55] CERT was developed and validated using continuous protocols.[23,24,40]

Fewer studies have applied effort production procedures in which children are requested to regulate their exercise output to match experimenter-prescribed effort ratings. These studies have included continuous exercise protocols (6–20 RPE Scale,[22] CERT[23,24,56]) and intermittent protocols (6 to 20 RPE Scale,[19–21] CERT[25,56]). It is fairly common to compare the objective indicators of effort with *expected* values derived from a previous estimation trial.[19,20,21,24] In effect, the ability of children to use perceptions of effort to *actively* self-regulate exercise intensity levels using predetermined RPEs has, in our opinion, been inappropriately compared to their ability to *passively* appraise exercise intensity from a previous test.

It is therefore difficult to appraise children's ability to reliably and accurately produce a given objective effort from these studies. For example, in the first full paper published on this theme,[19] it was concluded that 9–15 year old, overweight children could discriminate between four work rates based on predetermined RPE values (7, 10, 13 and 16). However, it was reported that the children produced work rates that were significantly different to expected (or 'criterion') values. It is necessary to point out that these criterion values were derived from a different perceptual process. Similar findings were reported in later studies.[20,21] These observations lead us to recommend that validity studies should focus on either production data only, or estimation data only, and not confound the issue by comparing data derived from a passive perceptual process on one occasion with an active perceptual process on a subsequent occasion. Noble's[45] argument that this involves two dissimilar psychophysical processes is highly pertinent. Furthermore, the disparity between the two psychophysical processes is most likely attenuated by the extent of children's limited perceptual experience. The issue is further confounded when data, collected during a passive, continuous estimation trial are compared to data from an active, intermittent production trial.

An indication of the *reliability* of effort production can be obtained from studies using RPE, CERT[21,22,24,25] and CALER.[46] Indirect evaluation of reliability was provided by Williams *et al.*[22] who reported that the mean heart rates produced by 11 to 14 year old children at levels 9, 13 and 17 were not significantly different over the course of three identical cycling trials. Furthermore, although they did not provide supporting analysis, Ward *et al.*[21] claimed that a sample of wheelchair-bound children and adults displayed an excellent retention over one month of an ability to regulate wheeling intensities using RPE. Eston *et al.*[24] also reported a seven-day intra-class reliability coefficient of $R = 0.91$ to 0.97 for power outputs, and $R = 0.65$ to 0.86 for heart rates produced at three levels of CERT during cycling in pre-adolescent children. More recently, however, results from Lamb[25] on a larger sample of children (aged nine to ten years) have proved less encouraging. In his study, seven day reliability coefficients ranging from 0.47–0.82 for heart rates and 0.10–0.74 for power outputs, were produced at four levels of CERT. Effort production using the RPE Scale was equally inconsistent, with reliability coefficients of $r = 0.48$–0.85 for heart rates and $0.08 - 0.76$ for power outputs. It is important to note, however, that these comparisons were based on a single test–retest scenario. As this is unlikely to provide the period of practice necessary to allow adequate learning to occur, the results are not that surprising.

The results from a recent study[46] bear testament to this assumption. Twenty children (aged seven to ten years) performed four trials of 3×3 minute intermittent bouts on a cycle ergometer at CALER 2, 5 and 8. Each bout was separated by 2.5 minutes rest and trials were separated by one week. Intra-class correlations between trials 1 and 2, 2 and 3, and 3 and 4 were 0.75, 0.86 and 0.98, respectively. The 95% levels of agreement procedure (bias $\pm 1.96 \times S.D$)[57] also indicated improved reliability with practice with no evidence of systematic bias between trials (12 ± 15 W between trials 1 and 2 and 0 ± 5 W between trials 3 and 4). As far as we are aware, this is the only study which has involved more than three repeated effort production protocols. It provides convincing evidence that the reliability of RPE to gauge exercise intensity is mediated by the number of periods of practice.

Much of our understanding of children's effort perceptions has evolved from measuring responses to a situation in which they realize that the exercise is getting progressively harder. Studies which have allowed rest periods between exercise bouts,[29,35,46,54,55,58] and thereby reduced the influence of fatigue on effort perceptions, have all been incremental in nature. Few studies have randomized the order of presentation of work loads.[19,33,56] Logically, the 'accuracy' and reliability of effort perceptions and objective markers of effort produced at specified effort ratings, will be influenced by test protocol (continuous or intermittent), the order of the load presentation (incremental or random) and the timing of the data collection. In a recent study by Lamb et al.[56] to assess the influence of exercise protocol on 66 children aged nine to ten years, we observed that the type of exercise protocol and the point at which the data were recorded influenced the heart rate response at specific effort ratings (CERT). The provision of three-minute recovery periods between exercise bouts produced higher relationships between CERT and heart rate ($r = 0.66$ c.f. $r = 0.46$, for the intermittent and continuous protocol, respectively). In addition, heart rates were significantly higher at three minutes compared to two minutes into the exercise. These results indicate that children may be more able to use effort ratings to control exercise intensity when the exercise is intermittent, rather than continuous in nature. Future investigations into children's effort perception should not disregard the manner in which the exercise is applied, nor the duration and number of the exercise bouts, as these two factors seem to have a bearing on the outcome measures.

Summary

As the importance of encouraging physical activity in children is recog-nized, it makes sense to study the accuracy and reliability of effort perception in this population. Studies should extend beyond the laboratory, take into account the respective cognitive abilities of each age group, and use appropriate methods of assessing the relationships between effort perception and objective markers of effort. This involves consideration of scales which are not semantically too advanced for the age group concerned and attention to issues involving exercise protocol, design and the nature of the perceptual process. Whatever scale is used, it is important to provide a period of practice to allow learning to occur and anchoring of the scale prior to data collection. Future studies should focus on the extent to which children of various ages and health status can learn to use effort perceptions in a variety of tasks.

References

1. Noble, B. J. and Robertson, R. J. *Perceived exertion.* Human Kinetics Publishers, Champaign, Il, 1996.
2. Carton, R. L. and Rhodes, E. C. A critical review of the literature on rating scales for perceived exertion. *Sports Medicine* 1985; 2: 198–222.
3. Watt, B. and Grove, R. Perceived exertion: Antecedents and applications. *Sports Medicine* 1993; 15: 225–41.
4. Williams, J. G. and Eston, R. G. Determination of the intensity dimension in vigorous exercise programmes with particular reference to the use of the rating of perceived exertion. *Sports Medicine* 1989; 8: 177–89.
5. Eston, R. G. and Connolly, D. A. Use of ratings of perceived exertion for exercise prescription in patients receiving beta-blocker therapy. *Sports Medicine* 1996; 21: 176–90.
6. Lamb, K. L. and Eston, R. G. Effort perception in children. *Sports Medicine* 1997; 23: 139–48.
7. Lamb, K. L. and Eston, R. G. Measurement of effort perception: time for a new approach. In *Children and exercise XIX volume II* (ed. J. Welsman, N. Armstrong and B. Kirby). Washington Singer Press, Exeter, 1997; 11–23.
8. Borg, G. Perceived exertion as an indicator of somatic stress. *Journal of Rehabilitation Medicine* 1970; 2: 92–8.
9. Borg, G. Psychophysical studies of effort and exertion: Some historical, theoretical, and empirical aspects. In *The perception of exertion in physical work* (ed. G. Borg and D. Ottoson). Macmillan, London, 1986; 3–14.
10. Borg, G. Psychophysical basis of perceived exertion. *Medicine and Science in Sports and Exercise* 1982; 14: 371–81.
11. Pandolf, K. B. Advances in the study and application of perceived exertion. *Exercise and Sport Sciences Reviews* 1983; 11: 118–58.
12. Eston, R. G., Davies, B. L. and Williams, J. G. Use of perceived effort ratings to control exercise intensity in young healthy adults. *European Journal of Applied Physiology and Occupational Physiology* 1987; 56: 222–4.
13. Eston, R. G. and Williams, J.G. (1988) Reliability of ratings of perceived effort for regulation of exercise intensity. *British Journal of Sports Medicine* 1988; 22: 153–4.
14. Dunbar, C. C., Robertson, R. J., Baun, R., Blandin, M. F., Metz., R. K., Burdett, R. and Goss, F. L. The validity of regulating exercise intensity by ratings of perceived exertion. *Medicine and Science in Sports and Exercise* 1992; 24: 94–9.
15. Glass, S., Knowlton, R. and Becque, M. D. Accuracy of RPE from graded exercise to establish exercise training intensity. *Medicine and Science in Sports and Exercise* 1992; 24: 1303–7.
16. Parfitt, G., Eston, R. G. and Connolly, D. A. Psychological affect at different ratings of perceived exertion in high- and low-active women: A study using a production protocol. *Perceptual and Motor Skills* 1996; 82: 1035–42.
17. Williams, J. G. and Eston, R. G. Exercise intensity regulation. In *Kinanthropometry and exercise physiology laboratory manual* (ed. R. G. Eston and T. Reilly). E. and F. N. Spon, London, 1996; 221–35.
18. Eston, R. G. and Thompson, M. Use of ratings of perceived exertion for predicting maximal work rate and prescribing exercise intensity in patients receiving atenolol. *British Journal of Sports Medicine* 1997; 31: 114–9.
19. Ward, D. S. and Bar-Or, O. Use of the Borg Scale in exercise prescription for overweight youth. *Canadian Journal of Sports Sciences* 1990; 15: 120–5.
20. Ward, D. S, Jackman, J. D. and Galiano, F. J. Exercise intensity reproduction: children versus adults. *Pediatric Exercise Science* 1991; 3: 209–18.
21. Ward, D. S., Bar-Or, O., Longmuir, P. and Smith, K. Use of ratings of perceived exertion (RPE) to prescribe exercise intensity for wheelchair-bound children and adults. *Pediatric Exercise Science* 1995; 7: 94–102.
22. Williams, J. G., Eston, R.G. and Stretch, C. Use of rating of perceived exertion to control exercise intensity in children. *Pediatric Exercise Science* 1991; 3: 21–7.
23. Williams, J. G., Eston, R. G. and Furlong, B. CERT: A perceived exertion scale for young children. *Perceptual and Motor Skills* 1994; 79: 1451–8.

24. Eston, R. G., Lamb, K. L., Bain, A., Williams, M. and Williams, J. G. Validity of a perceived exertion scale for children: A pilot study. *Perceptual and Motor Skills* 1994; **78**: 691–7.

25. Lamb, K. L. Exercise regulation during cycle ergometry using the CERT and RPE scales. *Pediatric Exercise Science* 1996; **8**:337–50.

26. Borg, G. *Physical work and effort*. Pergamon Press, Oxford, 1977; 289–93.

27. Bar-Or, O. Age-related changes in exercise perception. In *Physical work and effort* (ed. G. Borg). Pergamon Press, Oxford, 1977; 255–66.

28. Bar-Or, O. and Ward, D. S. Rating of perceived exertion in children. In *Advances in pediatric sports sciences, vol 3* (ed. O. Bar-Or). Human Kinetics Publishers, Champaign, Il, 1989; 151–68.

29. Kahle, C., Ulmer, H. V. and Rummel, L. The reproducibility of Borg's RPE scale with female pupils from 7 to 11 years of age. *Pflugers Archiv European Journal of Physiology* 1977; **368**: R26 (Abstract).

30. Davies, C. T. M., Fohlin, L. and Thoren, C. Perception of exertion in anorexia nervosa patients. In *Children and exercise IX* (ed. K. Berg and B. O. Eriksson). University Park Press, Baltimore, 1980; 327–32.

31. Eston, R. G. A discussion of the concepts: Exercise intensity and perceived exertion with reference to the secondary school. *Physical Education Review* 1984; **7**: 19–25.

32. Bar-Or, O. and Reed, S. Rating of perceived exertion in adolescents with neuromuscular disease. In *The perception of exertion in physical work* (ed. G. Borg and D. Ottoson). Macmillan Press, Basingstoke, 1986; 137–48.

33. Eston, R. G. and Williams, J. G. Exercise intensity and perceived exertion in adolescent boys. *British Journal of Sports Medicine* 1986; **20**: 27–30.

34. Miyashita, M., Onedera, K. and Tabata, I. How Borg's RPE scale has been applied to Japanese. In *The perception of exertion in physical work* (ed. G. Borg and D. Ottoson). Macmillan Press, Basingstoke, 1986; 27–34.

35. Van Huss, W. D., Stephens, K. E., Vogel, P., Anderson, D., Kurowski, T., Jones, J. A. and Fitzgerald, C. Physiological and perceptual responses of elite age group distance runners during progressive intermittent work to exhaustion. In *Sport for children and youth* (ed. M. Weiss and D. Gould). Human Kinetics Publishers, Champaign, Il, 1986; 239–46.

36. Ward, D. S., Blimkie, C. J. R. and Bar-Or, O. Rating of perceived exertion in obese adolescents. *Medicine and Science in Sports and Exercise* 1986; **18**: S72.

37. Nystad, W., Oseid, S. and Mellbye, E. B. Physical education for asthmatic children: The relationship between changes in heart rate, perceived exertion, and motivation for participation. In *Children and exercise XIII* (ed. S. Oseid and K. Carlsen). Human Kinetics Publishers, Champaign, Il, 1989; 369–77.

38. Lowry, A. The development of a pictorial scale to assess perceived exertion in school-children. *Unpublished Bachelor of Science thesis.* University College Chester, United Kingdom, 1995.

39. Williams, J. G., Furlong. B., MacKintosh, C. and Hockley, T. J. Rating and regulation of exercise intensity in young children. *Medicine and Science in Sports and Exercise* 1993; **25**: Suppl. S8 (Abstract).

40. Lamb, K. L. Children's ratings of effort during cycle ergometry: An examination of the validity of two effort rating scales. *Pediatric Exercise Science* 1995; **7**: 407–21.

41. Robertson, R. J. and Noble, B. J. Perception of physical exertion: Methods, mediators and applications. *Exercise and Sports Sciences Reviews* 1997; **25**: 407–52.

42. Robertson, R. J. Perceived exertion in young people: future directions of enquiry. In *Children and exercise XIX volume II* (ed. J. Welsman, N. Armstrong and B. Kirby). Washington Singer Press, Exeter, 1997; 33–9.

43. Yelling, M. and Swaine, I. Illustrated CERT Scale. Unpublished paper De Montfort University, Bedford, UK, 2000.

44. Robertson, R. J. Central signals of perceived exertion during dynamic exercise. *Medicine and Science in Sports and Exercise* 1982; **14**: 390–6.

45. Noble, B. J. Clinical applications of perceived exertion. *Medicine and Science in Sports and Exercise* 1982; **14**: 406–11.

46. Eston, R. G., Parfitt, G., Lamb, K. L. and Campbell, L. Reliability of effort perception for regulating exercise intensity: A study using the Cart and Load Effort Rating (CALER) Scale in children aged 7–10 years. *Pediatric Exercise Science* (in press).

47. Gillach, M. C., Sallis, J. F., Buono, M. L., Patterson, P. and Nader, P. The relationship between perceived exertion and heart rate in children and adults. *Pediatric Exercise Science* 1989; **1**: 360–8.

48. Alekseev, V. M. Correlation between heart rate and subjectively perceived exertion during muscular work. *Human Physiology* 1989; **15**: 39–44.

49. Eakin, B. L., Finta, K. M., Serwer, G. A. and Beckman, R. Perceived exertion and exercise intensity in children with or without structural heart defects. *Journal of Pediatrics* 1992; **120**: 90–3.

50. Mahon, A. D. and Marsh, M. L. Reliability of the rating of perceived exertion at ventilatory threshold in children. *International Journal of Sports Medicine* 1992; **13**: 567–71.

51. Stratton, G. and Armstrong, N. Children's use of RPE during indoor handball lessons. *Journal of Sports Sciences* 1994; **12**: 182–3.

52. Mahon, A. D. and Ray, M. L. Ratings of perceived exertion at maximal exercise in children performing different graded exercise tests. *Journal of Sports Medicine and Physical Fitness* 1995; **35**: 38–42.

53. Mahon, A. D., Duncan, G. E., Howe, C. A. and Del Corral, P. Blood lactate and perceived exertion relative to ventilatory threshold: boys versus men. *Medicine and Science in Sports and Exercise* 1997; **29**: 1332–7.

54. Tolfrey, K. and Mitchell, J. Ratings of perceived exertion at standard and relative exercise intensities in prepubertal, teenage and young adult males. *Journal of Sports Sciences* 1996; **14**: 101–2.

55. Ueda, T. and Kurokawa, T. Validity of heart rate and ratings of perceived exertion as indices of exercise intensity in a group of children while swimming. *European Journal of Applied Physiology* 1991; **63**: 200–4.

56. Lamb, K. L., Eston, R. G. and Trask, S. The effect of discontinuous and continuous testing protocols on effort perception in children. In *Children and exercise XIX* (ed. N. Armstrong, B. Kirby and J. Welsman). E. and F. N. Spon, London, 1997; 258–64.

57. Bland, J. M. and Altman, D. G. Statistical methods for assessing agreement between two methods of clinical measurement. *Lancet* 1986; i: 307–10.

58. Meyer, F., Bar-Or, O. and Wilk, B. Children's perceptual responses to ingesting drinks of different compositions during and following exercise in the heat. *International Journal of Sports Nutrition* 1995; **5**: 13–24.

PART II

Developmental Aspects of Paediatric Exercise Science

2.1 Growth and maturation: do regular physical activity and training for sport have a significant influence?

Robert M. Malina

Introduction

It is often assumed that regular physical activity is important to support normal growth and maturation.[1,2] Studies spanning nearly a century have suggested that regular physical activity, including training for sport, has a stimulatory influence on growth and sexual maturation.[3–8] Rarick[1] suggests:

> … certain minima of muscular activity are essential for supporting normal growth and for maintaining the protoplasmic integrity of the tissues. What these minima mean in terms of intensity and duration of activity has not been ascertained. (p. 459)

At the same time, concern has also been expressed about potentially negative influences, specifically of training for sport during childhood and adolescence.[9–12] Shephard,[10] for example, states:

> Some reports have described slow growth … , a retardation of bone development … and a delay of menarche … among child athletes. (p. 208.)

It is of interest that the specific studies cited to document this generalization are not consistent with the statement. For example, the report of Rowe[9] on interscholastic touch football (American) players is cited as indicating slow growth in association with sport; unfortunately, the qualifying observation of Rowe that the differences between the groups of boys in the study may have reflected differential maturation and timing of the adolescent spurt was not considered. The work of Shuck[13] was also cited as suggesting slower growth in junior high school (grades seven to nine) athletes in basketball, American football, baseball and track; according to the author, however:

> … there seems to be no retardation in growth due to participation in the athletic programme. … When comparisons were made between the original and final percentage differences in body sizes, body shapes, and speeds of growth of athletes and nonathletes, athletes in selected sports, and athletes in multiple sports, in the three grades, no pronounced retardation or acceleration appeared among the athletes due to athletic participation. (p. 290)

The references dealing with bone development are derived from marginally nourished children in a depressed region of Japan[14] and from an experimental running and dietary programme in rats.[15] Finally, all data dealing with later menarche are derived from retrospective studies of college age athletes, and it is not possible to

draw a cause–effect sequence from such data. More recently, concern for the growth and sexual maturation of active girls was highlighted in a recent report of the American Medical Association and the American Dietetic Association,[16] which cautions:

> Some fitness programmes may be detrimental to adolescents if they mandate prolonged, strenuous exercise and/or very low body fat to maximize their competitive edge. … These regimes may delay sexual maturation, decrease bone growth and ultimate height … (p. 4)

These comments focus largely on girls participating in sports requiring small body size, slender physiques and/or low body mass, i.e. gymnastics, figure skating, ballet.

The contrasting views and inconsistencies in interpretations of the literature highlight some of the difficulties in evaluating the role of physical activity and training in growth and maturation. Physical activity and training are variably defined constructs, activity and training are not synonymous, generalizations based upon select athletes may not apply to the general population, and so on. If physical activity and training for sport are important factors that may influence growth and maturation, can their potential effects be partitioned from changes associated with normal growth and maturation? It is only on the basis of longitudinal studies of children and youth regularly participating in programmes of physical activity or training for sport that such generalizations and others can be evaluated. What specific longitudinal data underlie these generalizations? How can the growth and maturation data for physically active youth and young athletes in a variety of sports be interpreted?

This chapter considers the growth and maturity characteristics of youth who are regularly active and/or who are regularly training for sport. The available data are evaluated in the context of the following question: Are the physical and physiological demands of habitual physical activity and/or intensive training for sport during childhood and adolescence capable of altering individual patterns of growth and maturation?

Physical activity and training

Physical activity is ordinarily viewed in the context of gross bodily movements associated with a significant increase in energy expenditure above resting levels.[17] Physical activity is, however, more complex. It involves at least four major components: energetic (METS, $\dot{V}O_2$

max), biomechanical (body mass bearing activities, ground reaction forces), strength (static, dynamic), and motor skill (economy, accuracy of movement). In addition, physical activities are carried out in specific contexts, which are variable and culturally determined.

Most discussions refer to a child's estimated level of habitual physical activity, e.g. h wk^{-1} or an activity score, ordinarily derived from questionnaires, interviews, diaries and heart rate integrators. Presently available techniques for estimating physical activity have measurement limitations (see Chapter 1.8).

Physical activity is not the same as regular training. Although activity is integral to training, the latter refers to systematic, specialized practice for a specific sport or sport discipline for most of the year or to specific short-term experimental programmes, e.g. 15 weeks of endurance training in running or resistance training. Although there is variation by sport or events within a sport, sport-specific training programmes routinely involve multiple components (aerobic, anaerobic, strength, skill, imagery, tactical), so that it may be difficult to specify training demands on the child or adolescent.

Patterns of participation in physical activity and sport

Estimated levels of activity increase from about five to six years of age into early or mid-adolescence, and then decline across adolescence, although the magnitude of the decline varies among studies. Adolescent changes in physical activity are apparently more related to intensity of activity rather than duration or frequency. The decline in habitual activity is more evident in medium (7 to 10 METS) and heavy (10 + METS) activities. Males are, on average, more active than females at all ages, but males also experience a greater decline in habitual physical activity in late adolescence.[18,19] Changes in physical activity during adolescence should be viewed in the context of developmental tasks related to social demands of adolescence and perhaps to career choices, i.e. the transition from high school to college or to the work force. Some evidence suggests that current youth spend less time in vigorous physical activity than those of only a few years ago, and that the decline is greater in females than males.

The pattern of participation in organized sport is similar to that for physical activity. The number of children involved in organized sport increases with age from about five to six years to about 12 to 13 years, and then declines. Changing interests associated with the onset of adolescence is a factor in the decline. However, it is also at these ages that many youth sports programmes become more selective and specialized, and, at the more specialized, elite levels, sport is extremely selective and exclusive, i.e. inequitable. Selection criteria and practices for specific sports vary with programmes.

Community based programmes emphasize mass participation; age and willingness to participate are the primary criteria. Programmes that emphasize the elite generally have as their objective the identification and subsequent training of young athletes with potential for success in regional, national and/or international competition high performance sports.[20,21] The selection/exclusion process begins early and is rather systematic. It may begin at five to six years of age in some sports, with gymnastics being perhaps the most visible example. Diving programmes in some countries, e.g. the Peoples' Republic of China, also select at these ages. Criteria and timing of evaluation for

other sports, including ballet, vary. Identifying and selecting the potentially talented athlete at an early age is the first step in a relatively long-term process. The perfection of talent is another matter which requires long hours of systematic and often repetitive training under the scrutiny of demanding coaches, dietary regulation and manipulation, social manipulation (control combined with preferential treatment, separation from family), and perhaps chemical manipulation in some sports.[22] Such programmes focus on the retention of a relatively small number of select athletes and the exclusion of others. Hence, a sample of elite young athletes is not representative of the general population of children and adolescents.

Growth and maturation

Growth refers to an increase in size, either of the body as a whole or of its parts. It involves increases in stature and mass, and related changes in physique, body composition and various systems. Maturation refers to the tempo (rate) and timing of progress to the mature state. The processes of growth and maturation are cellular, but it is not possible to systematically study these processes in children and adolescents. Rather, the study of growth and maturation is based largely on measurement and observation.[2]

In the subsequent discussion, stature and mass are the primary indicators of growth that are considered. Body mass is also considered in the context of body composition and its primary components, skeletal muscle, skeletal and adipose tissues. Skeletal muscle is the major work-producing and oxygen-consuming tissue, and is the producer of physical activity. The skeleton is the framework of the body and the main reservoir of mineral, while adipose tissue represents energy in stored form. Maturation is considered in the context of the timing and tempo of the adolescent growth spurt, skeletal age and secondary sex characteristics. Details of methods used to assess growth and maturity status are described in detail elsewhere[2] (and see Chapter 1.2).

Limitations

Inferences about the influence of regular physical activity and training for sport on indicators of growth and maturation are based largely on cross-sectional and relatively few longitudinal comparisons of children and adolescents classified as active and non-active, and athletes in specific sports and non-athletes. Longitudinal studies that span childhood and adolescence, and that control for physical activity and/or specify training, are few.

Although many talented young athletes train regularly for several years, especially in sports like gymnastics, figure skating and swimming, the selective nature of specific sports cannot be overlooked. Athletes as a group are highly select. They are selected for specific skills and in many sports for certain size and physique characteristics. Among female gymnasts and swimmers, for example, the former are already shorter than average and the latter are already taller than average prior to the start of the respective training programmes. Parents of gymnasts are also shorter than those of swimmers, which would imply a genotypic factor in stature. Successful young ballet dancers tend to have the thinness and proportional features of elite ballerinas. On the other hand, males who are successful in many sports at relatively young ages tend to be advanced in biological maturity status, especially in early adolescence, and are thus generally taller and heavier than their chronological age peers. The selectivity of sport thus limits the utility of comparisons of athletes and non-athletes in the context of specifying potential training effects. It cannot be assumed *a priori* that differences in growth and maturation between young athletes and non-athletes are due to regular training. The same applies to studies showing differences between adult athletes and non-athletes, which are often interpreted as reflecting the influence of training during childhood and adolescence.[23,24]

The subsequent discussion is based on healthy, adequately nourished children and youth. Intensive physical activity and training may be contraindicated in chronically undernourished individuals.

Stature and the adolescent growth spurt

Regular physical activity, sport participation and training for sport have no apparent effect on attained stature and rate of growth in stature. Longitudinal data on active and inactive boys followed from

late childhood through adolescence indicate no differences in stature (Fig. 2.1.1). Data for boys and girls regularly active in sport during childhood and adolescence indicate, with few exceptions, mean statures that either approximate or exceed reference medians (Table 2.1.1). Female gymnasts and figure skaters and male divers present, on average, statures that are shorter than reference medians. Several short-term longitudinal studies of athletes in several sports (volleyball, diving, distance running, basketball), indicate growth rates similar to those of reference data for non-athletes.[23,24]

Age at peak height velocity (PHV), the time of maximum velocity of growth in stature during the adolescent spurt, is not affected by regular physical activity and training for sport. Presently available data are limited largely to boys, with only few observations for girls (Table 2.1.2). Age at PHV tends to be earlier in male athletes, which is consistent with observations for other maturity indicators (see below). The magnitude of PHV in active and inactive boys, and in youngsters regularly training for sport is well within the range of variation associated with growth velocity at this stage of growth. By inference, peak velocity of growth in stature during the adolescent growth spurt is not affected by regular activity and training.

The lack of a normal adolescent growth spurt in female gymnasts has been suggested.[25] However, longitudinal data for female gymnasts that span late childhood and adolescence are extremely limited. This caution is based on results of a short-term longitudinal study of 22 Swiss female gymnasts[12] that spanned only two to 3.7 years in individual athletes (mean = 2.3 years). The resulting average velocity curve, which was plotted relative to skeletal age, indicated a somewhat blunted spurt which, however, was within the range reported for reference data. The blunting is in part a function of the cross-sectional treatment of the short-term mixed-longitudinal data.

Longitudinal observations for nine Polish female gymnasts[26,27] indicate an adolescent spurt, with a mean age at PHV of 13.1 ± 0.7 years and a peak velocity = 5.8 ± 0.5 cm y^{-1}. These estimates compare closely with a maximum increment of 5.5 ± 0.3 cm y^{-1} at a chronological age of 13 years and a skeletal age of 12.5 years in the Swiss gymnasts followed for periods of only two to 3.7 years.[28] The short-term nature of the Swiss data illustrate their limited utility in defining an adolescent growth spurt.

Nevertheless, the data indicate a later age at PHV in female gymnasts compared to non-athletes, but peak velocities, though somewhat lower, are within the range of normal variation during adolescence. For example, the mean peak velocity (based on smoothing splines) for Swiss girls[29] is 7.1 ± 1.1 cm y^{-1} with a range from 5 to 10.1 cm y^{-1}. Similar trends are apparent for male gymnasts (Table 2.1.2). The adolescent growth pattern of female and male gymnasts is similar to that of short, normal, slow maturing children, and/or late maturing children with short parents.[24,27]

In the context of the preceding, and allowing for individual differences in the timing and tempo of the adolescent growth spurt, it is difficult to establish causality from the evidence offered to indicate an influence of training for sport on the growth in stature and the timing of PHV of young gymnasts. The same applies to physically active youngsters and young athletes. When the literature is compiled and critically evaluated, taking into consideration the importance of controlling for variation in maturity status, it is reasonable to conclude that regular physical activity and training for sport have no apparent effect on stature in adequately nourished growing youth.

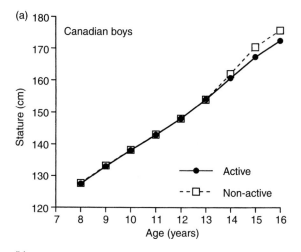

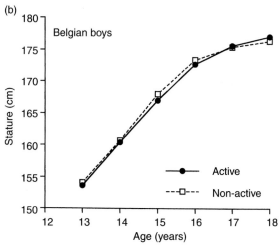

Fig. 2.1.1 Mean statures of active and non-active Canadian (a) and Belgian (b) boys. Drawn from data reported by Mirwald *et al.*[78] and Beunen *et al.*[48]

Table 2.1.1 Stature and mass of child and adolescent athletes relative to percentiles (P) of United States reference data

Sport	Males		Females	
	Stature	Mass	Stature	Mass
Basketball	P 50–>P 90	P 50–>P90	P 75–>P90	P 50–P 75
Volleyball			P 75	P 50–P 75
Soccer	P 50±	P 50±	P 50	P 50
Ice hockey	P 50±	P 50		
Distance runs	P 50±	≤P 50	≥P 50	<P 50
Sprints	≥P 50	≥P 50	≥P 50	≤P 50
Swimming	P 50–P 90	P 50–P 75	P 50–P 90	P 50–P 75
Diving	<P 50	≤P 50	≤P 50	P 50
Gymnastics	≤P 10–P 25	≤P 10–P 25	≤P 10–<P 50[1]	P 10–<P 50[1]
Tennis	P 50±	≥P 50	>P 50	P 50±
Figure skating	P 10–P 25	P 10–P 25	P 10–<P 50	P 10–<P 50
Ballet	<P 50	P 10–P 50	≤P 50	P 10–<P 50

[1]More recent samples of gymnasts are closer to P 10.

Adapted from Malina[23,24] which contain the references for individual studies.

Body mass and body composition

In contrast to stature, body mass can be influenced by regular activity and training, resulting in changes in body composition. The latter is most often viewed in a two-compartment model, body mass = fat-free mass plus fat mass. Activity and training are associated with a decrease in fatness in both sexes and occasionally with an increase in fat-free mass in boys. Males, athletes and non-athletes, show a decline in relative fatness during adolescence, but athletes also have less fatness. The decline in relative fatness during adolescence is due to the rapid gain in fat-free mass so that fat mass contributes proportionally less to body mass at this time. Relative fatness does not increase as much with age during adolescence in female athletes as it does in non-athletes. Thus, the difference between female athletes and non-athletes is greater than the corresponding trend in males.[2] Changes in fatness depend on continued, regular activity or training (or caloric restriction, which often occurs in sports like gymnastics, figure skating and ballet in girls, and wrestling in boys) for their maintenance. When activity or training are significantly reduced, fatness tends to accumulate.

It is often difficult to partition effects of training on fat-free mass from expected changes associated with growth and maturation, specifically during adolescence. Both sexes have a significant adolescent spurt in fat-free mass, males more so than females.[2] In the frequently cited study of Parizkova,[30–32] three groups of boys with different activity (training?) programmes were followed longitudinally from 11 to 18 years of age. The active boys ($n=8$, 6 h wk^{-1}) were selected primarily for basketball (6) and athletics (2). The other two groups had less regular physical activity, including school physical education. The active boys were taller than boys in the other two groups throughout the study, made greater gains in fat-free mass, and accumulated relatively less fat than boys in the two less active groups. The active group was also advanced in skeletal age and attained PHV at an earlier age, showing a growth pattern characteristic of early maturing boys. Their greater statures and larger gains in fat-free mass compared to the other groups could be related in part to their advanced maturity status, which was not statistically controlled in the comparison.

In a short-term study of nine boys during the course of a six month endurance training programme, Von Dobeln and Eriksson[33] noted significant gains in potassium concentration. The gain in potassium, an index of muscle mass, after the training programme was 6% greater than expected, while the gain in mass was 5% less than expected relative to linear growth. In addition, the boys gained an average of 3.5 cm in stature over the 16 week programme,[34] suggesting rather strongly that the adolescent growth spurt occurred in some boys during the course of the study. Hence, the observed changes in body composition could reflect in part those that accompany the adolescent spurt in boys, and not the effect of the training programme. Further, endurance programmes are not often associated with large gains in fat-free mass. Closer examination of the individual data shows the following: three boys had body masses above one standard deviation of Swedish reference data, five boys lost mass during the training programme, and with one exception the largest gains in estimated fat-free mass and stature were made by boys advanced in maturity status (based on testicular volume).

The studies of Parizkova[32] and Von Dobeln and Eriksson[33] illustrate the difficulties partitioning changes associated with activity/training from those that accompany normal growth and maturation during male adolescence. Are the changes in body composition associated with regular activity/training greater than those which accompany growth and maturation?

Skeletal muscle

Information on the effects of physical activity and training on skeletal muscle tissue is derived largely from short-term, specific training studies of small samples. Muscular hypertrophy is associated with high resistance

Table 2.1.2   Estimated mean ages ($\pm$ standard deviations) at peak height velocity (y) and peak velocities (cm y^{-1}) in active and non-active adolescents and in adolescent athletes in several sports

Activity status/sport	n	Age at PHV	PHV	Method[1]
Males—active versus non-active				
Active	14	14.3 ± 1.2	8.7 ± 1.1	PB
Inactive	11	14.1 ± 0.7	9.9 ± 1.4	PB
Active	32	14.2 ± 0.8	9.4 ± 1.5	P
Inactive	32	14.1 ± 0.8	8.9 ± 2.1	P
Moderate activity	19	14.5 ± 1.0	9.7 ± 1.5	G
Limited activity	12	14.6 ± 1.2	9.8 ± 1.5	G
Active[2]	7	13.3		G
Average activity[2]	43	13.3		G
Males—athletes				
Soccer	32	14.2 ± 0.9	9.5 ± 1.5	G, P
Soccer	8	14.2 ± 0.9		G
Basketball and athletics	8	14.1 ± 0.9	10.1 ± 1.2	G
Basketball and track[2]	16	11.1 ± 0.9		W
Cycling	6	12.9 ± 0.4		G
Rowing	11	13.5 ± 0.5		G
Ice hockey	16	14.5 ± 1.0		G
Ice hockey	11	12.8 ± 0.5	9.3 ± 3.0	G
Distance runs[2]	4	12.6		G
Gymnasts	14	15.0 ± 0.8	7.5 ± 1.1	P
	11	14.9 ± 0.8	7.4 ± 0.8	KR
Several sports[3]	25	13.6 ± 0.9	9.7 ± 1.1	PB
Several sports[4]	21	13.1 ± 1.0	9.3 ± 1.2	KR
Males—range of means for non-athletes[5]				
		13.8–14.4	8.3–10.3	
Females—athletes				
Gymnasts	9	13.1 ± 0.8	5.6 ± 0.5	P
	6	13.1 ± 0.7	5.8 ± 0.5	KR
Several sports[2]	13	12.3 ± 0.8	7.8 ± 0.6	PB
Several sports[3]	23	12.0 ± 0.8	8.0 ± 1.3	KR
Females—range of means for non-athletes[5]				
		11.6–12.2	7.0–9.0	

Adapted from Malina[24] which contains the references for individual studies. The data for a combined sample of basketball and track athletes[76] and for gymnasts[26,27] (Malina unpublished) were added.

[1] Methods for estimating ages at PHV and peak velocities: G, graphic interpolation; P, polynomials; PB, Preece-Baines model I; KR, kernel regression; W, wavelet interpolation. Some of the variation reflects differences among methods and precision of graphic interpolation.

[2] These are estimates for Japanese samples. Age at PHV occurs earlier, on average, in Japanese than in European adolescents.

[3] Several individual and team sports.

[4] Track and rowing with several in swimming.

[5] Range of mean ages at PHV and peak velocities, based on a variety of methods, reported in European longitudinal studies; 18 of the 20 estimated ages at PHV for boys are between 13.9 and 14.2 years, while 14 of 19 estimated ages at PHV for girls are between 11.9 and 12.2 years.[77]

programmes, such as weight or strength training in adolescent boys, and may not occur or may occur to a much lesser extent in prepubertal boys and girls.[2] Studies of adults indicate that gains in muscularity associated with resistance training revert to pre-training values when the resistance programme is stopped. A question of interest to growing and maturing individuals relates to the partitioning of training-related changes from those associated with normal growth and maturation, particularly in adolescent boys. Similarly, do the training-related changes in muscle mass in adolescents persist after the training programme has stopped? How much activity is needed to maintain the training-induced changes?

There is no strong evidence to suggest that fibre type distribution in youth can be changed as a result of training. Progressive strength training is associated with an increase in the relative area of Type II (fast twitch) fibres, while endurance training is associated with an increase in the relative area of Type I (slow twitch) fibres in young adults. Data for youth are variable. In 16 year old boys, three months of endurance training were associated with an increase in the areas of both Type I and II fibres, while three months of sprint training did not affect fibre areas.[35] Corresponding data for young females are not available. The limited data suggest that regular training has the potential to modify the metabolic capacity of muscle in children and youth. However, changes in response to short-term programmes are generally not permanent and depend upon regular activity for their maintenance.

Skeletal mineral and mass

Regular physical activity and training during childhood and adolescence are associated with increased bone mineral content, but the osteogenic influence of activity is generally specific to the skeletal sites at which the mechanical strains occur.[36] Beneficial effects are also more apparent in mass bearing than non-mass bearing activities. Of particular importance is the observation that bone mineral established during childhood and adolescence is a determinant of adult bone mineral status.

Similar trends are apparent both in boys and girls[37,38] and in young athletes from late childhood through young adulthood, although the latter data are derived largely from female athletes in gymnastics, figure skating, ballet, swimming and running.[39–43]

The long-term effect of early sport training on skeletal tissue is especially apparent in the dominant compared to the non-dominant arms of racket sport athletes (Fig. 2.1.2). The difference in the mineral content of the humerus and radius of the dominant and non-dominant arms of female tennis and squash players who began formal training three or more years before menarche was greater than that in athletes who began training near the time of menarche or after menarche.[44] The data suggest a dose-response effect.

There is generally more concern for the integrity of skeletal tissue of females, particularly athletes, than of males. This concern is in part related to later sexual maturation, which is often characteristic of female athletes (see below). Presumably later sexual maturation is related to reduced total oestrogen exposure and in turn potentially less accretion of bone mineral content and mass. However, adolescent female athletes in several sports tend to have greater bone mineral, specifically at the skeletal sites at which mechanical strains occur. Enhanced bone mineral accretion associated with training for sport may thus offset the reduced oestrogen exposure associated with later maturation.

In contrast to the positive influence of training on bone mineralization, excessive training associated with altered menstrual function in some, but not all, post-menarcheal athletes may be associated with

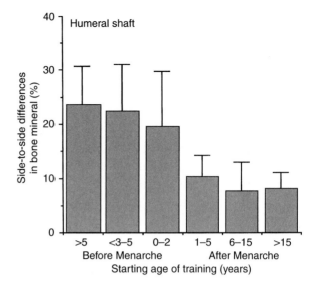

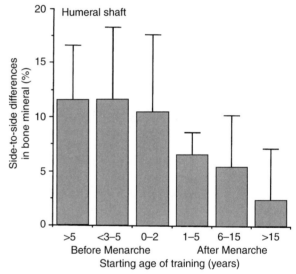

Fig. 2.1.2 Side-to-side differences in bone mineral content of the humeral (a) and radial (b) shafts of female tennis and squash players relative to the starting age of training. Drawn from data reported by Kannus *et al.*[44]

loss of bone mineral.[45,46] Restrictive diets and/or disordered eating are contributory factors. The interaction of disordered eating, cessation of regular menstrual cycles and osteoporosis in high performance athletes is of concern for some, but not all, adolescent athletes, and may impact the accretion of skeletal mineral during adolescence. An important question that needs careful consideration is: Can adolescent athletes at risk be identified in the context of normal variation in menstrual cycles for a year or two after menarche? Under conditions of altered menstrual function (secondary amenorrhea) and a deficient diet, physical activity/training may have a negative influence on the integrity of skeletal tissue.

Adipose tissue

In studies of children and youth, adipose tissue is most often measured in the form of skinfold thicknesses, which provide an estimate of subcutaneous adipose tissue. Cross-sectional data indicate thinner skinfolds in active children and young athletes compared to reference samples. However, longitudinal data for active and non-active boys and girls followed from 6 to 12 years[47] and adolescent boys followed from 13 to 18 years[48] do not differ from each other in skinfold thicknesses. Similarly, boys and girls active in sport and followed longitudinally from 8 to 18 years have skinfold thicknesses that do not differ from reference data.[49] The discrepancies between the cross-sectional and longitudinal observations should be noted. It is likely that more intensive physical activity is essential to modify skinfold thicknesses in children and especially adolescents. In addition, skinfolds change differentially during male adolescence, i.e. extremity but not trunk skinfolds ordinarily decline in thickness during adolescence.[50]

Data dealing with potential effects of training on subcutaneous fat distribution during growth are presently not available. In young adult males, intensive training for 15 and 20 weeks was associated with a greater reduction in trunk than in extremity skinfolds, while corresponding changes in young adult females were evenly distributed between trunk and extremity sites.[51,52] Information on the effects of regular training on adipose tissue cellularity during childhood and adolescence is also lacking. Adipose tissue cellularity increases gradually during childhood and then more rapidly with the onset of puberty.[2] The decrease in fatness associated with training in adults is attributable solely to a reduction in estimated adipocyte size.[53]

Biological maturation

Biological maturation is a highly individual characteristic which is variable in timing (when specific events/changes occur) and tempo (rate or progress). Skeletal maturation is the only system of maturity assessment that spans the period of growth prenatally to adulthood. The hand-wrist area is used most often. Assessment of skeletal maturation is based upon the radiographic appearance of ossification centres, characterization of these centres, and epiphyseal union (long ones) and adult morphology (carpals). Several methods of assessment are available (see Chapter 1.2). Although the methods of assessment vary, they each provide an estimate of skeletal age (SA), which is subsequently related to the individual's chronological age (CA). An SA > CA by more than one year indicates advanced or early maturation, while an SA < CA by more than one year indicates slower or late maturation.[2]

Sexual maturation is useful only when overt manifestations of the processes are evident, i.e. breast development in girls, genital development in boys, pubic hair in both sexes and menarche in girls. Breast, genital and pubic hair assessments are ordinarily made on clinical examination by trained personnel, although a number of studies use self-assessments (see Chapter 1.2).

Trends in the maturity status of child and adolescent athletes based on skeletal age and secondary sex characteristics (excluding menarche) are summarized in Table 2.1.3.

Skeletal maturation

Although regular activity and training functions to enhance bone mineralization, it does not influence skeletal maturation of the hand and wrist as it is radiographically assessed in growth studies. Active and non-active boys followed longitudinally from 13 to 18 years do not differ in SA.[48] Young athletes in several sports differ in skeletal maturity status, although skeletal maturation data for some sports are lacking. Boys successful in a variety of sports tend to have, on average, SAs in advance of CAs. The pattern for young ice hockey and soccer players, however, varies with chronological age. Among young male athletes in these two sports, the available data suggest that in late childhood and early adolescent athletes, SA and CA do not differ, on average. However, in older adolescent athletes SA is advanced over CA, indicating that early maturing boys appear to dominate these sports in later adolescence. Among girls, those in ballet, gymnastics and track tend to have SAs that lag behind CAs, while those in swimming tend to have SAs in advance of CAs.[23,24] The trend for gymnastics is especially evident in later adolescence, which suggests that later maturing girls persist in the sport, or conversely, that girls of early or average maturity status tend to drop out of the sport.[23,24,27,54]

Short-term longitudinal observations on young athletes indicate corresponding gains in CA and SA during the course of regular training, thus implying that the process of skeletal maturation is not influenced by training for sport.[23] It should be noted that during adolescence skeletal maturation generally proceeds in concert with indicators of sexual and somatic maturation, and that in late adolescence, differences between individuals of contrasting maturity status are reduced and eventually eliminated as skeletal maturity is attained.

Secondary sex characteristics

Longitudinal data on the development of secondary sex characteristics of either boys or girls regularly active or training for sport are not extensive. Cross-sectional observations on breast, genital and pubic hair development in young athletes are consistent with those for SA, while the limited longitudinal data indicate no effect of physical activity or training on the timing and progress of breast, genital and pubic hair development in boys and girls.[23] For example, in 23 girls who were actively training for sport (rowing, track, swimming) about 12 hours per week during the growth spurt and pubertal maturation, the interval between age at PHV and menarche, and the estimated duration of stages of breast and pubic hair development were the same as in non-athletes.[55] These results are consistent with those for a retrospective study of 13 girls who were active in several individual and team sports during childhood and adolescence, and also active in sport as adults.[49]

In contrast, a study of elite ballet dancers suggests normal progress of pubic hair, but very slow progress in breast development, with especially variable progression from breast stage three to stage four or five.[56] The latter may be influenced by the extreme linearity of build and thinness of elite ballet dancers, i.e. a deficiency in subcutaneous fat which may influence assessment of breast development. And, in the sample of ballerinas studied, mass-for-stature of the elite dancers decreased during puberty (it did not stabilize until after 17 years of age). Further, the criteria for the assessment of stage of breast development are in part physique and fat dependent, specifically stage four, and the areolar mound that characterizes stage four does not occur in all girls and may also be relatively slight in some girls.[57] Given the decline in mass-for-stature during puberty in elite ballet dancers, as well as the observation that significant numbers of young ballerinas have persistent problems with disordered eating related to concerns for body mass, the slow and variable progression of breast development may be related to low mass gain and low levels of fatness during puberty rather than to intensity of training.

Table 2.1.3 Trends in maturity status based on skeletal age and secondary sex characteristics (excluding menarche) in child and adolescent athletes (indicated ages are approximate)

Sport (males)	Childhood (<11 y)	Adolescence (11 to 15.9 y)	Late adolescence (>16 y)
Baseball	*	Advanced	No difference
Football	*	Advanced	No difference
Basketball	No difference	Average/advanced	No difference
Soccer	Average	Average	Advanced
Ice hockey	Average	Average/advanced	Advanced
Distance runs	*	Slightly later/average	No difference
Track and field	*	Advanced	No difference
Swimming	Average/advanced	Advanced	*
Gymnastics	Average	Later	*

Sport (females)	Childhood (<10 y)	Adolescence (10 to 14.9 y)	Late adolescence (>15 y)
Basketball	*	*	Average
Volleyball	*	*	Average
Distance runs	*	Slightly later/average	Slightly later/average
Track and field	*	Average	Average
Swimming	Average/advanced	Average/advanced	Average
Gymnastics	Average	Later/average	Later
Ballet	*	Later/average	Later

Adapted from Malina.[24] These are trends suggested in a review of data from a variety of studies of young athletes.[23] Characterizing maturity status in late adolescence is influenced by the early attainment of maturity in advanced maturers (who are in turn excluded from estimates of statistical parameters for skeletal age), and catch-up of average and later maturers (i.e. all youth eventually reach skeletal and sexual maturity). The upper limit of one skeletal maturity assessment system is 16 years (maturity) for girls.

*Satisfactory data are not available.

Age at menarche

Discussions of physical activity and training in the context of sexual maturation most often focus on females rather than on males. The specific concern is the age at menarche, which is a late event in the pubertal sequence. It is also a maturational event which has cultural and social significance in the lives of adolescent girls. It occurs, on average, a bit more than a year after PHV.[55] Later mean ages at menarche are commonly reported in athletes in many, but not in all sports.[58,59] It is often inferred that the later mean ages at menarche in athletes are a consequence of regular training before menarche, i.e. training 'delays' menarche. This inference is also made relative to physical activity in the epidemiological and auxological literature. Use of the term 'delay' in the context of physical activity and sport is, however, misleading; it implies that training for sport or regular physical activity 'causes' menarche to be later than normal.

The confusion associated with later ages at menarche in athletes is related, in part, to a rather narrow clinical definition of 'delayed' menarche, and to the different methods of estimating age at menarche. Clinically, 'delayed' menarche is defined as an age at menarche of 14 years or older.[60,61] Presumably, 14 years means that menarche is attained after the 14th birthday (> 14.0 years). This reflects a narrow view of normal human variability in ages at menarche reported in samples of adequately nourished, healthy girls worldwide.[62]

There are three methods for estimating age at menarche: prospective, status quo or retrospective. Prospective studies of young girls regularly training in a sport are generally short term and are limited to small, select samples. Since girls are seen at regular intervals in prospective studies, the recalled age at menarche by the girl (or her mother) is generally quite accurate. Status quo data for young athletes actively involved in systematic training for sport, on the other hand, provide an estimate only for the sample or population. In contrast, the vast majority of data for athletes are retrospective, and are often collected several years after menarche has occurred.

Prospective and status quo estimates of ages at menarche in adolescent athletes are summarized in Table 2.1.4. Retrospective estimates are reported elsewhere.[58,59] The estimates for gymnasts, ballet dancers, Junior Olympic divers and soccer players are generally consistent with the retrospective data. The limited prospective and status quo data for tennis players, rowers, track athletes, and more available data for age group swimmers indicate earlier mean ages at menarche than retrospective estimates for each sport respectively; i.e. late adolescent and young adult athletes (recall) in these sports tend to attain menarche later than those involved in the respective sports during the circumpubertal years (prospective and/or status quo). The differences probably represent the interaction of several factors, including the longer growth period associated with later maturation (some do not attain adult body size until the late teens or early 20s), selective success in sport of late maturing girls, selective drop-out of early maturing girls, and probably others.

Secular factors related to the opportunity for sport for girls and women also need to be considered. This is especially evident in data for swimmers. Age group, national and Olympic level swimmers from several countries in the 1950s to 1970s presented mean ages at menarche that approximated the means of the general population, and there were no differences between younger and older swimmers.[58] However, university level swimmers from elite programmes in the US in the mid-1980s to mid-1990s have mean ages at menarche of 14.3 and 14.4 years.[21] This trend is probably related to increased opportunities for girls in swimming. In the 1950s to 1970s, it was common for female swimmers to retire by 16 to 17 years of age. With the advent of Title IX legislation in the US, some high school and many university athletic programmes added and/or improved their swim programmes so that more opportunities were available for girls and women. Also, later maturing age group swimmers, catching-up to their peers in size and strength in late adolescence, now had an opportunity to persist in the sport and may have experienced success in swimming. Another factor may be change in the size and physique of female swimmers. A comparison of university level female swimmers in the late 1980s and early 1990s with swimmers in the mid 1970s indicated that the former were taller and more linear, a physique characteristic of later maturers. The more recent swimmers were also more androgynous in build.[63]

Training for sport is commonly indicated as the causative factor in the later mean ages at menarche observed in athletes, with the inference that training 'causes' the later onset of this late maturational event. Retrospective and cross-sectional data, of course, do not permit cause–effect statements, and results of consensus discussions indicate no presently available evidence to support the conclusion that physical activity and training influence the age at menarche. Correlating years of training before menarche and age at menarche is erroneous and misleading. Assume that two girls begin training at six years of age; one is an early maturer who will attain menarche at 11 years, while the other is a late maturer who will reach menarche at 16 years. A priori there will be a correlation between the two events; the early maturer will have five years of training before menarche, while the late maturer will have ten years of training before menarche.

Training is not ordinarily quantified in these studies, and no distinction between initial participation in a sport and systematic, formal training in the sport is made. Thus, years of sport participation may not be equivalent with years of training. Further, not all athletes experience late menarche, so that those who take up systematic training after menarche are excluded in discussions of the assumed training effect. The range of reported ages at menarche in 370 elite university athletes in seven sports (swimming, diving, tennis, golf, track and field, basketball and volleyball) is 9.2 to 17.7 years, and early and late maturers are found in all seven sports.[64] The range of ages in athletes completely overlaps that in 314 non-athlete students attending the same university, 9.1 to 17.4 years (Malina, unpublished).

There are other confounding and/or modifier variables that must be considered in discussions of menarche, physical activity and training. Other factors which are known to influence menarche are generally not included in analyses. For example, sister–sister and mother–daughter correlations for age at menarche in families of athletes are similar to those for the general population,[65] and the number of siblings in the family has a similar effect on the age at menarche in

Table 2.1.4 Estimated mean/median ages (± standard deviations) from prospective and status quo studies of menarche (years) in adolescent athletes[1]

Athletes—prospective	Age	Athletes—status quo	Age
Gymnasts, Polish	15.1 ± 0.9	Gymnasts, world[3]	15.6 ± 2.1
Gymnasts, Swiss	14.5 ± 1.2	Gymnasts, Hungarian	15.0 ± 0.6
Gymnasts, Swedish	14.5 ± 1.4	Swimmers, age group, US	13.1 ± 1.1
Gymnasts, British[2]	14.3 ± 1.4	Swimmers, age group, US	12.7 ± 1.1
Swimmers, British	13.3 ± 1.1	Divers, Junior Olympic, US	13.6 ± 1.1
Tennis players, British	13.2 ± 1.4	Ballet dancers, Yugoslavia	13.6
Track, Polish	12.3 ± 1.1	Ballet dancers, Yugoslavia	14.1
Rowers, Polish	12.7 ± 0.9	Track, Hungarian	12.6
Elite ballet dancers, US	15.4 ± 1.9	Soccer players, age group, US	12.9 ± 1.1
		Team sports, Hungarian	12.7
Range of means for non-athletes[4]	12.1–13.5		

[1] Prospective data report means, while status quo data report medians based on probit analysis.

[2] Among the British athletes, 13% had not yet attained menarche so that the estimated mean ages will be somewhat later. Small numbers of Swiss and Swedish gymnasts and ballet dancers also had not reached menarche at the time of the studies.

[3] This sample is from the 1987 world championships in Rotterdam. It did not include athletes under 13 years of age so that the estimate may be biased towards an older age.

[4] Status quo estimates for European girls from the mid 1960s through the 1980s. All except two of the 39 ages were between 12.5 and 13.5 years. There is a geographic gradient in the distribution of menarcheal ages within Europe, median ages decline from the north to south. The status quo estimate for United States girls is 12.8 years.

Adapted from Malina[24] which contains the references for individual studies.

athletes as in the general population.[64] Although data are not extensive, athletes tend to be from larger families than non-athletes.[64,66]

Menarche is also influenced by a number of socially or bioculturally mediated variables, e.g. socioeconomic differentials in some countries and positive secular changes in age at menarche in association with improved health and nutritional circumstances over time. Sport specific selective factors must be considered as a part of this biocultural matrix in athletes. Current female gymnasts, for example, are younger, shorter and lighter than those of 20 to 25 years ago.[67,68] Dietary concerns are a factor among athletes, not only gymnasts, ballet dancers and figure skaters, but also in distance runners, swimmers, divers and probably others. Additional factors may interact with marginal caloric status and altered eating habits, e.g. psychological and emotional stress associated with maintaining body mass when the natural course of growth is to gain, year long training (often before school in the morning and after school in the late afternoon), frequent competitions, altered social relationships with peers, and perhaps overbearing and demanding coaches.

Aspects of the home environment are also implicated in the timing of menarche. Results of several studies suggest a role for household composition and stress as factors associated with an earlier age at menarche.[64]

If training for sport is related to the age at menarche, it probably interacts with, or is confounded by, other factors, so that a specific effect of training or physical activity *per se* may be difficult to extract. Nevertheless, two reasonably comprehensive discussions of physical activity and female reproductive health have concluded as follows: 'although menarche occurs later in athletes than in nonathletes, it has yet to be shown that exercise delays menarche in anyone' (see Ref. 69, p. S288), and 'the general consensus is that while menarche occurs later in athletes than in nonathletes, the relationship is not causal and is confounded by other factors' (see Ref. 70, pp. 2–3).

Sexual maturation of boys

The effects of training for sport on the sexual maturation of boys has not generally been considered. This may not be surprising since early and average maturation are characteristic of the majority of young male athletes. Further, males do not have an outcome variable of pubertal maturation equivalent to menarche. With the exception of constant emphasis on weight regulation in some sports, environmental stresses related to sport, such as anxiety and sleep problems, probably affect boys as well as girls. Wrestling is the primary sport among males that has an emphasis on weight regulation, but the emphasis is short term; longitudinal observations over a season indicate no significant effects on maturation and hormonal profiles.[71] Other hormonal data for adolescent males indicate gonadotrophic hormone and testosterone responses to acute or chronic exercise which vary with pubertal status and which are equivocal.[72]

It has been proposed that males are ' … better prepared physically for metabolic demands during the development of reproductive maturity…' (see Ref. 73, p. 370). This proposition presumably includes the demands associated with rigorous physical activity and training. However, longitudinal studies of males indicate no effect of regular training for sport on the timing and tempo of indicators of somatic, skeletal and sexual maturation. In the context of Warren's[73] suggestion, it has also been proposed that ' … the significant gains in strength and muscle mass which are possible in prepubertal boys undergoing resistance training could accelerate pubertal onset' (see Ref. 74, pp. 56–7).

However, resistance training in prepubertal boys results in gains in muscular strength without muscular hypertrophy; pubertal boys, on the other hand, increase in both strength and muscle mass in response to resistance training[75] (see Chapter 2.11).

Summary

There is confusion about the specific role of physical activity or training for sport as factors which may significantly influence indicators of growth status and rate, and especially sexual maturation. The confusion derives in part from a loose or imprecise use of the terms physical activity and/or training; lack of adequate longitudinal observations that span the growth spurt and pubertal maturation and in which physical activity/training are controlled; a tendency to make inferences from highly select athletes to the general population; erroneous statistical inferences (e.g. correlation does not imply a cause – effect relationship); and failure to consider other factors that are known to influence indicators of growth and maturation.

Although regular physical activity and training for sport have traditionally been viewed as having a favourable influence on growth and maturation, adequately nourished children and adolescents will grow and mature whether or not they are physically active. Conversely, more recent suggestions of negative effects of intensive physical activity and training for sport on the growth spurt and sexual maturation of adolescent girls does not appear to be warranted in light of the currently available data. Evidence for active and non-active children and adolescents, and for young athletes training in a variety of sports indicates no apparent effects of regular activity and training on size attained and rate of growth in stature, and on indices of somatic, skeletal and sexual maturation. Menarche occurs, on average, later in athletes in many sports, but the presently available data do not warrant the conclusion that training 'delays' menarche. Other factors known to be associated with menarche (as well as other indicators of biological maturation during puberty—skeletal age, timing of PHV, secondary sex characteristics) need to be considered and statistically controlled in studies of athletes and regularly active adolescents.

Allowing for variation in methodology and sampling, the data appear to emphasize a primary role for constitutional factors in the selection and sorting processes of young athletes of both sexes. If intensive training is a factor of any consequence in the size attained and maturation of young athletes, its effects must be partitioned from constitutional factors, social and environmental factors, and components of the overall sport environment before causality can be established.

In contrast, regular activity and training are important in the regulation of body mass, particularly fatness, and skeletal mineralization. It is difficult to partition training effects from expected age- and maturity-associated changes in body composition, especially fat-free mass in adolescent boys, given the close association of biological maturation and adolescent gains in fat-free and specifically muscle mass. Regular physical activity and training for sport, especially of body-mass-bearing type, are associated with enhanced skeletal mineralization, although presently available data are derived largely from samples of females.

References

1. **Rarick, G. L.** Exercise and growth. In *Science and medicine of exercise and sports* (ed. W. R. Johnson). Harper and Brothers, New York, 1960; 440–65.
2. **Malina, R. M.** and **Bouchard C.** *Growth, maturation, and physical activity.* Human Kinetics Publishers, Champaign, Il, 1991.

3. **Beyer, H. G.** The influence of exercise on growth. *Journal of Experimental Medicine* 1896; **1**: 546–58.

4. **Godin, R.** *Growth during school age* (translated by S. L. Eby). Gorham Press, Boston, 1920.

5. **Schwartz, L., Britten, R. H.** and **Thompson, L. R.** Studies in physical development and posture. 1. The effect of exercise in the physical condition and development of adolescent boys. *Public Health Bulletin* 1928; **179**: 1–38.

6. **Jokl, E., Cluver, E. H. Goedvolk, C.** and **de Jongh T. W.** *Training and efficiency.* South African Institute for Medical Research, Johannesburgh, Report 303, 1941.

7. **Parizkova, J.** Functional development and the impact of exercise. In *Puberty: Biological and psychosocial components* (ed. S. R. Berenberg). Stenfert Kroese, Leiden, 1975; 198–219.

8. **Chen, J. D.** Growth, exercise, nutrition and fitness in China. In *Human growth, physical fitness and nutrition* (ed. R.J. Shephard and J. Parizkova). Karger, Basel, 1991; 119–32.

9. **Rowe, F. A.** Growth comparisons of athletes and non-athletes. *Research Quarterly* 1933; **4**: 108–16.

10. **Shephard, R. J.** Physical activity and child health. *Sports Medicine* 1984; **1**: 205–33.

11. **Laron, Z.,** and **Klinger B.** Does intensive sport endanger normal growth and development. In *Hormones and sport* (ed. Z. Laron and A. D. Rogol). Raven, New York, 1989; 1–9.

12. **Theintz, G. E, Howald H. Weiss U.** and **Sizonenko P. C.** Evidence for a reduction of growth potential in adolescent female gymnasts. *Journal of Pediatrics* 1993; **122**: 306–13.

13. **Shuck, G. R.** Effects of athletic competition on the growth and development of junior high school boys. *Research Quarterly* 1962; **33**: 288–98.

14. **Kato, S.,** and **Ishiko T.** Obstructed growth of children's bones due to exercise labor in remote corners. In *Proceedings of international congress of sport sciences, 1964* (ed. K. Kato). Japanese Union of Sport Sciences, Tokyo, 1966; 479.

15. **Suzuki, S.,** Experimental studies on factors in growth. *Monographs of the Society for Research in Child Development* 1970; **35**(serial no. 140): 6–11.

16. American Medical Association/American Dietetic Association. *Targets for adolescent health: Nutrition and physical fitness.* American Medical Association, Chicago, 1991.

17. **Bouchard, C.,** and **Shephard R. J.** Physical activity, fitness, and health: The model and basic concepts. In *Physical activity, fitness, and health* (ed. C. Bouchard, R.J. Shephard and T. Stephens). Human Kinetics Publishers, Champaign, Il, 1994; 77–88.

18. **Malina, R. M.** Growth, exercise, fitness, and later outcomes. In *Exercise, fitness, and health: A consensus of current knowledge* (ed. C. Bouchard, R. J. Shephard, T. Stephens and B. D. McPherson). Human Kinetics Publishers, Champaign, Il, 1990; 637–53.

19. **Malina, R. M.** Physical activity and fitness of children and youth: Questions and implications. *Medicine, Exercise, Nutrition, and Health* 1995; **4**: 123–35.

20. **Malina, R. M.** Youth sports: Readiness, selection and trainability. In *Kinanthropometry IV* (ed. W. Duquet and J. A. P. Day). Spon, London, 1993; 285–301.

21. **Malina RM.** The young athlete: Biological growth and maturation in a biocultural context. In *Children and youth in sport: A biopsychosocial perspective* (ed. F.L. Smoll and R.E. Smith). Brown and Benchmark, Dubuque, IA, 1996; 161–86.

22. **Franke, W. W.** and **Berendonk B.** Hormonal doping and adrogenization of athletes: A secret programme of the German Democratic Republic government. *Clinical Chemistry* 1997; **43**: 1262–79.

23. **Malina, R. M.** Physical growth and biological maturation of young athletes. *Exercise and Sports Science Reviews* 1994; **22**: 389–433.

24. **Malina, R. M.** Growth and maturation of young athletes—Is training a factor? In *Sports and children* (ed. K-M. Chan and L.J. Micheli). Williams and Wilkins, Hong Kong, 1998; 133–61.

25. **Mansfield MJ, Emans SJ.** Growth in female gymnasts: Should training decrease during puberty? *Journal of Pediatrics* 1993; **122**: 237–40.

26. **Ziemilska, A.,** Wplyw intensywnego treningu gimnastycznego na rozwoj somatyczny i dojrzewanie dzieci. Akademia Wychowania Fizycznego, Warsaw, 1981.

27. **Malina, R. M.** Growth and maturation of elite female gymnasts: Is training a factor. In *Human growth in context* (ed. F. E. Johnston, B. Zemel and P. B. Eveleth), Smith-Gordon, London, 1999; 291–301.

28. **Theintz, G. E, Howald. H.** and **Weiss, U. Sizonenko P. C.** Evidence for a reduction of growth potential in adolescent female gymnasts. *Journal of Pediatrics* 1993; **122**: 306–13.

29. **Largo, R. H. Gasser, Th. Prader, A. Stuetzle, W.** and **Huber P. J.** Analysis of the adolescent growth spurt using smoothing spline functions. *Annals of Human Biology* 1978; **5**: 421–34.

30. **Parizkova, J.,** Longitudinal study of the relationship between body composition and anthropometric characteristics in boys during growth and development. *Glasnik Antropoloskog Drustva Jugoslavije* 1970; **7**: 33–8.

31. **Parizkova, J.,** Particularities of lean body mass and fat development in growing boys as related to their motor activity. *Acta Paediatrica Belgica* 1974; **28**: 233–43.

32. **Parizkova, J.,** *Body fat and physical fitness.* Martinus Nijhoff, The Hague, 1977.

33. **Von Dobeln, W.** and **Eriksson B. O.** Physical training, maximal oxygen uptake and dimensions of the oxygen transporting and metabolizing organs in boys 11 to 13 years of age. *Acta Paediatrica Scandinavica* 1972; **61**: 653–60.

34. **Eriksson, B. O.** Physical training, oxygen supply and muscle metabolism in 11–15 year old boys. *Acta Paediatrica Scandinavica* 1972; **384**: 1–48.

35. **Fournier, G. B,** Ricci J, Taylor AW, Ferguson RJ, Montpetit RR, Chaitman BR. Skeletal muscle adaptation in adolescent boys: Sprint and endurance training and detraining. *Medicine and Science in Sports and Exercise* 1982; **14**: 453–6.

36. **Kannus, P,** Sievanen, H. and Vuori, I. Physical loading, exercise, and bone. *Bone* 1996; **18**: 1S-3S.

37. **Slemenda, C. W. Miller J. Z. Hui S. L, Reister T. K.** and **Johnston C. C.** Role of physical activity in the development of skeletal mass in children. *Journal of Bone and Mineral Research* 1991; **6**: 1227–33.

38. **Slemenda, C. W. Reister, T. K. Hui S. L. Miller, J. A, Christian, J. C.** and **Johnston C. C.** Influences on skeletal mineralization in children and adolescents: Evidence for varying effects of sexual maturation and physical activity. *Journal of Pediatrics* 1994; **125**: 201–7.

39. **Cassell C. Benedict M.** and **Specker B.** Bone mineral density in elite 7- to 9-yr-old female gymnasts and swimmers. *Medicine and Science in Sports and Exercise* 1996; **28**: 1243–6.

40. **Grimston, SK. Willows, N. D.** and **Hanley, D. A.** Mechanical loading regime and its relationship to bone mineral density in children. *Medicine and Science in Sports and Exercise* 1993; **25**: 1203–10.

41. **Robinson, TL. Snow-Harter C. Taaffe D. R. Gillis D. Shaw, J.** and **Marcus, R.** Gymnasts exhibit higher bone mass than runners despite similar prevalence of amenorrhea and oligomenorrhea. *Journal of Bone and Mineral Research* 1995; **10**: 26–35.

42. **Slemenda, C. W.** and **Johnston, C. C.** High intensity activities in young women: Site specific bone mass effects among female figure skaters. *Bone and Mineral* 1993; **20**: 125–32.

43. **Young, N. Formica, C. Szmukler, G.** and **Seeman E.** Bone density at weight-bearing and nonweight-bearing sites in ballet dancers: The effects of exercise, hypogonadism, and body weight. *Journal of Clinical Endocrinology and Metabolism* 1994; **78**: 449–54.

44. **Kannus, P. Haapasalo, H. Sankelo, M. Sievanen, H. Pasanen, M. Heinonen A. Oja,** and **P. Vuori, I.** Effect of starting age of physical activity on bone mass in the dominant arm of tennis and squash players. *Annals of Internal Medicine* 1995; **123**: 27–31.

45. **Drinkwater, B. L. Nilson K, Chesnut CH, Bremner WJ, Shainholtz S,** and **Southworth MB.** Bone mineral content of amenorrheic and eumenorrheic athletes. *New England Journal of Medicine* 1984; **311**: 277–81.

46. Okano, H. Mizunuma, H. Soda, M-Y, Matsui, H. Aoki I. Honjo S-I. and Ibuki, Y. Effects of exercise and amenorrhea on bone mineral density in teenage runners. *Endocrine Journal* 1995; **42** : 271–6.

47. Saris, W. H. M. Elvers, J. W. H. van't Hof M. A. and Binkhorst, R. A. Changes in physical activity of children aged 6 to 12 years. In *Children and exercise XII* (ed. J. Rutenfranz, R. Mocellin and F. Klimt). Human Kinetics Publishers, Champaign, Il, 1986; 121–30.

48. Beunen, G. P. Malina, R. M. Renson, R. Simons. J. Ostyn, M. and Lefevre J. Physical activity and growth, maturation and performance: A longitudinal study. *Medicine and Science in Sports and Exercise* 1992; **24**: 576–85.

49. Malina, R. M. and Bielicki, T. Retrospective longitudinal growth study of boys and girls active in sport. *Acta Paediatrica* 1996; **85**: 570–6.

50. Malina, R. M. Regional body composition: Age, sex, and ethnic variation. In *Human body composition* (ed. A.F. Roche, S.B. Heymsfield and T.G. Lohman). Human Kinetics Publishers, Champaign, Il, 1996; 217–55.

51. Despres, J.-P., Bouchard, C. Tremblay, A. Savard, R. and Marcotte, M. Effects of aerobic training on fat distribution in male subjects. *Medicine and Science in Sports and Exercise* 1985; **17**: 113–8.

52. Tremblay, A. Despres, J.-P. Bouchard, C. Alteration in body fat and fat distribution with exercise. In *Fat distribution during growth and later health outcomes* (ed. C. Bouchard and F.E. Johnston). Liss, New York, 1988; 297–312.

53. Bjorntorp, P. Grimby, C. Sanne, H. Sjostrom, L. Tibblin, G. and Wilhelmsen, L. Adipose tissue fat cell size in relation to metabolism in weight-stable physically active men. *Hormone and Metabolism Research* 1972; **4**: 178–82.

54. Beunen, G. P. Malina, R. M. and Thomis, M. Physical growth and maturation of female gymnasts. In *Human growth in context* (ed. F. E. Johnston, B. Zemel and P. B. Eveleth). Smith-Gordon, London, 1999; 281–9.

55. Geithner, C. A., Woynarowska, B. and Malina, R. M. The adolescent spurt and sexual maturation in girls active and not active in sport. *Annals of Human Biology* 1998; **25**: 415–23.

56. Warren, M. P. The effects of exercise on pubertal progression and reproductive function in girls. *Journal of Clinical Endocrinology and Metabolism* 1980; **51**: 1150–7.

57. Tanner, J. M. *Growth at adolescence* (2nd edn). Blackwell Scientific Publications, Oxford, 1962.

58. Malina, R. M. Menarche in athletes: A synthesis and hypothesis. *Annals of Human Biology* 1983; **10**: 1–24.

59. Beunen G, and Malina R. M. Growth and biological maturation: Relevance to athletic performance. In *The child and adolescent athlete* (ed. O. Bar-Or). Blackwell Science, Oxford, 1996; 3–24.

60. Constantini, N. W. and Warren, M. P. Physical activity, fitness, and reproductive health in women: Clinical observations. In *Physical activity, fitness, and health* (ed. C. Bouchard, R.J. Shephard and T. Stephens). Human Kinetics Publishers, Champaign, Il, 1994; 955–66.

61. Warren, M. P. Amenorrhea in ballet dancers. *Abstracts, Eleventh International Jerusalem Symposium on Sports Injuries.* Israel Society of Sports Medicine, Tel Aviv, 1995; 18.

62. Eveleth, P. B. and Tanner, J. M. *Worldwide variation in human growth* (2nd edn). Cambridge University Press, Cambridge, 1990.

63. Malina, R. M. and Merrett, D. M. S. Androgyny of physique of women athletes: Comparisons by sport and over time. In *Essays on auxology* (ed. R. Hauspie, G. Lindgren and F. Falkner). Castlemead Publications, Welwyn Garden City, Hertfordshire, 1995: 355–63.

64. Malina, R. M. Katzmarzyk, P. T. Bonci, C. M. Ryan, R. C. and Wellens, R. E. Family size and age at menarche in athletes. *Medicine and Science in Sports and Exercise* 1997; **29**: 99–106.

65. Malina, R. M. Ryan, R. C. and Bonci, C. M. Age at menarche in athletes and their mothers and sisters. *Annals of Human Biology* 1994; **21**: 417–22.

66. Malina, R. M. Bouchard, C. Shoup, R. F. and Lariviere, G. Age, family size and birth order in Montreal Olympic athletes. In *Physical structure of Olympic athletes: Part I. The Montreal Olympic games anthropological project* (ed. J. E.L. Carter). S. Karger, Basel, 1982: 13–24.

67. Claessens, A. L. Elite female gymnasts: a kinanthropometric view. In *Human growth in context* (ed. F. E. Johnston, B. Zemel and P. B. Eveleth). Smith-Gordon, London, 1999; 273–80.

68. Malina, R. M. Growth and maturation of female gymnasts. *Spotlight on youth sports*, Institute for the Study of Youth Sports, Michigan State University 1996; **19**: 1–3.

69. Loucks, A. B. Vaitukaitis, J. Cameron, J. L. Rogol, A. D. Skrinar, G. Warren, M. P. Kendrick, J. and Limacher, M. C. The reproductive system and exercise in women. *Medicine and Science in Sports and Exercise* 1992; 24:S288–93.

70. Clapp, J. F. and Little, K. D. The interaction between regular exercise and selected aspects of women's health. *American Journal of Obstetrics and Gynecology* 1995; **173**: 2–9.

71. Roemmich, J. N. Weight loss effects on growth, maturation, growth related hormones, protein nutrition markers, and body composition of adolescent wrestlers. Doctoral Dissertation, Kent State University, Kent, OH, 1994.

72. Malina, R. M. Darwinian fitness, physical fitness and physical activity. In *Applications of biological anthropology to human affairs* (ed. C.G.N. Mascie-Taylor and G.W. Lasker). Cambridge University Press, Cambridge, 1991; 143–84.

73. Warren MP. Effects of undernutrition on reproductive function in the human. *Endocrine Reviews* 1983; 4: 363–77.

74. Cumming, D. C. Wheeler, G. D. and Harber, V. J. Physical activity, nutrition, and reproduction. *Annals of the New York Academy of Sciences* 1994; **709**: 55–74.

75. Sale, D. G. Strength training in children. In *Youth, exercise, and sport* (ed. C. Gisolfi and DR. Lamb). Benchmark Press, Carmel, In, 1989; 165–216.

76. Fujii, K. An investigation regarding sequence of age at MPV in physique growth of male athletes. *Studies of growth and development, Japanese Society of Physical Education* 1998; **26**: 26–32.

77. Malina. R. M. and Beunen, G. Monitoring of growth and maturation. In *The child and adolescent athlete* (ed. O. Bar-Or). Blackwell Science, Oxford, 1996; 647–72.

78. Mirwald, R. L. Bailey, D. A. Cameron, N. and Rasmussen, R. L. Longitudinal comparison of aerobic power in active and inactive boys aged 7.0 to 17.0 years. *Annals of Human Biology* 1981; 8: 405–14.

2.2   Biomechanics of movement

James Watkins

Introduction

All movements and changes in movement are brought about by the action of forces. A force may be defined as that which alters or tends to alter an object's state of rest or type of movement. Human movement is brought about by the musculoskeletal system under the control of the nervous system. The musculoskeletal system consists of the skeletal muscles, the skeleton and joints. The skeleton consists basically of a number of fairly rigid components, the bones, joined together in a way which allows the bones to move in relation to each other. The skeletal muscles pull on the bones in order to control the movement of the joints and, thereby, the movement of the body as a whole. By coordinated activity between the various muscle groups, forces generated by the muscles are transmitted by the bones and joints to enable the individual to maintain an upright or partially upright posture and bring about voluntary controlled movements. Consequently, the musculoskeletal system, also referred to as the locomotor system, is essentially a machine, i.e. a powered mechanism for generating and transmitting forces in order to counteract the effects of gravity and bring about desirable movements of the body.[1]

Mechanics is the study of the forces acting on objects and the effects of the forces on the movement, size, shape and structure of the objects. Biomechanics is the study of the forces that act on, and within, biological systems and the effects of the forces on the size, shape and structure of the biological systems. Biomechanics of human movement is the study of the relationship between the external forces (due to body weight and physical contact with the external environment) and internal forces (active forces generated by muscles and passive forces exerted on other structures) which act on the body and the effect of these forces on the movement of the body.[2]

Forms of motion

There are two basic forms of motion, linear and angular. Linear motion, also referred to as translation occurs when all parts of an object move the same distance in the same direction in the same time. When the movement is in a straight line the motion is called rectilinear translation (Fig. 2.2.1(a)). When the movement follows a curved path the motion is called curvilinear translation (Fig. 2.2.1(b)).

Angular motion, also referred to as rotation, occurs when an object or part of an object moves in a circular path about a line in space such that all parts of the object move through the same angle in the same direction in the same time. The axis of rotation may be stationary or it may experience linear motion (Fig. 2.2.2).

Most whole body human movements involve a combination of linear and angular motion. For example, while walking the head and

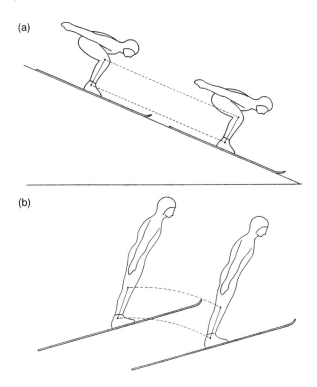

Fig. 2.2.1   Linear motion: a ski jumper is likely to experience rectilinear motion on the runway (a) and curvilinear motion during flight (b).

trunk experience more-or-less continuous linear motion and the other segments experience simultaneous linear and angular motion as the body as a whole moves forward (Fig. 2.2.3). Movement of a multi-segmented system involving linear and angular motion of one or more segments is usually referred to as general motion.

Kinematics

Kinematics is the branch of mechanics that describes the movement of an object in terms of the position and change in position with time of the object with respect to its spatial environment. A kinematic analysis describes the movement of the object in terms of distance (amount of change in position), speed (rate of change of position), and acceleration (variability in the rate of change of position). Distance and speed are scalar quantities, that is, like area, volume and temperature, they can be completely specified in terms of magnitude. Displacement, velocity, acceleration and force are vector quantities, i.e. they specify

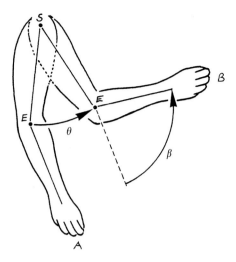

Fig. 2.2.2 Angular motion: as the arm swings forward from position A to position B the upper arm rotates through an angle of θ about a stationary transverse (side to side) axis S through the shoulder and the lower arm and hand simultaneously rotate through an angle β about a transverse axis E through the elbow joint. E experiences curvilinear motion.

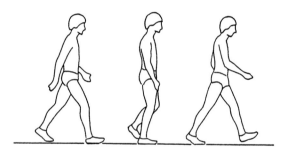

Fig. 2.2.3 General motion: during walking the trunk and head experience more-or-less continuous rectilinear motion and the other segments experience simultaneous linear and angular motion while the body as a whole moves forward.

magnitude and direction. Displacement indicates distance in a given direction. Similarly, velocity indicates speed in a given direction, i.e. rate of change of displacement. Acceleration is rate of change of velocity. There is no general term for the scalar equivalent of acceleration.

Linear kinematics

Linear kinematics describe linear motion. In the metric system of units linear distance is measured in centimetres (cm) or metres (m), linear speed is measured in centimetres per second ($cm\,s^{-1}$) or metres per second ($m\,s^{-1}$), and linear acceleration is measured in centimetres per second per second ($cm\,s^{-2}$) or metres per second per second ($m\,s^{-2}$). If a sprinter completes a 100 m race in 10.6 s his average linear velocity $\bar{v}$ is given by $\bar{v} = d/t$ where d = distance = 100 m and t = time = 10.6 s, i.e.

$$\bar{v} = \frac{100\,\text{m}}{10.6\,\text{s}} = 9.43\,\text{m}\,\text{s}^{-1}$$

Whereas the sprinter's average velocity is $9.43\,\text{m}\,\text{s}^{-1}$, his actual velocity is likely to vary considerably during the race. Following the start his velocity gradually increases up to maximum, achieved after approximately 50 m in elite sprinters, and then he tries to maintain maximum velocity till the end of the race. However, his velocity is likely to decrease during the latter part of the race. If, for example, he achieved a maximum velocity of $11\,\text{m}\,\text{s}^{-1}$ after 5.5 s his average acceleration $\bar{a}$ during this period is given by $\bar{a} = (v_2 - v_1)/(t_2 - t_1)$ where $t_1 = 0 =$ time at start of time period, $t_2 =$ time at end of time period = 5.5 s, $v_1 =$ velocity at $t_1 = 0$, and $v_2 =$ velocity at $t_2 = 11\,\text{m}\,\text{s}^{-1}$, i.e.

$$\bar{a} = \frac{11\,\text{m}\,\text{s}^{-1} - 0\,\text{m}\,\text{s}^{-1}}{5.5\,\text{s} - 0\,\text{s}} = \frac{11\,\text{m}\,\text{s}^{-1}}{5.5\,\text{s}} = 2\,\text{m}\,\text{s}^{-2}$$

The positive figure of $2\,\text{m}\,\text{s}^{-2}$ indicates that the sprinter's velocity increased by an average of $2\,\text{m}\,\text{s}^{-1}$ every second during the first 5.5 s of the race. Similarly, if the velocity of the sprinter at the finish of the race was $9.4\,\text{m}\,\text{s}^{-1}$ his average acceleration during the latter part of the race is given by:

$$\bar{a} = \frac{9.4\,\text{m}\,\text{s}^{-1} - 11\,\text{m}\,\text{s}^{-1}}{10.6\,\text{s} - 5.5\,\text{s}} = \frac{-1.6\,\text{m}\,\text{s}^{-1}}{5.1\,\text{s}} = -0.31\,\text{m}\,\text{s}^{-2}$$

The negative figure of $-0.31\,\text{m}\,\text{s}^{-2}$ indicates that the sprinter's velocity decreased by an average of $0.31\,\text{m}\,\text{s}^{-1}$ during the last 5.1 s of the race. Positive acceleration is usually referred to simply as acceleration, and negative acceleration is usually referred to as deceleration.

Angular kinematics

Angular kinematics describe angular motion. Figure 2.2.4 shows a gymnast rotating about a horizontal bar in an clockwise direction with respect to Fig. 2.2.4. In rotating from position (a) to position (d) the angular distance and angular displacement (angular distance in a clockwise direction) is 180°. In rotating from position (a) through (d) and back to (a) the angular distance is 360° but the angular displacement is zero.

In mechanics angular distance is usually measured in radians rather than degrees. A radian is defined as the angle subtended at the centre of a circle by an arc on the circumference equal in length to the radius of the circle (Fig. 2.2.5).

Angular speed is the rate of change of angular distance and angular velocity is the rate of change of angular displacement. If the angular displacement of the gymnast, with respect to position (a), changes from 1.04 radians (about 60°) at position (b) to 2.09 radians (about 120°) at position (c) in 0.3 s the average angular velocity $\bar{\omega}$ of the gymnast during this period is given by $\bar{\omega} = (\sigma_2 - \sigma_1)/(t_2 - t_1)$ where $t_1 =$ time at start of time period = 0 (for the example), $t_2 =$ time at end of time period = 0.3 s, $\sigma_1 =$ angular displacement at $t_1 = 1.04$ radians, and $\sigma_2 =$ angular displacement at $t_2 = 2.09$ radians, i.e.

$$\bar{\omega} = \frac{2.09\,\text{rad} - 1.04\,\text{rad}}{0.3\,\text{s} - 0\,\text{s}} = \frac{1.05\,\text{rad}}{0.3\,\text{s}} = 5.25\,\text{rad}\,\text{s}^{-1}$$

Angular acceleration is the rate of change of angular velocity. If the angular velocity of the gymnast changes from $3.8\,\text{rad}\,\text{s}^{-1}$ at position (b) to $6.1\,\text{rad}\,\text{s}^{-1}$ at position (c) in 0.3 s the average angular acceleration $\bar{\alpha}$ of the gymnast during this period is given by $\bar{\alpha} = (\omega_2 - \omega_1)/(t_2 - t_1)$

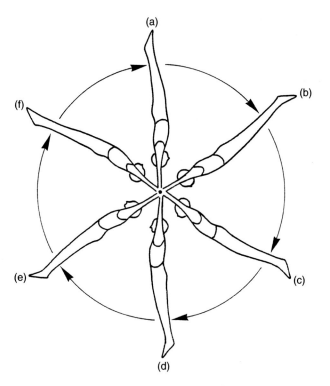

Fig. 2.2.4 A gymnast rotating about a high bar.

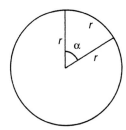

Fig. 2.2.5 A radian is the angle subtended at the centre of a circle by an arc on the circumference equal in length to the radius of the circle.

where t_1 = time at start of time period = 0 (for the example), t_2 = time at end of time period = 0.3 s, ω_1 angular velocity at t_1 = 3.8 rad s^{-1}, and $\bar{\omega}_2$ = angular velocity at t_2 = 6.1 rad s^{-1}, i.e.

$$\bar{\alpha} = \frac{6.1 \text{ rad s}^{-1} - 3.8 \text{ rad s}^{-1}}{0.3 \text{ s} - 0 \text{ s}} = \frac{2.3 \text{ rad s}^{-1}}{0.3 \text{ s}}$$

$$\bar{\alpha} = 7.67 \text{ rad s}^{-2}$$

Kinetics

Kinetics is the branch of mechanics that describes the forces acting on objects, i.e. the cause of the observed kinematics. Linear kinetics describes the causes and changes of linear motion. Angular kinetics describes the causes and changes of angular motion.

Linear kinetics

Force is a vector quantity and, as such, a force can be represented diagrammatically by a straight line with an arrowhead; the length of the line corresponds (with respect to an appropriate scale) to the magnitude of the force and the orientation of the line (with respect to an appropriate reference axis) and arrow head indicate the direction. Figure 2.2.6(a) represents a curling stone resting on a perfectly flat horizontal ice rink and acted on by three horizontal forces A, B and C which are shown as vectors. Assuming that the friction between the stone and the ice is negligible, the movement of the stone will depend entirely on the three forces. Each force will tend to move the stone in the direction in which the force is acting. However, the net effect of all of the forces is equivalent to a single resultant force. The forces A, B and C are called component forces of the resultant force. The resultant of two or more forces can be determined in two ways: vector chain method and parallelogram of vectors method. In the vector chain method the component vectors are linked together in a chain (in any order) and the resultant vector runs from the start of the first component vector in the chain to the end point of the last component vector. Figure 2.2.6(b) shows the vector chain determination of the resultant R of the component forces A, B and C. Consequently, the stone will move as if acted on by a single force R (Fig. 2.2.6(c)).

In the parallelogram of vectors method two component vectors form adjacent sides of a parallelogram. The resultant of the two component vectors is the vector consisting of the diagonal of the completed parallelogram. When there are three or more component vectors the resultant R_1 of any two components is determined and then the resultant of R_1 and another component vector is found and so on until the resultant of all of the vectors is found. Figures 2.2.6(d) and (e) show the determination of the resultant R of the three component vectors A, B and C using the parallelogram of vectors method.

Mass, inertia and linear momentum

The mass of an object is the quantity of matter comprising the object. Mass is the product of volume and density (mass per unit volume). For example, a golf ball and a table tennis ball have a similar volume

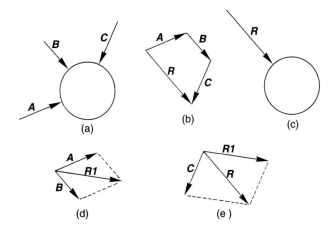

Fig. 2.2.6 Component forces and resultant forces acting on a curling stone; all forces are shown as vectors. (a) Three forces A, B and C acting on the stone; (b) vector chain determination of the resultant force R; (c) resultant force R acting on the stone; (d) determination of the resultant R_1 of A and B by the parallelogram of vectors method; (e) determination of the resultant of R_1 and C by the parallelogram of vectors method.

(occupy the same amount of space) but the density and, consequently, the mass of a golf ball is much greater than that of a table tennis ball. A stationary object, such as a rock resting on the ground, exhibits a reluctance to move, i.e. a certain amount of effort is needed to move it and the greater the mass the greater the effort required. The reluctance of a stationary object to move linearly is called its inertia and the greater the mass the greater the inertia.

Just as a stationary object exhibits a reluctance to start moving, a moving object exhibits a reluctance to change the way it is moving, i.e. a reluctance to change its linear velocity. The product of the mass (m) and the linear velocity (v) of an object is called its linear momentum (mv). The effect of a change in the resultant force acting on an object on the linear motion of the object depends on the amount of change (magnitude and direction) in the resultant force in relation to the mass (stationary object) or the linear momentum (moving object) of the object. The relationship between change in resultant force and change in linear motion is described in Newton's laws of motion (Isaac Newton 1642–1727). The three laws apply to linear motion and angular motion (see later section on angular kinetics).

Newton's laws of motion in relation to linear motion

The first law (law of inertia) incorporates the fundamental principle that a change in resultant force is necessary to bring about a change in movement, i.e. *an object will remain stationary or continue to move with constant linear velocity unless compelled to move and/or change its linear velocity by a change in the resultant force acting on it.*

Newton's second law (law of momentum) relates the change in linear momentum experienced by an object to the change in resultant force, i.e. *the change in linear momentum experienced by an object as a result of a change in the resultant force acting on it takes place in the direction of the change in resultant force and is directly proportional to the magnitude and duration of the change in resultant force.* The second law in relation to linear motion can be expressed algebraically as follows:

$$Ft = mv_2 - mv_1 \qquad (1)$$

where F = change in resultant force, t = duration of F, m = mass of object, v_1 = velocity of object in the direction of F at the start of time period, and v_2 = velocity of object in the direction of F at the end of the time period. The product of F and t is called the impulse of F. From equation (1), $F = m(v_2 - v_1)/t = ma$ since $(v_2 - v_1)/t = a$ = linear acceleration. Consequently,

(1) when the linear acceleration of an object is zero the resultant force acting on the object is zero, i.e. the object is stationary or moving with constant linear velocity;

(2) for a constant mass, which is usually the case in the analysis of human movement, the greater the change in the resultant force the greater the change in linear acceleration.

Newton's third law (law of interaction) incorporates the fundamental principle that *objects in contact exert equal and opposite forces on each other.*

Units of force

In the metric system the unit of force is the Newton (N) which is defined in accordance with Newton's second law of motion as the force which accelerates a mass of one kilogram at 1 m s^{-2}, i.e. $1 \text{ N} = 1 \text{ kg} \times 1 \text{ m s}^{-2} = 1 \text{ kg m s}^{-2}$. Since the acceleration due to gravity is 9.81 m s^{-2} it follows that the weight of a mass of 1 kg, often referred to as 1 kg wt, is given by $1 \text{ kg wt} = 1 \text{ kg} \times 9.81 \text{ m s}^{-2} = 9.81 \text{ kg m s}^{-2} = 9.81 \text{ N}$. The kg wt is a gravitational unit of force.

Contact forces and attraction forces

There are two types of forces, contact forces and attraction forces. Contact forces result from contact of one object with another. For example, the articular surfaces of the hip joint exert compression (pressing, pushing) forces on each other in postures where body weight is supported by the legs, as in standing upright. Similarly the muscles exert tension (pulling) forces on bones in order to control joint movements. Attraction forces tend to move objects towards each other (positive attraction) or away from each other (negative attraction). The human body is subjected to one considerable positive attraction force, i.e. body weight. The weight of an object is the pulling force exerted on the object by the earth, i.e. the force due to gravity. In accordance with Newton's second law of motion the weight W of an object is given by $W = mg$ where m = mass of the object, g = acceleration due to gravity = 9.81 m s^{-2}.

Centre of gravity

Whereas the mass and consequently the weight of an object is distributed throughout the whole of its volume, the object behaves, in terms of the effect of its weight on its movement, as if all of its weight is concentrated at a point called the centre of gravity of the object. Figure 2.2.7(a) shows the human body divided into ten segments (head and neck, trunk, upper arms, lower arms and hands, thighs, lower legs and feet) with the weight of each segment acting at its centre of gravity. Figure 2.2.7(b) shows the whole body centre of gravity.

Angular kinetics

Figures 2.2.8(a) and (b) represent a curling stone on a perfectly flat horizontal ice rink; the stone is acted on by a horizontal force F which is concentric, i.e. the line of action of F passes through the centre of gravity of the stone. A concentric force produces (or tends to produce) rectilinear translation. Assuming that the frictional force between the stone and the ice is negligible, the only horizontal force acting on the stone is the concentric force F and, as such, the stone will experience rectilinear translation in the direction of F. In Fig. 2.2.8(c) the force F is eccentric, i.e. its line of action does not pass through the centre of gravity of the stone. An eccentric force produces (or tends to produce) simultaneous rectilinear translation and rotation of an object about an axis which passes through the centre of gravity of the object and is perpendicular to the eccentric force. Consequently, in response to the eccentric force F the stone will experience simultaneous rectilinear translation and rotation about a vertical axis Y^G passing through its centre of gravity (Figs 2.2.8(c) and (d)).

In some situations the position of Y^G is fixed as, for example, in a child's roundabout which is designed to rotate about a fixed vertical support which passes through the centre of gravity of the roundabout. In response to a horizontal eccentric force F exerted on the roundabout the support exerts a force T on the roundabout which is equal and opposite to F (Fig. 2.2.8(e)). The tendency of F and T to translate the roundabout cancel each other out but the rotation effect of F

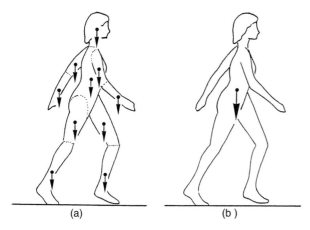

Fig. 2.2.7 Centre of gravity: (a) a ten-segment model of the human body showing the positions of the centres of gravity of the segments and the weights of the segments; (b) the centre of gravity of the whole body.

remains, i.e. the roundabout rotates about Y^G, but does not translate. The force system produced by F and T is called a couple; a couple produces (or tends to produce) rotation without translation.

Moment of a force and resultant moment

The tendency of a force to rotate an object about a particular axis depends upon the moment (also referred to as turning moment and torque) of the force about the axis of rotation. The moment of a force is the product of the magnitude of the force and the perpendicular distance between the line of action of the force and the axis of rotation. The latter is usually referred to as the moment arm of the force. In Figs 2.2.8(c) and (e) the moment of the force F is Fd where d is the moment arm of F about Y^G. In the metric system the moment arm of a force is measured in centimetres or metres and the moment of a force is measured in Newton centimetres (N cm) or Newton metres (N m).

When two or more eccentric forces act on an object the net effect of the forces on rotation of the object is determined by the resultant moment. For example, Fig. 2.2.9(a) represents a curling stone on a perfectly flat horizontal ice rink; the stone is acted on by two horizontal eccentric forces A and B which are shown as vectors. A exerts a clockwise moment on the stone about Y^G and B exerts an anticlockwise moment on the stone about Y^G. If clockwise moments are regarded as positive and anticlockwise moments are regarded as negative, the resultant moment RM exerted on the stone by A and B about Y^G is given by $RM = (A \times d_1) - (B \times d_2)$. If $A = 20$ N, $B = 25$ N, $d_1 = 4$ cm and $d_2 = 8$ cm then,

$$RM = (20 \text{ N} \times 4 \text{ cm}) - (25 \text{ N} \times 8 \text{ cm})$$
$$RM = 80 \text{ N cm} - 200 \text{ N cm}$$
$$RM = -120 \text{ N cm}$$

Consequently, the resultant moment exerted by A and B is an anticlockwise moment of 120 N cm. The resultant moment is equivalent to the moment of the resultant force, i.e. the resultant of A and B. The vector chain determination of the resultant R of A and B is shown in Fig. 2.2.9(b); $R = 24$ N. The moment arm d_3 of R about Y^G is given by $d_3 =$ resultant moment/resultant force $= 120$ N cm/24 N $= 5$ cm. (Fig. 2.2.9(c)).

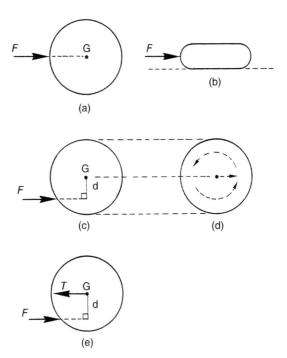

Fig. 2.2.8 Concentric force, eccentric force and couple. (a) Concentric force F acting on a curling stone (overhead view); (b) concentric force F acting on the curling stone (side view); (c) eccentric force F acting on the curling stone (overhead view); (d) effect of eccentric force F on the movement of the curling stone (overhead view); (e) couple (Fd) acting on a child's roundabout (overhead view). $G =$ centre of gravity.

Moment of inertia and angular momentum

As described earlier, a stationary object exhibits a certain reluctance (inertia) to translate. Similarly, a stationary object also exhibits a certain reluctance to rotate. The reluctance of an object to start rotating about a particular axis is called its moment of inertia. The moment of inertia of an object about a particular axis depends upon the mass of the object and the distribution of its mass around the axis. The more concentrated the mass around the axis the smaller the moment of inertia and vice versa. Just as a stationary object exhibits a reluctance to start rotating, a rotating object exhibits a reluctance to change the way it is rotating, i.e. a reluctance to change its angular momentum. The angular momentum ($I\omega$) of an object with respect to a particular axis of rotation is the product of the moment of inertia (I) of the object about the axis and the angular velocity (ω) of the object about the axis. Since the moment of inertia of an object about a particular axis depends upon the distribution of mass around the axis, the angular velocity of the object can be varied by changing the moment of inertia while the angular momentum stays the same. For example, when a gymnast performs a front somersault following a run-up the body rotates about a transverse (side to side) axis Z^G through the centre of gravity of the whole body (Fig. 2.2.10). Just after take-off the moment of inertia of the gymnast about Z^G is large due to the extended body position. In order to rotate faster the gymnast tucks her body which considerably reduces her moment of inertia about Z^G and simultaneously increases her angular velocity since, in accordance with Newton's first law of motion, angular momentum is conserved during the flight phase. Having completed the somersault the gymnast extends her body in preparation for landing which increases her moment of inertia about

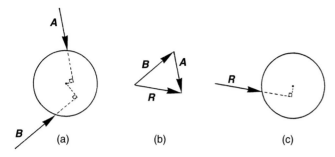

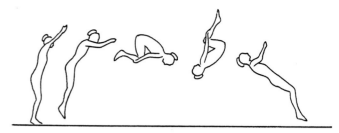

Fig. 2.2.9 Resultant moment. (a) Curling stone acted on by eccentric forces *A* and *B* (overhead view): *A* = 20 N, d_1 = moment arm of *A* = 4 cm; *B* = 25 N, d_2 = moment arm of *B* = 8 cm. (b) Vector chain determination of the resultant *R* of *A* and *B*. (c) Resultant R acting on the stone: *R* = 24 N, d_3 = moment arm of R = 5 cm.

Z^G and simultaneously decreases her angular velocity. The effect of a change in the resultant moment of force acting on an object on the angular motion of the object depends on the amount of change (magnitude and direction) in the resultant moment in relation to the moment of inertia (stationary object) or angular momentum (rotating object) of the object. The relationship between change in resultant moment and change in angular motion is described in Newton's laws of motion.

Newton's laws of motion in relation to angular motion

In relation to angular motion Newton's first law of motion may be expressed as follows: *with respect to a particular axis of rotation an object will remain stationary or continue to rotate with constant angular momentum unless compelled to rotate and/or change its angular momentum by a change in the resultant moment acting on it.*

Newton's second law of motion in relation to angular motion relates the change in resultant moment to the change in angular momentum and may be expressed as follows: *the change in angular momentum experienced by an object (about a particular axis of rotation) as a result of a change in the resultant moment acting on the object takes place in the direction of the change in resultant moment and is directly proportional to the magnitude and duration of the change in resultant moment.* The second law in relation to angular motion can be expressed algebraically as follows:

$$(Fd)t = I\omega_2 - I\omega_1 \qquad (2)$$

where *Fd* = change in resultant moment, *t* = duration of *Fd*, *I* = moment of inertia of the object, ω_1 = angular velocity of the object in the direction of *Fd* at the start of the time period, and ω_2 = angular velocity of the object in the direction of *Fd* at the end of the time period. The product of *Fd* and *t* is called the impulse of *Fd*. From equation (2), $Fd = I(\omega_2 - \omega_1)/t = I\alpha$ since $(\omega_2 - \omega_1)/t = \alpha$ = angular acceleration. Consequently,

(1) with respect to a particular axis of rotation, when the angular acceleration of the object is zero, the resultant moment acting on the object is zero, i.e. the object is stationary or rotating with constant angular momentum;

(2) for a particular moment of inertia the greater the change in resultant moment the greater the change in angular acceleration.

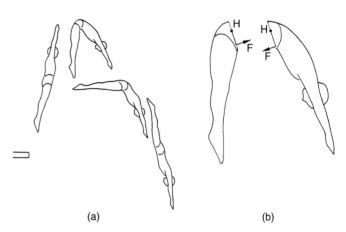

Fig. 2.2.10   A gymnast performing a front somersault following a run-up.

Fig. 2.2.11 Newton's third law of motion in relation to angular motion: (a) a diver performing a forward pike dive; (b) during the piking action the hip flexors (*F*) exert equal and opposite moments of force on the upper body and the legs. H = hip joint centre.

Figure 2.2.11(a) shows a diver performing a forward piked dive. Just after the take-off the body is in an extended position. The diver then flexes his hips to achieve the pike position. In doing so the hip flexor muscles pull equally on both of their attachments, the upper body and the legs. Furthermore the hip flexor muscles exert equal and opposite moments of force on the upper body and the legs (Fig. 2.2.11(b)). The effect of the hip flexor muscles in piking the hips illustrates Newton's third law in relation to rotation, i.e. *when two objects A and B are linked together and free to rotate about a common axis of rotation T, and object A exerts a moment of force on object B about T, then there will be an equal and opposite moment of force exerted simultaneously by object B on object A about T.*

Work and energy

In mechanics a force does work when it moves its point of application in the direction of the force and the amount of work done is the product of the force and the distance moved by its point of application. For example, in moving from a sitting to a standing position the work done on the body is equal to *FD*, where *F* is an upward force marginally greater than body weight and *D* is the vertical displacement of the whole body centre of gravity. *F* must be greater than body weight in order to create a resultant upward force. However, when speed of movement is not important it is reasonable to consider F to be equal to body weight. With this proviso, if the weight W of the man in Fig. 2.2.12 is 75 kg wt and D is 0.45 m, then the work done by his leg muscles is given by,

$$\text{Work done} = WD$$
$$= 75 \text{ kg wt} \times 0.45 \text{ m}$$
$$= 735.7 \text{ N} \times 0.45 \text{ m}$$
$$= 331 \text{ Nm}$$

One Newton metre (Nm) is the work done by a force of 1 N when it moves its point of application a distance of 1 m in the direction of the force. A Newton metre of work (rather than torque) is usually referred to as a Joule (J), i.e. in the above example the work done is 331 J.

In doing this work the leg muscles expend energy, i.e. chemical energy in the muscle cells is converted to mechanical energy in the form of work. A body (object) is said to have energy if it can do work. When a muscle contracts isometrically (no change in length) it expends energy but does no work. When a muscle contracts concentrically (shortens) it does work by pulling its skeletal attachments closer together. When a muscle contracts eccentrically (lengthens) it expends energy in creating muscle tension, but in contrast to a concentric contraction, work is done on the muscle–tendon unit, i.e. it lengthens and as it does so the elastic components of the muscle–tendon unit absorbs energy in the form of strain energy. Strain energy in a muscle–tendon unit is an example of potential energy, i.e. stored energy which, given appropriate conditions, may be used to do work. In the case of strain energy in a muscle–tendon unit, the extent to which the strain energy can be utilized to do work, rather than being completely dissipated as heat, depends largely on the speed of change-over from eccentric to concentric activity; in general, the faster the change-over the greater the proportion of the strain energy which is likely to be recycled in the form of work.

Conservation of energy

If a ball of mass m is dropped from a height h and hits the floor after time t, then in accordance with Newton's second law of motion,

$$mgt = mv \qquad (3)$$

where mg = weight of the ball and v = the velocity of the ball as it hits the floor.

The average velocity of an object acted on by a constant force for a time t is given by $(v_1 + v_2)/2$ where v_1 and v_2 are the velocities of the object at the start and end of the time period. The weight of the ball is a constant force and, consequently, its average velocity during its fall is equal to $v/2$ since its initial velocity is zero. The average velocity of the ball is also equal to h/t. Consequently, $v/2 = h/t$ and, therefore, $t = 2h/v$. By substitution of t from this expression into equation (3),

$$mg \times 2h/v = mv$$
i.e. $$mgh = (mv^2)/2$$

The term mgh is the work done (force $mg \times$ distance h) on the ball during its fall and the term $(mv^2)/2$ is referred to as the kinetic energy of the ball, i.e. the energy possessed by the ball by virtue of its linear

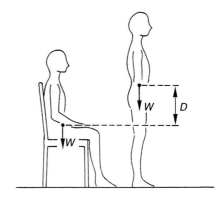

Fig. 2.2.12 Work done in moving from a sitting to a standing position: work done by leg muscles = WD, where W = body weight and D = upward vertical displacement of whole body centre of gravity.

motion. Consequently, the work done on the ball is equivalent to the kinetic energy gained by the ball. As well as representing the work done on the ball the term mgh also represents the gravitational potential energy of the ball, i.e. the potential energy possessed by the ball by virtue of its height above the floor. At the instant of release the gravitational potential energy of the ball is maximum and its kinetic energy is zero. At the instant that the ball hits the floor its gravitational potential energy is zero and its kinetic energy is maximum, i.e. the gravitational potential energy has been transformed into kinetic energy and the total amount of energy possessed by the ball remains unchanged throughout its fall. This illustrates the principle of conservation of energy, i.e. energy cannot be created or destroyed, it can only be converted from one form of energy to another, in the above example from gravitational potentisal energy to kinetic energy.

Total body energy

Just as an object moving with linear velocity possesses a certain amount of linear kinetic energy $(mv^2)/2$, where v is the linear velocity of the centre of gravity of the object, a rotating object possesses a certain amount of angular kinetic energy $(I\omega^2)/2$ where I is the moment of inertia of the object about an axis through its centre of gravity perpendicular to the plane of motion and ω is the angular velocity of the object about the axis. Consequently, at any particular point in time the total mechanical energy E of an object is given by $E = GPE + LKE + AKE$, where GPE = gravitational potential energy, LKE = linear kinetic energy and AKE = angular kinetic energy.[3]

Mechanical efficiency of the human body

The total mechanical energy E of a multisegmental system like the human body is the sum of the mechanical energies of all the segments, i.e.

$$E(t) = \sum_{i=1}^{n} PE(i, t) + \sum_{i=1}^{n} LKE(i, t) + \sum_{i=1}^{n} AKE(i, t)$$

where $E(t)$ = energy of body at time t; $PE(i, t)$ = gravitational potential energy of the ith segment at time t; $LKE(i, t)$ = linear kinetic energy of the ith segment at time t; $AKE(i, t)$ = angular kinetic energy of the ith segment at time t; n = number of segments.

In human movements net concentric muscular activity (positive work) increases $E(t)$ and net eccentric work (negative work) decreases $E(t)$. However, both positive and negative work contribute to the metabolic cost of the activity. Consequently, the work done W on the body during a particular period of time is the absolute sum of all the positive and negative changes in $E(t)$ during the time period, i.e.

$$W = \sum_{i=1}^{n} |\Delta E_c|$$

where ΔE_c = change (increase or decrease) in $E(t)$ during the ith change; n = the number of changes. Mechanical efficiency is given by,

$$\eta = \frac{W}{C} \times 100\%$$

where C = metabolic cost. W is the result of muscular activity (active work) and the utilization of strain energy in the musculoskeletal system (passive work). Consequently,

$$\eta = \frac{\text{active work} + \text{passive work}}{C} \times 100\%$$

Since C reflects active work, a decrease in C indicates a decrease in active work. Consequently, an increase in mechanical efficiency is likely to reflect greater utilization of strain energy.

Coordination and control of human movement

The brain coordinates and controls movement via muscular activity.[4] Coordination refers to the timing of relative motion between body segments and control refers to the optimization of relative motion between body segments, i.e. the extent to which the kinematics of segmental motion and, consequently, the motion of the whole body centre of gravity, matches the demands of the task.[5] For example, the mature form of coordination of the leg action in a countermovement vertical jump, as shown in Fig. 2.2.13, is characterized by simultaneous flexion of the hips, knees and ankles in the countermovement phase (Fig. 2.2.13(a–c)) followed by simultaneous extension of the hips, knees and ankles in the propulsion phase (Fig. 2.2.13(c–e)). This pattern of coordination normally occurs between three and four years of age.[5] However, whereas all normal mature individuals exhibit similar coordination in the standing vertical jump (and other whole body movements) there are considerable differences in the extent to which individuals can control the movement, i.e. optimize the relative motion of the body segments in order to match the task demands.

If the objective in performing a countermovement vertical jump is to maximize height jumped (upward vertical displacement of the whole body centre of gravity measured from the floor), then control of the movement is concerned with maximizing the height of the centre of gravity at take-off (h_1) and maximizing the upward vertical displacement of the centre of gravity after take-off (h_2) (Figs 2.2.13(e) and (f)). h_1 is determined by body position which, in turn, is determined by the range of motion in the joints and the extent to which the available range of motion is used. h_2 is determined by the vertical velocity of the centre of gravity at take-off, the greater the take-off velocity, the greater h_2. Take-off velocity is determined by the impulse of the ground reaction force (the force exerted between the feet and the floor) prior to take-off, the larger the impulse the greater the velocity. The impulse Ft of the ground reaction force F is determined by the magnitude of F and its duration t; the larger the force and the longer its duration the larger the impulse. The magnitude of F will depend upon the strength of the muscles, especially the extensor muscles of the hips, knees and ankles. The duration of F will depend upon the range of motion in the hips, knees and ankles and the extent to which the available range of motion is used. Clearly, restricted ranges of motion in any of the joints, especially hips, knees and ankles, and lack of strength in any of the muscles, especially the extensor muscles of the hips, knees and ankles will adversely affect an individual's ability to control the movement and, consequently, result in less than optimal performance.

There are numerous studies of jumping performance in adults, especially elite athletes.[6,7] However, there are relatively few studies on the development of coordination and control of jumping in young children. Jensen et al.[5] investigated coordination and control in the countermovement vertical jump in two groups of young children (mean $\pm$ SD age = 3.4 $\pm$ 0.5 y) and a group of skilled adults. The two groups of children ($n_1 = n_2 = 9$) were selected from a larger group ($n = 32$) on the basis of their take-off angle (angle of velocity vector of the whole body centre of gravity at take-off) into a high take-off group (HT0) and low take-off group (LT0). Take-off angle is a key control variable, since to maximize vertical displacement after take-off the take-off angle should be 90° (with respect to the horizontal). The criterion for inclusion in the HT0 and LT0 groups was a take-off angle at least one standard deviation greater or less than the total group mean, respectively. All jumps were performed on a force platform (to measure the ground reaction force) and to encourage maximum effort a suspended ball, just out of reach, was used as a visual target. Coordination was examined in terms of the timing of reversals (between the countermovement and propulsion phases of the jump) of the hip, knee and ankle joints and the timing of the peak extension velocities of the hip, knee and ankle joints. Control was examined in terms of the body position at three significant events in the propulsion phase; the time of maximum acceleration downwards (minimum ground reaction force), the time of maximum acceleration upwards (maximum ground reaction force), and take-off.

No significant differences were found between the three groups with regard to the coordination variables. This finding is consistent

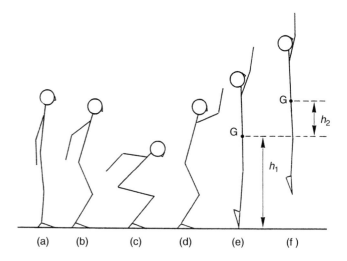

Fig. 2.2.13 Stick figure sequence of a countermovement vertical jump from a standing position: (a) to (c) = countermovement or dip phase; (c) to (e) = propulsion phase. G = whole body centre of gravity; h_1 = height of G above the floor at take-off; h_2 = upward vertical displacement of G after take-off.

with the results of a study by Clark et al.[8] of three, five, seven and nine year old children involving the same task and methodology. The mean take-off angles for the adults, HT0 and LT0 groups, $91.8 \pm 3.8°$, $82.0 \pm 3.5°$ and $61.2 \pm 5.6°$, respectively, were significantly different from each other and the mean of the adult group was closest to the theoretically desired angle of 90°. There were also significant differences between the groups in some of the other control variables (hip, knee and ankle angles) at one or more of the three events, in particular, ankle angle between adults and both child groups at take-off and knee angle between all three groups at take-off. The small angle of take-off of the LT0 group was found to be associated with a large (relative to the adults and HT0 groups) forward displacement of the centre of gravity (CG) during the countermovement and propulsion phases, i.e. the trajectory of the CG was V-shaped, downward and forward then upward and forward. In contrast, the trajectory of the CG of the adults was U-shaped, downward and very slightly forward then upward and very slightly forward. The trajectory of the CG of the HT0 group was in between those of the adult and LT0 groups. In general, the smaller the forward displacement of the CG the greater the take-off angle and vice versa. Whereas the HT0 and LT0 groups had smaller take-off angles than the adult group the HT0 and LT0 groups still accomplished a clearly recognizable vertical jump, the jumps were simply not optimized for maximum vertical displacement of the CG. Jensen et al.[5] concluded that the performances of the children were coordinated but poorly controlled, due perhaps to inadequate strength of the leg extensor muscles, especially during the braking period of the countermovement phase (the period when the downward velocity of the CG is reduced to zero).

Development of coordination and control

The human neuromusculoskeletal system consists of approximately 10^{11} neurons, 10^3 muscles and 10^2 moveable joints.[4,9] The way that the nervous system organizes movement in the face of such complexity has been viewed historically from two viewpoints: the neuromaturational perspective and the information-processing perspective.[9]

The neuromaturational perspective has been used primarily to explain motor development in infants and children. The neuromaturational perspective arose from the work of Gesell[10] and McGraw[11] who observed and described the gradual and sequential development of motor skills in infants, from apparently unintentional reflex movements through the development of intentional movements, such as crawling, sitting, standing and walking. Gesell and McGraw came to the view that the gradual development of motor skills reflected the gradual maturation of the nervous system. This view became widely held and the age norms for the emergence of motor skills in infants and children produced by Gesell and McGraw became, and still are, widely used.[12] Whereas neuromaturation is undeniably a major determinant of motor development in infants and children, it does not explain skill acquisition in adults where the nervous system is considered to be fully mature.[13]

Traditionally the information-processing perspective has dominated theories of skill acquisition in adults.[14] From the information-processing perspective, the brain is regarded rather like a computer with a very large number of motor programmes which can be executed at will to match the specific demands of each movement task as defined by the sensory information available. However, like the neuromaturational perspective, the information-processing perspective does not account for the great flexibility demonstrated by individuals in accommodating rapidly changing task demands, especially in the context of sports.

The deficiencies of the neuromaturational and information-processing perspectives were pointed out by Bernstein.[15] He argued that the complexity of the neuromusculoskeletal system was such that there could not be a one-to-one relationship between activity in the nervous system and actual movements. He also pointed out that a particular set of muscular contractions is not always associated with the same movement pattern, and that not all movements are controlled by the nervous system. For example, if you raise your arm to the side by activity in the shoulder abductor muscles and then relax the muscles, the arm will fall down under its own weight without any involvement of the nervous system. Similarly, if you hold your arm with the upper arm horizontal, the lower arm vertical and the wrist relaxed, and then alternately slightly flex and extend the elbow fairly rapidly, the hand will flail about the wrist due to its own inertia and the force exerted on the hand at the wrist by the movement of the lower arm, without any involvement of the nervous system. At any particular point in time each body segment may be acted on by four kinds of forces which can be classified in two ways; internal (muscle, articular) and external (weight, contact) forces, and active (muscle) and passive (articular, weight, contact) forces. Articular forces are passive forces exerted between articular surfaces and by joint support structures due to movement of adjacent segments. Contact forces are forces resulting from contact with surfaces external to the body, such as the floor.

Reference axes and degrees of freedom

In describing the movement of a joint it is useful to refer to three mutually perpendicular axes: anteroposterior, transverse and vertical (Fig. 2.2.14). With respect to the three reference axes there are six possible directions, called degrees of freedom, in which, a joint, depending upon its structure, may be able to move. There are three possible linear directions (along the axes) and three possible angular directions (about the axes). Most of the joints in the body have between one and three degrees of freedom. Most movements of the body involve simultaneous movement in a number of joints and the degrees of freedom of the whole segmental chain is the sum of the degrees of freedom of the individual joints in the chain. For example, if the wrist (which is comprised of eight small irregular shaped bones) is regarded as a single joint with two degrees of freedom (flexion–extension and abduction–adduction) then the arm has approximately 25 joints (joints of the shoulder, elbow, wrist and fingers) and approximately 35 degrees of freedom.

Coordination and degrees of freedom

Bernstein[15] described the development of coordination as a progressive increase in mastery of the very many degrees of freedom in a particular movement. He suggested that the development of skill in any particular task-oriented movement could be divided into two stages.

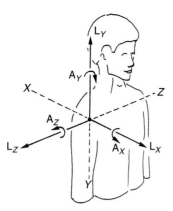

Fig. 2.2.14 Linear and angular degrees of freedom with respect to the shoulder joint. X = Anteroposterior axis; Y = vertical axis; Z = transverse axis; L_X = linear motion along X axis; L_Y = linear motion along Y axis; L_Z = linear motion along Z axis; A_X = angular motion about X axis; A_Y = angular motion about Y axis; A_Z = angular motion about Z axis.

The first stage involves the development of functional synergies between the muscle groups in the segmental chain, which is characterized by joint couplings between the joints in the segmental chain; the joint couplings result in reciprocal movement between the joints, i.e. coordinated movement of the linked segments, which effectively considerably reduces the number of degrees of freedom. In addition, coordination is further simplified, at least initially, by restricting the range of motion in the joints. The second stage involves the development of control, i.e. the functional synergies and ranges of motion in the joints gradually become optimized to maximize effectiveness in terms of task demands and maximize movement efficiency in terms of energy expenditure. This process involves neural integration of the active and passive forces in a manner which minimizes energy expenditure (the work done by muscles) and maximizes energy conservation (by facilitating energy transformation, potential to kinetic and vice versa, and energy transfer between segments).

Most of the muscles (muscle–tendon units) of the body cross over more than one joint. These muscles, such as the rectus femoris and hamstrings, are usually referred to as biarticular muscles, since muscles which cross over more than two joints function in the same way as muscles that cross over just two joints.[16] Biarticular muscles are too short to fully flex or fully extend all the joints that they cross over simultaneously. For example, the hamstrings are too short to fully extend the hip and fully flex the knee at the same time; indeed, hip extension is usually associated with knee extension and hip flexion is usually associated with knee flexion, as in a countermovement vertical jump (Fig. 2.2.13). Ingen Schenau[17] has suggested that correct use of biarticular muscles is of prime importance in the development of functional synergies (Fig. 2.2.15).

Research on Bernstein's ideas was fairly limited until recently (last ten years) due, it would appear, to a combination of factors including the hypothetical nature of some biomechanical concepts, such as resultant joint moment,[17] and difficulties associated with modelling the human body for the purpose of biomechanical analysis.[18,19] Recent advances in modelling capability and increased use of biomechanical analysis techniques by motor development researchers have resulted in more research on the biomechanics of coordination.[20,21] However, there would appear to be few studies which have related kinematics to kinetics, investigated the effects of practice, or involved children.

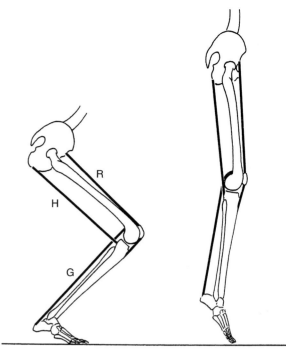

Fig. 2.2.15 Coupling of the trunk, upper leg and lower leg by the rectus femoris, hamstrings and gastrocnemius. The trunk is linked to the lower leg by the hamstrings (H) and the rectus femoris (R), and the upper leg is linked to the foot by the gastrocnemius (G). If the lengths of H, F and G are appropriately set, hip extension will result in simultaneous knee extension and ankle plantar flexion (adapted from Ingen Schenau[17]).

Kinematics of coordination

Whereas control of movement is essential to maximize performance, the development of coordination is a necessary precursor to the development of control. This was demonstrated by Anderson and Sidaway[22] in a study of the effects of practice on performance in kicking. A novice group of right foot dominant subjects, five males and one female (mean age 20.3 years, age range 18 to 22 years) was selected on the basis of no previous experience of organized soccer or soccer training. An expert group of three males (mean age 25.2 years, age range 22 to 30 years), each with more than ten years experience of organized soccer, was included in the study in order to determine if the coordination of the three experts was similar, and to compare the pre- and post-practice coordination of the novices with the experts. The task to be learned (only the novice group took part in the practice sessions) was a right-footed instep drive at a two metre square target placed five metres from the ball following a two step approach. The primary goal was to maximize the velocity of the ball while trying to hit the target. The subjects practised twice a week for ten weeks and had between 15 and 20 trials during each session. Prior to and after the practice period, three trials of each subject were videotaped with a single camera placed perpendicular to the plane of motion on the right side of the subject. By using markers on the right shoulder, right hip, right knee, right ankle and right small toe (Fig. 2.2.16), the angular displacement and angular velocity of the hip and knee and linear velocity of the foot (toe) was found for each subject at 60 Hz throughout each trial. From the linear and angular velocity data and angular displacement data three velocity measures, three timing measures and two ranges of motion were derived for each subject in each trial (as defined in Table 2.2.1). Since each subject exhibited a high degree of consistency with regard to the eight variables the data were averaged across the three trials.

Table 2.2.1 shows the group means and standard deviations for the eight variables for the novices, pre- and post-practice, and the experts, together with percentage changes pre- and post-practice for the novices, and percentage comparison of the novices, pre- and post-practice, with the experts. It is clear that the performance of the novices, in terms of maximum foot linear velocity (which reflects ball velocity) improved considerably with practice (47%) but was still well below that of the experts (85%) post-practice. However, the 47% increase in maximum foot linear velocity was associated with much smaller increases in maximum hip angular velocity (2.1%), maximum knee angular velocity (12.3%), hip range of motion (19.8%), and knee range of motion (14.5%). These changes, especially the angular velocity changes, suggest that improvement in performance resulted largely from a change in coordination rather than an increase in the speed of execution of the pre-practice movement pattern. This interpretation is supported by the change in the timing variables which were much closer to those of the experts post-practice than pre-practice (see Table 2.2.1). It is also supported by the change in relative motion of the thigh and lower leg as reflected in the representative knee angle–hip angle diagrams shown in Fig. 2.2.16. The post-practice pattern was similar to that of the experts which suggests that the novices had developed coordination. However, comparison of the novice post-practice and expert linear and angular velocities and

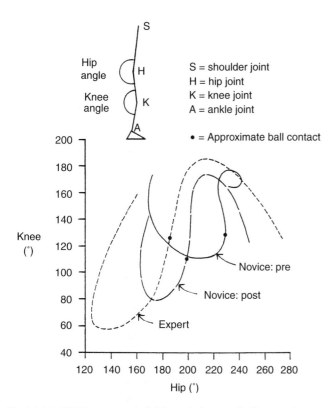

Fig. 2.2.16 Kicking a soccer ball: hip angle–knee angle diagrams for one representative novice's performance, pre- and post-practice, and one representative expert's performance (adapted from Anderson and Sidaway[22]).

ranges of motion in Table 2.2.1 indicates that control was less than optimal. The results of the study provide support for Bernstein's two-stage theory of skill acquisition, i.e. development of coordination followed by development of control.

Kinetics of coordination

A kinematic analysis describes the way an object moves. In order to understand why an object moves the way that it does it is necessary to carry out a kinetic analysis, i.e. an analysis of the impulses and timing of the impulses of the forces acting on the object during the movement. With regard to human movement this involves analysis of the active and passive forces acting on each segment.

Modelling

Each body segment is comprised of hard and soft tissues. Whereas the segment may deform to a certain extent during movement, the amount of deformation is usually very small and, as such, for the purpose of biomechanical analysis the body segments may be regarded as rigid.[23] Consequently, the human body may be regarded as a system of rigid segments with the main segments (head, trunk, upper arms, forearms, hands, thighs, lower legs, feet) linked by freely moveable joints.

Free body diagram

Jensen et al.[24] carried out kinetic analyses of spontaneous leg movements in infants while reclined at 45°, as shown in Fig. 2.2.17(a). Figures 2.2.17(b) and (c) show free body diagrams of the thigh and the combined lower leg and foot of the right leg, i.e. sketches of the segments showing all of the forces acting on them. It is assumed that the movement of the legs takes place in the sagittal plane (X–Y plane with respect to Fig. 2.2.17). There are no contact forces acting on the segments and, as such, the only forces shown are the weights of the segments acting at the segmental CGs, and the force distributions around the hip and knee joints. It can be shown that any force distribution is equivalent to the resultant force R acting at an arbitrary point P together with a couple C equal to the resultant moment of the force distribution about P. The combination of R (acting at P) and C is referred to as the equipollent of the force distribution. In a kinetic analysis of human movement it is usual to show the force distribution around a joint as the equipollent with respect to the joint centre. In Figs 2.2.17(b) and (c) the equipollent of the force distribution around the hip joint is shown as F_H and M_H, and the equipollent of the force distribution around the knee joint is shown as F_K and M_K. In Figs 2.2.17(d) and (e) the resultant forces through the hip and knee joint centres are replaced by their horizontal (F_{HX}, F_{KX}) and vertical (F_{HY}, F_{KY}) components.

Components of net joint moment

Each segment will move in accordance with Newton's laws of motion. Consequently, with respect to the lower leg and foot segment of mass m,

$$F_X = ma_X \qquad (4)$$

$$F_Y = ma_Y \qquad (5)$$

$$M_Z = I\alpha \qquad (6)$$

where F_X = resultant of horizontal forces acting on the segment; F_Y = resultant of vertical forces acting on the segment; a_X = horizontal

Table 2.2.1 Kicking a soccer ball: means, standard deviations and comparative data for velocity, timing and range of motion variables for novice and expert subjects (adapted from Anderson and Sidaway [22])

| | Novice | | | | | | | Expert | |
| | Pre-practice | | | Post-practice | | | | | |
	Mean	SD	%E	Mean	SD	%E	%pp	Mean	SD
MFLV ($\mathrm{m\,s^{-1}}$)	14.9	1.7	58	21.9	1.5	85	47	25.6	1.1
MHAV ($\mathrm{deg\,s^{-1}}$)	671	77	78	685	168	79	2.1	864	49
MKAV ($\mathrm{deg\,s^{-1}}$)	1146	213	77	1287	251	86	12.3	1494	115
SKE/IMHAV	1.02	0.06	117	0.89	0.05	102	−13	0.87	0.03
IMHAV/IMFLV	0.61	0.1	77	0.69	0.03	87	13	0.79	0.01
IMKAV/IMFLV	1.14	0.06	109	1.04	0.05	100	−8.7	1.04	0.03
HIP ROM (deg)	86	14	64	103	21	77	19.8	135	9.5
KNEE ROM (deg)	90	16	75	104	13	86	14.5	121	5.7

MFLV, maximum foot linear velocity; MHAV, maximum hip angular velocity; MKAV, maximum knee angular velocity; SKE, start of knee extension; I, instant of.

%E, per cent of expert value; %pp, per cent difference between pre- and post-practice.

component of the linear acceleration of the CG of the segment; a_Y = vertical component of the linear acceleration of the CG of the segment; M_Z = resultant moment about the Z axis through the CG of the segment; I = moment of inertia of the segment about the Z axis through the CG of the segment; α = angular acceleration of the segment about the Z axis through the CG of the segment.

From equations (4), (5) and (6) it follows that

$$F_{KX} = ma_X \tag{7}$$
$$F_{KY} - W_S = ma_Y \tag{8}$$
$$M_K - F_{KX}d_1 - F_{KY}d_2 = I\alpha \tag{9}$$

From equation (8)

$$F_{KY} = ma_Y + W_S \tag{10}$$

By substitution of F_{KX} from equation (7) and F_{KY} from equation (10) into equation (9),

$$M_K - ma_X d_1 - (ma_Y + W_S)d_2 = I\alpha$$
$$M_K - ma_X d_1 - ma_Y d_2 - W_S d_2 = I\alpha$$
$$M_K - (ma_X d_1 + ma_Y d_2) - W_S d_2 = I\alpha$$

M_K = Generalized Muscle Moment (MUS): the resultant moment of the force distribution about the Z axis through the knee joint centre, i.e. the moment exerted by the muscle and articular forces about the joint. $(ma_X d_1 + ma_Y d_2)$ = Motion Dependent Moment (MDM): the moment acting on the segment as a result of the motion of adjacent segments, i.e. the thigh. $W_S d_2$ = Gravitational Moment (GRAV): the moment acting on the segment due to its weight. $I\alpha$ Net Joint Moment (NET): the resultant of MUS, MDM and GRAV moments acting on the segment.

The relationship between MUS, MDM and GRAV is usually referred to as the dynamics of the system. With current technology it is not possible to directly measure the forces which contribute to MUS

or, therefore, to measure the separate contributions of muscle and articular forces to the MUS. However, since the MUS comprises the only active (muscle) component of the NET, the MUS is particularly important for understanding coordination. Whereas MUS cannot be measured directly it can be determined indirectly, i.e. MUS = NET − MDM − GRAV.

NET, MDM and GRAV can be calculated directly by kinematic analysis of the movement involving the following stages:

1. Digitization of film or videotape of the movement with respect to a suitable X–Y frame of reference to obtain joint centre displacement–time data.

2. Calculation of segmental angular displacement–time data and CG displacement–time data (by use of published data concerning location of segmental CG in relation joint centres, e.g. [25,26]).

3. Calculation of a_X and a_Y from CG displacement–time data.

4. Calculation of α from angular displacement–time data.

5. Calculation of moment arms of forces from the joint centre and CG displacement–time data.

6. Estimation of m and I values from published data (e.g. [18,19]).

This indirect method of determining MUS is referred to as indirect dynamics or inverse dynamics.[27] The converse of indirect dynamics, i.e. determination of kinematics from directly measured kinetic (forces and moments of force) data is referred to as direct dynamics.

In the study by Jensen et al.[24] of spontaneous leg movements in children reclined at 45° it was found that the infants naturally produced kicks of varying degrees of vigour and range of motion. In general, the infants exhibited a consistent pattern of relative motion between trunk, thigh and lower leg segments suggesting a high level of coordination. With regard to kinetics, the relationship between the MUS, MDM and GRAV profiles was similar at the hip and knee joints. At slow speeds of movement the MDM were very small and the MUS served mainly to counteract the GRAV (Fig. 2.2.18(a)). The GRAV profile, as expected, was similar at all kicking speeds. However, at fast speeds the MUS and MDM profiles were sinusoidal and out of phase

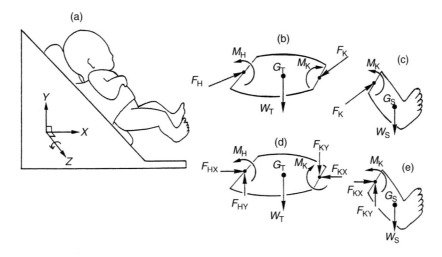

IF_H = force distribution (muscle and articular) about the hip joint
IF_K = force distribution (muscle and articular) about the knee joint
M_H = moment of IF_H about the Z axis through the hip joint centre
M_K = moment of IF_K about the Z axis through the hip joint centre
F_H = resultant of IF_H acting through the hip joint centre
F_{HX} = horizontal component of F_H
F_{HY} = vertical component of F_H
F_K = resultant of IF_K acting through the knee joint centre
F_{KX} = horizontal component of F_K
F_{KY} = horizontal component of F_K
G_T = centre of gravity of the upper leg
G_S = centre of gravity of the combined lower leg and foot
W_T = weight of upper leg
W_S = weight of combined lower leg and foot
d_1 = moment arm of F_{KX} about the Z axis through G_S
d_2 = moment arm of F_{KY} about the Z axis through G_S

Fig. 2.2.17 Free body diagrams of the thigh and combined lower leg and foot of the right leg of a three month old infant inclined at 45°: (a) infant inclined at 45°; (b) free body diagram of right upper leg; (c) free body diagram of combined right lower leg and foot; (d) free body diagram of right upper leg with resultant joint forces replaced by horizontal and vertical components; (e) free body diagram of combined right lower leg and foot with resultant joint force replaced by horizontal and vertical components.

by approximately 180° suggesting that as speed of movement increased the main function of the *MUS* was to counteract the *MDM* (Fig. 2.2.18(b)). The *MUS* profile was also found to be approximately 180° out of phase with the change in joint angle, i.e. the peaks of the *MUS* profile corresponded to changes in direction of movement of the segment. Since change in direction of movement is associated with eccentric muscle activity during the deceleration phase, the correspondence between the profiles of joint angle, *MUS* and *MDM* suggest that coordinated movement tends to exploit the capacity of muscle–tendon units to store energy (in the elastic components during eccentric contractions), which, in turn, is likely to enhance energy conservation and reduce the energy expenditure of the muscles. Schneider *et al.*[28] found similar correspondence between the profiles of joint angle (shoulder, elbow and wrist), *MUS* and *MDM* in adults performing a rapid reciprocal precision hand-placement task.

Energy generation and absorption by muscles

Just as it is not possible to directly measure the forces which contribute to *MUS* it is not possible to directly measure the work done by and on the individual muscles which contribute to *MUS*. However, the net work done by and on the muscles within *MUS* can be determined indirectly by integration of the power–time curve associated with the *MUS* around each particular joint. The power P at a joint is the product of the *MUS* and angular velocity ω, i.e. $P = MUS\omega$. Power is positive (power output) if *MUS* and ω are of the same polarity, i.e. net concentric activity; for example, hip flexion coinciding with a hip flexor moment. Power is negative (power absorption) if *MUS* and ω are of opposite polarity, i.e. net eccentric activity; for example, hip flexion coinciding with a hip extensor moment.

Winter[29] investigated the energy generated and absorbed by the muscles around the hip, knee and ankle in adult subjects while walking at fast ($n = 10$, mean cadence 125.4 steps min^{-1}), natural ($n = 9$, mean cadence 104.4 steps min^{-1}) and slow ($n = 9$, mean cadence 85.9 steps min^{-1}) speeds of walking. Figure 2.2.19 shows typical power–time curves at the hip, knee and ankle for one stride (heel contact to heel contact of the same foot) for one subject walking at a fast cadence. The net energy generated and absorbed by the muscles around each joint is represented by the positive and negative areas of the curves, respectively. The actual amounts of energy generated and absorbed in the various phases, as shown on the figure, indicate that over the complete stride the hip muscles ($+ 20$ J, -35 J) and knee muscles ($+20$ J, -60 J) were net energy absorbers and the ankle muscles ($+35$ J, -7 J) were net energy generators. Patterns of energy generation and absorption at the hip were not consistent, but the patterns at the knee (net energy absorbers) and ankle (net energy generators) were consistent across all subjects and all cadences. It is not possible to determine how much of the absorbed energy was subsequently released in energy generation. However, it is likely that greater utilization of stored energy, i.e recycling of absorbed energy, is made at a preferred (natural) cadence since energy expenditure (oxygen consumption) has been shown to be lowest at preferred cadence for the same speed of walking in adults and children.[30,31]

Dynamical systems approach to development of coordination

Studies of spontaneous kicking[24] and reaching[32] clearly indicate that infants have a high level of coordination in spontaneous (non-task oriented, non-intentional) multi-joint limb movements,

which suggests an intrinsic ability of the body segments to self-organize their relative motion.[33] Self-organization is a key feature of complex dynamical systems which, like the human body, have many degrees of freedom and are subject to a range of constraints.[34] Dynamical systems theory was developed nearly a 100 years ago to try to explain how physical systems including, for example, weather patterns, change over time.[9] The dynamical systems approach was first applied to coordination of human movement by Kugler et al.,[35] and since then concepts from dynamical systems have been increasingly used to illuminate problems of motor learning and motor development.[14]

The dynamical systems approach emphasizes the thermodynamic nature of biological systems and how thermodynamic laws guide behaviour.[36] Biological systems obey the second law of thermodynamics, i.e. all systems tend toward instability and disorder which, in the case of a living organism, culminates in death. However, during life a biological system can maintain an ordered state by a cyclical process of generation, transformation and dissipation of energy which occurs at all levels of the system including circadian rhythms, cardiac rhythms, respiratory rhythms and locomotion.[37] It is believed that the oscillatory nature of biological systems is analogous to inanimate self-organizing oscillatory systems.[38]

Harmonic oscillators

If the pendulum of a clock is stopped from swinging, it will hang vertically. This is the equilibrium position of the pendulum. If the pendulum is displaced from its equilibrium position and released, it will oscillate about the equilibrium position with a constant cycle time. The cycle time is determined by the distribution of the mass of the pendulum with respect to the point of support; the greater the distance of the centre of gravity of the pendulum from the point of support the

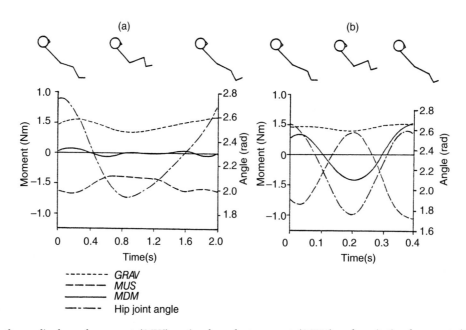

Fig. 2.2.18   Profiles of generalized muscle moments (*MUS*) motion dependent moments (*MDM*), and gravitational moments (*GRAV*) about the hip joint in relation to hip joint angle for an infant performing a spontaneous non-vigorous kick (a) and a vigorous kick (b) (adapted from Kamm *et al.*[13]).

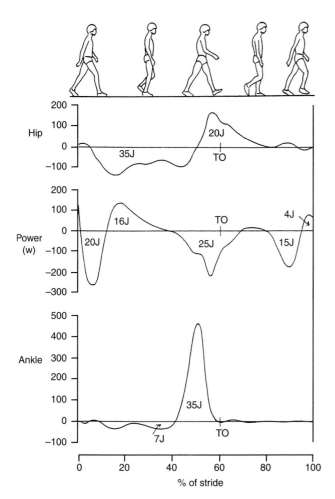

Fig. 2.2.19 Power generation and absorption at the hip, knee and ankle joints during one stride (heel strike to heel strike of the right leg; TO = toe off) while walking (adapted from Winter[29]).

governed largely by its physical properties, which is likely to simplify neural control of the movement.[34]

Force driven harmonic oscillators

A force driven harmonic oscillator (FDHO) is an oscillating system that is periodically forced to overcome any resistance that would otherwise cause the system to stop oscillating. Resonance frequency refers to the frequency at which the periodic force required to maintain the oscillation is minimal. There is evidence that adults and children naturally adopt a walking frequency which optimizes energy expenditure, symmetry between the left and right sides of the body, and stability in terms of the consistency of the movement pattern from cycle to cycle.[30,39] Furthermore, the preferred walking frequency can be predicted from the resonant frequency of an FDHO model of the leg swing.[31,39] Similarly, Ledebt and Breniere[40] found that in four to eight year old children, gait initiation (from the start of movement to maximum horizontal velocity in the first step) can be closely predicted from the resonant frequency of an FDHO model of the movement of the CG over the grounded foot. Even very young children appear to adopt movement patterns at resonant frequency in certain situations. For example, Goldfield et al.[41] showed that infants bouncing up and down in a jumper device tend to adopt resonant frequency as modelled by a FDHO mass–spring system.

Summary

Human movement is brought about by the musculoskeletal system under the control of the nervous system. By coordinated activity between the various muscle groups, forces generated by the muscles are transmitted by the bones and joints to enable the individual to maintain an upright or partially upright posture and bring about voluntary controlled movements. Biomechanics of human movement is the study of the relationship between the external forces (due to body weight and physical contact with the external environment) and internal forces (active forces generated by muscles and passive forces exerted on other structures) which act on the body and the effect of these forces on the movement of the body. Recent advances in modelling capability and increased use of biomechanical analysis techniques by motor development researchers has resulted in the current dynamical systems approach to research into the development of coordination.

longer the cycle time. An oscillator in which the cycle time is constant is called a harmonic oscillator. If the friction around the point of support of the pendulum was zero, the pendulum would oscillate with constant amplitude and the energy of the system would be entirely conserved at the level it had at the point of release. In practice, there would be a certain amount of friction around the point of support, such that a certain amount of energy would be dissipated (lost to the system) as heat during each oscillation. Consequently, the amplitude of oscillation would gradually decrease and the pendulum would eventually come to rest in its equilibrium position. The pendulum is a very simple example of a dynamical system, i.e. the movement of the system after release is self-organized (amplitude and frequency of oscillation), entirely predictable and energy is conserved (to a level determined by the friction around the point of support). Similarly, if a metal spring is stretched or compressed and then released the spring will oscillate in a predictable manner and come to rest at its equilibrium position; there is no brain controlling its movement which is determined completely by its physical properties of stiffness and damping. Just as the physical properties of the pendulum and spring determine their movement when allowed to oscillate freely, it is reasonable to assume that limbs might move in the same way, i.e. if the stiffness and damping levels of a limb are set, its movement will be

References

1. **Watkins, J.** *Structure and function of the musculoskeletal system.* Human Kinetics, Champaign, Il, 1999.
2. **Watkins, J.** *An introduction to mechanics of human movement.* MTP Press, Lancaster, England, 1983.
3. **Winter, D. A.** A new definition of mechanical work done in human movement. *Journal of Applied Physiology* 1979; **46**: 79–83.
4. **Turvey, M. T.** Coordination. *American Psychologist* 1990; **45**: 938–53.
5. **Jensen, J. L., Phillips, S. J.** and **Clark, J. E.** For young jumpers, differences are in movement's control, not in coordination. *Research Quarterly for Exercise and Sport* 1994; **65**: 258–68.
6. **Bobbert, M. F.** and **Ingen Schenau, G. J. V.** Coordination in vertical jump. *Journal of Biomechanics* 1988; **21**: 249–62.
7. **Hay, J. G.** Citius, altius, longius (faster, higher, longer): The biomechanics of jumping for distance. *Journal of Biomechanics* 1993; **26**: 7–21.

8. Clark, J. E., Phillips, S. J. and Petersen, R. Developmental stability in jumping. *Developmental Psychology* 1989; **25**: 929–35.

9. Clark, J. E. On becoming skillful: Patterns and constraints. *Research Quarterly for Exercise and Sport* 1995; **66**: 173–83.

10. Gesell, A. and Thompson, H. *The psychology of early growth including norms of infant behavior and a method of genetic analysis.* Macmillan, New York, 1938.

11. McGraw, M. G. *The neuromaturation of the human infant.* Columbia University Press, New York, 1943.

12. Thelen, E. Motor development: a new synthesis. *American Psychologist,* 1995; **50**: 79–85.

13. Kamm, K., Thelen, E. and Jensen, J. L. A dynamical systems approach to motor development. *Physical Therapy* 1990; **70**: 763–75.

14. Handford, C., Davids, K., Bennett, S. and Button, C. Skill acquisition in sport: some implications of an evolving practice ecology. *Journal of Sports Sciences* 1997; **15**: 621–40.

15. Bernstein, N. *The coordination and regulation of movements.* Pergamon, London, 1967.

16. Lieber, R. L. *Skeletal muscle structure and function.* Williams and Wilkins, Baltimore, 1992.

17. Ingen Schenau, G. J. V. From translation to rotation: constraints on multijoint movements and the unique action of biarticular muscles. *Human Movement Science* 1989; **8**: 301–37.

18. Schneider, K. and Zernicke, R. F. Mass, centre of mass, and moment of inertia estimates for infant limb segments. *Journal of Biomechanics* 1992; **25**: 145–8.

19. Sun, H. and Jensen, R. K. Body segment growth during infancy. *Journal of Biomechanics* 1994; **27**: 265–75.

20. Lockman, J. J. and Thelen, E. Developmental biodynamics: brain, body and behavior connections. *Child Development* 1993; **64**: 953–9.

21. Zernicke, R. F. and Schneider, K. Biomechanics and developmental neuromotor control. *Child Development* 1993; **64**: 982–1004.

22. Anderson, D. I. and Sidaway, B. Coordination changes associated with practice of a soccer kick. *Research Quarterly for Exercise and Sport* 1994; **65**: 93–9.

23. Andrews, J. G. Biomechanical analysis of human motion. In *Kinesiology IV.* American Alliance for Health, Physical Education and Recreation, Reston, VA, 1974; 32–42.

24. Jensen, J. L., Ulrich, B. D., Thelen, E., Schneider, K. and Zernicke, R. F. Reported as unpublished in Kamm, K., Thelen, E., and Jensen, J. L. A dynamical systems approach to motor development. *Physical Therapy* 1990; **70**: 763–75.

25. Dempster, W. T. Space requirements of the seated operator: geometrical, kinematic and mechanical aspects of the body with special reference to the limbs. WADT Technical Report No. 55–159. Wright Patterson Air Force Base, Ohio, 1955.

26. Hatze, H. A mathematical model for the computational determination of parameter values of anthropometric segments. *Journal of Biomechanics* 1980; **13**: 833–43.

27. Winter, D. A. *Biomechanics and motor control of human movement.* John Wiley, New York, 1990.

28. Schneider, K., Zernicke, R. F., Schmidt, R. A. and Hart, T. J. Changes in limb dynamics during the practice of rapid arm movements. *Journal of Biomechanics* 1989; **22**: 805–17.

29. Winter, D. A. Energy generation and absorption at the ankle and knee during fast, natural, and slow cadences. *Clinical Orthopaedics and Related Research* 1983; **175**: 147–54.

30. Holt, K. G., Hamill, J. and Andres, R. O. Predicting the minimal energy costs of human walking. *Medicine and Science in Sports and Exercise* 1991; **23**: 491–8.

31. Jeng, S.-F., Liao, H-F., Lai, J.-S. and Hou, J-W. Optimization of walking in children. *Medicine and Science in Sports and Exercise* 1997; **29**: 370–6.

32. Thelen, E., Corbetta, D., Kamm, K., Spencer, J., Schneider, K. and Zernicke, R. F. The transition to reaching: Mapping intention and intrinsic dynamics. *Child Development* 1993; **64**: 1058–98.

33. Jensen, J. L., Thelen, E. and Ulrich, B. D. Constraints on multijoint movements: from spontaneity of infancy to the skill of adults. *Human Movement Science* 1989; **8**: 393–402.

34. Kugler, P. N. and Turvey, M. T. *Natural law, and the self assembly of rhythmic movement.* Erlbaum, Hillside, NJ, 1987.

35. Kugler, P. N., Kelso, J. A. S. and Turvey, M. T. On the concept of coordinative structures as dissipative structure: I. Theoretical lines of convergence. In *Tutorials on motor behavior* (ed. G. E. Stelmach and J. Requin). North Holland, New York, 1980; 3–47

36. Holt, K. G. and Jeng, S. F. Advances in biomechanical analysis of the physically challenged child: Cerebral palsy. *Pediatric Exercise Science* 1992; **4**: 213–35.

37. Morowitz, H. J. *Foundations of bioenergetics.* Academic, New York, 1978.

38. Beek, P. J. and Wieringen, P. C. W. V. Perspectives on the relation between information and dynamics: An epilogue. *Human Movement Science* 1994; **13**: 519–33.

39. Holt, K. G., Hamill, J. and Andres, R. O. The force driven harmonic oscillator as a model for human walking. *Human Movement Science* 1990; **9**: 55–68.

40. Ledebt, A. and Breniere, Y. Dynamical implication of anatomical and mechanical parameters in gait initiation process in children. *Human Movement Science* 1994; **13**: 801–15.

41. Goldfield, E. C., Kay, B. A. and Warren, W. H. Infant bouncing: The assembly and tuning of action systems. *Child Development* 1993; **64**: 1128–42.

2.3   Motor development

Helen C. Wright and David A. Sugden

Introduction

The performance and the learning of motor skills is a lifelong process that challenges the individual in a rich variety of ways. Motor development, and changes in skill learning, and competencies are clear and obvious in the growing child, but both adolescents and adults continually adapt and refine their motor skills as they strive for the most proficient route to effective movement.[1] According to Keogh and Sugden[2] development is quite simply adaptive change towards competence, and these adaptations and alterations to our movements are constantly in flux even though the adaptations are not always apparent to the human eye. Changes occur in biological, physical and social environments to enable individuals and their surroundings to become congruous. Behaviour, including motor behaviour, is the cumulation of many influences, including psychological, sociological, biological, physiological, cognitive and mechanical changes, with their integration being the basis on which the understanding of behaviour is made.[1] The understanding of motor development is based on the integration of many behavioural changes that take place within and across phases of development.

Motor development begins with conception and continues through to adulthood. It is often considered age related, but as individuals and environments differ so extensively, development is best viewed as a continuous process of change, with age being an indicator of the amount of time we have been alive. Dramatic changes in individuals are seen as the new born baby develops into the young child with self-help skills and on into adult life as our movements adapt to meet the demands of our environment. This process involves the development of motor control, where the individual gains control of body movements in the context of the environmental conditions.

Early researchers concluded that the regularity of the emerging motor skills seen in children reflected the genetically driven process common to all normally developing children, namely that of brain maturation.[3–7] This view inferred, and offered findings to support such a claim, that it was autonomous changes in the nervous system that supported motor skill development. Dennis and Dennis[3] demonstrated that even when children had their movements restricted, as did the Hopi children on cradleboards, the genetically driven timetable for motor skill development, in this case walking, would continue unabated.

For many years a child's motor development has been traced through an account of their physical growth patterns (for reviews see Malina,[8] and Malina and Bouchard[9]) and the monitoring of the increasingly complex skills that they acquire (for a review see Haywood[1]). One can record the changes in height and weight of a baby, the disappearance of primitive reflexes, and the appearance of new features such as the ability to smile and react to the mother's presence. These changes mark the growth and development of a child as they mature both physically and socially. Of equal concern is the integrated process of how children learn to synthesize, blend and mix these developing physical and social functions as they evolve. The information offered by the physical monitoring and assessment of development is essential in charting what is considered normal, healthy development.[10] Children change drastically in the years preceding schooling, and the motor milestones that they achieve, in what order and at what level of competence, are used as indicators in one of the processes known as motor development. Motor development can be assessed by such tools as the Bayley scales,[11,12] the Denver Developmental Screening Test;[13] the Miller Assessment for Preschoolers[14] and so on. However this type of charting and assessment does not deal with the intriguing questions of how, or why do, infants and children adapt and alter their movements to better suit the requirements of their lives. In other words how do they develop the resources that are necessary to accomplish motor tasks? Descriptions of motor milestones are fascinating and relatively straightforward to obtain. A more complex and difficult task involves analysing how and why children change in their development towards some form of mature behaviour.

The scientific study of motor development can be traced back to the 1930s and 40s when pioneer developmental scientists such as Shirley,[7] Gesell and Amatruda[4] and McGraw[5,6] spent many years observing and reporting on how infants gain control of their movements. Shirley[7] compiled individual movement biographies cataloguing the movements of 25 babies from birth to two years of age through regular home visits of at least once per week. The child's movements were recorded graphically and by long hand. The detail amounted to an intensive, longitudinal study of early walking development. Gesell and Amatruda[4] also collected observations of child development, so much so, that their data were used to produce developmental scales on which a diagnosis of development could be based. McGraw[6] and the other early developmentalists were not only observers of children, they were also theorists. They noted that children universally pass through a series of motor milestones and that these movements occur in sequence. For example, McGraw[6] felt that the consistencies seen in the emerging motor skills of young children were due to a genetically driven process, that of the brain maturing. However, the conclusions and interpretations that she and others made are now being re-evaluated.

Theories of motor development have gone through many changes themselves. Haywood[1] neatly summarizes the changes in perspectives from the 1900s through to the 1990s in Fig. 2.3.1.

This chapter could attempt to outline and summarize the theories from Fig. 2.3.1, and in so doing trace the path from behavioural theory to the ecological perspective. Many other authors have dealt with the theories spanning the 1900s to the 1970s and the references for these approaches and explanations can be seen in Table 2.3.1. Rather, in this chapter, we would like to move the reader onto the perspective known by Haywood[1] as the ecological perspective. Other researchers (e.g. Thelen[15]) have coined the title the 'new synthesis'. This new and exciting perspective involves humans acting as dynamic systems with their perceptions and experiences interacting with their environment in a self-organizing manner.

Thelen,[15] a strong proponent of the new approach, disputes the genetically driven stance, concluding that it is too simplistic, and backs her claim with empirical evidence. As Gallahue[16] stated in the early 1980s:

> Current research is making it abundantly clear that infants are able to process a great deal more information than we ever suspected. (p. 157.)

The more recent views of motor development in the 1980s and 1990s stress the roles of exploration, and the selection of solutions to the demands of novel tasks. These new views contrast with the traditional maturational accounts of motor development by proposing that the so-called 'phylogenetic' skills, such as reaching, crawling and walking, are in fact learnt by adapting current dynamics through exploration and selection of possible movements to fit the new task.[15] Changes in behaviour are not brought about by prescribed genetic instructions as earlier thought, but rather are motivated by a task, such as moving across a room to join other people, and recruiting the available resources to do this. It is the matching of the internal resources of the child together with the challenging contextual demands and requirements which promote development.

An enormous amount of literature exists covering the motor development of children from birth to primary school age and further. The difference between the more traditional approach to motor development and the 'new synthesis', as Thelen[15] calls it, or dynamic approach, is that there is a move away from looking at performance variables, such as crawling, and relating those behaviours to age or stage of development, to moving towards investigating the processes by which a child develops and learns new skills.

Table 2.3.1 Theoretical perspectives in motor development

Perspective	Author	Basic principles
Maturation	Gessell	'Ontogeny recapitulates phylogeny.' Development is ultimately controlled by heredity. Central nervous system is the major rate-controlling system
Descriptive—normative branch	Espenschade, Glasgow, Rarick	Motor development can be described through age group norms
Descriptive—biomechanical branch	Glasgow, Halverson	Motor development can be described through sequential improvements in movement patterns
Behaviourism—social learning branch	Bandura	Behaviour is shaped by both direct and vicarious reinforcement
Cognitivism	Piaget	Development involves individuals acting upon the environment. Development occurs in stages
Information processing	Connolly	Information is manipulated in humans through a series of operations leading to a (movement) response
Ecological psychology— dynamic systems branch	Kugler, Kelso, Turvey	Body systems can spontaneously self-organize. Individuals are composed of cooperative systems. Development is discontinuous
Ecological psychology— perception–action branch	Gibson	Environment affords certain movements to individuals. Movement is perceived directly

Based on Clark and Whitall[56] and reproduced with permission.

Behavioural theory	Maturation approach	Normative/ descriptive approach	Cognitive theory (Piaget)		Information processing theory	Ecological perspectives (dynamic systems and perception–action)	
					Social learning theory		
Early 1900s	1930s	1940s	1950s	1960s	1970s	1980s	1990s

Fig. 2.3.1 Various theories and perspectives have emerged in the history of developmental psychology and motor development. Although a perspective may dominate only for a time, its influence can be felt even as other perspectives emerge. Reprinted from Haywood[1] with permission.

Through the imposition and presentation of novel tasks the new experimenters and researchers witness how an infant explores, discovers, adapts and remembers transitions from one behaviour to the next. The nervous system, in this new approach, is seen as dynamic and self-organizing, using repeated cycles of perception and action to facilitate new forms of behaviour. The new research represents a move away from explanations which rely alone upon internal mechanisms such as genes, programmes and cognitive structures suggesting a blueprint for behavioural change.[17] Many, many studies exist which exemplify the traditional view of motor development, we will not attempt to critique or discuss these studies in this chapter but rather refer the reader to Haywood[1] for a review.

The notion that another theory, other than a genetically driven theory, cognitive theory, information processing modelling or social learning theory, could exist to explain motor skill development is something at the heart of this chapter. As Thelen[15] notes:

> The study of the acquisition of motor skills, long moribund in developmental psychology, has seen a renaissance in the last decade. Inspired by contemporary work in movement science, perceptual psychology, neuroscience, and dynamics systems theory, multidisciplinary approaches are affording new insights into the processes by which infants and children learn to control their bodies … Studies are concerned less with how children perform and more with how the components cooperate to produce stability or engender change. Such process approaches make moot the traditional nature–nurture debates. (p. 79.)

From any chosen perspective it is clear that humans without a disability demonstrate similarities in motor skill development. It is true to say that children over two years old choose to walk, as a means to transport themselves from A to B on a flat surface when time is not an issue, rather than jump or hop, but each and every child has a different gait pattern. The issues that are to be addressed throughout this chapter attempt to show that gait is not genetically determined but rather is the result of another process. If gait is not genetically determined, does this apply to all our motor solutions? In our lifetime we are constantly involved in the solution, or development of answers, to motor questions: How should I catch that ball? Where should I run to? How fast should I move? When should I move? If he goes there and she moves closer, how much force should I use to throw this ball? How can I get my hands on that ice cream over there? And so the questions can continue… Could it be that as humans we basically have similar anatomies, similar goals, similar motivations, similar dynamics, and so take similar motor skill routes to achieve the answers to those motor skill questions, rather than genetics being in the driving seat?

Thelen, herself a leading disciple of this new synthesis, is far from being the only researcher or advocate. Keogh and Sugden[2] consider motor development from a multicausal perspective too as they regard motor development as not only the development of motor control over body movements, but also consider the inextricable link of development to the mover's resources. Their stance is explained by con sidering the demands of the task as it relates directly to the resources the mover has at that moment in time. The example quoted is buttoning a shirt, a task that an adult finds simple, yet a young child may possibly find beyond their control. The more difficult an individual finds a task, the less efficient they are in dealing with it and the more errors they make, so contributing to the higher task demands because of their lack of resources at the time. Even an adult when asked to button a shirt very quickly can fumble and make mistakes. The interaction of the mover–environment interplay as a transactional relationship is basic to Keogh and Sugden's[2] view of motor development. This notion of always relating motor skills to the situation in which they occur is a recurring theme in the explanation of motor skill development.

The newly emerging theories proposed by Adolph *et al.*,[18] Goldfield *et al.*,[19] Jensen *et al.*,[20] Sporns and Edelman,[21] Stroffregen *et al.*,[22] Thelen,[15] and Turvey and Fitzpatrick,[23] for example, bring together a new synthesis of information attempting to explain motor skill development from a multicausal perspective emphasizing the contextual and self-organizing nature of development through the roles of exploration–action–perception cycles, degrees of freedom equations and brain plasticity, working together with environmental constraints.

A greater emphasis is placed upon the role of the child, and the link of perception to the development of skills from the learner's explorations, in other words, there is a unity of perception, action and cognition through the process of exploration.[15] The more recent trend is, in effect, a move away from regarding the motor skill development of a child being solely at the hands of physical maturation, or solely at the hands of cognition or the ability to process information. Children are regarded as active participants in their own development as they attempt to recruit and use the resources they have at that time to solve the presented tasks.

This is different to previous work which while carefully documenting the changing motor skills seen in a growing child, chronicled these changes periodically as *fait accompli* with little or no explanation of how the changes occurred. The processes involved in how children alter their locomotor patterns to change from crawling to walking is not discussed, rather presumed to be a genetically determined pattern.

To summarize, the more recent findings on motor skill development argue against both a genetically driven timetable and cognitive explanations as to why children change in their motor skills. The questions trying to be answered by today's researchers are more to do with the processes involved in change, rather than a description of the changes. Research from the 1960s and 1970s had a tendency to concentrate upon stages of development, as time went on those so called stages became regarded as 'phases' as individual differences were more and more noted. This chapter will deal with the 'new synthesis' as labelled by Thelen,[15] with information available from studies conducted in the 1980s and 1990s, and as such will concentrate upon the debate surrounding the process of change and its explanation.

The new synthesis

The thrust of this new and alternative view of motor development is that through repeated cycles of perception and action, new behaviours emerge that are not explained by a pre-existing genetic plan. The notion that there is a relationship between cognition and action is not new, it being one of the basic assumptions of Piaget.[24] The difference is that this new synthesis of development views the growing human as a true dynamic system, rejecting the dualism of structure and function.[15] However, it is still possible to outline the types of motor skills that growing humans gain over time, for although we are all individuals we have much in common too. Given normal development, we all discover walking rather than jumping as a more efficient means of locomotion most of the time, but as mentioned earlier, the style with which we walk is quite idiosyncratic. Walking as a solution to moving from point A to point B is not just the result of preprogramming, but rather walking develops because of the constraints we as humans find anatomically, biomechanically and environmentally. These constraints can include those in the environment, those personal to the performer, the present state of the nervous and musculoskeletal system, the masses and lengths of limbs, the material properties of environmental objects and the ever present gravitational field.[19] Walking is viewed then as an inevitable solution to the demands of the task.

Many studies have now been published that examine the motor development of infants from a multicausal perspective. These studies reveal that the perception–action relationship, proposed by Gibson[25] and Gibson,[26] appears to play a major role in the control of movements through the repeated cycle of exploration–perception–action, with the child being an active participant in the process that affords change. As we perceive the environment, the activity of seeing, for example, creates an optical flow field providing both space and time information. The rate of image expansion given by the light hitting the retina offers us direct information about oncoming objects for instance. Gibson[25] believes that the information from the rate of image expansion offers direct perception of objects colliding or the timing of interceptions without the need for higher order cortical calculations. Gibson[26] demonstrated how infants of six months old possess functional depth perception, and are able to instantly judge that a 'visual' cliff is not passable even though their mothers called to them from across the other side of the 'visual' drop (the 'cliff' in real terms did not exist, it was covered by Plexiglas; nevertheless, the infant would regard it as a drop). By this experiment Gibson and Walk[27] demonstrated the use of direct perception and the relationship between affordances in the environment and personal affordances in the control of movements, even from this early age. The perception–action perspective is one of the integrated branches of the new synthesis.

Another branch of the new synthesis considers the question asked by Bernstein[28] about how humans, or indeed animals, control the many degrees of freedom possible in our movements. Degrees of freedom in this sense refer to the very many possibilities a person may have in their movements by the fixing or releasing of the limb joints. This grouping of degrees of freedom is referred to as synergies. The development of synergies to accomplish a task does not demand the use of higher cortically processed instructions to carry out a movement, rather the process relies to an extent on the physical properties of our dynamic system as we self-organize, such as the spring-like properties of our muscles, the nature of the performer's environment and the demands of the task. The more degrees of freedom used in a movement, in most cases, the finer the movement can be, provided that the person has control of these multiple joint movements. The fewer degrees of freedom used, the more fixed the movement is. A person reaching for an object with fixed elbow and wrist joints uses fewer degrees of freedom, so possibly making the reaching easier to control but allowing fewer options in the manner in which they reach. As the infant explores its environment, the movements they use change from simply exploratory to more refined and purposeful movements which result in an efficiency not seen earlier. The movements developing children use are seen to adapt to the degrees of freedom equation, altering and adapting these synergies to suit the task in hand and their changing resources. The self-assembly of the synergies required to meet the demands of the task in the case of the developing child is dependent upon the child's own resources, such as postural control, muscular strength and attractiveness of the task. This particular approach to the explanation of motor control and change examines development from a multicausal perspective, always looking for information on how our complex, dynamic and evolving system supports the environmental task.

The notion of exploration and selection as processes involved in development includes a view of the brain as a changing, developing organ that is itself moulded through experience. This is referred to as 'plasticity' of the brain, where individual perception and action act as fodder for brain change, which in turn opens new opportunities for experience. As Sporns and Edelman[21] write,

> There is overwhelming evidence that the emergence of coordinated movements is intimately tied both to the growth of the musculoskeletal system and to the development of the brain. Thus, neural development and learning cannot be considered outside of their biomechanical context. (p. 967)

Sporns and Edelman[21] refute the idea that development evolves from genetic instructions, and instead propose that through periods of instability, (where many options to solve a motor problem are experienced) and stability (where far fewer options are used to solve a motor problem) humans select solutions which strengthen certain connections or groups of neurones through use. Selection is experience dependent, with diversity providing the raw material. Sporns and Edelman[21] also believe that there are reciprocal and recursive signals from many areas of the brain that integrate messages from multiple senses to give a coordinated response. Thelen[15] has referred to this as a kind of mapping of maps. Basically this neural diversity and cross entries of sensory information allows the nervous system to recognize and categorize signals through a dynamic and self-organizing system. The brain develops through experiences, rather than through genetic maturation. Adopting this theory of development, individual differences can be accounted for. The reason for some children not crawling before they walk can be explained, for under these terms not every child is timetabled to go through certain inevitable motor milestones.

Studies from the ecological perspective or new synthesis are worthy of elaboration as they emphasize the notion of active learning from a multidiscipline, multicausal position. In addition these studies, whilst concentrating upon changes seen in infants and young children, offer a model for change throughout the lifespan not simply related to childhood. If experience and resources afford adaptation, if exploration leads to selection and further exploration develops into retention of preferred actions, the same model can be applied to the acquisition of new or adapted skills learnt by adults. If young children alter and adapt the degrees of freedom used to accomplish a task as they experiment with the nature of the task and their own constraints, then it may be possible for this process to be applied to the learning adult or older child too. Our resources and our ideas on solutions to the motor skill questions asked of us are continually evolving and self-organizing through our dynamic system.

Infant development and examples of 'new synthesis' research

At birth, a baby is completely reliant on adults and its movements are dictated by gravity. There are reflex mechanisms seen in the early months which stabilize joints and can, for instance, prevent possible damage by fast movements. In addition to these involuntary movements, Thelen[29] noted the seemingly random leg kicks, arm waves and body rolling of young babies. These movements, known as spontaneous movements, are not reflexes or involuntary movements, yet for a long time were viewed by researchers as apparently serving no purpose or use in the goal-directed sense. However, more recently researchers have viewed both reflexive movements and spontaneous movements as possible precursors to later voluntary movements. Thelen et al.[30] measured the spontaneous movements seen in young babies and, very interestingly, noted that the kinematics of the spontaneous kicking movements resemble the spatial and temporal components of mature walking patterns.

The early or primitive reflexes found in babies are related to infant survival and are nourishment-seeking as well as protective actions. These subcortically controlled reflex movements are present in all new born babies, and the rate and strength at which they appear and disappear are considered indicators of healthy development or early indicators of central nervous system disorders.[16] Some researchers also believe that there is a link between these subcortical reflex behaviours, such as the crawling, primary stepping and swimming reflexes, and later cortically processed voluntary movements such as actual walking, swimming and climbing.[31] This is despite there being a gap between the disappearance of the reflexive behaviours and the appearance of the voluntary movements. In the case of spontaneous leg movements however, there is no disappearance of the movements before the onset of locomotion. The reflexive movements seen in the stepping reflex disappear with time, but the spontaneous kicking of a child laid on his/her back remains.[15] This is significant because as noted earlier, the spontaneous leg movements have the same movement pattern as stepping.

It has been suggested that early and regular stimulation of reflexive behaviours may bring forward the onset of the corresponding voluntary movement.[16] It is also thought that as the cortex matures it is able to store information from the involuntary actions, and that this may aid the infant in the performance of later voluntary stepping or grasping. The same observation, of using information from previous behaviours, could well be made of the spontaneous leg movements mentioned earlier. Certainly the preservation of a reflex beyond a certain age or the absence of a reflex would lead a paediatrician to suspect damage in the central nervous system. For this reason alone, information about early involuntary movements has a very important role to play.

Thelen[15] proposes a different explanation for the disappearance of the so-called new-born stepping reflex. This stepping action occurs when a new-born infant is held upright with their feet on a support surface and they perform alternating steplike movements. Thelen[15] believes this appearance and subsequent disappearance of the stepping behaviour can be explained by looking at the multicausality of action rather than depending upon the maturation hypothesis.

Traditionally the disappearance of this so-called stepping reflex was attributed to maturation of the voluntary cortical centres which inhibited reflexive movements and then later facilitated the movements under a different and higher level of control.[6] This was a long-held view to explain the onset of this stepping 'reflex', its disappearance and its reappearance towards the end of the child's first year. Taking a multi-causal view of the disappearance of the so-called stepping reflex Thelen and Fisher[32,33] noted that firstly the random, spontaneous kicking actions that infants perform when laid on their backs had very similar movement patterns to the stepping 'reflex', but unlike the stepping 'reflex' these spontaneous kicks continued and did not disappear after a few months. The comment Thelen[15] makes is that these two movements, the so-called reflexive stepping and the spontaneous kicking, were the same movements performed in two different postures. So why would the cortex supposedly inhibit one movement, the stepping reflex, but not the other, the spontaneous kicking? The explanation according to Thelen and Fisher[32,33] lies not in a maturational timetable taking hold of the infant, but because of the dynamics of the situation for the infant at that moment in their lives. Considering the dynamics, such as the task demands, the resources of the infant at that particular age, and the development of the muscular–skeletal system, another explanation for the disappearing reflex was proposed.

At the same time as the stepping reflex disappears infants experience a rapid gain in mass, most of which is subcutaneous fat rather than muscle tissue. It was suggested, therefore, that in order for the infant to move their legs in a steplike movement they required the postural support from a prone or supine position, as quite simply, the legs had become too heavy for the infants to move them while upright.

In order to test out their hypothesis Thelen and Fisher[32] experimented with the infant's mass against gravity by either submerging the infant in warm water to 'restore' the stepping, or by adding weights to 'inhibit' stepping, thereby simulating the developmental changes by simple physical means. The relationship between gravity and weight gain was therefore seen to combine to afford or not afford the stepping actions from different support positions.

Other studies support Thelen's proposals demonstrating that the child's resources are brought to bear on the task in hand as they respond adaptively to the constraints within and before them. Goldfield et al.[19] monitored the development of infants learning to use a 'baby bouncer' as they adjusted their kicking to gain optimal bounce. The researchers predicted that two processes would occur when the infants, age six months, were placed in the baby bouncer. Firstly there would be an 'assembly' of the action system with low-dimensional dynamics as the child explored this new situation, followed by a tuning of the system to refine and adapt the movements to this particular condition. The early assembly, it was predicted, would be characterized by sporadic, irregular kicking, followed by more periodic kicking as the tuning took place. The third prediction suggested that once bouncing was optimized as a stable attractor, there would be a decrease in variability, an increase in amplitude, phase locking of kicking and bouncing, and stable limit-cycle and phase resetting in the face of perturbation. Lastly it was predicted that the child would be able to adapt to changing conditions, such as a new bouncer with different dynamics, using the experience from the previous bouncing. The results of the kinematic analysis provided evidence that:

> ...infants assemble and tune a periodic kicking system akin to a forced mass–spring, homing in on its resonant frequency (p. 1137)

Basically the infants in this study moved to an optimized attractor state where they got the maximal bounce for minimal energy input. It appears that through vision and perception, the infants sensed the timing and force necessary to get what Thelen[15] describes as 'the most bounce for the ounce'.

Adolph et al.[18] set up a study to investigate the perceived affordances of toddlers aged 14 months when presented with ascending or descending sloping walkways of differing angles. We have all seen how young children, and even adults, adapt their methods of locomotion to suit the terrain or explore the unknown. Developing children relatively new to locomotion have many new challenges presented to them, with the question of balance high on their agenda. The toddlers in this study were all able to walk unaided for ten feet (3 m), and initially they were required to walk towards one of their parents on a flat walkway. This walkway was then angled to form an ascending or descending slope in the middle of two flat pathways. The children were then beckoned by one of their parents again. The results of the study indicate that toddlers perceive affordances for walking over slopes. The children overestimated their ability to ascend slopes, falling often but picking themselves up, altering their style of locomotion to include climbing but continuing with the task to completion. On the descents the children chose alternative methods to get down the slope other than walking, they altered their locomotion to include sliding positions and it was noted that in contrast to their ascents the toddlers asked for help when descending. All in all the toddlers had few falls and actively explored alternative means to achieve the task so demonstrating their perception of affordance.

A similar experiment with infant crawlers, reported that younger children did not explore alternative means to descend the slopes before plunging down! Even though they had the ability to alter their method of locomotion to backward scooting, they did not make use of that option. This is in direct contrast to the toddlers who rarely fell because of their appropriately adapted movements. Adolph et al.[18] suggest that infant crawlers are less attentive to their own postural ability than are toddlers who are possibly more focused because of the demands of balancing on two legs. In addition it is suggested that the infant crawlers seeing the supportive nature of the flat walkway below the slope felt the descent would be safe and that at this moment in their development they were unable to relate the steepness of the descending slope to their own locomotor abilities.

Stoffregen et al.[22] undertook a study to determine whether young children with only a few weeks of standing experience, were able to maintain and adapt their standing posture to the constraints placed upon them by different support surfaces. The study set out to assess whether these children were successfully able to adapt their postural control according to the constraints of the surface; to determine whether the children would choose to use manual control, in this case holding a pole, as a strategy for maintaining their postural control; and to look at these adaptations in the absence of imposed perturbations. The prediction was that the children would demonstrate adaptive control on the differing surfaces and make use of manual control by holding the poles and making hip adjustments. The surfaces were a rigid high-friction surface, a soft mattress, a rigid low-friction surface (coated with baby oil) and a narrow wooden beam ($3 \times 60 \times 4$ cm) upon which the children stood crosswise. The children were encouraged to maintain a forward perspective by having their parent in front of them proffering toys and encouragement.

The children in this study were seen to exhibit remarkable adaptive postural control to the varying surfaces[22] with very few outright failures. The children used complex movements to maintain postural control including movements of the hips (not previously thought possible until three to four years of age) and the ankles, and use of the arms and hands. The children used a wide variety of coordination modes in the maintenance of their stance. They utilized the poles in manual control in a surface-specific manner, indicating, the authors believe, perception of and adaptive response to at least some of the constraints of the surfaces to their postural control. The children were able to spend most of their time engaged in suprapostural activities, which leads the researchers to suggest that future research should develop to examine the integration of posture with supra postural activities, as it seems clear that even these children have such capabilities.

In a study of three month old infants Thelen[34] found that babies were in fact able to direct movements towards a novel task; in this case, moving an overhead mobile. Her study suggests that, even at this early stage in life, learning processes are in place, once again supporting the view that new movements seen in infants are not simply the result of autonomous brain maturation. This study by Thelen[34] represents an excellent example of the evolving resources of the infant and the developing dynamic system used to find a solution to the presented motor problem. The babies were placed lying on their backs under an attractive overhead mobile. When the infants were allowed to control the movement of the mobile by their left ankles being tethered by soft elastic to the mobile, it was found that all the babies kicked more and faster as their kicks were reinforced by the mobile movement. This was not the only finding from the study. Thelen[34] decided to join the tethered left ankle to the right ankle so making it possible for the infant to alter their previous style of independent leg kicks to an in-phase pattern that would recruit the strength from both legs to move the mobile. Not only did Thelen[34] find that the babies kicked more when their movements made the mobile move but she also found that those babies with the right ankle yoked to the left increasingly kicked in a simultaneous or in-phase fashion. Thelen[34] states in her discussion:

> In everyday learning of new motor skills, tasks and constraints also appear and disappear. Opportunities for action depend on the presence of desired objects, suitable support surfaces, postures available to the infant, helping social support, and so on…Thus, in Gibsonian terms, a certain class of objects affords reaching or mouthing, or certain surfaces afford crawling upon. What is important for understanding development is how infants discover and learn new patterns in a specific situation, as demonstrated in this experiment: how those patterns are remembered: and then how classes of solutions are generalized to novel, but similar situations. (p. 284)

All the children in these studies demonstrated an awareness of their environment, its constraints and an ability to link their perceptions with their actions and develop solutions. The children's motor activities provided the means to explore their environment and the opportunity to learn about its properties. As each new solution was gained, it opened up opportunities for further perceptual motor exploration, and so the children built on their knowledge from the demands of the tasks. So once again this perspective of motor development disputes the notion of inevitable stages in motor development and emphasizes the dynamic and ecological nature of development.

Resources supporting change and motor development

From a dynamical perspective the fundamental skills that children develop from birth to around their second birthday, and onwards, have arisen because of the relationship that exists between the child's physical development and the ever changing action–perception cycles. These relationships have engendered stability and instability to produce change as the child has sought out solutions to the motor problems presented to them. For a review of these developing competencies and progressions of changes in the posture and locomotion of babies the reader may refer to Keogh and Sugden.[2]

New behaviours are seen in abundance in children from two to six years of age. Many developmentalists refer to the skills emerging during this period as fundamental movements,[1,16,35,36] and include activities such as running, hopping, jumping, skipping, climbing, throwing, catching, kicking, striking, rolling, twisting, turning and balancing, plus the manual grips needed for writing and drawing. Motor control improves drastically during this phase and the child's repertoire of skills increases substantially too. By six years of age most children have not only acquired the above skills but can also use them in combination, for example, running to kick a ball. The changes seen from the infant to the six year old child are dramatic.

Between the ages of two and six years children acquire and, in the case of some skills, refine these so-called fundamental skills. For example, skipping and hopping are acquired, while walking and running become more efficient and graceful as the child's experiences multiply. Despite more smoothness and consistency being evident in some of the normal six year old's motor skills, there is still much to discover and learn concerning the constraints that fast movements, lack of time or complex movements can exert. There are also difficulties experienced with movements in unpredictable and variable conditions.[2]

Taking the new approach to motor development these fundamental skills do not follow a predetermined plan of occurrence, rather they develop from the child finding new solutions to new tasks as their human resources afford them. Using the example of throwing, a baby soon learns how to get rid of an implement held in their hands. This develops into transporting hand-held objects to destinations further away than simply dropping them, often it seems, simply for the pleasure of seeing an adult retrieve it! As these developments take place, the child is learning categories of movements which can be applied to a constrained task. These constraints require the young child to freeze the degrees of freedom used in the act of throwing, and over time the synergies developed reveal how those degrees of freedom are freed as their experiences and resources expand (see Fig. 2.3.2).

The younger child tends to limit the throwing action to one mainly from the elbow with little rotary movement. The child's body mass is not really transferred into the throw and the feet tend to remain stationary. If the same child without the adult resources attempted to use a more mature technique to throw, they would probably end up in a heap on the floor, so the child freezes the degrees of freedom in order to keep control of the movement. This self-organizing system is demonstrating the resources the child has at this moment in time and how they are adapting to the internal and external constraints placed upon them. The coordinative structures or synergies seen in the developing child of fixed or locked joints later include greater flexibility enabling more adaptive movements. As the child learns that moving more of the arm is beneficial to the throw, and that the non-throwing arm can be used to stabilize the increased movement, so more rotation comes into play and a definite shift of body mass supports the additional movements. The child is freeing some degrees of freedom as their resources now enable them too. As Thelen[15] indicates, a new category of movements make a higher level association. So the story

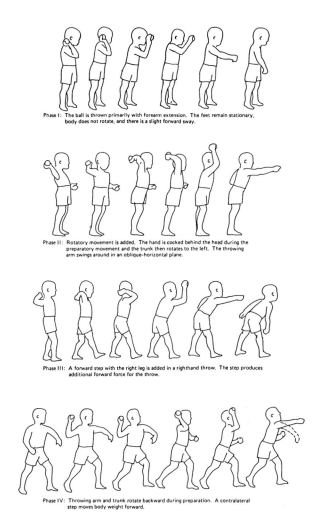

Phase I: The ball is thrown primarily with forearm extension. The feet remain stationary, body does not rotate, and there is a slight forward sway.

Phase II: Rotatory movement is added. The hand is cocked behind the head during the preparatory movement and the trunk then rotates to the left. The throwing arm swings around in an oblique-horizontal plane.

Phase III: A forward step with the right leg is added in a righthand throw. The step produces additional forward force for the throw.

Phase IV: Throwing arm and trunk rotate backward during preparation. A contralateral step moves body weight forward.

Fig. 2.3.2 Sequence pictures to illustrate differences in movement mechanics for four phases proposed by Wild.[37] Reproduced with permission.

continues, as the throwing action becomes more dynamic, the arm movements more extensive and there is a greater awareness of how these additional degrees of freedom can be controlled and used to produce a more efficient throw, in a variety of contexts. The child's movements are being tuned to their ever evolving resources. (Exactly the same argument can be made to explain how an ageing adult with arthritis, for example, redefines their actions to within their resources and the demands of the task.)

The six year old child normally uses many more degrees of freedom when throwing than the two year old would, but this is not always the case. The six year old can return to the status of the two year old when the constraints of the environment are such that the many degrees of freedom developed would lead to an inaccurate or inefficient movement. For example, if a child was running fast to throw a ball in an atmosphere of much excitement and tripped *en route*, he/she would be very likely to revert to the pattern of throwing seen in the two year old. So although the child learns to free their many degrees of freedom in order to produce more efficient movements, they also become aware of what conditions demand the freezing of them. Vereijken *et al.*[38] have demonstrated exactly this process of freeing and freezing degrees of freedom as a task is learnt, in this case a simulated ski task, where the novice first freezes at the knee and ankle joints and latterly frees the joints for a more efficient movement once previous constraints have been overcome. One would hypothesize that should the skier meet with a very steep slope, next to a vertical drop, scattered with moguls and bumps, that the actions from the easier ski runs would be seriously adapted to meet the demands of the task! At least for those human skiers! So demonstrating that actions alter not only as we acquire a skill but also upon the conditions in which the acquired task is performed.

Developmental coordination disorder

This brief section acknowledges that not all children are able to develop efficient motor solutions to the tasks placed before them, despite these children not having any diagnosable neurological disorder. Children who suffer from developmental coordination disorder (DCD) find every day functional tasks difficult as they struggle to perform skills their peers can easily master. These difficulties have been documented by DSM-IV,[39] Gubbay,[40] Henderson,[41] Wright and Sugden,[42,43] Wright *et al.*,[44] and many other authors (see Wright,[45] for a review of the literature). If children have a diagnosable neurological disorder or a physical disability which constrains their development, the new synthesis is able to explain the deficits seen in their movement solutions by reference to the impaired dynamics available as a resource to the children. Children with DCD have very different profiles within the course of their disorder making the explanation of their difficulties more complex.[43,46,47] It appears that whilst all the children with DCD may obtain a 'fail' score overall on normative or criterion referenced assessment tests their difficulties surface in different ways. Some children may be clumsy or awkward when presented with tasks demanding fine motor skills but not in any other area, some when gross skills are presented, some seem to have planning difficulties when attempting to execute motor movements in unstable and open environments, and so on. These children exhibit much variability in their solutions to motor problems. There does not appear to be a stability about their movement patterns as seen in their peers, and if there is a semblance of stability of movement pattern, it is often an awkward, stiff movement, inappropriate for the demands of the task. This leaves the child with DCD struggling to complete tasks in the time given, and the performance of motor skills is often accompanied by a feeling of failure and inadequacy.[48–51]

Whilst there is an ever growing amount of descriptive information and empirical evidence regarding the deficits seen in children with DCD, there is a paucity of empirical works explaining the causes or nominating the systems that do not function appropriately in DCD. If one attempts to explain the difficulties seen in children with DCD taking the new synthesis as a model, then one might hypothesize that the children's actions are subject to different (perhaps inappropriate) constraints, be they ones intrinsic to the movement patterns themselves, imposed by intention, or part of the essential task-specific coupling between perception and action. Children with DCD have been noted to experience perceptual difficulties, and this may be because these children do not pick up the same invariants in the environment as do normally developing children, so leading to a different coupling in the action–perception cycle. The child with DCD may intend to accomplish

the same task as his or her peers but their intrinsic dynamics appear to couple with the task differently than that seen in other children. The difficulties experienced by the child with DCD could emerge from difficulties in the self-organization of the low-level synergies that coordinate actions. As Rose[52] stresses, within the dynamical system theory importance is placed on the ability of the human system to produce highly sophisticated patterns of movement without resorting to cortical guidance as the major force behind the generation of movement. If the new synthesis is to be used as a model to explain development, or the lack of it, then the area of DCD is waiting for empirical testing to consider the systems that are functioning differently in children with DCD. A start has been made by Williams and Burke[53] and Raynor,[54,55] with these studies choosing to look at aspects of the patella tendon reflex[53–55] and visual reaction time[54,55] as an indicator of neuronal abnormalities in children with DCD, but more research in this area is necessary from dynamical and action–perception perspectives before any formal conclusions can be drawn as to why this group of children, thought to be approximately five to six per cent of the primary school population,[39,42] exhibit either a delay and/or a deviation from normal motor development.

Summary

The study of motor development has been seen to move away from phylogenetic and ontogenetic explanations and into a process orientated approach, where self-organizing dynamic systems are tuned to the constraints of the environment and the resources of the mover, through individual action and perception. The growing child is regarded far more as an intricate part of the evolution and development of the relationship between affordance and developing motor skills, and definitely not simply a product of a predetermined genetic map.

The latest research based on the ecological or new synthesis has rejuvenated and made exciting the topic of motor development. There is much yet to be discovered but the stage has been set to make a detailed account of the processes of change from a multicausal perspective.

References

1. **Haywood, K. M.** *Life span motor development* (2nd edn). Human Kinetics, Champaign, Il, 1993.

2. **Keogh, J. F.** and **Sugden, D. A.** *Movement skill development.* Macmillan, New York, 1985.

3. **Dennis, W.** and **Dennis, M.** The effect of cradling practices upon the onset of walking in Hopi children. *Journal of Genetic Psychology* 1940; **56**: 77–86.

4. **Gesell, A.** and **Amatruda, C. S.** *Developmental diagnosis.* Harper, New York, 1941.

5. **McGraw, M. B.** *Growth: A study of Johnny and Jimmy.* Appleton-Century, New York, 1935.

6. **McGraw, M. B.** *The neuromuscular maturation of the human infant.* Colombia University Press, New York, 1943.

7. **Shirley, M. M.** *The first two years: A study of twenty-five babies. Vol. 1: Postural and locomotor development.* University of Minnesota Press, Minneapolis, 1931.

8. **Malina, R. M.** *Social and biological predictors of nutritional status, physical growth, and neurological development.* Academic Press, San Diego, Ca, 1980.

9. **Malina, R. M** and **Bouchard, C.** *Growth maturation and physical activity.* Human Kinetics, Champaign, Il, 1991.

10. **Abernethy, B., Kippers, V., Mackinnon, L. T., Neal, R. J.** and **Hanrahan, S.** *The Biophysical foundations of human movement.* Human Kinetics, Champaign, Il, 1997.

11. **Bayley, N.** *Bayley scales of infant development.* Psychological Corporation, New York, 1969.

12. **Bayley, N.** *Bayley scales II.* Psychological Corporation, London, 1994.

13. **Frankenburg, W.** and **Dodds, J.** The Denver developmental screening test. *Journal of Pediatrics,* 1967; **71**: 181–7.

14. **Miller, L. J.** *Miller assessment for preschoolers.* Psychological Corporation, London, 1994.

15. **Thelen, E.** Motor development a new synthesis. *American Psychologist,* 1995; **50**: 79–95.

16. **Gallahue, D. L.** *Understanding motor development in children.* John Wiley and Sons, New York, 1982.

17. **Sugden, D. A.** and **Wright, H. C.** *Motor coordination disorders in children.* Sage, CA, USA, 1998.

18. **Adolph, K. E., Eppler, M. A.** and **Gibson, E. J.** Crawling versus walking infants' perception of affordances for locomotion over sloping surfaces. *Child Development,* 1993; **64**: 1158–74.

19. **Goldfield, E. C., Kay, B. A.** and **Warren, W. H., Jr.** Infant bouncing: The assembly and tuning of action systems. *Child Development,* 1993; **64**: 1128–42.

20. **Jensen, J. L., Thelen, E., Ulrich, B. D., Schneider, K.** and **Zernicke, R. F.** Adaptive dynamics of the leg movement patterns of human infants: III. Age-related differences in limb control. *Journal of Motor Behavior,* 1995; **27**: 366–74.

21. **Sporns, O.** and **Edelman, G. M.** Solving Bernstein's problem: A proposal for the development of coordinated movement by selection. *Child Development,* 1993; **64**: 960–81.

22. **Stoffregen, T. A., Adolph, K., Thelen, E., Gorday, K. M.** and **Sheng, Y. Y.** Toddlers' postural adaptations to different support surfaces. *Journal of Motor Control,* 1997; **1**: 119–37.

23. **Turvey, M. T.** and **Fitzpatrick, P.** Commentary: Development of perception–action systems and general principles of pattern formation. *Child Development,* 1993; **64**: 1175–90.

24. **Piaget, J.** *The origins of intelligence in children.* International Universities Press, New York, 1952.

25. **Gibson, J. J.** *The ecological approach to visual perception.* Houghton Mifflin, Boston, 1979.

26. **Gibson, E. J.** The concept of affordances in development: The renaissance of functionalism. In *The concept of development. Minnesota symposium on child psychology,* Vol. 15 (ed. W. A. Collins). Erlbaum, Hillsdale, NJ, 1982; 55–81.

27. **Gibson, E. J.** and **Walk, R. D.** The 'visual cliff'. *Scientific American,* 1960; **202**: 64–71.

28. **Bernstein, N.** *The coordination and regulation of movements.* Pergamon, London, 1967.

29. **Thelen, E.** Rhythmical stereotypes in normal human infants. *Animal Behaviour,* 1979; **27**: 699–715.

30. **Thelen, E., Bradshaw, G.** and **Ward, J. A.** Spontaneous kicking in month old infants: Manifestation of a human central locomotor program. *Behavioural and Neural Biology,* 1981; **32**: 45–53.

31. **Zelazo, P.** From reflexive to instrumental behavior. In *Developmental psychobiology: The significance of infancy.* (ed. L. P. Lipsitt). Lawrence Erlbaum, Hillsdale, N.J, 1976; 87–106.

32. **Thelen, E.** and **Fisher, D. M.** New-born stepping: An explanation for a 'disappearing reflex'. *Developmental Psychology,* 1982; **18**: 760–75.

33. **Thelen, E.** and **Fisher, D. M.** The organization of spontaneous leg movements in new-born infants. *Journal of Motor Behavior,* 1983; **15**: 353–77.

34. **Thelen, E.** Three-month-old infants can learn task-specific patterns of interlimb coordination. *Psychological Science,* 1994; **5**: 280–5.

35. **Roberton, M. A.** Changing motor patterns during childhood. In *Motor development during childhood and adolescence* (ed. J. R. Thomas). Burgess, Minneapolis, Minnesota, 1984; 48–90.

36. **Smoll, F. L.** Developmental kinesiology: toward a subdiscipline focusing on motor development. In *The development of movement control and co-ordination* (ed. S. J. A. Kelso and J. E. Clarke). John Wiley and Sons, Chichester, 1982; 319–54.

37. **Wild, M. R.** The behavior pattern of throwing and some observations concerning its course of development in children. *Research Quarterly,* 1938; **9**: 20–4.

38. **Vereijken, B., van Emmerik R. E. A., Whiting, H. T. A.** and **Newell, K. M.** Free(z)ing degrees of freedom in skill acquisition. *Journal of Motor Behavior,* 1992; **24**: 133–42.

39. **DSM-IV** *Diagnostic and statistical manual of mental disorders* (4th edn). American Psychiatric Association, Washington DC, 1994.

40. **Gubbay, S. S.** Clumsy children in normal schools. *The Medical Journal of Australia,* 1975; **1**: 233–6.

41. **Henderson, S. E.** Clumsiness or developmental coordination disorder: a neglected handicap. *Current Paediatrics,* 1992; **2**: 158–62

42. **Wright, H. C.** and **Sugden, D. A.** A two step procedure for the identification of children with developmental coordination disorder in Singapore. *Developmental Medicine and Child Neurology,* 1996a; **38**: 1099–105.

43. **Wright, H. C.** and **Sugden, D. A.** The nature of developmental coordination disorder: inter and intra group differences. *Adapted Physical Activity Quarterly,* 1996b; **13**: 358–74.

44. **Wright, H. C., Sugden, D. A, Ng, R.** and **Tan, J.** Identification of children with movement problems in Singapore: Usefulness of the movement ABC checklist. *Adapted Physical Activity Quarterly,* 1994; **11**: 150–7.

45. **Wright, H. C.** Developmental coordination disorder: A review. *European Journal of Physical Education,* 1997; **2**: 5–22.

46. **Dewey, D.** and **Kaplan, B. J.** Subtyping of developmental motor deficits. *Developmental Neuropsychology,* 1994; **10**: 265–84.

47. **Hoare, D.** Subtypes of developmental coordination disorder. *Adapted Physical Activity Quarterly,* 1994; **11**: 158–69.

48. **Cantell, M. H., Ahonen, T. P.** and **Smyth, M. M.** Clumsiness in adolescence: educational, motor, and social outcomes of motor delay detected at 5 years. *Adapted Physical Activity Quarterly,* 1994; **11**: 115–29.

49. **Losse, A., Henderson, S. E., Elliman, D., Hall, D., Knight, E.** and **Jongmans, M.** Clumsiness in children-do they grow out of it? A ten year follow-up study. *Developmental Medicine and Child Neurology,* 1991; **33**: 55–68.

50. **Schoemaker, M. M.** and **Kalverboer, A. F.** Social and affective problems of children who are clumsy: how early do they begin? *Adapted Physical Activity Quarterly,* 1994; **11**: 130–40.

51. **Wright, H. C.** and **Sugden, D. A.** A school based intervention programme for children with developmental coordination disorder. *European Journal of Physical Education,* 1998; **3**: 35–50.

52. **Rose, D.J.** *A multilevel approach to the study of motor control and learning.* Allyn and Bacon, Singapore, 1997.

53. **Williams, H. G.** and **Burke, J. R.** Conditioned patellar tendon reflex function in children with and without developmental coordination disorders. *Adapted Physical Activity Quarterly,* 1995; **12**: 250–61.

54. **Raynor, A. J.** *Neuromuscular performance of poorly and normally coordinated children.* Unpublished doctoral dissertation. The University of Western Australia, Perth, Australia, 1994.

55. **Raynor, A. J.** Fractionated reflex and reaction times in children with developmental coordination disorder. *Journal of Motor Control,* 1998; **2**: 114–24.

56. **Clark, J. E.** and **Whitall, J.** What is motor development? The lessons of history. *Quest,* 1998; **41**: 183–202.

2.4 Strength and muscle growth

David A. Jones and Joan M. Round

Introduction

Childhood is the time when the young person moves from physical dependence on its parents to a stage, with the arrival of puberty, when the adolescent comes to equal or challenge the physical ascendancy of its elders. The development of skeletal muscle strength is central to this process and the transition is so universal as to be generally unremarked. However, every parent with teenage children, and especially boys, will remember that moment when the physical strength and presence of their offspring reminds them they are living with a young adult who is no longer a child. It is also very poignant when normal development is disrupted by disease or deformity and the adult son or daughter continues to need the physical support of ageing parents.

There are three reasons for studying the growth of skeletal muscle. The first is as a matter of academic interest to complement and complete the pioneering work such as that of Jones[1] and others in the Fels Growth Study in North America and Tanner[2] in the UK, which did so much to document the normal patterns of growth and increasing strength in children. The second reason is to provide normal data against which to judge the progress or potential of children, whether they be training for some sporting event, recovering from injury or suffering a disability affecting their strength or mobility. The third reason is because childhood offers the opportunity to observe muscle as it undergoes the unique process of rapid growth, development and maturation. Very little is known about the stimulus for muscle growth and a young child is a living experiment where it is possible to observe growing muscle and, hopefully, to identify the factors that promote its growth and increase in strength.

Embryological origins of muscle and early development

There is a huge diversity in the adult population with respect to body shape, muscularity and the propensity for endurance or power events. The origins of this diversity occur early in fetal development when, at about the fifth week of gestation, pre-myoblastic mesodermal cells begin to express myogenic determination factors and differentiate into myoblasts. The myoblasts subsequently fuse to form multinucleate myotubes and attach to the developing skeletal structures to form the primordial muscles. Some myoblasts remain as single mono-nucleate cells with mitotic potential and these cells will form the satellite cells of mature muscle.[3] Within the developing myotube a central chain of nuclei forms (Fig. 2.4.1) surrounded by basophilic cytoplasm rich in polyribosomes. In the human fetus the transition from myoblast to primary myotube takes place between the seventh and ninth weeks of gestation and by the end of this period the primordia of most muscle groups are well defined. At this time the synthesis of the contractile proteins, actin and myosin, begins and the first signs of cross striations are visible. From 11 weeks onwards there is proliferation of myofibrils leading to hypertrophy of the muscle fibres, which also grow in length by the addition of sarcomeres at the ends. By 18 to 23 weeks the nuclei of the more mature myotubes begin to move to the periphery of the fibre. Under the light microscope it is very difficult to distinguish muscle fibre nuclei from the 10% to 20% of nuclei that belong to satellite cells, but the latter can be identified under the electron microscope where they are seen to lie between the basement membrane and the surface membrane of the muscle fibre. Myonuclei are incapable of mitosis, and if the muscle fibre is damaged, it is the satellite cells that are activated to divide and begin the process of regeneration.

At about ten weeks of gestation the developing muscle fibres become innervated by outgrowths from the spinal motor neurones. At first there are several attachments per muscle fibre, but as they mature so the number of innervating nerves decreases until there is only one surviving motor axon per fibre with a single neuromuscular junction, usually situated near the middle of the fibre.[4] It is the electrical activity dictated by the innervating motor neurone that largely determines the development of the contractile and metabolic characteristics of the fibre, the so called 'fibre type'. At first the fibres express fetal and embryonic myosins but as the fibres differentiate adult forms of myosin are expressed. In most muscles, about half of the developing fibres express slow myosin and half the fast myosin isoforms, together with the associated regulatory proteins and characteristic contents of sarcoplasmic reticulum and mitochondria. Muscle fibre differentiation, which is apparent by about 32 weeks of development, is not fully complete until some months after birth.

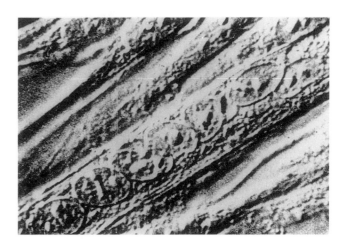

Fig. 2.4.1 Myotubes formed by the fusion of myoblasts and showing the characteristic chain of central nuclei.

The muscularity of any individual will depend on the size and number of muscle fibres. The number of fibres is determined largely by the number of fetal myoblasts and clearly has a large genetic component. The factors controlling the size of the fibres are dealt with in the sections that follow.

Muscle fibre growth

Muscle growth is thought to be by a process of fibre hypertrophy rather than hyperplasia. That is, growth in size of the anatomical muscle is due to an increase in size of the constituent fibres while the number remains constant. In the rat, fibre numbers have been shown not to change during life while the mean fibre cross-sectional area increases nearly tenfold from the newborn to adult animal.[5] There are considerable practical and ethical problems involved in making measurements of fibre size and number in children and adults, but the limited data available suggest that, as with rats, there is an increase in size without a change in fibre numbers (hypertrophy without hyperplasia) as the muscles grow in size and strength (Fig. 2.4.2). A comparison of quadriceps cross-sectional area and muscle fibre areas, in a limited number of subjects, showed that muscle fibre area was the main factor determining cross-sectional area of the whole muscle,[6] implying that fibre numbers are relatively constant.

Adult muscle fibre cross-sectional areas are reached some time after puberty (Fig. 2.4.2). In an adult man about 40 to 45% of the body mass is muscle and this figure is slightly lower in females. The mean cross-sectional area of fibres in a biopsy from the quadriceps muscle in a normal man is 3500 to 7500 μm^2 and in normal women from 2000 to 5000 μm^2 (Fig. 2.4.3).[7]

The average cross-sectional area (CSA) of the quadriceps muscle, measured at mid femur, is approximately 60 cm^2 in women and 80 cm^2 in men (i.e. women have about 75% of the male CSA) and the isometric force is in a similar ratio (Fig. 2.4.4).[8] Although there are limited data, it appears that the ratio of fibre areas in the sexes is similar to that of the muscle cross-sectional areas and strengths, and this is consistent with the notion that there are similar numbers of fibres in male and female muscle. Also shown in Fig. 2.4.4 are the values for muscle force and cross-sectional area for two prepubertal children, and it can be seen that they fall very much within the adult relationship indicating that the 'quality' of children's muscle is much the same as an adult of either sex.

In discussing growth of a complex structure such as muscle, it must be stressed that growth is not simply the accumulation of more and more protein as with bricks when building a house, but is a process of

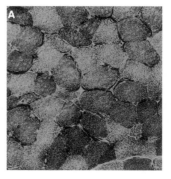
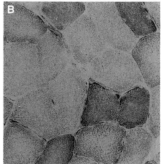

Fig. 2.4.3 Transverse sections (at the same magnification) of muscle biopsies from: (A) female and (B) male subject, showing differences in fibre size. Sections stained for NADH-TR, showing variations in mitochondrial density in the different fibre types.

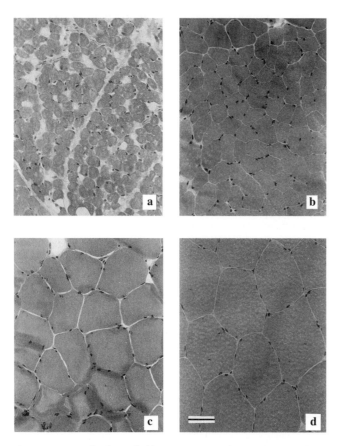

Fig. 2.4.2 Growth of muscle fibre cross-sectional area. (a) Biopsy from 8 month old baby; (b) 5 year old child; (c) 14 year old boy; (d) a large 23 year old man. Transverse sections of quadriceps muscle samples, stained with trichrome. Bar in (d) = 50 μm.

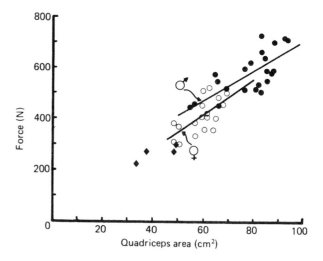

Fig. 2.4.4 The relationship between force and cross-sectional area (determined by CT scanning) of the quadriceps for adult male (•) and female (○) subjects and two boys (♦) aged 10 and 12. Data from Chapman *et al.*[8]

continual remodelling. Net growth of the tissue is the balance between protein synthesis and protein breakdown. Growth can be achieved by an increase in protein synthesis but, in theory at least, it can also be the result of a decrease in protein breakdown.

Muscle growth requires the deposition of new proteins and this can occur in two ways. The first is an increase in the amount of protein synthesized per unit of DNA, either by increasing transcription or translation. The second major mechanism for growth is by nuclear division. For skeletal muscle it is established that it is the satellite cell nuclei that divide[3] and in post-natal life, rather than forming new fibres, they are incorporated into existing fibres thereby increasing the nuclear material available within the fibre to support protein synthesis. The notion is that a muscle fibre nucleus can support a certain maximum volume of cytoplasm and that the fibre must, as a consequence, acquire more nuclei as a result of satellite cell division in order to gain in volume.

It is not known to what extent muscle growth is the result of increased protein synthesis based on existing nuclear material and how much is due to satellite cell division. Cheek[9] suggested that during the course of development in man there is a 14- to 20-fold increase in the DNA within the muscle mass but only a twofold increase in the DNA unit size. Histological data, such as in Fig. 2.4.2, show the density of nuclei to decrease about fourfold, rather more than suggested by Cheek.[9] Short-term fluctuations in size and strength, such as seen with dietary manipulation or as the result of atrophic muscle disease, may be the result of a change in the protein synthesis per unit DNA. Longer-term increases in muscle size, such as seen during growth and possibly prolonged strength training, certainly require nuclear proliferation. The precise details of which phase of growth depends on proliferation and which on expanding the DNA unit size remain to be elucidated.

Size and strength

In common with cardiac and smooth muscle, it is the contractile proteins actin and myosin that generate force and movement in skeletal muscle. The regular arrangement of the contractile proteins has functional implications for the relationship between muscle size, strength and power output and is an important consideration for those interested in scaling strength and body size.

The maximum force of an idealized muscle is determined by the number of sarcomeres arranged in parallel and is unaffected by the number in series, i.e. by the length of the muscle (Fig. 2.4.5). In such a muscle the force is, therefore, proportional to the cross-sectional area of the muscle or to the square of the linear dimensions (l^2). In contrast, because all sarcomeres contract together and each by a similar and fixed amount, the velocity of overall muscle shortening will depend on the number of sarcomeres in series, i.e. is directly proportional to the length of the muscle (l). Power is the product of force and velocity and consequently it can be seen that it is proportional to l^3, or the volume of the muscle.[10] Maximum power is usually obtained at about one-third Vmax so that although the maximum power may be the same in two muscles, one short and fat, the other long and thin, the velocity at which this occurs will be different and this has considerable implications for performance.

For a growing child, an increase in linear dimensions would be expected to result in an increase in strength to the power of two, provided the muscle increased in its linear dimensions in proportion to the rest of the body. It can be seen that, in this situation, strength would lag behind body mass which increases as the third power of the linear dimensions. In this model, therefore, strength would lag behind body mass.

In addition to the physical dimensions discussed above, there are a number of other factors that will influence the force generated for a given size or cross-sectional area of muscle. The packing of contractile material within the muscle fibre may vary, possibly as a result of changes in the separation of the actin and myosin filaments. More realistically there may be differences in the amount of non-contractile material in the fibre, such as mitochondria, sarcoplasmic reticulum, fat droplets and glycogen etc.

Fibre type composition

There is some evidence from both human and animal work that type two fibres are intrinsically stronger than type one,[11] but there is no evidence that during normal growth there is preferential development of any particular fibre type or change in fibre type proportions.

The angle of muscle fibre insertion

Individual muscles vary in the arrangement of their fibres between tendons and a change in this angle of insertion (or pennation) may alter the force measured between the ends of a muscle.[12] It is possible that during development the angle of pennation may change thus changing the force produced per volume of muscle, but there is no information available on this point.

Lever ratios

Muscle strength is measured indirectly through the lever system of the skeleton. Consequently the force measured with the strain gauge or dynamometer is the force of the muscle multiplied by the mechanical advantage (or usually disadvantage) of the lever system. For the quadriceps the schematic arrangement is shown in Fig. 2.4.6 and the force measured at the ankle is seen to be the force generated in the patella tendon multiplied by the ratio of, essentially, the size of the patella tuberocity and the length of the tibia. The tuberocity is small compared to the length of the bone, and it is evident that small changes in the width of the bone at this point could have a significant

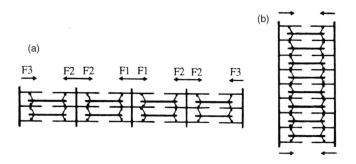

Fig. 2.4.5 Force generated by sarcomeres in series and in parallel. (a) Sarcomeres in series: the forces F1 and F2 are opposed, leaving only F3 to exert force at the ends of the muscle. (b) The same number of actin and myosin filaments arranged in parallel to give four times the isometric force of (a).

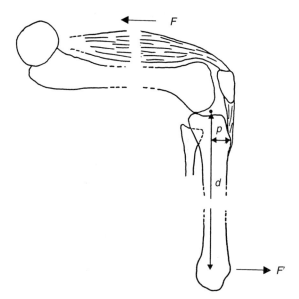

Fig. 2.4.6 Diagrammatic representation of the lever system for the quadriceps. The force measured, F', is derived from the force generated in the quadriceps, F, by multiplying it by the ratio p/d.

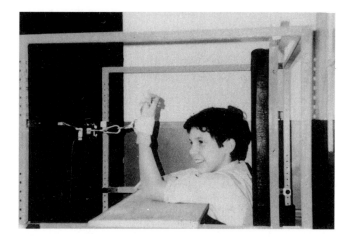

Fig. 2.4.7 Measuring the isometric strength of the forearm flexor muscle group (mainly biceps) in a 9 year old boy.

effect on the mechanical advantage and thus the force measured at the ankle. It has proved very difficult to obtain information about possible changes in the proportions or shapes of bones during development. However, Parker[13] examined museum specimens and found very little difference in the proportions (lengths to breadth) of the tibia in adult and juvenile bones. With the bones of the forearm, there was a suggestion of a change in the lever ratio of muscles attached to the radius such that the measured force would, if anything, decrease with age.

A change in force independent of any change in the size of a muscle can undoubtedly occur and probably for a variety of reasons, as outlined above. However, although there is little evidence, it is probably fair to assume that the major influence on strength during childhood and adolescence is growth in the quantity of muscle rather than changes in the quality.

Measurement of force

The practical and theoretical questions arising from the measurement of strength in children have been reviewed in Chapter 1.3. It will have become apparent that there is a multitude of ways in which strength can be assessed. There is also something of a conflict between the interests of coaches and sports scientists who need a measure that is 'relevant' to their sport or activity and the physiologist who is concerned to make measurements that reflect the structure and function of individual muscle groups. Thus conflict arises because the 'relevant' measurements involve complex muscle groups, where performance will depend not only on the size and strength of individual muscles but also on their coordinated activation. Even a simple test such as pushing or pulling (e.g. Fig. 2.4.7) requires the coordinated action of stabilizing muscles all over the body for optimal performance.

For the muscle physiologist concerned, as we are here, with questions of muscle growth, actions such as arm pull and arm thrust, vertical jump, leg lifts and bent arm hang are all too complex for simple

analysis. Even a widely used measure such as hand grip is complicated by the involvement of both the finger flexors in the forearm and the intrinsic hand muscles together with the complex biomechanics of muscles acting through long tendons and complex lever systems, where the mechanical advantage must be, at best, uncertain (see Chapter 2.2). For these reasons we believe that measurement of isometric force of major muscle groups, such as the knee extensors (quadriceps), the forearm flexors (mainly biceps) or plantar flexors (calf muscles), represents the best option for physiological assessment (Fig. 2.4.7). However, it is recognized that measurement of isometric force at one joint angle may fail to demonstrate changes in force/angle or force/velocity relationships if they occur with maturation.

Growth studies and the measurement of strength

There have been a number of longitudinal studies charting the development of strength during adolescence and a few that include younger children. Tanner[2] provides a comprehensive review of the earlier work and he also provides a brief history of growth studies,[14] although the latter does not include any information about strength. The most frequently quoted early work relating to strength is that of Jones[1] on the adolescent group in the University of California Child Welfare study. The static strength of hand grip, arm pull and arm thrust were measured using an isometric dynamometer and the most striking feature of the results is the clear separation in strength between boys and girls that occurs at the time of puberty (Fig. 2.4.8).

Stoltz and Stoltz[15] reported data on Californian boys during adolescence (part of the Fells Growth Study) and Faust[16] complemented the Stoltzs' work with her study of a group of Californian girls. Further reports of strength development include those of Carron and Bailey[17] on boys from the Saskatchewan Growth Study. All of these studies emphasize the fact that there is a major increase in strength of boys during puberty and that this is in sharp contrast to the girls. More recently, Beunen and co-workers[18] have measured static, dynamic and explosive strength in Belgian boys as part of the Leuven study of growth and motor performance, and similar tests have been used by Kemper[19,20] and his group on Dutch children in the Amsterdam growth study. Most recently, Round *et al.*[21] have reported the isometric strength of quadriceps and biceps in a longitudinal study of British children from north London.

It is generally agreed that during childhood there is a steady increase in strength with little difference seen between boys and girls until puberty when both sexes show a significant increase in the velocity of strength gain. At this time boys increase to a greater final strength than girls and show a disproportionate increase in the upper limb musculature, which reaches a final strength nearly double that of young women.

The only suggestions of a sex difference in strength before puberty involves muscular actions of the arms. Jones[1] reported greater handgrip strength and others have commented on the superiority of overarm throwing in boys (reviewed by Malina[22]). After puberty it is clear that boys' strength increases but Jones[1] remarked that girls seem to decrease in strength after menarche. This suggestion was supported by Faust[16] who commented that dynamometer strength testing might be unreliable as a measure of strength in teenage girls and that the decrease she found was most likely as a result of the teenage girls not trying so hard. Our own experience of post-menarchial girls in the mid 1990s is that they show no evidence of a loss of strength during this time, but we were using isometric strength testing which reduces the component of skill and coordination to a minimum.

Early reports on the timing of the adolescent spurt in strength suggested that it occurred around the time of the peak height velocity (PHV)[1,2] but more recent reports place it about one year after PHV and roughly coincident with peak weight velocity.[18]

The old adage that boys may outgrow their strength at some period during puberty was questioned by Tanner in the 1960s and finds no support from modern studies. Neither in the Leuven study[18] or the north London study[21] was there any period during puberty where strength failed to increase (but see discussion of data in Fig. 2.4.13).

It is interesting to speculate about the causes of greater strength in young men. Men are bigger, on average, than women as a result of the later (about two years) and larger growth spurts in stature and mass in boys compared to girls. Can the greater strength of young men be explained entirely by the differences in their physical dimensions or is there some other factor? In other words, would men and women be of the same strength if properly scaled to the same physical dimensions? This point is explored in the following sections.

Determinants of strength during development

Very little is known about growth of muscle and increase in strength during the first five or six years of life. The practical difficulties and ethical considerations make it difficult to perform biopsies or scan young children and, as discussed earlier, it is also difficult to obtain reliable strength measurements. After that age it becomes possible to make reliable measurements and therefore to speculate about the growth of muscle tissue.

Figure 2.4.9 shows the development of strength in boys and girls in two major muscle groups and it is clear that before puberty there is a steady increase in both sexes, and whilst the boys, on average, may be slightly stronger than the girls, there is little significance in this difference. The results are qualitatively very similar to those obtained 40 years earlier,[1] although the strengths reported by Jones[1] are somewhat larger than those measured by Parker *et al.*,[23] allowing for the fact that 1 kg force is equivalent to about 10 N. The difference is probably due to the fact that 'Arm Pull' measured by Jones[1] includes a variety of muscle groups acting around the shoulder, whilst the strength measurements of Parker *et al.*[23] represent the isolated action of the forearm flexors.

It is interesting to see how the development of strength relates to other parameters of growth during this prepubertal period when the sex steroids have no role to play. The relationships between stature and strength of the biceps for boys and girls is shown in Fig. 2.4.10.[23] For girls, there is a curvilinear relationship between strength and stature, with the more mature girls clustering at the higher end of the curve, showing strength to be proportional to the square of stature. For boys the relationship shows a clear discontinuity at around the time of puberty. Taking the values for boys below the age of 12, when it is fair to assume that the majority will be prepubertal, the relationship between strength and stature is very similar to that for girls with strength being proportional to the second power of stature. A similar

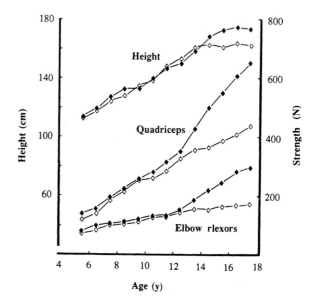

Fig. 2.4.9 Changes in strength with age. Cross-sectional study in which the isometric strength of the quadriceps and elbow flexors were measured in boys (filled symbols) and girls (open symbols). From Parker *et al.*[23]

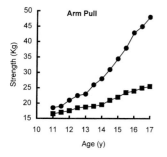
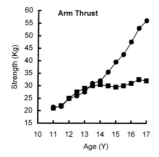

Fig. 2.4.8 Changes in arm strength with age. Data for 'arm pull' and 'arm thrust' taken from the mixed longitudinal study of Jones:[1] ■, girls; ●, boys. Note that strength is reported in kg force, equivalent to 9.81 N.

situation was found for the relationship between strength of the quadriceps and stature, except that strength in this case was proportional to the cube of stature for girls and prepubertal boys. The implications of these results has been anticipated in a previous section (*Size and strength*) and suggest that the biceps grow in size in proportion to the increase in linear dimensions. For the quadriceps the findings imply that the muscles increase in size to a greater extent than would be predicted from the increase in linear dimensions, but this is a very useful outcome since the quadriceps are clearly essential in supporting body mass which is proportional to length cubed.

Passive stretch of muscle imposed by longitudinal growth of the bones may well provide a stimulus for muscle growth[24,25] and this could regulate the growth of biceps muscles in the prepubertal children. The quadriceps muscles are body mass bearing and will consequently be subject to two stimuli, an increase in muscle length, as for the biceps, but also the increasing load of the body mass experienced during the course of normal daily activities.

The changes in strength in boys and girls found by Parker *et al.*[23] are comparable with the changes in width of the muscles determined radiologically in the Harpenden growth study.[26] In that study, arm muscle width increased by approximately 10% and 50% for girls and boys, respectively, from 13 to 18 years of age, indicating that cross sectional areas increased by 20% and 125%, respectively. These values compare with increases in biceps strength of 20% in girls and 95% in boys from 12 to 18 years found by Parker *et al.*,[23] suggesting that strength gains are mainly the result of increase in muscle bulk.

While the increase in muscle strength is very similar in boys and girls in the early childhood years, it is clear that puberty marks a clear divergence in patterns of growth (Figs 2.4.8 and 2.4.9), and the relationships between strength and stature, as shown in Fig. 2.4.10 for prepubertal children, no longer apply to the adolescent boy. The divergence from the growth pattern of prepubertal boys is most noticeable for the biceps muscle group and there is other evidence that upper and lower body musculature show different patterns of growth during adolescence. In a longitudinal study, Carron and Bailey[17] found that measures of upper body strength in boys increased 3.9-fold between the ages of 10 and 16 years, whilst for lower body strength the increase was 2.5-fold. Tanner *et al.*[26] estimated that peak growth velocity of arm

muscles in boys was about twice that in girls while there were no sex differences in the calf. Kemper and Verschuur,[19] in a longitudinal study measuring muscle volumes, showed that sex differences became apparent at puberty, with a suggestion of greater differences between boys and girls in the upper body musculature.

Tanner[2] speculated that the greater strength in boys seen after puberty was probably associated with the action of circulating sex steroids on the muscle, and it seems very likely that the differences in muscle development are due to the increase in circulating testosterone that is a feature of maturation in normal male adolescents at this time of testicular growth.[27,28] However, the association between testosterone and muscle growth, although widely accepted, is based largely on anecdotal reports of drug abuse in athletes and body builders, and the observation that major differences in muscular development appear around the time of puberty. Recently it has been shown that supra-physiological doses of testosterone, combined with specific training, stimulate muscle growth in adults,[29] but it is not clear how this action relates to normal patterns of growth. Testosterone is also known to restore muscle bulk in hypogonadal males[30] but, again, it is not clear how this situation relates to normal muscle development.

Recently Round and colleagues[21] completed a longitudinal study of muscle strength development in boys and girls that included measures of circulating sex hormones in addition to those of stature, mass and strength. Longitudinal studies allow growth curves, that may differ in their timing by as much as two or three years, to be aligned to the time of peak height velocity so that the relative timing of events, such as the increase in growth of muscle and changes in circulating hormone levels, can be seen with more precision than in cross-sectional surveys.

This type of study has also been helped by the development of a relatively new statistical method. Multilevel modelling of mixed longitudinal data effectively allows individuals to have their own growth curves, as well as fitting separate growth curves for specific groups within the sample, e.g. boys and girls[31] (and see Chapter 1.1). Thus group effects (i.e. comparing the boys' and girls' growth parameters) that are larger than the within-individual variation can be identified.

Figure 2.4.11 shows data for the development of boys' and girls' strength that have been aligned to the time of PHV. Before PHV, absolute strengths are higher in the boys compared to the girls for a

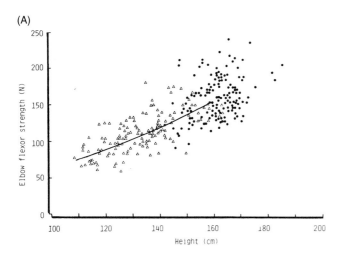

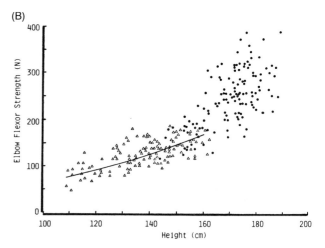

Fig. 2.4.10 Relationship between strength of the elbow flexors and height. Individual data from the study shown in Fig. 2.4.8. A: Data for girls, open triangles are girls under 12 years and the fitted line has the equation $N = m^{1.9} \times 10^{1.8}$ ($r = 0.69$). B: Data for boys, open triangles are boys under 13 years and the fitted line has the equation $N = m^{1.99} \times 10^{1.81}$ ($r = 0.71$).

given age relative to PHV as a consequence of the later occurrence of PHV in boys. The boys had been growing at a fairly constant rate for, on average, two years longer than had the girls before their growth spurt occurred. Increases in strength, as opposed to the absolute strength, were similar in the two sexes until about one year before PHV. For both muscle groups, clear differences between the sexes in the rate of increase in strength were evident up to two years after the time of PHV. Figure 2.4.12 shows the plasma testosterone measurements centred upon the time of PHV for boys. Circulating testosterone levels begin to rise one year before PHV and then increase steadily, reaching adult levels around three years after PHV. The increase in testosterone coincides with the divergence of strength between boys and girls seen in Fig. 2.4.11.

The multilevel modelling analysis for the quadriceps indicates that, for the girls during puberty, strength increases in proportion to the size of the body and that no other age-related factor is required to explain the increase in strength. For the boys, however, stature and mass alone are not sufficient to explain the increase in strength and an additional term is required, which is provided by circulating testosterone. The results of the modelling show that testosterone fully explains the differences between the sexes that remain after making allowance for body size (stature and mass). The analysis indicates that for every unit of circulating testosterone (nmol litre^{-1}), strength of

the quadriceps increases by 0.7%, so, taking the young adult male testosterone to be 20 to 30 nmol litre^{-1}, the young males are 15 to 20% stronger as a result of the circulating androgens than might be expected from their overall body stature.

A similar analysis of the results for the biceps shows interesting and complex results. The difference between boys' and girls' strength was greater than could be fully explained by the action of testosterone in the young men. There could be two explanations for this, the first is that there may be some inhibition of muscle growth in the girls as a consequence of increased levels of circulating oestrogen. Oestrogen is a potent promoter of skeletal maturation and will lead to a cessation of growth of stature and remove the lengthening stimulus for muscle growth. However, the quadriceps muscle does not seem to be affected in this way, and following the menopause oestrogen withdrawal is associated with decline in muscle function.[32] The explanation proposed by Round et al.[21] is that the linear measurement 'seen' by the developing biceps is the length of the upper arm, rather than stature as used in their data analysis. Selective development of various parts of the skeleton are well known features of the process of sexual maturation, the most obvious being the development of the pelvis in girls and of the upper limb girdle in boys. It is suggested that biceps development is greater in boys, firstly because of the direct action of testosterone on the muscle itself and secondly because the hormone causes a disproportionate increase in the length of the humerus and in so doing provides an additional stimulus for muscle growth.

It has to be acknowledged, however, that there may be other explanations for the preferential muscular development in boys. The difference might reflect cultural attitudes, with boys, at around the time of puberty, taking up sports and activities which train the upper body musculature, and Verschuur and Kemper[33] have shown that boys of this age spend significantly more time than girls undertaking 'heavy' activities. However, if this was the explanation we might expect to see an overlap in strength between the sexes with some of the less active boys in the cohort avoiding such exercise while some active girls defied the social norms for their sex. In practice, virtually no overlap is found between the sexes in strength of the biceps, while for the quadriceps there is appreciable overlap between large active women and small sedentary men. For many years standards for quadriceps strength have been used that relate strength to body mass, irrespective of sex.[34] The data for biceps strength in Fig. 2.4.11B shows a very clear separation between the sexes, with no suggestion of the increased variance that might be expected in the older age groups if habitual activity was an important determinant of strength. Of all the 16 year old children, only one boy had a biceps strength below 200 N, while no girl had a biceps strength greater than 199 N.

It is interesting, and sometimes entertaining, to speculate on the evolutionary significance of the differences in upper body strength between the sexes. In terms of hunting and gathering, there would seem to be little point in women not having the same strength in the upper body as men, and this leads to the conclusion that it may be a secondary sexual characteristic analogous to the shoulder girdle development seen in many mammalian species, including other primates and cattle. An unscientific survey of female staff and students suggests that excessive muscular development in men is not particularly attractive to the opposite sex, and consequently the upper body development seems to have served in the past as a way of asserting dominance over other males rather than attracting mates. Whether it still retains this function was not clear from the unscientific responses of male staff and students.

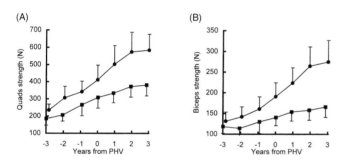

Fig. 2.4.11 Strength in relation to time of peak height velocity: A, Quadriceps; B, forearm flexors (biceps). Values are given as mean + or − SD of the values for children in each year for whom the age of PHV could be clearly identified: ● boys, ■ girls (Round et al.[21]).

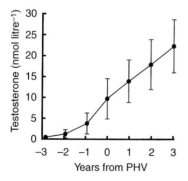

Fig. 2.4.12 Circulating testosterone in relation to time of peak height velocity. Plasma testosterone in boys plotted against the years before or after the time of peak height velocity. Values are given as mean + or − SD of the values for children in each year for whom the age of PHV could be clearly identified (Round et al.[21]).

Muscle growth, strength and performance

The development of motor performance has been reviewed by Malina[22,35] (and see Chapter 2.3), and it is important to consider the role that development of muscle strength plays in this vital process. As discussed in Chapters 2.2 and 2.3, even the simplest task such as jumping or running depends on an interplay of strength and coordination with the complex biomechanics of the musculoskeletal system. For running and explosive tasks such as jumping, the strength to body mass ratio would seem to be a critical factor, yet it is interesting to note that whilst running speed and jumping performance improve steadily throughout childhood, and often dramatically in teenage boys, the ratio of isometric strength to body mass remains remarkably constant or decreases somewhat until puberty (Fig. 2.4.13). This observation emphasizes the importance of other factors that contribute to performance.

One aspect of muscle function that has been overlooked so far in the discussion of changes in isometric strength is the influence of changing muscle length. As discussed earlier, isometric strength is not dependent on muscle length but the velocity of shortening is directly proportional to the number of sarcomeres in series, and this will increase roughly in parallel with stature. The consequence of changing muscle length is shown in Fig. 2.4.14. At low velocities of contraction, there is little difference in either the force or power output of the two muscles but it becomes progressively more important the higher the velocity. The longer, faster muscle will be able to impart a greater impulse to the ground during jumping or move a longer limb at the same angular velocity to impart a greater momentum to the hand or foot when throwing or kicking. Round et al.[21] measured only isometric strength, but it is possible to estimate the changes in power by multiplying the isometric strength by a factor proportional to the changes in stature of their subjects. The ratio of the estimated power to body mass (Fig. 2.4.15) increases in both boys and girls and it is probably this measure that is best related to the observed improvements in performance in running and jumping.

One of the consequences of the greater upper limb girdle development in the male is that performance in throwing events is very much better than that of female competitors. In most track events the differential between men and women is of the order of 10% which may be explained (albeit with some difficulty) by the differences in strength and length of male and female muscles. For the throwing events, however, the difference is so marked that women throw lighter javelins,

hammers and shots and still do not achieve the same distances as men. World class men will throw an 800 g javelin about 90 m while women throw 600 g but achieve only about 70 m. Although it is tempting for a muscle physiologist to ascribe these differentials to the preferential muscle development of the male upper limb girdle, it is notable that, of all performance indicators, overarm throwing is superior in boys, and is seen long before the time when sex hormones play their part in promoting upper limb girdle development.[22] Although prepubertal boys throw better than girls they are not noticeably stronger in the arms compared to girls at this stage (Figs 2.4.8 and 2.4.9). Tanner[2] mentions the possibility of a greater development of the forearm in boys that is apparent soon after birth, but another explanation is that boys acquire this skill very early in development and that it is one of the markers of maleness.

Muscle development is clearly central to normal growth and development and the growing child provides fascinating information about the factors that regulate muscle growth. When trying to account for changes in performance with increasing maturity, again, muscle strength has a central role to play, but the relationships are complex and muscle strength has to be seen in the context of many other changes, in development of the skeletal lever system, of skill acquisition and probably also social attitudes towards certain types of activity and exercise.

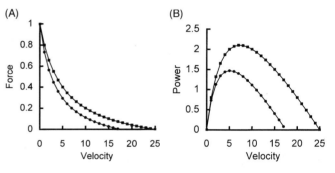

Fig. 2.4.14 The effect of increasing muscle length on the force/velocity (A) and power/velocity (B) relationships of a muscle. The effect of increasing muscle length by 40% (as may occur between the ages of 6 to 18 in normal children) on the force and power generated at different velocities. ● short and ■ long muscles data calculated from the Hill[36] equation, assuming the isometric strength remains constant; all arbitrary units.

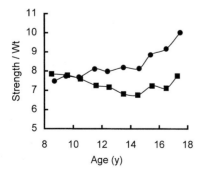

Fig. 2.4.13 Ratio of isometric strength to body weight for the quadriceps muscles: ● boys; ■ girls. Strength in Newtons, body weight in kg. From the data of Round et al.[21]

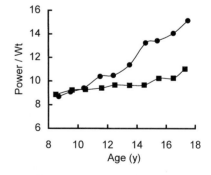

Fig. 2.4.15 Ratio of estimated power of the quadriceps to body weight: ● boys and ■ girls. Power is estimated from the data in Fig. 2.4.14, multiplying the strength by height. Power is given in arbitrary units.

Summary

Increases in skeletal muscle bulk and strength are characteristic of normal growth during childhood and adolescence. The major gains in strength are the result of increases in quantity of muscle rather than changes in the quality, since strength and muscle cross-sectional areas increase in parallel. The increase in muscle bulk is the result of muscle fibre hypertrophy and comes about largely as a result of satellite cell division and incorporation of daughter cells into existing fibres. There is, however, some increase in the volume of a muscle fibre that can be supported by a single myonucleus.

Muscle strength is similar in young boys and girls and, during the prepubertal years, strength increases in proportion to body size, with stretch on the muscle as a result of increasing bone length probably being an important stimulus for growth. The quadriceps muscles of the lower limb also receive an additional stimulus such that strength increases in proportion to body mass, an important consideration for body mass-bearing muscles. In addition to changes in muscle cross-sectional area and increase in isometric strength, the growth in length gives rise to an increase in shortening velocity and this leads to improvements in muscle power. The isometric strength/mass ratio changes relatively little during childhood and does not explain improvements in jumping and running speeds, but the power/ mass ratio probably gives a better explanation for improvements in performance.

Puberty is the time when major differences develop between the strength of boys and girls. Puberty in girls is marked by a cessation of muscle growth in the upper body, and in the year or so after PHV there are only minor increases in lower body strength, probably in response to continuing increases in body mass. In contrast, puberty in boys is associated with a rapid increase in strength, lasting for two to three years after the PHV. The difference in strength between boys and girls can be largely attributed to circulating testosterone levels in boys/young men, accounting for about a 15% increase in muscle strength compared to women, after taking into account differences in stature. Although differences between the sexes are seen in all muscle groups, they are particularly noticeable in the muscles of the upper limb girdle. The greater male muscle development may be due to a combination of a direct action of testosterone on the muscle together with an action stimulating bone growth in the shoulders and upper limbs.

The greater upper limb girdle development of the young male may account for the superior overarm throwing ability of men. However, it is interesting to note that young boys can throw further than young girls, although, in the prepubertal years, there are no differences in the measured strength of their muscles. It possible that, in addition to the advantage of increased muscular development, men also learn the skills of throwing at a very early age as part of a sexual stereotyping of behaviour.

References

1. **Jones, H. E.** *A developmental study of static dynamometric strength.* University of California Press, Berkley, 1949: 34–52.
2. **Tanner, J. M.** *Growth at adolescence.* Blackwell Scientific Publications, Oxford, 1962.
3. **Mauro, A.** Satellite cell of skeletal muscle fibres. *Journal of Biophysics, Biochemistry and Cytology* 1961; **9**: 493–4.
4. **Vrbova, G., Gordon, T.** and **Jones, R.** *Nerve-muscle interaction.* Chapman and Hall, London 1995.

5. **Rowe, R. W. D.** and **Goldspink, G.** Muscle fibre growth in five different muscles in both sexes of mice: I, normal mice. *Journal of Anatomy* 1969; **104**: 519–20.
6. **Jones, D. A., Round, J. M., Edwards, R. H. T., Grindrod, S. R.** and **Tofts, P. S.** Size and composition of the calf and quadriceps muscles in Duchenne muscular dystrophy. *Journal of the Neurological Sciences* 1983; **60**: 307–22.
7. **Round, J. M., Jones, D. A.** and **Edwards, R. H. T.** A flexible microprocessor system for the measurement of cell size *Journal of Clinical Pathology* 1982; **35**: 620–4.
8. **Chapman, S. J., Grindrod, S. R.** and **Jones, D. A.** Cross-sectional area and force production of the quadriceps muscle. *Journal of Physiology* 1984; **353**: 53P.
9. **Cheek, D. B.** The control of cell mass and replication. The DNA unit—a personal 20-year study. *Early Human Development* 1985; **12**: 211–39.
10. **Jones, D. A.** and **Round, J. M.** *Skeletal muscle in health and disease: A textbook of muscle physiology.* Manchester University Press, Manchester 1990.
11. **Grindrod, S., Round, J. M.** and **Rutherford, O. M.** Type 2 fibre composition and force per cross-sectional area in the human quadriceps. *Journal of Physiology* 1987; **390**: 154P.
12. **Alexander, R. Mc. N.** and **Vernon A.** The dimensions of the knee and ankle muscles and the forces they exert. *Journal of Human Movement Studies* 1975; **1**: 115–23.
13. **Parker, D. F.** *Factors controlling the development of strength of human skeletal muscle.* PhD Thesis, University of London 1989
14. **Tanner, J. M.** A brief history of the study of human growth. In *The Cambridge encyclopaedia of human growth and development* (ed. S. J. Ulijaszek, F. E. Johnston and M. A. Preece). Cambridge University Press, Cambridge 1998: 3–12.
15. **Stoltz, H. R.** and **Stoltz, L. M.** *The somatic development of adolescent boys.* Macmillan, New York 1951.
16. **Faust, M. S.** Somatic development of adolescent girls. *Monographs of the Society for Research in Child Development* 1977; **42**: 1–90.
17. **Carron, A. V.** and **Bailey, D. A.** Strength development in boys from 10 through 16 years. *Monographs of the Society for Research in Child Development* 1974; **39**: 1–37.
18. **Beunen, G. P., Malina, R. M., Van't Hof, M. A., Simons, J., Ostyn, M., Renson, R.** and **Van Gerven, D.** *Adolescent growth and performance. A longitudinal study of Belgian boys.* Human Kinetics Publishers, Champaign, Il, 1988.
19. **Kemper, H. C. G.** and **Verschuur, R.** Body build and composition. *Medicine and Sport Science* 1985; **20**: 88–95.
20. **Kemper, H. C. G.** and **Verschuur, R.** Motor performance fitness tests. *Medicine and Sport Science* 1985; **20**: 96–106.
21. **Round, J. M., Jones, D. A., Honour, J. W.** and **Nevill, A. M.** Hormonal factors in the development of differences in strength between boys and girls during adolescence: A longitudinal study. *Annals of Human Biology* 1999; **26**: 49–62.
22. **Malina, R. M.** Motor development and performance. In *The Cambridge encyclopaedia of human growth and development* (ed. S. J. Ulijaszek, F. E. Johnston and M. A. Preece). Cambridge University Press, Cambridge 1998: 247–50.
23. **Parker. D. F., Round, J. M., Sacco, P.** and **Jones, D. A.** A cross sectional survey of upper and lower limb strength in boys and girls during childhood and adolescence. *Annals of Human Biology* 1990; **17**: 199–211.
24. **Laurent, G. J., Sparrow, M. P.** and **Millward, D. J.** Turnover of muscle protein in the fowl. *Biochemical Journal* 1978; **176**: 407–17.
25. **Frankeny, J. R., Robert, M. A., Holly, G.** and **Ashmore, C. R.** Effects of graded duration of stretch on normal and dystrophic skeletal muscle. *Muscle and Nerve* 1983; **6**: 269–77.
26. **Tanner, J. M., Hughes, P. C. R.** and **Whitehouse, R. H.** Radiographically determined widths of bone, muscle and fat in the upper arm and calf from age 3–18 years. *Annals of Human Biology* 1981; **8**: 495–517.

27. Winter, J. S. D. and Faiman, C. Pituitary–gonadal relations in male children and adolescents. *Pediatric Research* 1972; **6**: 126–35.

28. Sizonenko, P. C. and Paunier, L. Hormonal changes in puberty III. *Journal of Clinical Endocrinology and Metabolism* 1975; **41**: 894–904.

29. Bhasin, S., Storer, T. W., Berman, N., Callegari, C., Clevenger, B., Phillips, J., Bunnell, T. J., Tricker, R., Shirazi, A. and Casaburi, R. The effects of supraphysiological doses of testosterone on muscle size and strength in normal men. *The New England Journal of Medicine* 1996; **335**: 1–7.

30. Grinspoons, S., Corcoran, C., Lee ,K., Burrows, B., Hubbard, J., Katznelson, L., Walsh, M., Guccione, A., Cannan, J., Heller, H., Basgoz, N. and Kilbanski, A. Loss of lean body and muscle mass correlates with androgen levels in hypogonadal men with acquired immunodeficiency syndrome and wasting. *Journal of Clinical Endocrinology and Metabolism* 1996; **81**: 4051–8.

31. Nevill, A. M., Holder, R. L., Baxter-Jones, A., Round, J. M. and Jones, D. A. Modelling developmental changes in strength and aerobic power in children. *Journal of Applied Physiology* 1998; **84**: 1963–70.

32. Rutherford, O. M. and Jones, D. A. The relationship of muscle and bone loss and activity levels with age in women. *Age and Ageing* 1992; **21**: 286–93

33. Verschuur, R. and Kemper, H. C. G. The pattern of daily physical activity. *Medicine and Sport Science* 1985; **20**: 169–86.

34. Edwards, R. H. T., Young, A., Hosking, G. P. and Jones D.A., Human skeletal muscle function: description of tests and normal values. *Clinical Science and Molecular Medicine* 1977; **52**: 283–90.

35. Malina, R. M. and Bouchard, C. *Growth, maturation and physical activity.* Human Kinetics Publishers, Champaign, Il, 1991.

36. Hill, A. V. The heat of shortening and the dynamic constants of muscle. *Proceedings of the Royal Society* 1938; **126**: 136–95.

2.5 Anaerobic performance

Anthony J. Sargeant

Introduction

'Anaerobic' performance is a convenient but misleading shorthand expression used to refer to the performance of short duration exercise lasting for seconds rather than minutes. Implicit in the expression is the fact that human performance depends upon the generation of external power rather than simply muscle force.

The rate at which work is done—that is, power is delivered—ultimately depends upon the rate of energy turnover in the muscle. It should be noted here, however, that power generation at the level of cross-bridges may be significantly modulated by the tendinous and other parallel elastic structures within and around the contractile elements of the muscle.

As described in Chapter 1.4 both anaerobic and aerobic pathways for energy supply contribute to maximum exercise performance of short duration, with the aerobic contribution increasing with duration, such that in exercise of two minutes duration aerobic energy supply will already account for ~50% of the total energy required. In exercise of shorter duration aerobic metabolism may make a significant minority contribution (see Chapter 1.4). In adults, and with present technology, quantitative measurements of the contribution of the different energy pathways in short-term high intensity exercise require highly invasive and technically extremely difficult experiments. In children, there are in addition serious ethical constraints on the nature of experiments that can be justified. As a consequence there is very little direct evidence, although much speculation, on the development of the major energy pathways and their contribution to total energy turnover in short-term exercise performed by children. Because of the technical and ethical constraints on the direct measurement of muscle energy turnover in children most investigators have adopted instead the approach of measuring the mechanical output in different forms of short-term exercise. Clearly it is not possible in these circumstances to say anything about the relative contribution of the different pathways. It is for these reasons that it might be considered preferable to refer to 'short-term power output' or 'short-duration exercise performance' for example rather than 'anaerobic power or performance'.

Maximum short-term athletic performance during growth

In seeking to understand the development of short-term exercise performance in children it is interesting to consider the athletic records in different age groups. Figure 2.5.1 shows data for sprint performance for the United States Junior Olympic championships.[1] In seeking to understand these data it should be remembered that it is cross-sectional and it cannot be assumed that the training status within the different age groups is the same—indeed it would be surprising if it were! Nevertheless, the data illustrate that performance of these short-term

maximum efforts improves in both boys and girls as body size continues to increase but that after puberty there is a plateau in performance. Consistent with the earlier onset of puberty the plateau in performance occurs earlier in the girls than the boys.

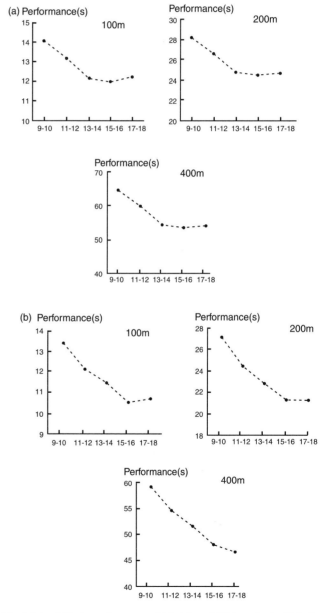

Fig. 2.5.1 Athletic performance of (a) girls and (b) boys in the United States Junior Olympic Championships (ages 9 to 18 years). Adapted with permission from Van Praagh and França.[1]

The nature of performance in these short-duration events is that the body mass has to be moved as fast as possible over the set distance by the locomotory muscles. Notwithstanding a minority aerobic contribution, most of the mechanical power delivered will be dependent upon anaerobic energy supply—that is from energy systems which are intrinsic to the muscle. At first sight therefore it may not seem surprising that as the muscle size increases so does performance in short-duration events. However, while muscle size and hence power will be increasing with age, so too will the size of the whole body which has to be moved. A great deal of energy and thought has been expended on scaling of whole body dimensions, such as stature and mass, to account for changes in performance with age (see Chapter 1.1), but often these analyses have neglected to consider basic muscle mechanics which ultimately determine the power output of muscle.

Determinants of short-duration power output from muscle and performance

In the following section the determinants of the mechanical output of muscle are described; the relationship of these to the performance of short-duration tasks is discussed; and the impact of growth on both is commented upon.

Length–force relationship

As shown in Fig. 2.5.2 the force that a muscle can generate depends upon the length at which it is activated.[2] This is generally believed to be due to the consequence of the degree of overlap between actin and myosin filaments within each sarcomere and the number of cross-bridges which may be formed between these filaments. In addition to active force there is, at long muscle lengths, an increasing element of passive force as structural elements both outside and within the muscle fibre are stretched.

To obtain the active length–force relationship the passive force is usually subtracted from the total recorded force. When this is done the resultant active force corresponds reasonably closely (although not exactly) to the degree of overlap of actin and myosin as predicted from the cross bridge theory of muscle contraction (see Woledge *et al.*[3]).

The length–force relationship has usually been characterized using isometric contractions but obviously the development of muscle power will also critically depend upon the length range over which the muscle is contracting in accordance with the length–force relationship.

There are a number of important considerations which should be taken into account in investigations of exercise performance where muscle length may play a critical role. The first is that even in a single joint movement there are usually a number of muscles which will contribute to torque about the joint and hence power output. Each of the muscles may have a different length–tension relationship in relation to joint angle. Equally within each muscle there may be variation in the length–tension relationships between motor units dependent upon task related recruitment patterns.[4]

The effect of this variation in length–tension relationship of the component units (muscles or motor units) acting around a joint is

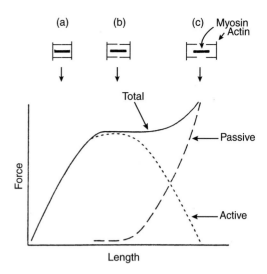

Fig. 2.5.2 Relationship between muscle length and the active (…) and passive (---) isometric tension. The amount of actin and myosin overlap which determines the active component is indicated for: (a) a short length where actin filaments from opposite ends of the sarcomere overlap and force is reduced; (b) optimum length where the greatest active force is generated due to the maximum number of cross-bridges; and (c) at a long length at which there is no overlap and no cross-bridges. Reproduced with permission from Sargeant.[2]

shown schematically in Fig. 2.5.3. If all three of the units are at optimum length for maximum force at the same joint angle there will be a maximum summation of forces. If on the other hand there is a range of length–tension relationships, then the maximum force will be lower but it will be sustained over a greater range of joint excursion.

A dramatic example of the latter case is shown in the example of a human muscle illustrated in Fig. 2.5.4.[5] In this maximally stimulated adductor pollicis muscle there is almost no change in the force developed by the muscle over almost the entire range of joint angle. Presumably this is due to the muscle being composed of fibres having a wide range of optimal lengths relative to the joint angle, which is quite probably related to task-related differences in the recruitment of different pools of motor units in manipulative movements using the hand.

There are few data on these effects in adult human muscle and none in children, although clearly they may have a profound effect on performance. There is, however, some evidence from studies of rat locomotory muscle that in young animals the degree of heterogeneity in force–length relationships may be greater than in adult muscle, and this may well contribute to reduction in the maximum force and hence power output of young muscle compared to adult.[6]

Force–velocity and power–velocity relationships

The relationship of muscle force and power to the velocity of contraction was first described in the 1920s and 1930s and the basic description remains much the same as that shown in Fig. 2.5.5. The figure illustrates that when making measurements of maximum power, it is vitally important that they are made at speeds that correspond to the

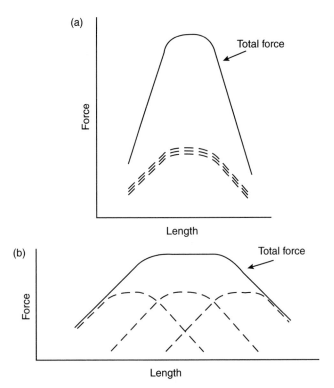

Fig. 2.5.3 Schematic to show the effect of variation in the length–tension relationship of three contributing muscle units to the total active force generated. (a) When all components have the same length–tension relationship with optimum length for maximum force at the same joint angle, the forces will summate. This gives high maximum force with steep ascending and decending arms. (b) In contrast, when there is a range of length–tension relationships, the maximum force is lower but will be sustained over a wider range of joint angle.

'global' optimum velocity for maximum power of the active muscles. The difficulty of controlling or identifying this optimum accounts for the relative neglect of this aspect of human performance over the years. The relatively recent development of isokinetic cycle ergometers and other techniques have, however, led to a renewal of interest in this aspect of human performance.

Using an isokinetic cycle ergometer Sargeant et al.[7] were able to characterize the power–pedalling rate relationship for maximum short-term power over a wide range of movement frequencies and hence contraction velocities. In both adult males and females and in 12 year old males, the optimum 'velocity' for maximum power was found to be in the range of 110–120 rev min^{-1} with no significant differences between the groups[8] (Fig. 2.5.6). It should be noted that this 'velocity' is pedal rate. It might be thought that, since the boys have shorter legs and are cycling using cranks of the same length as the adults, this might imply differences in fibre contraction velocity at the same angular velocity of the cranks. Due, however, to the complexity of the joint actions involved it is impossible and probably pointless to speculate on what the 'averaged' velocity is at the fibre level. Nevertheless, what is certain is that if reliable comparisons of performance are to be made between different groups with different body, limb or muscle size, then it is of critical importance that the optimum movement frequency for maximum power is identified for each group and that measurements are made at that frequency.

Muscle fibre type composition

The basis of the variability in muscle fibre type has been discussed in Chapter 2.4. In relation to the generation of muscle power, it should be emphasized that this is primarily determined by the particular isoform of the myosin heavy chain which is expressed—the so-called 'molecular motor'.[9] In human muscle there appear to be three main isoforms of this contractile protein in the mature muscle: type I (slow); type IIA (fast); and type IIX (the fastest). It should be noted that in older classification systems IIX is sometimes referred to as human type IIB

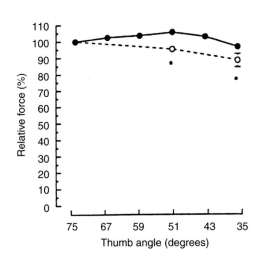

Fig. 2.5.4 Length–force relationship of adductor policis muscle. Active force (that is, total force minus passive force) (means ± S.E.M.) at different thumb angles as a percentage of force at the 74° thumb angle. Reproduced with permission from de Ruiter et al.[5]

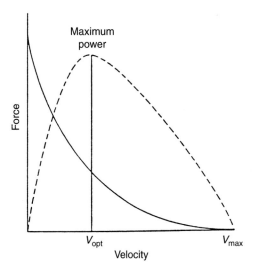

Fig. 2.5.5 Force–velocity and power–velocity relationship of skeletal muscle. Maximum power is generated at the optimum velocity (V_{opt}) which is about 30% of the maximum velocity of shortening (V_{max}) when force is zero. Reproduced with permission from Sargeant.[2]

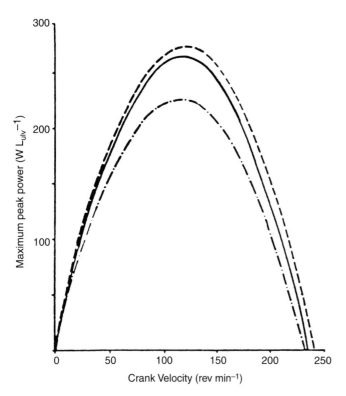

Fig. 2.5.6 The calculated relationship between maximum peak power and crank velocity for adult males (—), females (---), and children (—·—·). The calculation is based on experimental data collected during isokinetic cycling at pedal rates from 22 to 171 rev min[-1]. Maximum peak power is given in watts normalized for the volume of the upper leg muscle (W L_{ulv}^{-1}). Reproduced with permission from Sargeant and Dolan.[8]

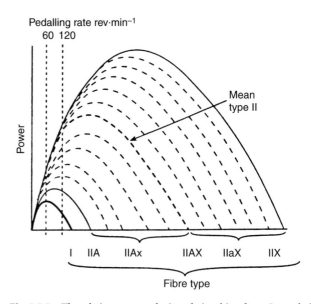

Fig. 2.5.7 The relative power–velocity relationship of type I muscle fibres compared to that for the *mean* of type II. In fact there is probably a continuum of properties for the type II fibres dependent upon the proportion of IIA and IIX myosin heavy-chain isoforms present. This is represented by the broken lines. The uppercase letter indicates a predominance of that isoform in the coexpressing fibres. The vertical lines are suggestions for how these contraction velocities might relate to cycling at 60 and 120 rev min[-1]. Reproduced with permission from Sargeant.[12]

(see Ennion *et al.*[10] for a discussion of this issue). These isoforms are associated with human muscle fibre types identified by traditional histochemical techniques which were, however, specifically designed to differentiate muscle fibres into three discrete groups. The reality is somewhat different. There is a continuum of muscle fibre properties and contractile protein expression. In type II fibres especially, it has been shown that many fibres coexpress both type IIA and IIX isoforms of the myosin heavy chain in variable proportions.[11] Thus, there is a continuum of power–velocity relationships depending upon the type and proportion of isoform present, as schematically suggested in Fig. 2.5.7.[12] As will be realized, it is possible that quite subtle changes in the isoform expression, especially in terms of the proportion of IIA and IIX isoform expressed, may have a large impact on the power generating capability of the fibre and therefore on whole muscle power and performance. It is not known whether subtle shifts in the myosin heavy chain isoform expression, and other contractile and regulatory protein isoforms, might occur during the later period of muscle growth in children.

Muscle size and geometry

As indicated earlier it might be expected that the power of the muscle would also increase as the size increases during growth. Nevertheless, even when normalized for the size of the active muscle, a number of authors have reported a significantly lower power output in children compared to adults.[13] The observed differences are seen in measurements

of instantaneous power which assuming adequate activation, suggest differences in the intrinsic power generating properties of children's muscle compared with adults.

In seeking to understand possible causes for these differences it might first be noted that appropriate measurements of muscle dimensions are very difficult to make and some of the reported differences may be due to systematic measurement errors and/or inappropriate normalization. It is possible now with magnetic resonance imaging to calculate the volume of each individual muscle in a limb.[14] Unfortunately, it is probably unrealistic to attempt to calculate the relative contribution of the different muscles to the total power delivered around one joint, let alone in relation to the 'whole limb' or 'whole body' performance.

Muscle force and muscle dimension

The force generated by skeletal muscle is generally believed to be the consequence of the attachment of cross-bridges between actin and myosin filaments. These filaments are organized in sarcomeres as shown in Fig. 2.5.8 with the cross-bridges in each half of the sarcomeres developing force in opposite directions.

The consequence is that the net force either side of a Z line separating two sarcomeres is theoretically zero. Therefore the total force of the system in Fig. 2.5.8(a) where the four sarcomeres are arranged in series is the force of only one sarcomere. In contrast the total force developed by the system shown in Fig. 2.5.8(b) where the sarcomeres are arranged in parallel is the sum of all four sarcomeres. Thus the isometric strength of muscle depends upon the number of sarcomeres

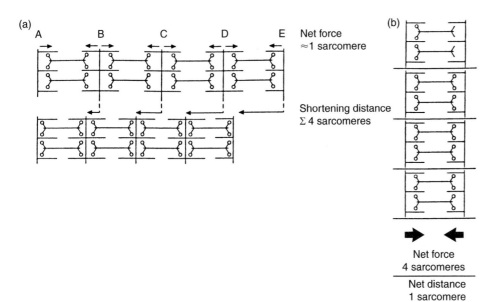

Net force
≈1 sarcomere

Shortening distance
Σ 4 sarcomeres

Net force
4 sarcomeres

Net distance
1 sarcomere

Fig. 2.5.8 Schematic illustration to show the force generated by four sarcomeres arranged (a) in series and (b) in parallel. (a) The forces either side of the Z lines B, C and D cancel one another out, thus the net force of the system is only the forces generated at A, and E, i.e. equivalent to one sarcomere. (b) The forces generated by all four sarcomeres add up to give four times the net force delivered by (a). [Note: conversely, the distance shortened (and hence velocity) will be four times greater in system (a) compared with system (b). Thus the maximum power (i.e. force × velocity) will be the same in both systems, although it will be achieved at different optimal velocities.] Reproduced with permission from Sargeant.[2]

arranged in parallel and this should most accurately be reflected by a measurement of the physiological cross-sectional area, that is, the area at right angles to the fibres that comprise the muscle(s). Unfortunately, this is a difficult measurement to make in the intact human, since the active muscles acting around the joint have a complex architecture with different angles of pennation. Furthermore, these angles may change as the muscle contracts even in the isometric situation.[15] A reasonable and pragmatic compromise has been to measure the anatomical cross-section of a muscle group at right angles to the axis of the limb segment about which it functions. Clearly, however, there could be systematic differences in the geomtry of the muscle between adults and children as well as differences in, for example, the compliance of the tendinous elements. Such differences might introduce artefactual differences when performance of whole body tasks is considered in relation to the intrinsic quality of the muscle.

Muscle power and muscle dimensions

Human performance depends upon the generation of muscle power either to move the body mass or to move another object. Muscle power is the product of force and velocity and is therefore determined by both the muscle cross-section, reflecting the number of sarcomeres in parallel (and hence total force as discussed in the previous subsection), and also the muscle length, because this will reflect the number of sarcomeres in series. It can be seen from Fig. 2.5.8(b) that the distance moved when four sarcomeres in series contract is four times greater than when the same number of sarcomeres are arranged in parallel. As a consequence the power of both systems is the same, although that power will be delivered at different velocities of contraction. From a practical point of view when seeking to normalize power data for muscles of different size a measurement of muscle volume might best reflect the number of sarcomeres in series and in parallel.

What would these considerations suggest about the increase in muscle power and performance consequent upon an increase in muscle size during growth?

Body circumferences increase during growth and these increases will presumably be reflected in proportional increases in the cross-section of all the component tissues including muscle. In addition, however, there will be an increase in the length of the limbs and their muscles. The increase in muscle length will occur by the addition of sarcomeres in series at the ends of the muscle fibres, and under otherwise constant conditions this will result in increased velocity, and hence increased power as indicated in Fig. 2.5.8.

Hence, it may well be that some of the increase seen in whole body performance during growth in children, and the differences in power output between children and adults might be related to differential increases in the body mass to be moved, muscle length and muscle cross-section. Unfortunately, no useful conclusion can be reached on this topic from studies in the intact human due to the many factors which determine the available power output—these will include:

(1) the complexity of the muscular geometry including pennation angles;

(2) unknown degrees of activation and contribution of different muscles acting around a joint;

(3) length of lever arms, length of fibres and their length–tension relations within the intact limb and in relation to joint angle;

(4) degree of activation of the different active muscles;

(5) the intrinsic speed of the active muscle fibres—in humans this may vary by a factor of up to 12 times, dependent primarily on the type of myosin heavy chain isoform expressed;[2]

(6) the modulation of mechanical output of the contractile elements through the tendons as well as other structural elements such as the intra-muscular collagen fibrils; and

(7) the prevailing muscle temperature which may vary depending on limb size, surface area to volume ratio, and subcutaneous fat thickness.

In conclusion, studies in the intact human are an inappropriate experimental model (a) to establish whether there is a difference in the intrinsic force and power generating capability of young prepubertal muscle compared to adult muscle and, if so, (b) to determine possible mechanisms. Other experimental models are needed to examine these issues. Recent work in our own laboratory has used isolated rat locomotory muscle.[16] In these experiments, muscle mass, physiological cross-sectional area and fibre cross-sectional area can be very accurately determined and related to isometric force and power production. Interestingly, in young rats in which fibre differentiation is complete, but which are still rapidly increasing in muscle fibre length, specific force (isometric force/physiological cross-sectional area) can be ~30% less than in the young mature animal in which rapid length changes have ceased. The reason for this difference remains unknown. There are a number of possibilities including: a difference in myofibrillar packing density; changes in connective tissue in the muscle; changes in cross bridge kinetics; or a compromise of the ability to transmit force directly related to the growth process itself.

Training induced changes in muscle power and size

Despite the many uncertainties it is clear that muscle power and volume should normally be expected to show concomitant increases as a consequence of training. In a study of 13 year old boys taking part in a special supplementary programme of fitness training in addition to normal school physical education lessons, there was a significant 10% increase in the upper leg muscle volume over an eight week period and this was reflected in a 9% increase in leg extension power measured on an isokinetic ergometer.[17]

Neural activation

If muscles are to develop the maximum power of which they are capable they must be fully activated. Whether children during development can, or do, fully activate their muscles is difficult to establish with certainty, and there are no longitudinal or even cross-sectional data available which examine the evidence in children over a wide age range.

A few investigators have used direct electrical stimulation to study muscle function in children under isometric conditions,[18] but these data do not enable any judgement to be made on whether in voluntary isometric contractions children are able, or willing, to fully activate their muscles. In any case, it could not be assumed, even were it demonstrated, that failure to activate fully a muscle under isometric conditions would necessarily imply that there would be a similar failure under dynamic conditions, where the maximum forces generated and the mechanical consequences seen by proprioceptors would be quite different.

Such evidence as we have is based upon studies in adults where electrical stimulation has been used to confirm maximum activation, or more properly stated, to exclude contractions in which activation is submaximal.

The technique commonly employed is developed from experiments first described by Merton in the 1950s. In these, subjects were asked to generate a maximal effort during which an electrical stimulation was applied to the nerve. If the muscle was not fully activated by the nervous system, then an increased force would be generated by the applied stimulation, and the size of the extra force would be inversely proportional to the level of activation as illustrated in Fig. 2.5.9.[19] It should be pointed out that properly applied this technique can only

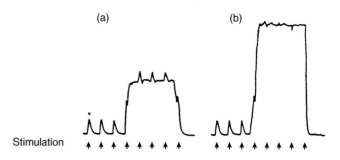

Fig. 2.5.9 Electrical stimulation superimposed on voluntary contractions. The muscle was stimulated with single twitches (arrows) while the subject made either submaximal (a) or maximal (b) contractions. During the maximal contraction there was no additional force on stimulation. Reproduced with permission from Jones and Round.[19]

exclude contractions which are submaximal, it cannot confirm maximality. This is because as full activation is approached the extra force that can be elicited decreases and may be difficult to detect in the total force signal.

Notwithstanding these difficulties, the technique has been used by many laboratories and the consensus of evidence, at least for the commonly used limb muscles in healthy adults, is that subjects can usually achieve maximal or near maximal contractions ($>95\%$) voluntarily in isometric contractions. Much less is known about the degree of voluntary activation in maximal dynamic contractions and almost nothing about the degree of activation achieved in whole body locomotory performance (but see[20,21]). Such evidence as there is suggests that in concentric contractions adults can fully activate voluntarily the major muscle groups during single contractions and during 10 to 20 s of repeated contractions (see Sargeant[2] for a recent review of this topic). Unfortunately, this evidence from adults cannot be used to assume that children undergoing tests of maximal short-term power output will behave in a similar fashion.

In the context of neural drive, it might be pointed out that there is evidence that the maturation process of the cortico-spinal tract continues into the second decade in humans. Thus, for example cortico-spinal conduction velocity continues to increase up to about 15 years of age. It is not clear what the functional significance of these surprisingly late changes might be. They may have no significant effect on muscle activation but further research is undoubtedly merited. Similarly, it is well recognized that the performance of even apparently simple tasks, such as lifting a bar with weights, can be dramatically improved as the subject learns the optimum pattern of muscle activation in order to generate and translocate useful power from proximal to distal limb muscles. It would not be surprising if these effects were greater in children with a still maturing neural system.

Even if there is maximal activation of an agonist muscle in a limb, if there is simultaneous antagonistic activation, the net torque around a joint will be reduced. Recent studies of the ankle dorsi- and plantar-flexors indicates that in adults this effect is most marked at extreme plantarflexions, where antagonistic muscle activation may reduce the net torque by 20–30%.[22] It is not known whether in the developing neuromuscular system of children such antagonist activation occurs or what the magnitude of such an effect might be.

Finally, it is perhaps worth commenting that, even in well-motivated adults, experience suggests that it becomes more difficult to maintain a maximum effort the longer the duration of the exercise—in our experience maximum power output in exercise lasting more than about 25 seconds requires considerable motivation and concentration from the subject. In population studies of children it may be unreasonable to expect similar levels of motivation.

Clearly, in the absence of objective evidence of maximal activation, measurements of maximal power output in children should be treated with caution, especially if conclusions are being drawn from such data about the intrinsic power generating capability of the muscles during development.

Temperature and fatigue effects

In investigations of short-duration exercise in which intrinsic power of the active muscles is the principal determinant of performance it is important to be aware of the profound effect that both temperature and fatigue can have.

Muscle fatigue

An important observation, first made in animal studies, but subsequently confirmed in humans is that muscle fatigue may lead to temporary transformation of the muscle towards slower properties.[23,24] Functionally this means that following fatiguing exercise there may be minor or no detectable reduction in maximum isometric force or muscle power at slow contraction velocities, but a very large reduction at the optimum velocity for power output,[24] as shown in Fig. 2.5.10.

It should be pointed out that these human observations were made on adults. There are no equivalent data for children and adolescents, although there is no reason to suppose that qualitatively the same acute transformation towards slower properties would not occur. However, it should be emphasized that the fatigue generated by other forms of exercise may have different origin and might lead to different effects[25] (for general review see Refs 26, 27).

Muscle temperature

Since the classic paper of Asmussen and Bøje[28] it has been known that short-duration human performance could be improved by increasing the muscle temperature. In a more recent paper, it has been shown that in human muscle the effect of muscle temperature on leg extension power is velocity dependent.[29] Increasing muscle temperature transforms muscle towards faster properties while cooling it has the opposite effect. The magnitude of the velocity dependent effect is shown in Fig. 2.5.11. In interpreting the significance of the effect of changes in muscle temperature on performance, it should be realized that there is often a marked gradient across muscle. Under normal laboratory conditions it is not unusual for the superficial layers of the quadriceps muscle to be 2 to 3°C lower than the muscle close to the femur and surprisingly this gradient may increase during exercise itself as a consequence of the movement of the limb through the air.[30] Great care therefore needs to be exercised in any study of short-duration exercise performance that measurements are made under similar temperature and metabolic conditions. Ideally muscle power should be measured at homogenous and known temperature and in a stable metabolic state, ideally from rest. In studies of children, where repeated measurement of deep muscle temperature are unacceptable, the best that might be done is to ensure that measurements are made under rigorously standardized conditions. Experimental protocols which include an exercise based warm-up in particular should be very carefully standardized.

The importance of the issue can be illustrated by the fact that in a longitudinal study of muscle power even a 1°C difference in mean muscle temperature—a difference that could easily occur as a consequence of seasonal change in the ambient temperature, or a different warm-up time or intensity—would be expected to lead to a systematic difference of 5% in the measured power at optimal velocity for maximum power.

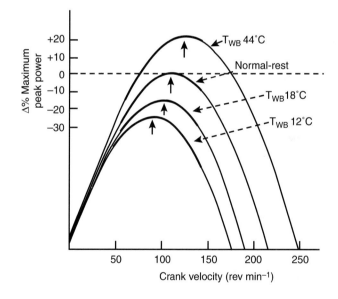

Fig. 2.5.11 The relationship of leg extension power generated in isokinetic cycling exercise to pedalling rate after immersion of the legs in water baths at different temperatures and under control conditions. The thicker sections of the lines represent the limits of the experimental data; the thinner sections are the theoretical extrapolations. Power is expressed as a percentage change from that obtained at optimal velocity under control conditions. Temperatures are for the water bath. The increase in the optimal velocity for maximal power with increasing temperature is indicated by the arrows. Reproduced with permission from Sargeant.[12]

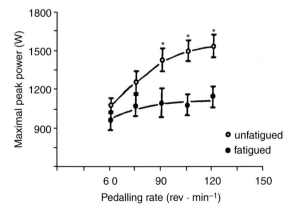

Fig. 2.5.10 Human maximum peak power cycling at five different pedalling rates in fatigued and unfatigued states. *p < 0.05 fatigued vs non-fatigued. Reproduced with permission from Beelen and Sargeant.[24]

Summary

Systematic data on the development of short duration exercise performance in children and adolescents are limited. In particular, very little is known with respect to how muscle dimensions and geometry change during growth. Equally, although fibre differentiation seems largely complete a few years after birth, changes that may occur in later childhood as a consequence of growth-related changes in the mechanical, metabolic or temperature environment in which the fibre operates, and which may modulate any genetic code have received little attention. It is recognized that the prevailing pattern of contractile activity plays an important role influencing the contractile and metabolic properties of muscle fibres (see, for example, the classic studies of Buller et al.,[31] and Salmons and Vrbová[32]). The nature of the signals which trigger modification of the molecular structure and function have yet to be fully elucidated, although mechanical events, energy status of the cell or excitation contraction coupling processes are all possible candidates.

At the level of whole body performance it is also worth commenting that many physical tasks involve complex contractions in which there is first a stretch of the active muscle before a subsequent shortening phase—the stretch–shortening cycle.[33] Despite its obvious importance for the performance of many tasks, little is known about how in childhood the mechanical output from the muscles is modulated through tendinous structures, and how these properties may change with age. In addition, the generation of mechanical power by large proximal muscles and the translocation of that power via bi-articular muscles from proximal to distal limb segments depends upon a coordinated sequence of activation of the limb muscles.[34] The nature of the development of optimal pattern in children has not yet received systematic attention.

References

1. **Van Praagh, E.** and **França, N. M.** Measuring maximal short-term power output during growth. In Pediatric anaerobic performance (ed. E. Van Praagh). Human Kinetics Publishers, Champaign, Il, 1997; 115–89.

2. **Sargeant, A. J.** Neuromuscular determinants of human performance. In P*hysiological determinants of human exercise tolerance.* Studies in Physiology No. 4 (ed. B. Whipp and A. J. Sargeant). Portland Press, London, 1999; 13–28.

3. **Woledge, R. C., Curtin, N. A.** and **Homsher, E.** *Energetic aspects of muscle contraction.* Academic Press, London, 1985.

4. **Kernell, D.** Organized variability in the neuromuscular system: a survey of task-related adaptations. *Archives Italiennes Biologie* 1992; **130**: 19–66.

5. **De Ruiter, C. J., de Haan. A., Jones, D. A.** and **Sargeant, A. J.** Shortening induced force depression in human adductor pollicis muscle. *Journal of Physiology* 1998; **507**: 583–91.

6. **Lodder, M. A. N., de Haan, A.** and **Sargeant, A. J.** The effect of growth on efficiency and fatigue in rat EDL muscle. *European Journal of Applied Physiology* 1994; **69**: 429–34.

7. **Sargeant, A. J., Hoinville, E.** and **Young, A.** Maximum leg force and power output during short-term dynamic exercise. *Journal of Applied Physiology: Respiratory, Environmental, and Exercise Physiology* 1981; **51**: 1175–82.

8. **Sargeant, A. J.** and **Dolan, P.** Optimal velocity of muscle contraction for short-term (anaerobic) power output in children and adults. In *Children and exercise XII* (ed. R. Mocellin, F. Klimt and J. Rutenfranz). Human Kinetics Publishers, Champaign, Il, 1986; 39–42.

9. **Goldspink, G.** Cellular and molecular aspects of adaption in skeletal muscle. In *Strength and power in sport* (ed. P. V. Komi). Human Kinetics Publishers, Champaign Il, 1992; 211–38.

10. **Ennion, S., Sant'Ana Pereira, J. A., Sargeant, A. J., Young, A.** and **Goldspink, G.** Characterization of human skeletal muscle fibres according to the myosin heavy chains they express. *Journal of Muscle Research and Cell Motility* 1995; **16**: 35–43.

11. **Sant'Ana Pereira, J. A., de Wessels, A., Nijtmans, L., Moorman, A. F. M.** and **Sargeant, A. J.** New method for the accurate characterization of single human skeletal muscle fibres demonstrates a relation between mATPase and MyHC expression in pure and hybrid fibres types. *Journal of Muscle Research and Cell Motility* 1995; **16**: 21–34.

12. **Sargeant, A. J.** The determinants of anaerobic muscle function during growth. In *Pediatric anaerobic performance* (ed. E. Van Praagh). Human Kinetics Publishers, Champaign, Il, 1998; 97–117.

13. **Van Praagh, E.** (ed.) *Pediatric anaerobic performance.* Human Kinetics Publishers, Champaign, Il, 1998.

14. **Narici, M. V., Binzoni, T., Hiltbrand, E., Fasel, J., Terrier, F.** and **Cerretelli, P.** *In vivo* human gastrocnemius architecture with changing joint angle at rest and during graded isometric contraction. *Journal of Physiology* 1996; **496**: 287–97.

15. **Maganaris, C. N., Baltzopoulos, V.** and **Sargeant, A. J.** *In vivo* measurements of the triceps surae complex architecture in man: implications for muscle function. *Journal of Physiology* 1998; **512**: 603–14.

16. **De Haan, A., de Ruiter, C. J., Lind, A.** and **Sargeant, A. J.** Growth-related change in specific force but not in specific power of fast rat skeletal muscle. *Experimental Physiology* 1992; **77**: 505–8.

17. **Sargeant, A. J., Dolan, P.** and **Thorne, A.** Effects of supplemental physical activity on body composition, aerobic and anaerobic power in 13 year old boys. In *Children and exercise XI* (ed. R. A. Binkhorst, H. C. G. Kemper and W. H. M. Saris). Human Kinetics Publishers, Champaign, Il. 1985; 135–9.

18. **Davies, C. T. M., Rutherford, I. C.** and **Thomas, D. O.** Electrically evoked contractions of the triceps surae during and following 21 days of voluntary leg immobilization. *European Journal of Applied Physiology* 1987; **56**: 306–12.

19. **Jones, D. A** and **Round, J. M.** *Skeletal muscle in health and disease: A textbook of muscle physiology.* Manchester University Press, Manchester, 1990.

20. **Beelen, A., Sargeant, A. J., Jones, D. A.** and **de Ruiter, C. J.** Fatigue and recovery of voluntary and electrically elicited dynamic force in humans. *Journal of Physiology* 1995; **484**: 227–35.

21. **James, C., Sacco, P.** and **Jones, D. A.** Loss of power during fatigue of human leg muscles. *Journal of Physiology* 1995; **484** :237–46.

22. **Maganaris, C. N., Baltzopoulos, V.** and **Sargeant, A. J.** Differences in human antagonistic ankle dorsiflexor coactivation between legs; can they explain the moment deficit in the weaker plantarflexor leg? *Experimental Physiology* 1998; **83**: 843–55.

23. **De Haan, A., Jones, D. A.** and **Sargeant, A. J.** Changes in power output, velocity of shortening and relaxation rate during fatigue of rat medial gastrocnemius muscle. *European Journal of Physiology* 1989; **413**: 422–8.

24. **Beelen, A.** and **Sargeant, A. J.** Effect of fatigue on maximal power output at different contraction velocities in humans. *Journal of Applied Physiology, Respiratory, Environmental and Exercise Physiology* 1991; **71**: 2332–7.

25. **Beelen, A.** and **Sargeant, A. J.** Human power output measured after fatiguing isometric vs dynamic exercise shows opposite velocity dependent effects. *Muscle and Nerve* 1996; **4**: S57.

26. **Sargeant, A. J.** and **Kernell, D.** (eds) *Neuromuscular Fatigue.* Academy Series. Royal Netherlands Academy of Arts and Sciences, Amsterdam, 1993; 1–95.

27. **Gandevia, S. C., Enoka, R. M., McComas, A. J., Stuart, D. G.** and **Thomas, C. K.** (eds) Fatigue: Neural and muscular mechanisms. *Advances in Experimental Medicine and Biology* 1995; **384**: 1–541.

28. **Asmussen, E.** and **Bøje, O.** Body temperature and capacity for work. *Acta Physiologica Scandinavica.* 1987; **10**: 1–22.

29. **Sargeant, A. J.** Effect of muscle temperature on leg extension force and short-term power output in humans. *European Journal of Applied Physiology* 1987; **56**: 693–8.

30. **Sargeant, A. J.** Acute plasticity—effects of temperature and fatigue on human locomotory performance. *Journal of Physiology* 1998; **6S**: 506P.

31. **Buller, A. J., Eccles, J. C. and Eccles, R. M.** Interactions between motorneurones and muscles in respect of the characteristic speeds of their responses. *Journal of Physiology* 1960; **150**: 417–39.

32. **Salmons, S. and Vrbová, G.** The influence of activity on some contractile characteristics of mammalian fast and slow muscles. *Journal of Physiology* 1969; **201**: 535–49.

33. **Alexander, R. Mc. N.** Elastic energy stores in running vertebrates. *American Zoology* 1984; **24**: 85–94.

34. **Soest, A. J., van., Bobbert, M. F. and van Ingen Schenau, G. J.** A control strategy for the execution of explosive movements from various starting positions. *Journal of Neurophysiology* 1994; **71**: 1390–1402.

2.6 Pulmonary function

Thomas W. Rowland

Introduction

Effective pulmonary responses to exercise are essential in the regulation of blood oxygen and carbon dioxide concentrations as well as maintaining body acid–base homeostasis. Yet the work of ventilation comes at a cost, as the increased mechanical work of breathing during physical activity must be paid for through added energy expenditure. Nonetheless, healthy individuals do not tax the lungs to their functional limits, even with exhaustive exercise.[1,2]

Put simply, the pulmonary response to exercise is increased minute ventilation ($\dot{V}_E$). That response, which is achieved both by augmenting tidal volume (V_T) and raising breathing rate (f_R), is dictated by the need to increase oxygen uptake ($\dot{V}O_2$) for aerobic metabolism and eliminate its by-product, carbon dioxide (CO_2). In addition, ventilation is stimulated by additional CO_2 produced by the buffering of lactic acid by bicarbonate as well as the metabolic acidosis that ensues at high exercise intensities when the buffering capacity of bicarbonate is exceeded.

The effectiveness of the lungs in performing these tasks is remarkable. Total body $\dot{V}O_2$ may increase over tenfold in a progressive exercise test, yet arterial oxygen pressure (P_aO_2) remains stable throughout (except in highly trained athletes at exhaustion). A slight dip in P_aCO_2 is observed (to about 35 mm Hg) and blood pH falls (usually to no less than 7.30), but only at high exercise intensities. Except perhaps in the most elite athletes, pulmonary function is not a limiting factor in exercise performance. The critical role of ventilation in maximizing such performance, however, is indicated by the decline in exercise tolerance observed in individuals with lung disease.[3]

The ventilatory responses to exercise demand increased mechanical work of breathing to distend the lung (overcome elastic forces) and overcome airway resistance to flow. That work elevates metabolic costs of breathing, which may become substantial (reaching approximately 14% of total $\dot{V}O_2$ at maximal exercise in normal, non-athletic subjects). The peak work of ventilation at exhaustive exercise is still far short (about 40%) of the work required at the maximal voluntary ventilation rate (MVV). $\dot{V}_E$ at peak exercise is typically no more than 60–70% of MVV, indicating that healthy subjects have considerable ventilatory reserve at maximal exercise.

These concepts hold true for children as they do for adults. Yet certain aspects of the ventilatory response to exercise appear to be different in growing subjects. These include:

1. Children hyperventilate during exercise compared to adults, manifest as a relative inefficiency of breathing (higher $\dot{V}_E/\dot{V}O_2$, or ventilatory equivalent for oxygen) and lower P_aCO_2. This may reflect greater neural drive in immature subjects.

2. Children breathe faster than adults during exercise, with a higher ratio of f_R to V_T to achieve the same $\dot{V}_E$. In addition, they may rely relatively more on V_T to achieve $\dot{V}_E$ at high exercise intensities.

3. Because children produce less lactic acid during progressive exercise, their ventilatory anaerobic threshold (VAT, when $\dot{V}_E$ accelerates in response to buffering of lactate) is higher (expressed as per cent of $\dot{V}O_2$ max) compared to that of adults.

The extent that the respiratory responses to exercise in children are influenced by a sedentary life style or can be modified with training is unclear. Most studies indicate that measures of resting pulmonary volumes and function in young athletes do not differ from non-athletes. However, $\dot{V}_E$ max increases in parallel with improvements in maximal metabolic rate ($\dot{V}O_2$ max) with endurance training.

As with other physiological variables, measures of ventilation must be related to body size to allow researchers to examine inter-individual differences and assess intra-individual changes over time. The appropriate anthropometric measure to normalize these variables to body size remains uncertain. The weaknesses of use of the ratio standard (mass, stature or body surface area raised to the power 1.0) have been recognized, and allometrically derived denominators may be more appropriate (see Chapter 1.1).

The task of the paediatric exercise physiologist—and this chapter—is to:

(1) identify and understand the unique aspects of pulmonary function with exercise that separate children from adults;

(2) recognize how ventilatory changes with exercise may be modified by changes in regular physical activity as well as athletic training; and

(3) appreciate the difficulties of expressing pulmonary function relative to body size in the paediatric age group.

Ventilation at rest

The total capacity of the lung increases from approximately 1400 to 4500 ml between ages 5 and 14 years. In their cross-sectional study of 438 children ages 6–14 years, Lyons and Tanner[4] found that total lung volume correlated closely with stature and even slightly better with stature cubed ($r=0.91$ and $r=0.86$ for boys and girls, respectively). Values were slightly but significantly greater in the males.

As might be expected, a child's $\dot{V}_E$ at rest changes during the growing years in parallel to resting metabolic rate. Thus, as resting $\dot{V}O_2$ relative to body mass or surface area steadily declines during the course of childhood, so does resting $\dot{V}_E$. A typical value for resting minute ventilation in a 10 year old boy, for instance, is 199 ml kg^{-1}min^{-1}, while 158 ml kg^{-1} min^{-1} might be observed in a 16 year old.[5]

An allometric analysis of resting $\dot{V}_E$ has not been reported in humans. In animal studies, minute ventilation relates to body mass by the exponent 0.80 (indicating that $\dot{V}_E$/kg decreases with increasing body size).[6] This exponent corresponds closely to that observed when resting $\dot{V}O_2$ is related to body mass (0.76), confirming the close coupling of ventilation with metabolic rate in the resting state.

Breathing rate at rest demonstrates a progressive decline throughout the childhood years. In a cross-sectional study, Robinson[7] reported a decrease in resting rate from 24 to 13 breaths min^{-1} between groups of boys aged 6 and 17 years old, respectively. When large groups of children spanning the childhood age range are studied, f_R relates to body mass by the allometric scaling exponent of −0.53.[8]

Tidal volume, of course, increases with lung growth during childhood, but resting V_T expressed relative to body size declines as a child ages. Over the age range of 6 to 17 years, a decrease of 13 $ml\,kg^{-1}$ to 9 $ml\,kg^{-1}$ has been described.[7] Cassels and Morse[9] reported mean V_T values of 321, 297 and 242 $ml\,m^{-2}$ body surface area in girls 6–8, 8–12 and 12–17 years, respectively. Thus, both a fall in f_R and V_T during childhood contribute to the decrease in $\dot{V}_E$ at rest adjusted for body size.

It is of interest that a child's vital capacity (VC), the greatest amount of air that can be expelled after a maximal inspiratory effort, increases with age in direct proportion to body mass. Scaling exponents of 0.98 and 0.94 for VC relative to body mass have been reported for boys and girls, respectively, meaning that VC per kg body mass remains stable as a child grows. Since V_T per kg decreases during this time, the proportion of VC used for tidal volume at rest diminishes with age. Robinson[7] noted that V_T/VC was 0.23 in 6 year old boys but 0.13 in 17 year olds. Values were 0.181 and 0.153 in the 6 to 12 and 13 to 17 year old subjects, respectively, described by Morse et al.[5]

Although the relationship between VC and body size is gender-independent in children, boys demonstrate greater VC values relative to body dimensions than girls. With body mass and stature considered, Armstrong et al.[10] reported a mean forced vital capacity (FVC) of 2.50 litre in 11 year old boys ($n=101$) and 2.19 litre in girls ($n=76$). DeMuth and Howatt[11] analysed allometric relationships with height and body mass in 147 children ages 4 to 18 years. The equation for boys was $VC = 0.00216 \times ht^{2.81}$ and for girls $VC = 0.00186 \times ht^{2.82}$. The observation that girls have a lower intercept value supports the concept that girls have smaller VC relative to body size than males. Whether this finding can be explained by gender-related differences in mechanical properties of the lungs is uncertain.[12]

Ventilation during submaximal exercise

The onset of exercise triggers increases in both f_R and V_T, resulting in a rise in $\dot{V}_E$. In exercise of low-to-medium intensity (less than 50% $\dot{V}O_2$ max) the increasing values of $\dot{V}_E$ parallel those of metabolic rate ($\dot{V}O_2$). At higher intensities, above the ventilatory anaerobic threshold, $\dot{V}_E$ climbs at a steeper rate than $\dot{V}O_2$, driven by the excessive CO_2 produced by bicarbonate buffering of lactic acid.

At intensities below VAT, then, changes in $\dot{V}_E$ with growth can be expected to parallel those of $\dot{V}O_2$. At a given treadmill running or walking speed, children demonstrate lower energy economy (greater $\dot{V}O_2$ per kg) than adults, and improvements in economy are observed in a continuum through the childhood years. The reason for this trend is not altogether clear but appears to largely reflect changes in stride frequency with increasing leg length (see Chapter 2.9).

$\dot{V}_E$ follows the same pattern. As a child ages, his or her $\dot{V}_E$ relative to body size at a given submaximal treadmill setting progressively declines. Rowland and Cunningham[13] examined longitudinal changes

in $\dot{V}O_2$ and $\dot{V}_E$ in 20 children annually over a period of five years beginning at age nine years. Metabolic requirement for walking, measured at a treadmill speed of 1.45 $m\,s^{-1}$ and 8% slope, decreased steadily with age, with $\dot{V}O_2$ per kg falling from 31.1 to 26.9 $ml\,kg^{-1}\,min^{-1}$ in the boys and 30.9 to 25.9 $ml\,kg^{-1}\,min^{-1}$ in the girls. Similarly, $\dot{V}_E$ relative to body mass steadily declined. The average value for the entire group was 0.97 $litre\,kg^{-1}\,min^{-1}$ at the beginning of study and 0.72 $litre\,kg^{-1}\,min^{-1}$ at its conclusion.

Cross-sectional investigations have demonstrated similar findings. Robinson[7] found that males 6 and 17 years had an average absolute $\dot{V}_E$ while walking at 1.56 $m\,s^{-1}$ of 21.2 and 48.6 $litre\,min^{-1}$, respectively. When expressed relative to body size, these values corresponded to 1.05 $litre\,kg^{-1}\,min^{-1}$ in the young boys and 0.67 $litre\,kg^{-1}\,min^{-1}$ in the adolescents.

This decline in size-relative minute ventilation at a given submaximal exercise intensity is entirely accounted for by a decrease in rate of breathing. In the longitudinal study of Rowland and Cunningham[13] the average submaximal f_R fell from 45 to 36 breaths min^{-1} over the five years of annual testing. Rutenfranz et al.[14] described longitudinal findings in two separate European groups between ages 8 and 17 years. These data assessed ventilatory findings at the same relative intensity (65 to 70% $\dot{V}O_2$ max) rather than identical submaximal workload. Breathing rate fell from an average 39 to 28 breaths min^{-1} in the boys and 36 to 26 breaths min^{-1} in the girls.

While submaximal f_R falls with age, increases in absolute V_T match body size, resulting in a stable submaximal V_T per kg body mass as a child grows. V_T per kg was approximately 0.021 $litre\,kg^{-1}$ throughout the five-year study of Rowland and Cunningham.[13] In the cross-sectional investigation by Robinson[7], values were 0.021 at age 6 years and 0.025 at age 17 years.

Armstrong et al.[10] described significant gender differences in ventilatory responses to submaximal exercise. Whether measured at the same absolute or relative (per cent $\dot{V}O_2$ max) treadmill exercise intensity, boys demonstrated greater size-relative values of both $\dot{V}_E$ and V_T.

Ventilation at maximal exercise

Minute ventilation at maximal exercise is influenced by factors which are not operative at lower exercise intensities. As the point of exhaustion is approached in a progressive test, rising levels of lactic acid are buffered by bicarbonate, resulting in production of CO_2 which is additive to that resulting from aerobic metabolism. This excessive CO_2, plus the metabolic acidosis that ensues when the buffering capacity of bicarbonate is exceeded, stimulates $\dot{V}_E$ beyond levels that parallel metabolic rate. Consequently, $\dot{V}_E/\dot{V}O_2$ increases at high levels of exercise intensity.

As expected, maximal $\dot{V}_E$ increases with age during childhood. This development of $\dot{V}_E$ max is an expression of growing lung dimensions that parallel the increase in size of other components of the oxygen delivery chain. In addition, there is evidence that developmental differences in lactate production and control of ventilatory drive during childhood may also influence changes in $\dot{V}_E$ max with age. It follows, then, that patterns of maximal $\dot{V}_E$ in respect to body size during the growing years might not necessarily parallel those of $\dot{V}O_2$ max.

Patterns of change in $\dot{V}_E$ max with age relative to body dimensions have been examined in both cross-sectional and longitudinal studies. Rutenfranz et al.[14] found that $\dot{V}_E$ max increased linearly with stature or the square of stature in both boys and girls, although values actually declined in females over 160 cm tall. In their five year longitudinal study, Rowland and Cunningham[13] described scaling exponents for $\dot{V}_E$ max to body mass of 0.92 and stature of 2.50. $\dot{V}_E$ max per kg decreased with age in the girls (1.90 to 1.71 litre kg^{-1}min^{-1}) but not in the boys (Fig. 2.6.1).

These data suggest that stature or stature^2 are both practical and accurate measures for normalizing maximal ventilation to body size in children and adolescents. However, when Armstrong et al.[10] combined mass and stature in the same allometric analysis of 11 year children, the adjusted exponents were 0.69 for stature and 0.48 for mass. They concluded that:

> the conventional approach of accounting for body size differences in the interpretation of children's ventilatory data, i.e., by dividing by either body mass or stature, is inappropriate. (p. 1558)

Two cross-sectional studies have also failed to find differences in mass-relative maximal minute ventilation with increasing age in boys. Robinson[7] described an average $\dot{V}_E$ max of 1.59 and 1.60 litre kg^{-1} min^{-1} in males 6 and 14 to 18 years old, respectively. Morse et al.[5] could detect no relationship between $\dot{V}_E$ max per kg and age in boys between the ages of 10 and 17 years.

Mercier et al.[15] reported that $\dot{V}_E$ max expressed relative to lean body mass was unchanged with age in a cross-sectional study of boys 10 to 15 years old. In that report, the allometric scaling factors of $\dot{V}_E$ max in respect to body mass and stature were 0.68 and 2.06, indicating that $\dot{V}_E$ max per kg decreased with age. The findings of Astrand[16] support that conclusion. He found that mean $\dot{V}_E$ max was 1.94 and 1.59 litre kg^{-1}min^{-1} in boys ages 4–6 and 14–15 years, respectively.

Given these conflicting data, the true relationship between $\dot{V}_E$ max and body size—and how this is influenced by age or biological development—remains uncertain. Consequently, identifying 'norms' for maximal ventilation in children is problematic. Most studies indicate values in children of 1.60 to 1.90 for $\dot{V}_E$ max per kg and about 0.50 for $\dot{V}_E$ max per cm stature. The variability in data among research studies suggests, however, that norms for ventilatory variables at maximal exercise in a particular laboratory are best based on those established by the experience of that laboratory.

The effect of testing modality and protocol may explain much of this variability. Boileau et al.[17] found a mean $\dot{V}_E$ max value of 67.4 litre min^{-1} when a group of 11 to 14 year old boys performed a maximal treadmill walking test. When the same boys underwent a maximal cycling test the average $\dot{V}_E$ max was 62.9 litre min^{-1}. Paterson et al.[18] recorded average $\dot{V}_E$ max values of 67.6 and 73.3 litre min^{-1} on the same boys with a walking and running treadmill protocol, respectively. In a similar study, Sheehan et al.[19] found that $\dot{V}_E$ max with treadmill running was 15% greater than with walking. Such differences in $\dot{V}_E$ max in respect to testing modality and protocol must reflect similar variations in metabolic demand, lactate production and metabolic acidosis.

While the pattern of maximal $\dot{V}_E$ relative to body size in children remains uncertain, f_R at exhaustive exercise clearly declines with age. In the longitudinal study of Rowland and Cunningham,[13] maximal rate during treadmill walking over the five years fell from 65 to 57 breaths min^{-1} in the boys and 63 to 57 breaths min^{-1} in the girls (Fig. 2.6.2).

Similar findings have been seen in cross-sectional studies. In the study by Robinson,[7] the six year old boys had a mean maximal breathing rate of 62 breaths min^{-1} compared to 46 breaths min^{-1} in the 18 year old subjects. Astrand[16] reported that over a similar age span, f_R decreased from an average of 70 breaths min^{-1} to 45 breaths min^{-1} in boys and 66 to 51 breaths min^{-1} in girls.

The decline in maximal f_R with age has been sufficiently consistent to be expressed mathematically. Morse et al.[5] described the relationship as f_R max $= 60.5 - 0.92$(age), and Mercier et al.[15] reported that maximal f_R could be expressed relative to body mass (M) by the allometric equation f_R max $= 137\ M^{-0.27}$ in children. There is no apparent gender influence on maximal f_R.[10,13,16]

The decline in maximal f_R with age is more than overcome by increases in maximal V_T. This results in the obligatory rise in maximal absolute $\dot{V}_E$ necessary to match $\dot{V}O_2$ max and expel excessive CO_2 from buffering of lactic acid. It follows, then, that the ratio of f_R (breaths min^{-1}) to V_T (litre) at exhaustive exercise progressively declines during the course of the childhood years. Between the ages of 9 and 13 years this value has been reported to fall from 60.7 to 29.2 in boys and 58.9 to 32.6 in girls.[13] While this study indicated no gender

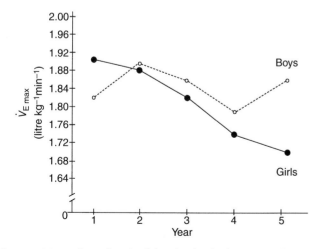

Fig. 2.6.1 Mean values of maximal $\dot{V}_E$ related to body mass in a five-year longitudinal study of boys and girls. Reprinted from Rowland and Cunningham[13] with permission.

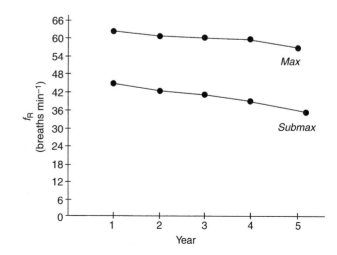

Fig. 2.6.2 Five year longitudinal assessment of maximal breathing rates at maximal and submaximal exercise in boys and girls. Reprinted from Rowland and Cunningham[13] with permission.

effect, Armstrong et al.[10] reported an average f_R to V_T ratio of 48.4 in boys and 60.0 in girls at maximal treadmill exercise ($p < 0.05$).

Increases in maximal V_T with age reflect the size of the growing lung, which, in turn, is closely linked to body size. Rowland and Cunningham[13] found that V_T max per kg was essentially unchanged over the five years of their longitudinal study. The mean value of approximately $30 \, ml \, kg^{-1}$ was not substantially different in the boys and girls. Similarly, Astrand[16] found that boys and girls ages 7 and 13 years had about the same mass-relative V_T (34 to 35 $ml \, kg^{-1}$). Supporting these findings, Mercier et al.[15] reported scaling exponents of 0.96 and 2.90 for maximal V_T relative to mass and stature, respectively. Armstrong et al.,[10] however, found that average maximal V_T adjusted for stature and mass was significantly greater in 11 year old boys than girls (1.10 litre versus 0.95 litre).

The same investigators observed that the V_T at maximal exercise represented the same per cent of VC in boys and girls (45%). Thus, while girls have a relatively smaller VC than boys, the use of lung capacity at maximal exercise is independent of gender.

Respiratory patterns during exercise

In the typical adult, increases in both V_T and f_R contribute to the rise of $\dot{V}_E$ that accompanies the onset of physical activity. As exercise intensity increases, however, the relative contribution of these two factors changes.[2] Above moderate intensity, V_T tends to plateau, and subsequent improvements in $\dot{V}_E$ are solely due to the influence of rising f_R.

Some information suggests that this pattern may be different in children. Rowland and Green[20] found that 10–14 year old boys had a decrease in the ratio of f_R to V_T at high intensity levels. Similarly, Boule et al.[21] showed that breathing rate plateaued at 67% of maximum work in 6–15 year old children, while V_T rose linearly to exhaustion.

Armstrong et al.,[10] however, demonstrated a steady increase of both V_T and f_R throughout a maximal treadmill test in 11 year old boys and girls. During this progressive test, the $f_R : V_T$ ratio rose, supporting the adult model of increasing importance of f_R at high exercise intensities. In addition, Rutenfranz et al.[14] described a linear response of f_R to maximal exercise in both children and adolescents.

It does seem clear, though, that children utilize f_R to a greater extent than V_T to achieve $\dot{V}_E$. Specifically, during the course of biological development an increasingly greater relative importance is placed on tidal volume—a size-dependent factor which parallels lung and total body dimensions—with a diminishing contribution of breathing rate, which is independent of size. [This pattern bears a striking resemblance to changes in heart output, the lung's geographical and functional neighbour, during growth. Like minute ventilation, cardiac output reflects the product of a size-dependent volume (stroke volume) and frequency (heart rate). During the course of childhood, heart rate at rest and at a given submaximal workload decrease while stroke volume increases in direct proportion to heart and body size (see Chapter 2.7).]

The decline in $f_R : V_T$ for a particular $\dot{V}_E$ is progressive with age and is evident both at rest and during exercise. As a child grows, V_T is closely linked to body size at rest, submaximal and maximal exercise. It seems, therefore, that variations in breathing rate, rather than V_T, mediate alterations in $\dot{V}_E$ dictated by changes in metabolic rate and lactate production, which cannot be explained simply by increasing body size.

The relative contributions of breathing depth and frequency in children have been viewed from the standpoint of optimizing mechanical efficiency.[22] Presumably the body 'chooses' a particular ratio of f_R and V_T to achieve a given $\dot{V}_E$ that minimizes respiratory work. The work of breathing is strongly influenced by the mechanical properties of the lung as well as the diameter of the airways, factors which both evolve during the course of childhood.

For instance, the stiffness of the lung, or elastance, created by connective tissue and alveolar surface forces, decreases with growth in children. That is, lung compliance improves with age.[23] During the same time period, the work needed to overcome airway resistance changes as the bronchioles enlarge. However, the rates of changes of these two factors are not identical, and presumably such differences affect the metabolic efficiency outcomes which dictate an optimal frequency:volume ratio. As noted by Godfrey:[22]

> the increase in tidal volume and fall in respiratory frequency are functions of the changing mechanical conditions of the lungs as they grow. With increased size there is a fall in airways resistance and a rise in compliance, and the [breathing] frequency of a child is that which minimizes the work of breathing for the given mechanical conditions. (p. 81)

The pattern of ventilation at high exercise intensities differs from that at low-to-moderate workloads. As noted above, with the onset of accumulation of blood lactate, buffering by bicarbonate produces excess CO_2, and respiratory drive is stimulated. The metabolic acidosis that occurs when buffering becomes insufficient results in a further increase in $\dot{V}_E$. These effects result in an upperward divergence of $\dot{V}_E$ from $\dot{V}O_2$. The point of this deflection (the ventilatory anaerobic threshold, VAT) can be identified by a rise in $\dot{V}_E / \dot{V}O_2$.

This process is no different in children than adults. Compared to mature individuals, however, VAT occurs at a relatively higher exercise intensity (i.e. per cent $\dot{V}O_2$ max) in children. VAT in prepubertal boys and girls is typically 65 to 70% $\dot{V}O_2$ max, while values of approximately 55 to 60% are observed in adults. Reybrouck et al.[24] found that VAT was 74 and 69% $\dot{V}O_2$ max in five to six year old boys and girls, respectively, but 61% and 54% in 15 to 16 year olds. Kanaley and Boileau[25] reported VAT values in males 8–11, 13–14 and 18–24 years old of 68.8%, 65.4% and 58.5%, respectively. The dampened anaerobic capacity and consequent lower blood lactate levels with exercise in prepubertal subjects is the most likely explanation for these findings.[26]

Hyperventilation in children

Children characteristically hyperventilate during exercise, with a greater $\dot{V}_E$ to achieve a given $\dot{V}O_2$ compared to adults. This ventilatory inefficiency, expressed both by a higher ventilatory equivalent for oxygen ($\dot{V}_E / \dot{V}O_2$) and lower alveolar and arterial PCO_2, has been described at all levels of exercise intensity. A progressive improvement in ventilatory efficiency over the course of childhood has been observed, which suggests that maturation of respiratory drive and/or mechanical factors related to anatomic growth of the lung may be responsible.

Cross-sectional studies have indicated higher maximal $\dot{V}_E / \dot{V}O_2$ values in prepubertal compared to mature subjects. Andersen et al.[27] demonstrated a progressive decline in $\dot{V}_E / \dot{V}O_2$ between the ages of 8 and 16 years. In males values fell from 33.3 to 24.5 over this age range, and females demonstrated a decline from 34.8 to 23.9. Similar trends were observed when subjects exercised at 50% $\dot{V}O_2$ max. Astrand[16] reported an average maximal $\dot{V}_E/\dot{V}O_2$ of 40.5 in boys four to six years and 32.0 at age 14 to 15 years.

Longitudinal studies have provided mixed findings. Rutenfranz et al.[14] failed to find any age trend in maximal $\dot{V}_E/\dot{V}O_2$ in either boys or girls 8 to 17 years old. Rowland and Cunningham[13] studied children annually for five years beginning at age eight years. In girls, submaximal $\dot{V}_E/\dot{V}O_2$ at the same treadmill settings steadily declined, from an initial value of 32.28 to 29.05 at the end of the study. The boys demonstrated a better submaximal efficiency than girls, with a similar decline over the five years (31.46 to 26.34). At maximal exercise mean $\dot{V}_E/\dot{V}O_2$ fell from 37.15 to 34.05 in the boys, but no change was observed in the girls (39.64 to 39.37) (Fig. 2.6.3).

The data from Godfrey[22] also indicate that girls ventilate more relative to metabolic requirements at maximal exercise than boys except at very young ages. Gender differences in maximal $\dot{V}_E/\dot{V}O_2$ were confirmed by Armstrong et al.,[28] who found that boys were more efficient than girls at maximal treadmill exercise (29.6 and 30.4 for boys and girls, respectively).

As Godfrey[22] pointed out, age or gender comparisons of $\dot{V}_E/\dot{V}O_2$ at maximal exercise may not be an appropriate means of assessing differences in ventilatory efficiency. Values at peak exercise are influenced by anaerobic metabolism, acidosis and lactate levels which drive $\dot{V}_E$ above levels which accommodate aerobic metabolism.

Prepubertal subjects typically demonstrate lower anaerobic capacity compared to mature individuals. Given, then, that the contribution of these anaerobic factors should be expected to be *less* in young children, their higher values of $\dot{V}_E/\dot{V}O_2$ are even more convincing of their relative hyperventilation compared to adults.

With their rapid respiratory rates, it might be expected that the ventilatory inefficiency observed in children during exercise might be due to shallow breathing. Such does not appear to be the case, as several studies assessing PCO_2 levels in children indicate a true hyperventilation.[7,29–32] Robinson[7] described a progressive rise across the paediatric age range in alveolar PCO_2 during treadmill walking. Mean values were 33.0 mm Hg in 6 year old boys and 39.6 mm Hg in 17 year olds. Children exercising at 80% of VAT in the report by Armon et al.[29]

demonstrated end-tidal PCO_2 values approximately 3 mm Hg lower than adults. Gadhoke and Jones[30] reported average submaximal end-tidal PCO_2 levels of 36.5 and 39.5 mm Hg in children with a body surface area of 1.05 to 1.19 and 1.50 to 1.89 m^2, respectively.

Two concepts have been advanced in attempts to explain the inverse relationship of age with relative hyperventilation and ventilatory inefficiency in children. The first holds that this phenomenon can be explained by a greater respiratory neural drive in the young child, the other that size-related differences in ventilation mechanics are responsible.

Neural respiratory drive can be assessed by the mouth pressure (P) generated 0.1 s after airways occlusion. Gaultier et al.[33] found that P decreased with age (A) by the relationship $P = 8.51A^{-0.62}$ between the ages of 4 to 16 years. They concluded that the higher pressures observed in the younger children indicated greater neural ventilatory drive.

Further support of this idea came from the work of Gratas-Delamarche et al.[34] They used ventilation responses to inhaled CO_2 during exercise to assess maturity-related differences in the sensitivity of respiratory drive centres. Nine prepubertal boys demonstrated a significantly lower CO_2 sensitivity threshold (the value of end-tidal CO_2 when ventilation rose above a steady state level) than ten young men. In addition, the boys demonstrated a steeper slope of the linear relationship between $\dot{V}_E$ and end tidal CO_2.

These findings are all indicative of a greater sensitivity of respiratory drive centres in children compared to adults. This suggests that ventilation during exercise is regulated to maintain a lower CO_2 set point in immature individuals. Why this should be so is unclear.

Alternatively, the greater $\dot{V}_E/\dot{V}O_2$ in children could reflect their greater f_R compared to adults. It has been argued that this higher f_R causes a relatively smaller V_T and consequently greater dead space ventilation (V_D) contribution to $\dot{V}_E$; total $\dot{V}_E$ will consequently be higher to maintain alveolar ventilation. Investigations of V_D in children, however, indicate a constant relationship to V_T with increasing age (i.e. V_D/V_T remains stable throughout childhood).

The relatively rapid breathing rate during exercise in small children might alter $\dot{V}_E/\dot{V}O_2$ by other mechanisms. Gratas-Delamarche et al.[34] suggested that these high breathing rates might (1) impair efficient washout of alveolar gas compared to the slower rates of adults or (2) increase the total work of breathing needed to overcome the elastance properties of the lungs.

Lung diffusion capacity during exercise

The ease with which gases cross the lung–blood capillary interface can be estimated by the diffusion capacity for carbon monoxide ($D_L CO$). Generally, diffusion capacity is not a limiting factor except in highly trained athletes at intense exercise, when circulatory transit time through the lung is very brief.

$D_L CO$ is directly related to stature in both children and adults. Data from Anderson and Godfrey[35] suggest that diffusion capacity at maximal exercise (expressed relative to stature) is greater in children, and the slope of the $D_L CO$–stature regression line is steeper. In that study, $D_L CO$ rose at low exercise intensities and then plateaued. When Shephard et al.[36] measured $D_L CO$ in 10 to 12 year old children, however, values rose linearly to exhaustive exercise. It was noted that the

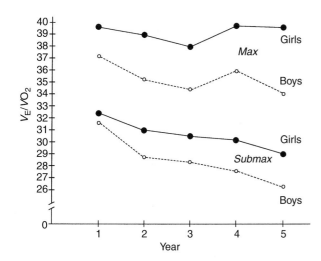

Fig. 2.6.3 Changes in ventilatory equivalent for oxygen ($\dot{V}_E/\dot{V}O_2$) with maximal and submaximal treadmill walking in a longitudinal study of boys and girls. Reprinted from Rowland and Cunningham[13] with permission.

slope of the D_LCO–$\dot{V}O_2$ relationship was approximately twice that observed in other studies of adults.

These findings suggest that lung diffusion capacity might be greater in children than adults. However, Johnson et al.[37] could find no differences in membrane diffusing capacity (a measure that eliminates red cell resistance from D_LCO) at maximal exercise in four children 8 to 12 years old and six subjects aged 15 to 28 years. Studies examining the importance of D_LCO in limiting blood oxygenation in trained child athletes have not been performed.

Submaximal ventilatory kinetics

$\dot{V}_E$ and $\dot{V}CO_2$ have been reported to rise 30% more rapidly at the onset of exercise in children 7 to 10 years old compared to 15 to 18 year old adolescents.[32] This maturity-related difference in ventilatory kinetics is difficult to explain given the observation that CO_2 production relative to metabolic expenditure is the same in children and adults. Lower storage of CO_2 in children might be responsible, but Armon et al.[29] found no significant differences in whole body CO_2 stores in adults and children at rest using [^{13}C]-bicarbonate tracer techniques.

However, such differences may occur with exercise. Zanconato et al.[38] measured CO_2 stores in 6 to 10 year old boys and young adults aged 21 to 39 years. No significant differences were observed in the two groups at rest. During exercise, CO_2 stores did not change in the children but rose 31% in the adults. They suggested that adults may store more CO_2 due to their greater amount of body fat (CO_2 has a greater solubility in adipose tissue) or higher haemoglobin levels (which binds CO_2).

Sustained exercise

Rowland and Rimany[39] compared ventilatory changes in 9 to 13 year old premenarcheal girls and young women (ages 20–31 years) during an extended period of submaximal exercise. Subjects cycled for 40 minutes at an intensity of 63% $\dot{V}O_2$ max. Increase in $\dot{V}_E$ between 10 and 40 minutes of exercise was similar in the two groups (7.1% and 11.7% in the girls and women, respectively). During this time the rate of breathing rose 15% in the girls and 14% in the women, while V_T fell by 6.0% and by 2.0%, respectively.

These patterns of ventilatory response mimic findings previously described in studies of adults[40] as well as those reported by Asano and Hirakoba[41] in a comparison of boys and men. Such responses are unusual, since most stimuli of ventilation (chemical, metabolic, progressive exercise) cause an increase in V_T rather than a decrease. It has been suggested that increases in body temperature are most likely responsible for this pattern of response to sustained steady state exercise.

Adaptations to physical training

Regular endurance exercise improves $\dot{V}O_2$ max (although less so in children than adults). Consequently, an aerobic training programme should be expected to enhance function of the various components of the oxygen delivery system, including ventilatory capacity. Insights into the 'plasticity' of lung function to physical training can be gained from (a) examining cross-sectional differences in ventilatory responses to exercise in child athletes and non-athletes, and (b)

assessing ventilatory function longitudinally in response to a period of endurance training. The value of the former approach is limited, of course, in that pre-selection characteristics, often genetic, cannot be differentiated from those which are induced by training.

Lakhera et al.[42] compared resting pulmonary spirometric variables in 20 Indian athletes, ages 13 to 16 years, with those of non-athletes on three occasions a year apart. The athletes participated in a variety of sports, including football, volleyball, middle distance running and cricket. The athletes had a greater forced expiratory volume (FEV_1) and maximal voluntary ventilation (MVV) than the non-athletes. Vital capacity, FEV_1, MVV, expiratory reserve volume and inspiratory capacity all improved significantly over the course of the study in both groups. The authors concluded that lung development during adolescence is influenced by the process of growth and only negligible additional effects can be expected from sports training.

Similar findings were observed in the TOYA (Training of Young Athletes) Study, a three year longitudinal investigation of young athletes training in gymnastics, swimming, soccer and tennis.[43] Age groups were overlapped to provide developmental data over an 11 year age span. Lung growth was assessed by FVC and FEV_1, controlled for both body size and level of sexual development. The athletes exhibited greater values for both of these variables at all ages. At the beginning of the study the VC of the female tennis players, gymnasts and swimmers was 20%, 21% and 34% greater than values in the non-athletes, respectively. In the male swimmers, average VC was consistently approximately 17% greater than that of non-athletic controls.

Values of both variables rose during the course of the study. The rate of increase in VC and FEV_1, however, was identical in the training athletes and controls. As noted by the authors:[43]

> this suggests that physical activity in itself does not influence lung growth and that the observed differences between the groups reflected a genetic predisposition towards superior lung function status in the athletes. (p. 319)

Other studies support that conclusion. Vaccaro and Poffenbarger[44] reported no significant differences in VC, FEV_1 or MVV in trained 10 to 14 year old runners compared to non-athletes. Bar-Or and Zwiren[45] described the same findings in nine to ten year old trained runners, and Cumming[46] found no correlation between either VC or MVV with performance on an 880-yard run in 13 to 17 year old boys who were participating in a track camp. Similarly, Vaccaro and Clarke[47] could observe no differences in changes in VC, FEV_1 or MVV after a season of swim training in 9 to 11 year old children compared to a group of non-training youngsters.

On the other hand, Andrew et al.[48] reported significantly greater values for VC and FEV_1 in both male and female swimmers ages 8 to 18 years compared to non-athletic control subjects. Courteix et al.[49] described improvements in both static and dynamic lung volumes after one year of swim training in five nine year old girls. Vital capacity, total lung capacity and FEV_1 all improved while values in a control group remained unchanged.

There is some evidence, too, that longer training periods than observed in the studies described above might effect change in resting pulmonary function. Sundberg and Elovainio,[50] for instance, found that VC and FEV_1 were not different in runners and controls at ages 12 and 14 years. Yet in a group of 16 year old runners, values for both of these variables were greater in the athletes. In reviewing these data both in children and adults, Cumming[46] concluded that any differences which might exist in resting pulmonary function between athletes and non-athletes are slight and 'not of great importance in the performance of athletics'.

Differences between child athletes and non-athletes have been observed in ventilatory responses during exercise. Again, it is difficult to ascertain if these characteristics represent a training effect, genetic pre-selection, or even advanced biological maturation of the athletes compared to control subjects. For instance, Rowland and Green[20] examined the patterns of V_T and f_R during a progressive treadmill running test in non-athletic boys and men and a group of trained child distance runners. At the same treadmill settings or at identical $\dot{V}_E$ per kg, the non-athletic boys exhibited a higher f_R/V_T than the non-athletic adults. That is, the adults relied less on f_R than V_T to achieve the same $\dot{V}_E$, a pattern typical of trained adult endurance athletes. Values for the trained child runners were intermediate between the two groups. It was impossible to determine whether this observation reflected:

(1) the effects of running training (i.e. conversion to a more adult ventilatory pattern);
(2) pre-selection for a more mature, advantageous breathing pattern; or
(3) a greater level of biological development in the runners.

Gratas et al.[51] also found that 11 to 13 year old child athletes (football, ice skating, table tennis) had lower submaximal values for breathing rate and $\dot{V}_E/\dot{V}O_2$ compared to non-athletes. Mouth occlusion pressures during exercise, however, were similar. They concluded that child athletes have a more economical breathing pattern but similar neural respiratory drive compared to non-athletes. When Ramonatxo et al.[52] studied 10 to 16 year old trained swimmers, however, both V_T and f_R were similar to non-athletic control children at the same exercising $\dot{V}_E$.

Child endurance athletes generally demonstrate a higher maximal $\dot{V}_E$ when compared to non-athletic subjects, but differences are often less dramatic and more variable than those for $\dot{V}O_2$ max. For instance, the 15 distance runners (mean age 11.7 years) studied by Unnithan et al.[53] had a $\dot{V}O_2$ max of 60.5 ml kg^{-1} min^{-1} compared to 51.1 ml kg^{-1} min^{-1} in controls. Average maximal $\dot{V}_E$ was greater in the runners (71.4 litre min^{-1} versus 64.7 litre min^{-1}) but the difference did not reach statistical significance. No significant differences were observed between the two groups in $\dot{V}_E/\dot{V}O_2$, V_T, f_R or $\dot{V}_E$ during submaximal running at 8.0 km h^{-1}.

Sundberg and Elovainio[50] found similar differences in 12 to 16 year old runners and non-athletic controls. In each age group $\dot{V}O_2$ max was significantly greater in the runners, usually by about 10 ml kg^{-1} min^{-1}. Maximal $\dot{V}_E$ was higher in the runners as well, but the differences did not reach statistical significance until age 16 years.

Longitudinal studies should provide better insight into the responses of ventilatory function of children to endurance training. In general, these have demonstrated increases in maximal $\dot{V}_E$ of a magnitude similar to that of $\dot{V}O_2$ max.[54,55] Such improvement in maximal $\dot{V}_E$ appears to be due entirely to increases in maximal V_T.

Rowland and Boyajian[56] trained 37 children, ages 10.9 to 12.8 years, in a 12 week aerobic programme. Mean $\dot{V}O_2$ max increased from 44.7 to 47.6 ml kg^{-1} min^{-1} (6.5% increase), while maximal $\dot{V}_E$ improved from 1.67 to 1.82 litre kg^{-1} min^{-1} (9.0% rise). No significant changes in these variables were seen during a 12 week pre-training control period. The rise in $\dot{V}_E$ max was due to an increase in V_T max (1.35 to 1.50 litre), as no significant change was observed in maximal f_R. No changes were observed with training in submaximal f_R, V_T, $\dot{V}_E$ or $\dot{V}_E/\dot{V}O_2$.

Summary

The essential role of the lung as the environmental interface for gas exchange during exercise is the same in the child as the adult. However, certain differences do exist, and these may reflect not only the obvious influence of body size but also level of functional maturity. The patterns of ventilatory response to exercise which separate the child from the adult typically evolve over the course of the childhood years. This suggests that these factors are influenced by size and biological development rather than the hormonal effects that mark the pubertal years.

It is disconcerting that inefficiency of ventilation (a greater $\dot{V}_E$ requirement for a given metabolic rate) is characteristic of younger children, as biological systems are expected to evolve toward processes which assume the greatest energy economy. It must be concluded, then, that the higher $\dot{V}_E/\dot{V}O_2$ in children reflects a 'best economy' given the influence of other factors, particularly the separate influences of changing airways resistance and lung compliance. It must be assumed, then, that the hyperventilation, higher neural respiratory drive and greater reliance on breathing rate during exercise in children can somehow be explained by such a compromise of mechanical characteristics of the lungs during the growing years. Understanding the interplay of these factors on ventilatory responses in children remains a challenge for future investigators.

Equally troublesome is the lack of a clear insight into the most appropriate means of adjusting measures of ventilation to changing body size during childhood. Allometric analysis may offer a better understanding of normalization for body dimensions, but how size-independent factors which develop during childhood (i.e. respiratory neural drive, breathing rate) can be compared between children still remains problematic.

Although information is limited, it appears that the role of pulmonary function during athletic performance and the response of ventilation to training in child athletes is similar to that observed in adults. Although lung function is critical to oxygen delivery and thus aerobic fitness, it does not normally limit $\dot{V}O_2$ max or endurance performance. (The only exception may be the elite athlete who demonstrates hypoxaemia at intense exercise levels. This phenomenon has not yet been assessed in highly trained children.)

Maximal ventilation is high both in child endurance athletes and following a period of aerobic training. Most data indicate that this does not reflect change in resting lung dimensions or function, however. It is likely that the higher $\dot{V}_E$ max of the athlete reflects only a greater utilization of lung capacity. Consequently, ventilatory reserve at maximal exercise is reduced in the athlete compared to the non-athlete. There is evidence in adults, however, that the ability to *sustain* high levels of $\dot{V}_E$ may be greater in trained athletes. Whether child athletes are similarly gifted remains to be investigated.

References

1. **Wasserman, K.** Breathing during exercise. *New England Journal of Medicine,* 1978; **298:** 780–5.

2. **Pardy, R. L., Hussain, S. N. A.** and **Macklem, P. T.** The ventilatory pump in exercise. *Clinics in Chest Medicine,* 1984; **5**: 35–49.

3. **Orenstein, D. M.** Exercise tolerance and exercise conditioning in children with chronic lung disease. *Journal of Pediatrics,* 1988; **112**: 1043–7.

4. **Lyons, H. A.** and **Tanner, R. W.** Total lung volume and its subdivisions in children: normal standards. *Journal of Applied Physiology,* 1962; **17**: 601–4.

5. **Morse, M., Schultz, F. W.** and **Cassels, D. E.** Relation of age to physiological responses of the older boy (10–17 years) to exercise. *Journal of Applied Physiology,* 1949; **1**: 683–709.

6. **Schmidt-Nielsen, K.** *Scaling. Why is animal size so important?* Cambridge University Press, Cambridge, 1984: 99–103.

7. **Robinson, S.** Experimental studies of physical fitness in relation to age. *Arbeitsphysiologie,* 1938; **10**: 318–23.

8. **Asmussen, E., Secher, N. H.** and **Andersen, E. A.** Heart rate and ventilatory frequency as dimension-independent variables. *European Journal of Applied Physiology,* 1981; **46**: 379–86.

9. **Cassels, D. E.** and **Morse, M.** *Cardiopulmonary data for children and young adults.* Charles C. Thomas, Springfield, Il, 1962: 52–7.

10. **Armstrong, N., Kirby, B. J., McManus, A. M.** and **Welsman, J. R.** Prepubescents' ventilatory responses to exercise with reference to sex and body size. *Chest,* 1997; **112**: 1554–60.

11. **DeMuth, G. R.** and **Howatt, W. F.** Pulmonary diffusion. *Pediatrics,* 1965; **35 Suppl**: 162–75.

12. **Taussig, L. M., Cota, K.** and **Kaltenborn, W.** Different mechanical properties of the lung in boys and girls. *American Review of Respiratory Disease,* 1981; **123**: 640–3.

13. **Rowland, T. W.** and **Cunningham, L. N.** Development of ventilatory responses to exercise in normal white children. *Chest,* 1997; **111**: 327–32.

14. **Rutenfranz, J., Andersen, K. L., Seliger, V., Klimmer, F., Ilmarinen, J., Ruppel, M.** and **Kylian, H.** Exercise ventilation during the growth spurt period: comparison between two European countries. *European Journal of Pediatrics,* 1981; **136**: 135–42.

15. **Mercier, J., Varray, A., Ramonatxo, M., Mercier, B.** and **Prefaut, C.** Influence of anthropometric characteristics on changes in maximal exercise ventilation and breathing pattern during growth in boys. *European Journal of Applied Physiology,* 1991; **63**: 235–41.

16. **Astrand, P. O.** *Experimental studies of physical working capacity in relation to sex and age.* Munksgaard, Copenhagen, 1952.

17. **Boileau, R. A., Bonen, A., Heyward, V. H.** and **Massey, B. H.** Maximal aerobic capacity on the treadmill and bicycle ergometer of boys 11–14 years of age. *Journal of Sports Medicine,* 1977; **17**: 153–62.

18. **Paterson, D. H., Cunningham, D. A.** and **Donner, A.** The effect of different treadmill speeds on the variability of VO₂max in children. *European Journal of Applied Physiology,* 1981; **47**: 113–22.

19. **Sheehan, J. M., Rowland, T. W.** and **Burke, E. J.** A comparison of four treadmill protocols for determination of maximal oxygen uptake in 10–12 year old boys. *International Journal of Sports Medicine,* 1987; **8**: 31–4.

20. **Rowland, T. W.** and **Green, G. M.** The influence of biological maturation and aerobic fitness on ventilatory responses to treadmill exercise. In *Exercise physiology. Current selected research* (ed. C. O. Dotson and J. H. Humphrey). AMS Press, New York, 1990: 51–9.

21. **Boule, M., Gaultier, C.** and **Girard, F.** Breathing pattern during exercise in untrained children. *Respiratory Physiology,* 1989; **75**: 225–34.

22. **Godfrey, S.** *Exercise testing in children.* Saunders, London, 1974.

23. **Lanteri, C. J.** and **Sly, P. D.** Changes in respiratory mechanics with age. *Journal of Applied Physiology,* 1993; **74**: 369–78.

24. **Reybrouck, T., Weymans, M., Stijns, H., Knops, J.** and **vander Hauwaert, L.** Ventilatory anaerobic threshold in healthy children. Age and sex differences. *European Journal of Applied Physiology,* 1985; **54**: 278–84.

25. **Kanaley, J. A.** and **Boileau, R. A.** The onset of the anaerobic threshold at three stages of physical maturity. *Journal of Sports Medicine,* 1988; **28**: 367–74.

26. **Rowland, T. W.** and **Cunningham, L. N.** Influence of aerobic and anaerobic fitness on ventilatory threshold in children [abstract]. *Medicine and Science in Sports and Exercise,* 1996; **28 Suppl**: S147.

27. **Andersen, K. L., Seliger, N., Rutenfranz, J.** and **Messel, S.** Physical performance capacity of children in Norway. Part III. Respiratory responses to graded exercise loadings–population parameters in a rural community. *European Journal of Applied Physiology,* 1974; **33**: 265–74.

28. **Armstrong, N., Kirby, B. J., Mosney, J. R., Sutton, N. C.** and **Welsman, J. R.** Ventilatory responses to exercise in relation to sex and maturation. In *Children and exercise XIX* (ed. N. Armstrong, B. J. Kirby and J. R. Welsman). E. and F. N. Spon, London, 1997: 204–10.

29. **Armon, Y., Cooper, D. M.** and **Zanconato, S.** Maturation of ventilatory responses to 1-minute exercise. *Pediatric Research,* 1991; **29**: 362–8.

30. **Gadhoke, S.** and **Jones, N. L.** The responses to exercise in boys 9–15 years. *Clinical Science ,* 1969; **37**: 789–801.

31. **Shephard, R. J.** and **Bar-Or, O.** Alveolar ventilation in near maximum exercise. Data on pre-adolescent children and young adults. *Medicine and Science in Sports,* 1970; **2**: 83–92.

32. **Cooper, D. M., Kaplan, M. R., Baumgarten, L., Weiler-Ravell, D.,** and **Whipp, B. J.** Coupling of ventilation and CO₂ production during exercise in children. *Pediatric Research,* 1987; **21**: 568–72.

33. **Gaultier, C., Perret, L., Boule, M., Buvry, A.** and **Girard, F.** Occlusion pressure and breathing pattern in healthy children. *Respiration Physiology,* 1981; **46**: 71–80.

34. **Gratas-Delamarche, A., Mercier, J., Ramonatxo, M., Dassonville, J., Prefaut, C.** Ventilatory response of prepubertal boys and adults to carbon dioxide at rest and during exercise. *European Journal of Applied Physiology,* 1993; **66**: 25–30.

35. **Anderson, S. D.** and **Godfrey, S.** Transfer factor for CO₂ during exercise in children. *Thorax,* 1971; **26**: 51–4.

36. **Shephard, R. J., Allen, C., Bar-Or, O., Davies, C. T. M., Degre, S., Hedman, R.** and **Ishi, K.** The working capacity of Toronto schoolchildren. Part II. *Canadian Medical Association Journal ,*1969; **100**: 705–14.

37. **Johnson, R. L., Taylor, H. F.** and **Lawson, W. H.** Maximal diffusing capacity of the lung for carbon monoxide *Journal of Clinical Investigation,* 1965; **44**: 349–55.

38. **Zanconato, S., Cooper, D. M. , Barstow, T. J.** and **Landaw, E.** ¹³CO₂ washout dynamics during intermittent exercise in children and adults. *Journal of Applied Physiology,* 1992; **73**: 2476–82.

39. **Rowland, T. W.** and **Rimany, T. A.** Physiological responses to prolonged exercise in premenarcheal and adult females. *Pediatric Exercise Science,* 1995; **7**: 183–91.

40. **Dempsey, J. A., Aaron, E.** and **Martin, B. J.** Pulmonary function and prolonged exercise. In *Perspectives in exercise science and sports medicine. Vol 1. Prolonged exercise* (ed. D. R. Lamb and R. Murray). Benchmark Press, Indianapolis, 1988: 75–124.

41. **Asano, K.** and **Hirakoba, K.** Respiratory and circulatory adaptation during prolonged exercise in 10–12 year old children and in adults. In *Children and sport* (ed. J. Ilmarinen and I. Valimaki). Springer-Verlag, Berlin, 1984: 119–28.

42. **Lakhera, S. C. Kain, T. C.** and **Bandopadhyay, P.** Changes in lung function during adolescence in athletes and non-athletes. *Journal of Sports Medicine and Physical Fitness,* 1994; **34**: 258–62.

43. **Baxter-Jones, A. D.** and **Helms, P. J.** Effects of training at a young age: A review of the Training of Young Athletes (TOYA) Study. *Pediatric Exercise Science,* 1996; **8**: 310–27.

44. **Vaccaro, P.** and **Poffenbarger, A.** Resting and exercise respiratory function in young female runners. *Journal of Sports Medicine,* 1982; **22**: 102–7.

45. **Bar-Or, O.** and **Zwiren, L.** Physiological effects of increased frequency of physical education classes and of endurance conditioning on 9–10 year old girls and boys. In *Pediatric work physiology: Proceedings of the Fourth International Symposium* (ed. O. Bar-Or). Wingate Institute for Physical Education, Wingate, Israel, 1973: 183–98.

46. **Cumming, G. R.** Correlation of athletic performance with pulmonary function in 13 to 17 year old boys and girls. *Medicine and Science in Sports,* 1969; **1**: 140–3.

47. **Vaccaro, P.** and **Clarke, D. H.** Cardiorespiratory alterations in 9 to 11 year old children following a season of competitive swimming. *Medicine and Science in Sports,* 1978; **10**: 204–7.

48. **Andrew, G. M., Backlake, M. R., Guleria, J. S.** and **Bates, D. V.** Heart and lung functions in swimmers and non-athletes during growth. *Journal of Applied Physiology,* 1972; **32**: 245–51.

49. **Courtiex, D., Obert, P., Lecoq, A.-M., Guenon, P.** and **Koch, G.** Effect of intensive swimming training on lung volumes, airway resistances and on the maximal expiratory flow-volume relationship in prepubertal girls. *European Journal of Applied Physiology,* 1997; **76**: 264–9.

50. **Sundberg, S.** and **Elovainio, R.** Cardiorespiratory function in competitive distance runners 12–16 years compared with ordinary boys. *Acta Paediatrica Scandinavica,* 1982; **71**: 987–92.

51. **Gratas, A., Dassonville, J., Beillot, J.** and **Rochcongar, P.** Ventilatory and occlusio-pressure responses to exercise in trained and untrained children. *European Journal of Applied Physiology,* 1988; **57**: 591–6.

52. **Ramonatxo, M., Mercier, J., Abdallah, El-Fassi-Ben, R., Vago, P.** and **Prefaut, C.** Breathing patterns and occlusion pressure during exercise in pre- and peripubertal swimmers. *Respiration Physiology,* 1986; **65**: 351–64.

53. **Unnithan, V. B., Timmons, J. A., Paton, J. Y,** and **Rowland, T. W.** Physiologic correlates to running performance in pre-pubertal distance runners. *International Journal of Sports Medicine,* 1995; **16**: 528–33.

54. **Eisenman, P. A.** and **Golding, L. A.** Comparison of effects of training on $\dot{V}O_2$ max in girls and young women. *Medicine and Science in Sports,* 1975; **7**: 136–8.

55. **Eriksson, B. O.** and **Koch, G.** Effects of physical training on hemodynamic response during maximal and submaximal exercise. *Acta Physiologica Scandinavia,* 1973; **87**: 27–39.

56. **Rowland, T. W.** and **Boyajian, A.** Aerobic response to endurance training in children: magnitude, variability, and gender comparisons. *Pediatrics,* 1995; **96**: 654–8.

2.7 Cardiovascular function

Thomas W. Rowland

Introduction

By the dictates of the Fick equation, the rate of aerobic metabolism (oxygen uptake, $\dot{V}O_2$) during exercise is the product of cardiac output ($\dot{Q}$) and peripheral arteriovenous oxygen difference. Consequently cardiac functional capacity should be expected to play a critical role in determining one's aerobic fitness, both in the testing laboratory ($\dot{V}O_2$ max) and during athletic performance (i.e. distance running, swimming, cycling). In fact, evidence from studies in both adults and children indicates the importance of maximal cardiac output as the limiting factor in the oxygen delivery chain.[1,2]

Circulation of blood acts not only to supply oxygen to exercising muscles. Augmented cardiac function during exercise is essential for dispelling body heat, transporting energy substrate, removing cellular metabolic wastes, circulating key hormonal responses (adrenaline, insulin), and controlling regional blood flow by selective changes in vascular tone. Given these critical multiple 'tasks', it is obvious that understanding the cardiovascular responses to exercise should help provide insight into the nature and limiting determinants of aerobic fitness.

Such an understanding has been hampered by lack of a simple means of assessing cardiac function during exercise. While determination of heart rate is both easy and accurate, measurement of stroke volume and cardiac output (the product of stroke volume and heart rate) is more problematic, particularly at high exercise intensities. As reviewed in Chapter 1.6, many techniques for assessing $\dot{Q}$ with exercise are invasive, while others require steady state, making them unsuited for obtaining maximal values. Direct determination of arteriovenous oxygen difference requires vascular catheterization and has therefore rarely been measured during exercise. Instead, values are calculated from the quotient of $\dot{V}O_2$ and $\dot{Q}$, causing any errors in the estimation of $\dot{Q}$ to be amplified. The investigator interested in assessing cardiac function with exercise in children is particularly hampered by ethical constraints, which limit use of vascular catheterization and radioactive materials in subjects who are minors.

These difficulties notwithstanding, recent advances in safe, non-invasive techniques, such as ultrasound and bioimpedance, have begun to provide informative data on the cardiac responses of children to exercise. Most of this information involves normal children and is purely descriptive in nature. Consequently, much remains to be learned concerning underlying mechanisms, particularly as they may differ from adults.

This chapter will review our current understanding of cardiac responses to exercise in the paediatric age group, focusing mainly on healthy children. It should be recognized, though, that characterizing cardiac responses in normal youngsters may have practical importance in managing young patients with heart disease. Appreciating how such responses in this group deviate from normal might permit not only a greater insight into a patient's prognosis, but also provide a means of appropriate timing of surgical intervention and interpreting response to medications.

It is also important to recognize normal cardiac findings and responses to exercise in children in comparison to those of trained child athletes. Many questions remain concerning the physiological effects and safety of intense training regimens for these young athletes. For example, whether cardiac findings such as left ventricular enlargement observed in adult endurance athletes (the 'athlete's heart') can be considered benign in child competitors is uncertain. Scant information is available regarding the cardiac responses to aerobic and resistance exercise in child athletes.

These research efforts should also improve our understanding of the basic physiological mechanisms behind the cardiac responses to exercise in children. Particularly important is the question of how these processes may be influenced by normal growth and development. Viewed superficially, the heart's work during exercise appears straight-forward—generating increased $\dot{Q}$ through a combination of stroke volume and heart rate—but, as outlined in this chapter, this apparent simplicity masks an extraordinarily complex set of physiological processes, most of which remain poorly understood both in adults and children.

The two-pump system

The traditional concept of the heart's role during exercise is that of a forward pump, a *supplier* of blood supply to contracting muscle. An alternative, more realistic view, however, considers the heart as part of a two-pump system in which heart function must respond to increases in blood flow returning from a second pump in the periphery. This idea places the heart in an equally important role as a *recipient* of circulating blood during exercise.

The propulsive effects of cardiac function are critical for blood flow *to* skeletal musculature, but other mechanisms must be responsible for blood *return* to the heart. In fact, the volume of blood returning to the heart must equal that being pumped forward; i.e. the mechanisms responsible for systemic venous return are equally important to circulation of blood during exercise.

The determinants of systemic venous return (termed the peripheral circulatory pump) are multiple and not well understood. Principal among these, however, is the contractile function of the exercising muscle itself. As noted by Rowell *et al.*,[3]

> the [skeletal] muscle pump can be viewed as a second heart on the venous return portion of the circuit, having a capacity to generate blood flow rivaling that of the left ventricle. (p. 779.)

The muscle pump has been observed to decrease venous pressures in the feet by 60 mm Hg during walking and running.[4] In animals, the contraction of leg muscles can produce a driving force for blood flow that will overcome a venous occlusive pressure of 90 to 100 mmHg.[3]

Venous return during exercise is also supported by contraction of the abdominal musculature and fall in intrathoracic pressure caused by increasing rate and depth of breathing. It is possible, too, that the pumping action of the heart itself may increase venous return, the ventricles creating a suction effect (increased atrial–ventricular pressure gradient) which augments diastolic filling.[5]

Considering its key role in blood circulation, an understanding of the peripheral pump may be important in identifying factors which limit aerobic fitness. That is, maximal heart systolic function, manifest as $\dot{Q}$, has traditionally been considered the principal determinant of $\dot{V}O_2$ max, but $\dot{Q}$ max is highly dependent on the function of the peripheral pump (i.e. it cannot pump 'out' what doesn't come 'in'). Therefore, characteristics of the peripheral pump might be equally or more important in limiting $\dot{Q}$ max than myocardial function itself. From the standpoint of the heart, this observation shifts attention from determinants of systolic function (i.e. the volume of blood it can expel) to diastolic function (the volume it can receive). As will be discussed later in this chapter, knowledge of diastolic function of the heart during exercise is limited; however, some information suggests that cardiac filling properties could be limiting to circulatory flow at high work loads.

Maturational differences in the two-pump system have not yet been evaluated. It is tempting to speculate, however, that development of components of the peripheral pump (i.e. skeletal muscle volume and endurance) might contribute to the growth of aerobic fitness during childhood.

The heart at rest

Not surprisingly, resting values for $\dot{Q}$ during childhood reflect those of metabolic rate (i.e. oxygen uptake). Basal metabolic rate relative to body size (either mass or surface area) steadily declines during the course of childhood, paralleled by a similar pattern in resting $\dot{Q}$. As a child grows, the resting stroke volume increases as a manifestation of greater heart size, while heart rate at rest progressively declines.

Cardiac output

Between the ages of 6 and 18 years, the mean basal metabolic rate in males falls from approximately 222 to 180 $kJ\,m^{-2}\,BSA\,h^{-1}$ (18.9% decrease).[6] Correspondingly, Rowland et al.[7] reported an 18.8% lower resting cardiac index in a group of 30 year old men (mean 3.05 litre $min^{-1}\,m^{-2}$) compared to 11 year old boys (mean 3.76 litre $min^{-1}\,m^{-2}$). In a cross-sectional study, Katori[8] found somewhat greater age differences when resting $\dot{Q}$ (determined using the earpiece dye dilution method) was related to body mass. Cardiac output per kg was approximately 220 $ml\,kg^{-1}\,min^{-1}$ at age five years and 140 $ml\,kg^{-1}\,min^{-1}$ in late adolescence. There were no gender influences on these values.

Normal values for resting $\dot{Q}$ in children, as well as heart rate and stroke volume, are dependent on body position. Pooling of blood in the lower extremities on assuming the sitting position is expected to decrease venous return, cardiac filling and stroke volume. Heart rate increases as a compensatory manoeuvre, with small overall decreases in $\dot{Q}$. Koch et al.[9] demonstrated an average increase in heart rate from 81 to 90 beats min^{-1} (11% rise) when 13 year old boys went from

supine to sitting. Average stroke volume fell from 69 to 51 ml (26% fall) and $\dot{Q}$ decreased from 5.6 to 4.6 litre min^{-1} (18%). Eriksson and Koch[10] reported a decrease in stroke volume from supine to sitting of 21% in a study of nine 11 to 13 year old boys. Rowland et al. (unpublished data) found an average decline in stroke index of 21% when 24 healthy 12 year old boys moved from supine to sitting. In these subjects, however, the resulting increase in heart rate (mean 75 beats - min^{-1} to 90 beats min^{-1}) was an effective compensation, as average cardiac index did not fall appreciably (3.90 to 3.84 litre $min^{-1}\,m^{-2}$).

These decreases in stroke volume when assuming the sitting position are similar to those previously reported in adults by Thadani et al.[11] (30%) and Higginbotham et al.[12] (28%). However, Buchberger and Koch[13] found a 41% decrease in supine–sitting stroke volume in 22 year old subjects using the same protocol as the study by Koch et al.[9] which indicated a 26% decline in children.

Given a consideration of body position, reported values for resting $\dot{Q}$ in children have generally been consistent. Mean resting cardiac index of 4.1 to 4.4 litre $min^{-1}\,m^{-2}$ (by the direct Fick and indicator dilution techniques) have been reported during cardiac catheterization in normal children who were sedated and supine.[14–16] Similar values have been described in supine children using impedance cardiography and Doppler echocardiography.[17,18] Studies in the sitting position have demonstrated an average resting cardiac index of 3.0 to 4.0 litre $min^{-1}\,m^{-2}$ in boys.[7,9,19,20]

Stroke volume

Resting stroke volume increases during childhood, corresponding to growth in heart size. Krovetz et al.[14] reported correlation coefficients of $r = 0.87$ and 0.90 between stroke volume (measured during cardiac catheterization) and body mass and surface area, respectively, in supine young people up to 20 years. Sproul and Simpson[16] found that supine stroke volume related equally well to body mass and surface area ($r = 0.83$ and $r = 0.81$, respectively).

No evidence exists that factors other than increasing left ventricular size (i.e. intrinsic contractility, afterload) contribute to resting stroke volume changes during growth. Using radionuclide angiography, Hurwitz et al.[21] could find no relationship between resting left ventricular ejection fraction (a measure of contractility) and age across the paediatric years (mean value approximately 65%). Similarly, left ventricular shortening fraction by echocardiography is essentially stable between age 4 and 20 years.[22] The ratio of resting left ventricular pre-ejection period to ejection time, another marker of contractility, was independent of age in the 0 to 19 year old subjects studied by Gutgesell et al.[23]

Reports of 'normal' values for resting stroke volume must be interpreted cautiously, since, besides body position, these values may be influenced by emotional state. Testing anxiety can increase resting heart rate, causing a reciprocal smaller stroke volume, particularly in the pre-exercise test situation. This phenomenon may partially explain the rather wide range of values reported for resting stroke volume. Most studies have indicated a mean stroke index at rest of 40 to 45 $ml\,m^{-2}$ in children,[7,14,16] but values ranging from 31 to 53 $ml\,m^{-2}$ have been described.[9,20]

Heart rate

Resting cardiac index declines with increasing age while stroke index is stable. It follows, then, that resting heart rate, a size-independent variable, must decline as the child grows. Mean heart rate obtained in a basal supine condition decreases from 85 beats min^{-1} at age four years to 60 beats min^{-1} at age 20 years, with values slightly greater in girls than boys.[24]

As noted above, resting heart rate is also strongly influenced by emotional state and body position. Seated resting heart rates are generally 15 beats higher than supine basal rates,[24] and 'resting' heart rates obtained immediately prior to exercise testing are likely to be even ten beats greater. It would be expected that significant inter-individual variability in anxiety surrounding such testing situations would affect these resting rates.

The mechanisms responsible for the decline in resting heart rate during childhood are not clear. Autonomic blockade studies indicate that children possess a higher intrinsic sinus node firing rate than adults.[25] Whether developmental changes in cardiac autonomic regulation might further influence heart rate in the childhood years is unknown.

Cardiac responses to exercise

The metabolic demands of exercise are accompanied by an increase in $\dot{Q}$, which reaches three to four times resting values at the point of maximal exercise. A rising heart rate is responsible for most of this increase, with limited contribution from stroke volume. Still, maximal stroke volume is the principal factor which separates individuals with high and low aerobic fitness. Such responses are qualitatively and quantitatively (relative to body size) similar in children and adults.

Heart rate

Studies in adults indicate that increases in heart rate with progressive exercise reflect parasympathetic withdrawal at low intensities and sympathetic stimulation (plus effects of circulating adrenaline) at high work loads. Whether this scenario is similar in children is unknown. Circulating noradrenaline levels (an index of sympathetic nervous activity) during exercise have been found to be greater in adults than children,[26,27] although such differences have not always reached statistical significance.[26] Lehmann et al.[27] reported similar serum adrenaline concentrations during exercise in boys and men.

A linear relationship is typically observed when mean group values for heart rate are plotted against increasing work loads. At high-intensity exercise, however, heart rate in individual subjects tends to decelerate in respect to work load (Fig. 2.7.1). Rowland and Cunningham[28] found that all 13 children in a treadmill walking study showed a tapering of heart rate at an exercise intensity above 60% $\dot{V}O_2$ max. A plateau (defined as less than a three-beat increase in the final stage) was observed in 38% of the subjects.

The explanation for this phenomenon, similar to that described in adults, is unclear. The fact that stroke volume remains constant during this time suggests that the heart rate taper might reflect a decrease in systemic venous return. Alternatively, baroreceptor response to increasing systemic blood pressure could play a role. It has been observed that the point at which the heart rate begins to decelerate corresponds with ventilatory markers of the anaerobic threshold.[29] It has been recognized, however, that onset of anaerobiosis is typically accompanied by an *increase* in heart rate.[30]

Heart rate at a given workload, either on the cycle ergometer or treadmill, decreases with age. For example, the average heart rate in a group of 10 year old boys during treadmill walking was

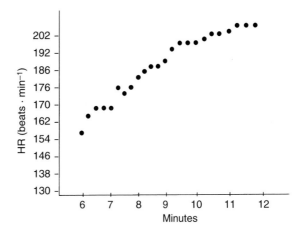

Fig. 2.7.1 Typical tapering of heart rate observed at high exercise intensity in an individual child.

167 beats min^{-1} but for 16 year olds the rate was 147 beats min^{-1}.[31] This fall in submaximal heart rate reflects increases in stroke volume with growth; that is, the metabolic rate and $\dot{Q}$ to perform a given level of work becomes increasingly satisfied through stroke volume rather than heart rate as a child grows.

Both longitudinal and cross-sectional studies have indicated that maximal heart rate during treadmill or cycling does not change over the course of the childhood years. Bailey et al.[32] showed that maximal treadmill running produced maximal heart rates that did not vary by more than 3 beats min^{-1} in an eight year longitudinal study of 51 boys. Mean maximal heart rate averaged 196 beats min^{-1}. Rowland et al.[33] reported stable maximal heart rates during treadmill walking (mean 202 and 204 beats min^{-1} for boys and girls, respectively) in a five year longitudinal study. The average for the 19 subjects on annual testing varied by 2 beats min^{-1} in the girls and 4 beats min^{-1} in the boys. These observations indicate that adult-based formulae to identify a target maximal rate (such as 220 minus age) are not appropriate for children, in whom maximal heart rate is independent of age.

Studies of maximal heart rates in children have generally demonstrated no significant gender effect. It is important to recognize, however, that maximal heart rate during exercise in children is influenced by testing modality.[34] Highest rates, usually approximately 200 to 205 beats min^{-1}, are achieved with treadmill running. Maximal rates with treadmill walking are often about 5 beats min^{-1} lower. Upright cycling protocols typically elicit maximal rates of about 195 beats min^{-1}, while values during semisupine cycling may be ten beats lower.[35] Cumming[36] described a maximal heart rate of 172 beats min^{-1} in children during supine cycling. Exercise tests with the rowing ergometer in children have demonstrated an average maximal heart rate of 190 beats min^{-1}.[37,38] Cumming and Langford[39] reported maximal heart rates in the same group of boys using different exercise protocols (Table 2.7.1).

Despite the fact that maximal heart rate is unchanged across the paediatric years, the rate of recovery following exhaustive exercise is inversely related to age. Washington et al.[40] described mean one minute recovery heart rates of 133, 138 and 148 beats min^{-1} after cycling in boys grouped by body surface area as <1.0 m^2, 1.0 to 1.19 m^2, and >1.2 m^2, respectively. Riopel et al.[41] reported similar findings, with a faster fall in heart rate in younger children after treadmill walking compared to older subjects, despite similar maximal

Table 2.7.1   Values for maximal heart rate and oxygen uptake in the same 23 children, ages 9 to 13 years, performing two different cycle protocols (James, Godfrey), treadmill running (Bruce protocol), and treadmill walking (Balke protocol)[39]

Protocol	Maximal heart rate (beat min^{-1})	$\dot{V}O_2$ max (ml kg^{-1}min^{-1})
Cycling		
James	197 (7)	48.5 (7.2)
Godfrey	195 (5)	47.9 (8.3)
Treadmill		
Bruce	204 (5)	54.0 (7.6)
Balke	198 (5)	48.2 (6.6)

Values are mean (standard deviation).

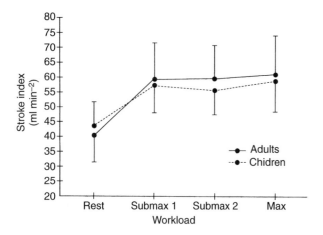

Fig. 2.7.2   Mean stroke index response during progressive cycling exercise in 15 boys (mean age 10.9 years) and 16 men (mean age 30.7 years). Reprinted by permission from Rowland et al.[7]

heart rates. Baraldi et al.[42] postulated that this pattern might be explained by lower catecholamine levels in young children.

Stroke volume

Cardiovascular variables typically demonstrate a steady rise during a progressive exercise test. Changes in stroke volume, on the other hand, are small and contribute little to increases in $\dot{Q}$ during exercise. Nonetheless, maximal stroke volume is the principal determinant of $\dot{Q}$ max, since peak heart rate is independent of level of aerobic fitness.[1] This fact highlights the importance of understanding the influences of cardiac filling, contractility and afterload on stroke volume during exercise.

When a healthy, untrained child on an upright cycle begins to pedal, stroke volume rises. At mild exercise intensities it reaches values which are 30 to 40% greater than resting. Stroke volume then changes little as work loads increase, demonstrating a plateau to the point of exhaustion.

This pattern has been consistently observed in studies of children, using thoracic bioimpedance,[9,43] Doppler echocardiography,[1,7,35,44] CO_2 rebreathing,[45–49] dye dilution[10] and acetylene rebreathing techniques.[18,19] In these reports, values for the ratio of maximal to resting

stroke volume have also been similar, with most between 1.30 and 1.38.[7,9,10,43,44] Similar patterns and values for stroke index are observed in young adults (Fig. 2.7.2).[7]

Boys have a greater stroke volume at the same submaximal $\dot{V}O_2$ or workload compared to girls, although differences have been small and in some cases statistically insignificant.[47,50–52] As noted by Turley and Wilmore[47] this trend probably reflects the larger values of left ventricular mass and volumes reported in boys. Scholz et al.[53] measured 200 autopsy specimens of normal hearts of persons between birth and age 19 years. Beyond early childhood, heart mass relative to body mass, stature or body surface area was consistently higher in males. For instance, the average boy and girl with an equal height of 150 cm had heart masses of 164 and 154 g, respectively. Such small but consistent gender differences in heart size are manifest by echocardiography[54] and chest X-ray.[55,56]

Most reports of maximal stroke index in children are in the range of 58 to 63 ml m^{-2} (see Table 2.7.2 below). Rowland et al. (unpublished data) studied 12 year old boys and girls who had mean values for $\dot{V}O_2$ max per lean body mass of 58.6 and 55.2 ml kg^{-1} min^{-1}, respectively ($p < 0.05$). Consistent with the effects of gender previously observed on submaximal stroke volume, the boys had a greater maximal stroke index relative to lean body mass than the girls (2.45 versus 2.33 ml m^{-2}), but the difference was not statistically significant ($p > 0.05$).

In the same study, allometric equations $Y = aX^b$ were created to identify the appropriate anthropometric denominator (X^b) for normalizing maximal stroke volume (Y) for body size in boys and girls. For the boys maximal stroke volume related to mass$^{0.55}$, stature$^{1.83}$ and BSA$^{1.03}$, while the respective b exponents for the girls were 0.55, 1.92 and 1.05. These findings suggest that, in this study population, indexing stroke volume to body surface area was an appropriate means of controlling values for body size.

The factors which can influence stroke volume with exercise are not only multiple but often interrelated. Consequently, no clear picture of the mechanisms and determinants of maximal stroke volume has emerged in either adults or children. Rowland et al.[1] showed that maximal stroke volume is related to resting values ($r = 0.67$), and subjects with high $\dot{V}O_2$ max demonstrate both higher maximal and resting stroke volumes compared to unfit children. This suggests that factors influencing resting stroke volume (larger left ventricular size, greater plasma volume) may play an important role in determining maximal stroke volume, cardiac output and $\dot{V}O_2$ max in children.

The pattern of stroke volume response to progressive exercise may reflect altered effects of preload, contractility and afterload in subjects other than healthy, non-trained children. Trained endurance athletes often demonstrate a progressive rise in stroke volume during such testing, suggesting either augmented diastolic filling or improved contractility.[57] Similar findings have been observed in child athletes. Rowland et al.[58] reported an average maximal stroke index in child distance runners of 69 ml m^{-2} compared to 58 ml m^{-2} in untrained but active control boys. Values were similar at rest (45 and 44 ml m^{-2}, respectively). The greater maximal stroke indices in the runners were achieved by a steady rise during the test, while values plateaued beyond a work intensity of 50 W in the controls.

Patients with myocardial dysfunction, on the other hand, often demonstrate a *decline* in stroke volume at moderate–high exercise intensities.[35,44] This pattern may reflect a lack of contractile reserve to accommodate increasing systemic venous return.

Cardiac output

During a progressive exercise test, a child will typically increase heart rate by a factor of approximately 2.4 and stroke volume by 1.3. Accordingly, $\dot{Q}$ max, the product of the two, typically rises threefold over resting levels. Published maximal indexed values are outlined in Table 2.7.2. It is interesting to note the consistency of reported values (generally 9.5 to 11.5 litre $min^{-1} m^{-2}$), despite issues concerning accuracy of the various methods employed.

Maximal cardiac index values in studies of young adult males have generally ranged from 10 to 13 litre $min^{-1} m^{-2}$.[59] Rowland et al.[7] could find no significant differences in maximal cardiac index by Doppler echocardiography in 11 year old boys and 30 year old men during upright cycling (mean 11.33 and 11.08 litre $min^{-1} m^{-2}$, respectively).

During the paediatric years maximal stroke volume increases in parallel with left ventricular size, while maximal heart rate values remain stable. It follows that $\dot{Q}$ max relative to body size should also be unchanged as a child grows. Experimental data bear this out. Miyamura and Honda[59] found no influence of age when they reported an average maximal cardiac index of 12.2 and 10.5 litre $min^{-1} m^{-2}$ in males and females aged 9 to 20 years. Yamaji and Miyashita[60] described no trends with age in $\dot{Q}$ max during cycle exercise in 10 to 18 year old boys. However, Gilliam et al.[61] found that maximal cardiac index fell from an average of 11.8 to 10.5 to 10.0 litre $min^{-1} m^{-2}$ in children ages 6 to 8, 9 to 10 and 11 to 13 years, respectively.

Limited data suggest that, as with stroke volume, maximal values of cardiac index are somewhat lower in female children than males. Miyamura and Honda[59] reported higher values for boys at every age between 9 and 20 years.

Rowland et al. (unpublished data) found maximal cardiac index values of 12.34 and 10.90 litre $min^{-1} m^{-2}$ in 12 year old boys and girls, respectively, almost identical to those described by Miyamura and Honda.[59]

At submaximal levels of exercise, cardiac output parallels the rise in oxygen uptake. The *exercise factor*, or ratio of change in cardiac output to that of $\dot{V}O_2$, has been used as an indicator of myocardial performance.

Values in paediatric studies have generally ranged from 5.7 to 6.5, mimicking those usually observed in populations of healthy adults.[62]

Ventricular dimensions

Studies utilizing echocardiography and nuclear angiography have demonstrated similar patterns of ventricular dimensional changes during progressive exercise: as exercise intensity increases, left ventricular end diastolic dimension (LVED) declines slightly while more exaggerated decreases occur in end systolic size (LVES). The result is a progressive increase in left ventricular shortening fraction [(LVED – LVES)/LVED].

Oyen et al.[63] demonstrated these trends echocardiographically during supine cycle exercise in children 6 to 14 years who exercised to a heart rate of 145 to 180 beats min^{-1}. In the youngest group, for example, average left ventricular end diastolic dimension fell from 3.81 cm at rest to 3.72 cm at the highest workload. At the same time, end systolic dimension decreased from 2.41 cm to 2.16 cm. Mean left ventricular shortening fraction increased from 37% to 46%, a change that was similar in all age groups.

Rowland et al.[35] studied 11 children and adolescents, ages 7 to 17 years, during maximal semisupine cycling (maximal heart rate 182 beats min^{-1}). Average left ventricular end diastolic dimension declined from 3.47 to 3.24 cm, while end-systolic diameter dropped from 2.18 to 1.55 cm. This resulted in a rise in shortening fraction from 37% to 53%.

These findings are similar to those reported in adults. Dickhuth et al.[64] demonstrated an increase in left ventricular shortening fraction from 34% to 42% in 21 to 35 year old subjects who pedalled to a heart rate of approximately 150 beats min^{-1}. End diastolic dimension did not change appreciably, while end systolic dimension declined from an average of 32.0 mm at rest to 28.9 mm at a work load of 150 W. These changes were observed with subjects exercising in both the sitting and supine positions.

Two radionuclide studies with children performing supine exercise support these findings. DeSouza et al.[65] found that end diastolic counts

Table 2.7.2 Maximal cardiac index and stroke index in studies of children

Study	Age (y)	N	Sex	Modality	Technique	$\dot{Q}$max (litre $min^{-1} m^{-2}$)	SV max (ml m^{-2})
Miyamura and Honda[59]	9–10	16	M	Upright cycle	CO_2 rebr	11.8	62
		16	F			10.0	54
	11–12	21	M			12.2	64
		17	F			11.5	61
Gilliam et al.[61]	6–8	22	MF	Upright cycle	CO_2 rebr	11.8	61
	9–10	36	MF			10.5	54
	11–13	24	MF			10.0	52
Eriksson and Koch[10]	12	9	M	Upright cycle	Dye dilution	9.1	49
Yamaji and Miyashita[60]	10–12	8	M	Upright cycle	CO_2 rebr	10.4	
Rowland et al.[43]	9–12	15	M	Upright cycling	Impedance	9.2	46
Rowland et al.[7]	10–11	15	M	Upright cycling	Doppler echo	11.4	59
Cortes et al.[44]	7–17	18	MF	Treadmill	Doppler echo	11.3	63
Rowland et al.[1]	12	39	M	Upright cycling	Doppler echo	12.0	61
Cyran et al.[20]	8–15	17	MF	Upright cycling	Acetylene rebr	10.8	62

changed little from rest to maximal exercise (heart rate 186 beats min^{-1}) in healthy subjects 8 to 18 years old. Systolic counts, however, fell by an average of 45%. In an investigation of 32 children 5 to 19 years old, Parrish et al.[66] described variable changes in left ventricular diastolic dimension during exercise but an overall 29% fall in systolic volume.

Myocardial function

Changes in intrinsic myocardial contractility are difficult to distinguish from the influences of ventricular preload (i.e. diastolic filling) and/or afterload. Given the relative stability of left ventricular diastolic size during exercise, however, any changes in markers of myocardial contractile force can be presumed to reflect alteration in intrinsic contractility (driven by sympathetic stimulation) and/or reduction in ventricular afterload (decline in systemic vascular resistance). In fact, such markers (left ventricular shortening fraction and ejection fraction, peak aortic velocity) are observed to steadily increase in children throughout the course of a progressive exercise test. Such responses of the myocardium to exercise are qualitatively and quantitatively similar to those seen in adults.

As noted above, echocardiographic studies have indicated a substantial rise in left ventricular shortening fraction during exercise. The expected rise is from approximately 37% at rest to 53% at maximal exercise, a reflection of decreased end systolic dimension. A similar magnitude of rise in ventricular contractile function with exercise has been observed in studies using radionuclide imaging. In the report of DeSouza et al.,[65] for instance, mean left ventricular ejection fraction in children increased from 63% at rest to 81% at maximal supine exercise. Studies in adults show similar findings, with a typical average increase of approximately 14%.[67]

Further evidence of augmented myocardial contractility during exercise is observed with Doppler flow measurements in the ascending aorta. Cyran et al.[68] reported that the acceleration time of aortic flow increased from 0.069 s standing to 0.057 s at maximal treadmill exercise in a group of 31 children and adolescents. Average peak systolic velocity rose from 129 cm s^{-1} at rest to 217 cm s^{-1} at exhaustion. In a similar study, Cortes et al.[44] described peak velocities of 95 and 182 cm s^{-1} at rest and maximal treadmill exercise (heart rate 178 beats min^{-1}), respectively. Rowland et al.[35] reported an increase in average peak velocity from 113 cm s^{-1} at rest to 180 cm s^{-1} at exhaustion in children and adolescents performing semisupine exercise.

Rowland et al.[7] could find no differences in peak aortic velocities during upright cycling exercise in a direct comparison of 12 year old boys and adult men. Average values were 98 and 82 cm s^{-1} at rest in the boys and men, respectively, increasing to 149 and 140 cm s^{-1} at maximal exercise.

Systolic ejection/diastolic filling periods

As the heart rate increases in response to exercise, systolic and diastolic time intervals necessarily shorten. The resulting time constraints may serve as critical determinants of cardiovascular function at high exercise intensities. Adequate diastolic time is important for both ventricular filling and coronary blood flow, while ejection volumes are dependent on sufficient systolic duration.

Not only do systolic and diastolic times shorten with exercise, but the relative contribution of each period to the cardiac cycle also

changes. Rowland et al.[35] identified systolic ejection time during semi-supine cycle exercise in 7 to 17 year old children using Doppler-derived aortic flow curves. Diastolic filling time was estimated by subtracting systolic ejection time from total cycle time (thereby overestimating diastolic time, as short isovolumic systolic and diastolic periods were ignored). At rest, the mean systolic and diastolic periods were 0.260 and 0.487 s, respectively. During progressive exercise both intervals decreased, with a greater rate of decline in diastolic period (69.4%) than systolic (30.4%). At maximal exercise (heart rate 182 beats min^{-1}), average systolic ejection time was 0.181 s, and estimated diastolic time was 0.149 s.

Other authors have described similar findings. Vavra et al.[69] showed, using measurement of systolic time intervals, that the systolic fraction of heart cycle length rose from 40% at a heart rate of 60 beats min^{-1} to over 65% when heart rate reached 160 beats min^{-1}. Moreover, these findings were similar in children and adults. In a second study, Rowland et al.[7] reported no significant differences in systolic ejection times between 12 year old boys and young men at rest or during exercise. Systole occupied approximately 33% of the cardiac cycle at rest and 63% at maximal exercise.

These data highlight the potential importance of factors influencing diastolic filling during exercise in limiting cardiac responses to exercise. The filling rate of the heart must equal $\dot{Q}$. Given the differences in intervals, diastolic filling at high exercise intensities must occur at a greater rate than that of forward ejection of the blood during systole.

That this review has addressed only the features of systolic function in children speaks to the dearth of information regarding diastolic function during exercise. Two studies have provided norms for mitral valve flows at rest in normal children using Doppler echocardiography.[70,71] A better understanding of the importance of diastolic function to cardiovascular fitness awaits improved techniques to characterize cardiac filling patterns during exercise.

Synthesis

Despite recent advances, the understanding of the cardiac responses to exercise in children is far from complete. Particularly needed are improved insights into the mechanisms for the observed cardiovascular changes as children grow. Nevertheless, it is possible to create a reasonable picture of the cardiac alterations during progressive exercise in young subjects.

At the onset of upright exercise the contractions of the skeletal muscle pump initiate augmented systemic venous return to the heart. The initial $\dot{Q}$ response is mediated by increases in both stroke volume and heart rate. It has been presumed that the initial rise in stroke volume represents a 'refilling' of the ventricles from the decrease in volume which occurs when one assumes the sitting position. By this concept, then, the 30 to 40% rise in stroke volume at low exercise intensities reflects a Frank–Starling mechanism, an increase in output in response to augmented diastolic filling. While this concept is intuitively attractive, it is possible that increases in peripheral vascular conductance at the onset of exercise (i.e. a fall in peripheral resistance) might also contribute.[72]

As exercise intensity increases to moderate and high levels, several phenomena are evident:

(1) systemic venous return increases;

(2) stroke volume remains constant;

(3) left ventricular end diastolic dimension is relatively stable; and

(4) heart rate rises.

These observations are consistent with the concept that the increase in heart rate matches the augmented cardiac filling, causing stroke volume to remain stable. That is, at least in healthy, non-athletic children, the heart rate appears to 'defend' a constant left ventricular size despite the rise in systemic venous return. The explanation for this phenomenon may lie in the heart's efforts to minimize wall tension. According to LaPlace's Law, wall tension or stress is minimized by an appropriate ratio of wall thickness to chamber diameter.[73]

From moderate to high exercise intensities, stroke volume plateaus, but markers of intrinsic contractility and/or changes in afterload (shortening fraction, ejection fraction, aortic velocity) continue to rise. This apparent contradiction may be explained by the fact that, as exercise intensity increases, the same stroke volume must be ejected in a shorter time. Rowland et al.,[7] for instance, described a fall in systolic ejection period of approximately 10% and increase in aortic peak velocity of 15% while stroke volume remained unchanged. The need to increase the *rate* of ejection may thus account for the improvement in contractile variables while stroke volume is stable.

Systemic blood pressure and peripheral vascular resistance

As observed in adults, systolic blood pressure rises in children with increasing exercise intensity. At the same time, diastolic pressure either remains stable or decreases slightly. Increases in mean blood pressure are modest, typically about 20 to 30 mm Hg from rest to maximal exercise.[10,74]

At maximal exercise systolic pressure is typically 40% greater than that at rest, and since resting pressure rises with age, so does systolic pressure at maximal exercise. There is some evidence that the magnitude of increase from rest to peak exercise, however, may be greater in older compared to younger children.[41] Normative values have been reported by several authors.[40,41,75] These data must be interpreted cautiously, however, given the technical difficulty of accurately measuring blood pressure at maximal exercise (see Chapter 1.6).

Changes in total body peripheral vascular resistance during exercise reflect the combined vasomotor responses in non-exercising tissues (vasoconstriction), cutaneous (vasodilation) and exercising muscle (vasodilation). Like adults, children demonstrate a decline in total peripheral resistance during a bout of progressive exercise. Eriksson and Koch[10] reported an average fall from 21.4 units at rest to 8.6 units at maximal cycle exercise in 11 to 13 year old boys. Similarly, Ensing et al.[19] described a decrease from 26 units to 12 units m^{-2} during maximal cycling in healthy children. Cyran et al.[20] found that peripheral resistance was reduced by 53% during a maximal cycle test in children 8 to 15 years old.

Prolonged exercise

Studies in adults indicate that during sustained constant-load exercise $\dot{V}O_2$ rises, heart rate increases, stroke volume falls and $\dot{Q}$ remains stable or increases slowly.[76] The explanation for this *cardiovascular drift* is unclear, but shifts of central circulation to the cutaneous vessels in response to increased body temperature may play an important role.

The same trends have been described in children. Asano and Hirakoba[77] reported cardiovascular responses of 10 to 12 year old boys and men 20 to 34 years during one hour of cycling at 60% $\dot{V}O_2$ max. No changes in $\dot{Q}$ were seen in either group, while heart rate rose from an average of 152 to 166 beats min^{-1} in the boys and 134 to 154 beats·min^{-1} in the men. Stroke volume (as estimated by bioimpedance) decreased from 58 to 54 ml in the boys and 98 to 86 ml in the men.

Rowland and Rimany[78] performed a similar study comparing responses to sustained exercise in premenarcheal girls and young adult females. During 40 min of steady-load cycling at 63% $\dot{V}O_2$ max, $\dot{Q}$, heart rate and $\dot{V}O_2$ rose similarly in both groups. The only significant difference was a greater magnitude of increase in heart rate in the adults. These studies suggest that the cardiovascular response of adults and children to prolonged exercise is similar.

Summary

The information presented in this chapter suggests that the cardiovascular responses to exercise in children are not unique compared to those of young adults. Small differences (i.e. maximal heart rate) do not seem to be translated into important functional differences in cardiac capacity during exercise. The pattern and magnitude of stroke volume and cardiac responses to progressive as well as sustained steady work are not different in children and young adults. Similarly, changes in myocardial function, systolic:diastolic intervals, blood pressure and peripheral vascular resistance during exercise also appear to be independent of maturation.

Several studies have indicated that children demonstrate a lower $\dot{Q}$ for a given $\dot{V}O_2$ during exercise compared to adults.[7,47,49,74] This does not, however, appear to reflect any age-related impairment of cardiac function. At a given workload, absolute $\dot{V}O_2$ is similar in children and adults (i.e. there are no maturational influences on metabolic efficiency). Absolute stroke volume will be smaller in the child (because of smaller ventricular dimensions), compensated only partially by a higher heart rate. Since children and adults do not normally exercise at the same absolute $\dot{V}O_2$, the lower $\dot{Q}/\dot{V}O_2$ in children appears to have no functional significance.

References

1. Rowland, T., Kline, G., Goff, D., Martel, L. and Ferrone, L. Physiological determinants of maximal aerobic power in healthy 12-year old boys. *Pediatric Exercise Science* 1999; **11**: 317–26.

2. Saltin, B. Oxygen transport during exercise. In *Biological effects of physical activity* (ed. R. S. Williams and A. G. Wallace). Human Kinetics Publishers, Champaign, Il, 1989: 3–24.

3. Rowell, L. B. O'Leary, D. S., and Kellogg D. L. Integration of cardiovascular control systems in dynamic exercise. In *Handbook of physiology,, exercise: Regulation and integration of multiple systems* (ed. L. B. Rowell and J.T. Shephard). American Physiological Society, Bethesda, MD, 1996; 778–81.

4. Rieckert, H. The beginning of applied physiology and sports medicine in ULM. In *The physiology and pathophysiology of exercise tolerance* (ed. J.M. Steinacker and S. A. Ward). Plenum Press, New York, 1996; 9–13.

5. Thomas, J. D. and Weyman, A. E. Echocardiographic doppler evaluation of left ventricular diastolic function. *Circulation* 1991; **84**:977–90.

6. Knoebel, L. K. Energy metabolism. In: Selkurt EE, ed. *Physiology*. Boston: Little, Brown, 1963; 564–79.

7. Rowland, T. W. Popowski B. and Ferrone L. Cardiac responses to maximal upright cycle exercise in healthy boys and men. *Medicine and Science in Sports and Exercise* 1997; **29**: 1146–51.

8. **Katori, R.** Normal cardiac output in relation to age and body size. *Tokohu Journal of Experimental Medicine* 1979; **128**: 377–87.

9. **Koch, G., Mobert J.** and **Oyen, E-M.** Cardiovascular adjustment to supine versus seated posture in prepubertal boys. In *Children and exercise XIX* (ed. N. Armstrong, B. Kirby and J. Welsman). E. and F. N. Spon, London, 1997; 424–8.

10. **Eriksson, B. O.** and **Koch, G.** Effect of physical training on hemodynamic response during submaximal and maximal exercise in 11–13-year old boys. *Acta Physiologica Scandinavia* 1973; **87**: 27–39.

11. **Thadani U.** and **Parker J. O.** Hemodynamics at rest and during supine and sitting bicycle exercise in normal subjects. *American Journal of Cardiology* 1978; **41**: 52–9.

12. **Higginbotham, M., Morris, K. G., Williams, R. S., McHale, P. A., Coleman, R. E.** and **Cobb F. R.** Regulation of stroke volume during submaximal and maximal upright exercise in normal man. *Circulation Research* 1986; **58**: 281–91.

13. **Buchberger, D.** and **Koch, G.** Adjustment of stroke volume and of left ventricular contractility during the initial phase of exercise in the supine versus seated posture. In *Pediatric work physiology* (ed. J. Coudert and E. Van Praagh). Masson, Paris 1992; 67–9.

14. **Krovetz, L. J., McLoughlin, T. G, Mitchell, M. B.** and **Schiebler, G. L.** Hemodynamic findings in normal children. *Pediatrics* 1967; **1**: 122–30.

15. **Locke, J. E., Einzig, S.** and **Moller J. H.** Hemodynamic responses to exercise in normal children. *American Journal of Cardiology* 1978; **41**: 1278–85.

16. **Sproul A.** and **Simpson E.** Stroke volume and related hemodynamic data in normal children. *Pediatrics* 1964; **33**: 912–18.

17. **Barbacki, M., Gluck, A., Sandhage, K.** and **Metzner, G.** Impedance cardiography in normal children. *Cor Vasa* 1981; **23**: 190–6.

18. **Sholler, G. F., Celermajer, J. M.** and **Whight, C. M.** Doppler echocardiographic assessment of cardiac output in normal children with and without innocent precordial murmurs. *American Journal of Cardiology* 1987; **59**: 487–8.

19. **Ensing, G. J, Heise, C. T.** and **Driscoll, D. J.** Cardiovascular response to exercise after the Mustard operation for simple and complex transposition of the great vessels. *American Journal of Cardiology* 1988; **62**: 617–22.

20. **Cyran, S. E., James, F. W., Daniels, S., Mays, W., Shukla, R.** and **Kaplan, S.** Comparison of the cardiac output and stroke volume response to upright exercise in children with valvular and subvalvular aortic stenosis. *Journal of the American College of Cardiology* 1988; **11**: 651–8.

21. **Hurwitz, R. A., Treves, S.** and **Kuruc, A.** Right ventricular and left ventricular ejection fraction in paediatric patients with normal hearts: first-pass radionuclide angiography. *American Heart Journal* 1984; **107**: 726–32.

22. **Colan, S. D., Parness, I. A., Spevak, P. J.** and **Sanders, S. P.** Developmental modulation of myocardial mechanics: age- and growth-related alterations in afterload and contractility. *Journal of the American College of Cardiology* 1992; **19**: 619–29.

23. **Gutgesell, H. P., Paquet, M., Duff, D. F.** and **McNamara, D. G.** Evaluation of left ventricular size and function by echocardiography. *Circulation* 1977; **56**: 457–62.

24. **Malina, R. M.** and **Bouchard, C.** *Growth, maturation, and physical activity.* Human Kinetics Publishers, Champaign, Il, 1991; 157.

25. **Marcus, B., Gillette, P. C.,** and **Garson A.** Intrinsic heart rate in children and young adults: an index of sinus node function isolated from autonomic control. *American Heart Journal* 1990; **112**: 912–6.

26. **Rowland, T. W., Maresh, C. M., Charkoudian. N., Vanderburgh, P. M., Castellani, J. W.** and **Armstrong, L. E.** Plasma norepinephrine response to cycle exercise in boys and men. *International Journal of Sports Medicine* 1995; **17**: 22–6.

27. **Lehmann, M., Keul, J.** and **Korsten-Reck, U.** The influence of graduated treadmill exercise on plasma catecholamines, aerobic, and anaerobic capacity in boys and adults. *European Journal of Applied Physiology* 1981; **47**: 301–11.

28. **Rowland, T. W.** and **Cunningham, L. N.** Heart rate deceleration during treadmill exercise in children [abstract]. *Pediatric Exercise Science* 1993; **5**: 463.

29. **Mahon, A. D.** and **Vaccaro, P.** Can the point of deflection from linearity of heart rate determine ventilatory threshold in children? *Pediatric Exercise Science* 1991; **3**: 256–62.

30. **Thimm, F.** Effect of local anaerobiosis on heart rate. In *Oxygen transport to tissue XII* (ed. J. Piper). Plenum Press, New York, 1990; 459–66.

31. **Cassels, D. E.** and **Morse, M.** *Cardiopulmonary data for children and young adults.* Charles C Thomas, Springfield, Il, 1962; 24–7.

32. **Bailey, D. A., Ross, W. D., Mirwald, R. L.** and **Weese C.** Size dissociation of maximal aerobic power during growth in boys. *Medicine in Sport* 1978; **11**: 140–51.

33. **Rowland, T., Vanderburgh, P.** and **Cunningham, L.** Body size and growth of maximal aerobic power in children: A longitudinal analysis. *Pediatric Exercise Science* 1997; **9**: 262–74.

34. **Rowland, T. W.** Aerobic exercise testing protocols. In *Pediatric laboratory exercise testing* (ed. T. W. Rowland). Human Kinetics Publishers, Champaign, Il, 1993; 19–42.

35. **Rowland, T. W., Potts, J., Potts, T., Son-Hing, J., Harbison, G.** and **Sandor G.** Cardiovascular responses in children and adolescents with myocardial dysfunction. *American Heart Journal* (in press).

36. **Cumming, G. R.** Hemodynamics of supine cycle bicycle exercise in 'normal' children. *American Heart Journal* 1977; **93**: 617–22.

37. **Wilson, B. A.** and **Chisholm, D.** Total body maximal aerobic power in children as measured by Concept II row ergometer [abstract]. *Pediatric Exercise Science* 1993; **5**: 487.

38. **Gibson, P. B., Szimonisz, S. M.** and **Rowland, T. W.** Rowing ergometry for assessment of aerobic fitness in children. *Pediatric Exercise Science*, (in press).

39. **Cumming, G. R.** and **Langford, S.** Comparison of nine exercise tests used in paediatric cardiology. In *Children and exercise XI* (ed. R. A. Binkhorst, H. C. G. Kemper and W. H. M. Saris). Human Kinetics Publishers, Champaign, Il, 1985; 58–68.

40. **Washington, R. L., van Gundy, J. C., Cohen, C., Sondheimer, H. M.** and **Wolfe, R. R.** Normal aerobic and anaerobic exercise data for North American school-age children. *Journal of Pediatrics* 1988; **112**: 223–33.

41. **Riopel, D. A., Taylor, A. B.** and **Hohn, A. R.** Blood pressure, heart rate, pressure-rate product, and electrocardiographic changes in healthy children during treadmill exercise. *American Journal of Cardiology* 1979; **44**: 697–704.

42. **Baraldi E, Cooper D. M, Zanconato S.** and **Armon Y.** Heart rate recovery from 1 minute of exercise in children and adults. *Pediatric Research* 1991; **29**: 575–9.

43. **Rowland, T.** and **Popowski, B.** Comparison of bioimpedance and Doppler cardiac output during exercise in children [abstract]. *Pediatric Exercise Science* 1997; **9**: 188.

44. **Cortes, R. G. S., Satomi, G., Yoshigi, M.** and **Momma, K.** Maximal hemodynamic response after the Fontan procedure: Doppler evaluation during the treadmill test. *Pediatric Cardiology* 1994; **15**: 170–7.

45. **Kirby, B. J., Armstrong, N.** and **Welsman, J. R.** Cardiac output response to submaximal exercise in adolescents [abstract]. *Medicine and Science in Sports and Exercise* 1997; **29 Suppl**: S2.

46. **Page, E., Perrault, H., Flore, P., Rossignol, A-M., Pironneau, S., Rocca, C.** and **Aguilaniu, B.** Cardiac output response to dynamic exercise after atrial switch repair for transposition of the great arteries. *American Journal of Cardiology* 1996; **77**: 892–5.

47. **Turley, K. R.** and **Wilmore, J. H.** Cardiovascular responses to submaximal exercise in 7- to 9-yr-old boys and girls. *Medicine and Science in Sports and Exercise* 1997; **29**: 824–32.

48. **Potter, C. R., Armstrong, N., Kirby, B. J.** and **Welsman J.** An exploratory study of cardiac output responses to submaximal exercise. In *Children and exercise XIX* (ed. N. Armstrong, B. Kirby and J. Welsman). E. and F. N. Spon, London, 1997; 440–5.

49. **Bar-Or, O., Shephard, R. J.** and **Allen, C. L.** Cardiac output of 10- to 13-year-old boys and girls during submaximal exercise. *Journal of Applied Physiology* 1971; **30**: 219–23.

50. Katsuura, T. Cardiac output of 10 to 11-year old children during exercise under different ambient conditions. *Journal of the Anthropological Society of Nippon* 1985; **93**: 303–15.

51. Godfrey, S., Davies, C. T. M., Wozniak, E. and Barnes, C. A. Cardio-respiratory responses to exercise in normal children. *Clinical Science* 1971; **40**: 419–31.

52. Anderson, S. D. and Godfrey, S. Cardio-respiratory response to treadmill exercise in normal children. *Clinical Science* 1971; **40**: 433–42.

53. Scholz, D. G., Kitzman, D. W., Hagen, P. T., Ilstrup, D. M. and Edwards, W. D. Age-related changes in normal human hearts during the first 10 decades of life. Part I (Growth): A quantitative anatomic study of 200 specimens from subjects birth to 19 years old. *Mayo Clinic Proceedings* 1988; **63**: 126–36.

54. Daniels, S. R., Meyer, R. A., Liang, Y. and Bove, K. Echocardiographically determined left ventricular mass index in normal children, adolescents and young adults. *Journal of the American College of Cardiology* 1988; **12**: 703–8.

55. Shephard, R. J., Allen, C., Bar-Or, O., Davies, C. T. M., Degre, S., Hedman, R., Ishii, K., Kaneko, M., LaCour, J. R., di Prampero, P. E. and Seliger, V. The working capacity of Toronto schoolchildren. *Canadian Medical Association Journal* 1969; **100**: 560–8.

56. Nagasawa, H., Arakaki, Y., Yamada, O., Nakajima, T. and Kamiya, T. Longitudinal observations of left ventricular end-diastolic dimension in children using echocardiography. *Pediatric Cardiology* 1996; **17**: 169–74.

57. Gledhill, N., Cox, D. and Jamnik, R. Endurance athletes' stroke volume does not plateau: major advantage is diastolic function. *Medicine and Science in Sports and Exercise* 1994; **26**: 1116–21.

58. Rowland, T., Goff, D., Popowski, B., DeLuca, P. and Ferrone, L. Cardiac responses to exercise in child distance runners. *International Journal of Sports Medicine*, (in press).

59. Miyamura, M. and Honda, Y. Maximum cardiac output related to sex and age. *Japanese Journal of Physiology* 1973; **23**: 645–56.

60. Yamaji, K. and Miyashita, M. Oxygen transport system during exhaustive exercise in Japanese boys. *European Journal of Applied Physiology* 1977; **36**: 93–9.

61. Gilliam, T. B., Sady, S., Thorland, W. G. and Weltman, A. C. Comparison of peak performance measures in children ages 6 to 8, 9 to 10, and 11 to 13 years. *Research Quarterly* 1977; **48**: 695–702.

62. Rowland, T. W. *Developmental exercise physiology.* Human Kinetics Publishers, Champaign, Il, 1996; 117–40.

63. Oyen, E. M., Ignatzy, K., Ingerfeld, G. and Brode, P. Echocardiographic evaluation of left ventricular reserve in normal children during supine bicycle exercise. *International Journal of Cardiology* 1987; **14**: 145–54.

64. Dickhuth, H. H., Simon, G., Heiss, H. W., Lehmann, M., Wybitul, K. and Keul, J. Comparative echocardiographic examinations in sitting and supine position at rest and during dynamic exercise. *International Journal of Sports Medicine* 1981; **2**: 178–81.

65. DeSouza, M., Schaffer, M. S., Gilday, D. L. and Rose, V. Exercise radionuclide angiography in hyperlipidemic children with apparently normal hearts. *Nuclear Medicine Communications* 1984; **5**: 13–7.

66. Parrish, M. D., Boucek, R. J., Burger. J., Artman, M. F., Partain, C. L. and Graham, T. P. Exercise radionuclide ventriculography in children: normal values for exercise variables and right and left ventricular function. *British Heart Journal* 1985; **54**: 509–16.

67. Rerych, S. K., Scholz, P., Newman, G., Sabiston, D. C. and Jones, R. H. Cardiac function at rest and during exercise in normals and patients with coronary heart disease. *Annals of Surgery* 1978; **187**: 449–64.

68. Cyran, S. E., Grzeszczak, M., Haas, J. H. and Baylen, B. G. Characterization of the aortic echo-Doppler profile in normal children during maximal treadmill exercise. *American Heart Journal* 1993; **126**: 1024–9.

69. Vavra, J., Sova, J. and Macek, M. Effect of age on systolic time intervals at rest and during exercise on a bicycle ergometer. *European Journal of Applied Physiology* 1982; **50**: 71–8.

70. Obert, P., Courteix, D., Germain, P., LeCoq, A. M. and Guenon P. Cardiac structure and function in highly-trained prepubertal gymnasts and swim-mers.In *Children and exercise XIX* (ed. N. Armstrong, B. Kirby and J. Welsman). E. and F. N. Spon, London, 1997; 494–500.

71. Ozer, S., Cil, E., Baltaci, G., Ergun, N. and Ozme, S. Left ventricular structure and function by echocardiography in childhood swimmers. *Japanese Heart Journal* 1994; **35**: 295–300.

72. Sheriff, D. D., Rowell, L. B. and Scher, A. M. Is rapid rise in vascular conductance at onset of dynamic exercise due to muscle pump? *American Journal of Physiology* 1993; **265**: H1227–34.

73. Martin, R. R. and Haines, H. Application of LaPlace's law to mammalian hearts. *Comparative Biochemistry and Physiology* 1970; **34**: 959–62.

74. Eriksson, B. O., Grimby, G. and Saltin, B. Cardiac output and arterial blood gases during exercise in pubertal boys. *Journal of Applied Physiology* 1971; **31**: 348–52.

75. Alpert, B. S., Flood, N. L., Strong, W. B., Dover, E. V., DuRant, R. H., Martin, A. M. and Booker, D. L. Responses to ergometer exercise in a healthy biracial population of children. *Journal of Paediatrics* 1982; **101**: 538–45.

76. Raven, P. B. and Stevens, G. H. J. Cardiovascular function and prolonged exercise. In *Perspectives in exercise science and sports medicine.* Vol. 1, (ed. D. R. Lamb and R. Murray). Benchmark Press, Indianapolis, 1988; 43–74.

77. Asano, K. and Hirakoba, K. Respiratory and circulatory adaptation during prolonged exercise in 10–12 year-old children and adults. In *Children and sport* (ed. J. Ilmarinen and I. Valimaki). Springer-Verlag, Berlin, 1984; 119–28.

78. Rowland, T. W. and Rimany, T. A. Physiological responses to prolonged exercise in premenarcheal girls and adult females. *Pediatric Exercise Science* 1995; **7**: 183–91.

2.8   Aerobic fitness

Neil Armstrong and Joanne R. Welsman

Introduction

Aerobic exercise depends upon pulmonary, cardiovascular and haematological components of oxygen delivery and the oxidative mechanisms of exercising muscle. Maximal oxygen uptake ($\dot{V}O_2$ max), the highest rate at which an individual can consume oxygen during exercise, limits the capacity to perform aerobic exercise and $\dot{V}O_2$ max is widely recognized as the best single measure of adults' aerobic fitness.[1–3] The conventional criterion for the attainment of $\dot{V}O_2$ max during an exercise test is a levelling-off or plateau in $\dot{V}O_2$ despite an increase in exercise intensity.[4–6] Both the theoretical[7–9] and the methodological bases[10–12] of the $\dot{V}O_2$ plateau phenomenon have been questioned, and it is well-documented that many young people can exercise to exhaustion without demonstrating a $\dot{V}O_2$ plateau.[13–15] The appropriate term to use with young people is therefore peak oxygen uptake (peak $\dot{V}O_2$), the highest $\dot{V}O_2$ elicited during an exercise test to exhaustion,[16–18] rather than $\dot{V}O_2$ max which conventionally implies the existence of a $\dot{V}O_2$ plateau. If a child or adolescent has been habituated to the laboratory environment and shows clear signs of intense effort supported by objective criteria (see Chapter 1.7), peak $\dot{V}O_2$ can be accepted as a maximal index of aerobic fitness.[17,19,20]

As submaximal $\dot{V}O_2$, $\dot{V}O_2$ kinetics and blood lactate responses to submaximal exercise are addressed elsewhere in this book (Chapters 2.9, 2.10 and 1.7, respectively) the present chapter will focus specifically on peak $\dot{V}O_2$.

Components of peak oxygen uptake

Pulmonary function

The development of pulmonary function is comprehensively reviewed in Chapter 2.6 and although there are clear age,[21–23] growth and maturation,[24–26] and sex[27–29] differences in ventilation at peak $\dot{V}O_2$ it appears that ventilation does not limit the peak $\dot{V}O_2$ of healthy young people. Pulmonary function will therefore not be considered further.

Cardiovascular function

The Fick equation establishes that $\dot{V}O_2$ can be expressed as the product of cardiac output and arteriovenous (AV) oxygen difference. Cardiac output is a function of heart rate and stroke volume but as its development is reviewed in detail in Chapter 2.7 only salient issues will be addressed here.

Heart rate

Heart rate at peak $\dot{V}O_2$ is subject to wide individual variations and varies with the ergometer used[30–32] and the exercise protocol.[13,33,34]

Progressive, incremental treadmill running protocols elicit the highest heart rates with typical mean and standard deviation values of 200 ± 7 beats min^{-1}.[35,37] Both cross-sectional and longitudinal data are consistent and demonstrate that, during childhood and adolescence, heart rate at peak $\dot{V}O_2$ is independent of age,[38–40] growth and maturation,[41–43] and sex.[44–46]

Stroke volume

Our understanding of the response of young people's stroke volume and cardiac output to exercise is subject to methodological limitations[47–49] (see Chapter 1.6). Nevertheless, the data are consistent and suggest that during exercise in the upright position stroke volume rises progressively to values about 40% greater than resting, and reaches this level at 40 to 60% of peak $\dot{V}O_2$. Stroke volume then demonstrates a plateau despite an increase in exercise intensity, with subsequent rises in cardiac output relying exclusively on heart rate.[50–52] Maximal stroke volume appears to increase in parallel with left ventricular size but data on stroke volume at peak $\dot{V}O_2$ are sparse (see Table 2.7.2).

Cardiac output

As heart rate at peak $\dot{V}O_2$ is independent of age, body size, maturation and sex it follows that during childhood and adolescence changes in cardiac output at peak $\dot{V}O_2$ reflect changes in stroke volume. In absolute values (litre min^{-1}) cardiac output at peak $\dot{V}O_2$ therefore increases with age.[53,54] Cross-sectional data indicate values rising from 12.5 to 21.1 litre min^{-1} in males and 10.5 to 15.5 litre min^{-1} in females, over the age range 9 to 20 years.[53] Rowland *et al.*[43] reported no significant differences in maximal cardiac index in 11 year old boys and 30 year old men during cycling whereas Gilliam *et al.*[55] noted a decline in cardiac index from 6 to 13 years (see Table 2.7.2). The influence of maturation, independent of body size and age, on cardiac output at peak $\dot{V}O_2$ is unknown but Rowland[49] reviewed data on the ratio change in cardiac output to change in $\dot{V}O_2$ and concluded that maturity-related differences in the cardiac response to exercise were not evident in the extant literature.

Arteriovenous oxygen difference

AV oxygen difference is a manifestation of a range of factors including blood haemoglobin concentration, blood volume, muscle blood flow, aerobic enzyme activity and mitochondrial density. It therefore serves as an index of haematological components of oxygen delivery and the oxidative mechanisms of exercising muscle. Ethical and methodological problems have clouded our understanding of AV oxygen difference during childhood and adolescence and few secure data are available.

Cardiac catheterization has been used to determine resting AV oxygen difference and data indicate wide individual variations around a mean value of about 44 ml of oxygen per litre of blood (ml litre^{-1}), with no relationship between resting AV oxygen difference and age during the period from birth to 20 years.[56,57]

AV oxygen difference during exercise is generally estimated from measurements of $\dot{V}O_2$ and estimates of cardiac output via the Fick equation. Within the limitations of this methodology, it appears that AV oxygen difference increases with progressive exercise,[52,58] and it has been reported both to have a linear relationship with exercise intensity[59] and to plateau at near-maximal exercise.[60] At the same submaximal $\dot{V}O_2$ and exercise intensity, no significant sex differences were demonstrated in either AV oxygen difference or cardiac output in a sample of 12 year old boys ($n = 61$) and girls ($n = 56$), although girls had significantly higher heart rates and lower stroke volumes than boys.[58] With the same group of children maturity, estimated from Tanner staging,[61] demonstrated an independent effect on both submaximal $\dot{V}O_2$ and AV oxygen difference but not on cardiac output, stroke volume or heart rate.[58]

Data on young people's AV oxygen difference at peak $\dot{V}O_2$ are limited and the available evidence is equivocal. Yamaji and Miyashita[54] observed no relationship between AV oxygen difference at peak $\dot{V}O_2$ and age in 77 boys aged 10 to 18 years, whereas others have demonstrated age-related increases.[43,53,55] Reported mean values of AV oxygen difference over the age range 6 to 18 years have varied between 103 and 146 ml litre^{-1}.[54,55,59] Data on girls' AV oxygen difference at peak $\dot{V}O_2$ are sparse.

Although data showing an age-related increase in AV oxygen difference at peak $\dot{V}O_2$ must be treated cautiously, the lower blood haemoglobin concentration in children than in adults supports the premise that adults have a greater arterial oxygen content. Blood haemoglobin concentration rises from 125 g litre^{-1} at age 2 years to 135 g litre^{-1} at 12 years and is independent of sex.[62] During the teen years boys experience a marked increase in haemoglobin concentration to about 152 g litre^{-1} at 16 years whereas girls' values tend to plateau and only rise to perhaps 137 g litre^{-1} at 16 years.[62] As 1 g of fully saturated haemoglobin will hold 1.34 ml of oxygen the oxygen carrying capacity of haemoglobin for girls rises from 168 ml litre^{-1} at 2 years to 184 ml litre^{-1} at 16 years, an increase of 9.5%, whereas boys' values rise by 21.4% over the same period. Children's mixed venous oxygen content at peak $\dot{V}O_2$ is unknown, but as adults can lower their mixed venous oxygen content to 20 to 30 ml litre^{-1} during heavy exercise, children inevitably have a lower AV oxygen reserve than adults.

Haemoglobin is essential for oxygen transport[63] and blood haemoglobin concentration has been demonstrated to be significantly correlated with peak $\dot{V}O_2$ in 11 to 16 year olds.[41] Blood volume rises through childhood and adolescence[23,64] and therefore total haemoglobin also increases, and has been shown to be linearly related to peak $\dot{V}O_2$ across all age levels and in both sexes.[23] The dissociation of oxygen from haemoglobin is, however, quite complex and influenced by factors such as temperature, acidity, carbon dioxide content and concentration of 2,3-diphosphoglycerate (2,3-DPG).[65] A greater facility for oxygen unloading at the tissues has been observed in young people compared with adults[66] and, as 2,3-DPG reduces haemoglobin's affinity for oxygen, this may be due to the decline in 2, 3-DPG with age.[67] Females have been reported to have significantly higher 2,3-DPG : haemoglobin

ratios than males of similar fitness[68] and differing levels of 2, 3-DPG may partially compensate for age and sex differences in haemoglobin concentration.

AV oxygen difference is dependent on muscle blood flow and, in adults, exercise results in a marked redistribution of blood away from non-exercising vascular beds to the muscles. The scale of blood redistribution may be different in young people[69] and lower noradrenaline levels at peak $\dot{V}O_2$[70,71] may be indicative of diminished sympathetic activity in children, which may result in less shunting of blood to exercising muscles. However, a study of nine 12 year old, trained boys examined muscle blood flow during exercise and indicated that the boys had a higher muscle blood flow immediately following exercise than adults studied using comparable techniques.[72] The child–adult differences diminished when the same boys were tested one year[64] and four years[73] later.

AV oxygen difference is not only a function of oxygen delivery to the muscles but also of the oxidative mechanisms of exercising muscles. Data are limited but consistent and suggest that the activity of aerobic enzymes in children's muscle is significantly higher than in adult muscle.[74–76] Children appear to have a higher proportion of type 1 fibres in the vastus lateralis muscle compared to untrained adults and, in fact, are more typical of adult endurance athletes.[77–79] The slightly greater mitochondrial volume, ratio of mitochondria to myofibrillar volume, and intramuscular lipid storage observed in six year old children compared with untrained adults[77] provide additional indications that children have an enhanced ability to generate energy from aerobic metabolism.

Oxygen delivery to muscle and subsequent oxidative metabolism in relation to age, growth, maturation and sex requires further exploration, and additional insights may be dependent on technological advances in non-invasive methodology.

Peak oxygen uptake and age

The peak $\dot{V}O_2$ of children and adolescents has been extensively documented[17,80,81] with data available from children as young as three years of age.[82] The validity of peak $\dot{V}O_2$ determinations in children younger than 8 years has been questioned,[83] as young children typically have short attention spans, poor motivation and lack sufficient understanding of experimental procedures therefore making it difficult to elicit genuine maximal efforts.[84] Equipment and protocols designed for adults make testing with young children problematic and the smaller the child the greater the potential problem (see Chapter 1.7). Reports of peak $\dot{V}O_2$ in very young children are difficult to interpret. Small sample sizes are common[85–87] and several studies have pooled data from boys and girls.[82,88,89] Whether the children exhibited maximal values is unclear in some reports in the absence of explicit exercise termination criteria,[21,90,91] and there is a tendency to report only mass-related data.[89,92] Data from young people aged 8 to 16 years are more secure and we will therefore focus on this age group.

Armstrong and Welsman[17] reviewed the extant literature and generated graphs representing over 10 000 peak $\dot{V}O_2$ determinations of untrained subjects, aged 8 to 16 years. Because of the ergometer dependence of peak $\dot{V}O_2$ (see Chapter 1.7) data from treadmill and cycle ergometry were graphed separately, and the treadmill-determined peak $\dot{V}O_2$ scores ($n = 4937$) are reproduced here as Fig. 2.8.1. The data must be interpreted cautiously, as means from both longitudinal and cross-sectional studies with varying sample sizes are included. No information is available on randomly selected groups of young people, and since volunteers are generally used as subjects, selection bias cannot be ruled out. Nevertheless, Fig. 2.8.1 clearly illustrates an almost linear increase in peak $\dot{V}O_2$ with age in both boys and girls. The regression equations indicate that peak $\dot{V}O_2$ increases from 1.25 to 2.24 litre min^{-1} between the ages of 8 and 16 years in girls and from 1.22 to 3.06 litre min^{-1} in boys over the same period. Several cross-sectional studies, however, have indicated a decline or at least a levelling-off in girls' peak $\dot{V}O_2$ between 13 and 15 years.[93–95]

There have been few longitudinal studies of young people's peak $\dot{V}O_2$ but the data are in general agreement with cross-sectional studies. Table 2.8.1 describes the published longitudinal studies from which appropriate data could be extracted, and unpublished data from large samples studied in the editors' laboratories. These studies provide a consistent picture of a gradual rise in boys' peak $\dot{V}O_2$ from 8 through 16 years of age. Mirwald and Bailey[96] tested 75 boys annually throughout this period and reported an average annual increase in peak $\dot{V}O_2$ of 11%, (with the greatest increase in absolute terms occurring between 13 and 14 years (0.31 litre min^{-1}) and 14 and 15 years (0.32 litre min^{-1})). Girls from the same study demonstrated a very similar trend from 8 to 13 years but further data are not available. Longitudinal studies with older girls indicate that from about 14 years of age girls' peak $\dot{V}O_2$ levels off or even declines.

Peak oxygen uptake, growth and maturation

Peak $\dot{V}O_2$ is strongly correlated with body size with coefficients describing its relationship with body mass or stature typically exceeding $r = 0.70$.[41,85] Thus, much of the age-related increase in aerobic fitness illustrated in Fig. 2.8.1 reflects the overall increase in body size during the transition from childhood through adolescence. It has also been suggested that peak $\dot{V}O_2$ is likely to be influenced by an interaction between body size and maturational effects.[97] There is some evidence from longitudinal studies that the greatest increase in peak $\dot{V}O_2$

accompanies the attainment of peak height velocity (PHV) in both boys and girls.[96,98] In contrast, however, Cunningham et al.[99] noted a consistent growth of peak $\dot{V}O_2$ in boys measured from three years before to two years after PHV. The separation and quantification of the independent contributions of age and maturity to the growth of peak $\dot{V}O_2$ therefore relies upon the appropriate removal of the effects of body size.

The vast majority of studies reporting growth-related changes in size-adjusted aerobic fitness have attempted to control for body size differences by expressing peak $\dot{V}O_2$ as the simple ratio ml kg^{-1}min^{-1}, and their results have been comprehensively reviewed elsewhere.[17,18,80] Collectively, these studies present patterns of change in aerobic fitness over the age range 8 to 16 years which can be summarized simply; mass-related peak $\dot{V}O_2$ in boys remains essentially unchanged (at around 50 ml kg^{-1} min^{-1}), whilst in girls over this same age range a progressive decline is apparent (from approximately 45 to 35 ml kg^{-1}min^{-1}).

In Chapter 1.1, compelling arguments were presented to refute the validity of simple ratio scaling to remove the influence of body mass effects from size-dependent performance measures, bringing into question the accuracy of this accepted interpretation. Studies in which the influence of body size has been removed using appropriate allometric techniques may provide a clearer, more accurate picture of growth-related peak $\dot{V}O_2$. Welsman et al.[100] used both traditional ratio and allometric scaling to partition size effects from peak $\dot{V}O_2$ data in groups of prepubertal, circumpubertal and adult subjects spanning the age range 11 to 23 years. The results of the traditional analyses conformed to the conventional interpretation described above, with mass-related peak $\dot{V}O_2$ consistent among the male groups, whilst in the females mass-related peak $\dot{V}O_2$ demonstrated a significant decrease between the circumpubertal and adult groups. In direct contrast, allometric scaling revealed significant, progressive increases in peak $\dot{V}O_2$ across male groups suggesting that, relative to body size, aerobic fitness is, in fact, improving during growth rather than remaining static. In females, peak $\dot{V}O_2$ increased significantly into puberty, subsequently remaining consistent with no decline into adulthood evident.

The application of allometry to longitudinal data is not straightforward but its use is increasing and evidence to support the cross-sectional findings described above is accumulating. In 51 boys tested annually from the age of 8 to 15 years, Bailey and Ross[38] reported changes in size related peak $\dot{V}O_2$ computed as both the simple ratio ml kg^{-1} min^{-1} and adjusted using the theoretically proposed mass exponents 0.67 and 0.75 (see Chapter 1.1). In contrast to the ratio standard findings, the latter two mass adjustments both yielded results indicating increasing aerobic fitness over the study period. Similar findings have been reported for 11 boys studied annually for five years from the age of nine years.[43] In the nine girls concurrently studied, correction of peak $\dot{V}O_2$ scores using the theoretical exponents altered the pattern of change from a decline in mass-related aerobic fitness evident in the final two years of the study into a relatively stable profile across the study period.

Although cross-sectional studies with large, well-defined subject populations have identified mass exponents approximating these theoretical values,[35,42] sample-specific values may deviate markedly from them[101] being influenced by factors such as sample size and homogeneity. Therefore, although providing results which may be a closer reflection of underlying patterns of change, indiscriminate application of theoretical exponents is imprecise and unlikely to provide an accurate representation of the true longitudinal changes within a specific sample.

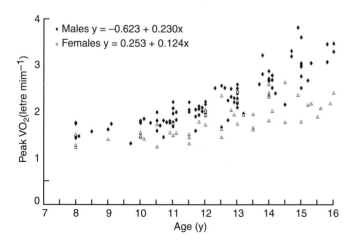

Fig. 2.8.1 Peak oxygen uptake by age. Redrawn from N. Armstrong and J. R. Welsman.[17] Reprinted with permission.

Table 2.8.1　Longitudinal studies of peak $\dot{V}O_2$

Citation	Country	Age (y)	N	Mode of exercise	Peak $\dot{V}O_2$ (litre min^{-1})
Boys					
Rutenfranz et al.[24]	Germany	12.7	28	CE	2.33 ± 0.32
		13.7	27	CE	2.50 ± 0.46
		14.7	26	CE	2.83 ± 0.49
		15.8	27	CE	3.05 ± 0.54
		16.7	23	CE	3.00 ± 0.34
Rutenfranz et al.[24]	Norway	8.4	28	CE	1.44 ± 0.19
		9.4	29	CE	1.59 ± 0.24
		10.4	31	CE	2.03 ± 0.30
		11.4	29	CE	2.07 ± 0.30
		12.3	30	CE	2.31 ± 0.34
		13.3	29	CE	2.70 ± 0.51
		14.5	27	CE	2.82 ± 0.41
		15.3	27	CE	3.14 ± 0.38
Cunningham et al.[99]	Canada	10.8	62	CE	1.72 ± 0.38
		11.8	62	CE	1.90 ± 0.28
		12.8	62	CE	2.16 ± 0.40
		13.8	62	CE	2.58 ± 0.55
		14.8	62	CE	2.88 ± 0.51
Mirwald and Bailey[96]	Canada	8	75	TM	1.42 ± 0.21
		9	75	TM	1.60 ± 0.20
		10	75	TM	1.77 ± 0.22
		11	75	TM	1.93 ± 0.25
		12	75	TM	2.12 ± 0.29
		13	75	TM	2.35 ± 0.38
		14	75	TM	2.66 ± 0.46
		15	75	TM	2.98 ± 0.48
		16	75	TM	3.22 ± 0.45
Amsterdam Growth and Health Study (unpublished data provided by Van Mechelen)	The Netherlands	13	83	TM	2.66 ± 0.39
		14	80	TM	3.07 ± 0.48
		15	84	TM	3.37 ± 0.43
		16	79	TM	3.68 ± 0.52
Armstrong and Welsman (unpublished data)	United Kingdom	11.1	71	TM	1.80 ± 0.25
		12.1	71	TM	2.15 ± 0.34
		13.2	71	TM	2.45 ± 0.47
Girls					
Rutenfranz et al.[24]	Germany	12.7	24	CE	2.19 ± 0.30
		13.7	24	CE	2.20 ± 0.22
		14.7	22	CE	2.26 ± 0.26
		15.7	22	CE	2.18 ± 0.29
		16.7	17	CE	1.97 ± 0.31
Rutenfranz et al.[24]	Norway	8.2	33	CE	1.25 ± 0.20
		9.3	33	CE	1.48 ± 0.19
		10.3	34	CE	1.79 ± 0.23
		11.2	34	CE	1.88 ± 0.22
		12.2	34	CE	2.26 ± 0.32
		13.3	33	CE	2.48 ± 0.46
		14.2	32	CE	2.35 ± 0.26
		15.2	30	CE	2.44 ± 0.30

Table 2.8.1 (*Continued*)

Citation (litre min^{-1})	Country	Age (y)	N	Mode of exercise	Peak $\dot{V}O_2$
Mirwald and Bailey[96]	Canada	8	22	TM	1.27 ± 0.14
		9	22	TM	1.39 ± 0.15
		10	22	TM	1.53 ± 0.20
		11	22	TM	1.72 ± 0.28
		12	22	TM	1.97 ± 0.36
		13	22	TM	2.20 ± 0.39
Amsterdam Growth and Health Study (unpublished data provided by Van Mechelen)	The Netherlands	13	97	TM	2.45 ± 0.31
		14	97	TM	2.60 ± 0.35
		15	96	TM	2.58 ± 0.34
		16	96	TM	2.65 ± 0.33
Armstrong and Welsman (unpublished data)	United Kingdom	11.1	61	TM	1.63 ± 0.28
		12.1	61	TM	1.93 ± 0.28
		13.1	61	TM	2.14 ± 0.30

Mode: CE is cycle ergometer, TM is treadmill; peak $\dot{V}O_2$ values are mean±standard deviation.

Table 2.8.2 Multilevel regression analysis for peak $\dot{V}O_2$ in 11 to 13 year olds

Fixed parameters:	Estimate (SE)	Random parameters	Estimate (SE)
Constant	-2.0094 (0.0874)	Level 2	
Log$_e$ mass	0.9146 (0.0287)	Constant	0.0028 (0.0004)
Log$_e$ skinfolds	-0.1819 (0.0129)	Age	0.0006 (0.0003)
Age*	0.0574 (0.0104)	Covariance	Ns
Sex	-0.1253 (0.0081)	Level 1	
Age·sex	-0.0189 (0.0064)	Constant	0.0029 (0.0004)

*Deviated around the group mean age of 12.0 years.
$N = 590$.

Multilevel modelling techniques[102] (see Chapter 1.1) represent a sensitive and flexible approach to the interpretation of longitudinal exercise data which enable body size, age and sex effects to be partitioned concurrently within an allometric framework. Using these methods to interpret peak $\dot{V}O_2$ in young elite athletes Nevill *et al.*[103] noted a significant positive effect of age upon aerobic fitness in both boys and girls, which was over and above increases explained by the growth in body mass and stature. The authors attributed this additional age effect partially to the athlete's trained status, but recent data from healthy untrained young people suggest that, rather than representing a training effect, a disproportionate increase in aerobic fitness relative to body size is a feature of normal growth during the pubertal years.[104]

Table 2.8.2 illustrates the results of applying multilevel regression modelling to the interpretation of peak $\dot{V}O_2$ in 11 to 13 year old boys and girls. The estimates for the fixed parameters reflect the group mean response whilst the random parameters describe the random variation between individuals (level 2), i.e. allowing individuals to have their own slope and intercept terms, and within individuals (level 1), i.e. variation around the individual growth trajectory. Key variables explaining the increase in peak $\dot{V}O_2$ during this period were body mass and skinfolds (sum of triceps and subscapular skinfolds), with an additional positive effect of age. Despite this evidence of a progressive growth in aerobic

fitness in both sexes, peak $\dot{V}O_2$ remained lower in girls than boys with the significant sex by age interaction term indicating that sex differences progressively diverged over the studied age range.

The frequent disparity between chronological age and true biological age during puberty combined with the differential effects of maturity on both body size and composition between the sexes make it imperative to consider independently the effects of age versus the effects of maturation upon size-related exercise performance.

Using simple ratio scaling (ml kg^{-1} min^{-1}), Armstrong *et al.*[42] found no additional effect of stage of sexual maturation[61] on peak $\dot{V}O_2$. However, when they re-analysed the data using log-linear regression to control for body mass, significant increases in peak $\dot{V}O_2$ were observed across the four maturational stages represented in both boys and girls. The same authors[104] introduced stage of maturation into a multilevel regression model of 11 to 13 year olds' peak $\dot{V}O_2$, so that the model reflected the responses of a prepubertal child from which any additional effects of later maturity could be quantified. A significant, incremental effect of stage of maturation, independent of age and body size, was demonstrated in both boys and girls (Table 2.8.3).

Clearly, the quantity of data available describing growth and maturational changes in peak $\dot{V}O_2$ using appropriate scaling techniques to partition body size effects is, to date, limited. However, the results of the studies presented provide convincing and consistent evidence that,

Table 2.8.3 Multilevel regression analysis for peak $\dot{V}O_2$ in 11 to 13 year olds, including stage of maturation

Fixed parameters	Estimate (SE)	Random parameters	Estimate (SE)
Constant	−1.2525 (0.0978)	Level 2	
Log$_e$ mass	0.4765 (0.0320)		
Log$_e$ stature	0.8105 (0.1172)	Constant	0.0042 (0.0005)
Age*	0.0428 (0.1160)	Age	0.0008 (0.0003)
Age^2	−0.0073 (0.0035)	Covariance	0.0004 (0.0003)
Sex	−0.1495 (0.0094)		
Age·sex	−0.0177 (0.0068)	Level 1	
Maturity 2	0.0382 (0.0090)		
Maturity 3	0.0548 (0.0106)	Constant	0.0024 (0.0003)
Maturity 4	0.0902 (0.0140)	Age	0.0004 (0.0005)
Maturity 5	0.0892 (0.0221)	Covariance	−0.0006 (0.0002)

*Deviated around the group mean age of 12.0 years.
$N = 590$. Modified from N. Armstrong, et al.[104]

relative to body size, peak aerobic fitness increases progressively in boys throughout childhood and adolescence into adulthood and in girls increases at least into puberty. The maturational process itself induces increases in aerobic fitness over and above those explained by size, body fatness and age. These patterns of change, although contrasting with traditional interpretation appear wholly consistent with the growth of the underlying physiological processes described in the previous sections.

Peak oxygen uptake and sex

Boys' peak $\dot{V}O_2$ values are consistently higher than those of girls by late childhood and the sex difference becomes more pronounced as young people progress through adolescence. The data presented in Fig. 2.8.1 indicate that peak $\dot{V}O_2$ is 12% higher in boys than girls at age 10 years, increasing to 23% higher at 12 years, 31% higher at 14 years, and 37% higher at 16 years of age. Longitudinal data (Table 2.8.1) support this trend, although with relatively small samples there is some variation in reported sex differences within the age range 12 to 14 years, which may be due to individual variations in rate of growth and maturation. The multilevel modelling approach described in the previous section has revealed age and maturity effects on peak $\dot{V}O_2$, independent of body size and this emphasizes the importance of incorporating both age and maturity into analyses of young people's peak $\dot{V}O_2$.[104]

Sex differences in peak $\dot{V}O_2$ during childhood and adolescence have been attributed to a combination of factors including habitual physical activity, body composition and blood haemoglobin concentration.

Boys are more physically active than girls[105–107] (see Chapter 3.1), but the evidence relating habitual physical activity to young people's peak $\dot{V}O_2$ is weak[108–110] and the issue is confounded by problems with accurately assessing children's and adolescents' physical activity patterns[18,111,112] (see Chapter 1.8). However, both boys' and girls' current physical activity patterns demonstrate that they rarely experience the levels of physical activity associated with increases in peak $\dot{V}O_2$[18,112,113] and habitual physical activity is therefore unlikely to contribute to sex differences in peak $\dot{V}O_2$.

Muscle mass increases through childhood and although boys generally have more muscle mass than girls, marked sex differences do not become apparent until the adolescent growth spurt. Girls experience an adolescent spurt in muscle mass but it is less dramatic than that of boys. Between 5 and 16 years boys' relative muscle mass increases from 42 to 54% of body mass, whereas in girls muscle mass increases from 40 to 45% of body mass between 5 and 13 years and then, in relative terms, it declines due to an increase in fat accumulation during adolescence (see Chapter 2.4). Girls have slightly more body fat than boys during childhood but during the adolescent growth spurt, girls' body fat increases to about 25% of body mass while boys' declines to about 12 to 14%.[83,114,115] These dramatic changes in body composition during puberty are highly likely to contribute to the progressive increase in sex differences in peak $\dot{V}O_2$ over this period. Boys' greater muscle mass will not only facilitate the use of oxygen during exercise but may also supplement the venous return to the heart, and therefore augment stroke volume, through the peripheral muscle pump[116] (see Chapter 2.7). Armstrong et al.[104] used multilevel modelling to analyse longitudinal data in 11 to 13 year olds and demonstrated that the introduction of sum of triceps and subscapular skinfold thicknesses to the baseline model, incorporating body mass, stature and age, reduced the sex difference in peak $\dot{V}O_2$ but could not explain fully the greater increase in boys' peak $\dot{V}O_2$ with growth. However, the authors concluded that sex, age and maturational differences in the increase in fat-free mass relative to body mass are the predominant influence on the differential growth of boys' and girls' peak $\dot{V}O_2$ during the age range 11 to 13 years.[104]

During puberty there is a marked increase in haemoglobin concentration and hence oxygen-carrying capacity in boys, whereas girls' values plateau.[62,83,117] It might therefore be expected that differences in haemoglobin levels between boys and girls, which are about 11% at 16 years, would be a contributory factor to the observed sex difference in peak $\dot{V}O_2$.[41,118,119] This has been demonstrated with 14 and 15 year olds,[41] and by the midteens boys' superior haemoglobin concentration augments their greater muscle mass in the attainment of higher peak $\dot{V}O_2$ than girls. However, haemoglobin concentration, which is independent of sex until about 12 years of age, is not a factor in sex differences in peak $\dot{V}O_2$ in younger children.[35,41,42] When haemoglobin concentration was investigated as an additional explanatory variable, to body mass, stature, skinfold thicknesses, age and maturity, in a multilevel regression model of peak $\dot{V}O_2$ a non-significant parameter estimate was obtained with 11 to 13 year olds.[104]

The multilevel modelling approach has revealed age and maturity effects, independent of body size, on peak $\dot{V}O_2$ but even with age, maturity and body mass controlled for and no significant sex difference in either skinfold thicknesses or haemoglobin concentration observed, sex differences in peak $\dot{V}O_2$ have been recorded. A large, representative sample ($n = 164$) of 11 year old prepubertal children (i.e. Tanner stage one for pubic hair and either breast or genitalia rating) demonstrated a 21.9% higher peak $\dot{V}O_2$ in boys than in girls.[35] With the removal of the influence of body mass using a log-linear adjustment model (see Chapter 1.1), the boys' peak $\dot{V}O_2$ remained significantly higher than the girls' with the difference now being 16.2%.

Explanations for girls' lower peak $\dot{V}O_2$ during the prepubertal period are speculative but may be due to a lower exercise stroke volume than boys. During submaximal exercise a consistent finding is boys' greater stroke volume compared with girls at the same exercise intensity or $\dot{V}O_2$,[48,120,121] although others have not reported this difference to be significant[122] (see Chapter 2.7). Comparative data at peak $\dot{V}O_2$ appear to be limited to one published study[53] which, using carbon dioxide rebreathing, reported boys' stroke index to be 15% higher than girls at 9 to 10 years and 5% higher at 11 to 12 years. However, recent work by Rowland, using doppler echocardiography (see Chapter 2.7), provides supportive data with 12 year old boys reported to have 13% higher stroke indices than similarly aged girls.

The trend for boys to have higher stroke volumes during exercise[123] has been attributed to their greater heart mass (or size) in relation to body mass (or size)[124–126] but conflicting data indicating no sex differences in relative heart size are available.[127–129] Exercise stroke volume is, however, not just a function of ventricular size and it is difficult to distinguish between the complex and interrelated effects of ventricular preload, myocardial contractility and ventricular afterload. Markers of contractility and/or afterload have been shown to rise during exercise[130–132] but sex differences remain to be established.

Summary

Data consistently show a progressive, almost linear, increase in the peak $\dot{V}O_2$ of young people with age, although some studies indicate that from about 14 years of age girls' peak $\dot{V}O_2$ levels off or even declines. Understanding of age-related changes in the components of peak $\dot{V}O_2$ is subject to methodological limitations and data on cardiac output and AV oxygen difference at peak $\dot{V}O_2$ are sparse. Studies demonstrating an age-related rise in AV oxygen difference must be interpreted cautiously, but the increase in total haemoglobin with age supports the premise that adults have a greater arterial oxygen content. Data on young people's mixed venous oxygen content at peak $\dot{V}O_2$ are not available but adult data indicate that children are likely to have a lower AV oxygen reserve than adults. Heart rate at peak $\dot{V}O_2$ is independent of age, and age-related increases in cardiac output at peak $\dot{V}O_2$ therefore reflect changes in stroke volume. Stroke volume at peak $\dot{V}O_2$ is related not only to left ventricular size but also to a complex interplay of ventricular preload, myocardial contractility and ventricular afterload, all of which may vary with growth and maturation.

The increase in peak $\dot{V}O_2$ with age is strongly correlated with body size and inappropriate analyses have clouded our understanding of the independent contributions of age and maturity to the growth of peak $\dot{V}O_2$. Traditional analyses, using the ratio standard (ml kg^{-1} min^{-1}), have reported mass-related peak $\dot{V}O_2$ to be unchanged in boys over the age range 8 to 16 years, whereas girls' values steadily decline. Studies using appropriate allometric techniques to remove the influence of body size have provided further insights and demonstrated that boys' peak $\dot{V}O_2$ improves during growth rather than remaining static, whereas girls' peak $\dot{V}O_2$ increases into puberty and then levels off into young adulthood. The emergence of multilevel modelling techniques has provided a valuable tool to facilitate the interpretation of longitudinal data. Data are limited to a few studies but the evidence is unequivocal and indicates that maturation induces increases in peak $\dot{V}O_2$ independent of those explained by body size, body fatness and age. Physiological explanations for these maturational effects have yet to be established fully, although the importance of incorporating both age and maturity into analyses of peak $\dot{V}O_2$ during growth is readily apparent.

Boys' peak $\dot{V}O_2$ is higher than girls' at least from late childhood and there is a progressive divergence in boys' and girls' values during the teen years. Girls are less physically active than boys from an early age[133–135] but there is no compelling evidence to suggest that habitual physical activity contributes to sex differences in peak $\dot{V}O_2$. Explanations for prepubertal boys' higher peak $\dot{V}O_2$ than prepubertal girls are speculative but there is a growing conviction that it may be related to girls' lower exercise stroke volume. During the early teens boys' progressively greater increase in muscle mass augments the sex difference in peak $\dot{V}O_2$, and from about 14 years of age the sex difference is enhanced further by the marked increase in haemoglobin concentration experienced by boys but not by girls.

References

1. Astrand, P. O. and Rodahl, K. *Textbook of work physiology.* McGraw-Hill, New York, 1986.
2. American College of Sports Medicine. *ACSM's guidelines for exercise testing and prescription.* Williams and Wilkins, Baltimore, 1995.
3. Wilmore, J. H. and Costill., D. L. *Physiology of sport and exercise.* Human Kinetics Publishers, Champaign Il, 1994.
4. Shephard, R. J. Tests of maximum oxygen intake. A critical review. *Sports Medicine* 1984; 1: 99–124.
5. Bassett, D. R. and Howley, E. T. Maximal oxygen uptake: 'Classical' versus 'contemporary' viewpoints. *Medicine and Science in Sports and Exercise* 1997; 29: 591–603.
6. Howley, E. T., Bassett, D. R. and Welch, H. G. Criteria for maximal oxygen uptake: review and commentary. *Medicine and Science in Sports and Exercise* 1995; 27: 1292–301.
7. Noakes, T. D. Implications of exercise testing for prediction of athletic performance: A contemporary perspective. *Medicine and Science in Sports and Exercise* 1988; 20: 319–30.
8. Noakes, T. D. Challenging beliefs: Ex Africa semper aliquid novi. *Medicine and Science in Sports and Exercise* 1997; 29: 571–90.
9. Noakes T. D. Maximal oxygen uptake: 'Classical' versus 'contemporary' viewpoints: a rebuttal. *Medicine and Science in Sports and Exercise* 1998; 30: 1381–98.
10. Myers, J. N. *Essentials of cardiopulmonary exercise testing.* Human Kinetics Publishers, Champaign, Il, 1996.
11. Myers, J., Walsh, D., Buchanan, N. and Froelicher, V. F. Can maximal cardiopulmonary capacity be recognised by a plateau in oxygen uptake? *Chest* 1989; 96: 1312–6.
12. Myers, J., Walsh, D., Sullivan, M. and Froelicher, V. Effect of sampling on variability and plateau in oxygen uptake. *Journal of Applied Physiology* 1990; 68: 404–10.

13. **Armstrong, N., Welsman, J.** and **Winsley, R.** Is peak $\dot{V}O_2$ a maximal index of children's aerobic fitness? *International Journal of Sports Medicine* 1996; **17**: 356–9.

14. **Rowland T. W.** Does peak $\dot{V}O_2$ reflect $\dot{V}O_2$ max in children? Evidence from supramaximal testing. *Medicine and Science in Sports and Exercise* 1993; **25**: 689–93.

15. **Rowland, T. W.** and **Cunningham, L. N.** Oxygen uptake plateau during maximal treadmill exercise in children. *Chest* 1992; **101**: 485–9.

16. **Armstrong, N.** and **Davies, B.** The metabolic and physiological responses of children to exercise and training. *Physical Education Review* 1984; **7**: 90–105.

17. **Armstrong, N.** and **Welsman, J. R.** Assessment and interpretation of aerobic fitness in children and adolescents. *Exercise and Sport Sciences Reviews* 1994; **22**: 435–76.

18. **Armstrong, N.** and **Welsman, J. R.** *Young people and physical activity.* Oxford University Press, Oxford, 1997.

19. **Armstrong, N.** and **Welsman, J.** The assessment and interpretation of aerobic fitness in children and adolescents: An update. In *Exercise and fitness—benefits and limitations* (ed. K. Froberg, O. Lammert, H. St. Hansen and C. J. R. Blimkie). University Press, Odense, 1997; 173–80.

20. **Rowland, T. W.** Aerobic exercise testing protocols. In *Pediatric laboratory exercise testing in children* (ed. T. W. Rowland). Human Kinetics Publishers, Champaign Il, 1993; 19–42.

21. **Robinson, S.** Experimental studies of physical fitness in relation to age. *Arbeitsphysiologie* 1938; **10**: 251–323.

22. **Morse, M., Schlutz, F. W.** and **Cassels, D. E.** Relation of age to physiological responses of the older boy to exercise. *Journal of Applied Physiology* 1949; **1**: 683–709.

23. **Astrand, P. O.** *Experimental studies of physical working capacity in relation to sex and age.* Munksgaard, Copenhagen, 1952.

24. **Rutenfranz, J., Andersen, K. L., Seliger, V., Klimmer, F., Ilmarinen, J., Ruppel, M.** and **Kylian, H.** Exercise ventilation during the growth spurt period: Comparison between two European countries. *European Journal of Pediatrics* 1981; **136**: 135–42.

25. **Mercier, J., Varray, A., Ramonatxo, M., Mercier, B.** and **Prefaut, C.** Influence of anthropometric characteristics on changes in maximal exercise ventilation and breathing pattern growth in boys. *European Journal of Applied Physiology* 1991; **63**: 235–41.

26. **Rowland, T. W.** and **Green, G. M.** The influence of biologic maturation and aerobic fitness on ventilatory responses to treadmill exercise. In *Exercise physiology. Current selected research* (ed. C. O. Dotson and J. H. Humphrey). AMS Press, New York, 1990; 51–9.

27. **Armstrong, N., Kirby, B. J., McManus, A. M.** and **Welsman, J. R.** Prepubescents' ventilatory responses to exercise with reference to sex and body size. *Chest* 1997; **112**: 1554–60.

28. **Armstrong, N., Kirby, B. J., Mosney, J. R., Sutton, N. C.** and **Welsman, J. R.** Ventilatory responses to exercise in relation to sex and maturation. In *Children and exercise XIX: Promoting health and well-being* (ed. N. Armstrong, B. J. Kirby and J. R. Welsman). E. and F. N. Spon, London, 1997; 204–10.

29. **Rowland, T. W.** and **Cunningham, L. N.** Development of ventilatory responses to exercise in normal caucasian children: a longitudinal study. *Chest* 1997; **111**: 337–2.

30. **Armstrong, N.** and **Davies, B.** An ergometric analysis of age group swimmers. *British Journal of Sports Medicine* 1981; **15**: 20–6.

31. **Boileau, R. A., Bonen, A., Heyward, V. H.** and **Massey, B. H.** Maximal aerobic capacity on the treadmill and bicycle ergometer of boys 11–14 years of age. *Journal of Sports Medicine and Physical Fitness* 1977; **17**: 153–62.

32. **Cumming, G. R.** and **Langford, S.** Comparison of nine exercise tests used in pediatric cardiology. In *Children and exercise XI* (ed. R. A. Binkhorst, H. C. G. Kemper and W. H. M. Saris). Human Kinetics Publishers, Champaign Il, 1985; 58–68.

33. **Sheehan, J. M., Rowland, T. W.** and **Burke, E. J.** A comparison of four treadmill protocols for determination of maximal oxygen uptake in 10 to 12 year old boys. *International Journal of Sports Medicine* 1987; **8**: 31–4.

34. **Riopel, D. A., Taylor, A. B.** and **Hohn, A. R.** Blood pressure, heart rate, pressure-rate product and electrocardiographic changes in healthy children during treadmill exercise. *American Journal of Cardiology* 1979; **44**: 697–704.

35. **Armstrong, N., Kirby, B. J., McManus, A. M.** and **Welsman, J. R.** Aerobic fitness of pre-pubescent children. *Annals of Human Biology* 1995; **22**: 427–41.

36. **Turley, K. R., Rogers, D. M., Harper, K. M., Kujawa, K. I.** and **Wilmore, J. H.** Maximal treadmill versus cycle ergometry testing in children: Differences, reliability, and variability of responses. *Pediatric Exercise Science* 1995; **7**: 49–60.

37. **Rivera-Brown, A. M.** and **Frontera, W. R.** Achievement of plateau and reliability of $\dot{V}O_2$ max in trained adolescents tested with different ergometers. *Pediatric Exercise Science* 1998; **10**: 164–75.

38. **Bailey, D. A.** and **Ross, W. D.** Size dissociation of maximal aerobic power during growth in boys. *Medicine in Sport* 1978; **11**: 140–51.

39. **Bale, P.** Pre- and post-adolescents' physiological response to exercise. *British Journal of Sports Medicine* 1981; **15**: 246–9.

40. **Tolfrey, K.** and **Armstrong, N.** Child-adult differences in whole blood lactate responses to incremental treadmill exercise. *British Journal of Sports Medicine* 1995; **29**: 196–9.

41. **Armstrong, N., Williams, J., Balding, J., Gentle, P.** and **Kirby, B.** The peak oxygen uptake of British children with reference to age, sex and sexual maturity. *European Journal of Applied Physiology* 1991; **62**: 369–75.

42. **Armstrong, N., Welsman, J. R.** and **Kirby, B. J.** Peak oxygen uptake and maturation in 12-year-olds. *Medicine and Science in Sports and Exercise* 1998; **30**: 165–9.

43. **Rowland, T. W., Popowski, B.** and **Ferrone, L.** Cardiac responses to maximal upright cycle exercise in healthy boys and men. *Medicine and Science in Sports and Exercise* 1997; **29**: 1146–51.

44. **Armstrong, N., Balding, J., Gentle, P., Williams, J.** and **Kirby, B.** Peak oxygen uptake and physical activity in 11 to 16 year olds. *Pediatric Exercise Science* 1990; **2**: 349–58.

45. **Welsman, J.** and **Armstrong, N.** Daily physical activity and blood lactate indices of aerobic fitness. *British Journal of Sports Medicine* 1992; **26**: 228–32.

46. **Andersen, K. L., Seliger, V., Rutenfranz, J.** and **Skrobak-Kaczynski, J.** Physical performance capacity of children in Norway. Part IV—The rate of growth in maximal aerobic power and the influence of improved physical education of children in a rural community. *European Journal of Applied Physiology* 1976; **35**: 49–58.

47. **Washington, R. L.** Measurement of cardiac output. In *Pediatric exercise testing* (ed. T. W. Rowland). Human Kinetics Publishers, Champaign, Il, 1993; 131–40.

48. **Driscoll, D. J., Staats, B. A** and **Beck, K. C.** Measurement of cardiac output in children during exercise: A review. *Pediatric Exercise Science* 1989; **1**: 102–15.

49. **Rowland, T. W.** *Developmental exercise physiology.* Human Kinetics Publishers, Champaign, Il, 1996.

50. **Eriksson, B. O., Grimby, G.** and **Saltin, B.** Cardiac output and arterial blood gases during exercise in pubertal boys. *Journal of Applied Physiology* 1971; **31**: 348–52.

51. **Sholler, G. F., Celermajer, J. M.** and **Whight, C. M.** Doppler echocardiographic assessment of cardiac output in normal children with and without innocent precordial murmurs. *American Journal of Cardiology* 1987; **59**: 487–8.

52. **Kirby, B. J., Armstrong, N.** and **Welsman, J. R.** Cardiac output response to submaximal exercise in adolescents (abstract). *Medicine and Science in Sports and Exercise* 1997; **29**: S2.

53. **Miyamura, M.** and **Honda, Y.** Maximum cardiac output related to sex and age. *Japanese Journal of Physiology* 1973; **23**: 645–56.

54. **Yamaji, K.** and **Miyashita, M.** Oxygen transport system during exhaustive exercise in Japanese boys. *European Journal of Applied Physiology* 1977; **36**: 93–9.

55. **Gilliam, T. B., Sady, S., Thorland, W. G.** and **Weltman, A. L.** Comparison of peak performance measures in children ages 6 to 8, 9 to 10, and 11 to 13 years. *Research Quarterly* 1977; **48**: 695–702.

56. **Krovetz, L. J., McLoughlin, T. G., Mitchell, M. B.** and **Schiebler, G. L.** Hemodynamic findings in normal children. *Pediatric Research* 1967; **1**: 122–30.

57. **Sproul, A.** and **Simpson, E.** Stroke volume and related hemodynamic data in normal children. *Pediatrics* 1964; **33**: 912–8.

58. **Potter, C. R., Armstrong, N., Kirby, B. J.** and **Welsman, J. R.** An exploratory study of cardiac output responses to submaximal exercise. In *Children and exercise XIX: Promoting health and well-being* (ed. N. Armstrong, B. J. Kirby and J. R. Welsman). E. and F. N. Spon, London, 1997; 440–5.

59. **Eriksson, B. O.** Physical training oxygen supply and muscle metabolism in 11–13 year old boys. *Acta Physiologica Scandinavica* 1972; **384**: 1–48.

60. **Rowland, T. W., Staab, J., Unnithan, V.** and **Siconolfi, S.** Maximal cardiac responses in prepubertal and adult males (abstract). *Medicine and Science in Sports and Exercise* 1988; **20**: S332.

61. **Tanner, J. M.** *Growth at adolescence* (2nd edn). Blackwell Scientific Publications, Oxford, 1962.

62. **Dallman, P. R** and **Siimes, M. A.** Percentile curves for hemoglobin and red cell volume in infancy and childhood. *Pediatrics* 1979; **94**: 26–31.

63. **Hsia, C. C. W.** Respiratory function of hemoglobin. *New England Journal of Medicine* 1998; **338**: 239–46.

64. **Koch, G.** Muscle blood flow in prepubertal boys. *Medicine in Sport* 1978; **11**: 39–46.

65. **McArdle, W. D, Katch, F. I.** and **Katch, V. L.** *Exercise physiology*. Williams and Wilkins, Baltimore, 1996.

66. **Cassels, D. E** and **Morse, M.** *Cardiopulmonary data for children and young adults*. Thomas, Springfield, Il, 1962.

67. **Kalafoutis, A., Paterakis, S., Koutselinis, A.** and **Spanos, V.** Relationship between erythrocyte 2, 3-diphosphoglycerate and age in a normal population. *Clinical Chemistry* 1976; **22**: 1918–9.

68. **Pate, R. R., Barnes, C.** and **Miller, W.** A physiological comparison of performance matched female and male distance runners. *Research Quarterly for Exercise and Sport* 1985; **56**: 245–50.

69. **Macek, M.** Aerobic and anaerobic energy output in children. In *Children and exercise XII* (ed. J. Rutenfranz, R. Mocellin and F. Klimt). Human Kinetics Publishers, Champaign, Il, 1986; 3–10.

70. **Berg, A.** and **Keul, J.** Biochemical changes during exercise in children. In *Young athletes* (ed. R. M. Malina). Human Kinetics Publishers, Champaign, Il, 1988; 61–78.

71. **Lehmann, M., Keul, J.** and **Korsten-Reck, U.** The influence of graduated treadmill exercise on plasma catecholamines, aerobic and anaerobic capacity in boys and adults. *European Journal of Applied Physiology* 1987; **47**: 301–11.

72. **Koch, G.** Muscle blood flow after ischemic work and during bicycle ergometer work in boys aged 12 years. *Acta Paediatrica Belgica* 1974; **28**: 29–39.

73. **Koch, G.** Aerobic power, lung dimensions, ventilatory capacity and muscle blood flow in 12–16 year old boys with high physical activity. In *Children and exercise IX* (ed. K. Berg and B. O. Eriksson). University Park Press, Baltimore, 1980; 99–108.

74. **Eriksson, B. O., Gollnick, P. D.** and **Saltin, B.** Muscle metabolism and enzyme activities after training in boys 11–13 years old. *Acta Physiologica Scandinavica* 1973; **87**: 485–99.

75. **Haralambie, G.** Enzyme activities in skeletal muscle of 13–15 year old adolescents. *Bulletin European Physiopathologie Respiratoire* 1982; **18**: 65–74.

76. **Berg A, Kim S. S., Keul J.** Skeletal muscle enzyme activities in healthy young subjects. *International Journal of Sports Medicine* 1986; **7**: 236–9.

77. **Bell, R. D., MacDougall, J. D., Billeter, R.** and **Howald, H.** Muscle fibre types and morphometric analysis of skeletal muscles in six year old children. *Medicine and Science in Sports and Exercise* 1980; **12**: 28–31.

78. **Gollnick, P. D., Armstrong, R. B., Saubert, C. W., Piehl, K.** and **Saltin, B.** Enzyme activity and fibre composition in skeletal muscle of untrained and trained men. *Journal of Applied Physiology* 1972; **33**: 312–9.

79. **Eriksson, B. O.** and **Saltin, B.** Muscle metabolism during exercise in boys aged 11 to 16 years compared to adults. *Acta Paediatrica Belgica* 1974; **28**: 257–65.

80. **Krahenbuhl, G. S., Skinner, J. S.** and **Kohrt, W. M.** Developmental aspects of maximal aerobic power in children. *Exercise and Sport Sciences Reviews* 1985; **13**: 503–38.

81. **Léger, L.** Aerobic performance. In *Measurement in pediatric exercise science* (ed. D. Docherty). Human Kinetics Publishers, Champaign, Il, 1996; 183–223.

82. **Shuleva, K. M., Hunter, G. R., Hester, D. J.** and **Dunaway, D. L.** Exercise oxygen uptake in 3-through 6 year old children. *Pediatric Exercise Science* 1990; **2**: 130–9.

83. **Malina, R. M.** and **Bouchard, C.** *Growth, maturation and physical activity*. Human Kinetics Publishers, Champaign, Il, 1991.

84. **Bar-Or, O.** *Pediatric sports medicine for the practitioner*. Springer-Verlag, New York, 1983.

85. **Davies, C. T. M, Barnes, C.** and **Godfrey, S.** Body composition and maximal exercise performance in children. *Human Biology* 1972; **44**: 195–214.

86. **Saris, W. H. M.** *Aerobic power and daily physical activity in children*. Kripps Repro, Meppel, Netherlands, 1982.

87. **Saris, W. H. M., Noordeloos, A. M., Ringnalda, B. E. M., Van't Hof, M. A.** and **Binkhorst, R. A.** Reference values for aerobic power of healthy 4 to 18 year old Dutch children: Preliminary results. In *Children and exercise XI* (ed. R. A. Binkhorst, H. C. G. Kemper and W. H. M. Saris). Human Kinetics Publishers, Champaign, Il, 1985; 151–60.

88. **Krahenbuhl, G. S., Pangrazi, R. P., Stone, W. J., Morgan, D. W.** and **Williams, T.** Fractional utilization of maximal aerobic capacity in children 6 to 8 years of age. *Pediatric Exercise Science* 1989; **1**: 271–7.

89. **Fenster, J., Freedson, P., Washburn, R. A.** and **Ellison, R. C.** The relationship between physical activity and peak $\dot{V}O_2$ in 6 to 8 year old children. *Pediatric Exercise Science* 1989; **1**: 127–36.

90. **Cumming, G. R.** Current levels of fitness. *Canadian Medical Association Journal* 1967; **88**: 351–5.

91. **Yoshizawa, S., Ishizaki, T.** and **Honda, H.** Physical fitness of children aged 5 and 6 years. *Journal of Human Ergology* 1977; **6**: 41–51.

92. **Forster, M. A., Hunter, G. R., Hester, D. J., Dunaway, D.** and **Shuleva, K.,** Aerobic capacity and grade-walking economy of children 5–9 years old: A longitudinal study. *Pediatric Exercise Science* 1994; **6**: 31–8.

93. **Chatterjee, S., Banerjee, P. K., Chatterjee, P., Maitra, S. R.** Aerobic capacity of young girls. *Indian Journal of Medical Research* 1979; **69**: 327–33.

94. **Nakagawa, A.** and **Ishiko, T.** Assessment of aerobic capacity with special reference to sex and age of junior and senior high school students in Japan. *Japanese Journal of Physiology* 1970; **20**: 118–29.

95. **Yoshizawa, S.** A comparative study of aerobic work capacity in urban and rural adolescents. *Journal of Human Ergology* 1972; **1**: 45–65.

96. **Mirwald, R. L.** and **Bailey, D. A.** *Maximal aerobic power*. Sports Dynamics, London, Ontario, 1986.

97. **Cunningham, D. A., Paterson, D. H.** and **Blimkie, C. J. R.** The development of the cardiorespiratory system with growth and physical activity. In *Advances in pediatric sport sciences*, Vol 1 (ed. R. A. Boileau). Human Kinetics Publishers, Champaign, Il, 1984; 85–116.

98. **Mirwald, R. L., Bailey, D. A., Cameron, N.** and **Rasmussen, R. L.** Longitudinal comparison of aerobic power in active and inactive boys aged 7.0 to 17.0 years. *Annals of Human Biology* 1981; **8**: 405–14.

99. **Cunningham, D. A., Paterson, D. H., Blimkie, C. J. R.** and **Donner, A. P.** Development of cardiorespiratory function in circumpubertal boys: A longitudinal study. *Journal of Applied Physiology* 1984; **56**: 302–7.

100. **Welsman, J. R., Armstrong, N., Kirby, B. J., Nevill, A. M.** and **Winter, E. M.** Scaling peak $\dot{V}O_2$ for differences in body size. *Medicine and Science in Sports and Exercise* 1996; **28**: 259–65.

101. **Welsman, J.** Interpreting young people's exercise performance: sizing up the problem. In *Children and exercise XIX: Promoting health and well-being* (ed. N. Armstrong, B. J. Kirby and J. R. Welsman). E. & F. N. Spon, London, 1997; 191–203.

102. **Goldstein, H., Rasbash, J., Plewis, I., Draper, D., Browne, W., Yang, M., Woodhouse, G.** and **Healy, M.** *A user's guide to MlwiN*. University of London, Institute of Education, London, 1998.

103. Nevill, A. M., Holder, R. L., Baxter-Jones, A., Round, J. M. and Jones, D. A. Modeling developmental changes in strength and aerobic power in children. *Journal of Applied Physiology* 1998; **84**: 963–70.

104. Armstrong, N., Welsman, J. R., Nevill, A. M. and Kirby, B. J. Modeling growth and maturation changes in peak oxygen uptake in 11–13 year olds. *Journal of Applied Physiology* 1999; **87**: 2230–6.

105. Armstrong, N., Balding, J., Gentle, P. and Kirby, B. Patterns of physical activity among 11 to 16 year old British children. *British Medical Journal* 1990; **301**: 203–5.

106. Armstrong, N. and Bray, S. Physical activity patterns defined by continuous heart rate monitoring. *Archives of Disease in Childhood* 1991; **66**: 245–7.

107. McManus, A. and Armstrong, N. Patterns of physical activity among primary schoolchildren. In *Children in sport* (ed. F. J. Ring). University Press, Bath, 1995; 17–23.

108. Armstrong, N., McManus, A., Welsman. J. and Kirby, B. Physical activity patterns and aerobic fitness among pre-pubescents. *European Physical Education Review* 1996; **2**: 7–18.

109. Armstrong, N., Welsman, J. and Kirby, B. Physical activity, peak oxygen uptake and performance on the Wingate anaerobic test in 12-year-olds. *Acta Kinesiologiae Universitatis Tartuensis* 1998; **3**: 7–21.

110. Morrow, J. R. and Freedson, P. S. Relationship between habitual physical activity and aerobic fitness in adolescents. *Pediatric Exercise Science* 1994; **6**: 315–29.

111. Armstrong, N. and Van Mechelen, W. Are young people fit and active? In *Young and active* (ed. S. Biddle, J. Sallis and N. Cavill). Health Education Authority, London, 1998; 69–97.

112. Armstrong, N. Young people's physical activity patterns as assessed by heart rate monitoring. *Journal of Sports Sciences* 1998; **16**: 1–9.

113. Armstrong, N. Physical fitness and physical activity during childhood and adolescence. In *Sports and children* (ed. K. M. Chan and L. Micheli). Williams and Wilkins, Hong Kong, 1998; 50–75.

114. Guo, S., Chumlea, W. C., Siervogel, R. M. and Roche, A. F. Tracking of body fatness from 9 to 21 years. *Medicine and Science in Sports and Exercise* 1992; **24**: S189.

115. Malina, R. M., Bouchard, C. and Beunen, G. Human growth: Selected aspects of current research on well-nourished children. *Annual Review of Anthropology* 1988; **17**: 187–219.

116. Rowell, L. B., O'Leary, D. S and Kellogg, D. L. Integration of cardiovascular control systems in dynamic exercise. In *Handbook of physiology, exercise: Regulation and integration of multiple systems* (ed. L. B. Rowell and J. T. Shephard). American Physiological Society, Bethesda, MD, 1996; 778–81.

117. Harrison, G. A., Weiner, J. S. and Tanner, J. M. *Human growth. An introduction to human evolution, variation and growth.* Clarendon Press, Oxford, 1964.

118. Kemper, H. C. G. and Verschuur, R. Maximal aerobic power in 13 and 14 year old teenagers in relation to biologic age. *International Journal of Sports Medicine* 1981; **2**: 97–100.

119. Cunningham, D. A. and Paterson, D. H. Physiological characteristics of young active boys. In *Competitive sports for children and youth* (ed. E. W. Brown and C. F. Branta). Human Kinetics, Champaign Il, 1988; 159–70.

120. Katsuura, T. Influences of age and sex on cardiac output during submaximal exercise. *Annals of Physiological Anthropology* 1986; **5**: 39–57.

121. Godfrey, S., Davies, C. T. M., Wozniak, E. and Barnes, C. A. Cardiorespiratory response to exercise in normal children. *Clinical Science* 1971; **40**: 419–31.

122. Turley, K. R. and Wilmore, J. H. Cardiovascular responses to submaximal exercise in 7- to 9-yr-old boys and girls. *Medicine and Science in Sports and Exercise* 1997; **29**: 824–32.

123. Turley, K. R. Cardiovascular responses to exercise in children. *Sports Medicine* 1997; **24**: 241–57.

124. Scholz, D. G., Kitzman, D. W., Hagen, P. T., Ilstrup, D. M. and Edwards, W. D. Age-related changes in normal human hearts during the first 10 decades of life. Part 1 (Growth): A quantitative anatomic study of 200 specimens from subjects birth to 19 years old. *Mayo Clinic Proceedings* 1988; **63**: 126–36.

125. Nagasawa, H., Arakaki, Y., Yamada, O., Nakajima, T. and Kamiya, T. Longitudinal observations of left ventricular end-diastolic dimension in children using echocardiography. *Pediatric Cardiology* 1996; **17**: 169–74.

126. Daniels, S. R., Meyer, R. A., Liang, Y. and Bove, K. Echocardiographically determined left ventricular mass index in normal children, adolescents and young adults. *Journal of the American College of Cardiology* 1988; **12**: 703–8.

127. Maresh, M. M. Growth of the heart related to bodily growth during childhood and adolescence. *Pediatrics* 1948; **2**: 382–404.

128. Nidorf, S. M., Picard, M. H., Triulzi, M. O., Thomas, J. D., Newell, J., King, M. E. and Weyman, A. E. New perspectives in the assessment of cardiac chamber dimensions during development and adulthood. *Journal of the American College of Cardiology* 1992; **19**: 938–88.

129. Gutin, B., Owens, S., Treiber, F. and Mensah, G. Exercise haemodynamics and left ventricular parameters in children. In *Children and exercise XIX: Promoting health and well-being* (ed. N. Armstrong, B. Kirby and J. Welsman). E. and F. N. Spon, London, 1997; 460–4.

130. Oyen, E. M., Ignatzy, K., Ingerfeld, G. and Brode, P. Echocardiographic evaluation of left ventricular reserve in normal children during supine bicycle exercise. *International Journal of Cardiology* 1987; **14**: 145–54.

131. Rowland, T. W., Potts, J., Potts, T., Son-Hing, J., Harbison, G. and Sandor, G. Cardiovascular responses in children and adolescents with myocardial dysfunction. *American Heart Journal* (in press).

132. DeSouza, M., Schaffer, M. S., Gilday, D. L. and Rose, V. Exercise radionuclide angiography in hyperlipidemic children with apparently normal hearts. *Nuclear Medicine Communications* 1984; **5**: 13–7.

133. Welsman, J. R. and Armstrong, N. Physical activity patterns of 5-to 7-year-old children and their mothers. *European Journal of Physical Education* 1998; **3**: 145–55.

134. DuRant, R. H., Baranowski, T., Rhodes, T., Gutin, B., Thompson, W. O., Carroll, R., Puhl, J. and Greaves, K. A. Association among serum lipid and lipoprotein concentrations and physical activity. physical fitness and body composition in young children. *Journal of Pediatrics* 1993; **123**: 185–92.

135. Welsman, J. R. and Armstrong, N. Physical activity patterns of 5 to 11-year-old children. In *Children and exercise XIX: Promoting health and well-being* (ed. N. Armstrong, B. J. Kirby and J. R. Welsman). E. and F. N. Spon, London, 1997; 139–44.

2.9 Economy of locomotion

Don W. Morgan

Introduction

Mobility is a quintessential human activity that promotes health, well-being and independence. Because nearly all locomotor activities are performed at less than maximal intensity, a useful index of the energy expenditure associated with movement is economy of locomotion, defined as the oxygen consumption ($\dot{V}O_2$) for a given submaximal speed or power output. To the extent that locomotion economy can be optimized, the capability to perform locomotor activities without undue fatigue is enhanced, leading to improved endurance performance in children and adults.[1-11] From a clinical standpoint, knowledge of variables influencing economy of locomotion might also be useful in designing and implementing therapeutic regimens aimed at reducing the metabolic cost of transport in individuals with physically-disabling conditions.

The intent of this chapter is to present and synthesize research findings related to economy of locomotion during childhood. Because the majority of research on children has focused on walking and running, material covered in this chapter will focus exclusively on these modes of gait. Topics to be addressed include:

(1) differences in economy among children, adolescents and adults;
(2) variability in economy;
(3) sex differences in economy;
(4) the influence of running instruction and training on running economy;
(5) the relationship between running economy and running performance;
(6) physical growth and changes in economy;
(7) the role of economy as a determinant of walking speed; and
(8) economy considerations in children with physical disabilities.

Where appropriate, summaries of each section are provided. The chapter will conclude by proposing future research questions designed to help sport scientists, coaches and clinicians identify and better understand factors associated with efficient paediatric locomotion.

Economy differences among children, adolescents and adults

Tables 2.9.1 and 2.9.2 display descriptive and longitudinal comparisons of body mass-based walking and running economy values between children and adults and between younger and older children.[4,8,9,12-25] Data in Table 2.9.1 reveal that children are less economical than adults, with the magnitude of economy differences varying substantially among studies. As shown in Table 2.9.2, younger children are also less economical than older children, and economy differences are more pronounced when children exhibit a greater disparity in chronological age.

The higher metabolic costs of paediatric locomotion may be attributable to a variety of factors. These include:

(1) less efficient ventilation (as evidenced by a higher ventilatory equivalent for oxygen);[21,26]
(2) faster stride rates;[13,18,20,24,27,28]
(3) immature running patterns (e.g. shorter strides, greater displacement of the centre of mass, less extension of the hip, knee and ankle during takeoff, a greater distance between the heel and the buttock during the forward swing phase, lower height of the forward knee during takeoff, a longer relative distance of the support foot in front of the centre of mass, less single-leg stance time, higher relative peak vertical ground reaction forces, greater cocontraction of lower extremity muscles);[29-35]
(4) larger surface area to body mass ratio;[13,18,36]
(5) shorter stature;[22,24]
(6) decreased ability to store and recoil elastic energy in the legs;[28,37]
(7) an imbalance between body mass and leg muscle contraction speed;[28,38]
(8) more distal distribution of mass in the lower extremities;[39,40] and
(9) a greater dependence on fat as a metabolic substrate and a diminished ability to utilize anaerobic energy sources.[35,41,42]

While each of these factors has been linked theoretically to higher aerobic demands, direct evidence confirming their relationship with or causative influence upon locomotion economy is limited.

In considering potential explanations for adult–child economy differences, the most consistent level of experimental support exists for the stride frequency and body surface area : body mass ratio hypotheses. In brief, the basic premise of the stride frequency hypothesis is that each gram of muscle uses a set amount of energy for each step taken.[43-45] Hence, children would be expected to consume more oxygen than adolescents or adults at any walking or running speed because their shorter legs would, of necessity, be required to turn over at a faster rate to cover a given distance. Evidence for this hypothesis can be found in a number of human studies, wherein comparable economy values have been reported for adults and children and for younger and older children when $\dot{V}O_2$ is expressed per stride ($ml\,kg^{-1}\,stride^{-1}$).[13,18,20,24,27,28] Similar results have also been reported when adult–child comparisons of gait transport costs are expressed relative to body surface area (e.g. $ml\,min^{-1}\,m^{-2}$).[13,18,36] This latter finding reflects both the need to maintain internal heat production to offset heat loss from the surface of the body and the progressive age-related drop in the body surface area to mass ratio. Taken together, these dual observations suggest that children also require a

Table 2.9.1   Comparison of walking and running economy values between children and adults

Authors	Age (y)		Sex	Speed (m s^{-1})	$\dot{V}O_2$ (ml kg^{-1}min^{-1})		% diff
	Child	Adult			Child	Adult	
Armstrong et al.[12]	11.0	21.7	F	2.50	38.2	36.3	5.2
Ebbeling et al.[13]	9.5	20.0	M	75% of mean walk speed in 1-mile walk	19.7	15.0	31.3
Krahenbuhl et al.[14]	8.0	Y&M	M	2.90	45.5	35.3–40.2	13–29
Van Mechelen et al.[15]	13.0	21.0	M	2.22	37.6	30.3	24.1
	13.0	21.0	F	2.22	36.5	29.8	22.5
Maliszewski and Freedson[16]	9.8	25.0	M	2.67	40.6	34.9	16.3
Martinez and Haymes[17]	9.1	24.4	F	2.00	32.9	27.6	19.2
Rowland et al.[18]	11.6	29.2	M	2.67	49.5	40.0	23.8
Rowland and Green[19]	11.3	28.7	F	2.03	35.8	30.9	15.9
Unnithan and Eston[20]*	10.4	20.8	M	2.67	47.5	40.0	18.8

% diff = percentage difference from adult value.

Y&M = young and middle-age adults.

* = data estimated from figures provided in the cited publication.

higher rate of oxygen use to move a unit of body mass because they have a larger relative surface area.[36]

The lack of age-associated differences in economy when aerobic demand is scaled to stride frequency or body surface area points to the growing popularity of alternative methods for standardizing $\dot{V}O_2$. Some authors, in fact, have questioned the validity of the ratio method of scaling aerobic power (i.e. absolute $\dot{V}O_2$ divided by total body mass) and suggested that regression or allometrically based scaling approaches may be more suitable for normalizing $\dot{V}O_2$ to body size in children.[46–48] Others, though, have argued that ratio scaling is an entirely appropriate method of accounting for growth-related changes in $\dot{V}O_2$, since the total body mass is lifted, lowered and supported during bipedal locomotion.[42,49,50] While an in-depth discussion of various scaling models and their applicability is beyond the scope of this chapter, the reader is referred to a number of papers on the subject[46–51] (and see Chapter 1.1 in this volume).

In summary, the body mass-related aerobic demands of walking and running are higher in children compared with adults, and younger children are less economical than older children. A host of physiological, biomechanical and structural factors have been linked to this elevation in submaximal $\dot{V}O_2$, but few studies have been conducted to validate these relationships. The limited data available suggest that a faster stride rate and a higher body surface to body mass ratio may contribute to the inefficient metabolic responses exhibited by children and adolescents when $\dot{V}O_2$ is expressed relative to total body mass. The manner in which aerobic power is scaled to account for differences in body structure can alter the interpretation of child–adult differences in locomotion economy.

Variability in economy

In order to determine the efficacy of manipulations designed to improve walking and running economy in children, it is essential to quantify the consistency of submaximal $\dot{V}O_2$ responses. To this end, recent studies have begun to document the stability of gait transport costs in children. No mean between-trial or between-day group differences in $\dot{V}O_2$ were reported by Frost and colleagues[52] in 24 children (mean age 9.1 ± 1.4 y) who completed six 6-min bouts of treadmill walking or running on two days following a minimal amount of exposure (<1 min) to treadmill walking. Individual economy responses, however, varied considerably across trials. Unnithan and colleagues[53] also demonstrated that a single exercise session yielded valid group measures of running economy among prepubertal boys (mean age 10.7 ± 0.7 y). Conversely, in a study of 42 children (mean age 8.9 ± 0.7 y) who were given varying time periods (5 to 15 min) to practise treadmill walking or running on each of two days, Rogers et al.[54] found that $\dot{V}O_2$ values measured while running for 5 min each at 2.23 and 2.68 m s^{-1} were lower on the second day of testing. In this study, between-day reliability estimates for $\dot{V}O_2$ were moderate to high in magnitude (range = 0.71 to 0.94) and the coefficient of variation (CV) in $\dot{V}O_2$ ranged from 7.4% to 8.4% across running speeds.

With respect to the issue of metabolic variability in children, it is possible that younger children, being structurally less mature, may exhibit greater variation in submaximal exercise $\dot{V}O_2$ compared to older, physically mature children. With respect to this question, findings from ongoing research conducted in our laboratory[55,56] have shown that after 10 to 15 min of treadmill accommodation, six year old children walking at 1.34 m s^{-1} ($n = 46$) and running at 2.23 m s^{-1} ($n = 30$) displayed stable within-day walking economy values and within- and between-day running economy values. Parenthetically, in our investigations, average CV values for $\dot{V}O_2$ were considerably lower (<3%) than those reported previously in the literature.[54]

In summary, the general tenor of these findings suggests that if some treadmill accommodation is provided, stable submaximal walking and running $\dot{V}O_2$ values can be obtained in a relatively short time period in younger and older prepubescent children. However, given

Table 2.9.2 Comparison of walking and running economy values between younger children and older children

Authors	Age (y)		Sex	Speed (m s⁻¹)	$\dot{V}O_2$ (ml kg⁻¹ min⁻¹)		% diff
	YC	OC			YC	OC	
Åstrand[21]**	4–6	16–18	M	2.78	47.0	38.0	23.7
	7–9	16–18	M	2.78	43.0	38.0	13.2
	10–11	16–18	M	2.78	42.0	38.0	10.5
	12–13	16–18	M	2.78	41.0	38.0	7.9
	14–15	16–18	M	2.78	39.0	38.0	2.6
	4–6	17	F	2.78	45.0	37.0	21.6
	7–9	17	F	2.78	43.0	37.0	16.2
	10–11	17	F	2.78	40.0	37.0	8.1
	12–13	17	F	2.78	40.0	37.0	8.1
	14–15	17	F	2.78	37.0	37.0	0.0
Cureton et al.[4]	7–10	15–17	M	2.22	39.3	32.6	20.6
	11–14	15–17	M	2.22	34.9	32.6	7.1
	7–10	15–17	F	2.22	36.9	30.2	22.2
	11–14	15–17	F	2.22	31.9	30.2	5.6
Daniels et al.[8]	10	12	M	3.37	53.9	45.7	17.9
	12	17	M	3.37	52.8	42.2	25.1
Forster et al.[22]	5.2	9.3	M,F	1.12, 10% grade	29.0	22.6	28.3
Kanaley et al.[23]	<8.99	13–15	M	1.61, 10% grade	35.1	31.9	10.0
	9–10.99	13–15	M	1.61, 10% grade	34.0	31.9	6.6
	11–12.99	13–15	M	1.61, 10% grade	33.2	31.9	4.1
Krahenbuhl et al.[9]*	9.9	16.8	M	2.23–2.90 (YC) 2.68–3.57 (OC)	234†	203†	15.3
MacDougall et al.[24]*	7–9	15–16	M,F	2.83	44.7	37.9	17.9
	10–12	15–16	M,F	2.83	41.8	37.9	10.3
	13–14	15–16	M,F	2.83	39.1	37.9	3.2
Shuleva et al.[25]	3–4	5–6	M,F	1.12, 10% grade	31.1	26.1	19.2

YC = younger children; OC = older children.

% diff = percentage difference from OC value.

*Data estimated from figures or regression equations provided in the cited publication.

** Data drawn from Krahenbuhl and Williams.[87]

† $\dot{V}O_2$ in ml kg⁻¹ km⁻¹.

the limited number of available studies and the possibility that individual $\dot{V}O_2$ responses may be somewhat inconsistent, future research documenting the minimum time required to achieve acceptable levels of within- and between-day $\dot{V}O_2$ stability in adequately sized, age-diverse samples of boys and girls performing treadmill locomotion at varying speeds and grades seems warranted. Moreover, while all of the previously mentioned investigations attempted to control some of the factors known or postulated to influence total exercise energy expenditure (e.g. ambient temperature, circadian variation, diet, fatigue, footwear, resting energy cost), more research is needed to assess the single and collective contribution of these variables in affecting the stability of children's economy responses.

Sex differences in running economy

Studies addressing the issue of sex differences in running economy have produced equivocal results, with some investigators observing poorer running economy in boys[4,21,40] and others reporting no sex variation in economy.[24,38,48,57] In an attempt to reconcile these disparate findings, we recently quantified measures of locomotion economy in

35 six year olds (15 boys and 20 girls) following 30 min of treadmill running practice.[58] Both sexes were similar in stature, body mass and leg length, but the girls exhibited a higher percentage of body fat and a lower fat-free mass (FFM). A comparison of sex differences in running economy demonstrated that absolute gross $\dot{V}O_2$ (litre min⁻¹) and body mass-related gross and net $\dot{V}O_2$ (the latter calculated by subtracting resting $\dot{V}O_2$ from gross $\dot{V}O_2$) were higher in the boys. However, when exercise $\dot{V}O_2$ was expressed relative to FFM, no sex difference in $\dot{V}O_2$ was present. Hence, compared to girls of similar age and body mass, young, prepubescent boys displayed higher absolute and mass-related $\dot{V}O_2$ values because of their greater leanness.

While our findings confirm results from other studies indicating that boys are less economical than girls,[4,21,40] it should be emphasized that only young, similarly aged children were tested. Because data collected in our project are part of an ongoing, large-scale tracking study examining how gait efficiency and gait function change with physical growth, future analyses will be able to determine if girls continue to exhibit better running economy throughout early childhood, and evaluate how yearly changes in resting energy expenditure and body composition affect sex differences in the aerobic demand of running.

Influence of running instruction and run training on economy

A topic of obvious practical importance to coaches and young athletes is whether children can be taught or trained to adopt a more economical running style. Petray and Krahenbuhl[59] addressed this issue by randomly selecting 50 ten year olds and assigning them to one of five treatment groups. These groups were:

(1) a no-treatment control group;

(2) a control group in which subjects received instruction on a topic (viz., throwing) unrelated to running;

(3) a running technique instruction group which received 5 min of weekly instruction on various aspects of running form for 11 weeks;

(4) a run training group which trained 3 to 30 min per day three days per week for 11 weeks; and

(5) a group which combined both running instruction and run training.

Data from their study indicated that none of the experimental manipulations altered running economy, stride rate, stride length or vertical displacement of the body. In support of these data, Lussier and Buskirk[60] reported no change in the running economy of ten year old boys and girls who completed a four days per week, 12 week programme incorporating running games and continuous running.

While the previously cited studies imply that economy in children is not easily perturbed by short-term training regimens or instruction on running technique, some researchers have demonstrated enhanced gait economy among boys involved in middle- and long-distance running programmes. Sjödin and Svedenhag,[61] for instance, reported that over an eight year period, mass-related $\dot{V}O_2$ measured at 4.17 m s^{-1} decreased in eight young male runners (mean age 12.5 y) who ran an average of 48 to 60 km wk^{-1}. $\dot{V}O_2$ submax values for the trained boys were also consistently lower compared to values obtained on age- and sex-matched controls. Work by Daniels and coworkers[7,8] has shown that extended periods (2 to 5 y) of middle- and long-distance run training can also improve running economy in 10 to 13 year old boys. In their study, absolute measures of $\dot{V}O_2$ max rose linearly across the yearly testing periods, but remained stable when expressed relative to body mass. $\dot{V}O_2$ submax, though, dropped by 15% in ten year olds who were studied for two years and by 19% in 12 year olds followed for five years. Because subjects were tracked over a number of years, the observed improvement in running economy may have been due partly to physical growth. However, because the relative reduction in oxygen uptake was greater than that observed in non-run trained boys who were tested when they were 10 and 17 years of age,[9] run training may have exerted an influence on economy over and above that produced solely by physical growth.

To summarize, limited attempts to improve economy using short-term interventions featuring run training and instruction have been unsuccessful in young boys and girls. On the other hand, data from a few studies have shown that extended periods of demanding long-term run training can lower submaximal energy demands in pre-, circum- and post-pubertal boys. More studies are needed to establish whether longer periods of running instruction and different types and combinations of long-distance and interval training are efficacious in yielding improvements in running economy.

Relationship between running economy and running performance

Since distance-running success has been linked to better running economy in adults,[1–3,5,6,10,11] a logical question to ask is whether the same relationship exists in children. Early cross-sectional work conducted by Krahenbuhl and associates[14,62] demonstrated that the $\dot{V}O_2$ of submaximal running at 2.23, 2.57 and 2.90 m s^{-1} was not different among 20 eight year old boys[14] and 21 ten year old boys[62] stratified by distance covered in 5-, 7- and 9-min runs or by time recorded for a 1.6 km run. Conversely, Mayers and Gutin[63] reported that eight 8–11 year old boys who were competitive cross-country runners exhibited lower energy costs at 2.68 m s^{-1} compared with an equal number of age- and mass-matched controls. When stature was covaried between the two groups, however, the difference in $\dot{V}O_2$ submax was not statistically significant. A lack of association ($r = -0.05$) between running economy and distance running performance was also reported by Cunningham[64] in a study of 24 female high school runners who competed in a 5-km race. However, Cureton et al.[4] found that age-related improvement in 1-mile run/walk performance among 92 boys and 53 girls aged 7 to 17 years of age was explained partly by an improvement in running economy.

Longitudinal studies, while few in number, have established a stronger link between distance-running performance and running economy in children. To wit, Daniels and coworkers[7,8] showed that marked decrements in submaximal $\dot{V}O_2$ were accompanied by significant reductions in one and two mile run times among 10 and 12 year olds who participated in middle- and long-distance run training for two and five years. Since mass-related $\dot{V}O_2$ max remained unchanged over time, it was speculated that improvements in running economy contributed to better running performance in their trained subjects. Using a different approach, Krahenbuhl et al.[9] documented changes in 9 min run performance and running economy in six young boys (mean age 9.9 y) who were tested initially and seven years later (mean age 16.8 y). During the intervening time span, none of the subjects had engaged in formal distance-run training, but all had been active in recreational or high-school sports. Congruent with the findings of Daniels and colleagues,[7,8] body mass-related $\dot{V}O_2$ did not change over the seven year period, but running performance and running economy improved by 29% and 16%, respectively, and the estimated percentage of $\dot{V}O_2$ max incurred during the 9 min run rose by 13%. Viewed collectively, these latter findings demonstrate that improvements in childhood distance-running performance can occur in the absence of run training. Since maximal lactate values and glycolytic enzyme activity increase with age,[21,35,65–69] the higher relative workload generated by the teenage boys may reflect a greater contribution of anaerobic energy mechanisms to the total exercise energy requirement. Alternatively, it is possible that the older boys exhibited more mental toughness, which would also enable them to exercise at a higher percentage of $\dot{V}O_2$ max.

In summary, the association between running economy and distance-running success in boys and girls remains generally unconfirmed in a limited set of descriptive studies, but has been reported in a small number of long-term tracking investigations. Results from these longitudinal studies suggest that age-related decreases in submaximal $\dot{V}O_2$ are a function of run training and physical growth. In acknowledging the link between temporal reductions in submaximal aerobic demand and better running performance, an enhanced ability to work at a higher relative exercise intensity, greater anaerobic energy contribution and a more intense psychological resolve are additional factors which may partially account for childhood improvements in distance-running performance.

Physical growth and changes in locomotion economy

As noted previously, longitudinal decreases in submaximal $\dot{V}O_2$ among boys aged 10 to 18 years of age have been attributed to physical growth.[9] Although similar findings have been observed for graded walking (10% and 12.5% grade) in younger boys and girls,[22] pertinent factors underlying this relationship have not been examined systematically in a large, mixed-sex sample of children. To address this issue, we are currently involved in a five year tracking study aimed at documenting yearly changes in gait efficiency in 40 untrained able-bodied boys and girls on whom annual data collection was begun at age six years following extensive treadmill accommodation (Morgan *et al.*, unpublished data). Preliminary analyses conducted on data gathered over the first two years of our study indicate that gross and net $\dot{V}O_2$ during level treadmill walking at 1.34 m s^{-1} fell by 10% and 13%, respectively, whereas gross and net $\dot{V}O_2$ each decreased by 5% while performing level treadmill running at 2.23 m s^{-1}. Accompanying these improvements in locomotion economy were increases in walking and running step length and walking stance time, and reductions in body surface area to mass ratio. Annual decreases in ventilatory equivalent for oxygen, mean relative vertical ground reaction force, and moment of inertia of the leg about the hip during walking and running have also been observed. These initial results suggest that yearly decreases in the aerobic transport costs of young healthy prepubescent boys and girls are linked to growth-related changes in specific physiological, structural and biomechanical variables postulated to influence ambulatory energy demands.

Do children choose walking speeds that minimize energy demands?

Research has shown that walking speeds typically selected by young and older adults (~1.3 m s^{-1}) are similar to speeds at which oxygen uptake per unit distance travelled is lowest.[70,71] It is not known, however, if locomotion economy is a primary determinant governing the choice of walking speed in children. To answer this question, we recently measured preferred and energetically-optimal walking speeds in a large cohort of six year olds who walked at speeds ranging from 0.67 to 1.79 m s^{-1}.[72] Data from our study revealed that walking at a freely chosen speed required the least amount of energy compared to the curvilinear rise in $\dot{V}O_2$ observed as speed varied away from the preferred condition. Further analyses revealed no difference between subjects' freely chosen walking speed (mean, 1.30 m s^{-1}) and their most economical walking speed (mean, 1.28 m s^{-1}). This affinity between preferred and most economical walking speeds supports the notion that minimizing energy demand is a key factor regulating the choice of walking speed in young healthy children.

Economy of locomotion in children with physical disabilities

The assessment of paediatric gait efficiency is important not only with regard to the general health and sport performance of able-bodied children, but also for children with physical disabilities. From a clinical perspective, energetic penalties resulting from inefficient locomotion patterns may limit the functional capabilities of children with neuromuscular disease or lower-extremity injuries, thus restricting their physical independence and involvement in family, school and recreational activities.

While limited research has shown that children with below-knee amputations and spina bifida display elevated walking energy demands compared to control or expected population values,[73,74] the most studied developmental disorder linked to excessive paediatric locomotor energy demands is cerebral palsy (CP), a condition resulting from perinatal injury to the immature brain and characterized by loss of selective motor control.[75] Unpublished work from our laboratory (Morgan *et al.*, unpublished data) and a handful of other researchers[76–79] has indicated that walking $\dot{V}O_2$ values for children with CP measured over a wide range of speeds (0.36 to 1.34 m s^{-1}) are approximately 22% to 88% higher compared to control subjects (note that some comparisons have been estimated from graphical presentations of data). The higher energy cost associated with CP has been ascribed to a variety of factors, including adoption of a 'crouched gait pattern' typified by exaggerated flexion at the knee and hip and excess lower limb muscle coactivation.[79–82] Because $\dot{V}O_2$ max values are much lower in children with CP compared to able-bodied controls,[79] the cerebral-palsied child operates at a higher relative percentage of $\dot{V}O_2$ max at any given speed of walking or running. In addition, cross-sectional data acquired from children with spastic CP indicate that the rate of walking energy expenditure increases with advancing age.[83] From a clinical standpoint, these observations have important functional relevance for children with spastic cerebral palsy who complain of fatigue or require frequent rest following walking bouts. As noted by Campbell and Ball,[83] this age-related decrease in gait efficiency may also help explain why older children with CP tend to walk less or use a wheelchair more often.

Even though a number of rehabilitative strategies have been employed to improve gait function in children with cerebral palsy, surprisingly few studies have examined their impact on locomotion economy. Results from these investigations have been mixed, with some demonstrating no change in $\dot{V}O_2$ or heart rate-based measures of energy expenditure following short-term periods of lower extremity strength training,[84,85] and another reporting a lower physiological cost index following electrical stimulation of lower extremity muscles.[86] Given the paucity of available data, additional studies are needed to document the potential impact of these and other therapeutic interventions, such as gait training, electromyographic biofeedback, body mass support, surgical and pharmacological treatments, assistive devices, and physical therapy on the aerobic demand of locomotion in physically disabled children.

Summary and future directions

While some progress has been made in identifying and manipulating factors affecting locomotion economy during childhood, a number of important issues remain unresolved. In view of the generally small cohort sizes and often narrow range of subject characteristics found in many studies of paediatric gait efficiency, more research featuring larger, age-diverse samples of boys and girls is needed to confirm, refute or refine current thinking and approaches. Against this backdrop, the following questions are posed in the hope of providing guidance to sport scientists, coaches and clinicians as they endeavour to improve movement efficiency in healthy and diseased children and adolescents:

1. What are the mechanisms associated with physical growth that lead to better gait economy during childhood?
2. Do children with good or inferior running economy display unique physiological, biomechanical or structural profiles?
3. What is the minimum amount of time required for children to attain stable and reproducible submaximal $\dot{V}O_2$ values while walking and running on a treadmill at various intensities and grades? Is less accommodation needed as children age?
4. Do young girls exhibit better body mass-related economy throughout childhood? If so, how do sex-related changes in resting $\dot{V}O_2$ and body composition influence this comparison?
5. What types of run training are best suited to improve running economy in children? What combination(s) of training intensity, frequency and duration is(are) most effective in improving economy? Is there a particular time period during childhood when training is most optimal in eliciting positive changes in economy? Are there time periods when training may be relatively ineffective in modifying economy? What is the long-term effect on running economy resulting from short-term exposure to training?
6. Can childhood economy be improved by manipulating certain biomechanical variables? Aside from speed, are there other gait descriptors which are naturally chosen to optimize locomotor energy use?
7. Which rehabilitative strategies and assistive devices are effective in improving gait economy in children with physical disabilities or lower extremity injuries? Is economy improved to greater extent by combining different therapeutic interventions? If better economy is observed after therapy, how long does this change persist and what effect does enhanced locomotion economy have on functional mobility?

Acknowledgement

Some of the research presented in this paper was supported by a grant from the National Institute of Child Health and Human Development (HD 30749).

References

1. Bransford., D. R., and Howley, E. T. Oxygen cost of running in trained and untrained men and women. *Medicine and Science in Sports* 1977; **9**: 41–4.
2. Conley, D. L. and Krahenbuhl, G. S. Running economy and distance running performance of highly trained athletes. *Medicine and Science in Sports and Exercise* 1980; **12**: 357–60.
3. Conley, D. L., Krahenbuhl, G. S. and Burkett, L. N. Training for aerobic capacity and running economy. *The Physician and Sportsmedicine* 1981; **9**: 107–15.
4. Cureton, K. J., Sloniger, M. A., Black, D. M., McCormack, W. P. and Rowe, D. A. Metabolic determinants of the age-related improvement in one-mile run/walk performance in youth. *Medicine and Science in Sports and Exercise* 1997; **29**: 259–67.
5. Daniels, J. T. Physiological characteristics of champion male athletes. *Research Quarterly* 1974; **45**: 342–8.
6. Daniels, J. T. A physiologist's view of running economy. *Medicine and Science in Sports and Exercise* 1985; **17**: 332–8.
7. Daniels, J. and Oldridge, N. Changes in oxygen consumption of young boys during growth and running training. *Medicine and Science in Sports* 1971; **3**: 161–5.
8. Daniels, J. and Oldridge, N., Nagle, F. and White, B. Differences and changes in $\dot{V}O_2$ among young runners 10 to 18 years of age. *Medicine and Science in Sports* 1978; **10**: 200–3.
9. Krahenbuhl, G. S., Morgan, D. W. and Pangrazi, R. P. Longitudinal changes in distance-running performance of young males. *International Journal of Sports Medicine* 1989; **10**: 92–6.
10. Morgan, D., Baldini, F., Martin, P. and Kohrt, W. Ten kilometer performance and predicted velocity at O_2 max among well-trained male runners. *Medicine and Science in Sports and Exercise* 1989; **21**: 78–83.
11. Morgan, D. W. and Craib, M. W. Physiological aspects of running economy. *Medicine and Science in Sports and Exercise* 1992; **24**: 456–61.
12. Armstrong, N., Kirby, B. J., Welsman, J. R. and McManus, A. M. Submaximal exercise in prepubertal children. In *Children and exercise XIX* (ed. N. Armstrong, B. J. Kirby and J. R. Welsman). Chapman and Hall, London, 1997; 221–7.
13. Ebbeling, C. J., Hamill, J., Freedson, P. S. and Rowland, T. W. An examination of efficiency during walking in children and adults. *Pediatric Exercise Science* 1992; **4**: 36–49.
14. Krahenbuhl, G. S., Pangrazi, R. P. and Chomokos, E. A. Aerobic responses of young boys to submaximal running. *Research Quarterly* 1979; **50**: 413–21.
15. Van Mechelen, W., Kemper, H. C. G. and Twisk, J. The development of running economy from 13–27 years of age. *Medicine and Science in Sports and Exercise* 1994; **26**: S205.
16. Maliszewski, A. F. and Freedson, P. S. Is running economy different between adults and children? *Pediatric Exercise Science* 1996; **8**: 351–60.
17. Martinez ,L. R. and Haymes, E. M. Substrate utilization during treadmill running in prepubertal girls and women. *Medicine and Science in Sports and Exercise* 1992; **24**: 975–83.
18. Rowland, T. W., Auchinachie, J. A., Keenan, T. J. and Green, G. M. Physiologic responses to treadmill running in adult and prepubertal males. *International Journal of Sports Medicine* 1987; **8**: 292–7.
19. Rowland, T. W. and Green, G. M. Physiological responses to treadmill exercise in females: Adult-child differences. *Medicine and Science in Sports and Exercise* 1988; **20**: 474–8.
20. Unnithan, V. B. and Eston, R. G. Stride frequency and submaximal treadmill running economy in adults and children. *Pediatric Exercise Science* 1990; **2**: 149–55.
21. Åstrand, P-O. *Experimental studies of physical working capacity in relation to sex and age.* Enjar Munksgaard, Copenhagen, 1952; 75, 80, 82, 94–5, 129, 132–3.
22. Forster, M. A., Hunter, G. R., Hester, D. J., Dunaway, D. and Shuleva, K. Aerobic capacity and grade-walking economy of children 5–9 years old: A longitudinal study. *Pediatric Exercise Science* 1994; **6**: 31–8.
23. Kanaley, J. A., Boileau, R. A., Massey, B. H. and Misner, J. E. Muscular efficiency during treadmill walking: the effects of age and workload. *Pediatric Exercise Science* 1989; **1**: 155–62.
24. MacDougall, J. D., Roche, P. D., Bar-Or, O. and Moroz, J. R. Maximal aerobic capacity of Canadian schoolchildren: Prediction based on age-related oxygen cost of running. *International Journal of Sports Medicine* 1983; **4**: 194–8.
25. Shuleva, K. M., Hunter, G. R., Hester, D. J. and Dunaway, D. L. Exercise oxygen uptake in 3- through 6-year-old children. *Pediatric Exercise Science* 1990; **2**: 130–9.

26. **Anderson, K. L., Seliger, V., Rutenfranz, J.** and **Messel, S.** Physical performance capacity of children in Norway. Part III. Respiratory responses to graded exercise loadings-population parameters in a rural community. *European Journal of Applied Physiology* 1974; **33**: 265–74.

27. **Waters, R. L., Hislop, H. J., Thomas, L.** and **Campbell, J.** Energy cost of walking in normal children and teenagers. *Developmental Medicine and Child Neurology* 1983; **25**: 184–8.

28. **Thorstensson, A.** Effects of moderate external loading on the aerobic demand of submaximal running in men and 10 year-old boys. *European Journal of Applied Physiology* 1986; **55**: 569–74.

29. **Wickstrom, R. L.** *Fundamental motor patterns.* Lea and Febiger, Philadelphia, 1983; 51.

30. **Kram, R.** and **Taylor, C. R.** Energetics of running: A new perspective. *Nature* 1990; **346**: 265–7.

31. **Alexander, R. Mc. N.** and **Ker, R. F.** Running is priced by the step. *Nature* 1990; **346**: 220–1.

32. **Taylor, C. R.** Force development during sustained locomotion: A determinant of gait, speed and metabolic power. *Journal of Experimental Biology* 1985; **115**: 253–62.

33. **Greer, N. L., Hamill, J.** and **Campbell, K. R.** Ground reaction forces in children's gait. *Pediatric Exercise Science* 1989; **1**: 45–53.

34. **Frost, G., Bar-Or, O., Dowling, J.** and **Dyson, K.** Explaining differences in the metabolic cost of locomotion among three age groups of children. *Medicine and Science in Sports and Exercise* 1996; **28**: S41.

35. **Rowland, TW.** *Developmental exercise physiology.* Human Kinetics Publishers, Champaign Il, 1996; 182, 184, 193–214.

36. **Rowland, T. W.** Oxygen uptake and endurance fitness in children: A developmental perspective. *Pediatric Exercise Science* 1989; **1**: 313–28.

37. **Moritani, T., Oddsson, L., Thorstensson, A.** and **Åstrand, P-O.** Neural and biomechanical differences between men and young boys during a variety of motor tasks. *Acta Physiologica Scandinavica* 1989; **137**: 347–55.

38. **Davies, C. T. M.** Metabolic cost of exercise and physical performance in children with some observations on external loading. *European Journal of Applied Physiology* 1980; **45**: 95–102.

39. **Martin, P. E.** and **Morgan, D. W.** Biomechanical considerations for economical walking and running. *Medicine and Science in Sports and Exercise* 1992; **24**: 467–74.

40. **Ariens, G. A. M., Van Mechelen, W., Kemper, H. C. G.** and **Twisk, J. W. R.** The longitudinal development of running economy in males and females aged between 13 and 27 years: The Amsterdam Growth and Health Study. *European Journal of Applied Physiology* 1997; **76**: 214–20.

41. **Martinez, L. R.** and **Haymes, E. M.** Substrate utilization during treadmill running in prepubertal girls and women. *Medicine and Science in Sports* 1992; **24**: 975–83.

42. **Bar-Or, O.** *Pediatric sport medicine for the practitioner.* Springer Verlag, New York, 1983; 12–5.

43. **Taylor, C. R., Heglund, N. C.** and **Maloiy, G. M. O.** Energetics and mechanics of terrestrial locomotion. I. Metabolic energy consumption as a function of speed and body size in birds and mammals. *Journal of Experimental Biology* 1982; **97**: 1–21.

44. **Heglund, N. C.** and **Taylor, C. R.** Speed, stride frequency and energy cost per stride: How do they change with body size and gait? *Journal of Experimental Biology* 1988; **138**: 301–18.

45. **Taylor, C. R.** Force development during sustained locomotion: a determinant of gait, speed and metabolic power. *Journal of Experimental Biology* 1985; **115**: 253–62.

46. **Armstrong, N.** and **Welsman, J. R.** Assessment and interpretation of aerobic fitness in children and adolescents. *Exercise and Sport Sciences Reviews* 1994; **22**: 435–75.

47. **Welsman, J. R., Armstrong, N.** and **Nevill, A. M., Winter, E. M.** and **Kirby, B. J.** Scaling peak $\dot{V}O_2$ for differences in body size. *Medicine and Science in Sports and Exercise* 1996; **28**: 259–65.

48. **Rogers, D. M., Turley, K. R., Kujawa, K. I., Harper, K. M.** and **Wilmore, J. H.** Allometric scaling factors for oxygen uptake during exercise in children. *Pediatric Exercise Science* 1995; **7**: 12–25.

49. **Krahenbuhl, G. S., Skinner, J. S.** and **Kohrt, W. M.** Developmental aspects of maximal aerobic power in children. *Exercise and Sport Sciences Reviews* 1985; 503–38.

50. **Rowland, T. R.** The case of the elusive denominator. *Pediatric Exercise Science* 1998; **10**: 1–5.

51. **Cooper, D. M.** and **Berman, N.** Ratios and regressions in body size and function: A commentary. *Journal of Applied Physiology* 1994; 2015–7.

52. **Frost, G., Bar-Or, O., Dowling, J.** and **White, C.** Habituation of children to treadmill walking and running: metabolic and kinematic criteria. *Pediatric Exercise Science* 1995; **7**: 162–75.

53. **Unnithan, V. B., Murray, L. A., Timmons, J. A., Buchanan, D.** and **Paton, J. Y.** Reproducibility of cardiorespiratory measurements during submaximal and maximal running in children. *British Journal of Sports Medicine* 1995; **29**: 66–71.

54. **Rogers, D. M., Turley, K. R., Kujawa, K. I., Harper, K. M.** and **Wilmore, J. H.** The reliability and variability of running economy in 7-, 8-, and 9-year-old children. *Pediatric Exercise Science* 1994; **6**: 287–96.

55. **Keefer, D. J., Tseh, W., Caputo, J. L., Craig, I. S.** and **Morgan, D. W.** Stability of running economy in young children. *Medicine and Science in Sports and Exercise* 1998; **30**:S56.

56. **Tseh, W., Caputo, J. L., Craig, I. S., Keefer, D. J.** and **Morgan, D. W.** Metabolic accommodation of young children to treadmill walking. *Medicine and Science in Sports and Exercise* 1997; **29**: S205.

57. **Maffeis, C., Schutz, Y., Schena, F., Zaffanello, M.** and **Pinelli, L.** Energy expenditure during walking and running in obese and nonobese prepubertal children. *Journal of Pediatrics* 1993; **123**: 193–9.

58. **Morgan, D. W., Tseh, W., Caputo, J. L., Craig, I. S., Keefer, D. J.** and **Martin, P. E.** Sex differences in running economy of young children. *Pediatric Exercise Science* 1999; **11**: 122–8.

59. **Petray, C. K.** and **Krahenbuhl, G. S.** Running training, instruction on running technique, and running economy in 10-year-old males. *Research Quarterly for Exercise and Sport* 1985; **56**: 251–5.

60. **Lussier, L.** and **Buskirk, E. R.** Effects of an endurance training program on assessment of work capacity in prepubertal children. *Annals of the New York Academy of Sciences* 1977; **301**: 734–41.

61. **Sjödin, B.** and **Svedenhag, J.** Oxygen uptake during running as related to body mass in circumpubertal boys: A longitudinal study. *European Journal of Applied Physiology* 1992; **65**: 150–7.

62. **Krahenbuhl, G. S.** and **Pangrazi, R. P.** Characteristics associated with running performance in young boys. *Medicine and Science in Sports and Exercise* 1983; **15**: 486–90.

63. **Mayers, N.** and **Gutin, B.** Physiological characteristics of elite prepubertal cross-country runners. *Medicine and Science in Sports* 1979; **11**: 172–6.

64. **Cunningham, L.** Relationship of running economy, ventilatory threshold, and maximal oxygen consumption to running performance in high school females. *Research Quarterly for Exercise and Sport* 1990; **61**: 369–74.

65. **Morse, M., Schultz, F. W.** and **Cassels, D. E.** Relation of age to physiological responses of the older boy (10–17 years) to exercise. *Journal of Applied Physiology* 1949; **1**: 683–709.

66. **Eriksson, B. O., Gollnick, P. D.** and **Saltin, B.** Muscle metabolism and enzyme activities after training in boys 11–13 years old. *Acta Physiologica Scandinavica* 1973; **87**: 485–97.

67. **Eriksson, B. O., Karlsson, J.** and **Saltin, B.** Muscle metabolites during exercise in pubertal boys. *Acta Paediatrica Scandinavica* 1971; **217**: 154–7.

68. **Cumming, G. R., Hastman, L., McCort, J.** and **McCullough, S.** High serum lactates do occur in young children after maximal work. *International Journal of Sport Medicine* 1980; **1**: 66–9.

69. **Zanconato, S., Buchtal, S., Barstow, T. J.** and **Cooper, D. M.** 31P-magnetic resonance spectroscopy of leg muscle metabolism during exercise in children and adults. *Journal of Applied Physiology* 1993; **74**: 2214–8.

70. **Corcoran, P. J.** and **Brengelmann, G. L.** Oxygen uptake in normal and handicapped subjects, in relation to speed of walking beside velocity-controlled cart. *Archives of Physical Medicine and Rehabilitation* 1970; **51**: 78–87.

71. Ralston, H.J. Energy-speed relation and optimal speed during level walking. *Internationale Zeitschrift fur angewandte Physiologie einschlieblich Arbeitsphysiologie* 1958; **17**: 277–83.

72. Morgan, D. W., Martin, P. E., Tseh, W., Caputo, J. L., Craig, I. S. and Keefer, D. J. Relationship between preferred and energetically optimal walking speeds in young children. *Medicine and Science in Sports and Exercise* 1997; **29**: S16.

73. Evans, E. P. and Tew, B. The energy expenditure of spina bifida children during walking and wheelchair ambulation. *Zeitschrift feur Kinderchirurgie* 1981; **34**: 425–7.

74. Herbert, L. M., Engsberg, J. R., Tedford, K .G. and Grimston, S. K. A comparison of oxygen consumption during walking between children with and without below-knee amputations. *Physical Therapy* 1994; **74**: 943–50.

75. Gage, J. R. *Gait analysis in cerebral palsy.* MacKeith Press, London, 1991: 1,129.

76. Rose, J., Gamble, J. G., Medeiros, J., Burgos, A. and Haskell, W. L. Energy cost of walking in normal children and in those with cerebral palsy: Comparison of heart rate and oxygen uptake. *Journal of Pediatric Orthopaedics* 1989; **9**: 276–9.

77. Rose, J., Gamble, J. G., Burgos, A., Medeiros, J. and Haskell, W. L. Energy expenditure index of walking for normal children and for children with cerebral palsy. *Developmental Medicine and Child Neurology* 1990; **32**: 333–40.

78. Rose, J., Haskell, W. L. and Gamble, J. G. A comparison of oxygen pulse and respiratory exchange ratio in cerebral palsied and nondisabled children. *Archives of Physical Medicine and Rehabilitation* 1993; **74**: 702–5.

79. Unnithan, V., Dowling, J., Frost, G. and Bar-Or, O. Role of cocontraction in the O_2 cost of walking in children with cerebral palsy. *Medicine and Science in Sports and Exercise* 1996; **28**: 1498–504.

80. Falconer, K. and Winter, D. Quantitative assessment of co-contraction at the ankle joint in walking. *Electromyography and Clinical Neurophysiology* 1985; **25**: 135–49.

81. Jeng, S., Holt, K., Fetters, L. and Certo, C. Self-optimization of walking in nondisabled children and children with spastic hemiplegic cerebral palsy. *Journal of Motor Behavior* 1996; **28**: 15–27.

82. Winter, D. A. *Biomechanics and motor control of human movement.* John Wiley and Sons, New York, 1990: 115.

83. Campbell, J. and Ball, J. Energetics of walking in cerebral palsy. *Orthopedic Clinics of North America* 1978; **9**: 374–7.

84. Wiley, M. E. and Damiano, D. L. Lower-extremity strength profiles in spastic cerebral palsy. *Developmental Medicine and Child Neurology* 1998; **40**: 100–7.

85. MacPhail, H. E. A. and Kramer J. F. Effect of isokinetic strength-training on functional ability and walking efficiency in adolescents with cerebral palsy. *Developmental Medicine and Child Neurology* 1995; **37**: 763–75.

86. Carmick, J. Clinical use of neuromuscular electrical stimulation for children with cerebral palsy, Part 1: Lower extremity. *Physical Therapy* 1993; **73**: 505–13.

87. Krahenbuhl, G. S. and Williams, T. J. Running economy: changes with age during childhood and adolescence. *Medicine and Science in Sports and Exercise* 1992; **24**: 462–6.

2.10 Kinetics of pulmonary oxygen uptake

J. Alberto Neder and Brian J. Whipp

Introduction

With respect to the physical activity patterns of children engaged in spontaneous play or even organized games, the steady-state may be considered to be a contrivance of investigative convenience. It is important therefore to consider the physiological responses of children to increased metabolic demands with respect to their dynamic features. Furthermore, the bulk of the information regarding the control of physiological function relies in its transient, or non-steady state, response to an appropriate forcing regime. In addition, although the work rate challenges utilized in laboratory investigations of system-response dynamics are themselves typically remote from those of every day activity, they do offer the advantage of a standardized means of characterizing the response kinetics.

The analysis of the transient response characteristics of an organ system of interest can be used as a basis for assembling a physiological model of the system's control. This is exemplified by consideration of the oxygen uptake ($\dot{V}O_2$) response to constant-load exercise. In the steady state the amplitude of this response as a function of the work rate increment is largely independent of gender, age, physical 'fitness' or training status[1]—at least over the work-rate range within which there is not a sustained metabolic acidaemia (i.e. below the subject's lactate threshold, θ_L).[2,3] The transient behaviour, however, can be appreciably different, such that the $\dot{V}O_2$ increases more rapidly in 'fit' or endurance-trained subjects, whereas the transient response is slower in healthy, but non-trained subjects[4] (especially in the aged),[5–7] and also in patients with various cardiopulmonary disorders.[8–14] Even at this simplified level of characterization, these response differences provoke four important questions:

1. What are the physiological control mechanisms which produce this pattern of response in the non-steady state?
2. Why are these responses affected by sedentary, training or disease?
3. What are the consequences of the different response profile for the demands on the energy transfer mechanisms?
4. Do the responses dynamics exhibit maturational characteristics?

Fundamentals of pulmonary gas exchange dynamics

In order to sustain muscular activity, the lungs must transfer O_2 into the blood at rates commensurate with the mean rate of muscle utilization ($\dot{Q}O_2$) and also clear the consequent carbon dioxide at rates appropriate to regulate acid–base status.

The oxygen uptake by the lungs ($\dot{V}O_2$) is determined by the pulmonary blood flow (which, in absence of right-to-left intra-cardiac shunt, is equal to the cardiac output) and the mixed-venous to arterial O_2 content difference. However, it is only in the steady state that the increase in $\dot{V}O_2$ equals that of $\dot{Q}O_2$. In the non-steady state phase $\dot{V}O_2$ is dissociated from muscle $\dot{V}O_2$:

(1) temporally, as a result of the muscle-to-lung transit delay;
(2) in its rate of change, as any given value for the arterio-venous O_2 content difference established in the muscle will be associated with a higher blood flow at the lungs (that is, the cardiac output will have increased during the transit delay); and
(3) in magnitude, as a result of the muscle's utilization of stored O_2.[15]

The rate of $\dot{V}O_2$ increase during the transient will therefore depend upon:

(1) the dynamics of the cardiac output and pulmonary blood flow responses;
(2) the dynamics of tissue metabolic exchange; and
(3) the wash-in or wash-out of the gas in the accessible body stores.[15]

These complexities must be considered when interpreting the kinetics of pulmonary gas exchange.

However, interpretations of the response dynamics can be misleading, unless considered with respect to the intensity of the exercise. For example, the response profile of the pulmonary gas exchange variables differs in different intensity domains of aerobic function. In this respect, it is useful to consider four domains which are partitioned by three important parameters of functional capacity for work. These parameters are:

(1) the lactate threshold (θ_L), which is defined as the highest $\dot{V}O_2$ that can be achieved without a sustained metabolic acidosis associated with increased muscle and blood lactate;[2]
(2) the critical power or 'fatigue threshold' (θ_F), this is the asymptote of the power-duration curve for high-intensity exercise.[16] It has been found to coincide with the highest supra-θ_L work rate for which a steady-state of $\dot{V}O_2$ and blood lactate is attainable, even though delayed compared with the sub-θ_L profile;[17] and
(3) the maximum $\dot{V}O_2$ ($\mu\dot{V}O_2$), commonly agreed to represent the upper limit of the body's current ability for O_2 utilization.

The range of work rates for which the required $\dot{V}O_2$ is less than θ_L will be considered to be of *moderate* intensity; between θ_L and θ_F as *heavy* intensity; work rates requiring $\dot{V}O_2$ greater than θ_F but lower than $\mu\dot{V}O_2$ as *very heavy* intensity; and work rates requiring $\dot{V}O_2$ in excess of $\mu\dot{V}O_2$ as *severe* intensity (Fig. 2.10.1).[15,18]

Moderate exercise

The oxygen equivalent of the energy which was utilized during the exercise but which did not derive from reactions fuelled by atmospheric O_2 (i.e. taken into the body *after* the start of the exercise) has been termed the oxygen deficit (O_2def). It should be noted that quantifying the O_2def requires both a precise characterization of the

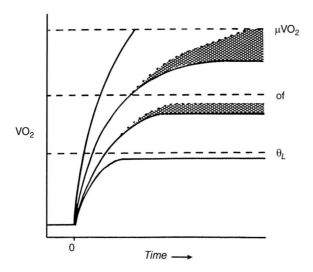

Fig. 2.10.1 Pulmonary oxygen uptake ($\dot{V}O_2$) response to constant work rates (WR) of different intensities. θ_L is the lactate threshold that separates moderate from heavy intensity; θ_f is the fatigue threshold or 'critical power' that separates heavy from very heavy exercise; and $\mu\dot{V}O_2$ is the maximum oxygen uptake, typically attained in response to severe exercise. Note that all WR above θ_L elicit $\dot{V}O_2$ requirements higher than the projected by the sub-θ_L VO_2 – WR relationship (slow phase of $\dot{V}O_2$ kinetics, stippled area); above θ_f, if time is sufficient, $\mu\dot{V}O_2$ can actually be attained. In the severe domain, the slow phase may not have time to develop and so the exponential response is truncated by $\mu\dot{V}O_2$.

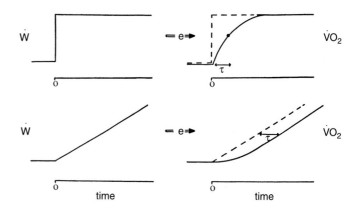

Fig. 2.10.2 Schematic representation of a mono-exponential $\dot{V}O_2$ profile in response to constant-load (*upper panel*) and ramp-incremental (*lower panel*) exercising protocols. The $\dot{V}O_2$ response to ramp exercise lags the actual $\dot{V}O_2$ requirement for a given WR by the time constant (τ) of the system. Reproduced from Whipp,[79] with permission.

non-steady-state O_2 response, and also a major assumption. For constant-load exercise, the assumption is that the energy demands throughout the non-steady state phase are precisely equivalent to those which obtain during the aerobic steady state.

Muscle $\dot{Q}O_2$ is expected to increase exponentially during exercise in proportion to the rate of decrease in creatine phosphate (PCr) concentration (details of the competing theories for this control process can be found in references 19 to 22). In fact, the transient time course of response for these variables are often implicitly taken to be surrogates of each other. This provides the basis for the exponential profile of pulmonary $\dot{V}O_2$. That is, its instantaneous rate of change ($d\dot{V}O_2/dt$) will be proportional to the difference between the steady-state requirement ($\dot{V}O_2(SS)$) and the instantaneous $\dot{V}O_2$ value ($\dot{V}O_2(t)$), i.e.

$$d\dot{V}O_2/dt \propto (\dot{V}O_2(SS) - \dot{V}O_2(t)) \tag{1}$$

or

$$d\dot{V}O_2/dt = k(\dot{V}O_2(SS) - \dot{V}O_2(t)) \tag{2}$$

The proportionality constant (k) is termed the rate constant: its inverse, as shown in Fig. 2.10.2, being the time constant (τ, i.e. the time to reach 63% of the asymptotic value). The time constant is therefore a crucial determinant of the response dynamics, i.e.:

$$\Delta \dot{V}O_2(t) = \Delta \dot{V}O_2(SS)(1 - e^{-t/\tau}) \tag{3}$$

Consequently, over the range in which steady states may be attained, the magnitude of the O_2def is exclusively determined by the steady state requirement and the time constant, i.e.:

$$O_2 def = \Delta \dot{V}O_2(SS)\tau \tag{4}$$

In reality, however, $\dot{V}O_2$ during constant-load exercise does not change with the simple exponential characteristics showed in the upper panel of Fig. 2.10.2. Rather, there is an early phase of $\dot{V}O_2$ (ϕI), which is closely associated with the increase in cardiac output, which occurs prior to blood with greater O_2 extraction (as a result of the muscle contraction) reaching the lung. During this period, the increase in $\dot{V}O_2$ can be considered to be 'cardiodynamic' as it is predominantly a reflection of the increase in cardiac output or pulmonary blood flow.[23]

Before the steady state (ϕIII) response is reached, a second phase (ϕII) develops as a result of an additional effect of the increased O_2 extraction in the blood perfusing the contracting muscles (Fig. 2.10.3). This two-phased feature of the non-steady-state $\dot{V}O_2$ response introduces a delay-like component (δ) into the response characterization, i.e.

$$\Delta \dot{V}O_2(t) = \Delta \dot{V}O_2(SS)(1 - e^{t - \delta/\tau}) \tag{5}$$

This equation, provides a 'better' characterization of the response dynamics than equation (3) and still allows an accurate quantification of the O_2def, i.e.

$$O_2 def = \Delta \dot{V}O_2(SS)(\tau + \delta) \tag{6}$$

The sum of $\tau + \delta$, as in equation (6) has been termed the mean response time (MRT) or the 'effective' time constant (τ') to the system response. As discussed below, the distinction between the actual τ and the τ' or MRT for the entire response has significant implications for the physiological inferences which can be drawn from the transient response. This τ' is not an accurate depiction of the real non-steady-state response dynamics, as schematized in Fig. 2.10.3. Furthermore, it is important to recognize that from a physiological standpoint, this δ is entirely factitious—it is *not* the limb-to-lung transit delay.

Consequently, those interested in using the response parameters to quantify the O_2def may use either equations (4) or (6) for accurate quantification. Those interested in the control of the non-steady state $\dot{V}O_2$ dynamics, however, need a more precise characterization of the response.

Two approaches have been made to this problem. Both Hughson[24] and Barstow et al.[25] have attempted to characterize the entire non-steady response with a six parameter model (i.e. two delays, two

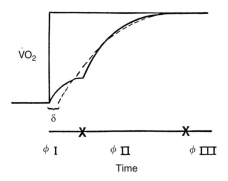

Fig. 2.10.3 Schematic representation of the actual $\dot{V}O_2$ response to sub-θ_L constant-load exercise (*solid line*): after the muscle-to-lung transit delay (ϕI), $\dot{V}O_2$ increases mono-exponentially (ϕII), towards the steady-state requirement (ϕIII). The best-fit mono-exponential (*dashed line*) with a delay term (δ) is also depicted: note that this mathematical representation is not the same as the physiological ϕI duration. Reproduced from Whipp,[79] with permission.

time constants and two proportional gains). However, Whipp *et al.*[26] have proposed the strategy of deleting the 'cardiodynamic' ϕI $\dot{V}O_2$ component from the exponential fit, arguing that there is no sufficiently sound evidence to support the exponentiality of the ϕI component. Both these approaches, however, support the concept that inferences for the control of $\dot{V}O_2$ during the non-steady state of muscular exercise require fitting procedures that appropriately characterize the τ of the $\dot{V}O_2$ response.

The energy transfer throughout the transient therefore can be considered to be the constant sum of a progressively increasing measured $\dot{V}O_2$ and a proportionally decreasing component from the O_2def mechanisms. It is therefore instructive to consider the source and potential magnitude of the physiological determinants of the O_2def. Over the moderate work-rate range, the O_2def is determined to a large extent by the available high-energy phosphate stores and the usable O_2 stores. In a typical adult, for example, the intramuscular PCr stores are approximately $20-22$ mmol kg^{-1} (wet weight); at maximum exercise this may fall to levels as low as 2 mmol kg^{-1}. Taking the muscle mass at the knee extensors to be some 5 kg,[27] a value double this for the muscle mass utilized during cycle ergometry would seem reasonable. Consequently, a 10 kg muscle mass with its PCr pool being depleted by some 20 mmol kg^{-1} results in approximately 200 mmol of a high-energy phosphate being available for the deficit. The muscles' ATP concentrations, which are normally only one-quarter or less that of PCr in human muscle, do not decrease appreciably until extremely high work rates. Consequently, as $\sim P{:}O_2 \cong 6$, this results in approximately 33 mmol of O_2 equivalent. Therefore, as each mmol of O_2 is equal to 22.4 ml, then the O_2 equivalent of the total depletable high-energy phosphate pool is approximately 750 ml. Naturally, only a small fraction of this will be utilized during moderate exercise.

The other alactic source of the O_2def is that taken from the O_2 stores: this is manifest predominantly as a decreased mixed-venous O_2 content. Considering an adult with a 3 litre venous blood volume, and a reduction in CvO_2 from 150 ml litre^{-1} at rest to some 50 ml litre^{-1} during high-intensity exercise, then the deficit equivalent of the usable O_2 stores will be 300 ml (i.e. 3 litre $\times$ 100 ml litre^{-1}). The O_2 solubility is low in plasma and muscle water (approximately 0.6 ml litre^{-1} muscle water/20 mmHg reduction in muscle tissue PO_2). Consequently, this component can be considered to be a trace quantity compared with respect to the total amount of O_2 used in the transient. Also, as the myoglobin, in the red muscle fibres, has a P50 of approximately 2.5 to 3.0 mmHg at physiological temperatures,[28] this is unlikely to contribute to any appreciable extent until extremely high levels of exercise. Even then, assuming that half of the total available myoglobin, at 25 mg g^{-1} dry weight,[29] is depleted of its O_2, this would only contribute to approximately 40 ml of the O_2def.

The total O_2def available from these sources at high levels of exercise in the adult, therefore, is only of the order of approximately 1.1 litre (750 + 300 + 40 ml). In a subject with an τ' of 30 s, this is equivalent to a work rate of approximately 200 W before the depletable alactic sources of O_2def are, in fact, depleted. For those with a τ' of 1 min, such as normal elderly subjects or younger subjects detrained as a result of cardiopulmonary disease, it would naturally occur at an appreciably lower work rate, approximately 100 W. Obviously, in children the available alactic sources will be reduced in proportion to the smaller muscle and venous blood volume (see below).

Heavy and very heavy exercise

In order to calculate a valid O_2def the actual steady-state O_2 requirement of the exercise must be known. This poses no problems for moderate exercise as the steady-state value serves as an appropriate frame of reference for the dynamic $\dot{V}O_2$ response profile. On the other hand, for heavy and very-heavy exercise intensities, recent literature consistently confirms that the asymptotic value of $\dot{V}O_2$ may not be constant but can vary as a function of time.[15,30–32] It is crucial, therefore, to consider the role of the intensity domain within which the $\dot{V}O_2$ kinetics are determined. For example, there is general agreement (for adults, at least) that first-order kinetics for $\dot{V}O_2$ are only manifest at work rates which do not engender a sustained lactic acidaemia.[33] At higher work rates (heavy-intensity exercise), the steady state for $\dot{V}O_2$ in response to constant-load exercise is delayed as a consequence of the addition of a 'slow' component, which causes $\dot{V}O_2$ to increase to values greater than those predicted from extrapolation of the sub-θ_L $\dot{V}O_2$–WR relationship.

Typically, this slow phase appears to develop only some 80 to 120 seconds after exercise onset and subsequently this component of the response is superimposed upon the 'fundamental' exponential.[15,25,30–34] Although the precise mechanisms which contribute to the slow component are largely speculative, the primary origin appears to be the working limbs,[34] with a magnitude and time course closely *correlated* with the rise in the arterial blood lactate.[33] Therefore, the supra-θ_L work-rate range within which steady states of $\dot{V}O_2$ can be attained has been shown to be commensurate with the work-rate range over which blood [lactate] and [H^+] do not continue to increase as the work continues.[17] The upper limit of this intensity domain has been termed the maximum lactate steady state (MLSS). Interestingly, the data of Poole *et al.*[17] suggest that the work-rate equivalent of the MLSS coincides with the power asymptote (θ_F) of the hyperbolic power–duration relationship for high-intensity dynamic exercise, i.e.:

$$W' = (W - \theta_F)t \qquad (7)$$

where t is time in seconds and W' is equivalent to a constant amount of work that can be performed above the asymptote, regardless its rate of performance. This relationship can be resolved for W and transformed into its linear formulation by taking the reciprocal of time[17]:

$$W = W'/t + \theta_F \qquad (8)$$

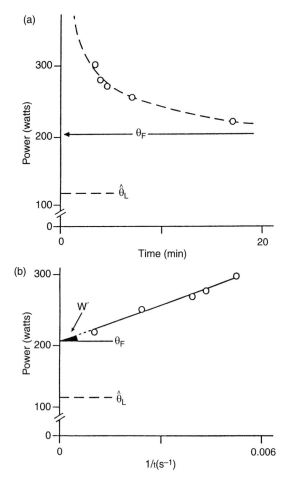

Fig. 2.10.4 (a) The power–duration (b) (W–t) relationship for five exhausting exercise bouts in a single subject. The relationship after linearization using the reciprocal of time as the abscissa. The hyperbolic shape of W–t is reflected by the constancy of the slope W′ (with units of work). The critical power (θ_f) is the y-intercept and corresponds to the asymptote of the W–t relationship. This typically lies above the subject's anaerobic threshold (θ_L).

in which W' and θ_F are the slope and intercept, respectively (Fig. 2.10.4). Although the precise physiological equivalents of those parameters remains to be elucidated, θ_F may be considered to represent the maximum sustainable rate of aerobic ATP repletion and W' equivalent to a finite store of accessible energy.

At work rates above MLSS, therefore, steady states of $\dot{V}O_2$ are not attained; $\dot{V}O_2$ typically continues to increase towards $\mu\dot{V}O_2$. In other words, with exercise of very-heavy intensity neither $\dot{V}O_2$ nor blood [lactate] and [H^+] can be stabilized. Rather they continue to increase until fatigue ensues, usually at, or close to, $\mu\dot{V}O_2$[35,36] as schematized in Fig. 2.10.1.

Severe exercise

In this domain, the exponential response profile is typically maintained up to a limiting maximal $\dot{V}O_2$ such that a steady state cannot be obtained and therefore the dynamic response is truncated by $\mu\dot{V}O_2$.

Under these conditions, the O_2 deficit is determined by the product of the $\dot{V}O_2$ max and the time constant, i.e.:

$$O_2 def = \mu\dot{V}O_2\tau \qquad (9)$$

In the moderate intensity domain, therefore, the O_2def increases as a linear function of work rate (equation (4)). Interestingly, however, in the severe domain the O_2def becomes constant for all work rates in which the mono-exponential kinetics project to $\dot{V}O_2 > \mu\dot{V}O_2$ (equation (9)).

Other dynamic work rate profiles have also been used to establish the features of the control of O_2 uptake kinetics, these include the ramp, impulse, sinusoid and pseudo-random binary sequences. The ramp is by far the most commonly used of those profiles. The ramp work-rate protocol[37] allows, in theory, the four key parameters that establish a subject's aerobic profile to be determined from a single exercise bout ($\mu\dot{V}O_2$, θ_L, work efficiency or η and τ'). In contrast to a square-wave protocol in which a constant work rate is imposed, a constant *rate of change* of work rate is produced by the ergometer in the ramp format—with the time to also achieve a constant *rate of change* of response being relevant. The ramp can be considered the limiting condition of the incremental test, in which the increments of power are imposed over such a short interval of time that their small instantaneous amplitude makes them indiscernible by the subject. In response to this type of test, $\dot{V}O_2(t)$ lags $\dot{V}O_2(SS)$. Eventually, however, the lag becomes constant (as $t >> \tau'$), with the measured $\dot{V}O_2$ being delayed from the steady-state requirement by τ' but with the same slope (Fig. 2.10.2, lower panel), i.e.

$$\Delta\dot{V}O_2(t) = \Delta\dot{V}O_2(SS) \text{ at } (t - \tau') \qquad (10)$$

Above θ_L the additional slow and delayed component of $\dot{V}O_2$, is virtually undetectable during ramp and rapid-incremental tests. However, the additional cost of supra-θ_L exercise becomes evident in incremental exercise tests when the duration of each increment is relatively long,[38] and even on ramp tests with slow rates of work-rate change.[39] The result is a curvilinear response of $\dot{V}O_2$ in this region, which is concave upwards, manifesting a reduced work efficiency for heavy exercise—even disregarding the simultaneous anaerobic energy transfer.

Oxygen uptake kinetics in children

Moderate exercise

A high degree of technical rigour is required to establish the characteristic features of the kinetic responses from the non-steady-state profile of $\dot{V}O_2$ in children. This is because the confidence with which the $\dot{V}O_2$ kinetics can be estimated is dependent in large part on the response amplitude ($\Delta\dot{V}O_2(SS)$).[40] This is, naturally, smaller in children than in adults, especially within the domain for which first-order kinetics are likely to obtain. In addition, the available high-energy phosphate stores are less in the paediatric group than in adults as a result of the smaller muscle mass. Similarly, the O_2 stores are less, as a result of the smaller blood and hence venous blood volume. It is reasonable to hypothesize, therefore, that as the depletable alactic deficit stores will be smaller, anaerobiosis will become obligatory at relatively low work rates unless the $\dot{V}O_2$ kinetics are appropriately rapid (i.e. a faster τ).

Cooper and his associates,[41] using ramp-incremental exercise, attempted to characterize the four aerobic parameters as a function of body size during growth in 109 healthy children in the age range 6 to 17 y (51 girls and 58 boys). They found that θ_L, as a fraction of $\mu\dot{V}O_2$, was independent of body mass in both sexes. Others,[42–45] however, have found that this ratio was high in young children and decreases with age (e.g. Fig. 2.10.5). With respect to the kinetics of $\dot{V}O_2$, Cooper et al. found that the τ was independent of body mass in children and adolescents, with a mean value of 43 ± 15 s. This is not significantly different from that for healthy young adults.[26]

These authors further investigated the kinetics of the $\dot{V}O_2$ response to dynamic exercise in children utilizing the averaged results of multiple repetitions of identical sub-θ_L constant-load exercise bouts.[46] This is an important procedure, as it improves the confidence with which the time constant can be estimated.[40] They demonstrated in this group that there was no differernce between the on-transient τ (i.e. they deleted the ϕI response from their model fit) for the ϕII $\dot{V}O_2$ kinetics for 7 to 9 year old children and 15 to 18 year old teenagers (τ $\dot{V}O_2$ values of 26.5 and 28 s, respectively; Fig. 2.10.6.). Although the older girls had significantly higher τ $\dot{V}O_2$ values than the other groups, their lower maximum aerobic power suggests that the longer time constants were reflective of lower 'fitness' than the other groups, as aerobic fitness is well-known to be associated with faster $\dot{V}O_2$ kinetics.[4]

The findings of Cooper et al.[46] are in agreement with those of Sady et al.[47] who found that the half-times for the $\dot{V}O_2$ response to constant load exercise, at approximately 40% of the $\mu\dot{V}O_2$ (i.e. plausibly sub-θ_L), were not significantly different between children and adults. The values for the half-times averaged 18.5 and 17.4 s, respectively. This is equivalent to 26.6 and 25.5 for the response time constants (for a mono-exponential process $\tau = 1.44 \times t_{1/2}$), and agrees closely with the values reported by Cooper et al.[46] Freedson et al.[48] also did not find a difference in the dynamics of the $\dot{V}O_2$ response to constant-load exercise in 28 children (mean age of 10.2 y) compared to other data for adults exercising ostensibly at the same intensity. However, the children all cycled at a work rate of 59 W. This represented 60.8% of the $\mu\dot{V}O_2$, which is close to the expected θ_L for this age group (Fig. 2.10.5). These studies therefore provide consistent support for the hypothesis that the kinetics of $\dot{V}O_2$ for sub-θ_L exercise are independent of size and age during growth.

While Zanconato et al.[49] were unable to discern differences in the $t_{1/2}$ of the $\dot{V}O_2$ response between children (7 to 11 y) and adults (26 to 42 y) to 1 min exercise bouts, the off-transient kinetics were faster in children than in adults, but only in response to supramaximal work rates. The cumulative O_2 cost for both exercise and recovery was lower in adults (mlO$_2$ J^{-1}): a consequence of the high $\Delta\dot{V}O_2$(SS) in children at this intensity (Fig. 2.10.7). However, inferences for the on-transient from the off-transient should be made with caution since Paterson and Whipp,[50] Gerbino et al.[31] and Hughson[24] have all found dynamic asymmetries of the $\dot{V}O_2$ kinetics between the on- and off-transient in adults. Whether this also obtains in children remains to be determined.

Heavy and very heavy exercise

In children, as for adults, the kinetics of $\dot{V}O_2$ are likely to be different in these work-intensity domains than for moderate exercise. However,

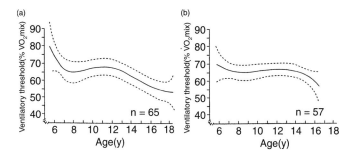

Fig. 2.10.5 Estimated anaerobic threshold (% of $\dot{V}O_2$ max) in a cross-sectional evaluation of 65 boys (a) and 57 girls (b). Dashed lines are the 95% confidence intervals. Higher values were found in younger children, notably boys, and declined non-linearly with age. Reproduced from Reybrouck et al.,[43] with permission.

detailing these kinetic responses presents a formidable technical challenge. As the ratio of the θ_L to $\mu\dot{V}O_2$ has been shown to be either independent of size and growth[41] or is even higher in younger children[42–45] (e.g. Figs 2.10.5 and 2.10.8), the absolute difference (Δ) between θ_L and $\mu\dot{V}O_2$ will be progressively less the younger and smaller the child. The absolute work-rate equivalents of these intensity domains, therefore, will be very small, and hence will present a challenge to the technique for discriminating the kinetic features. Elucidating finer details of the dynamic $\dot{V}O_2$ response may therefore require precise placement of the particular work rate into a given intensity domain (which is small, absolutely, in children), and also require that confidence limits on the estimated dynamic parameters be established to ensure that a statistically justifiable discrimination is used to corroborate apparent differences.

Several features of the dynamics of the $\dot{V}O_2$ response at high work rates in children are emerging, however. Beneke et al.,[51] for example, have carefully determined the MLSS throughout the second decade of life. The results are consistent with the MLSS being independent of age (Fig. 2.10.9) and occurring at a value of approximately 4 mmol litre^{-1}. This is similar to the average value found in adults, although marked individual differences are apparent in both groups. The absolute work rate at which the maximum lactate steady state occurred, however, increased as a linear function of age. In contrast, other authors have found that a 4 mmol litre^{-1} value is excessively high for a representative MLLS in children. Williams and Armstrong[52] proposed 2.5 mmol litre^{-1} to be a better value for children, i.e. consistent with their previous demonstration that the 4 mmol litre^{-1} value occurred, on average, at greater than 90% of $\mu\dot{V}O_2$ in 103 boys and girls, aged 11 to 13 y[53] (see Chapter 1.7). These issues underscore the importance of the intensity domain within which the $\dot{V}O_2$ kinetics are considered for a particular subject, rather than for the mean or modally-representative child or adult.

Asano and Hirakoba,[54] Macek and Vavra[55] and Rowland and Rimany[56] have all considered the slow phase of the O_2 kinetics. At work rates equivalent to some 60 to 65% of $\mu\dot{V}O_2$, there was no difference in the magnitude of the slow phase between boys and adult men, and between premenarcheal girls and adult women. The mean increase in $\dot{V}O_2$ between boys aged 10 y and men aged 40 to 60 y was 8 to 11% among the studies, with no differences between the children and adults. However, these results should be interpreted with caution since the magnitude of the slow phase is strongly influenced by

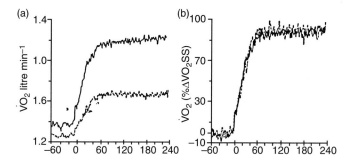

Fig. 2.10.6 Mean $\dot{V}O_2$ responses to sub-θ_L constant-load exercise grouped by age in children (7 to 9 y, dashed lines) and teenagers (15 to 18 y, solid lines): absolute (a) and normalized (b) responses relative to the steady-state asymptotic values (SS). Reproduced from Cooper et al.,[46] with permission.

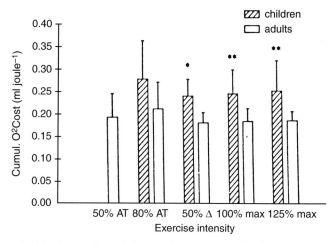

Fig. 2.10.7 Comparison of the cumulative O_2 cost (ml J^{-1}) at different work intensities between children and adults. AT is the anaerobic threshold and Δ is the difference between $\dot{V}O_2$ max and AT (*$P < 0.001$, **$P < 0.01$). Reproduced from Armon et al.,[57] with permission.

whether a particular work rate is sub- or supra-θ_F (Fig. 2.10.1). As discussed below, there is some evidence that the work rate at which θ_F occurs relative to $\mu\dot{V}O_2$ is different between children and adults, i.e. higher in children.

In contrast, Armon et al.[57] have demonstrated that the amplitude of the early exponential increase in $\dot{V}O_2$ during high-intensity exercise is actually greater in children than in adults. However, this was associated with a smaller additional increment in $\dot{V}O_2$ in children ('excess' $\dot{V}O_2$) (Fig. 2.10.10). Their finding of a high O_2 cost of work in children supports the previous results of Zanconato et al.[49]

The intramuscular determinants of $\dot{V}O_2$ during exercise were also addressed in another study by Zanconato et al.[58] Here, they compared the profiles of inorganic phosphate (Pi) to PCr (Pi/PCr) and pH in the calf muscle of children and adults performing incremental plantar-flexion exercise using ^{31}P magnetic resonance (MR) spectroscopy. They demonstrated a slow and a fast phase of both the Pi/PCr increase and the pH decrease as shown in Fig. 2.10.11 in 75% of the adults and 50% of the children. The slopes of the initial linear phase, however, were not different between groups: this is consistent with the determinants of the early $\dot{V}O_2$ kinetics not being discernibly different between the children and the adults in the moderate intensity domain. However, the subsequent more-rapid rate of change was appreciably greater in the adults, such that at high work rates the intramuscular pH was higher and the Pi/PCr ratios lower in children than in adults. These findings are consistent with the numerous reports of the relatively low blood lactate response to high-intensity exercise (Fig. 2.10.8), and also with reduced anaerobic enzymatic activity, in children compared with adults.[59-63] Pianosi et al.,[62] for example, demonstrated that the lactate/pyruvate ratio (L:P) during exercise at 70% of $\mu\dot{V}O_2$ increased as a linear function of age in 28 children and teenagers between 7 and 17 y. Kuno and his associates[64] have also presented ^{31}P-MR spectroscopic evidence of a reduced muscle glycolytic ability during exhausting exercise in children compared with adults.

It is interesting to note that although the results from the classical study of Eriksson et al.[65] and, subsequently, Tanaka and Shindo[66] and Mero[67] are all consistent with maturational features in both PCr and muscle glycolytic enzymatic content, subsequent studies failed to show a close relationship between hormonal markers of pubescence and improvement in anaerobic capacity.[68,69] The postulated low glycolytic ability in children and adolescents could be related to differences in muscle fibre type i.e. a lower population of the fast twitch

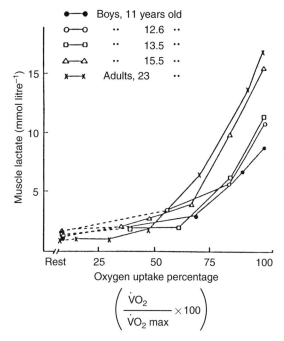

Fig. 2.10.8 Muscle lactate increase as a function of exercise intensity during incremental exercise in children and adults. Note that the inflection point is earlier and the absolute level higher the older the subject. Reproduced from Rowland,[80] with permission.

glycolytic (FT) fibres in children compared to the more oxidative slow twitch (ST) fibres (see Chapters 2.4 and 2.5). In fact, Fournier et al.[70] and Jansson and Hedberg[71] have both demonstrated a positive association between the population of FT fibres and age in adolescents. In this regard, it is of particular interest that Mizuno et al.,[72] using ^{31}P-MR spectroscopy found that forearm exercise in adults induced a pH reduction which was inversely related to the percentage of ST fibres. Since a smaller slow component is likely to be evident in a subject with

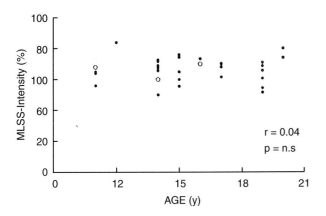

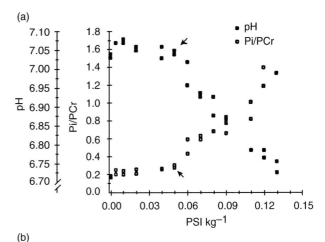

Fig. 2.10.9 The maximal lactate steady state value (MLSS, % of maximum exercise intensity) as a function of age. Reproduced from Beneke et al.,[51] with permission.

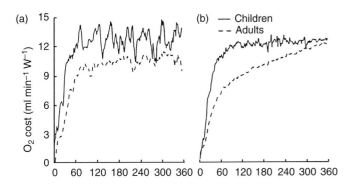

Fig. 2.10.10 Group mean O_2 cost for constant-load exercise at sub_θ_L (a) and supra-θ_L (b) in children (solid lines) and adults (dashed lines). Note (i) the higher cost of the work in children in both domains and (ii) the amplitude of the early exponential at supra_θ_L work rates being greater in children but with a smaller 'excess' $\dot{V}O_2$. Reproduced from Zanconato et al.,[49] with permission.

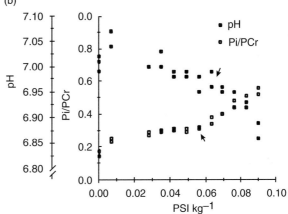

Fig. 2.10.11 Response profile of intramuscular Pi/PCr ratio and pH to incremental exercise as measured by ^{31}P magnetic resonance spectroscopy in an adult (a) and a child (b). Note that the inflection points (arrows) are of delayed-onset and the overall response is blunted in the child. Reproduced from Zanconato et al.,[58] with permission.

high ST/FT fibres ratio[73] (Fig. 2.10.12), these differences in fibre types could account, at least partially, for both the small magnitude of the slow component of $\dot{V}O_2$ and also the reduced glycolytic ability in the paediatric group.[74] On the other hand, Bell et al.[75] suggested that the higher availability of fat and intramuscular lipid stores in prepubescent children could reduce the proportional contribution of glycogen metabolism. While the precise mechanisms controlling the different response profiles remain to be definitively established, Cooper and Barstow[74] were able to conclude, on the basis of the available evidence on both gas exchange dynamics and intramuscular high-energy phosphate kinetics, that children do seem to rely less on anaerobic glycolytic metabolism than adults during high-intensity exercise.

As discussed previously, the limit between heavy and very heavy exercise is of fundamental importance to the capacity for sustaining endurance exercise. The detailed kinetic analysis of Armon et al.[57] provides evidence for children having a smaller proportional range between their θ_F or MLSS and their $\mu\dot{V}O_2$ than adults. These results confirm those of Gildein et al.[60] and Williams and Armstrong[52] who both found that the MLSS occurred at an average of 90% of $\mu\dot{V}O_2$ in

children. The issue of subject 'effort' is naturally of concern here. The small difference between both θ_L and θ_F and the maximum $\dot{V}O_2$ in children, coupled with the low level of maximal blood lactate are consistent with what may be termed 'lack of effort'. It seems unlikely, however, that this would be such a consistent finding from different laboratories. Furthermore, Armstrong et al.[76] have shown that there is no significant difference among the highest $\dot{V}O_2$ attained with incremental and two different high-intensity work rates (Fig. 2.10.13). This and the similar results found by Rowland,[77] while naturally not conclusive, is highly suggestive of similarly maximum effort among the tests. In summary, the available evidence is highly suggestive of maturational features of the anaerobic potential in children,[78–80] although the relationship between this maturational process and sexual hormonal levels seems to be remote.[68–69]

Severe exercise

Interestingly, the conclusions about the response profiles of the $\dot{V}O_2$ kinetics in children during severe exercise differ from those obtained in studies performed in the moderate domain. At work rates requiring supramaximal $\dot{V}O_2$, Macek and Vavra,[55] for example, demonstrated

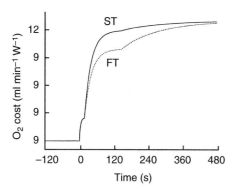

Fig. 2.10.12 Oxygen cost for exercise in two subjects with different muscle fibre proportions. The subject with predominantly slow-twitch (ST or type I) fibres in vastus lateralis presents higher amplitude in the initial response, but with less of a slow component of the kinetics compared to the subject with a high percentage of fast-twitch fibres (FT or type II). Reproduced from Coopes and Barstow,[74] with permission.

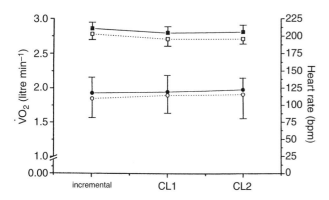

Fig. 2.10.13 Oxygen uptake (circles) and heart rate (squares) responses at exhaustion induced by an incremental protocol and two different bouts of constant-load (CL) exercise. Note that there was no significant difference among the maximum values for either peak $\dot{V}O_2$ or heart rate in either boys (filled symbols) and girls (open symbols). Data extracted from Armstrong et al.,[76] with permission.

that the $\dot{V}O_2$ on-transient during constant-load exercise was faster in 10 to 11 year old boys than in 20 to 22 year old men; Riner et al.[81] found that prepubescent boys and girls had faster $\dot{V}O_2$ kinetics ($t_{1/2}$) than adolescents; and Sady[82] demonstrated that ten year old boys had a faster $\dot{V}O_2$ response at the onset of exercise than adult men ($t_{1/2}$ of 17.2 and 28.5 s, respectively). On the other hand, Zanconato et al.[49] were unable to demonstrate differences in the $t_{1/2}$ of the $\dot{V}O_2$ response for very short exercise bouts (1 min) between children and adults at intensities up to 125% $\mu\dot{V}O_2$. Important methodological differences between studies performed at moderate or severe domains could account, at least partially, for the observed discrepancies. As described, the data of Cooper et al.,[46] Freedson et al.[48] and Sady et al.[47] considered the dynamic response to the steady state (moderate intensity domain) rather than the response to the system-limited maximum. In this context, it is important to recognize that a response to a system-limited value (i.e. $\mu\dot{V}O_2$) is fraught with complexities regarding the model assumptions. The asymptotic requirement for $\dot{V}O_2$ naturally increases

Table 2.10.1 Child–adult differences in the main parameters of aerobic function

Parameter	Child/adult
$\mu\dot{V}O_2$/lean body mass	>
$\theta_F/\mu\dot{V}O_2$	>
$\theta_L/\mu\dot{V}O_2$	>
A_{mod}	=
A_1	>
A_2	<
τ_1	<
τ_2	(?)

$\mu\dot{V}O_2$ = maximal oxygen uptake; θ_F = critical power or 'fatigue threshold'; θ_L = lactate threshold; τ = time constant; A = amplitude or gain; mod = moderate, sub-θ_L work rate; (1) = relative to the primary component of the $\dot{V}O_2$ kinetics (at supra-θ_L work rates); (2) = relative to the second component of the $\dot{V}O_2$ kinetics (at supra-θ_L work rates).

as a function of work rate even beyond $\mu\dot{V}O_2$: if the on-transient $\dot{V}O_2$ kinetics were independent of work rate, as was evident at the off-transient,[46] then the $t_{1/2}$ towards $\mu\dot{V}O_2$ would also necessarily increase with work rate, as the $\dot{V}O_2$ trajectory will be towards the *requirement* and not the attained maximum $\dot{V}O_2$.

Summary

We have attempted in this chapter to characterize current knowledge regarding the key features of the $\dot{V}O_2$ kinetics in response to dynamic exercise in children. As summarized in Table 2.10.1, there is strong evidence to suggest that the slow phase of the $\dot{V}O_2$ kinetics is less prominent in children than in adults and that the anaerobic potential seems to develop with age in the paediatric group, although at a different rate from the sexual maturation. On the other hand, the data are conflicting regarding the $\dot{V}O_2$ kinetics in the moderate-intensity exercise domain: some studies suggest that this response is faster in children than in adults, while others contend that there are no significant differences. Studies designed to elucidate further the mechanisms that control the $\dot{V}O_2$ kinetics in children require careful attention to the intensity domain under consideration, as small differences in work rate can shift the exercise to different intensity domain with major consequences for the analysis of the response kinetics.

References

1. **Wasserman, K.** and **Whipp, B. J.** Exercise physiology in health and disease. *American Review of Respiratory Diseases* 1975; **112**: 219–49.
2. **Wasserman, K., Beaver, W. L.** and **Whipp, B. J.** Gas exchange theory and the lactic acidosis (anaerobic) threshold. *Circulation* 1990; **81**: 14–36.
3. **Wasserman, K., Hansen, J. E., Sue, D. Y., Casaburi, R.** and **Whipp, B. J.** *Principles of exercise testing and interpretation* (2nd edn). Lea and Febiger, Philadelphia, 1994; 1–479.
4. **Henson, L. C., Poole, D. C.** and **Whipp, B. J.** Fitness as a determinant of oxygen uptake response to constant-load exercise. *European Journal of Applied Physiology* 1989; **59**: 21–8.

5. **Babcock, M. A., Paterson, D. H., Cunningham, D. A. and Dickinson, S. R.** Exercise on-transient gas exchange kinetics are slowed as a function of age. *Medicine and Science in Sports and Exercise* 1994; **26**: 440–6.
6. **Babcock, M. A., Paterson, D. H. and Cunningham, D. A.** Effects of aerobic endurance training on gas exchange kinetics of older men. *Medicine and Science in Sports and Exercise* 1994; **26**: 447–52.
7. **Chilibeck, P. D., Paterson, D. H., Cunningham, D. A., Taylor, A. W. and Noble, E. G.** Muscle capilarization, O_2 diffusion distance and $\dot{V}O_2$ kinetics in old and young individuals. *Journal of Applied Physiology* 1997; **82**: 63–9.
8. **Nery, L. E., Wasserman, K., Andrews, J. D., Huntsman, D. J., Hansen, J. E. and Whipp, B. J.** Ventilatory and gas exchange kinetics during exercise in chronic obstructive pulmonary disease. *Journal of Applied Physiology* 1982; **53**: 1594–602.
9. **Palange, P., Galassetti, P., Mannix, E. T., Farber, M. O., Manfredi, F. and Serra, P.** *et al.* Oxygen effect on O_2 deficit and $\dot{V}O_2$ kinetics during exercise in obstructive pulmonary disease. *Journal of Applied Physiology* 1995; **78**: 2228–34.
10. **Sietsema, K. E., Cooper, D. M., Rosove, M. A., Perloff, J. K., Chilo, J. S. and Canobbio, M. M.** *et al.* Dynamics of oxygen uptake during exercise in adults with cyanotic congenital heart disease. *Circulation* 1986; **73**: 1137–44.
11. **Sietsema, K. E., Ben-Dov, I., Zhang, Y. Y., Sullivan, C. and Wasserman, K.** Dynamics of oxygen uptake for submaximal exercise and recovery in patients with chronic heart failure. *Chest* 1994; **105**: 1693–700.
12. **Chelismeky-Fallick, C., Stenvenson, L. W., Lem, V. and Whipp, B. J.** Excessive oxygen deficit during low-level exercise in heart failure. *American Journal of Cardiology* 1995; **76**: 799–802.
13. **Cohen-Solal, A., Laperche, T., Morvan, D., Geneves, M., Caviezel, B. and Gourgon, R.** Prolonged kinetics of recovery of oxygen consumption after maximum graded exercise in patients with chronic heart failure. Analysis with gas exchange measurements and NMR spectroscopy. *Circulation* 1995; **91**: 2924–32.
14. **de Groote, P., Millaire, A., Decoulx, E., Nugue, O., Guimier, P. and Ducloux, D.** Kinetics of oxygen consumption during and after exercise in patients with dilated cardiomyopathy. New markers of exercise intolerance with clinical implications. *Journal of the American College of Cardiology* 1996; **28**: 168–75.
15. **Whipp, B. J. and Ward, S. A.** Physiological determinants of pulmonary gas exchange kinetics during exercise. *Medicine and Science in Sports and Exercise* 1990; **22**: 62–71.
16. **Moritani, T., Nagata, A., deVries, H. A. and Muro, M.** Critical power as a measure of physical work capacity and anaerobic threshold. *Ergonomics* 1981; **24**: 339–50.
17. **Poole, D. C., Ward, S. A., Gardner, G. W. and Whipp, B. J.** Metabolic and respiratory profile of the upper limit for prolonged exercise in man. *Ergonomics* 1988; **31**: 1265–79.
18. **Whipp, B. J. and Ozyener, F.** The kinetics of exertional oxygen uptake: assumptions and inferences. *Medicina dello Sport* 1998; **51**: 139–49.
19. **Chance, B., Leigh, Jr J. S., Clark, B. J., Maris, J., Kent, J. and Nioka, S.** *et al.* Control of oxidative metabolism and oxygen delivery in human skeletal muscle: a steady-state analysis of the work/energy cost transfer function. *Proceedings of the National Academy of Science* 1985; **82**: 8384–8.
20. **Funk, C. I., Clark, A. Jr and Connett, R. J.** A simple model of aerobic metabolism: applications to work transitions in muscle. *American Journal of Physiology* 1990; **258**: C995–1005.
21. **Kushmerick, M. J., Meyer, R. A. and Brown, T. R.** Regulation of oxygen consumption in fast- and slow-twitch muscle. *American Journal of Physiology* 1992; **263**: C598–606.
22. **Kemp, G. J., Taylor, D. J., Thompson, C. H., Haras, I. J., Rajagopalan, B. and Styles, P.** *et al.* Quantitative analysis by 31P magnetic resonance spectroscopy of abnormal mitochondrial oxidation in skeletal muscle during recovery from exercise. *NMR in Biomedicine* 1993; **6**: 302–10.
23. **Krogh, A. and Lindhard, J.** The regulation of respiration and circulation during the initial stages of muscular work. *Journal of Physiology (London)* 1913; **47**: 112–36.
24. **Hughson, R. L.** Exploring cardiorespiratory control mechanisms through gas exchange dynamics. *Medicine and Science in Sports and Exercise* 1990; **22**: 72–9.
25. **Barstow, T. K., Casaburi, R. and Wasserman, K.** O_2 uptake kinetics and the O_2 deficit as related to exercise intensity and blood lactate. *Journal of Applied Physiology* 1993; **75**: 755–62.
26. **Whipp, B. J., Ward, S. A., Lamarra, N., Davis, J. A. and Wasserman, K.** Parameters of ventilatory and gas exchange dynamics during exercise. *Journal of Applied Physiology* 1982; **52**: 1506–13.
27. **Andersen, P. and Saltin, B.** Maximal perfusion of skeletal muscle in man. *Journal of Physiology (London)* 1985; **366**: 233–49.
28. **Schenkman, K. A., Marble, D. R., Burns, D. H. and Feigl, E. O.** Myoglobin oxygen dissociation by multiwavelength spectroscopy. *Journal of Applied Physiology* 1997; **68**: 2369–72.
29. **Terrados, N., Jansson, E., Sylven, C. and Kaijser, L.** Hypoxia as a stimulus for synthesis of oxidative enzymes and myoglobin? *Journal of Applied Physiology* 1990; **68**: 2369–72.
30. **Gaesser, G. A. and D. C. Poole.** The slow component of oxygen uptake kinetics in humans. *Exercise and Sport Sciences Reviews* 1996; **24**: 35–71.
31. **Gerbino, A., Ward, S. A. and Whipp, B. J.** Effects of prior exercise on pulmonary gas exchange kinetics during high-intensity exercise in humans. *Journal of Applied Physiology* 1996; **80**: 99–107.
32. **Bohnert, B, Ward, S. A. and Whipp, B. J.** Effects of prior exercise on pulmonary gas exchange kinetics during high-intensity leg exercise in humans. *Experimental Physiology* 1998; **83**: 557–70.
33. **Poole, D. C., Barstow, T. J., Gaesser, G. A., Willis, W. T. and Whipp, B. J.** $\dot{V}O_2$ slow component: Physiological and functional significance. *Medicine and Science in Sports and Exercise* 1994; **26**: 1354–8.
34. **Poole, D. C., Schaffartzik, W., Knight, D. R., Derion, T. and Kennedy, B. and Guy, H.** *et al.* Contribution of exercising legs to the slow component of oxygen uptake kinetics in humans. *Journal of Applied Physiology* 1991; **71**: 1245–53.
35. **Sloniger, M. A., Cureton, K. J., Carrasco, D. I., Prior, B. M., Rowe, D. A. and Thompson, R. W.** Effect of the slow-component rise in oxygen uptake on $\dot{V}O_2$ max. *Medicine and Science in Sports and Exercise* 1996; **28**: 72–8.
36. **Roston, W. L., Whipp, B. J., Davis, J. A., Effros, R. M. and Wasserman, K.** Oxygen uptake kinetics and lactate concentration during exercise in humans. *American Review of Respiratory Diseases* 1987; **135**: 1080–4.
37. **Whipp, B. J., Davis, J. A., Torres, F. and Wasserman, K.** A test to determine the parameters of aerobic function during exercise. *Journal of Applied Physiology* 1981; **50**: 217–21.
38. **Hesser, C. M., Linnarson, D. and Bjursted, H.** Cardiorespiratory and metabolic responses to passive, negative and minimum-load dynamic leg exercise. *Respiration Physiology* 1977; **30**: 51–67.
39. **Hansen, J. E., Casaburi, R., Cooper, D. M. and Wasserman, K.** Oxygen uptake as related to work rate increment during cycle ergometer exercise. *European Journal of Applied Physiology* 1988; **57**: 140–5.
40. **Lamarra, N., Whipp, B. J., Ward, S. A. and Wasserman, K.** Breath-to-breath 'noise' and parameter estimation of exercise gas exchange kinetics. *Journal of Applied Physiology* 1987; **62**: 2003–12.
41. **Cooper, D. M., Weiler-Ravell, D., Whipp, B. J. and Wasserman, K.** Aerobic parameters of exercise as a function of body size during growth in children. *Journal of Applied Physiology* 1984; **56**: 628–34.
42. **Girandola, R. N., Wisewell, R. A., Frishe, E. and Wood, K.** $\dot{V}O_2$ and anaerobic threshold in pre- and post-pubescent girls. *Medicine and Sports* 1981; **14**: 151–61.
43. **Reybrouck, T., Weymans, M., Stijns, H., Knops, J. and Hauwert, L.** Ventilatory anaerobic threshold in healthy children: Age and sex differences. *European Journal of Applied Physiology* 1985; **54**: 278–84.
44. **Kanaley, J. A. and Boileau, R. A.** The onset of the anaerobic threshold at three stages of physical maturity. *Journal of Sports Medicine and Physical Fitness* 1988; **28**: 367–74.
45. **Rowland, T. W. and Green, G. M.** Physiological responses to treadmill exercise in females: Adult-child differences. *Medicine and Science in Sports and Exercise* 1988; **20**: 447–8.

46. Cooper, D. M., Berry, C., Lamarra, N. and Wasserman, K. Kinetics of oxygen uptake and heart rate at onset of exercise in children. *Journal of Applied Physiology* 1985; **59**: 211–7.

47. Sady, S. P., Katch, V. L., Villanacci, J. E. and Gilliam, T. B. Children-adult comparisons of oxygen uptake and heart rate kinetics during submaximum exercise. *Research Quarterly* 1983; **54**: 55–9.

48. Freedson, P. S., Gillian, T. B., Sady, S. P. and Katch, V. L. Transient $\dot{V}O_2$ characteristics in children at the onset of steady-state exercise. *Research Quarterly* 1981; **52**: 167–73.

49. Zanconato, S., Cooper, D. M. and Armon, Y. Oxygen cost and oxygen uptake dynamics and recovery with one minute of exercise in children and adults. *Journal of Applied Physiology* 1991; **1**: 993–8.

50. Paterson, D. H. and Whipp, B. J. Asymmetries of oxygen uptake transients at the on- and off-set of heavy exercise in humans. *Journal of Physiology (London)* 1991; **443**: 575–86.

51. Beneke, R., Heck, H., Schwartz, V. and Leithauser, R. Maximal lactate steady-state during the second decade of age. *Medicine and Science in Sports and Exercise* 1996; **28**: 1474–8.

52. Williams, J. R. and Armstrong, N. Relationship of maximal lactate steady state to performance at fixed blood lactate reference values in children. *Pediatric Exercise Science* 1991; **3**: 333–41.

53. Williams, J. R., Armstrong, N. and Kirby, B. J. The 4 mM blood lactate level as an index of exercise performance in 11–13 year old children. *Journal of Sports Science* 1990; **8**: 139–47.

54. Asano, K. and Hirakoba, K. Respiratory and circulatory adaptation during prolonged exercise in 10–12 year old children and in adults. In *Child and sport* (ed. J. Ilmarinen and I. Valimaki). Springer-Verlag, Berlin, 1984; 119–28.

55. Macek, M. and Vavra, J. The adjustment of oxygen uptake at the onset of exercise: A comparison between prepubertal boys and young adults. *International Journal of Sports Medicine* 1980; **1**: 75–7.

56. Rowland, T. W. and Rimany, T. A. Physiological responses to prolonged exercise in premenarcheal and adult females. *Pediatric Exercise Science* 1995; **7**: 183–91.

57. Armon, Y., Cooper, D. M., Flores, R., Zanconato, S. and Barstow T.J. Oxygen uptake dynamics during high-intensity exercise in children and adults. *Journal of Applied Physiology* 1991; **26**: 841–8.

58. Zanconato, S., Buchtal, S., Barstow, T. J. and Cooper, D. M. ^{31}P-magnetic resonance spectroscopy of leg muscle metabolism during exercise in children and adults. *Journal of Applied Physiology* 1993; **74**: 2214–8.

59. Gaul, C. A., Docherty, D. and Cicchini, R. Differences in anaerobic performance between boys and men. *International Journal of Sports Medicine* 1995; **16**: 451–5.

60. Gildein, H. P., Kaufmehl, K., Last, M., Leititis, J., Wildberg, A. and Mocellin, R. Oxygen deficit and blood lactate in prepubertal boys during exercise above the anaerobic threshold. *European Journal of Paediatrics* 1993; **152**: 226–31.

61. Mahon, A. D., Duncan, G. E., Howe, C. A. and Del Corral, P. Blood lactate and perceived exertion relative to ventilatory threshold: Boys versus men. *Medicine and Science in Sports and Exercise* 1997; **29**: 1332–7.

62. Pianosi, P., Seargeant, L. and Haworth, J. C. Blood lactate and pyruvate concentrations, and their ratio during exercise in healthy children: developmental perspective. *European Journal of Applied Physiology* 1995; **1**: 518–22.

63. Paterson, D. H., Cunningham, D. A. and Bumstead, L. A. Recovery O_2 and blood lactic acid: longitudinal analysis in boys aged 11–15 years. *European Journal of Applied Physiology* 1986; **55**: 93–9.

64. Kuno, S., Takahashi, H., Fujimoto, K., Akami, H., Miyamaru, M., Nemoto, I., Itai, Y. and Katsuta, S. Muscle metabolism during exercise using phosphorus-31 nuclear magnetic resonance spectroscopy in adolescents. *European Journal of Applied Physiology* 1994; **70**: 301–4.

65. Eriksson, B. O., Karlsson, J. and Saltin, B. Muscle metabolites during exercise in pubertal boys. *Acta Paediatrica Scandinavica* 1971; **217**: 154–7.

66. Tanaka, H. and Shindo, M. Running velocity at blood lactate threshold of boys aged 6–15 years compared with untrained and trained young males. *International Journal of Sports Medicine* 1985; **6**: 90–4.

67. Mero, A. Blood lactate production and recovery from anaerobic exercise in trained and untrained boys. *European Journal of Applied Physiology* 1988; **57**: 60–6.

68. Williams, J. and Armstrong, N. The influence of age and sexual maturation on children's blood lactate responses to exercise. *Pediatric Exercise Science* 1991; **3**: 111–20.

69. Welsman, J. R., Armstrong, N. and Kirby, B. J. Serum testosterone is not related to peak $\dot{V}O_2$ and submaximal lactate responses in 12- to 16-year old males. *Pediatric Exercise and Science* 1994; **6**: 120–7.

70. Fournier, M., Ricca, J., Taylor, A. W., Ferguson, R. J., Montpetit, R. R. and Chairman, B. R. Skeletal muscle adaptation in adolescent boys: Sprint and endurance training and detraining. *Medicine and Science in Sports and Exercise* 1982; **14**: 453–6.

71. Jansson, E. and Hedberg, G. Skeletal muscle fibre types in teenagers: Relationship to physical performance and activity. *Scandinavian Journal of Medicine Science in Sports* 1991; **1**: 31–44.

72. Mizuno, M., Secher, N. H. and Quistorff, B. ^{31}P-NMR spectroscopy, rsEMG, and histochemical fibre types of human wrist flexor muscles. *Journal of Applied Physiology* 1994; **76**: 531–8.

73. Barstow, T. J., Jones, A. M., Nguyen, P. H. and Casaburi, R. Influence of muscle fibre and pedal frequency on oxygen uptake kinetics of heavy exercise. *Journal of Applied Physiology* 1996; **81**: 1642–50.

74. Cooper, D. M. and Barstow, T. J. Magnetic resonance imaging and spectroscopy in studying exercise in children. *Exercise and Sports Science Reviews* 1996; **24**: 475–99.

75. Bell, R. D., MacDougall, J. D., Billeter, R. and Howard, H. Muscle fibre types and morphometric analysis of skeletal muscle in six-year-old children. *Medicine and Science in Sports* 1980; **12**: 28–31.

76. Armstrong, N., Welsman, J. and Winsley, R. Is peak $\dot{V}O_2$ a maximal index of children's aerobic fitness? *International Journal of Sports Medicine* 1996; **17**: 356–9.

77. Rowland, T. W. Does peak $\dot{V}O_2$ reflect $\dot{V}O_2$ max in children?: Evidence from supramaximal testing. *Medicine and Science in Sports and Exercise* 1993; **25**: 689–93.

78. Cooper, D. M. Development of the oxygen transport system in normal children. In *Advances in pediatric sport sciences*, Vol. 3 (ed. O. Bar-Or). Human Kinetics Publishers, Champaign, Il, 1989; 67–100.

79. Whipp, B. J. Developmental aspects of oxygen uptake kinetics in children. In *Children and exercise XIX* (ed. N. Armstrong, B. Kirby and J. Welsman). E. and F. N. Spon, London, 1997; 233–47.

80. Rowland, T. W. Short-burst activities and the development of anaerobic fitness. In *Developmental exercise physiology* (ed. T. W. Rowland). Human Kinetics Publishers, Champaign, Il, 1996; 193–214.

81. Riner, W. F., McCarthy, M., De Cillis, L. V. and Ward, D. S. Response of children and adolescents to onset of exercise. In *Children and exercise XIX* (ed. N. Armstrong, B. Kirby and J. Welsman). E. and F. N. Spon, London, 1997; 248–52.

82. Sady, S. P. Transient oxygen uptake and heart rate responses at the onset of relative endurance exercise in prepubertal boys and adult men. *International Journal of Sports Medicine* 1981; **2**: 240–4.

2.11   Exercise training

Anthony D. Mahon

Introduction

With the proliferation of team sport opportunities, junior Olympic style competitions, age-group swimming, youth triathlons and distance running races, many children are participating in intense exercise training programmes at very young ages. Additionally, extensive emphasis has been placed on developing and maintaining acceptable levels of physical activity and fitness during childhood. Knowledge of the child's adaptations to exercise is necessary for the formulation of developmentally acceptable, safe and effective exercise prescription and training practices.[1] In addition, recognition of the healthy child's adaptation to regular exercise training may be important in developing strategies for the use of exercise as a means to enhance the functional capacity for children with disease.[1–3] Perhaps even more important is the notion that promoting proper exercise habits during childhood may have a positive impact on activity and exercise patterns during the adult years, which then may lessen the risk for inactivity related disorders such as coronary artery disease.[4,5]

In order to understand adaptations to exercise training in children, there are several factors that must be kept in mind when designing and interpreting research protocols involving this age group. Cross-sectionally designed studies compare trained and untrained age-matched subjects, but do not permit the establishment of cause and effect. However, in this type of study, one may be able to study a group of subjects who are presently engaged in a high volume of training; a volume greater than that which could be achieved in a typical longitudinal study. Longitudinal studies permit the establishment of cause and effect because of the access to pre- and post-training measurements, although this type of study is time intensive for both the researcher and the subject. Moreover, it may be difficult in short periods of time (two to six months) to achieve a high volume of training. Control subjects are necessary in longitudinal studies in order to separate physiological changes attributed to normal growth, maturation and learning from those which are obtained from training. Examples of growth related changes are the increase in maximal oxygen uptake ($\dot{V}O_2$ max, litre min^{-1}), the decrease in submaximal $\dot{V}O_2$ (ml kg^{-1} min^{-1}) during treadmill exercise, and the increase in muscle strength.[6,7] Matching children for development within and between groups also is desirable in order to minimize the confounding influence of maturation.

There are other factors to consider when using children in exercise training studies which will affect the research design. For ethical reasons, measurements often are non-invasive in nature which limits identification of mechanisms of adaptations.[1,2,6] A number of non-invasive technologies, such as computerized tomography, magnetic resonance imaging (MRI) and echocardiography, are gaining widespread acceptance, but in many instances the use of this technology is not practical. The volume of training is an important consideration as adaptations to exercise follow a dose-response pattern (at least up to a point).[8] However, in establishing an appropriate training volume for children, the amount of training must minimize the physiological and psychological risk. Children who volunteer to participate in exercise training research studies may already be physically active via activities in the community, at school or at home. Thus, the confounding effect of activity outside of the training programme may make it difficult to determine the precise impact of a training programme. Recommending that children limit their physical activity outside of the training programme, however, cannot be justified. Consequently finding truly 'untrained' children to serve as subjects in exercise training studies can be challenging. Finally, many child participants in exercise training studies are volunteers and little effort has been made to randomly assign subjects to training and experimental groups.[2]

Aerobic adaptations

Adults

Maximal oxygen consumption

It is well established that aerobic training programmes adhering to the recommendations established by the American College of Sport Medicine (ACSM)[9] will result in significant improvements in $\dot{V}O_2$ max. Typically, $\dot{V}O_2$ max will increase approximately 15 to 20%,[10] although there may be a large intra-subject variation owing to genetic factors.[11] The change in $\dot{V}O_2$ max is also inversely related to the initial level indicating that those individuals with a high $\dot{V}O_2$ max at the beginning of an endurance training programme will demonstrate less increase compared to those with a low $\dot{V}O_2$ max at the start of training.[10] The increase in $\dot{V}O_2$ max is directly related to adaptations in oxygen transport and utilization. In particular cardiac output ($\dot{Q}$) increases due to an increase in stroke volume (SV), while maximal heart rate (HR) remains unchanged or decreases slightly.[10,12] The rise in SV is attributed to a number of factors including increases in left ventricular diameter, end-diastolic volume, contractility and blood volume as well as a reduction in pericardial restraint.[10,12,13] Despite the increase in $\dot{Q}$, mean arterial pressure is unchanged suggesting that peripheral adaptations in vascular conductance are also apparent.[10] The rise in vascular conductance and corresponding decrease in peripheral resistance prevents an increase in systemic blood pressure and ventricular afterload as a result.[10] The combined effect of an increase in $\dot{Q}$ and vascular conductance will increase blood flow and oxygen delivery to the exercising muscle.[10] In addition, an increase in capillary density reduces both the oxygen diffusion distance and the velocity of blood flow.[10,14] This will permit a greater extraction of oxygen as reflected by an increase in the arteriovenous oxygen difference ($a-vO_2$diff).[10,13]

Submaximal exercise

From a cardiovascular standpoint, there are fewer adaptations at the same absolute submaximal intensity compared to the adaptations at maximal exercise. $\dot{V}O_2$, $\dot{Q}$ and $a-vO_2$diff are usually unchanged in healthy adults.[13] However, HR is lower after training, and increases less from resting level to a given submaximal intensity. Stated another way, the intercept and slope of the HR–$\dot{V}O_2$ relationship are lower in the trained state. The decline in HR is usually attributed to a reduction in sympathetic activity.[13] In contrast to the HR reduction, SV increases in order to maintain a constant $\dot{Q}$. Similar to maximal exercise the rise in SV is attributed to an increase in both the capacity to fill and eject.[13] As a result of less sympathetic activation, splanchnic blood flow may be higher. Since $\dot{Q}$ is unchanged, the increase in splanchnic blood flow will reduce the amount of blood available to the exercising muscle.[13] To insure an adequate availability of oxygen in the exercising muscle, trained muscle $a-vO_2$diff will increase.[13,15] The increase in capillary density and more homogeneous distribution of blood facilitate the increased extraction.[14,15]

A number of other skeletal muscle adaptations alter substrate utilization and metabolite accumulation as a result of endurance training. Mitochondrial volume increases[14] thereby enhancing cellular oxidation.[16] Many of these adaptations are mediated by increases in the activity of various mitochondrial enzymes including those of the Krebs cycle, electron transport chain and beta oxidation.[16] The corresponding effect of these enzymatic adaptations is a reduction in the production and subsequent accumulation of lactate in the muscle and blood at any given submaximal intensity, and a rightward shift in the lactate threshold curve.[16] Additionally, the ability to use fatty acids to a greater extent promotes glycogen sparing, an adaptation which is particularly important during prolonged exercise.[15]

Children

For a number of reasons already mentioned, there are far fewer reports on the child's responses to exercise training. Furthermore, those studies that have examined the influence of training on children have been limited with respect to determining the underlying mechanisms of change. This is likely due to the difficulties associated with obtaining invasive measurements. For these reasons it is not surprising that many studies have focused primarily on changes in $\dot{V}O_2$ max and adaptations in submaximal responses.

Maximal oxygen consumption

Cross-sectional comparisons of age-matched trained and untrained children indicate that $\dot{V}O_2$ max is substantially higher in trained children. For example, Mayers and Gutin[17] reported that $\dot{V}O_2$ max was 23.3% higher (56.6 versus 45.9 ml kg^{-1} min^{-1}) in a group of elite male distance runners 8.3 to 11.8 years of age compared to an age-matched control group. The runners trained an average of three to five days per week running distances ranging from three to ten miles per day. Similarly, van Huss et al.[18] reported that $\dot{V}O_2$ max was 19% higher (61.8 versus 51.9 ml kg^{-1} min^{-1}) in trained boys and girls 8 to 15 years

of age versus a control group; details regarding the training history were not provided. Sundberg and Elovaino[19] analysed male runners of three different ages (12, 14 and 16 years) compared to untrained boys of the same ages. In all three age groups, $\dot{V}O_2$ max per kilogram body mass in the runners was significantly higher (13 to 18%) than in the control subjects. When $\dot{V}O_2$ max in litre min^{-1} was compared, only the 16 year old group was significantly higher than their control group suggesting that the superior aerobic power of the two younger groups was due to differences in body mass. However, as $\dot{V}O_2$ max in litre min^{-1} is directly related to body mass,[6] children with a smaller body mass should also have a lower absolute $\dot{V}O_2$ max. As this was not the case in Sundberg and Elovaino's study, it is conceivable that the similar absolute $\dot{V}O_2$ max is indicative of a training adaptation. Others have also reported that children involved in sports training programmes have a higher $\dot{V}O_2$ max than children not involved in similar pursuits.[20]

$\dot{V}O_2$ max has also been studied in well-trained children without comparison to control subjects. Vaccaro et al.[21] reported an average $\dot{V}O_2$ max of 56.8 ml kg^{-1}min^{-1} in a group of swimmers with a mean age of 15.1 years. At the time of study the swimmers had been training for six years and were swimming 3600–6400 m per day, four days per week. Butts[22] measured $\dot{V}O_2$ max in 127 female cross-country runners (13 to 18 years of age) and reported a mean value of 50.8 ml kg^{-1} min^{-1}. The girls had been training an average of 25.5 miles per week for 2.2 years. Substantially higher $\dot{V}O_2$ max values were reported by Cunningham[23] in his examination of male and female high-school cross-country runners (mean age ~16 years) who were participants in their state's high school cross-country championship. The group $\dot{V}O_2$ max ranged from 66.1 ml kg^{-1} min^{-1} in the females to 74.6 ml kg^{-1} min^{-1} in the males. In young hockey players 10 to 15 years of age, $\dot{V}O_2$ max has been shown to range from 56.0 to 68.0 ml kg^{-1} min^{-1}.[24,25] Although using a control group is preferred, the $\dot{V}O_2$ max values reported in these studies are well above what is expected for children of this age and gender.[2,6]

From this information it is apparent that trained children have a significantly higher $\dot{V}O_2$ max than age-matched untrained children; however, the cross-sectional design of these studies makes it impossible to separate the effect of exercise training from genetic endowment. It is possible that children with a very high $\dot{V}O_2$ max seek out competitive sport opportunities and are successful in these endeavours because of their superior aerobic ability. It also is interesting to note that the differences between trained and untrained children are somewhat smaller than what is observed between well-trained and untrained adults. This could be due to a variety of factors including the quantity and quality of training, the number of years in training, the relatively high $\dot{V}O_2$ max in comparison groups, and a maturational influence on the child's ability to adapt.[26] Nonetheless, these studies provide preliminary support regarding the aerobic trainability of children.

Although more difficult to conduct, a number of investigations have examined the effects of exercise training on $\dot{V}O_2$ max in children in a longitudinal manner. Table 2.11.1 displays a total of 39 studies involving children ranging from 5 to 17 years of age. The studies are arranged from the youngest mean age to the oldest and include information regarding the nature of the training programme and the percent improvement in $\dot{V}O_2$ max (regardless of statistical significance). Not all the studies involved endurance training, but all did examine the effect of some form of exercise training on $\dot{V}O_2$ max in children.

It also is apparent that length of the training programme (four weeks to 32 months), the type of training, and aspects related to the frequency, intensity and duration of training vary widely among these studies, which further complicates interpretation of the results. In some instances, information about the training regimen is lacking. This should be avoided in future studies in order to better understand the dose–response relationship in children. Most, but not all studies, employed control groups which were examined at the same time.

For obvious reasons there are only few investigations detailing the effect of exercise training on $\dot{V}O_2$ max in children younger than eight years of age. Difficulties with respect to obtaining valid measures of $\dot{V}O_2$ max as well as administering an effective training programme probably account for the paucity of data. Nonetheless there are three studies presented in Table 2.11.1 that describe the effect of exercise training on $\dot{V}O_2$ max in children between four and six years of age. Yoshida et al.[27] was unable to document an increase in $\dot{V}O_2$ max in five year old boys and girls following 14 months of training involving groups that were running 750 to 1500 m per day. One group of children was to train five days per week and another group was to train one day per week. However, due to difficulties, the children scheduled to train five days per week only trained about two days per week, while the children scheduled to train once a week actually ran approximately once every two weeks on average. Both the frequency and the duration of training were probably not sufficient to stimulate an adaptation in $\dot{V}O_2$ max[9]. Furthermore, $\dot{V}O_2$ max was measured during an overground run, rather than on a treadmill raising some doubt about the accuracy of the measurement. Two studies by Yoshizawa and his colleagues[28,29] found that $\dot{V}O_2$ max increased significantly in young children following a period of training. However, in their first study[29] the $\dot{V}O_2$ max increase, although statistically significant, was of a smaller magnitude in the experimental group versus the control group. In the later study,[28] however, a substantial increase in $\dot{V}O_2$ max was observed in the experimental group, but not in the control group. Although the children were running relatively short distances, it was apparently sufficient to elicit an adaptation in $\dot{V}O_2$ max. Presumably the frequency of training and possibly the intensity (not reported) were able to compensate for any deficiency in duration.

In contrast to the limited information on exercise training adaptations in very young children, the majority (28 of 39) of studies presented in Table 2.11.1 employed children between 8 and 13 years of age. In many instances pubertal status was not determined, so the potentially confounding effect of growth and training cannot always be determined. Nine of the 28 studies in this age range reported exercise training had essentially no effect (<4.0% increase) on $\dot{V}O_2$ max.[30–38] The study by Benedict et al.[31] used jump rope training, but did not appear to meet the recommendations of ACSM.[9] In three other studies,[30,35,36] interval running was used. It may be that the duration of this type of training is not a sufficient overload since it tends to mimic the child's usual pattern of activity, although increases in $\dot{V}O_2$ max ranging from 8.2% to 10% have been reported by other studies using interval training.[39,40] Haffor et al.[41] also found $\dot{V}O_2$ max per kilogram body mass to increase; however, the change was not statistically significant nor was it accompanied by an increase in $\dot{V}O_2$ max expressed in litre min[−1].

Gilliam and Freedson[33] examined the impact of a specific physical education programme conducted four days per week. The programme was designed to increase children's fitness level and the authors reported that HR averaged between 165 to 172 beats min[−1] over the final 20 min of a 25 min session. Although the guidelines recommended by the ACSM[9] appear to have been satisfied, $\dot{V}O_2$ max was unaffected by this programme. A similar programme conducted three days per week, but in after-school hours, also failed to increase $\dot{V}O_2$ max in children.[34] Although the frequency and the intensity of training appeared sufficient, it seems that the duration was too brief to elicit a cardiovascular adaptation. In contrast to these reports, two studies by Rowland and his colleagues[42,43] utilizing a variety of activities, found modest increases (5 to 7%) in $\dot{V}O_2$ max in children 10.8 to 12.9 years of age. There were no changes in $\dot{V}O_2$ max in the same group of subjects serving as their own controls in the 12 to 13 week period prior to training.

Two other studies that relied on continuous training and were conducted within the guidelines proposed by the ACSM[9] failed to increase $\dot{V}O_2$ max in children in this age range.[37,38] In contrast to these reports McManus et al.,[39] using a training protocol very similar to that which was used by Welsman's group,[38] reported a significant increase (10%) in $\dot{V}O_2$ max in nine year old girls.

Other investigations that have used more rigorous training programmes consistently report increases in $\dot{V}O_2$ max. Ekblom[44] used a variety of training methods and reported that $\dot{V}O_2$ max per kilogram body mass increased by 10% in the training group with no change in a control group over a six month period. When the training programme was extended an additional 26 months, there was a substantial difference between control and experimental subjects in the amount of improvement in $\dot{V}O_2$ max expressed in litre min[−1], but not when expressed relative to body mass. Eriksson and Koch[45] also employed a variety of training methods and found that $\dot{V}O_2$ max increased from 1.85 to 2.21 litre min[−1]. In a follow-up investigation Eriksson et al.[46] noted a modest increase in $\dot{V}O_2$ max. However, both studies by Eriksson and his colleagues did not use a control group so the influence of learning, growth and maturation cannot be easily separated from training induced adaptations.

Four studies which employed continuous running for 20 or more minutes for some or all of their training programmes reported increases in $\dot{V}O_2$ max relative to body mass.[47–50] In contrast, Daniels and Oldridge[32] found no increase in $\dot{V}O_2$ max expressed relative to body mass in boys (average age of 12.1 years) taking part in a 22 month running programme. Although $\dot{V}O_2$ max in litre min[−1] increased, a corresponding increase in body mass nullified any improvement in mass-related $\dot{V}O_2$ max. Two possible explanations for the failure to increase $\dot{V}O_2$ max per kilogram include the relatively high $\dot{V}O_2$ max at the onset of the training programme (59.5 ml kg[−1] min[−1]) and the wide variation in reported training volume. Moreover, no details regarding exercise intensity or frequency were provided, so it is unclear as to how these factors affected the outcome.

Swim training has also been shown to be effective in raising $\dot{V}O_2$ max in children. Vaccaro and Clarke[51] found that treadmill $\dot{V}O_2$ max increased from 47.3 to 55.4 ml kg[−1] min[−1] in a group of 9 to 11 year old boys and girls taking part in a seven month swimming programme. A small increase in $\dot{V}O_2$ max (46.8 to 49.0 ml kg[−1] min[−1]) also was observed in the control group; however, the difference between groups following training was significant. A very large increase in $\dot{V}O_2$ max occurred in the swim-trained girls in the study by Obert et al.[52] who used a swimming ergometer to make their assessment. Maximal HR also increased suggesting that $\dot{V}O_2$ max measurement prior to training, may not have been a 'true' $\dot{V}O_2$ max. However, the same effect was also noted in the control group, and the increase in

Table 2.11.1 Summary of exercise training studies and the effect on $\dot{V}O_2$ max

Study	Group	Age (y)	Gender	Length	Training programme Mode	F-I-D	Change in $\dot{V}O_2$ max (ml kg^{-1} min^{-1})	(litre min^{-1})
Children <8 years of age								
Yoshizawa et al.[28]	E	4.6	F	18 mths	Cont. run	F=6 d wk^{-1}; I=?; D=915 m d^{-1}	19.4%	48.5%
	C	4.5	F				8.3%	27.6%
Yoshizawa et al.[29]	E	5.8	M	6 mths	Cont. run	F=6 d wk^{-1}; I=?; D=915 m d^{-1}	5.8%	NR
	C	5.6	M				7.0%	NR
Yoshida et al.[27]	E	5.0	M/F	14 mths	Cont. run	F=~2 d wk^{-1}; I=HR at 190 beats min^{-1}; D=750−1500 m d^{-1}	NC	6.2%
	E	5.0	M/F	14 mths	Cont. run	F=~1 d 2 wk^{-1}; I = HR at 190 beats min^{-1}; D=750−1500 m d^{-1}	NC	10.1%
	C	5.0	M/F				NC	14.4%
Children 8–13 years of age								
Weltman et al.[57]	E	8.2	M	14 wks	Wt. train	F=3 d wk^{-1}; I=?; D=3×10 stations	13.8%	19.4%
	C	8.5	M/F				NC	NC
Gilliam and Freedson[33]	E	8.5	M/F	12 wks	PE fitness programme	F=4 d wk^{-1}; I=HR at 165–172 beats min^{-1}; D=25 min d^{-1}	NC	NC
	C	8.5	M/F				NC	4.5%
Clarke et al.[55]	E	8.5	M	3 mths	Wrestling	F=3 d wk^{-1}; I=?; D=90 min d^{-1}	14.7%	NR
	C	8.7	M				NC	NR
Mocellin and Wasmund[35]	E	8.4*	M/F	6 wks	Cont. run	F=1 d wk^{-1}; I=95% $\dot{V}O_2$max; D=800 m d^{-1}	NC	NC
	E	9.4*	M/F	7 wks	Cont. run	F=2 d wk^{-1}; I=95% $\dot{V}O_2$max; D=1000 m d^{-1}	NC	NC
Obert et al.[52]	E	9.3	F	11 mths	Swim	F=5 d wk^{-1}; I=HR at 170–180 beats min^{-1}; D=2000−4000 m d^{-1}	29.0%	39.2%
	C	9.3	F				NC	13.0%
McManus et al.[39]	E	9.3	F	8 wks	Cont. cycle	F=3 d wk^{-1}; I=80−85% HRmax; D=20 min d^{-1}	NR	10.0%
	E	9.8	F	8 wks	Int. run	F=3 d wk^{-1}; I=Max. speed; D=[3−6×10 and 30 s sprints]d^{-1}	NR	8.4%
	C	9.6	F				NR	NC

Study	Group	Age	Sex	Duration	Exercise	Protocol		
Ignico and Mahon[34]	E	9.7	M/F	10 wks	After school fitness programme	$F=3\,d\,wk^{-1}$; I=HR at 160–180 beats min^{-1} D=3–20 min d^{-1}	NC	NC
	C	9.8	M/F				NC	NC
Becker and Vaccaro[53]	E	9.5	M	8 wks	Cont. cycle	$F=3\,d\,wk^{-1}$; I=HR at 50% between VT and $\dot{V}O_2max$; D=40 min d^{-1}	20.5%	NR
	C	10.0	M				5.5%	NR
Vaccaro and Clarke[51]	E	9.7	M/F	7 mths	Swim and wt. train	$F=4\,d\,wk^{-1}$; I=?; D=3000–10 000 yd wk^{-1}	17.2%	NR
	C	10.0	M/F				4.7%	NR
Bar-Or and Zwiren[30]	E	9.9	M/F	9 wks	Int. run	$F=2, 3,$ or $4\,d\,wk^{-1}$; I=?; D=5–10 × 145 min d^{-1}	NC	NC
	C	NR	M/F				NC	NC
Benedict et al.[31]	E	10.0	M/F	8 wks	Jump rope	$F=2–3\,d\,wk^{-1}$; I=80% HRmax; D=8–15 min	NC	NC
Welsman et al.[38]	E	10.1	F	8 wks	Cont. cycle	$F=3\,d\,wk^{-1}$; I=80% HRmax; D=20 min d^{-1}	NR	NC
	E	10.2	F	8 wks	Aerobics	$F=3\,d\,wk^{-1}$; I=HR at 160 beats min^{-1} D=40 min d^{-1}	NR	NC
	C	10.2	F				NR	NC
Lussier and Buskirk[48]	E	10.3	M/F	12 wks	Cont. run and games	$F=4\,d\,wk^{-1}$; I=80%$\dot{V}O_2max$; D=2.0–5.4 km d^{-1}	6.8%	11.4%
	C	10.5	M/F				NC	7.1%
Mahon and Vaccaro[50]	E	10.6	M	14 wks	Cont. and int. run	$F=3\,d\,wk^{-1}$; I=70–80% and 90–100% $\dot{V}O_2max$; D=10–35 min d^{-1} and 1.5–4.0 km d^{-1}	12.9%	16.3%
	C	10.2	M				NC	NC
Brown et al.[47]	E	10.5	F	12 wks	Cont. and int. run	$F=4–5\,d\,wk^{-1}$; I=?; D=1–2 h d^{-1}	25.5%	NR
	C	NR	F				NC	NR
van Blaak et al.[37]	E	10.7	M	4 wks	Cont. cycle	$F=5\,d\,wk^{-1}$; I=55–67% $\dot{V}O_2max$; D=45 min d^{-1}	NC	NC
Rotstein et al.[40]	E	10.8#	M	9 wks	Int. run	$F=3\,d\,wk^{-1}$; I=?; D=1–2 × [3×600 m, 5×400 m, 6×150 m] d^{-1}	8.2%	NR
	C		M				NC	NR
Haffor et al.[41]	E	10.8	M	6 wks	Int. run and games	$F=5\,d\,wk^{-1}$; I=25–50%>VT; D=50 min d^{-1}	8.5%	NC

Table 2.11.1 (*Continued*)

Study	Group	Age (y)	Gender	Length	Training programme Mode	F–I–D	Change in $\dot{V}O_2$ max (ml kg^{-1} min^{-1})	(litre min^{-1})
Stewart and Gutin[36]	E	11.0*#	M	8 wks	Int. run	F=4 d wk^{-1}; I=Max speed and paced; D=[5−8 × 1 min, 3−4 × 3 min] d^{-1}	NC	NR
	C		M				NC	NR
Ekblom[44]	E	11.0	M	6 mths	Cont. and int. run, games	F=2 d wk^{-1}; I=HR at 130−max beats min^{-1}; D=45−60 min d^{-1}	10.2%	15.3%
	C	11.0	M				NC	NC
	E	11.0	M	26 mths	Sports training	F=3 d wk^{-1}; I=?; D=?	NC	38.6%
	C	11.0	M				NC	24.3%
Eriksson et al.[46]	E	11.2	M	6 wks	Cont. cycle	F=3 d wk^{-1}; I=HR at 180−max beats min^{-1}; D=20−50 min d^{-1}	NR	6.2%
Eriksson and Koch[45]	E	11.7	M	4 mths	Cont. run, gymnastics, X-C ski	F=3 d wk^{-1}; I=?; D=60 min d^{-1}	NR	19.5%
Rowland and Boyajian[42]	E	11.9	M/F	12 wks	Aerobic activities	F=3 d wk^{-1}; I=HR at 156−184 beats min^{-1}; D=20−30 min d^{-1}	6.5%	10.9%
	C¹		M/F				NC	NC
Rowland et al.[43]	E	11.9	M/F	13 wks	Aerobic activities	F=3 d wk^{-1}; I=HR at 153−192 beats min^{-1}; D=25−30 min d^{-1}	5.4%	7.8%
	C¹		M/F				NC	NC
Mahon and Vaccaro[49]	E	12.4	M	8 wks	Cont. and int. run	F=4 d wk^{-1}; I=70−80% and 90−100% $\dot{V}O_2$max; D=10−30 min d^{-1} and 100−800 m d^{-1}	7.6%	9.1%
	C	12.3	M				NC	NC
Daniels and Oldridge[32]	E	12.5	M	22 mths	Cont. run	F=?; I=?; D=7 Subjs. avg. 1114 mi y^{-1}, 7 subjs. avg. 336 mi y^{-1}	NC	21.8%
Docherty et al.[56]	E	12.4#	M	4 wks	Wt. train and cycle	F=3 d wk^{-1}; I=High resistance, low velocity; D=[2 × 6 stations (20 s on 20 s off)] d^{-1}	18.44%	21.6%
	E		M	4 wks		F=3 d wk^{-1}; I=Low resistance, high velocity; D=[2 × 6 stations (20 s on 20 s off)] d^{-1}	17.2%	18.0%
	C		M				4.3%	4.7%

Study	Group	Age	Sex	Duration	Type	F, I, D	%	%
Massicotte and Macnab[54]	E	12.5#	M	6 wks	Cont. cycle	F = 3 d wk^{-1}; I = HR at 170 − 180 beats min^{-1}; D = 12 min d^{-1}	10.9%	15.0%
	E		M	6 wks	Cont. cycle	F = 3 d wk^{-1}; I = HR at 150–160 beats min^{-1}; D = 12 min d^{-1}	NC	5.6%
	E		M	6 wks	Cont. cycle	F = 3 d wk^{-1}; I = HR at 140–150 beats min^{-1}; D = 12 min d^{-1}	NC	5.9%
	C		M				NC	NC
Children >13 years of age								
Burkett et al.[58]	E	15.6#	F	20 wks	Cont. and int. run	F = 5 d wk^{-1}; I = 70 and 90% HRmax; D = 9.7 − 32.2 km wk^{-1}	9.5%	NR
	C		F				NC	NR
Rowland et al.[62]	E	15.7	M/F	11 wks	Walking	F = 3 d wk^{-1}; I = ?; D = 27 min d^{-1}	9.9%	8.7%
	C^1		M/F				NC	NC
Fripp and Hodgson[65]	E	15.7	M	9 wks	Wt. train	F = 3 d wk^{-1}; I = ?; D = 60 − 80 min d^{-1}	NC	NR
	C	15.9	M				NC	NR
Stansky et al.[63]	E	15.8	F	7 wks	Swim	F = 4 d wk^{-1}; I = ?; D = 12 806 yd wk^{-1}	16.1%	14.3%
	C	15.9	F				NC	NC
Hagberg et al.[61]	E	16.0	M/F	6 mths	Cont. run	F = 3 d wk^{-1}; I = 60 − 65% $\dot{V}O_2$max; D = 30 − 40 min d^{-1}	9.7%	9.5%
	C	15.5	M/F				NR	NR
Eliakim et al.[59]	E	16.0*	F	5 wks	Cont. run, aerobics and sports	F = 5 d wk^{-1}; I = ?; D = 2 h d^{-1}	NR	10.1%
	C		F				NR	NC
Eliakim et al.[64]	E	16.0*	M	5 wks	Cont. run, aerobics, wt. train and sports	F = 5 d wk^{-1} I = ?; D = 2 h d^{-1}	NR	NC
	C		M				NR	NC
Fournier et al.[60]	E	16.3	M	3 mths	Int. run	F = 3 d wk^{-1}; I = ?; D = Repeated 50−250 m d^{-1}	6.2%	9.6%
	E	16.8	M	3 mths	Cont. run	F = 3 d wk^{-1}; I = 60−96% HRmax; D = 2 × 10 min d^{-1}−2 × 30 min d^{-1}	10.1%	11.6%

F = frequency of training; I = intensity of training; D = duration of a training session; E = experimental group; C = control group; M = male; F = female; Cont. = continuous; Int. = interval; NC = $\dot{V}O_2$ max change <4.0%; NR = not reported; VT = ventilatory threshold; change $\dot{V}O_2$ max = [(pre$\dot{V}O_2$ max − post$\dot{V}O_2$ max)/pre$\dot{V}O2$ max] × 100.

* Age corresponding to the middle of the reported range when mean age not reported.

\# Average age of all subjects.

C^1 = Subjects served as own controls prior to training programme.

$\dot{V}O_2$ max in the trained subjects far exceeded the increase in $\dot{V}O_2$ max in the control group.

As the result of an eight week cycle ergometer training programme $\dot{V}O_2$ max increased from 39.0 to 47.0 ml kg^{-1} min^{-1} in a group of 9 to 11 year old boys, while in a control group $\dot{V}O_2$ max increased only slightly, from 41.7 to 44.0 ml kg^{-1} min^{-1}.[53] Although the difference between groups following training was not statistically significant, the increase in $\dot{V}O_2$ max was rather large. Massicotte and Macnab[54] studied the effect of three different training intensities on $\dot{V}O_2$ max in 11 to 13 year old boys. Following the training programme only the children in the highest intensity group significantly increased $\dot{V}O_2$ max (litre min^{-1} and ml kg^{-1} min^{-1}), despite the relatively short duration of each training session. Consistent with the recommendations of the ACSM[9] there appears to be an intensity threshold for children under which cardiovascular adaptations are less likely to occur.

Three other studies using non-aerobic forms of training have also resulted in increases in $\dot{V}O_2$ max in experimental subjects without changes in control groups.[55–57] Clarke et al.[55] studied the effect of wrestling training on aerobic capacity in seven to nine year old boys. Although $\dot{V}O_2$ max increased by nearly 15%, the difference between the treatment and control groups post-training was not statistically significant. This was probably due to the fact that $\dot{V}O_2$ max in the control group was approximately 8% higher on the pre-training assessment. Docherty et al.[56] and Weltman et al.[57] used resistance training and reported significant increases in $\dot{V}O_2$ max (litre min^{-1} and ml kg^{-1} min^{-1}) in their experimental groups.

Fewer studies have examined the influence of exercise training on children older than 13 years of age. This seems surprising in light of the fact that older children may have a better recognition of the importance of exercise and fitness, and may have the maturity necessary for optimal compliance with the testing and training procedures. Nonetheless, examination of the information provided in Table 2.11.1 indicates that $\dot{V}O_2$ max increased from 6.2% to 17% in six of the eight studies listed.[58–63] Although a wide variety of training methods, including running, swimming and walking, were used, all these studies appear to satisfy the ACSM[9] recommendations. In addition to this, the study by Fournier et al.[60] indicated that sprint training significantly increased $\dot{V}O_2$ max, although to a lesser extent than endurance training. Moreover, with the exception of the interval trained group in the study by Fournier and colleagues, the amount of improvement noted in these studies is in line with what is typically reported in adults.[10]

In contrast, two studies listed in this section of Table 2.11.1 found no increase in $\dot{V}O_2$ max in adolescent males. In one study[64] $\dot{V}O_2$ max was unchanged following a short period of endurance training that was similar to that used in an earlier investigation.[59] Although the earlier study by Eliakim and colleagues[59] was successful in raising $\dot{V}O_2$ max in females, the higher pre-training $\dot{V}O_2$ max in the later study may have affected the ability of $\dot{V}O_2$ max to change. The other study reporting no change in $\dot{V}O_2$ max used resistance training as the mode of exercise.[65] While this type of training has been shown to significantly increase $\dot{V}O_2$ max in prepubertal children, apparently it does not have a similar effect on more mature children, which is consistent with the specificity of training principle.[8]

The aerobic trainability of the child

There are several factors, including the nature of the training programme, the $\dot{V}O_2$ max at the onset of training and the age of the subject, that may account for discrepancies regarding $\dot{V}O_2$ max adaptability in children. In general, many of the studies reporting an increase in $\dot{V}O_2$ max appear to satisfy the recommendations of the ACSM.[9] Despite the fact that these guidelines have been derived from adult responses to exercise training, they appear to apply to children.[3,66] However, the interaction of the frequency, intensity and duration of exercise in developing cardiorespiratory fitness in children is a very fruitful area of future research. It is also worth reiterating that while many studies outlined in Table 2.11.1 used endurance training programmes, other forms of training including high intensity, short-duration interval training, resistance training and wrestling have produced substantial increases in $\dot{V}O_2$ max in children. Inasmuch as children are not metabolic specialists,[2,67] it is not surprising that non-aerobic forms of training can increase $\dot{V}O_2$ max in paediatric subjects. However, as children mature, non-aerobic forms of training may have less influence on $\dot{V}O_2$ max.[60,65]

In adults, there is an inverse relationship between pre-training $\dot{V}O_2$ max and the amount of improvement.[10] Although Rowland[26] has suggested this may also apply to children, Pate and Ward[68] did not come to the same conclusion in their review of 15 studies. Similarly, no association between pre-training $\dot{V}O_2$ max and the amount of increase in children between 8 and 12 years of age has been reported.[42,48] In contrast, Eliakim et al.[59] found a significant correlation ($r = -0.68$) between per cent change in $\dot{V}O_2$ max versus predicted $\dot{V}O_2$ max in adolescent females. To better examine this issue, carefully designed training studies involving a large number of males and females with a wide range in pre-training $\dot{V}O_2$ max and representing different stages of maturation are needed. Alternatively, improvements in $\dot{V}O_2$ max may be influenced by the relationship between the child's level of habitual physical activity and the volume of training,[68] although the evidence for such a relationship is relatively weak.[42] Nonetheless, future studies should consider this potentially confounding influence as well.

Whether or not there is a critical age representing the onset of adaptability has been a source of considerable debate. In 1983 Katch[69] proposed the 'trigger hypothesis' which suggested that prior to puberty, the child may be less susceptible to exercise training adaptations. One reason for this maturational effect is that prepubertal children may lack certain hormonal responses to exercise that are necessary to stimulate tissue development and adaptations; a viewpoint shared by others.[26,66,70] Further evidence of the prepubertal child's blunted ability to increase $\dot{V}O_2$ max as a result of exercise training is provided in the meta-analysis performed by Payne and Morrow.[71] From an analysis of 28 studies, many of which are included in Table 2.11.1, they concluded that endurance training produced small increases ($< 5\%$) in $\dot{V}O_2$ max in children under 13 years of age. Similar conclusions have been drawn from the results of longitudinal studies which report large increases in $\dot{V}O_2$ max in active and trained children during the period corresponding to the attainment of peak height velocity.[72,73] Prior to this phase of development, training-induced changes in $\dot{V}O_2$ max are blunted.

Others have examined the trainability of various age-groups more directly, albeit in a cross-sectional manner (Table 2.11.2). Two of these studies[74,75] compared children to adults and found that the percent improvement in $\dot{V}O_2$ max was similar regardless of age. In both studies the respective training programmes were identical for both the children and the adults. In a third study, Weber et al.[76] compared training adaptations in 10, 13 and 16 year old monozygous twins. $\dot{V}O_2$ max (per kilogram) increased significantly in the youngest and oldest age-groups, but not in the middle age-group, and the largest per cent change in $\dot{V}O_2$ max was observed in the youngest age-group. The results of these studies appear to conflict with the idea that adaptations in the oxygen transport chain may be dependent on the maturational level of the child.

At this point it is difficult to determine the precise impact of the influence of maturation on aerobic trainability. More research, in which the volume of training is carefully regulated and reported, subjects are randomized into exercise and control groups, initial levels of $\dot{V}O_2$ max and habitual level of physical activity are accounted for, and maturation is accurately determined, will be required before any firm conclusions can be made. As a final note of consideration it also should be realized that many of the longitudinal training programmes involving children are at the minimal level recommended by the ACSM.[9] Thus, it is reasonable to expect the extent of the adaptations to be minimal as well.

Mechanism of adaptation in $\dot{V}O_2$ max

In order for $\dot{V}O_2$ max to increase, an increase in either $\dot{Q}$, a$-$vO$_2$diff or both is necessary in order to satisfy the Fick Equation. The increase in $\dot{Q}$ is usually attributed to a rise in SV, as maximal HR either is unchanged or declines slightly.[10] Studies examining these parameters in children are very limited, which is probably due to the difficulties in obtaining these measurements at maximal exercise. Eriksson and Koch[45] used the dye-dilution method to measure circulatory responses at maximal exercise. Following training $\dot{Q}$ and SV increased ~19% which was similar to the increase in $\dot{V}O_2$ max, while a$-$vO$_2$diff was unchanged. However, unlike the results observed in adults,[10] the increase in $\dot{Q}$ was not balanced by a reduction in peripheral resistance, and as a result mean arterial pressure increased from 105 to 115 mmHg.

Other investigations have measured $\dot{Q}$ and a$-$vO$_2$diff at the same relative submaximal intensities (percentage of $\dot{V}O_2$ max) before and after training. Because an increase in $\dot{V}O_2$ max would mean that the $\dot{V}O_2$ is higher at any given percentage of maximum, the results from these studies might also provide some insight to the mechanism of adaptation in $\dot{V}O_2$ max in children. In general, these studies report increases in SV and $\dot{Q}$ ranging from 10 to 15% in trained subjects.[48,50,76] Although, in some instances, the increases in SV and $\dot{Q}$ accounted for 50% or more of the increase in $\dot{V}O_2$ in trained subjects, the increases were not statistically significant and in some cases similar to changes in the control groups. Thus, the results from these studies are inconclusive with regard to adaptations in cardiac function. In contrast, a statistically significant increase (~6%) in a$-$vO$_2$diff at 50% and 75% of $\dot{V}O_2$ max was reported by Mahon and Vaccaro,[50] suggesting this parameter has an influence on the increase in $\dot{V}O_2$ max.

The underlying mechanisms mediating changes in SV are uncertain. Eriksson and Koch's[45] finding of a greater SV post-training along with an increase in mean arterial pressure is suggestive of an increase in cardiac contractility. Additionally, there are some cross-sectional and longitudinal data suggesting a larger SV may be due to adaptations in heart size and function.[44,45,77–79] However, in view of evidence to the contrary[80,81] as well as a variety of methodological considerations, including the research design, maturation levels of the subjects under investigation, differences in body size, assessment methods and measurement resolution, and the amount of training, these results must be viewed cautiously.

Likewise the mechanism mediating an adaptation in a$-$vO$_2$diff is uncertain. Rowland[70] has suggested that the lower arterial oxygen concentration in young children may limit the extent to which the a$-$vO$_2$diff can increase unless the arterial carrying capacity can increase. However, Mahon and Vaccaro[50] found a small, but statistically significant increase in resting haemoglobin concentration along with an increase in a$-$vO$_2$diff at two submaximal relative intensities. Thus, there is a mechanism accounting for the increase in a–vO$_2$diff.

Based on this information, it appears that endurance training, as well as other forms of exercise training, will increase $\dot{V}O_2$ max in children. However, it is very difficult to ascertain the precise influences of the training programme, pre-training $\dot{V}O_2$ max and the age or maturational stage of the subject on the amount of improvement in aerobic capacity. Moreover, there is a paucity of information regarding the specific adaptations in the oxygen transport system that underlie the increase in $\dot{V}O_2$ max in children at different stages of development.

Adaptations at submaximal intensities

Researchers have examined the physiological adaptations to endurance exercise training at submaximal intensities as well. One major advantage in assessing adaptations at a submaximal rather than at a maximal intensity is that the subject's willingness and motivation are less likely to affect the measurement. Studies that have examined submaximal adaptations in children have looked at adaptations in both the cardiorespiratory and metabolic responses to exercise.

A well-established finding in the adult literature is that the HR at a given submaximal work rate is decreased as a result of endurance training.[13] Similarly, in paediatric populations, a decline in submaximal HR has been observed in many investigations.[30,36,42,45,54,58,82,83] Moreover, the decline in submaximal HR can occur in the absence of any change in $\dot{V}O_2$ max as indicated in the studies by Stewart and Gutin[36] and Bar-Or and Zwiren,[30] and does not appear to be a function of age as children as young as nine to ten years old experience a reduction in HR with exercise training.[30] The mechanism behind the training induced reduction in submaximal HR in children is not certain. Gutin et al.[83] were unable to document any changes in autonomic function via heart rate variability assessment despite a small but statistically significant reduction in submaximal HR following training. However, these authors were able to demonstrate a decline in the sympathetic to parasympathetic ratio at rest suggesting a favourable adaptation in autonomic balance. More research is warranted with respect to establishing the influence of changes in autonomic activity and the reduction in submaximal HR in children.

In order to maintain $\dot{Q}$, the decrease in HR must be offset by a reciprocal increase in SV. Cross-sectional observations comparing trained and untrained children have provided inconsistent results with respect to the potential effect of training on submaximal SV. Andrew et al.[84] demonstrated that SV was similar in trained (swimmers) and untrained children between 8 and 18 years of age. Hamilton and Andrew[85] studied pre- and post-pubertal hockey players and found that HR and SV were similar in prepubertal control and hockey playing subjects. However, in postpubertal hockey players HR was lower and SV higher in comparison to their age-matched control group. In contrast to these findings, Soto et al.[86] reported that SV when exercising at a HR of 170 beats min^{-1} was higher in a group of prepubertal (9 to 13 year old) swimmers versus control subjects.

Table 2.11.2 Summary of studies examining the effects of exercise training on $\dot{V}O_2$ max in different age-groups

Study	Group	Age (y)	Gender	Length	Training programme Mode	F-I-D	Change in $\dot{V}O_2$ max (ml kg^{-1} min^{-1})	(litre min^{-1})
Weber et al.[76]	E	10.0	M	10 wks	Run, step and cycle	F=3d wk^{-1}; I=HR at 160 beats min^{-1}–HRmax; D=1 mile (run), 8.5 min (step) and 3 min (cycle [1 d wk^{-1}])	NR	23.2%
	E	13.0	M	10 wks	(all groups)		NR	13.7%
	E	16.0	M	10 wks			NR	20.3%
	C	10.0	M				NR	12.0%
	C	13.0	M				NR	15.1%
	C	16.0	M				NR	NC
Savage et al.[75]	E	8.5	M	11 wks	Cont. walk and run	F=3d wk^{-1}; I=40% $\dot{V}O_2$max; D=2.4–4.8 km d^{-1}	4.6%	NR
	E	36.6	M	11 wks	(all groups)	F=3d wk^{-1}; I=40% $\dot{V}O_2$max; D=2.4–4.8 km d^{-1}	NC	NR
	E	8.0	M	11 wks		F=3d wk^{-1}; I=75% $\dot{V}O_2$max; D=2.4–4.8 km d^{-1}	4.7%	NR
	E	36.6	M	11 wks		F=3d wk^{-1}; I=75% $\dot{V}O_2$max; D=2.4–4.8 km d^{-1}	7.9%	NR
	C	9.0	M				NC	NR
	C	36.7	M				NC	NR
Eisenman and Golding[74]	E	12.7	F	14 wks	Cont. run and bench step (both groups)	F=3d wk^{-1}; I=?; D=30 min d^{-1}	16.2%	25.0%
	E	19.6	F	14 wks			17.6%	17.4%
	C	12.7	F				NC	NC
	C	19.6	F				NC	NC

Abbreviations and calculations are the same as in Table 2.11.1.

The effect of exercise training on submaximal SV has been studied in a longitudinal manner as well. Gatch and Byrd[82] found that, in addition to the reduction in submaximal HR, SV increased following nine weeks of cycle interval training in nine to ten year old boys. Cardiac output, $\dot{V}O_2$ and a–vO_2diff were unchanged with training; adaptations consistent with adult responses.[13] In contrast, Eriksson and Koch[45] found $\dot{Q}$ to increase at two of three submaximal intensities. The rise in $\dot{Q}$ was due to the increase in SV (~18%) being greater than the decrease in HR (~2 to 4%). Correspondingly, $\dot{V}O_2$ increased significantly at the highest of the three work rates, while a–vO_2diff was unchanged at all levels of exercise.

Although cross-sectional comparisons provide equivocal results, longitudinal studies are suggestive that submaximal SV may increase with training. As previously noted, the effect of exercise training on myocardial structure and function is controversial, so it is not clear as to what aspects related to cardiac filling and ejection are adaptable to exercise training. Moreover, alterations in autonomic function during exercise have not been clearly established, so it is uncertain how this factor may affect adaptations in submaximal SV.

Ventilatory threshold (VAT), defined as the $\dot{V}O_2$ corresponding to the point when pulmonary ventilation begins to increase out of proportion to the increase in $\dot{V}O_2$ during incremental exercise,[87] also is adaptable to endurance training in children. Mahon and Vaccaro[49] examined changes in VAT in 10 to 14 year old boys before and after training, and reported that VAT increased by 19.4%, while no changes were observed in a control group. Becker and Vaccaro[53] also reported a large increase in VAT (28.1%); however, the 13.4% increase in VAT in the control group nullified a significant difference that could be attributed to training. Similarly, Haffor et al.[41] reported a large increase in VAT (27.8%) after interval training. Interestingly, in all three studies, the increase in VAT was greater than the increase in $\dot{V}O_2$ max, suggesting that VAT is more sensitive to exercise training. Whether other forms of exercise training, such as those outlined in Table 2.11.1, will have a positive impact on VAT, and the specific neural and humoral factors mediating the increase in VAT remain to be established.

Only six studies listed in Table 2.11.1 examined changes in blood lactate at submaximal work intensities.[29,40,44–46,54] Both Eriksson and Koch[45] and Ekblom[44] did not find a reduction in submaximal blood lactate concentration, although this probably can be attributed to the relatively low lactate values consequent to a low exercise intensity. In contrast, others have found significant reductions in blood lactate concentration following a period of exercise training.[46,54] Although it should be noted that the reduction in submaximal exercise blood lactate level in the Massicotte study[54] was only apparent in the high intensity training group.

Two studies examined the effect of training on changes in physiological function at fixed blood lactate concentrations. Rotstein et al.[40] found a significant increase in the running velocity corresponding to a blood lactate level of 4.0 mmol litre^{-1}, which would indicate that at a given running speed lactate level would be lower. However, the percentage of $\dot{V}O_2$ max corresponding to 4.0 mmol litre^{-1} actually declined as did the percent of $\dot{V}O_2$ max corresponding to lactate threshold. On the other hand, Yoshizawa et al.[29] were unable to document any changes in HR, $\dot{V}O_2$ or running velocity at two blood lactate concentrations (3.0 and 4.0 mmol litre^{-1}) following their training programme.

Several factors could account for a reduction in blood lactate concentration at a given submaximal work rate including a decline in lactate production and an increase in lactate clearance, although these factors have not been studied extensively in children. Muscle lactate concentration at two submaximal exercise work rates was unchanged in a group of 11 year old boys following six weeks of training suggesting that alterations in blood levels are not the result of reduced production.[46] Although muscle oxidative capacity, as determined from increases in muscle succinate dehydrogenase (SDH) activity, increases,[46,60] this apparently does not affect muscle lactate concentration. Eriksson et al.[46] observed a significant increase in phosphofructokinase (PFK) activity which may have counteracted any increase in oxidative capacity. In light of this information it may be tempting to speculate that a reduction in blood lactate concentration may be mediated by a greater hepatic clearance. At present time, however, there are apparently no data on children to support such a conclusion.

Similar to the ability for maximal aerobic power to adapt with exercise training, a number of submaximal adaptations are also apparent in children. These include a decline in HR and increase in SV at a given submaximal intensity, although the factors responsible for the increase in SV are uncertain. While evidence is available suggesting that training reduces the sympathetic to parasympathetic ratio at rest, similar alterations were not observed during exercise. The $\dot{V}O_2$ corresponding to VAT increases with training, often in greater magnitude than the increase in $\dot{V}O_2$ max. As a result, VAT expressed as percentage of $\dot{V}O_2$ max increases as well. Reductions in submaximal blood lactate concentration have been reported, but the effect of training on changes in lactate production and clearance remain uncertain.

Anaerobic adaptations

Adults

Although not as well studied as endurance training, anaerobic or sprint training will induce a number of physiological adaptations in the adult. Unlike aerobic training, however, anaerobic adaptations are primarily restricted to the skeletal muscle and perhaps the nervous system, with far less impact on the cardiovascular system. Exercise performance during anaerobic training usually increases,[88–90] although Jacobs et al.[91] reported that six weeks of training did not increase mean and peak power during the Wingate anaerobic test (WAnT). Enzymatically, increases in creatine kinase, phosphorylase and PFK activity have been noted as a result of anaerobic training.[88–92] Presumably these adaptations lead to an increased capacity to synthesize ATP via anaerobic pathways. However, anaerobic performance can also be improved in the absence of enzymatic adaptations, suggesting that other adaptations are also important.[88] Buffer capacity, which is calculated as the ratio between the change in lactate concentration and the change in pH before and after a bout of anaerobic exercise, increases with anaerobic training.[90] This will permit higher levels of lactate in the blood[91] and in the muscle[90] as a consequence of anaerobic exercise, which is suggestive of a greater degree of glycolytic ATP production prior to achieving a critical pH in the muscle. Other adaptations that may be taking place following anaerobic training include modest increases in oxidative ability[88,90,91] as well as muscle hypertrophy.[89] It is also possible that neurological adaptations associated with increased muscle force production also take place.

Children

In comparison to studies examining the effect of exercise training on $\dot{V}O_2$ max in children, there are far fewer reports regarding the adaptability of anaerobic exercise capacity. This is somewhat surprising in light of the fact that many child activities, both recreational and in competitive sport, involve brief bursts of activity performed at a high intensity. Studies that have examined anaerobic capacity in children before and after a period of exercise training indicate the ability to adapt. Sady and his colleagues[20] were able to demonstrate that well-trained prepubescent wrestlers had significantly greater peak power and mean power on a modified WAnT. Inasmuch as wrestling is a sport involving repeated, short bursts of high intensity activity, it is not surprising that well trained wrestlers have superior anaerobic ability compared to age-matched peers.

Changes in anaerobic ability have also been examined in several longitudinal studies. Grodjinovsky et al.[93] measured WAnT performance in a group of 50 boys between 11 and 13 years of age. The children were divided into two training groups and one control group. Training took place three days per week for six weeks. One group trained by performing repeated sprints on a cycle ergometer while the other group trained by sprint running. Following training, small (3.7 to 4.9%) but statistically significant increases in peak power expressed in absolute terms (W) and relative to body mass (W kg^{-1}) were found. The cycle-trained group also demonstrated a significant increase in both absolute (5.3%) and relative (3.9%) measures of anaerobic capacity as did the run-trained group, although the improvement in the latter group did not achieve statistical significance. No changes in peak power and anaerobic capacity were observed in the control group; nor were there differences between the two trained groups. In a follow-up investigation, Grodjinovsky and Bar-Or[94] examined anaerobic trainability in 12 to 13 year old boys and girls. Training was conducted over a seven month period and consisted of six physical education classes per week and after-school training (three days per week) specific to European handball. Following training, mean and peak power relative to body mass significantly increased in the experimental subjects and performance on the post-test was significantly higher than that observed in a control group.

Larger increases in absolute peak power (8.5 to 9.7%),[39,95] relative peak power (14.1%) and mean power (10%)[40] have been demonstrated in several other investigations employing high-intensity, short-duration training. However, it should be noted that mean power did not increase in the study by McManus et al.[39] nor did relative peak power in the study by Sargeant et al.[95] The lack of an increase in relative peak power in the Sargeant et al. study may have been due to the larger increase in lean body mass and leg volume observed in the trained group compared to the control group.

Not all studies that have examined the effect of exercise training on anaerobic ability have used measurements of muscle power. Mosher et al.[96] examined the effect of high-intensity training on anaerobic ability in prepubertal (10 to 11 years old) soccer players by using an all-out run performed on a treadmill set at 3.29 m s^{-1} (7 miles h^{-1}) and 18% grade. Following 12 weeks of soccer training, the experimental subjects increased their performance from 51.5 to 62.3 s, while no changes in treadmill duration were noted in another group of soccer players serving as control subjects. In a similar manner, Cadefau et al.[97] reported that eight months of various forms of anaerobic training significantly improved both 60 m and 300 m run time in a group of adolescent boys and girls.

Other forms of exercise training have also been examined for their effect on anaerobic ability in children. McManus et al.[39] found peak power increased by 20.1% in a group of ten year old girls involved in an eight week endurance training programme. Interestingly, the increase in peak power in the endurance-trained subjects was twice as great as the increase observed in a sprint-trained group of girls. In contrast to the studies reporting a significant effect of training on indices of anaerobic ability, Docherty and his group[56] were unable to detect any change in peak power in two groups of children participating in a four-week resistance training programme described in Table 2.11.1. However, the subjects in the study by Docherty et al.[56] had just completed a season of competitive hockey or soccer; thus, they may have already exhibited a relatively high anaerobic ability prior to the start of the resistance training programme.

Although exercise training can have a positive impact on various indices of anaerobic performance, the underlying adaptations in skeletal muscle are largely uncertain, especially in prepubertal children. Previously, Eriksson et al.[46] reported that exercise training increased both SDH and PFK activity in 11 to 13 year old boys. Fournier et al.[60] found PFK activity to increase in sprint-trained, but not endurance-trained, adolescents. More extensive biochemical adaptations are reported by Cadefau et al.[97] who found increases in muscle glycogen and a number of glycolytic and oxidative enzyme concentrations in 16 year old boys and girls. Changes in muscle size have also been linked to an increase in anaerobic performance in adults[88,89] and there is evidence of similar changes in adolescent children.[95,97] Adaptations in buffering capacity, muscle strength and in the nervous system apparently have not been systematically studied in young subjects.

Based on this information, it appears that indices of anaerobic ability (peak power, mean power and anaerobic capacity) will be increased with specific and non-specific types of exercise training in children ranging from age 10 to 13 years. There is some evidence that the adaptations may be mediated by increases in muscle glycolytic activity and muscle size, at least in adolescent children. Whether or not other factors contribute to the increase in anaerobic ability remain the subject of future research as does the effect of maturation on anaerobic adaptability.

Muscle strength adaptations

Adults

Muscle strength in adults typically increases as a result of weight lifting or resistance training provided the training protocol is of sufficient intensity. Similar to other forms of training, there is a dose–response relationship between training volume and strength adaptation. Although there is no one specific recommendation on how much training is necessary, a general guideline is to perform two to five sets of a given exercise with each set consisting of repetitions ranging from the two to ten repetition maximum (RM).[98] Improvements in muscle strength can be attributed to adaptations in both the nervous system and muscle fibre. In the nervous system an increase in motor unit recruitment and a reduction in inhibitory influences such as Golgi tendon organ activity and co-contraction of antagonist muscles will lead to increased muscle force production.[99,100] Indeed rapid increases in the amount of weight that can be lifted after only a few training sessions suggests the rapidity to which neural adaptations take place.[99] It is believed that these neural adaptations are necessary for strength development and precede changes in muscle size.[100] On the other hand, muscular enlargement is a somewhat slower process,[101] may require a longer period of time than is necessary to stimulate neural adaptations, and may not become apparent until neural adaptations have fully developed.[100]

Muscle enlargement is usually attributed to hypertrophy of already existing muscle fibres, although there is a tendency for fast twitch fibres to hypertrophy more than slow twitch fibres.[102] The hypertrophy is thought to be triggered by myofibril splitting and subsequent increase in the synthesis of actin and myosin. As a result of more actin and myosin, muscle enlargement occurs as does the potential for cross-bridge formation.[99,102] The formation of new actin and myosin is regulated by factors associated with protein synthesis, such that rate of synthesis exceeds rate of breakdown. The exact events regulating protein synthesis and breakdown are not entirely clear, but alterations in testosterone and cortisol activity as well as other hormones such as growth hormone and insulin-like growth factor I may be involved.[99,103–105] However, the precise contribution of all these hormones is difficult to ascertain since age, gender, and the volume and intensity of training influence the specific endocrine responses to resistance exercise.[105]

Muscle fibre hyperplasia has also been proposed as a mechanism of muscle enlargement;[106] however, there is considerable controversy surrounding this viewpoint and whether or not it is apparent in humans.[101,102] Support for muscle hyperplasia comes from studies that observed an increase in muscle fibre number in animals following a period of strength training.[107,108] Although these experiments have been challenged for methodological limitations,[106] they indicate that some animal species may rely on hyperplasia as an adaptive strategy to chronic stress from resistance exercise. In contrast to what has been observed in animals, evidence for hyperplasia in humans is less compelling. One investigation suggested muscle fibre number is greater in elite bodybuilders compared to control subjects who were resistance trained for six months.[109] Fibre number was estimated from arm circumference and average fibre area. However in a follow-up study,[110] estimated fibre number (based on fibre area and computerized tomograph scans) in bodybuilders and untrained control subjects were similar. The limitations in determining muscle fibre number directly in humans, as well as the inconsistent results, raise a question as to whether hyperplasia is a mechanism of resistance training induced muscle enlargement in humans.

Children

The evidence suggesting that resistance training will increase muscle strength in adults is well established. Fewer studies have examined training induced muscle strength adaptations in children. Concerns related to injury risk, the belief in the child's inability to adapt and strength training equipment limitations have probably contributed to the limited amount of information that is presently available. A list of studies, arranged by subject age, examining muscle strength adaptations in children is provided in Table 2.11.3. Details regarding the training programmes and the significant findings are also indicated.

Studies involving children eight years of age and younger are not very abundant. Moreover, several of these investigations did not use traditional forms of strength training, but nonetheless assessed muscle strength changes as a result of exercise training or sports participation. Falk and Mor[111] examined strength adaptations in six to eight year old boys and girls participating in a programme that employed martial arts training with upper and lower body strengthening activities. Sit-up and long jump performance improved in the experimental group significantly more than in the control group. Coordination also increased significantly in both groups, although the increase in the training group appeared to be larger than the increase in the control group. Increases in leg press strength and arm endurance, but not back lift, in seven to nine year old boys were observed by Clarke et al.[55] following a three-month wrestling programme. The resistive nature of a sport such as wrestling appears to be a sufficient stimulus for strength adaptations in some muscle groups. Siegel et al.[112] examined the effects of various forms of resistance training in young boys and girls as well. Using several different activities and exercises, they found relatively modest improvements in some, but not all, measures of strength.

Strength training utilizing more traditional methods has also been shown to increase muscle strength in young boys. Weltman et al.[57] examined prepubertal boys before and after a 14 week resistance training programme using hydraulic resistive machines in a circuit-training manner. Resistance was progressively increased over the course of the training period. Statistically significant interactions for a number of isokinetic strength and torque measurements revealed that muscle strength in the experimental group increased to a much greater extent than in the control group.

Five studies listed in Table 2.11.3 employed children with a mean age of approximately 10 to 11 years and used some form of traditional resistance training.[113–117] Sewall and Micheli[117] found that isometric knee extension, shoulder extension and shoulder flexion strength increased by 30.3%, 32.9% and 95.7%, respectively, with the latter finding being statistically significant. Changes in the control group ranged from −4.1% to 17.9% over the same three exercises. In a study by Ozmun et al.,[115] significant increases in muscle strength were also observed. Isokinetic elbow flexion strength increased nearly twice as much (27.8%) as the increase noted in the control group (15.5%), while isotonic elbow flexion strength increased 22.6% in the experimental group compared to 3.8% in the control group. The strength increases in the experimental subjects were significant while the changes observed in the control group were not. Resistance training also resulted in a large increase (26.1 to 40.1%) in knee extension strength in three subjects in the study by Mersch and Stoboy,[114] while much smaller increments were observed in three control subjects (4.5 to 9.8%).

Ramsey et al.[116] reported that the 1 RM for bench and leg press significantly increased by 34.6% and 22.1%, respectively, following 20 weeks of training. Although a significant increase in 1 RM bench press was also observed in the control group, the increase was of a smaller magnitude (12.3%). Training also significantly increased isokinetic elbow flexor and knee extensor peak torque by 25.8% and 21.3%, respectively, while no significant changes were noted for the control group. In addition, increases in isometric elbow flexor torque (37.3% collapsed across four joint angles) and knee extensor torque at 90° (25.3%) and 120° (13.3%) were greater than the changes noted in the control subjects.

Impressive increases in muscle strength were also observed by Faigenbaum and his colleagues,[113] but unlike the four previously mentioned studies in this age-group, Faigenbaum et al. trained their

214

Table 2.11.3 Summary of exercise training studies and the effect on muscle strength

Study	Group	Age (y)	Gender	Length	Training programme F-I-D-T	Significant results
Falk and Mor[111]	E	6.4	M	12 wks	F=2 d wk^{-1}; I=?; D=40 min d^{-1}; T=push-ups, sit-ups, stance/kicking, martial arts, & flexibility	Sit-ups reps and long jump distance↑ more in E versus C
	C	7.1	M			
Weltman et al.[57]	E	8.2#	M	14 wks	F=3 d wk^{-1}; I=all-out; D=30 min d^{-1} (3 sets × 10 stations [exer/rest: 30/30 s]); T=concentric hydraulic resistance	Isokinetic knee flexion/extension, elbow flexion/extension strength and vertical jump↑ more in E versus C
	C		M			
Siegel et al.[112]	E	8.4	M	12 wks	F=3 d wk^{-1}; I=?; D=30 min d^{-1} (exer/rest: 30/30 s to 45/15 s); T=hand wts, stretch tubing and self-supported movement	Rt. handgrip strength↑ E (M/F) but not C; isometric elbow flexion/extension strength↓ F; chin-up and flex arm hang↑ in E but not C
	E	8.5	F			
	C	8.6	M			
	C	8.4	F			
Clarke et al.[55]	E	8.5	M	3 mths	F=3 d wk^{-1}; I=?; D=90 min d^{-1}; T=wrestling training	Isometric leg press↑ more in E versus C
	C	8.4	M			
Ramsey et al.[116]	E	10.0*	M	20 wks	F=3 d wk^{-1}; I=70–75% 1 RM 1st 10 wks; 80–85% 1 RM 2nd 10 wks; D=3–5 sets × 5–12 reps × 5 exercises	1 RM bench and leg press, isometric and isokinetic elbow flexion and knee extension strength↑ more in E versus C
	C	10.0*	M			
Ozmun et al.[115]	E	10.0	M/F	8 wks	F=3 d wk^{-1}; I=?; D=3 sets × 7–11 reps	Isokinetic and isotonic elbow flexion strength↑ more in E versus C
	C	10.5	M/F			
Faigenbaum et al.[113]	E	10.8	M/F	8 wks	F=2 d wk^{-1}; I=50%, 75% and 100% 10 RM; D=35 min d^{-1} (3 sets × 10–15 reps × 5 exercises); T=child-size equipment	10 RM leg extension and curl, chest press, biceps curl and overhead press strength↑ more in E versus C
	C	9.9	M/F			
Sewall and Micheli[117]	E	10.5*	M/F	9 wks	F=3 d wk^{-1}; I=50%, 80% and 100% of 10 RM; D=25–30 min d^{-1} (3 sets × 10–max reps × 3 exercises); T=Nautilus and Cam II	Isometric shoulder flexion strength↑ more in E versus C
	C	10.5*	M/F			

Study	Group	Age	Sex	Duration	Training		Results
Docherty et al.[119]	E	12.4#	M	4 wks	F=3 d·wk⁻¹; I=high resistance, low reps; D=2×6 exercises [exer/rest = 20/20 s]		No significant training effect in either E group
	E		M	4 wks	F=3 d·wk⁻¹; I=low resistance, high reps; D=2×6 exercises [exer/rest: 20/20 s]		
	C		M				
Komi et al.[120]	E	14.0	M/F	12 wks	F=4 d·wk⁻¹; I=maximal; D=5×3–5 s; T=isometric knee extension		Isometric knee extension strength↑ more in E versus C
	C	14.0	M/F				
Blimkie et al.[121]	E	16.3	F	23 wks	F=3 d·wk⁻¹; I=max. effort; D=3–4 sets×10 reps×13 exercises; T=hydraulic resistance		Hydraulic resistance biceps curl, knee extension/flexion, triceps press and squat press strength↑ more in E versus C
	C	16.1	F				
Gillam[122]	E	HS	M	9 wks	F=1 d·wk⁻¹	I=1 RM; D=18 sets×1 RM; T=barbell	1 RM bench press strength↑ more in 5 d group versus all others; bench press strength↑ more in 4 d group versus 1 d group; bench press strength↑ more in 3 d group versus 1 and 2 d groups
	E	HS	M	9 wks	F=2 d·wk⁻¹		
	E	HS	M	9 wks	F=3 d·wk⁻¹		
	E	HS	M	9 wks	F=4 d·wk⁻¹		
	E	HS	M	9 wks	F=5 d·wk⁻¹		

E = experimental group; C = control group; F = frequency of training; I = intensity of training; D = duration of a training session; T = type of training; M = male; F = female; RM = repetition maximum.

⋆ Age corresponding to the middle of the reported range when mean age not reported.

Average age of all subjects.

subjects only two days per week. Increases in muscle strength ranged from 64.1% to 87.0% across five different exercises and were significantly greater than the increases in the control group (12.2% to 14.1%). Provided the training intensity is appropriate, it appears that a training frequency of two days per week is sufficient to promote the development of muscle strength in this age-group. Training only two days per week offers several advantages over more frequent training including a reduction in the risk for injury and less stress on equipment use, scheduling and supervisory requirements.

The effects of swim training on muscle strength has also been examined in 9 to 11 year old children.[118] However, unlike other studies examining sports training adaptations in muscle strength in children,[111,118] this type of training had no impact on muscle strength (handgrip, back lift or leg lift), although arm endurance increased significantly in the swim trained group compared to the control subjects. The fact that most of the training was endurance in nature may partially explain the lack of adaptation in muscle strength. Additionally, the muscle strength tests were not specific to the type of training, further confounding the outcome. However, the arm endurance test was also not specific to the training mode, but nonetheless increased; so it is unclear how the testing and training modalities interacted to influence the results of this study.

Although most of the studies examining muscle strength adaptations in children younger than 12 years of age seem to suggest that muscle strength is trainable, there are some studies involving older children that are less compelling, but methodological limitations must be considered. For example, Grodjinovsky and Bar-Or[94] reported that seven months of special sports training significantly increased handgrip strength in 12 to 13 year old boys and girls, while no significant changes were observed in the control group. However, close inspection of the results suggests little difference in the percent improvement in handgrip strength in the experimental (boys 11.8% and girls 6.8%) and control (boys 12.2% and girls 9.4%) groups. The lack of specific resistance training probably accounts for the modest results. Docherty et al.[119] also failed to demonstrate a significant effect of resistance training on muscle strength in boys with a mean age of 12.6 years. Measurements consisted of leg flexion/extension and arm adduction/abduction which were performed at 30 and 180 degrees s^{-1}. These movement speeds corresponded to the speed of training used by a low velocity and high velocity group, respectively. Reasons for the lack of improvement in the two training groups are not clear, but it is possible that the four to six weeks used for training was not long enough for strength adaptations to become apparent. The subjects also had just completed playing soccer or hockey, so it is possible that the strength training programme did not provide a sufficient overload necessary for adaptation. Another possible explanation proposed by the authors is that the neurological adaptations involved in the initial increase in strength may have occurred as a result of the children's specific sports training, and that muscular adaptations leading to increased strength were unable to occur because of subjects' immaturity, the relatively short duration of training, or a combination of the two.

In adolescent children, Komi et al.[120] reported that 12 weeks of isometric knee extension training significantly increased knee extensor strength to a greater extent in boys and girls participating in the exercise programme (19.9%), compared to a control group of a similar age and gender (−1.6%). Blimkie et al.[121] found that concentric muscle strength across five different exercises increased significantly more so in the group of 16 year old girls who participated in a 26 week pro-

gramme compared to age- and gender-matched control subjects. For the trained girls the increase in muscle strength ranged from 21.4% to 52.8% while in the control group the range was −14.1% to 13.1%. Increases in 1 RM bench press strength ranging from 19.5% to 40.7% were noted by Gillam[122] in an examination of American high-school students (grades 9 to 12). Sixty-eight boys were randomly assigned to train one, two, three, four or five days per week. Statistically, the increase in muscle strength in the five day per week group (40.7%) was greater than in the other four groups, the increase in the four day per week group (29%) was greater than the one day per week group (19.5%), and the increase in the three day per week group (32.3%) was greater than the two day per week (24.2%) and one day per week groups. No control groups were employed in this investigation; however, the increase in muscle strength was consistent with what has been observed by others.[116,121]

Strength trainability of children

Katch's[69] trigger hypothesis can also be applied to strength training adaptations in children. In that circulating androgens are very low in prepubertal children, the hormonal responses necessary to induce muscle hypertrophy may be lacking. Nonetheless the evidence presented above suggests that strength is trainable in children across various stages of maturation. More important though, is whether or not there is a difference in the degree of strength trainability across different levels of maturation. Several studies have examined this question and are outlined in Table 2.11.4. One of the early investigations into the effect of maturation on strength trainability was performed by Vrijens[123] who studied pre- and post-pubertal boys before and after eight weeks of isotonic training. Following training, isometric strength in four of six exercises increased more so in the older boys than in the younger boys, leading Vrijens to conclude that pubertal maturation was necessary to maximize strength increases. However, as Blimkie[124] has noted the strength training programme was relatively modest, and testing involved isometric muscle action while training involved isotonic muscle action. These limitations may have confounded the results.

More recent studies comparing strength adaptability across different stages of maturation provide contrasting results to those of Vrijens[123] and indicate that lesser and more mature subjects gain strength in a similar manner. Sailors and Berg[125] examined strength adaptations in prepubescent boys and young adult males. Although the absolute increase in muscle strength was greater in the men, relative increases in squat, bench press and biceps curl strength were similar between the groups. In addition, the increases in both training groups were statistically significant while the changes in each age-respective control group were not. Similar results were obtained by Pfeiffer and Francis[126] in their study involving prepubescent, pubescent and postpubescent males randomly assigned to training and control groups. The training groups performed a similar progressive resistance exercise programme. Significant increases in elbow and knee flexion and extension performed at two movement speeds were apparent in the training groups, but not the control groups. With just two exceptions, there were no significant differences in strength development between the three maturation groups. In the two exercises where significant differences were noted, the prepubescent group demonstrated a greater, not lesser, increase in strength than the older two groups. Nielsen et al.,[127] in examining strength training in girls 7 to 19 years of age, found a larger percent increase in isometric knee strength in the

Table 2.11.4 Summary of studies examining the effects of exercise training on muscle strength in different age-groups

Study	Group	Age (y)	Gender	Length	Training programme F-I-D-T	Significant results
Vrijens[123]	E	10.4	M	8 wks	$F=3$ d wk^{-1}; $I=75\%$ max; $D=1$ set × 8–12 reps × 8 exercises; $T=$concentric isotonic (both groups)	Isometric elbow flexion/extension, knee flexion/extension, abdomen and back strength↑ in older group; abdomen and back strength↑ in younger group
	E	16.7	M	8 wks		
Pfeiffer and Francis[126]	E	10.3	M	9 wks	$F=3$ d wk^{-1}; $I=50$–100% of 10 RM; $D=3$ sets × 10 reps for 4 primary exercises; 1 set × 10 reps for 5 secondary exercises (all E groups)	Isokinetic elbow flexion/extension strength↑ more in all E versus all C; isokinetic elbow flexion/extension strength↑ more in young E versus two older E groups
	C	9.7	M			
	E	13.1	M	9 wks		
	C	12.5	M			
	E	19.8	M	9 wks		
	C	19.6	M			
Nielsen et al.[127]	E	6 grps based on ht	F	5 wks	$F=3$ d wk^{-1}; $I=$maximal; $D=18$–20 min d^{-1}; $T=$each height group was divided into: isometric knee extension, vertical jump or sprint training	Isometric knee extension and vertical jump↑ more in E versus C; isometric knee extension↑ more in isometric group than other groups
	C		F			
Sailors and Berg[125]	E	12.6*	M	8 wks	$F=3$ d wk^{-1}; $I=50$–100% of 5 RM; $D=3$ sets × 5–10 reps; $T=$barbell/dumbbell (both E groups)	5 RM squat, bench press and biceps curl↑ in E groups versus C groups; no difference between E groups
	C		M			
	E	24.0*	M	8 wks		
	C		M			

* Age corresponding to the middle of the reported range when mean age not reported.

youngest girls (< 13.5 years) compared to the entire group. Finally, two recent meta-analyses also seem to support the concept that strength is as trainable in young children as in more mature subjects.[127,128]

Although there may be some limitations in the research design, training programmes and testing procedures, the results of these studies are certainly suggestive that relative strength trainability is similar between children across different levels of maturation. Differences in absolute strength gains can probably be attributed to differences in muscle mass between young and older subjects.

Mechanism of increased muscle strength

In prepubertal children, a number of studies have failed to show morphological changes in muscle despite successfully demonstrating increases in muscle strength, although some of these studies are limited by the methods utilized to assess changes in muscle size. For example, Ozmun et al.[115] found no change in upper arm circumference and skinfold thickness following isotonic biceps training. Likewise, Weltman et al.[57] reported that skinfold thickness and upper arm or upper leg circumferences were unchanged following training, although small, but significantly greater increases in chest, shoulder and abdomen circumferences were noted in their experimental group. Thigh circumference measurements did not change in the study by Faigenbaum and colleagues[113]. Sailors and Berg[125] were unable to document changes in biceps or calf circumference in early-pubertal boys; however, it is worth noting that there were no changes in the same girth measurements in young men. Siegel et al.[112] failed to demonstrate any changes in the sum of three circumferences (upper arm, chest and waist). Ramsey et al.[116] used computerized tomography and reported that cross-sectional area of the elbow flexors and knee extensors did not change with training. Finally, Vrijens,[123] using soft tissue radiography, found no change in upper arm and thigh cross-sectional area in prepubertal children. However, he also was unable to demonstrate much of a strength training effect in this age-group, so it is difficult to ascertain whether the lack of hypertrophy was related to maturation or to an inadequate training stimulus.

One exception to the failure to observe muscle size changes are the results provided by Mersch and Stoboy.[114] They used nuclear magnetic resonance tomography to examine changes in thigh cross-sectional area in two boys who underwent ten weeks of unilateral isometric knee extensor training. Muscle cross-sectional area increased 4 to 9% in the trained limb of two of the boys. Data on the third subject who dropped out after six weeks of training was not provided. No changes were observed in the untrained contralateral limb of the trained subjects or in the control subjects.

Only limited information is available concerning muscle enlargement in more mature children. Komi et al.[120] were unable to document any change in thigh muscle circumference in young adolescent children following strength training. However, Vrijens,[123] in opposition to the lack of hypertrophy demonstrated in prepubertal boys, found both increases in strength and muscle size in adolescent boys following training. Although hypertrophy was evident, the underlying hormonal events mediating the adaptive responses were not investigated. In a cross-sectional study involving female adolescent athletes (gymnasts, figure skaters and ballet dancers) compared with untrained age-matched females, Peltonen et al.[130] noted the following: psoas cross-sectional area and psoas and erector spinae and multifidius muscles cross-sectional area relative to body weight were greater in the

athletes. The larger muscle cross-sectional area also was related to greater trunk extension and flexion strength. Although these results are suggestive of training induced hypertrophy, the cross-sectional design ultimately limits cause and effect determination.

With the exception of the results of Mersch and Stoboy[114] muscle hypertrophy appears to be limited in young children. Thus, adaptations in muscle strength may be accounted for by neural mechanisms, which have been the topic of several investigations. Ozmun et al.[115] investigated this issue and found that integrated electromyographic (IEMG) amplitude significantly increased (16.8%) in the biceps during isokinetic elbow flexion in trained prepubertal children, but not in a control group. Ramsey et al.[116] utilized a technique known as the interpolated twitch technique which can be used to assess the degree of motor unit activation. This technique uses a supramaximal stimulation of the motor neurone during a maximal voluntary effort. An increase in muscle force production represents an increase in motor unit activation. Although not statistically significant, elbow flexor motor unit activation increased 13.2% and knee extensor activity increased 17.4% over the 20 week training programme. Collectively, the results of the studies by Ramsey et al.[116] and Ozmun et al.[115] suggest that the degree of motor unit activation increases with resistance training. However, in both instances the change in the neurological measurement was less than the change in strength. This would indicate that other neurological factors, such as coordination and firing frequency, may also be involved. In contrast to these findings, Komi et al.[120] reported an increase in IEMG activity that was nearly twice as large as the increase in knee extensor isometric strength in young adolescent children. The authors did not speculate as to why the neural adaptations exceeded the strength increase.

In contrast to the literature examining adaptations in $\dot{V}O_2$ max, there does not seem to be a difference between the degree of strength training adaptability in younger and older children. The mechanism of adaptation, however, appears to be primarily neurological, at least in young children, as there is only little evidence that muscle size actually increases. At this point it is not clear whether this represents an inability of young children to enlarge muscle mass beyond that which occurs naturally with growth, or whether resistance training programmes are insufficient from an intensity and/or duration (length of training programme) standpoint to stimulate muscle hypertrophy. In older and more mature children, neural adaptations have also been reported as has evidence of muscle hypertrophy, but it should be clear that these conclusions are based on an extremely small number of studies.

Summary

This chapter examined the exercise induced adaptations in children across different stages of maturation. While aerobic capacity appears to be trainable in children of all ages, some evidence suggests that it may be less responsive to training in young children compared to older children and adults. However, this notion should be viewed with caution when one considers that in the few studies conducted to date making direct comparisons between lesser and more mature subjects, little or no difference was observed in the per cent change in $\dot{V}O_2$ max. Less understood are the specific cardiovascular adaptations leading to a higher $\dot{V}O_2$ max, and the role of maturation in eliciting adaptations in these parameters. Adaptations in submaximal exercise responses have been observed, but are very limited in scope and in the determination of the mechanisms of adaptation. Measures of anaerobic ability, such as peak and mean power and anaerobic capacity, appear trainable in children, but there are apparently no reports examining the anaerobic trainability across different stages of maturation. Beyond a few reports detailing metabolic changes in anaerobically trained muscle, there is virtually no information regarding other adaptations leading to the child's enhanced ability to perform anaerobic exercise. Muscle strength is trainable in children, and unlike changes in aerobic capacity, there does not appear to be a maturational influence with respect to the relative increase in strength, although the underlying neural and muscular adaptations mediating strength adaptations are less established.

In closing, understanding the physiological adaptations in children as a result of regular exercise training has important implications from a fitness and health standpoint as well as from a sports training and performance standpoint. Identifying specific adaptations, the underlying mechanisms involved, and the role of maturation on both of these factors remain important topics of research in paediatric exercise physiology.

References

1. **Sady, S. P.** Cardiorespiratory exercise training in children. *Clinics in Sports Medicine* 1986; **5**: 493–514.
2. **Bar-Or, O.** *Paediatric sports medicine for the practitioner.* Springer-Verlag, New York, 1983.
3. **Vaccaro, P.** and **Mahon, A. D.** Cardiorespiratory responses to endurance training in children. *Sports Medicine* 1987; **4**: 352–63.
4. **Simons-Morton, B, G., Parcel, G. S., O'Hara, N. M., Blair, S. N.** and **Pate, R. R.** Health-related physical fitness in childhood: Status and recommendations. *Annual Review of Public Health* 1988; **9**: 403–25.
5. **Vaccaro, P.** and **Mahon, A. D.** The effects of exercise on coronary heart disease risk factors in children. *Sports Medicine* 1989; **8**: 139–53.
6. **Armstrong, N.** and **Welsman, J. R.** Assessment and interpretation of aerobic fitness in children and adolescents. *Exercise and Sport Sciences Reviews* 1994; **22**: 435–76.
7. **Bar-Or, O.** Trainability of the prepubescent child. *The Physician and Sportsmedicine* 1989; **17**: 65–82.
8. **Wilmore, J. H.** and **Costill, D. L.** *Physiology of sport and exercise.* Human Kinetics Publishers, Champaign, Il, 1994.
9. American College of Sports Medicine. The recommended quantity and quality of exercise for developing and maintaining cardiorespiratory and muscular fitness, and flexibility in healthy adults. *Medicine and Science in Sports and Exercise* 1998; **30**: 975–91.
10. **Rowell, L.** *Human cardiovascular control.* Oxford University Press, New York, 1993.
11. **Bouchard, C., Dionne, F. T., Simoneau, J. A.** and **Boulay, M. R.** Genetics of aerobic and anaerobic performances. *Exercise and Sport Sciences Reviews* 1992; **20**: 27–58.
12. **Blomqvist, C. G.** and **Saltin, B.** Cardiovascular adaptations to physical training. *Annual Review of Physiology* 1983; **45**: 169–89.
13. **Clausen, J. P.** Effect of physical training on cardiovascular adjustments to exercise in man. *Physiological Reviews* 1977; **57**: 779–816.
14. **Saltin, B.** and **Gollnick, P. D.** Skeletal muscle adaptability: significance for metabolism and performance. In *Handbook of physiology: skeletal muscle, section 10* (ed. L. D. Peachey, R. H. Adrian and S. R. Geiger). American Physiological Society, Bethesda, MD, 1983; 555–631.
15. **Kiens, B., Essen-Gustavsson, B., Christensen, N. J.** and **Saltin, B.** Skeletal muscle substrate utilization during submaximal exercise in man: Effect of endurance training. *Journal of Physiology* 1993; **469**: 459–78.
16. **Holloszy, J. O.** and **Coyle, E. F.** Adaptations of skeletal muscle to endurance exercise and their metabolic consequences. *Journal of Applied Physiology: Respiratory. Environmental. Exercise Physiology* 1984; **56**: 831–8.
17. **Mayers, N.** and **Gutin, B.,** Physiological characteristics of elite prepubertal cross-country runners. *Medicine and Science in Sports* 1979; **11**: 172–6.
18. **van Huss, W. D, Stephens, K. E., Vogel, P., Anderson, D., Kurowski, K., Janes, J. A.** and **Fitzgerald, C.** Physiological and perceptual responses of elite age group distance runners during progressive intermittent work to exhaustion. In *The 1984 Olympic scientific congress proceedings (Vol. 10), sport for children and youth* (ed. M. Weiss and D. Gould). Human Kinetics Publishing, Champaign, Il, 1986; 239–46.
19. **Sundberg, S.** and **Elovaino, R.** Cardiorespiratory function in competitive endurance runners aged 12–16 years compared with ordinary boys. *Acta Paediatrica Scandinavica* 1982; **71**: 987–92.
20. **Sady, S.** Physiological characteristics of high-ability prepubescent wrestlers. *Medicine and Science in Sports and Exercise* 1984; **16**: 72–6.
21. **Vaccaro, P., Clarke, D. H.** and **Morris, A. F.** Physiological characteristics of young well-trained swimmers. *European Journal of Applied Physiology* 1980; **44**: 61–6.
22. **Butts, N. K.** Physiological profiles of high school female cross country runners. *Research Quarterly for Exercise and Sport* 1982; **53**: 8–14.
23. **Cunningham, L. N.** Physiological comparison of adolescent female and male cross-country runners. *Pediatric Exercise Science* 1990; **2**: 313–21.
24. **Cunningham, D. A., Telford, P.** and **Swart, G. T.** The cardiopulmonary capacities of young hockey players: Age 10. *Medicine and Science in Sports* 1976; **8**: 23–5.
25. **Paterson, D. H, McLellan, T. M., Stella, R. S.** and **Cunningham , D. A.** Longitudinal study of ventilation threshold and maximal O_2 uptake in athletic boys. *Journal of Applied Physiology* 1987; **62**: 2051–7.
26. **Rowland, T. W.** Trainability of the cardiorespiratory system during childhood. *Canadian Journal of Sport Science* 1992; **17**: 259–63.
27. **Yoshida, T., Ishiko, I.** and **Muraoka, I.** Effect of endurance training on cardiorespiratory functions of 5-year-old children. *International Journal of Sports Medicine* 1980; **1**: 91–4.
28. **Yoshizawa, S., Honda, H., Nakamura, N., Itoh, K.** and **Watanbe, N.** Effect of an 18-month endurance run training programme on maximal aerobic power in 4- to 6-year-old girls. *Pediatric Exercise Science* 1997; **9**: 33–3.
29. **Yoshizawa, S., Honda, H., Urushibara, M.** and **Nakamura, N.** Effects of endurance run on circulorespiratory system in young children. *Journal of Human Ergology* 1990; **19**: 41–52.
30. **Bar-Or, O.** and **Zwiren, L. D.** Physiological effects of increased frequency of physical education class and of endurance conditioning on 9 to 10 year-old girls. In *Pediatric work physiology, proceedings of the fourth international symposium* (ed. O. Bar-Or). Wingate Institute, Tel Aviv, 1973; 279–85.
31. **Benedict, G. J., Vaccaro, P.** and **Hatfield, B. D.** Physiological effects of an eight-week precision jump rope program on children. *American Corrective Therapy Journal* 1985; **39**: 108–11.
32. **Daniels, J.** and **Oldridge, N.** Changes in oxygen consumption of young boys during growth and running training. *Medicine and Science in Sports* 1971; **3**: 161–5.
33. **Gilliam, T. B.** and **Freedson, P. S.** Effects of a 12-week school physical fitness program on peak $\dot{V}O_2$, body composition and blood lipids in 7 to 9 year old children. *International Journal of Sports Medicine* 1980; **1**: 73–8.
34. **Ignico, A. A.** and **Mahon, A. D.** The effects of a physical fitness program on low-fit children. *Research Quarterly for Exercise and Sport* 1995; **66**: 85–90.
35. **Mocellin, R.** and **Wasmund, U.** Investigation on the influence of a running training programme on the cardiovascular and motor performance capacity in 53 boys and girls of a second and third primary class. In *Pediatric work physiology, proceedings of the fourth international symposium* (ed. O. Bar-Or). Wingate Institute, Tel Aviv, 1973; 279–85.
36. **Stewart, K. J.** and **Gutin, B.** Effects of physical training on cardiorespiratory fitness in children. *Research Quarterly* 1976; **47**: 110–20.

37. van Blaak, E. F., Westerterp, K. R., Bar-Or, O., Wouters, L. J. M., and Saris, W. H. M. Total energy expenditure and spontaneous activity in relation to training in obese boys. *American Journal of Clinical Nutrition* 1992; **55**: 777–82.

38. Welsman, J., Armstrong, N. and Withers, S. Responses of young girls to two modes of aerobic training. *British Journal of Sports Medicine* 1997; **31**: 139–42.

39. McManus, A., Armstrong, N. and Williams, C.A. Effect of training on the aerobic and anaerobic performance of prepubertal girls. *Acta Paediatrica* 1997; **86**: 456–9.

40. Rotstein, A., Dotan, R., Bar-Or, O. and Tennenbaum, G. Effect of training on anaerobic threshold, maximal aerobic power and anaerobic performance of preadolescent boys. *International Journal of Sports Medicine* 1986; **7**: 281–6.

41. Haffor, A. A., Harrison, A. C. and Catledge Kirk , P.A. Anaerobic threshold alterations caused by interval training in 11-year-olds. *Journal of Sports Medicine and Physical Fitness* 1990; **30**: 53–6.

42. Rowland, T. W. and Boyajian, A. Aerobic response to endurance exercise training in children. *Pediatrics* 1995; **96**: 654–8.

43. Rowland, T. W., Martel, L., Vanderburgh, P., Manos, T. and Charkoudian, N. The influence of short-term aerobic training on blood lipids in healthy 10–12 year old children. *International Journal of Sports Medicine* 1996; **17**: 487–92.

44. Ekblom, B. Effect of physical training on adolescent boys. *Journal of Applied Physiology* 1969; **27**: 350–5.

45. Eriksson, B. O. and Koch, G. Effect of physical training on hemodynamic response during submaximal and maximal exercise in 11–13- year old boys. *Acta Physiologica Scandinavica* 1973; **87**: 27–39.

46. Eriksson, B. O., Gollnick, P. D. and Saltin, B. Muscle metabolism and enzyme activities after training in boys 11–13 years old. *Acta Physiological Scandinavica* 1973; **87**: 485–97.

47. Brown, C. H., Harrower, J. R. and Deeter, M. F. The effects of cross-country training on pre-adolescent girls. *Medicine and Science in Sports* 1972; **4**: 1–5.

48. Lussier, L. and Buskirk, E. R. Effects of an endurance training regimen on assessment of work capacity in pre-pubertal children. *Annals of the New York Academy of Sciences* 1977; **301**: 734–47.

49. Mahon, A. D. and Vaccaro, P. Ventilatory threshold and $\dot{V}O_2$ max changes in children following endurance training. *Medicine and Science in Sports and Exercise* 1989; **21**: 425–31.

50. Mahon, A. D. and Vaccaro, P. Cardiovascular adaptations in 8- to 12-year-old boys following a 14-week running program. *Canadian Journal of Applied Physiology* 1994; **19**: 139–50.

51. Vaccaro, P. and Clarke, D. H. Cardiorespiratory alterations in 9 to 11 year old children following a season of competitive swimming. *Medicine and Science in Sports* 1978; **10**: 204–7.

52. Obert, P., Courteix, D., Lecoq, A. M. and Guenon P. Effect of long-term intensive swimming training on the upper body peak oxygen uptake of prepubertal girls. *European Journal of Applied Physiology* 1996; **73**: 136–43.

53. Becker, D. M. and Vaccaro, P. Anaerobic threshold alterations caused by endurance training in young children. *Journal of Sports Medicine and Physical Fitness* 1983; **23**: 445–9.

54. Massicotte, D. R. and Macnab, R. B. J. Cardiorespiratory adaptations to training at specified intensities in children. *Medicine and Science in Sports* 1974; **6**: 242–6.

55. Clarke, D. H., Vaccaro, P. and Andersen, N. Physiological alterations in 7- to 9-year-old boys following a season of competitive wrestling. *Research Quarterly for Exercise and Sport* 1984; **55**: 318–22.

56. Docherty, D., Wenger, H. A. and Collis, M. L. The effects of resistance training on aerobic and anaerobic power in young boys. *Medicine and Science in Sports and Exercise* 1987; **19**: 389–92.

57. Weltman, A., Janney, C., Rains, C. B., Strand, K., Berg, B., Tippitt, S., Wise, J., Cahill, B. R. and Katch, F. I. The effect of hydraulic resistance strength training in pre-pubertal males. *Medicine and Science in Sports and Exercise* 1986; **18**: 629–38.

58. Burkett, L. N., Fernhall, B. and Walters, S. C. Physiologic effects of distance running training on teenage females. *Research Quarterly for Exercise and Sport* 1985; **56**: 215–20.

59. Eliakim, A., Barstow, T. J., Brasel, J. A., Ajie, H., Lee, W. N. P., Renslo, R., Berman, N. and Cooper, D. M. Effect of exercise training on energy expenditure, muscle volume and maximal oxygen uptake in female adolescents. *Journal of Pediatrics* 1996; **129**: 537–43.

60. Fournier, M., Ricci, J., Taylor, A. W., Ferguson, R. J., Montpetit, R. B. and Chaitmen, B. R. Skeletal muscle adaptation in adolescent boys: Spring and endurance training and detraining. *Medicine and Science in Sports and Exercise* 1982; **14**: 453–6.

61. Hagberg, J. A., Goldring, D., Ehsani, A., Heath, G., Hernandez, A., Schechtman, K. and Holloszy, J. O. Effect of exercise training on the blood pressure and hemodynamic features of hypertensive adolescents. *American Journal of Cardiology* 1983; **52**: 763–8.

62. Rowland, T. W., Varzeas, M. R. and Walsh, C. A. Aerobic responses to walking training in sedentary adolescents. *Journal of Adolescent Health* 1991; **12**: 30–4.

63. Stansky, A. W., Mickelson, R. J., van Fleet, C. and Davis, R. Effects of a swimming training regimen on hematological, cardiorespiratory, and body composition changes in young females. *Journal of Sports Medicine and Physical Fitness* 1979; **19**: 347–54.

64. Eliakim, A., Raisz , L. G., Brasel, J. A. and Cooper, D. M. Evidence of increased bone formation following a brief endurance-type training intervention in adolescent males. *Journal of Bone and Mineral Research* 1997; **12**: 1708–13.

65. Fripp, R. R. and Hodgson, J. L. Effect of resistive training on plasma lipid and lipoprotein levels in male adolescents. *Journal of Pediatrics* 1987; **111**: 926–31.

66. Rowland, T. W. Aerobic response to endurance training in prepubescent children: A critical analysis. *Medicine and Science in Sports and Exercise* 1985; **17**: 493–7.

67. Falk, B. and Bar-Or, O. Longitudinal changes in peak aerobic and anaerobic mechanical power in circumpubertal boys. *Pediatric Exercise Science* 1993; **5**: 318–31.

68. Pate R. R. and Ward, D. S.. Endurance exercise trainability in children and youth. In *Advances in medicine and fitness*, Vol. 3 (ed. W. A. Grana, J. A. Lombardo, B. J. Sharkey and J. A. Stone). Year Book Medical Publishers, Chicago, 1990: 37–55.

69. Katch, V. I. Physical conditioning in children. *Journal of Adolescent Health Care* 1983; **3**: 241–6.

70. Rowland, T. W. The 'trigger hypothesis' for aerobic trainability: A 14-year follow-up. *Pediatric Exercise Science* 1997; **9**: 1–9.

71. Payne, V. G. and Morrow, J. R. Exercise and $\dot{V}O_2$ max in children: A meta-analysis. *Research Quarterly for Exercise and Sport* 1993; **64**: 305–13.

72. Kobayashi, K., Kitamura, K., Miura, M., Sodeyama, H., Murase, Y., Miyashita, M. and Matsui, H. Aerobic power as related to body growth and training in Japanese boys: A longitudinal study. *Journal of Applied Physiology: Respiratory. Environmental. Exercise Physiology* 1978; **44**: 666–72.

73. Mirwald, R. L., Bailey, D. A., Cameron, N. and Rasmussen, R. L. Longitudinal comparison of aerobic power on active and inactive boys aged 7.0 to 17.0 years. *Annals of Human Biology* 1981; **8**: 405–14.

74. Eisenman, P. A., and Golding, L. A. Comparison of the effects of training on $\dot{V}O_2$ max in girls and young women. *Medicine and Science in Sports* 1975; **7**: 136–8.

75. Savage, M. P., Petratis, M. M., Thomson, W. H., Berg, K., Smith, J. L. and Sady, S. P. Exercise training effects on serum lipids of prepubescent boys and adult men. *Medicine and Science in Sports and Exercise* 1986; **18**: 197–204.

76. Weber, G., Kartodihardjo, W. and Klissouras, V. Growth and physical training with reference to heredity. *Journal of Applied Physiology* 1976; **40**: 211–5.

77. Gutin, B., Mayers, N., Levy, J. A. and Herman, M. V. Physiologic and echocardiographic studies of age group runners. In *Competitive sports for*

children and youth (ed. E. W. Brown and C. F. Branta). Human Kinetics Publishers, Champaign, Il, 1988: 117–28.

78. **Obert, P., Stecken, F., Courteix, D., Lecoq, A. M. and Guenon, P.** Effect of intensive endurance training on left ventricular structure and diastolic function in prepubertal children. *International Journal of Sports Medicine* 1998; **19**: 149–54.

79. **Oyen, E. M., Schuster, S. and Brode, P. E.** Dynamic exercise echocardiography of the left ventricle in physically trained children compared to untrained healthy children. *International Journal of Cardiology* 1990; **29**: 29–33.

80. **Rowland, T. W., Unnithan, V. B., MacFarlane, N. G., Gibson, N. G. and Paton, J. Y.** Clinical manifestations of the 'athlete's heart' in prepubertal male runners. *International Journal of Sports Medicine* 1994; **15**: 515–9.

81. **Telford, R. D., McDonald, I. G., Ellis, L. B., Chennells, M. H. D., Sandstrom, E. R. and Fuller, P. J.** Echocardiographic dimensions in trained and untrained 12-year-old boys and girls. *Journal of Sports Sciences* 1988; **6**: 49–57.

82. **Gatch, W. and Byrd, R.** Endurance training and cardiovascular function in 9- and 10-year-old boys. *Archives of Physical Medicine and Rehabilitation* 1979; **60**: 574–7.

83. **Gutin, B., Owens, S., Slavens, G., Riggs, S. and Treiber, F.** Effect of physical training on heart-period variability in obese children. *Journal of Pediatrics* 1997; **130**: 938–43.

84. **Andrew, G. M., Becklake, M. R., Guleria, J. S. and Bates, D. V.** Heart and lung functions in swimmers and nonathletes during growth. *Journal of Applied Physiology* 1972; **32**: 245–51.

85. **Hamilton, P. and Andrew, G. M.** Influence of growth and athletic training on heart and lung functions. *European Journal of Applied Physiology* 1976; **36**: 27–38.

86. **Soto, K. I., Zauner, C. W. and Otis, A. B.** Cardiac output in preadolescent competitive swimmers and in untrained normal children. *Journal of Sports Medicine and Physical Fitness* 1983; **23**: 291–9.

87. **Davis, J. A.** Anaerobic threshold: A review of the concept and directions for future research. *Medicine and Science in Sports and Exercise* 1985; **17**: 6–18.

88. **Costill, D. L., Coyle, E. F., Fink, W. J., Lesmes, G. R. and Witzmann, F. A.** Adaptations in skeletal muscle following strength training. *Journal of Applied Physiology: Respiratory. Environmental. Exercise Physiology* 1979; **46**: 96–9.

89. **Linossier, M. T, Dormois, D., Geyssant, A. and Denis, C.** Performance and fibre characteristics of human skeletal muscle during short sprint training and detraining on a cycle ergometer. *European Journal of Applied Physiology* 1997; **75**: 491–8.

90. **Sharp, R. L., Costill, D. L., Fink, W. J. and King, D. S.** Effects of eight weeks of bicycle ergometer sprint training on human muscle buffer capacity. *International Journal of Sports Medicine* 1986; **7**: 13–7.

91. **Jacobs, I., Esbjornsson, M., Sylven, C., Holm, I. and Jansson, E.** Sprint training effects on muscle myoglobin, enzymes, fibre types, and blood lactate. *Medicine and Science in Sports and Exercise* 1987; **19**: 368–74.

92. **Thortsensson, A.** Enzyme activities and muscle strength after sprint training in man. *Acta Physiologica Scandinavica* 1975; **94**: 313–8.

93. **Grodjinovsky, A., Inbar, O., Dot an, R. and Bar-Or, O.** Training effect on the anaerobic performance of children as measured by the Wingate Anaerobic Test. In *Children and exercise IX* (ed. K. Berg and B. O. Eriksson). University Park Press, Baltimore, 1990: 139–45.

94. **Grodjinovsky, A. and Bar-Or, O.** Influence of added physical education hours upon anaerobic capacity, adiposity, grip strength in 12–13-year-old children enrolled in a sports class. In *Children and sport* (ed. J. Ilmarinen and I. Valimaki). Springer-Verlag, Berlin, 1984: 162–9.

95. **Sargeant, A. J., Dolan, P. and Thorne, A.** Effects of supplemental physical activity on body composition, aerobic and anaerobic power in 13-year-old boys. In *Children and exercise XI* (ed. R. A. Binkhorst, H. C. G. Kemper and W. H. M. Saris). Human Kinetics Publishers, Champaign, Il, 1985: 135–9.

96. **Mosher, R. E., Rhodes, E. C., Wenger, H. A. and Filsinger, B.** Interval training: the effects of a 12-week programme on elite, pre-pubertal male soccer players. *Journal of Sports Medicine and Physical Fitness* 1985; **25**: 5–9.

97. **Cadefau, J., Casademont, J., Grau, J. M., Fernandez, J., Balaguer, A., Vernet, M., Cusso, R. and Urbano-Marquez, A.** Biochemical and histochemical adaptations to sprint training in young athletes. *Acta Physiologica Scandinavica* 1990; **140**: 341–51.

98. **Fleck, S. J. and Kraemer, W. J.** *Designing resistance training programs.* Human Kinetics Publishers, Champaign, Il, 1985.

99. **Kraemer, W. J., Deschenes, M. R. and Fleck, S. J.** Physiological adaptations to resistance exercise: implications for athletic performance. *Sports Medicine* 1988; **6**: 246–56.

100. **Sale, D. G.** Neural adaptations to resistance training. *Medicine and Science in Sports and Exercise* 1988; **20**: S135–45.

101. **McComas, A. J.** *Skeletal muscle: Form and function.* Human Kinetics Publishers, Champaign, Il, 1996.

102. **MacDougall, J. D.** Morphological changes in human skeletal muscle following strength training and immobilization. In *Human muscle* (ed. N. L. Jones, N. McCartney and A. J. McComas). Human Kinetics Publishers, Champaign, Il, 1986: 269–88.

103. **Hakkinen, K., Pakarinen, A., Alen, M. and Komi, P. V.** Serum hormones during prolonged training of neuromuscular performance. *European Journal of Applied Physiology* 1985; **53**: 287–93.

104. **Hakkinen, K., Pakarinen, A., Alen, M., Kauhanen, H. and Komi, P. V.** Relationship between training volume, physical performance capacity, and serum hormone concentrations during prolonged training in elite weight lifter. *International Journal of Sports Medicine* 1987; **8**: 61–5.

105. **Kraemer, W. J.** Endocrine responses to resistance exercise. *Medicine and Science in Sports and Exercise* 1988; **20**: S152–7.

106. **Antonio, J. and Gonyea, W. J.** Skeletal muscle hyperplasia. *Medicine and Science in Sports and Exercise* 1993; **25**: 1333–45.

107. **Gonyea, W. J.** Role of exercise in inducing increases in skeletal muscle fibre number. *Journal of Applied Physiology: Respiratory. Environmental. Exercise Physiology* 1980; **48**: 421–6.

108. **Gonyea, W. J., Sale, D. G., Gonyea, F. B. and Mikesky, A.** Exercise induced increases in muscle fibre number. *European Journal of Applied Physiology* 1986; **55**: 137–41.

109. **MacDougall, J. D., Sale, D. G., Elder, G. C. B. and Sutton, J. R.** Muscle ultrastructural characteristics of elite bodybuilders. *European Journal of Applied Physiology* 1982; **48**: 117–26.

110. **MacDougall, J. D., Sale, D. G, Alway, S. E. and Sutton, J. R.** Muscle fibre number in biceps brachii in bodybuilders and control subjects. *Journal of Applied Physiology: Respiratory. Environmental. Exercise Physiology* 1984; **57**: 1399–403.

111. **Falk, B. and Mor, G.** The effects of resistance and martial arts training in 6- to 8-year-old boys. *Pediatric Exercise Science* 1996; **8**: 48–56.

112. **Siegel, J. A, Camaione, D. N. and Manfredi, T. G.** The effects of upper body resistance training on prepubescent children. *Pediatric Exercise Science* 1989; **1**: 145–54.

113. **Faigenbaum, A. D., Zaichkowsky, L. D., Westcott, W. L., Micheli, L. J. and Fehlandt, A. F.** The effects of a twice-a-week strength training program on children. *Pediatric Exercise Science* 1993; **5**: 339–46.

114. **Mersch, F. and Stoboy, H.** Strength training and muscle hypertrophy in children. In *Children and exercise XIII* (ed. S. Oseid and K. H. Carlsen). Human Kinetics Publishers, Champaign Il, 1989: 165–82.

115. **Ozmun, J. C., Mikesky, A. E. and Surburg, P. R.** Neuromuscular adaptations following prepubescent strength training. *Medicine and Science in Sports and Exercise* 1994; **26**: 510–4.

116. **Ramsey, J. R., Blimkie, C. J. R., Smith, K., Garner, S., MacDougall, J. D. and Sale, D. G.** Strength training effects in prepubescent boys. *Medicine and Science in Sports and Exercise* 1990; **26**: 605–14.

117. **Sewall, L. and Micheli, L. J.** Strength training for children. *Journal of Pediatric Orthopedics* 1986; **6**: 143–6.

118. **Clarke, D. H. and Vaccaro, P.** The effect of swimming training on muscular performance and body composition in children. *Research Quarterly* 1979; **50**: 9–17.

119. Docherty, D., Wenger, H. A., Collis, M. L. and Quinney, H. A. The effects of variable speed resistance training in strength development in prepubertal boys. *Journal of Human Movement Studies* 1987; **13**: 377–82.

120. Komi, P. V., Viitasalao, J. T., Rauramaa, R. and Vihko, V. Effect of isometric strength training on mechanical, electrical and metabolic aspects of muscle function. *European Journal of Applied Physiology* 1978; **40**: 45–55.

121. Blimkie, C. J. R., Rice, S., Webber, C. E., Martin, J., Levy, D. and Gordon, C. L. Effects of resistance training on bone mineral content and density in adolescent females. *Canadian Journal of Physiology and Pharmacology* 1996; **74**: 1025–33.

122. Gillam, G. M. Effects of frequency of weight training on muscle strength enhancement. *Journal of Sports Medicine and Physical Fitness* 1981; **21**: 432–6.

123. Vrijens, J. Muscle strength development in the pre- and post-pubescent age. *Medicine and Sport* 1978; **11**: 152–8.

124. Blimkie, C. J. R. Resistance training during pre- and early puberty: Efficacy, trainability, mechanisms, and persistence. *Canadian Journal of Sport Science* 1992; **17**: 264–79.

125. Sailors, M. and Berg, K. Comparison of responses to weight training in pubescent boys and men. *Journal of Sports Medicine and Physical Fitness* 1987; **27**: 30–7.

126. Pfeiffer, R. D. and Francis, R. S. Effects of strength training on muscle development in prepubescent, pubescent, and postpubescent males. *The Physician and Sportsmedicine* 1986; **1499**: 134–43.

127. Nielsen, B., Nielsen, K., Behrendt Hansen, M. and Asmussen, E. Training of 'functional muscle strength' in girls 7–19 years old. In *Children and exercise IX* (ed. K. Berg and B. O. Eriksson).University Park Press, Baltimore, 1980: 69–78.

128. Falk, B. and Tenenbaum, G. The effectiveness of resistance training in children: A meta-analysis. *Sports Medicine* 1996; **22**: 176–86.

129. Payne, V. G., Morrow , J. R., Johnson, L. and Dalton, S.N. Resistance training in children and youth: A meta-analysis. *Research Quarterly for Exercise and Sport* 1997; **68**: 80–8.

130. Peltonen, J. E., Taimela, S., Erkintalo, M., Salminen, J. J., Oksanen, A. and Kujala, U. M. Back extensor and psoas muscle cross-sectional area, prior physical training, and muscle strength—a longitudinal study in adolescent girls. *European Journal of Applied Physiology* 1998; **77**: 66–71.

2.12   Temperature regulation

Bareket Falk

Introduction

Humans live in a broad range of environmental conditions, yet can regulate their body temperature within a relatively narrow range (35 to 41°C). The ability to thermoregulate is essential to preserve normal physiological function. During exercise, the metabolic heat produced by the working muscles can be 15 to 20 times that produced during rest, depending on the intensity of exercise and the working muscle mass. In a hot environment, this heat production places an added stress on the thermoregulatory mechanisms, while in a cold environment, the metabolic heat produced relieves some of the thermal stress.

Heat is exchanged between the body and the environment via evaporation or via dry heat exchange (radiation, convection and conduction). In a hot environment, physiological means to dissipate heat include sweating, to enhance evaporation, increased skin blood flow and dilation of superficial veins, to enhance heat loss from the body core to the periphery and from there to the environment. In a cold environment, physiological means to conserve body heat include increased metabolic rate, to enhance heat production, and peripheral vasoconstriction, to minimize heat loss from the body to the environment.

Thermoregulation is affected by environmental conditions as well as by physical and physiological characteristics of the body. Depending on the medium (e.g. air versus water), environmental factors that affect thermoregulation include temperature, velocity and humidity. Physical factors that can affect thermoregulation include body dimensions, body composition and body surface area-to-mass ratio, which can affect the evaporative and dry heat exchange. Physiological factors affecting thermoregulation include the sensitivity of various organ systems to thermal stimuli, as well as the individual's state of acclimatization, aerobic fitness or hydration. These factors affect the thermoregulatory response to heat and to cold, although their unique effect in the respective environment is not always clear.

This chapter outlines the physical and physiological changes that occur during growth and maturation and the possible effect that these changes can have on thermoregulation. The physiological response to heat stress is discussed in terms of the changes in body temperatures and the metabolic, circulatory, hormonal and sweating response to heat. Additionally, fluid regulation, which can affect the effectiveness of thermoregulation in the heat is also discussed. The physiological response to cold stress is considered in terms of the metabolic and circulatory responses and their possible influence on the effectiveness of thermoregulation. The discussion does not outline the thermoregulatory response *per se*, but rather emphasizes the differences in that response between children and adults. Finally, differences between children and adults in the acclimatization- and training-induced adaptations to thermal stress are discussed.

Most studies characterize their subjects by chronological age, and rarely by maturational stage, although the latter may affect thermoregulation. For the purpose of this discussion, the term *children* is used for girls and boys younger than 10 and 11 years, respectively. When maturational stage is not mentioned, children in this age category are considered to be prepubescents. The term *adolescents* is used for older children and, when not specifically mentioned, adolescents are considered to be mid- or late-pubescents.

Physical and physiological changes which occur during growth and maturation and are related to thermoregulation

Many physical and physiological characteristics change during growth and maturation, and these affect the ability to dissipate or preserve body heat. The changes which occur do so at different rates. Therefore, their unique and overall effect on the thermoregulatory response is difficult to evaluate. Nevertheless, Table 2.12.1 summarizes the physical and physiological changes which occur during growth and maturation and how they may be associated with thermoregulation.

Physical changes

Body surface area-to-mass ratio

Heat transfer between the body and the environment is related to the exposed body surface area. Metabolic heat production during exercise, on the other hand, is proportional to the active muscle mass, which in turn is related to body mass. The body surface area-to-mass ratio of a ten year old child (e.g. 135 cm, 30 kg, 1.07 m², ratio = 356 cm² kg⁻¹) can be over 30% greater than that of an adult (e.g. 180 cm, 70 kg, 1.89 m², ratio = 269 cm² kg⁻¹). During growth and maturation, there is a proportionally greater increase in body mass than in body surface area. Therefore, the body surface area-to-mass ratio decreases.

In a thermoneutral or warm environment, children's greater body surface area-to-mass ratio allows them to rely more on dry heat loss (radiation, convection and conduction) and less on evaporative cooling.[1-4] In more extreme hot or cold conditions the skin-to-air temperature gradient is large, and more heat is exchanged between the body and the environment. In a hot environment, the child's body absorbs heat from the surroundings and may not be able to compensate sufficiently with evaporative cooling. In a cold environment, the body dissipates heat to the surroundings and may not be able to compensate with

Table 2.12.1 Physical and physiological changes occurring during growth and maturation and their effect on thermoregulation*

Change	Effect on thermoregulation
Physical	
Decrease in body surface area-to-mass ratio	Decrease in heat gain in hot environments
	Decrease in heat loss in warm and cold environments
Decrease in body density (in girls versus women)	Decrease in the specific heat of the body
Increase in blood volume per unit body-surface area	Decrease in the proportion of blood volume necessary for the perfusion of the periphery or the central nervous system
Increase in sweat gland size	Increase in sweat gland output
Physiological	
Decrease in the oxygen cost of locomotion	Decrease in the metabolic heat production per unit body mass
Increase in submaximal and maximal cardiac output	Possible increase in the perfusion of the periphery, or the central nervous system
Increase in sweat gland sensitivity	Decrease in sweating threshold
	Decrease in time to sweating onset
	Increase in sweating rate
Increase in sweat gland anaerobic metabolism	Increase in sweating rate
Increase in prolactin response to exercise in the heat	Possible change in sweat electrolyte composition

*Modified from Falk.[31,32]

metabolic heat production. The decrease which occurs in the body surface area-to-mass ratio results in reduced heat gain during extreme heat and greater heat preservation during cold exposure.

Body composition

The specific heat of fat is much lower than that of fat-free mass (1.67 versus 3.35 kJ kg^{-1} °C^{-1}, respectively). Thus, the specific heat of the body depends on its level of adiposity. Generally, the level of adiposity is similar in boys and in men. In girls, on the other hand, per cent body fat increases early during adolescence and continues to increase into adulthood.[5] That is, per cent body fat in girls prior to puberty is generally lower than that of women. The lower adiposity in girls compared with women results in a slightly higher specific heat. That is, theoretically, given a similar body mass, a larger 'amount' of heat is needed to elevate girls' core temperature compared with women. During cold exposure, the lower adiposity of girls compared with women provides lower insulation and therefore, presents a disadvantage in heat preservation.

Blood and fluid volume

Children have a smaller absolute blood volume compared with adults. Mean volumes of 2.4 litre and 4.0 litre have been reported for 10 and 16 year old boys, respectively.[6] The difference is also evident when blood volume is expressed relative to body surface area (e.g. 2.18 versus 2.35 litre m^{-2}). That means that a larger proportion of the child's blood volume must be routed to the periphery for adequate perfusion and heat transfer. Therefore, the child's potential for heat transfer from the body core to the periphery and, subsequently, to the environment may be limited. Additionally, the larger fraction of total blood volume necessary to maintain adequate cooling by peripheral flow in children, may result in inadequate perfusion of the central nervous system and muscles during exercise in the heat. The latter may explain the lower heat tolerance sometimes reported in children[7] and their different subjective response to exercise in the heat.[8,9]

In a cold environment, provided that adequate peripheral vasoconstriction takes place, the smaller blood volume does not appear to affect the effectiveness of thermoregulation.

Physiological changes

Metabolic changes

The oxygen cost of locomotion (walking, running) per unit mass can be 15 to 20% higher in children compared with adults,[10] resulting in a higher metabolic heat production. The decrease in the cost of locomotion occurs during adolescence, as persuasively demonstrated recently in the Amsterdam Growth, Health and Fitness Study which followed children from the age of 13 to 27 years[11] (see Chapter 2.9). The higher energy expenditure is converted into metabolic heat and places an added strain on the thermoregulatory system during exercise in the heat. In the cold, the elevated metabolic heat production may be advantageous in the short run but has been argued to leave children with smaller reserves for long-term exercise.[12]

Circulatory changes

At any given exercise intensity, children are characterized by a lower cardiac output compared with adults[13] (see Chapter 2.7). This, coupled with the larger proportion of blood volume which is routed to the periphery, may hinder the transfer of body heat from the working muscles to the environment, and be especially evident while exercising in a hot environment.[7]

In boys, haemoglobin concentration increases during growth and maturation.[14] This increase, along with the increase in the dimensions of the heart and vascular system, is likely to contribute to an enhancement of cardiovascular function during adolescence and, thus, reduce the cardiovascular strain during exercise in the heat.

The lower cardiac output and lower haemoglobin concentration in children compared with adults do not present a disadvantage during cold exposure. That is, they are unlikely to contribute to an added heat loss and do not affect the increase in oxygen consumption and metabolism in the cold.[12]

Changes in hormonal status

Basal activity of aldosterone and vasopressin, hormones associated with fluid and electrolyte regulation, are not known to differ between children and adolescents compared with adults.[15] Additionally, there is no evidence to suggest that the sensitivity to these hormones changes during growth and maturation.

Several of the hormones which change during growth and which are associated with physical and sexual development have been implicated in thermoregulation, and particularly in the sweating mechanism. These include testosterone, oestrogen, prolactin and growth hormone.

As early as 1960, Kawahata[16] argued that testosterone has a sudorific effect. He based this argument on the observation of enhanced sweating rate in 70 to 81 year old men following injections of testosterone propronate. Indeed, androgen receptors have been detected on the secretory coils of sweat glands.[17] However, Rees and Shuster[18] could not demonstrate any sudorific effect of testosterone in adult men and women. Thus, they suggested that androgens may initiate but not maintain the increased sweating rate which occurs during maturation.

In women, the menstrual cycle has been shown to influence the thermoregulatory response to exercise in the heat (see Bar-Or[19] for review). Although an oestrogen receptor-related protein has been described in human sweat ducts,[20] the thermoregulatory differences between the menstrual phases have not been directly linked to any of the hormonal changes (mainly oestrogen and progesterone) that occur during these phases. Furthermore, it is unknown what if any effect the change in concentration of these hormones may have on thermoregulation during maturation.

Prolactin has been associated with osmoregulation and is suggested to influence sweat electrolyte concentration among adults,[21,22] as well as among adolescents.[23] However, its exact influence on sweat gland function and its possible differential role in children and adults is unclear.

Finally, several studies have described a reduced local sweating rate in patients with growth hormone (GH) deficiency[24,25] and patients with Laron Syndrome (undetectable to low IGF-I levels with normal GH levels).[26] Additionally, GH receptors and binding protein have been observed in the human sweat duct.[27,28] The mechanism with which the GH–IGF-I axis may affect sweat gland function and the possible differential effect of this axis on thermoregulation during growth and maturation needs to be examined.

Changes in the sweating mechanism

When ambient temperature is higher than skin temperature, the only means of heat dissipation is sweat evaporation. Several changes occur in the sweating mechanism during growth and maturation, and these may explain the increase in the sweating response to environmental heat which occurs from childhood to adulthood. (see Bar-Or;[29,30] Falk[31,32] for review). A summary of the changes which occur in the sweating mechanism during growth and maturation appears in Table 2.12.2. A discussion of the sweating response to thermal stress in children and adults follows.

Types of sweat glands

Traditionally, two types of sweat glands have been recognized: eccrine and apocrine.[33] The eccrine glands are abundantly distributed and are the main contributors to thermoregulation. The apocrine glands are found mainly in the axilla and mars pubis, and therefore contribute very little to thermoregulation. Additionally, they begin secretory function only during puberty. A third type of sweat gland has been observed in the axilla and is termed 'apoeccrine' because it shares physical and functional characteristics with the eccrine and apocrine glands. These glands appear to develop only during puberty. In view of their limited distribution, their role in thermoregulation is believed to be minimal. For a detailed description of the three types of glands the reader is referred to Sato et al.[33] The following discussion refers only to eccrine sweat glands.

Sweat gland size

Sweat glands are smaller in children compared with adults,[34,35] and during childhood, their size appears to be directly related to age ($r = 0.77$) and to stature ($r = 0.81$).[34] In vitro experiments demonstrated that, among adults, sweat gland size was directly related to sweating rate and to the gland's cholinergic sensitivity.[36] In the same study, subjects who described themselves as 'heavy sweaters' were characterized by larger and more sensitive glands compared with subjects who described themselves as 'poor sweaters'. Thus, the increase in the size of the sweat gland which likely occurs during growth and maturation is suggested to partly explain the increase in the sweating response to heat stress which occurs at that time.

Heat-activated sweat glands population density

The total number of eccrine sweat glands is determined by the age of two to three years[37] and during growth, there is a decrease in the

Table 2.12.2 Changes occurring in the sweating mechanism and pattern during growth and maturation and their contribution to the change in thermoregulation*

Variable	Change with growth and maturation	Contribution to thermoregulation
Sweating rate	Increase	Increase potential evaporative cooling
Sweat gland types:		
Eccrine	No change	Increase in local sweating rate (axila,
Apocrine	Begin to function during puberty	mars pubis) with no substantial effect
Apoeccrine	Appear and begin to function during puberty	on thermoregulation
Sweat gland size	Increase	Increase in sweating rate and potential evaporative cooling
Heat-activated sweat glands density	Decrease	No effect
Sensitivity to:		
Thermal stimuli	Increase	Increase in sweating rate and shortening
Cholinergic stimuli	Increase	of the time to onset of sweating. Thus, increase in potential evaporative cooling
Sweat gland metabolism (anaerobic capacity)	Increase	Increase in sweating rate and potential evaporative cooling

*Modified from Falk.[31]

number of sweat glands per unit area (population density).[38,39] Thus, the increase in sweating rate which is observed during growth and maturation occurs *in spite* of the decrease in heat-activated sweat glands (HASG) population density. Different body regions grow at different rates during growth and maturation, and this can affect the proportion of sweat glands on the extremities versus the central body regions. It is unknown how the possible change in the proportion of HASG population density on the central body regions and the extremities may affect the effectiveness of evaporative cooling.

Shibasaki *et al.*[40] recently demonstrated a lower sweating rate per gland on the back of boys compared with men who immersed their lower legs in hot water for 60 min. Additionally, Falk *et al.*[41] demonstrated a decrease in the population density of HASG on the lower back among pre-, mid- and late-pubertal boys exercising in the heat (Fig. 2.12.1). The younger boys had smaller sweat beads compared with the older boys. However, the percentage of skin area covered by sweat was similar in all groups (Fig. 2.12.1, bottom), suggesting similar evaporative cooling per unit area. In view of the similar skin area covered by sweat and the lower sweating rate on the back of boys compared with men,[40] it is possible that the boys' pattern of sweat distribution may facilitate more efficient cooling. This is supported by Shibasaki *et al.*[42] who demonstrated that following the onset of sweating, skin temperatures in boys exercising in a warm environment were lower, compared with men. The lower skin temperature was apparent despite greater vasodilation and lower local sweating rate in the boys. The authors argue that this may reflect a more effective cooling.

Sweating sensitivity

The sensitivity to thermal stress appears to be lower in children compared with adults. Shibasaki *et al.*[40] measured the frequency of sweat expulsions as an indicator of central sudomotor activity. The authors reported that, at a given heat stress (lower leg immersion in a hot bath), the slope of the sweating rate on the chest and thigh versus the

sweat expulsion frequency was lower in 7 to 11 year old boys compared with 21 to 25 year old men. That is, the boys displayed a lower sweating response to a given central thermal stimulus.

The sweating sensitivity can also be reflected by the change in body temperature which elicits a sweating response, or by the sweating rate associated with each degree rise in rectal temperature. Araki *et al.*[43] demonstrated that during exercise in the heat, boys began to sweat after a greater rise in rectal temperature, compared with adults (0.7 versus 0.2 °C, respectively). Likewise, Inbar[44] demonstrated a lower sweat production per degree rise in rectal temperature in eight to ten year old children compared with adults. Several studies have also reported a greater elevation in skin temperature in children compared with adults at a given thermal stress.[2,4,7,43,45,46] The higher skin temperature may be due to a delay in the onset of sweating in children compared with adults.

Although sweating results as a response to thermal stimuli, the sensitivity of the sweating apparatus can also be reflected in the sweating response to a pharmacological stimulus. The pharmacological stimuli to the sweating apparatus may be cholinergic or adrenergic in nature, although *in vivo*, eccrine glands respond mainly to cholinergic stimulation.[43,47] Sweat glands' sensitivity to intradermally injected adrenaline appears to reach its peak at the age of 14 years of age and decreases in old age.[48] Additionally, as previously mentioned, among adults, the *in vitro* response to metacholine is related to sweat gland size, as well as to the *in vivo* response.[36] This suggests that during growth and maturation, the increase in the size of sweat glands is accompanied by an increase in the sweating mechanism's sensitivity to cholinergic and to adrenergic stimuli. This enhancement in sensitivity likely contributes to an increase in the sweating rate.

Sweat gland metabolism

An additional contribution to the observed lower sweating rate in children compared with adults may be the lower metabolic capacity of their sweat glands. Sweat production is achieved mainly through

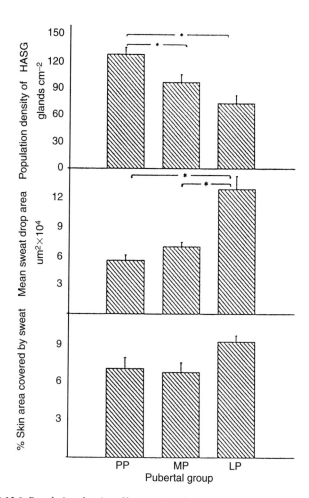

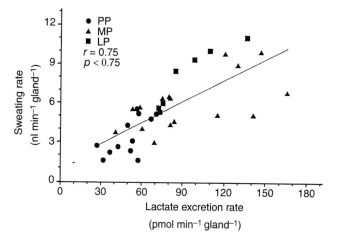

Fig. 2.12.2 The relationship between lactate excretion rate per gland and sweating rate per gland among pre-, mid- and late-pubertal boys (PP, MP, LP, respectively) exercising in the heat (50% peak $\dot{V}O_2$; 42 °C, 20% relative humidity). Reproduced from Falk *et al.*[49]

Fig. 2.12.1 Population density of heat activated sweat glands, sweat bead area and the percentage of skin area covered by sweat among pre-, mid- and late-pubertal boys (PP, MP, LP, respectively) exercising in the heat (50% peak $\dot{V}O_2$; 42 °C, 20% relative humidity). Modified from Falk *et al.*[41]

anaerobic glycolysis at the sweat gland, and the rate of the gland's lactate excretion has been used as an index of sweat gland metabolism.[35,49] In fact, sweating rate per gland was shown to be directly related to the lactate excretion rate per gland.[49] Additionally, both sweating rate and lactate excretion rate per gland appear to increase with the level of physical maturity (Fig. 2.12.2). The increase in the anaerobic metabolism of the sweat gland with growth and maturation is in line with the increase in glycolytic enzyme activity in muscle[50] and the increase in anaerobic muscle power[51] observed during adolescence.

Therefore, the higher sweating response observed in adults compared with children may be explained by:
(1) an increase in the size of the sweat glands;
(2) an increase in the glands' sensitivity; and
(3) an enhancement of the glands' anaerobic capacity.
Further research is needed to elucidate the unique contribution of each of these factors, as well as possible contributions of other factors.

Physiological response to thermal stress

Thermal stress, with or without exercise, is accompanied by changes in body temperatures, metabolic, circulatory and hormonal responses, as well as an activation of the sweating mechanism. This section focuses on the differences in the physiological responses to heat and to cold stress between children and adults, and the changes that may take place in this response during growth and maturation. Table 2.12.3 summarizes the available information on the differential physiological response to rest and exercise in the heat and in the cold between children and adults. It is clear that there is still a wide gap in our knowledge, especially with regard to cold stress.

Physiological response to heat stress

Changes in body temperatures in response to heat stress

Environmental heat stress, especially when accompanied by physical exercise, brings about an increase in core and peripheral temperatures. In children and adolescents, the core temperature has been examined through the measurement of rectal temperature, although oesophageal or tymphanic temperatures have also been used in adults. The temperature of the periphery is reflected by measurement of skin temperature at various sites.

Studies which investigated the thermoregulatory response to exercise in a thermoneutral or warm environment, reported similar or even lower rectal temperature in children than in adults.[1–3,52] In warm conditions (30 °C, 45% relative humidity), Shibasaki *et al.*[42] found that exercising boys and men displayed a similar rise in rectal temperature. This agrees with previous findings comparing girls with women in similar conditions (28 °C, 45% relative humidity).[7] That is, under thermoneutral or warm conditions, the effectiveness of thermoregulation,

Table 2.12.3   Differences in the physiological response to heat and cold exposure among children and adults*

	Response		Children compared with adults	
			Heat	**Cold**
Body temperature	Rectal	Rest	Similar or higher	Similar or lower
		Exercise	Higher	Similar
	Skin	Rest	Higher	Lower
		Exercise	Higher	Lower
Metabolism	$\dot{V}O_2$	Rest	Higher	Higher
		Exercise	Similar or higher	Higher
Circulation	Cardiac output	Rest	Lower	?
		Exercise	Lower	?
	Stroke volume	Rest	Lower	?
		Exercise	Lower	?
	Heart rate	Rest	Higher	Lower or higher
		Exercise	Higher	?
	Skin blood flow	Rest	?	?
		Exercise	Higher	?
	Blood pressure	Rest	Lower	?
		Exercise	?	?
Endocrine system	Fluid and electrolyte	Rest	Similar or lower	?
	Regulation	Exercise	Similar or lower	?
	Stress hormones	Rest	Similar or lower	?
		Exercise	Similar	?
Sweating rate	Per unit surface area	Rest	Lower	–
		Exercise	Lower	–
	Per gland	Rest	Lower	–
		Exercise	Lower	–
Sweating composition	Sodium chloride		Similar or lower	–
	Potassium		Similar or higher	–
	Lactate		Higher	–
Fluid regulation	Rate of dehydration		Similar	–

*Reproduced from Falk.[31]

? = no available information; – = not applicable.

as reflected by rectal temperature, is similar among children and adults. Bar-Or[29,30] pointed out that this is because under such conditions, children use a different 'strategy' to dissipate body heat. That is, compared with adults, children dissipate a greater proportion of body heat via radiation and convection than via sweat evaporation. This strategy has been implicated in thermoneutral[2,3,53] as well as in warm conditions.[7,54]

Despite the similar rectal temperatures under these conditions, skin temperature is reported to be higher in the children compared with adults in most,[1,2,7,46,52,55,56] although not all,[42] studies. The higher skin temperature in the children results in a smaller core-to-skin temperature gradient, which limits heat conduction from the core to the periphery. In view of the fact that children rely more on dry cooling than on evaporation, the smaller temperature gradient may contribute to a greater strain on the cardiovascular system.

When ambient temperature is high, and when high ambient temperature is accompanied by high humidity, mean body temperature[45,46,57–60] or heat storage per kg body mass[7,55,61] has been reported to be higher in children compared with adults. In these studies, children and adults either rested or walked. Falk et al.[8] on the other hand, found similar rectal temperatures in children and adoles-

cents of different pubertal stages (and ages) who cycled in hot, dry conditions (42 °C, 20% relative humidity). Furthermore, a longitudinal follow-up of these boys did not demonstrate any change in the rate of rise of rectal temperature.[62] This discrepancy may be explained by the fact that the oxygen cost of walking and running, but not of cycling,[63] is higher in children compared with adults. That is, during walking or running the mass-specific metabolic heat produced, and the heat that needs to be dissipated, is higher in children compared with adults.

Figure 2.12.3 schematically describes the effectiveness of thermoregulation in children versus adults in varying environmental stress conditions. In accordance with the above, in thermoneutral and warm conditions, children appear to thermoregulate as effectively as adults. However, when the heat stress becomes more extreme, thermoregulation in children appears to be somewhat deficient to that of adults. Further discussion of the effectiveness of thermoregulation can be found in Bar-Or[30] and in Falk.[32]

Surprisingly, there are not many epidemiological reports of heat illness in children. Danks et al.[64] reported on 47 cases of heat illness in infants and children during the heat wave in Melbourne, Australia in January 1959. Most of the children were below three years of age.

Thermoregulation has also been implicated in sudden infants' death.[65] The authors argue that during the first two to three months of life, there is an increase in the metabolic rate (relative to body mass), an increase in subcutaneous fat and, therefore, in tissue insulation, and an improvement in vasomotor control in response to cold stimuli. Additionally, the body's surface area-to-mass ratio decreases. All of these shift the thermal balance in favour of heat conservation. In other words, the infant becomes less vulnerable to cold stress but may be more vulnerable to heat stress. The authors argue further that a disturbance to the thermal balance could affect other physiological systems, such as respiration, which may be of importance in sudden unexpected death in infancy. Further research is needed to examine the relationship between environmental heat stress and heat-related illness or injury at various developmental stages.

The metabolic response to heat stress

The higher cost of locomotion previously mentioned, implies that while walking or running at identical speeds, children are under a greater metabolic strain compared with adults. This is the case in both thermoneutral and hot conditions.

The effect that heat stress has on the metabolic response to rest or to exercise is reflected mainly by changes in $\dot{V}O_2$. Most studies which compare the physiologic response between children and adults standardize the metabolic load. That is, all subjects exercise at the same load relative to peak $\dot{V}O_2$ or to kg body mass in the same environmental stress and no comparison is made to thermoneutral conditions. Therefore, the differential effect that environmental heat may have on the metabolic response of children and adults is difficult to evaluate.

Two studies compared the metabolic response of children and adults in varying environmental conditions. No change was seen in $\dot{V}O_2$ among prepubertal girls or adult women walking for one hour (30% peak $\dot{V}O_2$) in dry (48 °C, 10% relative humidity) and in humid (35 °C, 65% relative humidity) heat compared with warm conditions (28 °C, 45% relative humidity).[7] However, a significant increase in $\dot{V}O_2$ in the hot conditions in the girls but not in the women was observed during the second hour of exercise. Carlson and Le Rossignol[60] observed no effect of radiation ($T_g = 37$ °C versus 49 °C) on $\dot{V}O_2$ in ten year old boys, nor in adults cycling at 50% peak $\dot{V}O_2$ for 40 min in humid heat (31 °C, 73% relative humidity). Thus, it is clear

that further research is needed to clarify the metabolic response to heat stress in children and in adolescents and to determine whether this response is different from adults.

The circulatory response to heat stress

The circulatory response to thermal stress can be reflected by changes in cardiac output, stroke volume and heart rate, by changes in peripheral blood flow and possibly, by changes in blood pressure. Very limited information on the cardiovascular response to heat stress is available in children and adolescents.

Cardiac output during exercise of a given intensity is known to be lower in children compared with adults.[13] This, added to their smaller blood volume relative to body surface area, places an added strain on the cardiovascular system in children compared with adults exercising in the heat. During walking (30% peak $\dot{V}O_2$) in various environmental heat conditions, prepubertal girls' cardiac output was consistently lower compared with that of women, and likely contributed to their lower heat tolerance. Additionally, the girls' heart rate was consistently higher.[7] Likewise, Jokinen et al.[66] reported that children younger than five years, resting for 10 min in a Finnish sauna (70°C, 20% relative humidity), displayed a higher heart rate and greater decrease in stroke volume compared with older children, adolescents and adults. Cardiac output increased in the latter but not in the younger children (Fig. 2.12.4), possibly affecting their heat tolerance.

Hebestreit et al.[67] reported that children's heart rate at a given exercise intensity increased linearly with ambient temperature. No comparison was made with adults. Other studies[45] have reported a higher heart rate during exercise in the heat in children compared with adults. On the other hand, Falk et al.[8] reported no difference in the heart rate response to cycling (50% peak $\dot{V}O_2$) in the heat (42 °C, 20% relative humidity) in pre-, mid- and late-pubertal boys. The discrepancy may be due to differences in exercise mode (walk/run versus cycle) or intensity, as noted earlier.

In spite of the reduced cardiac output, peripheral blood flow has been reported to be higher among children compared with adults during or immediately following exercise in the heat.[7,8,42,45] In support of this, a faster rise in skin temperature was observed in 6 to 11 year old boys compared with adults during heat exposure.[4,68] Additionally, Yoshida et al.[69] recently reported that skin blood flow depends more on body temperature than on sweating. This observation was made in adults, although it may be true for children as well. Thus, the higher body temperatures observed in children compared with adults during thermal stress may partly explain their higher skin blood flow. This higher peripheral blood flow implies that a greater proportion of the already lower cardiac output is diverted to the periphery which places an added strain on the cardiovascular system. The higher strain may be partly compensated for by a greater increase in plasma volume in girls compared with women exercising in the heat, as reported by Drinkwater et al.[7]

Shibasaki et al.[42] recently reported higher skin blood flow, as measured by laser Doppler flowmetry, on the trunk but not the forearm of children compared with adults during moderate exercise (46% peak $\dot{V}O_2$) in warm conditions (30 °C, 45% relative humidity) (Fig. 2.12.5). Furthermore, no difference in regional skin blood flow was observed in the children, while in the men, skin blood flow in the forearm was higher than on the trunk. The authors suggested that regional differences exist in the maturation-related change in peripheral blood flow

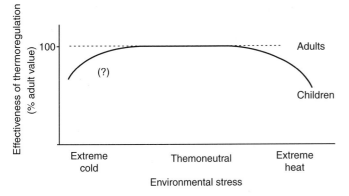

Fig. 2.12.3 Schematic representation of the effectiveness of thermoregulation among children, compared with adults, in relation to the environmental stress. Modified from Bar-Or.[30]

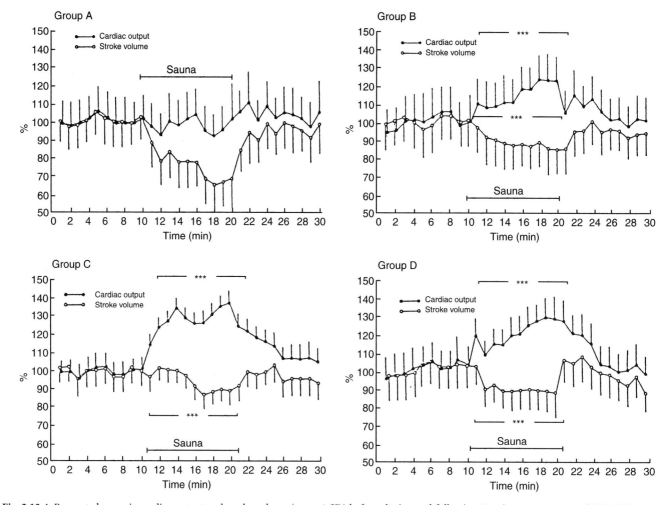

Fig. 2.12.4 Per cent changes in cardiac output and stroke volume (mean ± SD) before, during and following 10 min sauna exposure (70 °C, 20% relative humidity) in four groups. Group A, two to five year old children; group B, five to ten year old children; group C, 10 to 15 year old children and adolescents; group D, 15 to 40 year old adolescents and adults. The mean of the pre-sauna values was used as 100%. Reproduced from Jokinen *et al.*[59]

in response to exercise in the heat. The authors further suggested that these differences may be explained by structural changes in the cutaneous vasculature or by different sensitivity to vasoactive peptides.

It is suggested that the sometimes-reported lower subjective exercise tolerance in children exercising in the heat[7,8,70] may be due to maladjustment of the cardiovascular system, resulting in reduced blood flow to the working muscles and to the central nervous system. In fact, Jokinen *et al.*[59] reported two cases of vasovagal collapses immediately following exposure to a Finnish sauna in children younger than ten years, but not in older children, adolescents or adults. The same group[71] also reported extrasystoles among children as well as a reversible sinus arrest in a five year old girl during and following 10 min in a sauna. In both cases, the authors emphasized that extreme heat places an added demand on the cardiovascular system in young children.

The hormonal response to heat stress

The hormonal response to exercise in the heat has traditionally been studied in relation to hormones associated with fluid and electrolytes balance. Few studies have examined this response in children. An increase in aldosterone has been reported in pre- to late-pubertal boys following rest and exercise in the heat.[23,66] This is similar to the response generally described in adults. No change in vasopressin, cortisol or catecholamines concentration was observed in children following a 10 min exposure to a Finnish sauna, although an increase was observed among adults.[66]

Of the hormones associated with puberty, only the prolactin response to heat stress was investigated in children and adolescents, probably due to its association with osmoregulation. Heat stress, whether accompanied by exercise or not, has been reported to result in an increase in prolactin concentration in children and adolescents[23,66] as well as in adults.[21,72] Prolactin has also been implicated in sweat electrolyte composition in adults[21,22] and adolescent boys.[23] However, its differential influence on sweat gland function in children and adults is unknown. To the author's knowledge, no studies have examined the effect of thermal stress on other hormones associated with puberty or growth among children and adolescents. Therefore, it is unclear whether and how these hormones may modify the thermoregulatory response and what may be the differential response in children compared with adults.

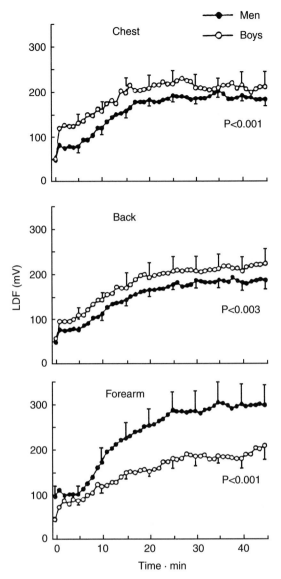

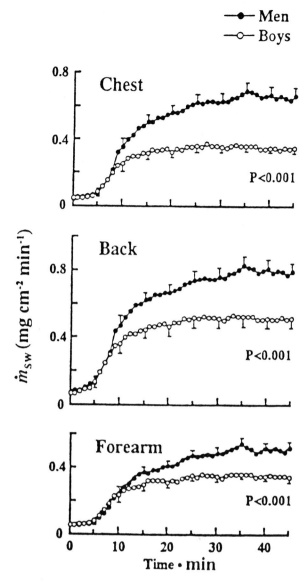

Fig. 2.12.5 Skin blood flow (LDF), as measured by laser Doppler flowmetry, on the chest, back and forearm of 10 to 11 year old prepubertal boys and 20 to 25 year old men cycling in the heat (40% peak $\dot{V}O_2$; 30 °C, 45% relative humidity). *P* values are for an overall effect of age during exercise. Reprinted from Shibasaki *et al.*[42]

Fig. 2.12.6 Local sweating rate ($\dot{m}_{sw}$) on the chest, back and forearm of 10 to 11 year old prepubertal boys and 20 to 25 year old men, cycling in the heat (40% peak $\dot{V}O_2$; 30 °C, 45% relative humidity). P values are for an overall effect of age during exercise. Reprinted from Shibasaki *et al.*[42]

The sweating response to heat stress

As previously mentioned, the sweating apparatus and mechanism is quantitatively and qualitatively different in children and adults. These dissimilarities are reflected in differences in the sweating rate, as well as in the sweat composition between children and adults.

Sweating rate

In any given environmental and metabolic load the sweating rate in prepubertal boys is consistently and distinctly lower compared with men (see Bar-Or;[29,30] Falk[32] for review), even when expressed per body surface area.[1,7,16,26,42–45,73] In contrast, the difference in the sweating rate between girls and women is much smaller[7,73] or even non-existent.[26]

Most studies comparing children and adults measure whole-body sweating rate. Shibasaki *et al.*[42] recently demonstrated a lower local sweating rate on the chest, back and forearm of 10 to 11 year old boys compared with men cycling (40% peak $\dot{V}O_2$) in a warm environment (30 °C, 45% relative humidity) (Fig. 2.12.6). Tochihara *et al.*[4] also reported a lower local sweating rate on the back of six to eight year old boys and girls compared with adults during legs immersion in hot water. However, the total sweating rate was similar in the two groups. The discrepancy between the two studies may be related to the different environmental stress (climatic chamber versus hot water leg immersion) or to the different metabolic load (exercise versus rest). Nevertheless, the findings indicate that differences in sweating rate between children and adults may depend on whether sweating rate is measured locally (and on the site measured), or whether it is assessed for the whole body. Furthermore, Tsuzuki-Hayakawa et al.[46] reported that nine months to 4.5 year old boys and girls resting in a warm and humid environment (35 °C, 70% relative humidity) displayed a higher sweating rate compared with their mothers. Thus, differences between children and adults may not be so apparent at a very young age.

Sweating rate per gland can be estimated given the sweating rate and the population density of HASG. The calculated sweating rate per gland has been shown to be much lower in children compared with adults during rest, as well as during exercise in the heat.[16,42,44,74] Similarly, Foster et al.[74] estimated a threefold lower sweating rate per gland in newborn babies compared with adults, when sweat was induced by an intradermal injection of acetylcholine. It is interesting to note that Shibasaki et al.[42] observed a lower sweating rate per gland in boys compared with men at all sites measured (back, chest and forearm). However, in the men, sweating rate per gland was lower in the forearm compared with the chest and back, while in the boys there were no regional differences. The authors suggested that the increase in sweat gland output which occurs during growth takes place at dissimilar rates over the different body parts.

The differences between children and adults described above were extended by comparing pre-, mid- and late-pubertal boys who exercised (50% peak $\dot{V}O_2$) in the heat (40 °C, 20% relative humidity).[41] The authors observed an increase in the sweating rate per body surface area and per gland with increasing maturity (Fig. 2.12.7). Furthermore, within an 18 month follow-up of these boys, sweating rate increased with age.[62] However, it could not be determined whether the increase was progressive, or whether it coincided with the physical growth spurt and hormonal changes which occur during puberty.

Gender differences in sweating rate have been reported in adults,[75] but these differences are not so clear among prepubescents and adolescents. Several studies reported a greater sweating rate in boys compared with girls in response to thermal stimuli[16,76] or pharmacological stimuli.[26] However, others reported similar sweating rates, or only a tendency toward a greater rate in boys compared with girls.[18,55,61,73,77]

The sweating rate is considered an index of the capacity for evaporative heat dissipation. However, in any given environmental stress condition there is an upper limit to the rate of evaporation above which the sweat will drip and any additional sweating will only lead to fluid loss. The maximal sweating rate in children and in adults is unknown. Therefore, it cannot be determined whether or not it is a limiting factor in thermoregulation. When previously reported sweating rates in children and adults were related to metabolic load (standardized for peak $\dot{V}O_2$ and body mass), no clear age-related differences were observed (Falk and Dotan, unpublished). Furthermore, Meyer and Bar-Or[78] could not ascertain differences in the sweat loss per kg body mass among children, adolescents and adults in similar environmental conditions. Thus, it is possible that in warm environments, children sweat less in comparison with adults because they take advantage of their greater body surface area-to-mass ratio and, thus, rely more on dry heat loss. In hot environments, children may sweat less than adults because they take advantage of a possibly higher evaporative cooling efficiency (many small sweat beads versus fewer, larger sweat beads).

Sweat composition

Dill et al.[77] examined sweat electrolyte concentration in children and adults during walks in the desert and came to the conclusion that

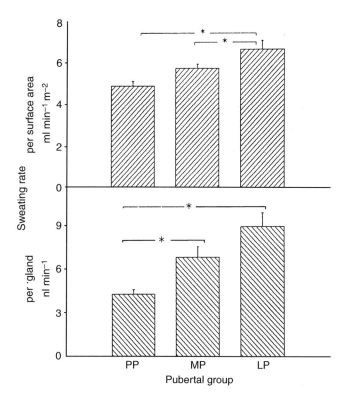

Fig. 2.12.7 Sweating rate per skin surface area and per gland among pre-, mid- and late-pubertal boys (PP, MP, LP, respectively) cycling in the heat (50% peak $\dot{V}O_2$; 42 °C, 20% relative humidity). Modified from Falk et al.[8,41]

sweat composition varies widely between and within individuals. Reviewing later studies, it appears that in general, the concentration of sodium and chloride in children's sweat while exercising in a hot environment is lower than that of adults (30 to 60 versus 60 to 90 mmol litre^{-1}, respectively). This difference is apparent in boys versus men[43] as well as in young children (boys and girls) compared with their mothers.[46] On the other hand, potassium concentration appears to be higher in children's sweat compared with that of adults.[73] It should be noted that while the above differences emerge in response to a thermal stress, they are not so clear when a pharmacological stimulus (e.g. pilocarpine iontophoresis) is used to induce sweat.[79]

In both children and adults, sweat chloride and sodium concentrations appear to increase with an increase in sweating rate. A possible explanation may be the shorter time the secretory fluid spends in the sweat duct, where electrolyte reabsorption occurs. However, in view of the shorter duct length reported in children, other mechanisms are needed to explain the lower thermal sweat salt concentration observed in children compared with adults.[43,46,73]

The neutral ionic balance in sweat is attained via sodium and potassium on the one hand and chloride and lactate on the other hand. While chloride concentration is lower in children compared with adults, lactate concentration is higher.[49] The latter appears to contradict the finding of increased lactate excretion rate per gland with growth and maturation[49] discussed earlier. The contradiction can be explained by the lower population density of HASG in adults compared with children. Thus, the lactate concentration in sweat collected from a *given* area *decreases* with growth and maturation.[49]

Finally, it is interesting to note that proteins which are seen in pharmacologically induced sweat in men but not in women, were observed in pubertal boys but not in prepubertal boys and girls.[80] The authors suggested that the protein profile of sweat may be related to the degree of sexual maturity in young males.

Among adults, differences in sweat electrolyte, lactate and protein concentrations have been attributed to differences in sweating rate, differences in metabolic load or differing hormonal status. However, these explanations cannot fully explain the observed difference in sweat composition between children and adults. Further research is needed to elucidate the mechanisms explaining these differences.

Fluid regulation during heat stress

During exercise in the heat, hypohydration may develop due to fluid losses through sweating. Studies have shown that when water is available *ad libitum*, both children[81,82] and adults[83] do not replace fluid loss sufficiently. This phenomenon, termed 'voluntary dehydration', was recently demonstrated also in late- to post-pubertal adolescent athletes during a simulated duathalon.[76] All subjects finished the duathalon in a state of dehydration, although rehydration was complete within 15 min.

Nursery school (two to six years old) and elementary school (eight to ten years old) children living in a hot climate were recently shown to be in a state of chronic voluntary dehydration, as reflected by high urine osmolality.[84,85] Additionally, among the nursery school children, urine osmolality increased with age.[85] This state of prolonged periods of concentrated urine is associated with an increased risk of development of renal stones. Recent observations suggest that one way to prevent the phenomenon of voluntary dehydration among children is to provide a beverage which is flavoured and enriched with NaCl and carbohydrates.[86–88]

The rise in heart rate and the reduction of stroke volume during exercise is directly related to the degree of hypohydration.[89] This places an added strain on the cardiovascular system. The cardiovascular strain, in turn, may result in reduced skin blood flow[90,91] and be accompanied by a lower sweating rate.[90,92] Although these phenomena have not been clearly demonstrated in children,[81] it should be noted that the added cardiovascular strain may be more detrimental in children than in adults. This is explained by the fact that children appear to rely more on dry heat loss, and therefore on elevated skin blood flow, than on evaporation in order to dissipate body heat. In fact, Bar-Or *et al.*[81] demonstrated that the same degree of voluntary dehydration, expressed as a percentage of body mass, will result in a greater rectal temperature rise in children than in adults exercising in the heat (Fig. 2.12.8). Thus, children's ability to thermoregulate effectively is more dependent on their body water and therefore, even a small reduction in body fluids can be detrimental.

Once hypohydration has set in it is very difficult to reverse during exercise. Thus, the above findings emphasize the need for sound hydration practices before, during and following physical activity in children and adolescents, as well as in adults. Specific recommendations for children include drinking flavoured beverages (especially grape[93]), enriched with carbohydrates (6%) and NaCl (18.0 mmol litre^{-1}).[86–88] Although the latter beverage composition was not shown to influence thirst, electrolyte balance, the thermoregulatory responses, aerobic performance or the perceptual response in children

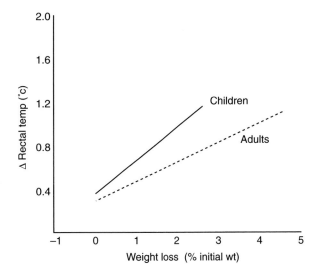

Fig. 2.12.8 The change in rectal temperature in relation to body-mass loss in children and adults. Reproduced from Bar-Or.[29]

exercising in the heat,[93–96] it did prevent dehydration when drink consumption was *ad libitum*.[86,88] Recommendations for the prevention of hypohydration in children can be found in several recent reviews.[31,78,97]

Physiological response to cold stress

Changes in body temperature in response to cold stress

Environmental cold stress results in a decrease in peripheral temperature, often accompanied by a decrease in core temperature. The latter can be prevented or delayed by an increase in the metabolic rate, which occurs during exercise or with shivering, as well as by peripheral vasoconstriction. There are very few studies which have reported upon the thermoregulatory response to cold stress in children.

Among 8 to 18 year old children swimming (30 m min^{-1}) in cool water (20.3 °C), oral temperature was found to decrease at a slower rate with an increase in age.[98] That is, in spite of the fact that the younger children swam at a faster speed relative to their size and assumed potential, their rate of cooling was faster than the older children. The rate of cooling was also found to be directly related to the surface area-to-mass ratio, and to the level of adiposity. These results indicate the importance of body dimensions, as well as body adiposity, in maintaining body temperatures in the cold.

The faster rate of cooling in the younger children reported above, was recently supported by Inoue *et al.*[99] who compared the thermoregulatory response of prepubertal boys with that of young men at rest during a linear decrease in environmental temperature (28 to 15 °C). The boys' skin temperature was lower compared with the men, reflecting greater vasoconstriction. This is in line with other reports of lower skin temperature in children and adults resting in cool conditions (15 to 20 °C).[68,100] Nevertheless, rectal temperature decreased in the boys while it remained stable in the men.

Different results were reported by Smolander *et al.*[12] who compared the body temperature response in children and adults during exercise in a cold environment (5 °C). Pre- and early-pubescent boys were able to maintain their body temperature as effectively as adults while cycling (30% peak $\dot{V}O2$) in the cold. In fact, the children's rectal temperature slightly (insignificantly) increased while exercising. The children's skin temperature was significantly lower at several sites, indicating a greater peripheral vasoconstriction, compared with the adults. The authors argued that the children were able to maintain their core temperature during exercise, by increasing their metabolic rate and constricting peripheral vessels to a greater extent than the adults. This age-related difference was observed when comparing two boys and two men with similar surface area-to-mass ratios, indicating that the different strategy is apparently related to maturation and not only to body size.

We recently studied 11 to 12 year old boys during rest and exercise (50 min rest, 10 min cycle, 50 min rest) in a cold (7 °C), cool (13 °C) and thermoneutral (22 °C) environment.[101] Rectal temperature decreased during the first 50 min of rest and continued to decrease in the subsequent rest period, in spite of the fact that the boys were dressed in sweat pants and shirts (Fig. 2.12.9). Following the 10 min of exercise rectal temperature slightly increased in the cool and neutral but not in the cold conditions. It should be stressed that rectal temperature did not return to pre-exposure levels even following 30 min of rest in a thermoneutral environment (21 to 23 °C). Skin temperature on the hand, which was exposed, decreased in the cold and cool environment, while there was no apparent change in chest temperature which was covered by two layers of clothes. The decrease in rectal temperature observed in this study are in contrast to the ability of boys to maintain their body temperature while exercising in 5 °C, and wearing only shorts.[12] The discrepancy may be explained by the fact that in the latter study exercise duration was much longer (40 versus 10 min) and rest duration was much shorter (20 versus 50 min). The difference in the results demonstrate the importance of the increase in metabolic rate during cold exposure for the maintenance of body temperature among children. The importance of the elevated metabolic rate during exercise in the cold was also demonstrated by the 0.5 to 0.6 °C increase in rectal temperature in 12 year old boys exercising at 50% peak $\dot{V}O_2$ for 60 min in effective temperatures of 25 °C and 10 °C.

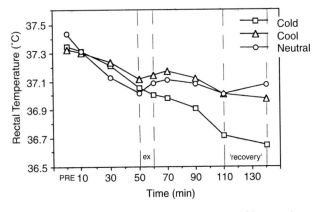

Fig. 2.12.9 Mean rectal temperature in 11 to 12 year old boys resting and exercising (50 min rest, 10 min cycle, 50 min rest) in a cold (7 °C), cool (13 °C) and thermoneutral (22 °C) environment and following 30 min 'recovery' in a thermoneutral environment. Modified from Falk *et al.*[101] (ex = exercise.)

The studies described above suggest that during rest, the effectiveness of thermoregulation is lower in children compared with adults, as schematically illustrated in Fig. 2.12.3. During exercise, children may maintain their core temperature by markedly increasing their metabolic rate. However, it is unclear how long this higher metabolic rate can be sustained.

The metabolic response to cold stress

As argued above, the metabolic response to cold stress, is very instrumental for maintaining body temperature in both children and adults. In adults, rest or submaximal exercise in the cold is accompanied by a marked increase in $\dot{V}O_2$ as a result of overt shivering or a possible decrease in the mechanical efficiency during exercise. An increase in $\dot{V}O_2$ was also reported in most studies,[12,100,102,103] although not all,[99,104] investigating children during rest or exercise in the cold. In fact, in studies where a comparison with adults was made, the increase in $\dot{V}O_2$ was greater in the boys. Ueda *et al.*[103] comment that the increase in $\dot{V}O_2$ during swimming in cold water (20 and 25 °C) among 10 to 12 year old boys was largely attributed to shivering, although it is unclear how this was measured. This is in line with children's higher subjective sensitivity to cold compared with adults.[12] Most studies do not report on shivering nor on mechanical efficiency. Therefore, it is impossible to determine the mechanisms responsible for the increase in metabolic rate and the possible differences between the boys and men. Nevertheless, in view of the greater body surface area-to-mass ratio in children, it is expected that at a given cold stress, children would have to elicit a greater metabolic rate compared with adults in order to maintain body temperatures.

The circulatory response to cold stress

Very little is known about the cardiovascular response to cold in children. Lower skin temperatures or a faster decrease in skin temperature was reported in children compared with adults resting or exercising in the cold.[12,68,99,100] The authors argue that the lower skin temperatures reflect a greater vasoconstriction in the children than in the adults. However, no study has reported peripheral blood flow in children during cold stress.

In adults, heart rate generally decreases in response to cold stress during rest or submaximal exercise. A lower heart rate was observed in 12 year old boys cycling at an effective temperature of 10 °C compared with 25 °C.[104] Additionally, the decrease in heart rate following exercise was more rapid in the lower temperature. Similarly, 11 to 12 year old boys cycling in 7 °C and 13 °C displayed a lower heart rate compared with that at 22 °C.[101] On the other hand, Marsh *et al.*[102] reported higher heart rates in 11 year old children cycling in 5 °C versus 22 °C. While no explanation is given for this discrepancy, it is clear that further research is needed to examine the cardiovascular response to exercise in the cold in children.

Adaptation to thermal stress

Repeated exposures to heat result in an adaptation to heat stress and is termed acclimatization or acclimation. On the other hand, repeated cold exposures result in limited adaptation in adults. The adaptation process to cold exposure in children has not been investigated. Thus, the following section discusses only the differences in the adaptation processes to heat between children and adults. Additionally, training-induced adaptations enable the body to better cope with heat stress, but not necessarily with cold stress. A discussion of the effects of training and of fitness on the response to heat and to cold stress in children and adolescents follows.

Acclimatization and acclimation to heat

The process of heat acclimation is similar in children, adolescents and adults, although the rate of acclimation may differ. Children and adults were shown to reach a similar acclimation level following a two-week, three times per week, acclimation protocol which involved exercising in the heat (43 °C, 21% relative humidity).[44] However, the rate of acclimation in the early stages was slower in the children than in the adults (Fig. 2.12.10). These findings are in line with the lower level of acclimation demonstrated among 11 to 16 year old boys compared with men following an eight day acclimation protocol involving exercise in the heat (48 °C, 17% relative humidity).[45]

One of the major changes which characterizes the process of heat acclimation is an increase in sweating rate. This has been demonstrated in children,[44,105] as well as in adults.[106] In adults, five daily exercise-in-the-heat sessions were found to provide only a minimal stimulus for sudomotor adaptation.[107] In children, six exercise-in-the-heat sessions over a two week period did not have an effect on total sweating rate. However, sweating rate during exercise increased, while during rest, a decrease in sweating rate was observed.[108] Although the acclimation protocol in the latter study was of a similar frequency and duration as that utilized by Inbar,[44] a different effect was demonstrated on sweating rate. The discrepancy may be explained by the different environmental conditions used in the two studies. That is, a two week, three times per week acclimation period in a hot and dry environment, where the only avenue of heat dissipation was sweat evaporation, resulted in an increase in sweating rate.[44] While a similar

protocol in a warm, more humid environment, where dry heat exchange can also be used for heat dissipation, had little effect on the sweating mechanism.[108]

From the above studies it is clear that added precaution is warranted during the early days of summer or during sudden climate changes in adults, and more so in children. The added precaution is emphasized especially in view of the finding that during acclimation to heat the subjective difficulty at any given heat-and-exercise stress decreases faster in children than in adults.[109] That is, the children are less likely to match their behaviour to the actual physiological strain.

In spite of the apparent slower rate of acclimation in children mentioned above, it should be noted that less stringent acclimation regimens (e.g. exercise in a thermoneutral environment or passive rather than active exposure to heat) have been shown to result in sufficient acclimation in children.[105] Thus, it is clear that much more research is needed to elucidate the mechanism of acclimation in children.

Training-induced adaptations and the response to heat stress

Physical training results in numerous physiological adaptations, some of which can affect the response to heat stress. For example, enhanced cardiovascular function can improve heat tolerance. The relationship between physical training or physical fitness and heat tolerance has been clearly demonstrated in adults, although not so consistently in children.

In adults, peak $\dot{V}O_2$ has been associated with an enhanced heat tolerance. On the other hand, in prepubertal boys, Delmarche et al.[2] could not demonstrate such a relationship. Similarly, peak $\dot{V}O_2$ was found to account for only 16% of the variance in the rectal temperature response to exercise in the heat among prepubertal boys.[54]

Intervention training studies in children have demonstrated inconsistent effects on the body temperature response to heat load. For example, Araki et al.[68] found no effect of training on the body temperature response to passive heat stress. On the other hand, Inbar et al.[105] observed that a two-week training programme involving cycling (85% of maximal heart rate) in a hot environment, as well as in a thermoneutral environment, resulted in a lower rectal temperature and heart rate response to exercise in the heat in eight to ten year old boys.

Training has been shown to result in an increased sweating rate in adults. Cross-sectional comparisons of trained and untrained boys revealed a higher sweating rate at any given rectal temperature in trained compared with untrained boys resting in a warm and humid environment (30 °C, 70% relative humidity).[110] However, a two week training programme did not result in any change in sweating rate.[105] Clearly, further research is needed to investigate the relationship between fitness and training-induced adaptations on the one hand, and the response to heat stress on the other hand.

Training-induced adaptations and the response to cold stress

Very little is known about training-induced adaptations and the thermoregulatory response to cold stress in adults. In children, two studies investigated the effect of training on the response to a relatively cool environments (18 to 20 °C), with inconsistent results. A smaller decrease in rectal temperature during rest in a cool environment

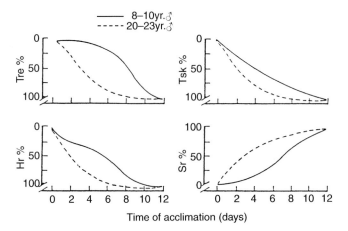

Fig. 2.12.10 Physiological adaptations during the course of heat acclimation among eight to ten year old boys and 20 to 23 year old men. Adaptations in rectal and skin temperatures, heart rate and sweating rate are expressed as per cent of final acclimation value, where baseline values are 0%. Schematic representation from Bar-Or;[29] modified from Bar-Or.[53]

(18 °C) was observed in trained compared with untrained prepubertal boys.[110] On the other hand, no difference in the rectal temperature response to exposure to a cool environment (20 °C) was observed in four prepubertal boys before and following 40 days of physical training.[68] Thus, there is a wide gap in our knowledge regarding the possible effects of training on the thermoregulatory response to cold stress in children, as in adults.

Summary

Thermoregulation during exposure to hot or cold environments differs between children and adults. The physical and physiological differences between children and adults may explain the dissimilar response to thermal stress.

The main physical differences between children and adults which affect thermoregulation are the larger surface area-to-mass ratio and the smaller blood volume in the children. These differences affect the children's strategy of thermoregulation, allowing them to rely more on dry heat loss and less on evaporative cooling in a warm environment. However, in extreme conditions, hot or cold, the greater surface area-to-mass ratio results in a higher rate of heat absorption or heat loss, respectively. The smaller blood volume in children, even when corrected for body surface area, may compromise their exercise performance in the heat and potentiate the effects of hypohydration.

The main physiological difference between children and adults is the lower sweating rate characteristic of children. Calculations have demonstrated that the lower sweating rate is due to a lower sweating rate per gland and not to a smaller number of sweat glands. The lower sweating rate per gland may be explained by the smaller sweat gland size, a lower sensitivity of the sweating mechanism to thermal stimuli and, possibly, a lower sweat gland metabolic capacity.

Metabolic, circulatory and hormonal differences between children and adults may also affect thermoregulation. Children are characterized by a higher metabolic cost of locomotion which places an added strain on the thermoregulatory system during heat exposure but may be advantageous during an acute cold exposure. The lower cardiac output at any given exercise intensity and the lower haemoglobin concentration in boys compared with men, contribute to an added cardiovascular strain during exercise in the heat. Finally, testosterone, oestrogen, prolactin and growth hormone differ in their baseline concentration between children and adults, and may affect sweat gland function and sweat composition.

During exercise in thermoneutral or warm environments, children thermoregulate as effectively as adults. In extreme environmental conditions, children's thermoregulation appears to be somewhat deficient compared with that of adults.

Heat stress often results in higher body temperatures, while cold stress can result in lower body temperatures, especially skin temperatures, in children compared with adults. In children, the changes in body temperature are accompanied by a greater increase in the metabolic cost of exercise in the heat, and especially in the cold. The cardiovascular system appears to be strained more in children when compared with adults exposed to heat, possibly explaining the greater subjective intolerance to heat stress sometimes reported in children. On the other hand, relatively little is known about the circulatory response to cold stress in children and adolescents. The few reports on the endocrine response to heat stress demonstrate a similar or sometimes lower response in children compared with adults, while the hormonal response to cold stress has not been investigated in children or in adolescents.

Voluntary dehydration is a phenomenon which occurs in both children and adults while exercising in the heat. This state of hypohydration, and the resultant added cardiovascular strain, is apparently more detrimental in children than in adults, probably because children rely more on dry heat loss and therefore on elevated skin blood flow to dissipate body heat. Dehydration in children can be prevented by providing a flavoured beverage, enriched with NaCl and carbohydrates.

A wide gap still exists in our understanding of the thermoregulatory response in children and how it changes during adolescence. Additionally, very little is known about acclimation, as well as training-induced adaptations and their effect on the response to heat or to cold in children and adolescents. Finally, gender differences in prepubertal children and differences between girls and women need to be studied further.

References

1. Davies, C. T. M. Thermal responses to exercise in children. *Ergonomics* 1981; **24**: 55–61.
2. Delmarche, P., Bittel, J., Lacour, J. R. and Flandrois, R. Thermoregulation at rest and during exercise in prepubertal boys. *European Journal of Applied Physiology* 1990; **60**: 436–40.
3. Gullestad, R. Temperature regulation in children during exercise. *Acta Paediatrica Scandinavica* 1975; **64**: 257–63.
4. Tochihara, Y., Ohnaka, T. and Nagai, Y. Thermal responses of 6- to 8-year old children during immersion of their legs in a hot water bath. *Applied Human Science* 1995; **14**: 23–8.
5. Forbes, G. B. Body composition in adolescence. In *Human growth*, Vol. 2 (ed. F. Falkner and J. M. Tanner). Plenum Press, New York, 1986; 119–45.
6. Koch, G. Muscle blood flow in prepubertal boys. *Medicine in Sport* 1978; **11**: 39–46.
7. Drinkwater, B. L., Kupprat, I. C., Denton, J. E., Christ, J. L. and Horvath, S. M. Response of prepubertal girls and college women to work in the heat. *Journal of Applied Physiology* 1977; **43**: 1046–53.
8. Falk, B., Bar-Or, O. and MacDougall, J. D. The thermoregulatory response of pre-, mid- and late-pubertal boys to exercise in dry heat. *Medicine and Science in Sports and Exercise* 1992; **24**: 688–94.
9. Orenstein, D. M., Henke, K. G., Costill, D. L., Doershuk, C. F., Lemon, P. J. and Stern, R. C. Exercise and heat stress in cystic fibrosis patients. *Pediatric Research* 1983; **17**: 267–9.
10. Unnithan, V. B. and Eston, R. G. Stride frequency and submaximal treadmill running economy in adults and children. *Pediatric Exercise Science* 1990; **2**: 149–55.
11. Arens, G. A. M., van Mechelen, W., Kemper, H. C. G. and Twisk, J. W. R. The longitudinal development of running economy in males and females aged between 13 and 27 years: The Amsterdam growth and health study. *European Journal of Applied Physiology* 1997; **76**: 214–20.
12. Smolander, J., Bar-Or, O., Korhonen, O. and Ilmarinen, J. Thermoregulation during rest and exercise in the cold in pre- and early pubescent boys and in young men. *Journal of Applied Physiology* 1992; **72**: 1589.
13. Turley, K. R. and Wilmore, J. H. Cardiovascular responses to treadmill and cycle ergometer exercise in children and adults. *Journal of Applied Physiology* 1997; **83**: 948–57.
14. Dallman, P. R. and Siimes, M. A. Percentile curves for haemoglobin and red cell volume in infancy and childhood. *Journal of Pediatrics* 1979; **94**: 26–31.
15. Soldin, S. J. and Hicks, J. M. *Pediatric reference ranges*. AACC Press, Washington, DC, 1995; 1589–94.

16. Kawahata, A. Sex differences in sweating. In *Essential problems in climatic physiology* (ed. H. Yoshimura, K. Ogata and S. Itoh). Nankodo, Kyoto, 1960; 169–84.

17. Choudhry, R., Hodgins, M. B., Van der Kwast, T. H., Brinkmann, A. O. and Boersma, W. J. A. Localization of androgen receptors I human skin by immunohistochemistry: Implications for the hormonal regulation of hair growth, sevaceous glands, and sweat glands. *Journal of Endocrinology* 1992; 133: 467–75.

18. Rees, J. and Shuster, S. Pubertal induction of sweat gland activity. *Clinical Science* 1981; 60: 689–92.

19. Bar-Or, O. Thermoregulation in females from a life span perspective. In *Perspectives in exercise science and sports medicine, Volume 9: Exercise and the female—A life span approach* (ed. O. Bar-Or, D. R. Lamb and P. M. Clarkson). Cooper Publishing Group, Indianapolis, 1996; 250–85.

20. Fraser, D., Padwick, M. L., Whitehead, M., Coffer, A. and King, R. J. B. Presence of an oestradiol receptor-related protein in the skin: Changes during the normal menstrual cycle. *British Journal of Obstetrics and Gynaecology* 1991; 98: 1277–82.

21. Kaufman, F. L., Mills, D. E., Hughson, R. L. and Peake, G. T. Effects of bromocriptine on sweat gland function during heat acclimatization. *Hormone Research* 1988; 29: 31–8.

22. Robertson, M. T., Boyajian, M. J., Patterson, K. and Robertson, W. V. B. Modulation of the chloride concentration of human sweat by prolactin. *Endocrinology* 1986; 119: 2439–44.

23. Falk, B., Bar-Or, O. and MacDougall, J. D. Aldosterone and prolactin response to exercise in the heat among circum-pubertal boys. *Journal of Applied Physiology* 1991; 71: 1741–5.

24. Juul, A., Main, K., Nielsen, B. and Skakkebaek, N. E. Decreased sweating in growth hormone deficiency: Does it play a role in thermoregulation? *Journal of Pediatric Endocrinology* 1993; 6: 39–44.

25. Juul, A., Hjortskov, N., Jepsen, L. T., Neilsen, B., Halkjaer-Kristensen, J., Vahl, N., Jorgensen, J. O., Christiansen, J. S. and Skakkebaek, N. E. Growth hormone deficiency and hypothermia during exercise: A controlled study of sixteen GH-deficient patients. *Journal of Clinical Endocrinology and Metabolism* 1995; 80: 3335–40.

26. Main, K., Nilsson, K. O. and Skiakkebaek, N. E. Influence of sex and growth hormone deficiency on sweating. *Scandinavian Journal of Clinical and Laboratory Investigation* 1991; 51: 475–80.

27. Lobie, P. E., Breipohl, W., Lincoln, D. T., Garcia-Aragon J. and Waters, M. J. Localization of the growth hormone receptor/binding protein in skin. *Journal of Endocrinology* 1990; 126: 467–72.

28. Oakes, S.R., Haynes, K. M., Waters, M. J., Herington, A.C. and Wether, G.A. Demonstration and localization of growth hormone receptor in human skin and skin fibroblasts. *Journal of Clinical Endocrinology and Metabolism* 1992; 75: 1368–73.

29. Bar-Or, O. Climate and the exercising child—A review. *International Journal of Sports Medicine* 1980; 1: 53–65

30. Bar-Or, O. Temperature regulation during exercise in children and adolescents. In *Perspectives in exercise science and sports medicine Vol. 2. Youth, exercise and sport* (ed. C. V. Gisolfi and D. R. Lamb). Benchmark Press, Indianapolis, 1989; 335–62.

31. Falk, B. Physiological and health aspects of exercise in hot and cold climates. In *Encyclopaedia of sports medicine: The child and the adolescent athlete* (ed. O. Bar-Or). Blackwell Scientific, Oxford, 1996; 326–52.

32. Falk, B. Effects of thermal stress during rest and exercise in the pediatric population. *Sports Medicine* 1998; 25: 221–40.

33. Sato, K., Leidal. R. and Sato, F. Morphology and development of an apoeccrine sweat gland in human axillae. *American Journal of Physiology* 1987; 252: R166–80.

34. Landing, B. H., Wells, T. R. and Wiliamson, M. L. Studies on growth of eccrine sweat glands. In *Human growth: Body composition, cell growth, energy and intelligence* (ed. D. G. Cheek). Lea and Febriger, Philadelphia, 1968; 382–94.

35. Wolfe, S., Cage, G., Epstein, M., Tice, L., Mitler, H. and Gordon, R. G. Jr. Metabolic studies on isolated human eccrine sweat glands. *Journal of Clinical Investigation* 1970; 49: 1880–4.

36. Sato. K. and Sato. F. Individual variations in structure and function of human eccrine sweat glands. *American Journal of Physiology* 1983; 245: R203–8.

37. Kuno, Y. *Human perspiration*. Charles C Thomas, Springfield, Il, 1956.

38. Bar-Or, O., Lundegren, H. M. and Buskirk, E. R. Distribution of heat-activated sweat glands in obese and lean men and women. *Journal of Applied Physiology* 1969; 26: 403–9.

39. Szabo, G. The number of eccrine sweat glands in human skin. *Advanced Biology of the Skin* 1962; 3: 1–5.

40. Shibasaki, M., Inoue, Y. and Kondo, N. Mechanisms of underdeveloped sweating responses in prepubertal boys. *European Journal of Applied Physiology* 1997; 76: 340–5.

41. Falk, B. Bar-Or, O. MacDougall, J. D. and Calvert, R. Sweat gland response to exercise in the heat among pre-, mid- and late-pubertal boys. *Medicine and Science in Sports and Exercise* 1992; 24: 313–19.

42. Shibasaki, M., Inoue. Y., Kondo, N. and Iwata, A. Thermoregulatory responses of prepubertal boys and young men during moderate exercise. *European Journal of Applied Physiology* 1997; 75: 212–8.

43. Araki, T., Toda, Y., Matsushita, K. and Tsujino, A. Age differences in sweating during muscular exercise. *Japanese Journal of Fitness and Sports Medicine* 1979; 28: 239–48.

44. Inbar, O. *Acclimatization to dry and hot environment in young adults and children 8–10 years old*. Ed.D. dissertation, Columbia University, 1978.

45. Wagner, J. A., Robinson, S., Tzankoff, S.W. and Marino RP. Heat tolerance and acclimatization to work in the heat in relation to age. *Journal of Applied Physiology* 1972; 33: 616–22.

46. Tsuzuki-Hayakawa, K., Tochihara, Y. and Ohnaka T. Thermoregulation during heat exposure of young children compared to their mothers. *European Journal of Applied Physiology* 1995; 72: 12–7.

47. Collins, K. J., Sargent, F. and Weiner J.S. Excitation and depression of eccrine sweat glands by acetylcholine, acetyl-B-methylcholine and adrenaline. *Journal of Physiology* 1959; 148: 592–614.

48. Wada, M. Sudorific action of adrenaline on the human sweat glands and determination of their excitability. *Science* 1950; 111: 376–7.

49. Falk, B., Bar-Or, O., MacDougal, J. D., McGillis. L., Calvert, R. and Meyer F. Sweat lactate in exercising children and adolescents of varying physical maturity. *Journal of Applied Physiology* 1991; 71: 1735–40.

50. Eriksson, B. O. and Saltin B. Muscle metabolism during exercise in boys aged 11 to 16 years compared to adults. *Acta Paediatrica Belgica* 1974; 28: 257–65.

51. Falk, B. and Bar-Or, O. Longitudinal changes in peak aerobic and anaerobic mechanical power of circumpubertal boys. *Pediatric Exercise Science* 1993; 5: 318–31.

52. Bittel J. and Henane R. Comparison of neutral exchanges in men and women under neutral and hot conditions. *Journal of Physiology (London)* 1975; 250: 475–89.

53. Bar-Or, O. *Pediatric sports medicine for the practitioner*. Springer-Verlag, New York, 1983; 259–99.

54. Docherty. D., Eckerson, J. D. and Hayward J. S. Physique and thermoregulation in prepubertal males during exercise in a warm, humid environment. *American Journal of Physical Anthropology* 1986; 70: 19–23.

55. Haymes, E. M., McCormick, R. J. and Buskirk, E. R. Heat tolerance of exercise in lean and obese prepubertal boys. *Journal of Applied Physiology* 1975; 39: 457–61.

56. McCormick, R. J. and Buskirk, E. R. Heat tolerance of exercising lean and obese middle-aged men. *Federal Proceedings* 1974; 33: 441.

57. Sohar, E. and Shapira, Y. The physiological reactions of women and children marching during heat. *Proceedings of the Israel physiology and pharmacology society* 1965; 1: 50.

58. Leppaluoto, J. Human thermoregulation in sauna. *Annals of Clinical Research* 1988; 20: 240–3.

59. Jokinen, E., Valimaki. I., Antila, K., Seppanen, A. and Tuominen, J. Children in sauna: Cardiovascular adjustment. *Pediatrics* 1990; 86: 282–8.

60. Carlson, J. S. and Le Rossignol, P. Children and adults exercising in hot wet climatic conditions with different levels of radiant heat.

North American society of pediatric exercise medicine, ninth annual meeting, Pittsburgh, PA, 1994; August 11–14, abstract.

61. Haymes, E. M., Buskirk, E. R., Hodgson, J. L., Lundegren, H. M. and Nicholas, W. C. Heat tolerance of exercising lean and heavy prepubertal girls. *Journal of Applied Physiology* 1974; **36**: 566–71.

62. Falk, B., Bar-Or, O., MacDougall, J. D., Goldsmith, C. and McGillis, L. A longitudinal analysis of the sweating response of pre-, mid- and late-pubertal boys during exercise in the heat. *American Journal of Human Biology* 1992; **4**: 527–35.

63. Rowland, T. W., Staab, J. S., Unnithan, V. B., Rambusch, J. M. and Sicondolfi, S. F. Mechanical efficiency during cycling in prepubertal and adult males. *International Journal of Sports Medicine* 1990; **11**: 452–5.

64. Danks, D. M., Webb, D. W. and Allen, J. Heat illness in infants and young children. *British Medical Journal* 1962; 287–92.

65. Fleming, P. J., Azaz, Y. and Wigfield, R. Development of thermoregulation in infancy: possible implications for SIDS. *Journal of Clinical Pathology* 1992; **45**: 17–9.

66. Jokinen, E., Valimaki, I., Marniemi, J., Seppanen, A., Irjala, K. and Simkell, O. Children in sauna: hormonal adjustments to intensive short thermal stress. *Acta Physiolgica Scandinavica* 1991; **80**: 370–4.

67. Hebestreit, H., Bar-Or, O., McKinty, C., Riddell, M. and Zehr, P. Climate-related corrections for improved estimation of energy expenditure from heart rate in children. *Journal of Applied Physiology* 1995; **79**: 47–54.

68. Araki, T., Tsujita, J., Matsushita, K. and Hori, W. Thermoregulatory responses of prepubertal boys to heat and cold in relation to physical training. *Journal of Human Ergonomics* 1980; **9**: 69–80.

69. Yoshida, R., Nagashima, K., Nose, H., Kawabata, T., Nakai, S. Torimoto A, et al. Relationship between aerobic power, blood volume, and thermoregulatory responses to exercise-heat stress. *Medicine and Science in Sports and Exercise* 1997; **29**: 867–73.

70. Mackie, J. M. *Physiological responses of twin children to exercise under conditions of heat stress.* MSc. Thesis, University of Waterloo, 1982.

71. Jokinen, E. and Valimaki, I. Children in sauna: Electrocardiographic abnormalities. *Acta Paediatrica Scandinavica* 1991; **80**: 370–4.

72. Brisson, G. R., Audet, A., Ledoux, M., Matton, P., Pellerin-Massicotte, J. and Perronet, F. Exercise-induced blood prolactin variations in trained adult males: A thermic stress more than an osmotic stress. *Hormone Research* 1986; **23**: 200–6.

73. Meyer, F., Bar-Or, O., MacDougall, D. and Heigenhauser, G. H. Sweat electrolyte loss during exercise in the heat: Effects of gender and matura-tion. *Medicine and Science in Sports and Exercise* 1992; **24**: 776–81.

74. Foster, K. G., Hey, E. N. and Katz, G. The response of the sweat glands of the new-born baby to thermal stimuli and intradermal acetylcholine. *Journal of Physiology* 1969; **203**: 13–29.

75. Shapiro, Y., Pandolf, K. B., Arellini, B. A., Pimental, N. A. and Goldman, R. F. Physiological responses of men and women to humid and dry heat. *Journal of Applied Physiology* 1980; **49**: 1–8.

76. Iuliano, S., Naughton, G., Collier, G. and Carlson, J. Examination of the self-selected fluid intake practices by junior athletes during a simulated duathlon event. *International Journal of Sport Nutrition* 1998; **8**: 10–23.

77. Dill, D. B., Horvath, S. M., Van. Beaumont, W., Gehlsen, G. and Burrus, K. Sweat electrolytes in desert walks. *Journal of Applied Physiology* 1967; **23**: 746–51

78. Meyer, F. and Bar-Or, O. Fluid and electrolyte loss during exercise: the paediatric angle. *Sports Medicine* 1994; **18**: 4–9.

79. Shwachman, H. and Mahmoodian, A. The sweat test and cystic fibrosis. *Diagnostic Medicine* 1982; June: 61–77.

80. Sens, D. A., Simmons, M. A., Spicer, S.S. The analysis of human sweat proteins by isoelectric focusing. I. Sweat collection utilizing the macroduct system demonstrates the presence of previously unrecognized sex-related proteins. *Pediatric Research* 1985; **19**: 873–8.

81. Bar-Or, O., Dotan, R., Inbar, O., Rotshtein, A. and Zonder, H. Voluntary hypohydration in 10- to 12-year-old boys. *Journal of Applied Physiology* 1980; **48**: 104–8.

82. Bar-Or, O., Blimkie, C. J. R., Hay, J. A., MacDougall, J. D., Ward, D. G. and Wilson, W. M. Voluntary dehydration and heat intolerance in cystic fibrosis. *Lancet* 1992; **339**: 696–9.

83. Pugh, L. G. C., Crobett, J. L. and Johnson, R. H. Rectal temperatures, weight losses and sweat rates in marathon running. *Journal of Applied Physiology* 1967; **23**: 347–52.

84. Bar-David, Y., Landau, D., Bar-David, Z., Pilpel, D. and Phillip, M. Voluntary dehydration among elementary school children living in a hot climate. *Child Ambulatory Health* 1998; **4**: 393–7.

85. Phillip, M., Singer, A., Chaimovitz ,C. and Golinsky, D. Urine osmolality in nursery school children in a hot climate. *Israel Journal of Medical Sciences* 1993; **29**: 104–6.

86. Wilk B. and Bar-Or, O. Effect of drink flavour and NaCl on voluntary drinking and hydration in boys exercising in the heat. *Journal of Applied Physiology* 1996; **80**: 1112–7.

87. Rivera-Brown, A., Gutiérrez, R., Gutiérrez, J. C., Padro, C., Frontera, W. and Bar-Or, O. Effect of drink composition on voluntary drinking and fluid balance in active boys exercising in hot outdoors climate. *Medicine and Science in Sports and Exercise* 1997; **29**: S170.

88. Wilk, B., Kriemler, S., Keller, H. and Bar-Or, O. Consistency in preventing voluntary dehydration in boys who drink a flavoured carbohydrate-NaCl beverage during exercise in the heat. *International Journal of Sport Nutrition* 1998; **3**: 1–9.

89. Heaps, C. L., Gonzalez,-Alonso, J. and Coyle, E. F. Hypohydration causes cardiovascular drift without reducing blood volume. *International Journal of Sports Medicine* 1994; **15**: 74–9.

90. Fortney, S. M., Wenger, C. G., Bove, J. R. and Nadel, E. R. Effect of hyperosmolality on control of blood flow and sweating. *Journal of Applied Physiology* 1984; **57**: 1688–95.

91. Kenney, W. L., Tankersley, C. G., Newswanger, D. L., Hyde, D. E., Puhl, S. M. and Turner, N. L. Age and hypohydration independently influence the peripheral response to heat stress. *Journal of Applied Physiology* 1990; **68**: 1902–8.

92. Sawka, M. N., Young, A. J., Francesconi, R. B., Muza ,S. R. and Pandolf, K. B. Thermoregulation and blood responses during exercise at graded hypohydration levels. *Journal of Applied Physiology* 1985; **59**: 1394–1401.

93. Meyer, F., Bar-Or, O., Salsberg, A. and Passe, R. Hypohydration during exercise in children: Effect on thirst, drink preferences, and rehydration. *International Journal of Sport Nutrition* 1994; **4**: 22–35.

94. Meyer, F., Bar-Or, O., MacDougall, J. D. and Heigenhauser, G. J. F. Drink composition and the electrolyte balance of children exercising in the heat. *Medicine and Science in Sports and Exercise* 1995; **27**: 882–7.

95. Meyer, F., Bar-Or, O. and Wilk, B. Children's perceptual responses to ingesting drinks of different compositions during and following exercise in the heat. *International Journal of Sports Nutrition* 1995; **5**: 13–24.

96. Gutiérrez, R., Rivera-Brown, A., Guiterrez, J. C., Padro, C., Frontera, W. and Bar-Or, O. Effect of drink composition on thermoregulation and perceptual responses in active boys exercise in hot outdoors climate. *Medicine and Sciences in Sports and Exercise* 1997; **29**: S170.

97. Bar-Or, O. and Wilk, B. Water and electrolyte replenishment in the exer-cising child. *International Journal of Sports Nutrition* 1996; **6**: 93–9.

98. Sloan, R. E. and Keatinge, W. R. Cooling rates of young people swimming in cold water. *Journal of Applied Physiology* 1973; **35**: 371–5.

99. Inoue, Y., Araki, T. and Tsujta, J. The thermoregulatory responses of prepubertal boys and young men in changing temperature linearly from 28 to 15 °C. *European Journal of Applied Physiology* 1996; **72**: 204–8.

100. Wagner, J. A., Robinson, S. and Marino, R. P. Age and temperature reg-ulation of humans in neutral and cold environments. *Journal of Applied Physiology* 1974; **37**: 616–22.

101. Falk, B., Bar-Eli, M., Dotan, R., Yaaron, M., Weinstein, Y., Epstein, S. et al. Physiological and cognitive responses to cold exposure in 11–12 year-old boys. *American Journal of Human Biology* 1997; **9**: 39–49.

102. Marsh, M. L., Mahon, A. D. and Naftzger, L. A. Children's physiological responses to exercise in a cold and neutral temperature. *Proceedings of the North American society of pediatric exercise medicine meeting.* Miami, Florida, 1992.

103. **Ueda, T., Choi, T. H.** and **Kurokawa, T.** Ratings of perceived exertion in a group of children while swimming at different temperatures. *Annals of Physiological Anthropology* 1994; **13**: 23–31.

104. **Mackova, J., Sturmova, M.** and **Macek, M.** Prolonged exercise in prepubertal boys in warm and cold environments. In *Children and sports* (J. Illmarinen and I. Valimaki). Springer-Verlag, Heidelberg, 1984; 135–41.

105. **Inbar, O., Bar-Or, O., Dotan R.** and **Gutin, B.** Conditioning versus exercise in heat as methods for acclimatizing 8–10 year old boys to dry heat. *Journal of Applied Physiology* 1981; **50**: 406–11.

106. **Armstrong, L. E.** and **Maresh, C. M.** The induction and decay of heat acclimatization in trained athletes. *Sports Medicine* 1991; **12**: 302–12.

107. **Cotter, J. D., Patterson, J. J.** and **Taylor, N. A.** Sweat distribution before and after repeated heat exposure. *European Journal of Applied Physiology* 1997; **76**: 181–6.

108. **Wilk, B.** and **Bar-Or, O.** Heat acclimation and sweating pattern in prepubertal boys. *Pediatric Exercise Science* 1997; **7**: 92.

109. **Bar-Or, O.** and **Inbar, O.** Relationship between perceptual and physiological changes during heat acclimatization in 8- to 10-year-old boys. In *Frontiers of activity and child health* (ed. H. Lavalee and R. J. Shephard). Pelican, Quebec, 1977: 205–14.

110. **Matsushita, K.** and **Araki, T.** The effect of physical training on thermoregulatory responses of preadolescent boys to heat and cold. *Japanese Journal of Physical Fitness* 1980; **29**: 69–74.

PART III
Physical Activity, Physical Fitness and Health

3.1 Physical activity, physical fitness and children's health: current concepts

Chris Riddoch and Colin Boreham

Introduction

With regard to children and physical activity, we live in a world of contrasts and contradictions. On the one hand, teenage world record holders in swimming are commonplace, many Olympic female gymnasts can be defined as prepubescent, and a 13 year old boy has run the marathon in 2 hours and 55 minutes. On the other hand, we have a widespread decline of school physical education, there is a perception that children's freedom to cycle, walk and play outdoors is curtailed, and that too much time is spent watching television and playing video games. Such contrasts beg the question: 'is there a happy medium of physical activity for the child that will ensure optimum growth and health into adulthood?' The question is difficult to answer. Despite widespread acceptance of the notion that physical activity is generally beneficial for children, relatively little scientific research has been carried out in this complex field, and methodological and conceptual discrepancies abound. It is therefore rather difficult to distil available information with a view to establishing absolute recommendations for activity and/or fitness levels that are optimal for health in this population.

This is in stark contrast to available evidence relating to adults. In adults, we are now undoubtedly much clearer about the general strength and direction of the relationships between activity, fitness and health. In particular, there exists a large measure of consistency between the results of many large studies that lead us to conclude that virtually any increase in activity from a state of sedentariness is beneficial to health. We now know that sedentary living is an element of contemporary lifestyle that impacts significantly, and adversely, upon health.

Given the current epidemic of lifestyle-related chronic diseases, contemporary lifestyles of developed nations have become a matter of some concern.[1] The increasing prevalence of sedentary living in adults has received particular attention.[2,3]

There is also concern that children may be as much at risk from sedentary living—either during childhood, in terms of adverse effects on growth and development, or later as an adult. Despite the fact that the Surgeon General's report on physical activity[3] contained no section specifically relating to children, there continues to be much current interest in children's levels of physical activity and fitness, and in their perceived decline.[4,5] Teachers of physical education are concerned that fitness levels in children appear to be falling, and recruits to the armed forces are believed to have lower fitness levels than in previous times.

However, despite such widespread perceptions and beliefs, there is surprisingly little hard evidence to support the contention that activity and/or fitness levels are either inadequate or declining in children. Thus, the activity and fitness levels of children will undoubtedly remain important issues and it is important to establish a conceptual framework within which we can work. We need to ascertain exactly why we consider childhood activity to be so important. In this respect, Blair *et al.*[6] have hypothesized a number of possible relationships between activity levels, health and stage of life (Fig. 3.1.1).

The hypothesized relationships within this model suggest three main beneficial effects which might derive from adequate childhood activity:

1. Enhancement of physiological and psychological development during childhood—directly improving childhood health status and quality of life (A).
2. Delay in the onset, or retardation of the rate of development of health risk factors—directly improving adult health status (B).
3. Improved likelihood of maintaining adequate activity levels into adulthood, thus indirectly enhancing adult health status (C).

Considering these possible relationships, it is interesting to note that the only strong evidence we have relates to adult activity and adult health (D). Relationships between child activity and either child health (A), adult health (B) or adult activity (C) are extremely weak by comparison. Further, as a cautionary note, it is important to note that increased activity may also carry a measure of increased health risk, through trauma and overuse, which must be balanced against the potential benefits.

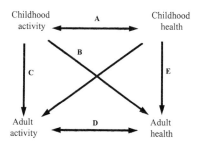

Fig. 3.1.1 Hypothetical relationships between physical activity and health in children and adults. Reproduced with permission from Blair *et al.*[6]

The purpose of this chapter is to draw together some of the more compelling evidence in the field of activity, fitness and health, and to relate it to the childhood period. Subsequent chapters will focus more closely on different dimensions of activity/fitness–health relationships. This chapter will provide a theoretical framework within which subsequent chapters can be interpreted.

Physical activity and physical fitness

Physical activity is a behaviour, and indeed a very complex behaviour. Activity behaviour can vary within a range of dimensions: the type of activity, the duration of activity sessions, the intensity, both absolute (energy cost) and relative (proportion of maximal capacity), and the frequency of sessions. Alternatively, we can think of activity in terms of energy expenditure, in other words the metabolic cost of performing all the day's physical activities. We can further consider whether the activity is *unavoidable*, e.g. for subsistence or work, or *voluntary*, e.g. for sport and recreation.

Because activity behaviour is so complex and variable it is extremely difficult to measure. No valid method of measuring physical activity exists which reflects all, or even most, of its dimensions. An obvious difficulty we have when a behaviour is so difficult to assess (i.e. carries a high capacity for measurement error) is that a high degree of misclassification of individuals is likely. For example, a questionnaire concentrating on sports and fitness training is likely to miss much activity performed through work and travel. An individual who plays no sport, but who walks a lot and does large amounts of housework, can potentially be misclassified as a sedentary person. When assessing relationships between activity levels and other parameters, for example health status, misclassification in terms of activity will weaken the observed relationships.

Fitness on the other hand is an attribute, and generally refers to one's capacity to undertake physical work. Like physical activity, there are many dimensions of fitness, for example, cardiovascular fitness, strength, flexibility, speed, power and anaerobic endurance. Many of these dimensions are not only related to performance, but also to health. Fitness is partly genetically determined, but can also be improved by regular appropriate physical activity. In contrast to physical activity, fitness can be accurately measured, leading to less misclassification of individuals and observed relationships that may be nearer to reality.

Activity and health in adults

Relationships between activity and health

In order to understand potential activity/health relationships in children, it is first necessary to look at the equivalent relationships in adults, where the picture is much clearer. In fact, the evidence that activity is beneficial to health comes almost exclusively from studies of adults. The question that arises is: 'What are the implications of the strong adult data—which clearly demonstrate that physical activity promotes improved health—to children?'

In adults, both physical activity and physical fitness levels are inversely related to mortality.[7,8] A strong, independent, inverse relationship between activity and/or fitness and health has now been established. Prospective population studies of adults have shown that higher levels of physical activity lead to reduced risk of coronary heart disease (CHD),[9,10] stroke,[11] hypertension,[12] non-insulin-dependent diabetes mellitus (NIDDM),[13] osteoporotic fractures,[14] depression[15] and some cancers.[16] Meta-analyses of data from more than 40 studies indicate that CHD is 1.9 times more likely to develop in physically inactive adults compared to active adults, independent of other risk factors.[9,10] This level of individual risk is comparable with the risk associated with the other main CHD risk factors (hypertension, cigarette smoking and cholesterol levels). Blair *et al.*[17] have reported similar data for low fitness, which carries a relative risk for all-cause mortality of 1.52 in men and 2.10 in women.

From a public health perspective, it is important to note that whereas inactivity carries equal *risk* as the other major CHD risk factors, the *prevalence* of inactivity is far higher—maybe up to three times as high.[18] This is of crucial importance, because it indicates that on a population basis, sedentary living may be the most significant health-compromising behaviour because of the high level of risk combined with the large proportion of the population exposed to that risk. Expressed in a different way, the greatest *scope* for population health gain may lie in preventing and reversing sedentary living habits.

Dose-response relationships

There appears to exist a graded dose-response relationship between activity level and mortality, with mortality being greatest at the lower end of the activity distribution, and lowest at the more active end.[7] Importantly, *increments* of risk reduction are greatest between activity groups at the low end of the activity distribution with a 'law of diminishing returns' as one moves along the distribution from low activity to high activity. There is also some evidence of a 'levelling off' of benefit at a certain point, which is suggestive of an *optimum* level of activity, above which few further health benefits can be gained. However, this level may vary—or not exist—depending on the health outcome selected. Similar relationships can be identified between fitness and health, with the greatest difference in cardiovascular risk being observed between individuals in the least fit groups and those who are slightly fitter. Increments of benefit between these groups and subsequent groups are smaller.[8]

At the higher end of the activity spectrum, where activity levels may be taken to the extreme, some body systems react adversely, even when the body has been conditioned gradually to these physical stresses, compared with more moderate levels of activity. For example, high levels of activity can cause musculo-skeletal injuries, renal abnormalities, gastrointestinal disturbances, immune system suppression and menstrual irregularities. Although these conditions are not necessarily serious, they are undoubtedly troublesome, and may partly offset any health benefits accruing from higher levels of activity. They may also have an adverse effect on adherence to activity. This again leads us towards the conclusion that an optimal level of activity—for health purposes—may exist.

An optimal level for health?

From the above, we might conclude that there exists a level of activity, lying somewhere between the couch potato and the trained athlete, which is *optimal* for health. Indeed it is likely that in evolutionary terms we have developed the biological equipment necessary for the lifestyle of a hunter/gatherer—daylong intermittent activities of varying intensity—but we are now forced by cultural, technological and environmental circumstances into a far more sedentary lifestyle. The current epidemic of sedentary living may be a significant contributory factor in the increased prevalence of degenerative, lifestyle-related disease, most notably coronary heart disease and stroke.

Changing this propensity for a sedentary lifestyle will not be easy. To go some way towards returning people to a more active lifestyle, health-related activity guidelines have been formulated for adults. The central message of the recommendation is the accumulation of 30 minutes of moderate intensity activity (equating to brisk walking for the majority of people), on at least 5 days of the week.[2] A stepping-stone of 30 minutes on one day per week is suggested for those who are initially totally sedentary, and a more distant goal of taking three sessions of more vigorous activity per week—approximating cardiovascular fitness training guidelines—is provided for people who are more ambitious or more motivated.

These guidelines balance what is known to be beneficial to health and what is likely to be *achievable* by the majority of people. It should be noted that the majority of health benefits should accrue with the moderate message, but there is some evidence to suggest that more vigorous activity may be necessary for certain improvements to take place, most notably normalization of blood pressure. However, such high levels of activity, are *not* necessary to improve the majority of the dimensions of health,[19] and the widely held view that running three times a week is in some way a health-related *threshold*, has now been rightly discarded.

We can therefore conclude that (a) avoiding the low end of the activity or fitness spectrum is the 'healthiest' scenario, and (b) high levels of activity are probably unnecessary for the achievement of most health benefits. In this respect, examples of activities which have been shown to confer a significant reduction in risk of CHD risk include gardening,[20] lawn mowing,[20] walking[7,20] and stair climbing.[7] While such activities may not be so attractive for children, these data do support the view that total activity energy expenditure, irrespective of the type, intensity, duration or frequency, may be the key dimension of activity for the improvement of health in a predominantly sedentary population. The important question is, however, do these adult data hold for children?

Activity and health in children

It is clear that young children enjoy active play. Given a free choice, most young children will play or invent active ways of passing time which involve jumping, dancing, skipping, hopping, chasing, running, climbing and cycling. Older children might play more organized sports, either formally, in clubs and teams, or informally, in parks and playgrounds. Generally speaking, these forms of play provide a large volume of activity incorporating a wide variety of movements, using many muscle groups, and promoting cardiorespiratory development, muscular strength, muscular endurance, speed, power and flexibility. In the mid and later teenage years these relatively high levels of activity decline as more sedentary alternatives are chosen. This decline is not necessarily problematical, and can be seen in other animal species. However, if activity levels decline to levels which are too low—and we should remember that adult levels are undoubtedly too low—then this may constitute a 'problem in the making'.

The question is, therefore, 'do children's activity levels decline over the teenage years to such an extent that either their current or future health is compromised?' To answer this question we must scrutinize the evidence relating activity to indicators of health status—or health risk factors—in children.

Unfortunately, for children, scrutiny of this evidence is not encouraging. Although there are indications of beneficial associations in some areas, there is no compelling evidence which unambiguously relates childhood physical activity or fitness to either childhood health, a more favourable childhood risk profile, or to later adult health.[21–23] Despite this, we have a growing body of literature on children's activity levels, which is predicated on the conventional wisdom that activity is beneficial for children. We should therefore more closely examine the evidence relating to each of the three hypothesized relationships suggested by Fig. 3.1.1.

Activity and current health status

It has been reported that relationships between activity levels and various health parameters—bone health, blood pressure, lipid profile and obesity—are hard to find in children.[23] A summary of relevant evidence follows.

Overweight and obesity

Bar-Or and Baranowski[24] have concluded that both controlled trials and cross-sectional studies indicate small but significant beneficial effects of activity for both non-obese and obese adolescents. However, no effect was observed in prospective observational studies. Some weak associations were evident, but no threshold 'dose' of activity could be identified. In a review of more recent evidence, Riddoch[23] has pointed out that only two studies[25,26] observed no effect, while others[27–31] observed some effect. These data must therefore be treated as suggestive rather than definitive. Must and colleagues[32] have emphasized the importance of avoiding overweight during adolescence. In this large, prospective study with 55 years of follow-up, overweight in adolescence predicted a broad range of adverse health effects in adulthood that were independent of adult weight. Overweight during adolescence is therefore concluded to be a more significant predictor of a range of future diseases than being overweight as an adult.

We can suggest three reasons why an increased prevalence of childhood obesity might be a major source of concern. Firstly, obesity is a major risk factor for insulin resistance and diabetes, hypertension, cancer, gall bladder disease and atherosclerosis.[33,34] Secondly, obesity tends to track into adulthood,[35] and thirdly, adults who were obese children have increased morbidity and mortality, irrespective of adult weight.[32] For these reasons, despite the lack of compelling evidence, childhood obesity might be a major target for intervention from both primary prevention and treatment perspectives, and physical activity should feature strongly in this.

Blood pressure and cholesterol

Armstrong and Simons-Morton[36] have reported that data suggesting a beneficial effect of activity on lipids and lipoproteins are minimal, although there is some evidence that high density lipoprotein cholesterol (HDL-C) concentrations might be enhanced. Alpert and Wilmore[37] concluded that exercise training had only a weak relationship with blood pressure within the normal range; however, aerobic-type training consistently reduced both systolic and diastolic blood pressure in hypertensive adolescents, but not to normal levels. Riddoch[23] reviewed more recent studies and reported that, for lipids and lipoproteins, six studies[38–43] show no association with measures of activity, whereas five studies[27,44–47] show a limited measure of association. For blood pressure, two studies[38,48] report no association, and six studies[27,39,40,42,43,49] report a beneficial association.

Bone health

Osteoporosis is a major public health problem, affecting more than 25 million people in the United States, mainly women. As osteoporosis, and the fractures that are associated with it, are largely a feature of old age, the scale of the problem is certain to grow as the population ages. It is estimated, for example, that the 6.26 million hip fractures currently recorded annually on a worldwide basis will increase four-fold by the year 2050.[50] Although osteoporosis is principally a condition of the elderly, attainment of a strong, dense skeleton during the growing years may be the best way to prevent osteoporosis in later life.[51,52]

Peak bone mass, which is achieved in the majority of people by the third decade,[53,54] appears to be largely under the control of genetic influences. Approximately 70–85% of the inter-individual variance in bone mass is genetically determined, with several candidate genes involved in the regulation and metabolism of collagen (*COLIA 1* gene), vitamin D (*VDR*-gene), oestrogen (*ER* gene) and nitric oxide (*ec NOS* gene) being strongly implicated.[55] However, the residual variance in bone mass is under environmental influences which are amenable to early intervention. The most important environmental factors appear to be diet—notably calcium intake[56]—and the amount and type of physical activity taken throughout childhood and adolescence.

Investigations examining the relationship between physical activity in childhood and adolescence and bone mineral acquisition have been reviewed in detail by Bailey *et al.*[51] Studies of representative populations have, in the main, been conducted retrospectively,[57–59] although longitudinal or prospective studies have reported recently.[60–62] These studies indicate that weight-bearing physical activity in childhood and adolescence is an important predictor of bone mineral density, while non-weight bearing activity (such as swimming or cycling) is not.[63] The size of the effect of physical activity (difference in BMD between the high and low fitness or activity groups) is, typically, between 5–15%. In his review, Vuori[52] estimates that physical activity, which is feasible for large numbers of young people, increases peak bone mass somewhat less than one standard deviation, or 7–8% approximately. This would be sufficient, if maintained into old age, to substantially reduce the risk of osteoporotic fracture.[64] However, more research on the optimal type and volume of physical activity required for bone health in young people is required. Based on available information[65] it is likely that activities which involve high strains, developed rapidly and distributed unevenly throughout the movement pattern, may be particularly osteogenic. Thus, activities such as aerobics, disco dancing, volleyball, basketball and racket sports may be effective, and need not necessarily be of prolonged duration, as the osteogenic response to such movement appears to saturate after only a few loading cycles.[65] It is also interesting to note that the natural play activities of young children do provide a significant element of high impact movement, and may be optimal—in type—for health.

Further work also needs to be done to establish the optimal period within childhood in which to perform such activities to promote bone growth. While, at one end of the spectrum, adult bone seems relatively unresponsive to all but the most vigorous of exercise regimes,[66–68] there is some evidence[62] that physical activity during the immediate prepubescent and pubescent years may be crucial for maximizing peak bone mass.

Therefore, physical activity is an essential stimulus for bone structure, and has the potential to increase peak bone mass in children and adolescents within the limits set by genetic, hormonal and nutritional influences. Such enhanced bone mass has considerable potential to reduce risk of osteoporosis and associated fracture in later life, particularly if the increase can be maintained throughout adulthood by exercise.

Other risk factors

It may be of particular importance to note the existence of studies[34,69–70] which show a beneficial effect of physical activity on parameters related to insulin metabolism. 'Metabolic syndrome' or 'syndrome X',[71] encompassing obesity, hypertension, hypertriglyceridaemia, depressed HDL-C, and glucose intolerance or hyperinsulinaemia, is now a recognized clinical condition, and it may be that this clustering of metabolic parameters—in both adults and children—will be an important aspect of future physical activity research.

From the above, we must acknowledge that significant relationships between activity levels and the various health parameters can rarely be seen in children. However, it is important to consider that absence of evidence may not indicate evidence of absence. In other words, subtle relationships and effects may exist, but we may not currently be able to detect them. In particular, very few well-conducted, large-scale studies exist, in particular longitudinal studies, which, critically, may link childhood risk with clinical outcomes in adulthood.

Activity and future health status
Direct effects

It has been hypothesized that degenerative biological processes are initiated during infancy and childhood that will manifest as chronic disease in later life. In fact, there is evidence to suggest that adult health status may be determined, at least in part, by biological events that occur *in utero*.[72] It is argued that early biological events trigger a morphological and/or functional change that subsequently becomes a chronic and worsening condition, ultimately leading to overt signs and symptoms, chronic illness and death. The individual is effectively 'programmed' for susceptibility to a disease through an early biological event. Crucially, the biological event may itself be triggered by an environmental influence (inadequate maternal nutrition, smoking) and it is in this respect that adequate physical activity may be important. It should be stressed that these assertions are currently hypothetical—and remain to be fully tested—but nevertheless, we have one further argument that physical activity during the early part of the lifespan is important, despite the fact that morbidity and mortality are features of the later years.

Indirect effects

It seems reasonable to presume that if high activity as a child increases the likelihood of being a more active adult—which we know enhances health—then childhood activity can be considered to indirectly influence adult health status. It is often presumed that this link exists, but the evidence is again rather sparse. The persistence of a behaviour, or attribute, over time is called 'tracking', and refers to the short-, medium- or long-term maintenance of a rank order position compared to one's peers. Our main concern, therefore, might be whether inactivity in childhood would lead to inactivity in adulthood, and subsequent elevated risk of adult disease.[73] Conversely, does high activity as a child predict high activity as an adult?

Levels of tracking though all stages of the lifespan have been comprehensively reviewed by Malina.[74] He concludes that activity tracks at weak to moderate levels during adolescence, from adolescence into adulthood, and across various ages during adulthood.

It is disappointing that tracking of activity from childhood to adulthood is not strong, but it might be the case that substantial tracking should not be expected in the case of physical activity. A multitude of factors can influence this behaviour from day to day, between seasons of the year, and because of various 'life events'. Examples of life events which can disturb activity patterns include changing schools, school-to-work transition, leaving home, moving house, moving to a new neighbourhood, biological and psychological development (especially puberty and adolescence), illness, marriage and child rearing. Any one of these can significantly affect activity levels, and therefore it is to be expected that activity levels will fluctuate greatly within any one individual over all stages of the lifespan. Measuring activity levels at any two points in time may detect an activity level, but this might be under the influence of any combination of life events. Linked with this is the fact that both active children and active adults are likely to change the dimension of activity they favour. As we grow older, we move from play, through sport, to social and recreational activities and the level of 'background' or lifestyle activity we do, for example walking to work and housework, confounds the whole scenario. We might therefore expect tracking coefficients to be weak or moderate.

The methodological and conceptual problems are therefore considerable in our quest to assess the stability of this complex and fundamentally changeable behaviour. Interestingly, there is some evidence to suggest[75] that how 'comfortable' an adult is about physical activity ('psychological readiness') is positively correlated with *how* active the adult is. Additionally PE grade at the age of 15 years is positively associated with psychological readiness at 30 years. This suggests, therefore, encouraging in children actual and perceived competence in sports and physical recreation—which may not promote higher *childhood* activity levels—might actually have long-lasting effects on adult attitudes towards activity and subsequently higher adult activity levels.

Prevalence of activity/inactivity

Cale and Almond[76] have reviewed 15 studies conducted on British children, and reported that children seldom participate in activity at a level which would have a cardiovascular training effect, or a health benefit. On the other hand, Sallis[77] examined nine studies and concluded that the average child is sufficiently active to meet the adult recommendations for conditioning activities, with the exception of the average female in mid to late adolescence. It has been argued that young children are highly and spontaneously active.[8,79] 'Simple observation tells us that toddlers are constantly on the move, exploring the environment, playing, and moving apparently for the sheer joy of it.'[21] Blair[80] has noted that children are generally fitter and more active than adults, and most of them are active enough to receive important health benefits from their activity.

Saris *et al.*[81] have reported physical activity level (PAL = total energy expenditure/resting metabolic rate) values of 1.95 in 9 year old boys and 1.71 in 8 year old girls, and Davies *et al.*[82] have reported PAL values of 1.84 for 9 year old boys and 1.65 in 9 year old girls. Using energy intake as an indirect measure of activity Boreham *et al.*[83] have reported energy intakes for 12 and 15 year old British children equating to average daily PAL values of 1.8–1.9. These results compare favourably with defined PAL values of 1.7 (moderately active) and 1.9 (very active).[84]

On the other hand, there is some evidence that activity levels may be falling, because children now have a lower daily caloric intake compared to previous generations,[85] and yet appear to be getting fatter in both the USA and the UK.[86–89] If true, the only logical explanation of this phenomenon is that activity levels have declined in children at a greater rate than the reported decline in energy intake. Compared to the strong data suggesting an increase in children's fatness, data relating to energy intake are more suspect. However, we do have supporting evidence from adult studies.[90]

From the above, it is clear that we are currently undecided about:

(1) how much activity children take;
(2) whether activity levels are falling; and
(3) whether activity levels are sufficient to promote health.

To exemplify this, Armstrong and colleagues[91] have reported an extremely low prevalence of activity which equates to the intensity, frequency and duration which is recommended for developing cardiopulmonary fitness. In their study only 2% of boys and 0% of girls achieved three sessions of 20 minutes of sustained activity at a heart rate above 139 beats min^{-1}. On the other hand, Blair *et al.*[6] have reported that 94% of boys and 88% of girls achieve an energy expenditure greater than 3 kcal $kg^{-1}day^{-1}$—known to be a health-related level in adults. At a stricter level, more than 75% of children achieve a standard that is 33% higher (4 kcal $kg^{-1}day^{-1}$).

How is it that such diverse conclusions can be reached by experienced researchers on the basis of well-conducted studies? This is one of the most important, and interesting, questions currently facing us. There are various explanations, for example, measurement error, different measurement methodologies, population differences, age-group differences and measurement of different dimensions of physical activity. However, one of the most compelling explanations is that these and other investigators adopt radically different criterion levels of activity against which they base their judgements. Criterion levels for developing cardiovascular fitness might be very different from levels that promote health.

To further demonstrate this important point, Welk[92] has reported that in his study only 17% of children achieved a single session with a heart rate in excess of 140 beats min^{-1}. However, when the *same data* were reanalysed according to health-related criteria—achieving 4 kcal $kg^{-1}day^{-1}$ of activity energy expenditure—99% of children achieved this. This demonstrates vividly that the selection of differing criteria for a health-related threshold can lead to substantial variations in the estimates of how much activity children take, and whether children are active 'enough'.

Guidelines for activity

Guidelines for health-related activity in children have been formulated, as the result of two international consensus conferences.[93,94] Despite the lack of unequivocal evidence suggesting that activity is related to health status,[27] and also that children are insufficiently active,[95] there are intuitive biological and behavioural arguments in favour of promoting physical activity to all children. Guidelines tend to reinforce the concept of a health-related threshold, but the amount and type of physical activity during childhood which is appropriate for optimal health is very difficult to ascertain.

Earlier criteria, or thresholds, were generally based on the amount of activity required for the development of cardiovascular fitness. However, they may not only have been too stringent for the majority of children to achieve, but may also have been unrelated to the amount of activity necessary to achieve a health benefit. Cale and Harris[96] have pointed out that from a behavioural perspective physical activity needs to be seen by children as an achievable and positive experience, and that adult fitness training guidelines, emphasizing continuous bouts of vigorous exercise, do not fulfil this. In this respect, recent criteria[93,94] are based more upon the existing evidence of activity/health relationships in children, the stronger adult data, and also take account of behavioural issues, in terms of activity adoption and maintenance. The most recent guidelines[94] propose the accumulation of 60 minutes of moderate intensity activity every day, including activities which promote strength, flexibility and bone health.

Fitness and health in children

Before examining relationships between children's fitness and health, it is worth defining and delimiting the two terms. Although several categories of physical fitness have been identified, the component that is most strongly associated with health is cardiovascular (C-V) endurance, defined as 'the ability to sustain moderate intensity, whole-body activity for extended time periods'.[97] It can be measured objectively in the laboratory setting using a variety of ergometers (cycle, treadmill, etc.) with or without respiratory gas analysis, or more simply in the field by maximal running tests or submaximal cycle or step tests. Health is also multifactorial, but, possibly owing to its pre-eminence as a cause of mortality in the developed world, coronary heart disease (CHD) and the risk factors predisposing to CHD are the most extensively studied in relation to physical fitness. Many of the studies investigating associations between fitness and health have been large-scale, cross-sectional population surveys, using multivariate analysis to adjust for potential confounding variables. More powerful evidence for causal links between fitness and health come from rarer longitudinal population studies, or from training studies in which changes in the two variables can be compared over time. Irrespective of study design, one important distinction between adult and child studies is that the former has the advantage of examining associations between fitness and mortality, whereas children's studies in this field are restricted to examining risk factors for CHD rather than death arising from the disease. Finally, recent work on the genetics of fitness[98] may improve our understanding of how fitness and health are predetermined and interrelated.

Numerous adult population studies[8,99–103] have shown strong and consistent relationships between C-V fitness and mortality from CHD and all causes, independent of possible confounding variables. Even more compelling has been evidence from prospective studies[104] which indicate that risk of mortality may be reduced substantially in middle-aged men who improve their fitness over a number of years.

The situation with children appears to be less clear-cut, partly because the outcome measure—'health'—cannot, for obvious reasons, be judged by mortality statistics. Rather, the investigator must rely upon risk factors for CHD mortality, such as high blood pressure, elevated blood lipids and fatness. However, such risk factors may only account for 50% of eventual coronary mortality and are therefore a relatively crude yardstick for coronary health.[105] Furthermore, as a result of maturation, these biological risk factors are constantly changing throughout adolescence, and may or may not relate to adult values.[106] Despite these limitations, some population studies have shown an independent relationship between C-V fitness and levels of risk factors for CHD.[107,108] Further evidence of a causal relationship between fitness and coronary risk status in children comes from long-term fitness training studies that report concomitant improvements in individual risk factors.[109,110]

One consistent finding in children's studies is the very strong relationship observed between C-V fitness and fatness.[27,111,112] It is thus not surprising that several studies indicate that fatness is a major confounding variable in the relationship between fitness and other CHD risk factors. In at least four population studies,[113–116] robust associations between C-V fitness and level of risk were abolished after accounting statistically for body fatness, while one other study[107] reported much reduced relationships. It is worth noting that this feature has also been observed in an adult study[117] investigating fitness and coronary risk factors, and so the confounding influence of body fatness on coronary risk does not seem to be confined to paediatric populations.

Therefore, although strong relationships between cardiovascular fitness and CHD risk status exist in children, these appear to be largely mediated by the level of fatness. Thus, any initiative to improve the health of children should ideally involve measures that simultaneously improve fitness and lower fatness, namely increased physical activity and dietary control.

Which is more important—activity or fitness?

It has been argued[118–120] that physical training adaptations may not be directly related to, nor necessary for, good health. We have discussed the evidence regarding both activity and fitness in relation to health, but the interesting question of whether physical activity level or fitness level is most strongly related to health status remains open for discussion. For example, does an individual who has genetically high fitness, but who is inactive, achieve health benefits from the high fitness level?. Conversely, can the genetically low-fit individual gain health benefits through being active? These questions are largely unanswered.

As we have discussed, reduction in risk of CHD in adults is associated with both higher levels of physical fitness[8,102,121,122] and physical activity.[7,9,10,20] Interestingly, the strength of the relationship appears to be stronger for fitness than for activity, but whether this is a result of higher levels of misclassification inherent in activity measurement, compared with fitness measurement,[123] is unclear.

It may be that high fitness, especially cardiorespiratory fitness, is directly related to improved health status. The morphological and functional condition of the heart and circulatory system may lead directly to a reduced risk of, for example, CHD. In this scenario, a genetically high-fit individual would automatically be blessed with better health status. Recent studies on the relationship between polymorphisms of the angiotensin-converting enzyme (ACE) and C-V fitness[98] give some credence to this hypothesis. An alternative explanation might be that fitness acts as a marker for high activity levels. This activity might not only produce an improved cardiovascular system, but might also promote other biochemical and haemodynamic changes (lower blood pressure, higher HDL cholesterol, lower triglycerides, improved glucose tolerance, modified clotting factors and post-prandial lipaemia) which are the 'real' mechanisms which promote improved health. What we are considering is, by common understanding, almost a 'spin-off' effect of activity that might be termed 'metabolic fitness'. It is entirely possible that this type of fitness is the true health related dimension of the generic term 'fitness'.

The jury is undoubtedly still out on all this, but the implications are of crucial importance because until we obtain a more fundamental understanding of the mechanisms, and the effects of different types of activity upon those mechanisms, it is difficult to establish appropriate and effective activity messages.

Physical activity and risks to the child

It should not go without mention that physical activity can carry its own inherent risk to both adults and children. Van Mechelen[124] has highlighted the potential for childhood injury when free play in various physical activities is replaced by competitive participation in just one or two sports. Whereas all activities carry increased risk of traumatic (acute) injury, too strong a focus on training for competition in a limited range of activities can result in the additional risk of overuse (chronic) injury. Whereas both types of injury normally heal without permanent disability, the costs must be considered in terms of activity time lost, school time lost, predisposition to reoccurrence, the risk of permanent damage, and the financial cost of treatment. Baxter-Jones et al.[125] have reported for elite child athletes an estimated one-year incidence rate of 40 injuries per 100 children, equating to less than one injury per 1000 hours of training. In these elite child athletes, about one third of injuries were overuse injuries, which were in turn more severe than the traumatic injuries (20 days lay-off versus 13 days, respectively).

It should be emphasized that all sports and active recreational pursuits carry increased injury risk. In both adults and children, the risks and benefits must be carefully balanced. However, we should not forget the moral issue of when, or at what age or stage of development, a child is capable of making such important judgements. The roles and responsibilities of teachers, parents, sports governing bodies and coaches in this matter are considerable.

Summary

Although evidence between activity/fitness and health status in children is weak, this could be due to (a) lack of large scale, longitudinal studies, and (b) difficulties inherent in measuring health, fitness and activity over the adolescent period (e.g. naturally occurring shifts in blood pressure, lipids, activity patterns, adiposity etc.). Also, given the strong and consistent relationships between activity/fitness and health in adults, it is highly likely that ensuring adequate activity and fitness in children will be of ultimate benefit. However, we must be clear that we are basing this judgement largely on limited paediatric data, strong adult data, a good measure of common sense and educated guesswork, and some basic physiological principles.

There exists no prospective work that can link, with any degree of certainty, health in adult years with childhood activity patterns. However, it is intuitively logical that preventive measures, i.e. the fostering of active lifestyles, should begin early in life, and that 'the public health goal of physical education is to prepare children for a lifetime of regular physical activity'.[126]

We must not forget that physical activity is our evolutionary heritage, we were 'designed' as a species for physical activity, and yet we are now living in an environment which is toxic to activity, where the opportunities for children—and adults—to be physically active are fast disappearing. Only enlightened public policy regarding school curricula, school transportation and youth sports clubs can change this situation for tomorrow's adults.

References

1. Department of Health and Social Services, *The Health of the Nation.* HMSO, London, 1992.

2. Department of Health and Social Services, *Strategy statement on physical activity.* Department of Health, London, 1996.

3. US Department of Health and Human Services, *Physical activity and health: a report of the surgeon general.* Department of Health and Human Services, Centers for Disease Control and Prevention, National Center for Chronic Disease Prevention and Health Promotion, Pittsburgh, PA, 1996.

4. **Reiff, G. G., Dixon, W. R., Jacoby, D., Ye, G. X., Spain, G. G.** and **Hunsicker, P. A.** (eds.) *The President's Council on Physical Fitness and Sports national school population fitness survey.* University of Michigan, Ann Arbor, 1986.

5. **Armstrong, N.** Children are fit but not active! *Education and Health* 1989; **7**: 28–32.

6. **Blair, S. N., Clark, D. G., Cureton, K. J.** and **Powell, K. E.** Exercise and fitness in childhood: implications for a lifetime of health. In *Perspectives in exercise science and sports medicine* (ed. C. V. Gisolfi and D. R. Lamb). McGraw-Hill, New York, 1989; 401–30.

7. **Paffenbarger, R. S., Hyde, R. T., Wing, A. L.** and **Hsieh, C.** Physical activity, all-cause mortality, and longevity of college alumni. *New England Journal of Medicine* 1986; **314**: 605–13.

8. **Blair, S. N., Kohl, H. W., Paffenbarger, R. S. J., Clark, D. G., Cooper, K.H.** and **Gibbons, L. W.** Physical fitness and all-cause mortality: a prospective study of healthy men and women. *Journal of the American Medical Association* 1989; **262**: 2395–401.

9. **Powell, K. E., Thompson, P. D., Caspersen, C. J.** and **Kendrick, K. S.** Physical activity and the incidence of coronary heart disease. *Annual Review of Public Health* 1987; **8**: 281–7.

10. **Berlin, J. A.** and **Colditz, A.** A meta-analysis of physical activity in the prevention of coronary heart disease. *American Journal of Epidemiology* 1990; **132**: 612–27.

11. **Wannamethee, G.** and **Shaper, A. G.** Physical activity and stroke in British middle-aged men. *British Medical Journal* 1992; **304**: 597–601.

12. **Paffenbarger, R. S., Wing, A. L., Hyde, R. T.** and **Jung ,D.** Chronic disease in former college students. XX. Physical activity and incidence of hypertension of college alumni. *American Journal of Epidemiology* 1983; **117**: 245–57.

13. **Helmrich, S. P., Ragland, D. R., Leung, R. W.** and **Paffenbarger, R. S.** Physical activity and reduced occurence of non-insulin dependent diabetes mellitus. *New England Journal of Medicine* 1991; **325**: 147–52.

14. **Wickham, C. A. C., Walsh, K., Cooper, C., Parker, D. J. P., Margetts, B. M., Morris, J.** and **Bruce , S. A.** Dietary calcium, physical activity, and risk of hip fracture: a prospective study. *British Medical Journal* 1989; **299**: 889–92.

15. **Stephens, T.** Physical activity and mental health in the United States and Canada: evidence from four population surveys. *Preventive Medicine* 1988; **17**: 35–47.

16. **Lee, I-M.** Physical activity, fitness and cancer. In *Physical activity, fitness and health: International proceedings and consensus statement* (ed. C. Bouchard, R. J. Shephard and T. Stephens). Human Kinetics Books, Champaign, Il, 1994; 814–31.

17. **Blair, S. N., Kampert, J. B., Kohl III, H. W., Barlow, C. E., Macera, C. A., Paffenbarger, R. S.** and **Gibbons, L. W.** Influences of cardiorespiratory fitness and other precursors on cardiovascular disease and all-cause mortality in men and women. *Journal of the American Medical Association* 1996; **276**: 205–10.

18. **White, A., Nicholaas, G., Foster, K.** and **Browne, F.** and **Carey S.** *Health Survey for England: OPCS health survey no. 1.* HMSO, London, 1993.

19. **Blair, S. N., Kohl, H. W., Gordon, N. F.** and **Paffenbarger R. S. J.** How much physical activity is good for health? *Annual Review of Public Health* 1992; **13**: 99–126.

20. **Leon, A. S., Connett, J., Jacobs, D. R. J.** and **Raurama R.** Leisure-time physical activity levels and risk of coronary heart disease and death: Multiple Risk Factor Intervention Trial. *Journal of the American Medical Association* 1987; **258**: 2388–95.

21. **Blair, S. N.** and **Meredith, M. D.** The exercise-health relationship: does it apply to children and youth? In *Health and fitness through physical education* (ed. R. R. Pate and R. C. Hohn). Human Kinetics, Champaign, Il, 1994; 11–9.

22. **Rowland, T.** Is there a scientific rationale supporting the value of exercise for the present and future cardiovascular health of children? The con argument. *Pediatric Exercise Science* 1996; **8**: 303–9.

23. **Riddoch, C. J.** Relationships between physical activity and physical health in young people. In *Young and active?* (ed. S. Biddle and J. F. Sallis). Health Education Authority, London, 1998; 17–48.

24. **Bar-Or, O.** and **Baranowski T.** Physical activity, adiposity and obesity among adolescents. *Pediatric Exercise Science* 1994; **6**: 348–60.

25. **Durant, R. H., Baranowski, T., Johnson, M.** and **Thompson, W. O.** The relationship among television watching, and body composition of young children. *Pediatrics* 1994; **94**: 449–55.

26. **Durant, R. H., Thompson, W. O., Johnson, M.** and **Baranowski, T.** The relationship among television watching, physical activity, and body composition of 5- or 6-year old children. *Pediatric Exercise Science* 1996; **8**: 15–26.

27. **Boreham, C. A. G., Strain, J. J., Twisk, J. W. R., Van Mechelen, W., Savage, J. M.** and **Cran, G. W.** Aerobic fitness physical activity and body fatness in adolescents. In *Children and exercise* (ed. N. Armstrong, B. Kirby and J. Welsman). E. and F. N. Spon, 1997; 69–74.

28. **Robinson, T. N., Hammer, L. D., Killen, J. D., Kraemer, H. C., Wilson, D. M.** and **Hayward, C.** Does television viewing increase obesity and reduce physical activity? Cross-sectional and longitudinal analyses among adolescent girls. *Pediatrics* 1993; **91**: 273–80.

29. **Wolf, A. M., Gortmaker, S. L., Cheung, L., Gray, H. M., Herzog, D. B.** and **Colditz, G. A.** Activity, inactivity, and obesity: racial, ethnic, and age differences among schoolgirls. *American Journal of Public Health* 1993; **83**: 1625–7.

30. **Durant, R. H., Baranowski, T., Rhodes, T., Gutin, B., Thompson, W. O., Carroll, R., Puhl, J.** and **Greaves, K. A.** Association among serum lipid and lipoprotein concentrations and physical activity: physical fitness and body composition in young children. *Journal of Pediatrics* 1993; **123**: 185–92.

31. **Gutin, B., Cucuzzo, N., Islam, S.** and **Smith, C.** *et al.* Physical training improves body composition of black obese 7- to 11- year old girls. *Obesity Research* 1995; **3**: 305–12.

32. **Must, A., Jacques, P. F., Dallal, G. E., Bajema, C. J.** and **Dietz ,W. H.** Long-term morbidity and mortality of overweight adolescents. *New England Journal of Medicine* 1992; **327**: 1350–5.

33. **Schonfeld-Warden, N., Warden, C. H.** Pediatric obesity. An overview of etiology and treatment. *Pediatric Clinics of North America* 1997; **44**: 339–61.

34. **Vanhala, M., Vanhala, P., Kumpusalo, E., Halonen, P.** and **Takala, J.** Relation between obesity from childhood to adulthood and the metabolic syndrome: population based study. *British Medical Journal* 1998; **317**: 319.

35. **Clarke, W. R.** and **Lauer, R. M.** Does childhood obesity track into adulthood? *Critical Reviews in Food Science and Nutrition* 1993; **33**: 423–30.

36. **Armstrong, N., Simons-Morton, B.** Physical activity and blood lipids in adolescents. *Pediatric Exercise Science* 1994; **6**: 381–405.

37. **Alpert, B. S.** and **Wilmore, J. H.** Physical activity and blood pressure in adolescents. *Pediatric Exercise Science* 1994; **6**: 361–80.

38. **de Visser, D. C., van Hooft, I. M., van Doorren, L. J., Hofman, A., Orlebeke, J. F.** and **Grobbee DE.** Anthropometric measures, fitness and habitual physical activity in offspring of hypertensive parents. Dutch hypertension and offspring study. *American Journal of Hypertension* 1994; **7**: 242–8.

39. **Dwyer, T.** and **Gibbons L. E.** The Australian Schools Health and Fitness Survey. Physical fitness related to blood pressure but not lipoproteins. *Circulation* 1994; **89**: 1539–44.

40. **Al-Hazzaa, H. M., Sulaiman, M. A., Al-Matar, A. J.** and **Al-Mobaireek, K. F.** Cardiorespiratory fitness, physical activity patterns and coronary risk factors in preadolescent boys. *International Journal of Sports Medicine* 1994; **15**: 267–72.

41. **Rowland, T. W., Martel, L., Vanderburgh, P., Manos T.** and **Charkoudian, N.** The influence of short-term aerobic training on blood lipids in healthy 10–12 year old children. *International Journal of Sports Medicine* 1996; **17**: 487–92.

42. **Harrell, J. S., McMurray, R. G., Bangdiwala, S. I., Frauman, A. C., Gansky, S. A.** and **Bradley, C. B.** Effects of a school-based intervention to reduce cardiovascular disease risk factors in elementary-school children: The Cardiovascular Health in Children (CHIC) Study. *Journal of Pediatrics* 1996; **128**: 797–805.

43. **Webber, L. S., Osganian, S. K., Feldman, H. A., Wu, M., Mckenzie, T. L., Nichaman, M., Lytle, L. A., Edmundson, E., Cutler J., Nader, PR.** and **Luepker, R. V.** Cardiovascular risk factors among children after a two and a half year intervention—The CATCH Study. *Preventive Medicine* 1996; **25**: 432–41.

44. **Craig, S. B., Bandini, L. G., Lichtenstein, A. H., Schaefer, E. J.** and **Dietz, W. H.** The impact of physical activity on lipids, lipoproteins and blood pressure in preadolescent girls. *Pediatrics* 1996; **98**: 389–95.

45. **Bistritzer, T., Rosenzweig, L., Barr, J., Mayer, S., Lahat, E., Faibel, H., Schlesinger, Z.** and **Aladjem, M.** Lipid profile with paternal history of coronary heart disease before age 40. *Archives of Disease in Childhood* 1995; **73**: 62–5.

46. **Suter, E.** and **Hawes, M. R.** Relationship of physical activity, body fat, diet and blood lipid profile in youths 10–15 Years. *Medicine and Science in Sports and Exercise* 1993; **25**: 748–54.

47. **Gutin, B., Cucuzzo, N., Islam, S., Smith, C.** and **Stachura, M. E.** Physical training, lifestyle education and coronary risk factors in obese girls. *Medicine and Science in Sports and Exercise* 1996; **28**: 19–23.

48. **Anderson, L. B.** Blood pressure, physical fitness and physical activity in 17-year-old Danish adolescents. *Journal of Internal Medicine* 1994; **236**: 323–30.

49. **Jenner, D. A., Vandongen, R.** and **Beilin, L. J.** Relationships between blood pressure and measures of dietary energy intake, physical fitness, and physical activity in Australian children aged 11–12 years. *Journal of Epidemiology and Community Health* 1992; **46**: 108–13.

50. **Cooper, C., Campion, G.** and **Melton, L. J.** Hip fractures in the elderly: a world-wide projection. *Osteoporosis International* 1992; **2**: 285–9.

51. Bailey, D. A., Faulkner, R. A. and McKay, H. A. Growth, physical activity and bone mineral acquisition. *Exercise and Sport Sciences Reviews* 1996; **24**: 233–66.

52. Vuori, I. Peak bone mass and physical activity: A short review. *Nutrition Reviews* 1996; **54**: S11–S14.

53. Theintz, G., Buchs, B., Rizzoli, R., Slosman D., Clavien, H., Sizonenko, P. C. and Bonjour, J. P. Longitudinal monitoring of bone mass accumulation in healthy adolescents : evidence for a marked reduction after 16 years of age at the levels of the lumbar spine and femoral neck in female subjects. *Journal of Clinical Endocrinology and Metabolism* 1992; **75**: 1060–5.

54. Lu, P. W., Brody, J. N. and Ogle, G. D. Bone mineral density of total body, spine and femoral neck in children and young adults: A cross-sectional and longitudinal study. *Journal of Bone and Mineral Research* 1994; **9**: 1451–8.

55. Ralston, S. H. Osteoporosis. *British Medical Journal* 1997; **315**: 469–72.

56. Cadogan, J., Eastell, R., Jones, N. and Barker, M. Milk intake and bone mineral acquisition in adolescent girls: randomised, controlled intervention trial. *British Medical Journal* 1997; **315**: 1255–60.

57. Tylavsky, F. A., Anderson, J. J. B., Talmage, R. V. and Taft, T. N. Are calcium intakes and physical activity patterns during adolescence related to radial bone mass of white college-age females? *Osteporosis International* 1992; **2**: 232–40.

58. Ruiz, J. C., Mandel, C. and Garabedian, M. Influence of spontaneous calcium intake and physical exercise on the vertebral and femoral bone mineral density of children and adolescents. *Journal of Bone and Mineral Research* 1995; **10**: 675–82.

59. Teegarden, D., Proulx, W. R., Kern, M., Sedlock, D., Weaver, C. M., Johnston, C. C. and Lyle, R. M. Previous physical activity relates to bone mineral measures in young women. *Medicine and Science in Sports and Exercise* 1996; **28**: 105–13.

60. Gunnes, M. and Lehmann, E. H. Physical activity and dietary constituents as predictors of forearm cortical and trabecular bone gain in healthy children and adolescents. A prospective study. *Acta Paediatrica* 1996; **85**: 19–25.

61. Slemenda, C. W., Reister, TK., Hui, S. L., Miller, J. Z., Christian, J. C. and Johnston, C. C. Influences on skeletal mineralization in children and adolescents: Evidence for varying effects of sexual maturation and physical activity. *Journal of Pediatrics* 1994; **125**: 201–7.

62. Morris, F., Naughton, G. A., Gibbs, J. L., Carlson, J. and Wark, J. G. Prospective ten-month exercise intervention in premenarcheal girls: positive effects on bone and lean mass. *Journal of Bone and Mineral Research* 1997; 1453–62.

63. Grimston, S. K., Willows, N. D. and Hanley, D. A. Mechanical loading regime and its relationship to bone mineral density in children. *Medicine and Science in Sports and Exercise* 1993; **25**: 1203–10.

64. Recker, R. R., Davies, K. M., Hinders, S. M. *et al.* Predictors of axial and peripheral bone mineral density in healthy children and adolescents, with special attention to the role of puberty. *Journal of Pediatrics* 1993; **123**: 863–70.

65. Lanyon, L. E. Using functional loading to influence bone mass and architecture: objectives, mechanisms and relationship with estrogen of the mechanically adaptive process in bone. *Bone Mineral* 1996; **18**: 37S–43S.

66. Friedlander, A. L., Genant, H. K., Sadowsky, S., Byl, N. N. and Gluer, C. C. A two-year program of aerobics and weight training enhances bone mineral density of young women. *Journal of Bone and Mineral Research* 1995; **10**: 574–85.

67. Lohman, T., Going, S., Pamenter, R., Hall, M., Boyden, T., Houtkooper, L., Ritenbaugh, C., Bare, L., Hill, A. and Aickin, M. Effects of resistance training on regional and total bone mineral density in premenopausal women: a randomized prospective study. *Journal of one and Mineral Research* 1995; **10**: 1015–24.

68. Skerry, T. M. Mechanical loading and bone: what sort of exercise is beneficial to the skeleton? *Bone Mineral* 1997; **20**: 179–81.

69. Saito, I., Nishino, M., Kawabe, H., Wainai, H., Hasegawa, C., Saruta, T., Nagano, S. and Sekihara, T. Leisure time physical activity and insulin resistance in young obese students with hypertension. *American Journal of Hypertension* 1992; **5**: 915–18.

70. Kahle, E. B., Zipf, W. B., Lamb, D. R., Horswill, C. A. and Ward, K. M. Association between mild, routine exercise and improved insulin dynamics and glucose control in obese adolescents. *International Journal of Sports Medicine* 1996; **17**: 1–6.

71. Reaven, G. M. Role of insulin resistence in human disease. *Diabetes* 1988; **37**: 1595–607.

72. Barker, D. J. P. The fetal and infant origins of adult disease. *British Medical Journal* 1990; **301**: 1111.

73. Riddoch, C. J., Savage, J. M., Murphy, N., Cran, G. W. and Boreham C. Long term health implications of fitness and physical activity patterns. *Archives of Disease in Childhood* 1991; **66**: 1426–33.

74. Malina, R. M. Tracking of physical activity and physical fitness across the lifespan. *Research Quarterly for Exercise and Sport* 1996; 67(Suppl to No. 3): S1–S10.

75. Engstrom, L-M. The process of socialisation into keep-fit activities. *Scandinavian Journal of Sports Science* 1986; **8**: 89–97.

76. Cale, L. and Almond, L. Children's activity levels: a review of studies conducted on British children. *Physical Education Review* 1992; **15**: 111–18.

77. Sallis, J. F. Epidemiology of physical activity and fitness in children and adolescents. *Critical Reviews in Food Science and Nutrition* 1993; **33**: 403–8.

78. Astrand, P.-O. Physical activity and fitness: evolutionary perspective and trends for the future. In *Physical activity, fitness, and health: international proceedings and consensus statement* (ed. C. Bouchard, R. J. Shephard and T. Stephens). Human Kinetics, Champaign, Il, 1994; 98–105.

79. Rowland, T. W (ed.) *Exercise and children's health.* Human Kinetics, Champaign, Il, 1990.

80. Blair, S. N. Are American Children and Youth Fit? The Need for Better Data. *Research Quarterly for Exercise and Sport* 1992; **63**: 120–3.

81. Saris, W. H. M., Emons, H. J. G., Groenenboom, D. C. and Westerterp, K. R. Discrepancy between FAO/WHO energy requirements and actual energy expenditure levels in healthy 7–11 year old children. In *Children and exercise* (ed. G. Beunen, J. Ghesquiere, T. Reybrouck and A. L. Claessens). Enke, Stuttgart, 1990: 119.

82. Davies, P. S. W., Day, J. M. E. and Lucas, A. Early energy expenditure and later body fatness. *International Journal of Obesity* 1991; **15**: 727–31.

83. Boreham, C., Savage, M., Primrose, D., Cran G. and Strain, J. Coronary risk factors in school children. *Archives of Disease in Childhood* 1993; **68**: 182–6.

84. Department of Health, *Dietary reference values for food energy and nutrition for the United Kingdom. Report on health and social subjects. 41.* HMSO, London, 1991.

85. Durnin, J. V. G. A. Physical activity levels—past and present. In *Physical activity and health: symposium of the Society for the Study of Human Biology* (ed. N. G. Norgan). Cambridge University Press, Cambridge, 1992; 20–7.

86. Freedman, D. S., Srinivasan, S. R., Valdez, R. A., Williamson, D. F. and Berenson, G. S. Secular increases in relative weight and adiposity among children over two decades: the Bogalusa Heart Study. *Pediatrics* 1997; **99**: 420–6.

87. Campaigne, B. N., Morrison, J. A., Schumann, B. C., Falkner, F., Lakatos, E., Sprecher, D. and Schreiber, G. B. Indexes of obesity and comparisons with previous national survey data in 9- and 10-year-old black and white girls: the National Heart, Lung, and Blood Institute Growth and Health Study. *Journal of Pediatrics* 1994; **124**: 675–80.

88. Troiano, R. P., Flegal, K. M., Kuczmarski, R. J., Campbell, S. M., and Johnson, C. L. Overweight prevalence and trends for children and adolescents. The National Health and Nutrition Examination Surveys 1963 to 1991. *Archives of Pediatrics and Adolescent Medicine* 1995; **149**: 1085–91.

89. Chinn, S. and Rona, R. J. Trends in weight-for-height and triceps skinfold thickness for English and Scottish children, 1972–82 and 1982–1990. *Paediatric and Perinatal Epidemiology* 1994; **8**: 90–106.

90. Prentice, A. M. and Jebb, S. A. Obesity in Britain: gluttony or sloth? *British Medical Journal* 1995; **311**: 437–9.

91. Armstrong, N., Williams, J., Balding, J., Gentle, P. and Kirby, B. Cardiopulmonary fitness, physical activity patterns, and selected coronary risk factor variables in 11-to 16-year-olds. *Pediatric Exercise Science* 1991; **3**: 219–28.

92. Welk, G. J. *A comparison of methods for the assessment of physical activity in children.* Ph.D. Dissertation. Arizona State University, Tempe, 1994.

93. Sallis, J. F. and Patrick, K. Physical activity guidelines for adolescents: consensus statement. *Pediatric Exercise Science* 1994; **6**: 302–14.

94. Biddle, S., Cavill, N. and Sallis, J. Policy framework for young people and health-enhancing physical activity. In *Young and active? Young people and health-enhancing physical activity—evidence and implications* (ed. S. Biddle, J. Sallis and N. Cavill). Health Education Authority, London, 1998; 3–16.

95. Riddoch, C. J. and Boreham, C. A. The health-related physical activity of children. *Sports Medicine* 1995; **19**: 86–102.

96. Cale, L. and Harris, J. Exercise recommendations for children and young people. *Physical Education Review* 1993; **16**: 89–98.

97. Baranowski, T., Bouchard, C., Bar-Or, O., Bricker, T., Heath, G., Kimm, SYS., Malina, R., Obarzanek, E., Pate, R., Strong, W. B., Truman, B. and Washington, R. Assessment, prevalence, and cardiovascular benefits of physical activity and fitness in youth. *Medicine and Science in Sports and Exercise* 1992; **24**: S237–47.

98. Montgomery, H. E., Marshall, R., Hemingway, H., Myerson, S., Clarkson, P. and Dollery, C., *et al.* Human gene for physical performance. *Nature* 1998; **393**: 221–2.

99. Cooper, K. H., Pollock, M. L., Martin, R. P., White, S. R., Linnerrud, A. C. and Jackson, A. Physical fitness levels vs selected coronary risk factors. *Journal of the American Medical Association* 1976; **236**: 166–9.

100. Gibbons, L. W., Blair, S. N., Cooper, K. H. and Smith, M. Association between coronary heart disease factors and physical fitness in healthy adult women. *Circulation* 1983; **67**: 977–83.

101. Van Saarse, J., Noteboom, W. M. P. and Vandenbrouke, J. P. Longevity of men capable of prolonged vigorous physical exercise: a 32 year follow-up of 2259 participants in the Dutch eleven cities ice skating tour. *British Medical Journal* 1990; **301**: 1409–11.

102. Sandvik, L., Erikssen J., Thaulow, E., Eriksson, G., Mundal, R. and odahl, K. Physical fitness as a predictor of mortality among healthy, middle-aged Norwegian men. *New England Journal of Medicine* 1993; **328**: 533–7.

103. Farrell, S. W., Kampert, J. B., Kohl III, H. W., Barlow, C. E., Macera, C. A., Paffenbarger, R. S., Gibbons, L. W. and Blair, S. N. Influences of cardiorespiratory fitness levels and other predictors on cardiovascular disease mortality in men. *Medicine and Science in Sports and Exercise* 1998; **30**: 899–905.

104. Blair, SN., Kohl III, H. W., Barlow, C. E., Paffenbarger, R. S., Gibbons, LW. and Maccra, C. A. Changes in physical fitness and all-cause mortality: a prospective study of healthy and unhealthy men. *Journal of the American Medical Association* 1995; **273**: 1093–8.

105. Thompson, G. R. and Wilson, P. W. *Coronary risk factors and their assessment.* London Science Press, London, 1982.

106. Raitakari, O. T., Porkka, K. V. K., Rasenen, L., Ronnemaa, T. and Viikari, J. S. A. Clustering and six-year cluster-tracking of serum total cholesterol, HDL-cholesterol and diastolic blood pressure in children and young adults. *Journal of Clinical Epidemiology* 1994; **47**: 1085–93.

107. Tell, G. S. and Vellar, O. D. Physical fitness, physical activity and cardiovascular disease risk factors in adolescents: The Oslo Youth Study. *Preventive Medicine* 1988; **17**: 12–24.

108. Hofman, A. and Walter, H. J. The Association between Physical Fitness and Cardiovascular Disease Risk Factors in Children in a Five-Year Follow-up Study. *International Journal of Epidemiology* 1989; **18**(4): 830–5.

109. Hansen, H. S., Froberg, K., Hyldebrandt, N. and Nielson, J. K. A controlled study of eight months of physical training and reduction of blood pressure in children: the Odense schoolchild study. *British Medical Journal* 1991; **303**: 682–5.

110. Eriksson, B. O. and Koch, G. Effects of physical training on hemodynamic response during submaximal and maximal exercise in 11–13 year old boys. *Acta Physiologica Scandanavica* 1973; **87**: 27–39.

111. Gutin, B., Islanm, S., Manos, T., Cucuzzo, N., Smith, C. and Stachura, ME. Relation of percentage of body fat and maximal aerobic capacity to risk factors for atherosclerosis and diabetes in black and white seven to eleven year-old children. *Journal of Pediatrics* 1994; **125**: 847–52.

112. Hager, R. L., Tucker, L. A. and Seljaas, G. T. Aerobic fitness, blood lipids and body fat in children. *American Journal of Public Health* 1995; **85**: 1702–6.

113. Fripp, R. R., Hodgson, J. L., Kwiterovich, P. O., Werner, J. C., Schuler, H. G., and Whitman, V. Aerobic capacity, obesity and atherosclerotic risk factors in male adolescents. *Pediatrics* 1985; **75**: 813–8.

114. Sallis, J. F., Patterson, T. L., Buono, M. J. and Nadder, P. R. Relation of cardiovascular fitness and physical activity to cardiovascular disease risk factors in children and adults. *American Journal of Epidemiology* 1988; **127**: 933–41.

115. Hansen, H. S., Hyldebrandt, N., Froberg, K. and Nielsen, J. R. Blood pressure and physical fitness in a population of children–the Odense Schoolchild Study. *Journal of Human Hypertension* 1990; **4**: 615–20.

116. Bergstrom, E., Hernall, O. and Persson, L. A. Endurance running performance in relation to cardiovascular risk indicators in adolescents. *International Journal of Sports Medicine* 1997; **18**: 300–7.

117. Haddock, B. L., Hopp, H. P. and Mason, J. J. Cardiorespiratory fitness and cardiovascular disease risk factors in postmenopausal women. *Medicine and Science in Sports and Exercise* 1998; **30**: 893–8.

118. Cureton, K. J. Commentary on 'children and fitness: A public health perspective'. *Research Quarterly* 1987; **58**: 315–20.

119. Haskell, W. L., Montoye, H. J. and Orenstein, D. Physical activity and exercise to achieve health-related physical fitness components. *Public Health Reports* 1985; March-April: 202–13.

120. Seefeldt, V. and Vogel P. Children and fitness: A public health perspective. *Research Quarterly* 1987; **58**: 331–3.

121. Peters, R. K., Cady, L. D. J., Bischoff, D. P., Bernstein, L. and Pike, M. C. Physical fitness and subsequent myocardial infarction in healthy workers. *Journal of the American Medical Association* 1983; **249**: 3052–6.

122. Sobolski, J., Kornitzer, M., De Backer, G., Dramaix, M., Abramowicz, M., Gegre, S. and Denolin, H. Protection against ischemic heart disease in the Belgian fitness study: physical fitness rather than physical activity? *American Journal of Epidemiology* 1987; **125**: 601–10.

123. Blair, S. N. Physical activity, fitness and coronary heart disease. In *Physical activity, fitness and health: international proceedings and consensus statement* (ed. C. Bouchard, R. J. Shephard and T. Stephens). Human Kinetics, Champaign, Il, 1994; 579–90.

124. van Mechelen, W. Etiology and prevention of sports injuries in youth. In *Children and exercise XVIII: Exercise and fitness—benefits and risks* (ed. K. Froberg, O. Lammert, H. Steen Hansen and J. R. Blimkie). Odense University Press, Odense, 1997; 209–27.

125. Baxter-Jones, A., Maffulli, N. and Helms, P. Low injury rates in elite athletes. *Archives of Disease in Childhood* 1993; **68**: 130–2.

126. Sallis, J. F. and McKenzie, T. L. Physical Education's Role in Public Health. *Research Quarterly for Exercise and Sport* 1991; **62**: 124–37.

3.2 Physical activity, physical fitness and cardiovascular health

Jos W. R. Twisk

Introduction

Cardiovascular disease (CVD) is one of the greatest causes of death in Western societies, and it probably will be in the future also in developing countries. It is now recognized that CVD is partly a paediatric problem; i.e. the onset of CVD lies in early childhood, even though the clinical symptoms of this disease do not become apparent until much later in life. The ideal study to answer the question whether high levels of physical activity and physical fitness during childhood and adolescence lower the risk of developing CVD later in life is a randomized controlled trial with a lifetime follow-up, in which a large group of children and adolescents is assigned to either a sedentary or an active lifestyle; a study which will probably never take place. The most classical and probably the only study investigating the relationship between physical activity in relatively young people and the occurrence of CVD at later age is the Harvard Alumni Study, performed by Paffenbarger et al.[1] In one part of this extensive observational study, physical activity levels during the student period (gathered from university archives) were related to the occurrence of CVD later in life. Regarding their physical activity levels, the students were divided into three groups:

(1) athletes;
(2) intramural sports play for more than five hours per week; and
(3) intramural sports play for less than five hours (usually none at all) per week.

The three groups did not differ regarding the occurrence of CVD later in life. Student athletes who discontinued their activity levels after college encountered a CVD incidence similar to the risk of alumni classmates who never had been athletes. In fact subjects who became physically active later in life had the same health benefits than the subjects who were active all along the observation period.

The incidence of morbidity and mortality related to CVD is rather low in a paediatric population. Studies investigating the relationship between physical activity, physical fitness and cardiovascular health in children and adolescents are therefore mostly limited to CVD risk factors as outcome measure. For this reason this chapter will focus on the association of physical activity and physical fitness with CVD risk factors in children and adolescents. These risk factors can be divided into the so called traditional CVD risk factors, i.e. lipoproteins (total cholesterol, low density lipoprotein cholesterol (LDL), high density lipoprotein cholesterol (HDL), triglycerides), blood pressure, body fatness and diabetes, and 'new' CVD risk factors, i.e. other lipoproteins (lipoprotein(a) (Lp(a)), apolipoprotein (Apo) B, and ApoA-1), fibrinogen, homocysteine and heart rate variability.

Traditional CVD risk factors

Lipoproteins

It is known that lipoprotein levels are directly related to the process of atherosclerosis and therefore to the occurrence of CVD. Although total serum cholesterol has been found to be related to CVD, its atherogenic effect merely depends on the structure of the cholesterol; or in other words on the ratio between low density lipoprotein cholesterol (LDL) and high density lipoprotein cholesterol (HDL). It is assumed that LDL may act directly or indirectly to cause endothelial damage, with subsequent proliferation of arterial smooth muscle cells resulting in an accumulation of lipids and a progression to atherosclerotic plaque formation. HDL on the other hand is assumed to be protective against CVD; HDL seems to be responsible for carrying cholesterol from peripheral tissue, including the arterial walls back to the liver where it is metabolized and excreted. Besides HDL and LDL, also very low density lipoprotein cholesterol (VLDL) and plasma triglycerides (TG) need to be considered, although the atherogenic effects of VLDL and TG are not firmly established yet. It is further assumed that during exercise, fatty acids are freed from their storage sites to be burned for energy production. Several studies suggest that human growth hormone may be responsible for this increased fatty acid mobilization. Growth hormone levels increase sharply with exercise and remain elevated for up to several hours in the recovery period. Other research has suggested that, with exercise, the adipose tissue is more sensitive to either the sympathetic nervous system or to rises in circulating catecholamines. Either situation would increase lipid mobilization.

From epidemiological studies among adults there is (some) evidence that physical activity and physical fitness are associated with favourable lipid profiles. However, for children and adolescents there is not much evidence that physical activity and physical fitness have beneficial effects on lipids (Table 3.2.1). From cross-sectional, longitudinal, as well as experimental studies there is ambiguous evidence that physical activity and/or physical fitness have some beneficial effects on any of the lipid levels. For an extensive overview regarding this topic one is referred to Armstrong and Simons Morton.[2]

One of the problems is that most of the studies in this field are cross-sectionally designed. Sallis et al.[3] for instance did not find any relation between activity and HDL in children aged 11–12 years. In the Beaver County Lipid Study,[4] a positive cross-sectional relation was found between daily physical activity and HDL in young adults. However, in multivariate analysis (correcting for smoking, alcohol consumption and body mass index) this positive relation disappeared.

Table 3.2.1 Overview regarding relationships between physical activity (PA) and physical fitness (PF) and total serum cholesterol (TC), high density lipoprotein cholesterol (HDL), low density lipoprotein cholesterol (LDL), the TC:HDL ratio and serum triglycerides (TG) in normal populations of children and adolescents

			TC	HDL	LDL	TC:HDL	TG
Observational	Cross-sectional	PA	±	−	±	±	±
		PF	−	±	±	±	±
	Longitudinal	PA	−	±	±	±	±
		PF	±	−	±	±	±
Intervention			±	±	±	±	±

++ = strong evidence; + = moderate evidence; ± = ambiguous evidence; − = no evidence.

There are only a few longitudinal studies investigating this problem. In the Amsterdam Growth and Health Study, for instance, an observational longitudinal study covering a period of 15 years from adolescence into young adulthood, the longitudinal development of daily physical activity (assessed by a structured interview covering three months prior to the interview, and expressed as a weighted activity score in METs/week) was positively related to the development of HDL. No relations were, however, found between the development of daily physical activity and the development of TC and the TC:HDL ratio.[5] In the Cardiovascular Risk in Young Finns Study,[6] boys with an initial age of 12 years who remained active over a period of six years showed lower values of the TC:HDL ratio at the age of 18 years than boys who had a sedentary lifestyle over that period. However, for boys no differences were found in TC and HDL values separately, while females did not show any significant differences for all three parameters. Also no relationships were found between the change in physical activity over the six-year period and the change in any of the lipoprotein levels for both boys and girls.

Intervention studies also show contradictory results. A problem with intervention studies is the fact that they are mostly carried out on very few subjects. An exception is the Child and Adolescent Trial for Cardiovascular Health (CATCH). In this large study, among more than 4000 children and adolescents, a multidisciplinary intervention was carried out, i.e. a 30 month diet, exercise and non-smoking programme. No significant differences were found in TC and HDL.[7] The same result was found in the Cardiovascular Health in Children Study after eight months of aerobic training.[8] Casanovas et al.[9] on the other hand found an increase in TC and a decrease in HDL after a programme in which the daily physical activity was decreased. These relations were shown in more than 400 young adults over a period of eight months.

So there is some evidence that physical activity and physical fitness are related to favourable HDL-levels. This positive effect is probably caused by an increased activity of lipoprotein lipase (LPL) and lecithinin:cholesterol acyltransferase (LCAT). Both activities are increased by high levels of cardiopulmonary work and both are known to increase the levels of HDL.[10,11]

Blood pressure

In adults it is shown that endurance training can reduce both systolic and diastolic blood pressure by approximately 10 mm Hg in individuals with moderate essential hypertension, but exercise does not seem to have an effect in subjects with severe hypertension.[12] However, the mechanisms responsible for the decrease in blood pressure with physical activity and endurance training have yet to be determined. A reduced cardiac output is mentioned as a reason for the fact that activity lowers blood pressure, although this cardiac output reducing effect of physical activity and fitness is not found in all studies.[13] If there is no influence on cardiac output, then the blood pressure decreasing effect may be caused by a reduction in peripheral vascular resistance, which may be due to an overall reduction of sympathetic nervous system activity.[13] In addition, the relation between physical activity and blood pressure can be caused by the anxiety reducing effect of physical activity.[14] It is questionable, however, if this mechanism is present in children and adolescents.

It appears that essential hypertension may begin early in life and that detection and treatment of possible blood pressure abnormalities at young ages is important. There is, however, no direct evidence that elevated blood pressure in children is related to CVD later in life. There is also not much evidence that physical activity and physical fitness have beneficial effects on blood pressure in children and adolescents. The studies analysing these relationships are extensively reviewed by Alpert and Wilmore.[15] There are many cross-sectional studies investigating this relationship, but again the best evidence comes from longitudinal and well-controlled intervention studies. In the Amsterdam Growth and Health Study, for instance, daily physical activity during adolescence was not significantly related to both SBP and DBP at young adult age,[5] and besides that the longitudinal development of physical activity was also not related to both systolic and diastolic blood pressure (Twisk, unpublished results). The latter was also reported in the Cardiovascular Risk in Young Finns Study.[16] In the CATCH study, the 30-month multidisciplinary intervention among more than 4000 children and adolescents did not have any effect on blood pressure.[7] Baranowski et al.[17] argued that, as in adults, the possible lowering effect of physical activity on blood pressure only holds for children and adolescents with hypertension and not for youngsters with normal values of blood pressure. This implies that this effect is difficult to observe in population studies in children with low incidence of hypertension. It should also be kept in mind that this effect is probably only true for high intensity aerobic type training and not for 'normal' habitual daily physical activity.[15] In Table 3.2.2 an overview is given regarding the relationships between physical activity and physical fitness and diastolic and systolic blood pressure in children and adolescents.

Table 3.2.2 Overview regarding relationships between physical activity (PA) and physical fitness (PF) and diastolic and systolic blood pressure (BP) in normal populations of children and adolescents

			Systolic BP	Diastolic BP
Observational	Cross-sectional	PA	−	−
		PF	±	±
	Longitudinal	PA	−	−
		PF	±	−
Intervention			−	−

+ + = strong evidence; + = moderate evidence; ± = ambiguous evidence; − = no evidence.

Table 3.2.3 Overview regarding relationships between physical activity (PA) and physical fitness (PF) and body fatness and body fat distribution in normal populations of children and adolescents

			Body fatness	Body fat distribution
Observational	Cross-sectional	PA	±	±
		PF	+	±
	Longitudinal	PA	±	−
		PF	±	−
Intervention			++	NA

+ + = strong evidence; + = moderate evidence; ± = ambiguous evidence; − = no evidence; NA = no studies available.

Body fatness and body composition

High body fatness (i.e. obesity) is known to be a risk factor for CVD in adults.[18] Not only directly, but also indirectly through other CVD risk factors, like lipoprotein levels and blood pressure. From prospective studies it is known that in adulthood also a central pattern of body fat is associated with CVD morbidity and mortality.[19] It has been suggested that adolescence is a sensitive period for the development of a central pattern of body fat.[20] Therefore adolescent body fat patterns may be of consequence for the development of CVD morbidity and mortality later in life. The etiology of childhood obesity is very complex. Besides heredity, which is regarded to be a major contributing factor in the development of childhood obesity, also neuro-endocrine and metabolic disturbances contribute significantly to one's propensity for fatness. Environmental factors, such as cultural background, socio-economic status, nutrition and physical activity, have also been recognized as causes for childhood obesity.

In the light of energy balance, it is obvious that the relationships between physical activity, physical fitness and body fatness and body fat distribution cannot be separated from the influence of food (i.e. energy) intake. There is a theory which states that a certain minimum level of physical activity is necessary for the body to precisely regulate energy intake to balance energy expenditure. A sedentary lifestyle may reduce this regulatory ability, resulting in a positive energy balance and an increase in body fatness.[21] Another theory states that exercise is a mild appetite suppressant; this is based on research in which the total number of calories consumed did not change after a training programme was started, although there was an increase in energy expenditure because of the training programme.[21] It is also suggested that resting metabolic rate is increased because of physical activity and/or aerobic training; some

studies have shown that this is true, while other studies failed to show this.[22,23]

Table 3.2.3 presents an overview of studies investigating the relationship between physical activity, physical fitness and body fatness and body fat distribution in children and adolescents. In general, it can be concluded that there is some evidence for a relationship between physical activity, physical fitness and body fatness in children and adolescents. This was also the conclusion of an extensive review performed by Bar-Or and Baranowski.[24] The evidence not only comes from several cross-sectional studies,[17,25] longitudinal studies also show the same results. In the Amsterdam Growth and Health Study, for instance, it was found that 'long term exposure' to daily physical activity during adolescence was inversely related to the sum of four skinfolds at adult age.[5] In another study with data from the Amsterdam Growth and Health Study, it was shown that the longitudinal development (from 13 to 27 years of age) of both daily physical activity and physical fitness (operationalized as $\dot{V}O_2$ max) was strongly inversely related to the development of the sum of four skinfolds.[26]

The evidence for a positive effect of physical activity and/or physical fitness on body fat distribution is, in contrast to the results for body fatness, very weak and the results are very ambiguous. In the Amsterdam Growth and Health Study, for instance, it was found that the amount of daily physical activity during adolescence was positively related to the waist to hip ratio (WHR) at adult age. This relation was found for females and not for males.[5] This finding is difficult to explain; firstly because WHR is found to be primarily under genetic control[27] and secondly, if there exists a relationship between physical activity and WHR, this relationship is assumed to be inverse.[28,29] An explanation for this paradoxical finding in the Amsterdam Growth and Health Study could be that in females' inactivity leads to a greater accumulation of fat in the thighs, which would give a lower WHR.[5] In another study with data from the Amsterdam Growth and Health Study, van Lenthe et al.,[30] however, did not found a longitudinal relationship between physical activity and body fat distribution (operationalized as the ratio between the thickness of the triceps skinfold and the subscapular skinfold and not as the WHR).

A major problem in the investigation of the relationship between physical activity, physical fitness and body fatness or obesity is the fact that it is difficult to make a distinction between cause and effect (Fig. 3.2.1). Physical activity, physical fitness and body fatness are associated with one another and this cluster of factors is assumed to be a risk factor for CVD. It is difficult to investigate what comes first.

Another problem in the investigation of the relationship between activity and body fatness is the operationalization of body fatness. Most commonly body fatness is operationalized as body mass index (BMI). BMI is easy to measure and therefore widely used as indicator for body fatness. Another option is using the sum of two or more skinfold thicknesses as indicator for body fatness. Although both operationalizations are used as indicator for the same parameter, they are not the same and analyses with both operationalizations can lead to different results; especially when one is interested in the relationship between physical activity and physical fitness and body fatness. This difference in results was shown in a paper by Twisk et al.[26] Based on data from the Amsterdam Growth and Health Study, a highly significant negative relationship was found between the sum of four skinfolds and $\dot{V}O_2$ max (directly measured by a treadmill test), while for BMI no relationship was found. In the same way, the amount of daily physical activity was found to be negatively related to the sum of four skinfolds, but not to BMI. One of the reasons for these different results is the fact that BMI is not only an indicator of fat mass, but also of lean body mass or muscle mass. Subjects with high muscle mass and moderate fat mass will have high values for BMI, but only moderate values for the sum of four skinfolds. When BMI is used as indicator of body fatness, the negative relationships between body fatness and $\dot{V}O_2$ max and between daily physical activity and body fatness can be more or less counterbalanced by the opposite relationships with lean body mass. The same phenomenon was observed by Bergström et al.[31] in an observational cross-sectional study, in which physical fitness (measured by a 3 km running test) was related to body fatness. In more than 1000 adolescents it was shown that running performance was highly related to the sum of four skinfolds in both boys and girls. Only for

girls, and with much lower levels of significance, was running performance related to BMI. This indicates that results obtained with BMI as the indicator for body fatness should be interpreted cautiously; especially in children and adolescents, because in this particular population the variables concerned are also influenced by natural growth and biological development.

Diabetes

Diabetes mellitus is a disorder of carbohydrate metabolism characterized by high blood sugar levels. It is known to be an important CVD risk factor. It develops when there is inadequate production of insulin by the pancreas, or inadequate utilization of insulin by the cells. A distinction must be made between insulin dependent diabetes mellitus (IDDM), type-I diabetes, also known as juvenile onset diabetes, and non-insulin dependent diabetes (NIDDM), type-II diabetes, also known as adult-onset diabetes. NIDDM is rare in children, but IDDM is much more common and presents a significant problem in youth. Also an adolescent version of type-II diabetes is known as maturity onset diabetes in the young (MODY).

In adults physical activity has many desirable effects for people with diabetes, particularly those with type-II diabetes.[32] Glycemic control is improved, possibly due to the insulin like effect of muscle contractions on translocating glucose from the plasma into the cell.[33] Exercise leads to an increase in muscle mass (lean body mass) and therefore to lower blood glucose levels, assisting in better glycemic and blood sugar control. The latter can reduce insulin resistance. Some researchers believe that physical activity can have an effect on glycemic control in children with IDDM, but in other studies this is not confirmed.[34]

The outcome variables most commonly used in studies relating physical activity and physical fitness to insulin metabolism disorders are glucose and insulin concentrations of blood serum. When reviewing the literature there are not many studies investigating the relationships between physical activity, physical fitness and serum insulin and glucose concentrations in children and adolescents; Table 3.2.4 gives an overview. For insulin levels the results are ambiguous. In the Cardiovascular Risk in Young Finns Study, for instance, for males an inverse cross-sectional relationship was observed between physical activity and insulin levels, while for females this relationship was not found.[35] For blood glucose, the few studies carried out did not show any influence of physical activity and physical fitness in children and adolescents. More consistent results are found in the even more limited number of studies among obese children and adolescents. In these studies, a positive effect was found of physical activity on parameters related to insulin metabolism.[36]

Multiple risk factors

It is known that biological CVD risk factors tend to occur together more frequently than expected by chance. This clustering of risk factors was not only shown in adults, but also in children and adolescents.[37–39] Clustered biological CVD risk factors give a higher risk for the development of CVD than just the sum of the risks of the separate biological risk factors. There seems to be a positive interaction between the risk factors in relation to the risk of developing CVD.[40,41] The clustering of dyslipidemia, hypertension, hyperinsulinemia and obesity has been recognized in children and adolescents and has been termed as 'syndrome X', or 'the deadly quartet'.[42] Although it seems to be important to investigate clustered CVD risk factors in addition to

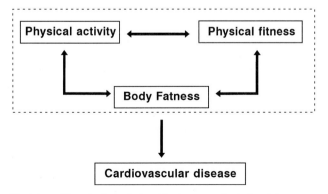

Fig. 3.2.1 Hypothetical relationships between physical activity, physical fitness and body fatness.

Table 3.2.4 Overview regarding relationships between physical activity (PA) and physical fitness (PF) and serum insulin and serum glucose concentrations in normal populations of children and adolescents

			Insulin	Glucose
Observational	Cross-sectional	PA	±	−
		PF	±	−
	Longitudinal	PA	NA	NA
		PF	NA	NA
Intervention			±	NA

+ + = strong evidence; + = moderate evidence; ± = ambiguous evidence; − = no evidence; NA = no studies available.

the study of single risk factors, the relationship between this clustering of CVD risk factors and physical activity and physical fitness has only been investigated in a few studies. In the longitudinal Amsterdam Growth and Health Study clustering concerned the TC:HDL ratio, mean arterial blood pressure, the sum of four skinfolds and $\dot{V}O_2$ max. Daily physical activity was found to be strongly inversely related to this cluster of CVD risk factors.[43] In contrast in the Northern Ireland Young Hearts Project in 12 and 15 year old boys and girls, no relationship was observed between daily physical activity and a cluster score based on the TC:HDL ratio, diastolic blood pressure, sum of four skinfolds and cardiopulmonary fitness (number of laps on a shuttle run test).[44] In the Cardiovascular Risk in Young Finns Study[39] clustering concerned total serum cholesterol, high density lipoprotein cholesterol and diastolic blood pressure. A large cohort with an initial age between 3 and 18 years was followed for a period of 6 years. At the initial measurement, as well as at the follow-up measurement, a 'high risk cluster' was defined as the subjects who belong to the high risk (age and gender specific) tertiles of all three risk factors. A shift from not belonging to this 'high risk cluster' at the initial measurement to belonging to this 'high risk cluster' at the follow-up measurement, was associated with a decrease in physical activity.

Other lifestyles

Physical inactivity is more or less independently related to CVD risk factors. Physical inactivity is also often found to be associated with other unhealthy lifestyles like smoking behaviour, alcohol consumption and unhealthy dietary habits. This clustering of unhealthy lifestyles may introduce a health risk that is greater than one would expect from the individual unhealthy lifestyles.[45] It is unlikely that these unhealthy lifestyles are related to each other in a causal chain. It is more likely that there is one or more underlying mechanism(s) (caused by genetic variables, psychosocial variables, socio-economic class, environmental factors, etc.) which is case related to the construct of 'unhealthy behaviour' (i.e. inactivity, smoking behaviour, alcohol consumption and unhealthy diet). In the Cardiovascular Risk in Young Finns Study, physical inactivity was found to be associated to smoking behaviour, alcohol consumption and having a diet with an excess of fat.[46] This finding was not confirmed in the Amsterdam Growth and Health Study where physical inactivity was not found to be associated with any of the other unhealthy lifestyles.[47] In a cross-sectional study among 18-year old Australians (301 males and 282 females) smoking, drinking alcohol and unhealthy dietary habits were related to each

other for males and females; for females also a low level of physical activity was associated with the other 'unhealthy' behaviours.[48] Terre et al.[49] also showed correlations between unhealthy behaviours and argued that a multidimensional view should be used in the prevention of chronic diseases in childhood. As a consequence there is nowadays the belief that prevention should not focus on a particular lifestyle, but that a multidisciplinary, healthy behaviour oriented preventive programme should be developed in order to prevent CVD. Such programmes would be not only beneficial for the prevention of CVD, but also for the prevention of many other chronic diseases.[50]

New CHD risk factors

Lipoproteins (Lp(a), ApoB, ApoA-1)

Due to progress in lipid biochemistry in the late 1970s and early 1980s, it was shown that the lipoprotein levels are not as such the most important factor in relation to the onset of CVD, but more the protein parts of the lipoproteins (apolipoproteins).[51] The two most important apolipoproteins (Apo) are: ApoA-1, which is the major protein content of HDL and which is therefore assumed to be protective against CVD; and ApoB, which is the major protein content of LDL, and which is therefore assumed to be atherogenic.[52–54] Later on lipoprotein(a) (Lp(a)) was detected. Lp(a) is comparable to LDL and was found to be an independent risk factor for CVD.[55,56] Lp(a) is, unlike LDL, inherited as a quantitative genetic trait.[57]

There are not many studies investigating the relationships between physical fitness and physical activity and ApoA-1, ApoB and Lp(a) among children and adolescents. Table 3.2.5 gives an overview of the results of different studies, which shows that the results are ambiguous. In a cross-sectional study based on data from the Cardiovascular Risk in Young Finns Study, among more than 2000 children, adolescents and young adults, physical activity was found to be inversely related to ApoB for males, but not for females. No relationship was observed with ApoA-1.[16] In a longitudinal study with the same data, however, subjects who remained active over a period of six years showed no difference in their ApoB and ApoA-1 levels compared with subjects who remained inactive over the same time period.[6] In the earlier mentioned CATCH study, the large multidisciplinary intervention had no effect on ApoB levels.[7] Regarding Lp(a), in a population based study among more than 4000 young adults, aged between 23 and 35 years, Lp(a) was not associated with daily physical activity; suggesting that Lp(a) levels are largely

Table 3.2.5 Overview regarding relationships between physical activity (PA) and physical fitness (PF) and apolipoprotein (Apo A-1, Apo B) and lipoprotein (a) (Lp(a)) in normal populations of children and adolescents

			ApoB	ApoA-1	Lp(a)
Observational	Cross-sectional	PA	±	±	±
		PF	−	−	−
	Longitudinal	PA	NA	NA	NA
		PF	NA	NA	NA
Intervention			±	±	NA

+ + = strong evidence; + = moderate evidence; ± = ambiguous evidence; − = no evidence; NA = no studies available.

genetically determined.[58] In the Cardiovascular Risk in Young Finns Study,[59] however, an inverse cross-sectional relationship was observed between physical activity and Lp(a) levels, i.e high levels of Lp(a) (>25 mg/dl) were less frequent in the physically most active subjects.

Fibrinogen

Fibrinogen is a main determinant of plasma viscosity and red cell aggregation. Both phenomena reduce blood fluidity especially in the microcirculation. Fibrinogen plays further a central role in platelet aggregation and performs as an essential substrate in the coagulation cascade. High fibrinogen levels may therefore favour a hypercoagulable state resulting in final thrombic events of CVD. In adults, the evidence linking physical activity and physical fitness to fibrinogen levels is unclear. Koenig et al.[60] showed, for instance, that leisure-time physical activity was (independently of other risk factors for CVD) inversely associated with plasma viscosity, whereas work related activity did not show this effect. In the Northern Ireland Health and Activity Survey, in older subjects (16+) an inverse relationship was observed between fibrinogen and physical activity, but this relation disappeared after correcting for possible confounders. In this survey an inverse relationship was also observed between cardiopulmonary fitness and fibrinogen, which remained significant after correction for possible confounders.[61]

There are only a few studies in which this relationship is investigated in children and adults. In the cross-sectional Coronary Artery Risk Development in Young Adults (CARDIA) Study, for instance, fibrinogen levels were inversely associated with physical activity levels.[62] Stratton et al.,[63] however, did not find a positive effect of a six months intensive endurance training programme among 10 subjects (24–30 years of age) on fibrinogen levels (where $\dot{V}O_2$ max increased significantly), while in an older group (60–82 years) there was an effect. In the Petah Tikva Project[64] a low but statistically significant inverse cross-sectional relationship was observed between sports activity and plasma fibrinogen levels. This was observed in 9 to 18 year old boys and girls. To conclude, like for many other CVD risk factors, the evidence for a possible inverse relationship between physical activity, physical fitness and fibrinogen levels in children and adolescents is rather weak.

Other risk factors (homocysteine and heart rate variability)

Just recently it has been recognized that hyperhomocysteinaemia is related to CVD morbidity and mortality. Homocysteine levels are

assumed to be independent of the traditional risk factors (lipoproteins, age, gender, blood pressure and smoking). In a large cross-sectional study among 16 000 middle-aged subjects an inverse relation was found between homocysteine level and physical activity.[65] Until now no studies investigating the relationship between physical activity and physical fitness and homocysteine levels in children and adolescents have been reported in the literature.

Another CVD risk factor which received attention recently is heart rate variability, which seems to be impaired in chronic artery disease. The biological mechanisms behind this phenomenon are not yet fully understood. The possible influence of physical activity and physical fitness on heart rate variability in children and adolescents has yet to be determined. It is assumed that the adaptive responses of the cardiovascular system to regular physical activity includes a reduction in sympathetic and an increase in parasympathetic activity during rest and at different absolute intensities of exercise. This assumption was not confirmed in a cross-sectional study in young subjects, where it was shown that both sympathetic and parasympathetic activity were not different in trained versus non-trained subjects.[66] In adults there is limited conflicting evidence of the influence of physical activity and physical fitness on heart rate variability. In a cross-sectional study among 88 middle-aged subjects, no relationship could be shown between heart rate variability and physical activity (assessed by a two-month diary follow-up).[67] In another study among 19 middle-aged subjects, it was found that after a training period of 30 weeks heart rate variability was increased in the training group compared to the control group.[68]

New developments
Gene–environment interactions

With the development of genetic epidemiology and the discovery of certain polymorphisms which are found to be related to CVD risk factors (especially related to lipoproteins and body fatness), there is a lot of scientific interest in the so called gene–environment interactions. Or in other words, one is trying to get an answer to the question: Is the relationship between physical activity, physical fitness and CVD risk factors different for different genotypes? Up to now, to the author's knowledge, the only study investigating the interaction between physical activity and genetic predisposition in a young population is the Cardiovascular Risk in Young Finns Study, which focused on apolipoprotein (Apo)E. ApoE determines serum total cholesterol and LDL and is therefore associated with CVD. In plasma three major ApoE isoforms can be determined (E2, E3 and E4) which are coded by three codominant alleles (2, 3 and 4), resulting in six major ApoE phenotypes (E2/2, E3/2, E4/2, E3/3, E4/3 and E4/4). In a cross-sectional sample of 1498 boys and girls (aged between 9 and 24 years), the relationship between daily physical activity (a weighted activity score assessed by a questionnaire) and TC and LDL was analysed for different subgroups with different ApoE phenotypes. It was shown that the influence of physical activity differed for the different subgroups. No associations were found in E4/4, moderate associations were found in E4/3 and E3/3, and much stronger associations were observed in E3/2 phenotype.[69] From these results it appears that ApoE phenotype partly determines the association between physical activity and TC and LDL, i.e. that there exists some degree of gene–environment interaction. However, much more research is needed in this field.

Pre-clinical atherosclerosis

Up to now research regarding the relationship between physical activity and physical fitness among children and adolescents and CVD mortality and morbidity later in life has been limited to the analysis of the associations between physical activity and physical fitness and biological CVD risk factors. Recently alternative ways have become available with which it is possible to 'assess' the degree of atherosclerosis before clinical symptoms occur. With non-invasive ultrasonographic methods it is possible to measure *in vivo* artery wall thickness, which provides a direct measure of the degree of atherosclerosis.[70] The relative simplicity of these new methods makes it possible to use them not only in small clinical trials, but also in large epidemiologic studies. Another new innovation is the assessment of endothelial dysfunction. With high resolution ultrasound the diameter of certain arteries can be measured under different conditions, from which endothelial dysfunction can be determined.[71] Also this endothelial dysfunction can be seen as an indicator of preclinical atherosclerosis. With these new techniques it will be possible to analyse the relationship between physical activity and physical fitness during childhood and adolescence and the actual degree of atherosclerosis, before clinical symptoms occur. This will definitely improve the knowledge about the causal pathway according the development of CVD and the possible beneficial effects of physical activity and physical fitness in children and adolescents.

General comments
Possible reasons for the lack of evidence

In analysing the effect of physical activity and physical fitness on CVD risk factors in children and adolescents, one must realize that almost all risk factors have a (large) genetic component; so the changes in CVD risk factors observed as a result of physical activity and/or physical fitness are generally small. Furthermore it must be taken into account that the development of CVD risk factors during childhood and adolescence can also be the result of normal growth and development. Especially during adolescence, the rate of maturation can be a very important factor. A nice example to illustrate the importance of this factor is the so called 'adolescent dip' in total serum cholesterol levels,[72] which can highly bias the results of studies investigating the relationship between physical activity and physical fitness and total serum cholesterol in adolescents.

A third important issue is the problem of assessing the amount of physical activity. There are many different ways described to measure physical activity;[73] they vary from direct measurements (i.e. observation, diary, questionnaires, interview) to indirect measurements (i.e. physiological measurements, mechanical devices, 'doubly labelled' water). First of all the use of different methods to assess physical activity in different studies can lead to ambiguous results, and secondly the definition of physical activity is often different between studies. Sometimes physical activity is defined as total habitual physical activity, while in other studies physical activity is limited to sports activity. Also proxy measures such as the time an individual watches television are used. However, whatever method is used it is impossible to measure the amount of physical activity in children and adolescents exactly. The best one can do is to get a crude indication of habitual physical activity (probably achieved by a combination of different methods). The measurement error related to the assessment of physical activity is in general non-differential, i.e. not related to the health outcome. This non-differential misclassification will lead to bias towards the null, which causes relationships to be underestimated; a phenomenon which exists both for under-reporting as for over-reporting.

Another important issue concerns the intensity of different activities. One is often interested in the total energy expenditure of a certain individual. With questionnaires or interviews (the methods mostly used in large population based studies) it is very difficult to assess the intensity of the different activities carried out by a particular subject. Data from questionnaires are often converted to an activity measure using standard tables in which a particular activity is related to a certain amount of energy expenditure. This certain amount of energy expenditure is often seen as an indicator of intensity. This method introduces a new source of bias; not only can the intensity of the same activity be extremely different for different individuals, but also different absolute levels of aerobic fitness between individuals can have important implications for the translation of certain activities into energy expenditure.

Finally when $\dot{V}O_2$ max is used as indicator for physical fitness, there is the problem that $\dot{V}O_2$ max is highly related to body composition and body mass. Therefore $\dot{V}O_2$ max is often expressed per kg body mass or per kg body mass to the 2/3 power. It is however known that in children and adolescents the relationship between $\dot{V}O_2$ max and body mass is not that straightforward. Furthermore the relationship with body mass is changing over time, i.e. is different for different age groups (see chapter 1.1). This can also be a possible reason for ambiguous results.

Cardiovascular health importance

To evaluate the importance of relationships between physical activity, physical fitness and CVD risk factors in childhood and adolescence it is important to realize that a high level of a risk factor during childhood and adolescence is not health threatening *per se*, i.e. it is mostly not directly related to disease. In fact the value of a particular CVD risk factor measured at an early age is a (less than perfect) predictor of that CVD risk factor in middle age, which is a (less than perfect) predictor of the occurrence of CVD events. So 'high risk' values for CVD risk factors in childhood or adolescence are a risk factor for 'high risk' values for CVD risk factors in adulthood, which are a risk factor for the development of CVD. In Fig. 3.2.2 this problem is

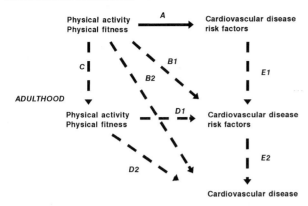

Fig. 3.2.2 Hypothetical relationships between physical activity, physical fitness and cardiovascular disease risk factors and cardiovascular disease throughout life (characters (*A*) to (*E2*) are explained in the text).

illustrated, and it shows that the situation is much more complicated than just the analysis of the relationships between physical activity or physical fitness and CVD risk factors in childhood and adolescence. Figure 3.2.2 is an extension of the hypothesized relationships between activity, health and stage of life by Blair *et al.*[74]

Looking at the different arrows in Fig. 3.2.2, there is no evidence that physical activity and/or physical fitness during childhood and adolescence are related to CVD risk factors in adulthood (*B1*). There is no evidence that physical activity and/or physical fitness during childhood and adolescence are related to the occurrence of CVD in adulthood (*B2*). There is (as has been shown earlier) weak evidence that physical activity and/or physical fitness in childhood and adolescence are related to CVD risk factors in childhood and adolescence (*A*), and there is (better) evidence that physical activity and/or physical fitness in adulthood are related to both CVD risk factors and to the occurrence of CVD[1,75] (*D1* and *D2*). So in fact the only two pathways involved in the potential benefits of physical activity and physical fitness for cardiovascular health concern the predictability of CVD risk factors in adulthood from the values of the same risk factors measured in childhood and adolescence (*E1*), and the predictability of physical activity and physical fitness in adulthood from the amount of physical activity and physical fitness measured in childhood and adolescence (*C*).

The issue of the predictability of a certain variable measured at young age for the value of the same variable later in life is called tracking. For several CVD risk factors this predictability is rather high; especially for the lipoproteins and for body fatness. For blood pressure this predictability is quite low. This is also the case for the predictability of physical activity and physical fitness.[76] Figures 3.2.3 and 3.2.4 show data from the Amsterdam Growth and Health Study, in which tracking was analysed for biological CVD risk factors as well as for physical activity and physical fitness from adolescence into young adulthood.

A few remarks must be made regarding the interpretation of the results of studies investigating tracking. First of all many authors are satisfied with a statistically significant tracking coefficient.[77] However, a significant tracking coefficient does not mean that the predictive value of measurements during childhood or adolescence for values

later in life is high. Suppose that tracking is calculated for subjects in a particular 'risk' quartile in a longitudinal study with two measurements in time, and that 50% of the initial 'high risk' quartile maintain their position at the follow-up measurement. In this situation the initial measurement had a predictive value of 50% and an a highly significant odds ratio of 5.0 would be found (an OR of 5.0 calculated for 'risk' quartiles translates to a predictive value of the initial measurement of 50%). This method to assess tracking was applied to the data-set of the Amsterdam Growth and Health Study.[76] A summary of the results is shown in Fig. 3.2.4. From Fig. 3.2.4 it can be seen that odds ratios >5.0 were only observed for lipoproteins and body fatness, while for blood pressure and physical activity and physical fitness much lower values were found.[76]

The second problem is that tracking concerns the relative position of a certain individual within a group of subjects over time. When

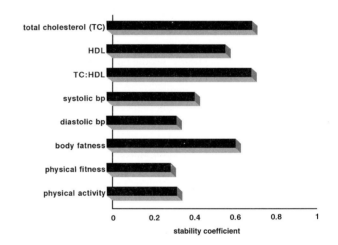

Fig. 3.2.3 Stability coefficients, which are interpretable as correlation coefficients varying between 0 and 1, calculated with generalized estimating equations over a period of 15 years from 13 to 27 years of age. Results from the Amsterdam Growth and Health Study.[76]

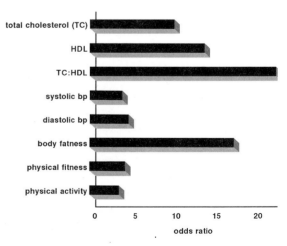

Fig. 3.2.4 Odds for subjects at risk at an initial measurement at the age of 13 years to stay at risk over a period of 15 years compared with the odds for subjects not at risk at the initial measurements. Results from the Amsterdam Growth and Health Study.[76]

tracking for a certain variable over time is high, it does not necessarily mean that the absolute level of that variable does not change over time. Especially for daily physical activity, it is known that the amount of physical activity in the total population is decreasing dramatically from childhood into adolescence and from adolescence into adulthood.[78] So when everybody is becoming inactive to the same degree tracking of physical activity will be high, while from a health perspective this is an undesirable situation. Thirdly, one must also take into account that tracking coefficients are highly influenced by measurement error. The assessment of physical activity for instance is not very accurate, i.e. the reproducibility of the measurement of physical activity is rather low. Consequently, the low tracking coefficients for physical activity are partly caused by this low reproducibility of the assessment method.

How much activity/fitness is good for cardiovascular health?

Although there is not much evidence for a strong relationship between physical activity and/or physical fitness during childhood and adolescence and cardiovascular health at adult age, there is much discussion about the amount of physical activity which should be recommended to young people from a health perspective. These guidelines vary from 30 minutes of light intensity physical activity most of the days of the week, to one hour of moderate intensity physical activity all days of the week.[79] When looking critically at these guidelines from the perspective of cardiovascular health, there is no direct scientific evidence for these guidelines. The argument against the 'old' guideline of 30 minutes of moderate physical activity on most days of the week was that although the majority of young people are currently meeting this old criterion, childhood overweight and obesity are increasing and that many young people have been shown to possess at least one modifiable CVD risk factor.[79] Although there is some rationale behind these two arguments, they ignore the facts that there is almost no evidence that physical activity is related to CVD risk factors in children and adolescents and that the aetiology of cardiovascular problems is multidimensional. In other words, there is no real scientific rationale for these guidelines.

If there is a relationship between physical activity, physical fitness and CVD risk factors in children and adolescents, this relationship will probably be some sort of S-shaped curve; i.e. at least in a large area of physical activity this relationship will be more or less a continuum; even above and beyond these guidelines an increase in physical activity will have beneficial effects. Maybe the proposed guidelines are equivalent with the sharpest increase in this S-shaped curve, which then can be seen as the optimal level of physical activity for cardiovascular health benefits. Although on a population level these guidelines can be of importance, on an individual level this importance is rather doubtful. Another issue related to these guidelines is the identification of so called 'high risk' individuals, i.e. individuals who do not meet the physical activity criterion. These 'high risk' individuals are the primary focus of preventive strategies. However, based on the lack of scientific evidence for the guidelines, this is a debatable approach. Preventive strategies to improve physical activity in our young population should aim at the entire young population. If there are beneficial effects of physical activity and/or physical fitness in children and adolescents, there will be a benefit for all.

Summary

There is only little evidence that physical activity and physical fitness are related to a healthy CVD risk profile in children and adolescents. The best evidence is found for a positive relationship with body fatness. One must bear in mind that most research is limited to the so called 'traditional' risk factors and that the outcome of most studies is hampered by the poor methods to measure physical activity. Regarding the new developments in CVD research (i.e. 'new' risk factors, gene–environment interaction, preclinical atherosclerosis), the influence of physical activity and physical fitness in children and adolescents is yet to be determined.

References

1. Paffenbarger, Jr. R. S. Contributions of epidemiology to exercise science and cardiovascular risk. *Medicine and Science in Sports and Exercise* 1988; **20**: 426–38.

2. Armstrong, N. and Simons-Morton, B. Physical activity and blood lipids in adolescents. *Pediatric Exercise Science* 1994; **6**: 381–405.

3. Sallis, J. F., Patterson, T. L., Buono, M. J. and Nader, P. R. Relation of cardiovascular fitness and physical activity to cardiovascular disease risk factors in children and adults. *American Journal of Epidemiology* 1988; **127**: 933–41.

4. Donahue, R. P., Orchard, T. J., Becker, D. J., Kuller, L. H. and Drash, A. L. Physical activity, insulin sensitivity, and the lipoprotein profile in young adults: The Beaver County Study. *American Journal of Epidemiology* 1988; **127**: 95–103.

5. Twisk, J. W. R., Mechelen, W. van, Kemper, H. C. G. and Post, G. B. The relation between 'long term exposure' to lifestyle during youth and young adulthood and risk factors for cardiovascular disease. *Journal of Adolescent Health* 1997; **20**: 309–19.

6. Raitakari, O. T., Porkka, K. V. K., Taimela, S., Telama, R., Räsänen, L. and Viikari, J. S. A. Effects of physical activity and inactivity on coronary risk factors in children and young adults: The Cardiovascular Risk in Young Finns Study. *American Journal of Epidemiology* 1994; **140**: 95–205.

7. Webber, L. S., Osganian, S. K., Feldman, H. A., Wu, M., McKenzie, T. L., Nichaman, M., Lytle, L. A., Edmunson, E., Cutler, J., Nader, P. R. and Luepker, R. V. Cardiovascular risk factors among children after a two and a half year intervention—The CATCH study. *Preventive Medicine* 1996; **25**: 432–41.

8. Harrel, J. S., McMurray, R. G., Bangdiwala, S. I., Frauman, A. C., Gansky, S. A. and Bradley, C. B. Effects of a school-based intervention to reduce cardiovascular disease risk factors in elementary-school children: The Cardiovascular Health in Children (CHIC) Study. *Journal of Pediatrics* 1996; **128**: 797–805.

9. Casanovas, J. A., Lapetra, A., Puzo, J., Pelegrin, J., Hermosilla, T., De Vicente, J., Garza, F., Del Rio, A., Giner, A. and Ferreira, I. J. Tobacco, physical exercise and lipid profile. *European Heart Journal* 1992; **13**: 440–5.

10. Nikkilä, E. A., Taskinen, M. R., Rehunen, S. and Harkonen, M. Lipoprotein lipase activity in adipose tissue and skeletal muscle of runners: relation to serum lipoproteins. *Metabolism* 1978; **27**: 1661–71.

11. Berg, A., Frey, I, Baumstark, M. W., Halle, M. and Keul, J. Physical activity and lipoprotein lipid disorders. *Sports Medicine* 1994; **17**: 6–21.

12. Tipton, C. M. Exercise training and hypertension: an update. *Exercise and Sport Sciences Reviews* 1991; **19**: 447–505.

13. Hagberg, J. B. Exercise, fitness and hypertension. In *Exercise, fitness, and health* (ed. C. Bouchard, R. J. Sheppard, T. Stephens, J. R. Sutton, and B. D. McPherson). Human Kinetics, Champaign, Il, 1990; 455–66.

14. Petruzzello, S. J., Landers, S. M., Hatfield, B. D., Kubitz, K. A. and Salazar, W. A meta-analysis on the anxiety-reducing effects of acute and chronic exercise. Outcomes and mechanisms. *Sports Medicine* 1991; 11: 143–82.

15. Alpert, B. and Wilmore, J. H. Physical activity and blood pressure in adolescents. *Pediatric Exercise Science* 1994; 6: 361–80.

16. Raitakari, O. T., Taimela, S., Porkka, K. V. K., Telama, R., Välimäki, I., Åkerblom, H. K. and Viikari, J. S. A. Associations between physical activity and risk factors for coronary heart disease: The Cardiovascular Risk in Young Finns Study. *Medicine and Science in Sports and Exercise* 1997; 29: 1055–61.

17. Baranowski, T., Bouchard, C., Bar-Or, O., Bricker, T., Heath, G., Kimm, S. Y., Malina, R., Obarzanek, E., Pate, R. and Strong, W. B. Assessment, prevalence, and cardiovascular benefits of physical activity and fitness in youth. *Medicine in Science and Sports and Exercise* 1992; 24: S237–7.

18. Hubert, H. B., Feinleib, M., McNamara, P. M. and Castelli, W. P. Obesity as an independent risk factor for cardiovascular disease: a 26-year follow-up of participants in the Framingham Heart Study. *Circulation* 1983; 67: 968–77.

19. Lapidus, L., Bengtsson, C., Larsson, B., Pennert, K., Rybo, E. and Sjöström, L. Distribution of adipose tissue and risk for cardiovascular disease and death: a 12 year follow-up of participants in the population study of women in Gotenburg, Sweden. *British Medical Journal* 1984; 289: 1257–61.

20. Donahue, R. P., Abbott, R. D., Bloom, E., Reed, D. M. and Yano, K. Central obesity and coronary heart disease in men. *Lancet* 1987; 8537: 821–4.

21. Björntorp, P. and Brodoff, B. N. *Obesity.* Lipincott, Philadelphia, 1992.

22. Poehlman, E. T. A review: exercise and its influence on resting energy metabolism in man. *Medicine and Science in Sports and Exercise* 1989; 21: 515–25.

23. Broeder, C. E., Burrhus, K. A., Svanevik, L. S. and Wilmore, J. H. The effects of either high intensity resistance or endurance training on resting metabolic rate. *American Journal of Clinical Nutrition* 1992; 55: 802–10.

24. Bar-Or, O. and Baranowski, T. Physical activity, adiposity, and obesity among adolescents. *Pediatric Exercise Science* 1994; 6: 348–60.

25. Moussa, M. A. A., Skaik, M. B., Selwanes, S. B., Yaghy, O. Y. and Bin-Othman, S. A. Factors associated with obesity in school children. *International Journal of Obesity* 1994; 18: 513–5.

26. Twisk, J. W. R., Kemper, H. C. G., Mechelen, W. van., Post, G. B. and Lenthe, F. J. van. Body fatness: longitudinal relationship of body mass index and the sum of four skinfolds with other risk factors for coronary heart disease. *International Journal of Obesity* 1998; 22: 915–22.

27. Stern, M. P. and Haffner, S. M. Body fat distribution and hyperinsulinemia as risk factors for diabetes and cardiovascular disease. *Atherosclerosis* 1986; 6: 123–30.

28. Marti, B., Tuomilehto, J., Salomaa, V., Kartovaara, L., Korhonen, H. J. and Pietinen, P. Body fat distribution in the Finnish population: environmental determinations and predictive power for cardiovascular risk factor levels. *Journal of Epidemiology and Community Health* 1991; 45: 31–7.

29. Seidell, J. C., Cigolini, M., Deslypere, J. P., Charzewski, J. and Ellsinger, B. M. Body fat distribution in relation to physical activity and smoking habits in 38-year old European men. *American Journal of Epidemiology* 1991; 133: 257–65.

30. van Lenthe, F. J., Mechelen, W. van., Kemper, H. C. G. and Post, G. B. Behavioral variables and development of body fat from adolescence into adulthood in normal-weight whites: The Amsterdam Growth and Health Study. *American Journal of Clinical Nutrition* 1998; 67: 846–52.

31. Bergström, E., Hernell, O. and Persson, L. A. Endurance running performance in relation to cardiovascular risk indicators in adolescents. *International Journal of Sports Medicine* 1997; 18: 300–7.

32. Helmrich, S. P., Ragland, D. R., Leung, R. W. and Paffenbarger, R. S. Physical activity and reduced occurrence of non-insulin-dependent diabetes mellitus. *New England Journal of Medicine* 1991; 325: 147–52.

33. Ivy, J. L. The insulin-like effect of muscle contraction. *Exercise and Sport Sciences Reviews* 1987; 15: 29–51.

34. Vitug, A., Schneider, S. H. and Ruderman, N. B. Exercise and Type I diabetes mellitus. *Exercise and Sport Sciences Reviews* 1988; 16: 285–304.

35. Raitakari, O. T., Porkka, K. V. K., Rasanen, L. and Viikari, J. S. Relations of life-style with lipids, blood pressure and insulin in adolescents and young adults. The Cardiovascular Risk in Young Finns Study. *Atherosclerosis* 1994; 111: 237–46.

36. Riddoch, C. J. Relationships between physical activity and health in young people. In *Young and active? Young people and health-enhancing physical activity—evidence and implications* (ed. S. Biddle, J. Sallis, and N. Cavill). Health Education Authority, London, UK, 1998; 17–48.

37. Webber, L. S., Voors, A. W., Srinivasan, S. R., Frerichs, R. P. and Berenson, G. S. Occurrence in children of multiple risk factors for coronary heart disease: The Bogalusa Heart Study. *Preventive Medicine* 1979; 8: 407–18.

38. Khoury, P., Morrison, J. A., Kelly, K., Mellies, M., Horvitz, R. and Glueck, C. J. Clustering and interrelationships of coronary heart disease risk factors in schoolchildren, ages 6–19. *American Journal of Epidemiology* 1980; 112: 524–38.

39. Raitakari, O. T., Porkka, K. V. K., Räsänen, L., Rönnemaa, T. and Viikari, J. S. A. Clustering and six year cluster-tracking of serum total cholesterol, HDL-cholesterol and diastolic blood pressure in children and young adults. The Cardiovascular Risk in Young Finns Study. *Journal of Clinical Epidemiology* 1994; 47: 1085–93.

40. Genest, J. J. and Cohn, J. S. Clustering of cardiovascular risk factors: targeting high-risk individuals. *American Journal of Cardiology* 1995; 76: 8A–20A.

41. Jousilahti, P., Tuomilehto, J., Vartiainen, E., Korhonen, H. J., Pitkäniemi, J., Nissinen, A. and Puska, P. Importance of risk factor clustering in coronary heart disease mortality and incidence in eastern Finland. *Journal of Cardiovascular Risk* 1995; 2: 63–70.

42. Bao, W., Srinivasan, S. R., Wattigney, W. and Berenson, G. S. Persistence of multiple cardiovascular risk clustering related to syndrome × from childhood to young adulthood. The Bogalusa Heart Study. *Archives of Internal Medicine* 1994; 154: 1842–7.

43. Twisk, J. W. R., Kemper, H. C. G., Mechelen, W. van. and Post, G. B. Clustering of risk factors for coronary heart disease. The longitudinal relationship with lifestyle. *Annals of Epidemiology* 2000; (under review).

44. Twisk, J. W. R., Boreham, C., Cran, G., Savage, J. M., Strain, J. and Mechelen, W. van. Clustering of biological risk factors for cardiovascular disease and the longitudinal relationship with lifestyle in an adolescent population: The Northern Ireland Young Hearts Project. *Journal of Cardiovascular Risk* 1999; 6: 355-62.

45. Hulshof, K. F. A. M., Wedel, M., Löwik, M. R. H., Kok, F. J., Kistemaker, C., Hermus, R. J. J., Hoor, F. ten. and Ockhuizen, Th. Clustering of dietary variables and other lifestyle variables (Dutch Nutritional Surveillance System). *Journal of Epidemiology and Community Health* 1992; 46: 417–24.

46. Raitakari, O. T., Leino, M., Räikkönen, K., Porkka, K. V. K., Taimela, S., Räsänen, L. and Viikari, J. S. A. Clustering of risk habits in young adults, The Cardiovascular Risk in Young Finns Study. *American Journal of Epidemiology* 1995: 142: 36–44.

47. Kilkens, O. J. E., Gijtenbeek, B. A. J., Twisk, J. W. R., Mechelen, W. van. and Kemper, H. C. G. Clustering of lifestyle CVD risk factors and its relationship with biological CVD risk factors. *Pediatric Exercise Science* 1999; 11: 169–77.

48. Burke, V., Milligan, R. A., Beilin, L. J., Dunbar, D., Spencer, M., Balde, E. and Gracey, M. P. Clustering of health-related behaviours among 18-year-old Australians. *Preventive Medicine* 1997; 26: 724–33.

49. Terre, L., Drabman, R. S. and Meydrech, E. F. Relationships among children's health related behaviours: a multivariate developmental perspective. *Preventive Medicine* 1990; 19: 134–46.

50. Berenson, G. S., Arbeit, M. L., Hunter, S. M., Johnsson, C. C. and Nicklas, T. A. Cardiovascular health promotion for elementary school children. The Heart Smart Program. *Annals of the New York Academy of Sciences* 1991; 623: 299–313.

51. Breslow, J. L. Human apolipoprotein molecular biology and genetic variation. *Annual Review of Biochemics* 1985; 54: 699–727.

52. Riesen, W. F., Mordasini, R., Salzmann, A., Theler, A. and Gurtner, H. P. Apoproteins and lipids as discriminators of severity of coronary heart disease. *Atherosclerosis* 1980; **37**: 152–62.

53. De Backer, G., Rosseneu, M. and Deslypere, J. P. Discriminative value of lipids and apoproteins in coronary heart disease. *Atherosclerosis* 1982; **42**: 197–203.

54. Hamsten, A., Walldius, G., Dahlén, G., Johansson, B. and Faire, U. de. Serum lipoproteins and apolipoproteins in young male survivors of myocardial infarction. *Atherosclerosis* 1986; **59**: 223–35.

55. Armstrong, V. W., Cremer, P., Eberle, E., Manke, A., Schulze, F., Wieland, H., Kreuzer, H. and Seidel, A. The association between serum Lp(a) concentrations and angiographically assessed coronary atherosclerosis: dependence on serum LDL levels. *Atherosclerosis* 1986; **62**: 249–57.

56. Marai, A., Miyahara, T., Fujimoto, N., Matsuda, M. and Kameyama, M. Lp(a) lipoprotein as a risk factor for coronary heart disease and cerebral infarction. *Atherosclerosis* 1986; **59**: 199–204.

57. Hasstedt, S. J. and Wiliams, R. R. Three alleles for quantitative Lp(a). *Genetic Epidemiology* 1986; **3**: 53–5.

58. Howard, B. V., Le, N. A., Belcher, J. D., Flack, J. M., Jacobs, D. R. Jr, Lewis, C. E., Marcovina, S. M. and Perkins, L. L. Concentrations of Lp(a) in black and white young adults: relations to risk factors for cardiovascular disease. *Annals of Epidemiology* 1994; **4**: 341–50.

59. Taimela, S., Viikari, J. S., Porkka, K. V. and Dahlen, G. H. Lipoprotein (a) levels in children and young adults: the influence of physical activity. The Cardiovascular Risk in Young Finns Study. *Acta Paediatrica* 1994; **83**: 1258–63.

60. Koenig, W., Sund, M., Doring, A. and Ernst, E. Leisure time physical activity but not work related physical activity is associated with decreased plasma viscosity. Results from a large population sample. *Circulation* 1997; **95**: 335–41.

61. MacAuley, D., McCrum, E. E., Stott, G., Evans, A. E., McRoberts, B., Boreham, C. A., Sweeney, K. and Trinick, T. R. Physical activity, physical fitness, blood pressure, and fibrinogen in the Northern Ireland Health and Activity Survey. *Journal of Epidemiology and Community Health* 1996; **50**: 258–63.

62. Folsom, A. R., Qamhieh, H. T., Flack, J. M., Hilner, J. E., Liu, K., Howard, B. V. and Tracy, R. P. Plasma fibrinogen: levels and correlates in young adults. The Coronary Artery Risk in Young Adults (CARDIA) Study. *American Journal of Epidemiology* 1993; **138**: 1023–36.

63. Stratton, J. R., Chandler, W. L., Schwartz, R. S., Cerqueira, M. D., Levy, W. C., Kahn, S. E., Larson, V. G., Cain, K. C., Beard, J. C. and Abrass, I. B. Effects of physical conditioning on fibrinolytic variables and fibrinogen in young and old healthy adults. *Circulation* 1991; **83**: 1692–7.

64. Zahavri, I., Yaari, S., Salman, H., Creter, D., Rudnicki, C., Brandis, S., Ferrara, M., Marom, R., Katz, M., Canetti, M., Hart, J. and Goldbourt, U. Plasma fibrinogen in Israeli Moslem and Jewish school-children: distribution and relation to other cardiovascular risk factors. The Petah Tikva project. *Israel Journal of Medical Sciences* 1996; **32**: 1207–12.

65. Nygard, O., Vollset, S. E., Refsum, H., Stensvold, I., Tverdal, A., Nordrehaug, J. E., Ueland, M. and Kvale, G. Total plasma homocysteine and cardiovascular risk profile. The Hordaland Homocysteine Study. *Journal of the American Medical Association*, 1995; **274**: 1526–33.

66. Gregoire, J., Tuck, S., Yamamoto, Y. and Highson, R. L. Heart rate variability at rest and exercise: influence of age, gender and physical training. *Canadian Journal of Applied Physiology* 1996; **21**: 455–70.

67. Kupari, M., Virolainen, J., Koskinen, P. and Tikkanen, M. J. Short-term heart rate variability and factors modifying the risk of coronary heart disease in a population sample. *American Journal of Cardiology* 1993; **72**: 897–903.

68. Seals, D. R. and Chase, P. B. Influence of physical training on heart rate variability and baroflex circulatory control. *Journal of Applied Physiology* 1989; **66**: 1886–95.

69. Taimela, S., Lehtimaki, T., Porkka, K. V., Rasanen, L. and Viikari, J. S. The effect of physical activity on serum total and low-density lipoprotein cholesterol concentrations varies with apolipoprotein E phenotype in male children and young adults. The Cardiovascular Risk in Young Finns Study. *Metabolism: Clinical and Experimental* 1996; **45**: 797–803.

70. Crouse III, J. R. and Thompson, C. J. An evaluation of methods for imaging and quantifying coronary and carotid lumen stenosis and atherosclerosis. *Circulation* 1993; **87** (suppl): II-17–33.

71. Celermajer, D. S., Sorensen, K. E., Gooch, V. M., Spiegelhalter, D. J., Miller, O. I., Sullivan, I. D., Lloyd, J. K. and Deanfield, J. E. Non-invasive detection of endothelial dysfunction in children and adults at risk of atherosclerosis. *Lancet* 1992; **340**: 1111–5.

72. Twisk, J. W. R., Kemper, H. C. G. and Mellenbergh, G. J. Longitudinal development of lipoprotein levels in males and females aged 12–28 years: The Amsterdam Growth and Health Study. *International Journal of Epidemiology* 1995; **24**: 69–77.

73. Montoye, H. J., Kemper, H. C. G., Saris, W. H. M. and Washburn, R. A. (eds). *Measuring physical activity and energy expenditure.* Human Kinetics, Champaign, Il, 1996.

74. Blair, S. N., Clark, D. G., Cureton, K. J. and Powell, K. E. Exercise and fitness in childhood: implications for a lifetime of health: In *Perspectives in exercise science and sports medicine* (ed. C. V. Gisolfi and D. R. Lamb). Benchmark Press, Indianapolis, Ind, 1989; 401–430.

75. Blair, S. N., Kohl, H. W., Barlow, C. E., Paffenbarger, R. S., Gibbons, L. W., and Maccra, C. A. Changes in physical fitness and all-cause mortality: a prospective study of healthy and unhealthy men. *Journal of the American Medical Association* 1995; **273**: 1093–8.

76. Twisk, J. W. R., Kemper, H. C. G., Mechelen, W. van. and Post, G. B. Tracking of risk factors for coronary heart disease over a 14 year period: a comparison between lifestyle and biological risk factors with data from the Amsterdam Growth and Health Study. *American Journal of Epidemiology* 1997; **145**: 888–98.

77. Twisk, J. W. R., Kemper, H. C. G. and Mellenbergh, G. J. The mathematical and analytical aspects of tracking. *Epidemiological Reviews* 1994; **16**: 165–83.

78. Riddoch, C. J. and Boreham, C. A. G. The health related physical activity of children. *Sports Medicine* 1995; **19**: 86–102.

79. Biddle, S., Sallis, J. and Cavill, N. Policy framework for young people and health-enhancing physical activity. In *Young and active? Young people and health-enhancing physical activity—evidence and implications* (ed. S. Biddle, J. Sallis, and N. Cavill). Health Education Authority, London, UK, 1998; 3–16.

3.3 Physical activity, physical fitness and bone health

Han C. G. Kemper

Introduction

Most people think that the skeleton is a passive structure; this is certainly not true. Bone is a vital, dynamic connective issue, which adapts its structure to its function. To fulfil these structure–function relations adequately, bone is continuously being broken down and rebuilt in a process called remodelling.

Bone mass increases at the same rate during growth and development in boys and girls, but at the beginning of puberty a sexual dimorphism occurs and bone mass increases faster in boys than girls (Fig. 3.3.1). Maximal bone mass is reached in the late teens and early twenties, whereafter it gradually declines, this decrease is accelerated in women after the menopause. The average woman has a higher risk of osteoporosis than the average man for at least two reasons: first women reach a lower maximal bone mass in their youth, and secondly women loose bone at a higher rate after the menopause.

This chapter reviews the development of bone mass in youth and the effects of physical activity as one of the important lifestyle factors for prevention of osteoporosis at older age.

Growth of bone

Physical growth and development have been extensively investigated from prenatal growth to birth and from postnatal growth to adulthood by many longitudinal studies all over the world. In 1955 J. M. Tanner published the first edition of his book *Growth at adolescence*,[1] and in 1981 *A history of the study of human growth*.[2] Both books are used as state of the art publications about human growth and development. The methods that are used in general to measure growth changes are mainly based on simple anthropometric measurements of the total body (body height, body mass) or of body segments (trunk height, limb lengths). Also breadth measurements (shoulder, hip, wrist and knee), circumferences (head, trunk, hip, waist and limbs) and skinfold measurements at different sites of the body are applied according to standard methods.[3] All of these measurements estimate different dimensions of the body but do not take into consideration changes in the composition of these body parts. Radiographic methods are used to indicate calcified cartilage and ossified bone and to estimate skeletal maturation. Different methods are developed to assess the rate of maturation or biological age from X-rays at wrist and knee. From a comparison of skeletal age with calendar age the child can be characterized as early or late maturer[4] (and see chapter 1.2).

In recent years, new methods have been developed to measure the bone mass by energy absorption from gamma radiation of calcium in the bone. The methods most described in the literature are single photon absorptiometry (SPA), dual photon absorptiometry (DPA), dual energy X-ray absorptiometry (DEXA) and quantitative computed tomography (QCT).

In the reviewed literature, bone mass is measured in different parts of the human skeleton, such as arm, hip, spine and heel, or in the total body mass. The details of method and place of measurement will only be mentioned if necessary and if they have important consequences for the interpretation of the outcomes.

Since not much is known about the natural development during youth of bone mass, the literature will be reviewed on:

(1) the changes in bone mass during prepubertal, circumpubertal and postpubertal development;
(2) the differences in bone development between boys and girls; and
(3) the point in time at which the maximal amount of bone mass, or the so called peak bone mineral density (PBMD), is reached.

Most of the BMD studies are aimed at prevention and retardation of bone loss in postmenopausal women. An important question remains: whether it is possible to increase the bone mass during the growing years by exercise, in order to attain higher maximal bone mass at young adult age.[5] Although there are only a few experimental studies in this respect, the main results will be summarized.

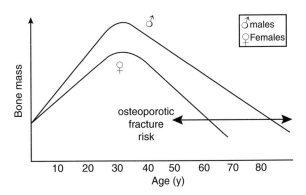

Fig. 3.3.1 The development of bone mass in males and females with age: the osteoporotic fracture risk is usually reached at an earlier age in females than in males.

Methods of measurement of bone mass

Anthropometrics

Von Döbeln[6] proposed a measure for the estimation of the skeletal weight from height and four breadth measurements (left and right femur condyli and radio-ulnar width). This is sound as long as it is used for estimating total weight of bone mass in comparison with estimates of muscle and fat mass, estimated by skinfolds and circumferences in combination with height and weight. In the Netherlands, this concept is used to correct the body weight to body height relationship: The Dutch Heart Foundation constructed a reference scale (for ideal body weight) based on the Quetelet Index or Body Mass Index (Ql or BMI: weight height^{-2}) that included the possibility of calculating the ideal body weight taking the breadth of the femur condyle into consideration. However, this is a misuse of the skeletal component of this algorithm, because an adjustment is made for the least variable of the three component model of body composition, with lean and fat mass being the other components.

Radiographics

In November 1895, over a hundred years ago, the German physicist Wilhelm Conrad Röntgen discovered gamma radiation and demonstrated a radiogram showing the bones of his own hand. He called this X-radiation. The anatomist Albert von Kölliker connected Röntgen's name to this kind of radiation. Since then, X-rays are widely used in medicine for detection of infectious diseases, pathologic neoplasmata and traumatology.

Another field in radiographics is its use as a measure of biological age with respect to skeletal growth and development. Skeletal maturation begins as a process when rudiments of bones appear during embryonic life, and is completed when skeletal form becomes comparatively stable in young adulthood. During maturation there are increases in the types and numbers of specialized cells, including cartilage and fibrous tissue cells, that form parts of bone.[7] In 1950 Greulich and Pyle published their radiographic atlas of skeletal development of the hand and wrist, with a second edition in 1959. Roche et al.,[8] from their Longitudinal Study, used the knee joint as bones of interest for determination of skeletal maturation (Roche–Wainer–Thissen method, RWT); however, most assessments of skeletal maturity are made from radiographs of the hand and wrist, because this site has considerable advantages over other parts of the skeleton. These advantages stem from the little irradiation required, the ease of radiographic positioning and the large number of bones included in the area. Therefore, the RWT method using the knee joint as a biological indicator for growth was extended with the hand–wrist method. In Europe, Tanner et al.,[9] from the Institute of Child Health in London, published their Tanner–Whitehouse II (TW2) method for the determination of growth also using X-ray photographs of the left hand including 20 bones of the hand and wrist.

All these skeletal maturity scales are used to estimate the developmental or biological age of children, correcting for children who mature faster or slower than the average child with the same calendar age. In paediatrics it can be used to predict adult height of children (mostly girls) who, or whose parents, expect that they will end up very tall, in consideration of whether to intervene in their growth by using hormones to close their endplates earlier.

Dual energy X-ray absorptiometry (DEXA)

Radiographs cannot easily quantify changes in bone density, because 30% of it has to be lost before it can be detected by X-ray. However, recent technical advances have made it possible to measure bone mass by energy absorption from gamma radiation in the bone. DEXA is now the most precise and widely used method of assessing bone density, and the preferred method because scanning time is shorter than with dual photon absorptiometry (DPA). Also resolution has been improved, and measurements can be made of the lumbar spine, femoral neck, forearm and for the total body.

From the DEXA method, two measures are calculated: the bone mineral content (BMC) and the bone mineral density (BMD). The BMC is the total amount of minerals in the selected bone in g, and the BMD is the amount of bone mineral, in g, divided by the area of the selected bone (g cm^{-2}). The BMD, however, is not a real measure of bone density (g cm^{-3}), and is therefore called areal density.

In growth bones not only increase their area but also their volume. These size changes influence the real BMD. Therefore, attempts have been made to estimate the volume of the bone of interest and to correct for this bone size effect by an additional measure of bone mineral apparent density (BMAD).[10]

Quantitative computed tomography (QCT)

QCT systems have been adapted for estimation of bone mineral content allowing cortical bone to be separated from trabecular bone. Furthermore, it provides us with a true measure of total, cortical or trabecular bone mineral volumetric density (mg mm^3). However, the equipment is more expensive, and exposes patients to high radiation doses. A peripheral QCT system is now available for the forearm with a lower dose of radiation.

Ultrasound

Ultrasound measurements have been available since 1984 for the calcaneus, and have the potential for widespread clinical applications.

Mechanisms of bone formation

Movement is the result of electric impulses being passed from the central nervous system to the skeletal muscles. These muscles contract (shorten) in order to move body parts with respect to each other (arms, legs, head and trunk) and/or the whole body with respect to the surroundings (walking, cycling, swimming). Exercise is not necessarily dynamic; sometimes muscles contract without causing movements, but increase their tension as in static exercises, such as standing, active sitting or pushing against a wall.

Both the duration and intensity of exercise play a role in the physical load placed on the body. Low-intensity, long-lasting exercise increases ventilation and circulation to meet oxygen demand for energy delivery to the active muscles. This is important for a better capillarization and oxygen delivery to the muscle. High-intensity, short-lasting exercise is important for the development of muscle and bone mass. Results show that of these two factors it is not the duration of exercise which is the key factor affecting bone health, but the intensity of the forces that act upon the bones. Weight-bearing activities, such as walking, running and dancing, have more effect on bone health of the legs and vertebrae of the lower back than have swimming and bicycling, although all activities need approximately the same amount of energy when performed for identical lengths of time. This difference in effect on bone health is in contrast to the effects of these activities on the lungs, heart and circulation: if performed with the same intensity and duration, swimming has the same effect as running on the oxygen transport system.

Two different mechanisms seem to act on bone mass: central hormonal factors, such as oestrogen production, and local mechanical factors, such as the muscle forces exerted on the bones of the skeleton during contraction and the forces of gravity that act on the entire body during standing and other weight-bearing activities.[11]

Central hormonal factors maintain serum calcium concentrations within a limited range. Calcium is one of the most common ions in the human body, and almost 99% of body calcium is deposited in the skeleton. Oestrogens suppress the activity of osteoclasts, the bone-resorbing cells, and thus help to maintain bone mass. During exercise, serum concentrations of testosterone and oestrogen are elevated, influencing calcium homeostasis and the activity of osteoclasts and osteoblasts. Hormonal replacement therapy in women after the menopause makes use of this action of oestrogen.

The local mechanical forces of exercise cause (1) strain on the bone and calcium accumulation on the concave side of the bending bone, and (2) microtraumata which are removed by osteoclasts and repaired by osteoblasts. The supposed mechanisms behind the local mechanical forces are as follows.

First, during flexion the bone acts like a piezo-electric crystal while accumulating calcium at the concave (=negative loaded) side. Secondly, mechanical demands, occurring by overload, are sensed in the bone by osteocytes via strain-derived flows of interstitial fluid. They stimulate the osteoclasts in removing the damaged structures and at the same time the osteoblasts repair the structure of the bone matrix.[12] In the case of a too strong or too often damaged bone, the process of repairing falls behind the process of removal and microfracture will occur. When the mechanical load falls below the fracture intensity remodelling activities are stimulated and result in bone hypertrophy. Remodelling of the bone after a change in mechanical load by weight bearing activities (including experiments with added extra weights) has been proved in experimental studies in a great number of animals.[13] Moreover, in some of these experiments it has been shown that the effects are proportional to the intensity of the (extra) load. The amount of hypertrophy seems also to depend on the difference between the extra load and the load to the bone before the extra load was added.

Not much is known about the interaction between central-hormonal and local mechanical factors. However, physical activity leads to an increase of serum oestrogen levels, and this diminishes the sensitivity of the bone for the parathyroid hormone and the activity of the osteoclasts. When bone mass thus increases, more calcium (Ca^{2+}) and phosphorus (P) are resorbed from the blood, and this lowering of Ca^{2+} and P concentrations in the blood then stimulates the parathyroid hormone; the latter inhibits vitamin D production, stimulates calcium absorption and decreases calcium secretion.

As long as the forces exerted on the bones remain weaker than those needed to cause a macro fracture (referred to as the fracture limit), this remodelling process is able to adapt the bone to the external biomechanical stress and bring about bone thickening (hypertrophy). During long periods of inactivity, such as prolonged bed rest, the

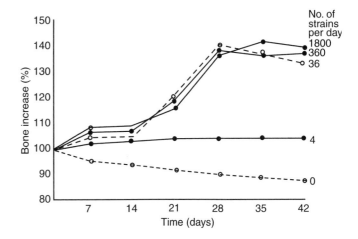

Fig. 3.3.2 Experiments in animals show that loading bones at a frequency of four times a day over a period of 42 days is sufficient to maintain bone mass and that an optimal rate is 36 times a day, which increases bone mass by 40%. A further increase in frequency to 360 or 1800 times a day did not have more effect (after Rubin and Lanyon[14]).

bone becomes atrophic as a result of relatively higher osteoclast activity compared to osteoblast activity. The central hormonal system and the local mechanical system interact to optimize the function of the skeletal system. In the case of exercise, mechanical factors seem to be most important for affecting bone mass.

Animal experiments[14] in an ulna-model of roosters have shown that loading of bone a few times (four times) a day can prevent bone loss, and that a certain frequency of loading (36 per day) results in an optimal increase in bone mass. Bone mass is not further increased by increasing the frequency of bone loading to 360 or even 1800 times per day (Fig. 3.3.2). Therefore in humans short bursts of explosive exercise, such as skipping, stair climbing and jumping, are supposedly more effective for bone development than popular forms of exercise, such as walking, jogging, bicycling and swimming.

Bone, therefore, appears to react best to exercise that is characterized by a pattern of unexpected and irregular high loads with a relatively low frequency and short duration. This is quite different from endurance exercise aimed at the moving aerobic function, which needs a load of long duration (or high frequency) and low intensity. For comparison, Fig. 3.3.3 shows an example of a typical and effective exercise for loading bone (skipping) and an effective exercise for loading the oxygen transport system (jogging). Extrapolated from the results of animal studies, skipping for one minute a day (six times for 10 seconds) seems effective for maintaining bone mass, whereas jogging for one hour a day (two times for 30 minutes) is more effective for the development of the oxygen transport system. Exercise that is effective in maintaining bone mass seems to take a lot less time than endurance exercise![15]

Natural course of bone mass development

Although in Fig. 3.3.1 the general course of bone mass was outlined, not much is known about the exact timing of the age at which the maximal amount of bone mass is reached. Therefore, firstly, the literature about bone development in boys and girls before puberty is reviewed. Secondly, an estimation is made about the importance of the

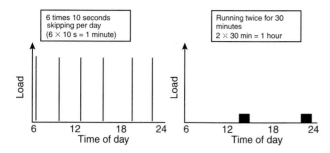

Fig. 3.3.3 Comparison of two types of exercise with different effects on the musculoskeletal and the cardiorespiratory system. Short explosive exercise (A), such as skipping six times a day for 10 seconds (total exercise time per day is 60 seconds), is effective for bone and muscle strength, whereas low-intensity exercise (B) of long duration, such as jogging two times a day for 30 minutes (total exercise time is 60 minutes), is more effective for the development of the oxygen transport system (after Kemper).[15]

pubertal period in the total development of bone mass. Thirdly, the question regarding the age at which maximal or peak bone mineral density occurs in males and females is answered.

Development of bone density before puberty

Six cross-sectional studies[16–22] and one longitudinal study[23] conclude that between boys and girls there is no significant difference between the bone mineral density of the radius and the lumbar spine. This indicates that the development of BMD before puberty is not dependent of steroids. Although there is a trend for a gradual increase from birth to puberty in bone mass, from seven reviewed publications it is not possible to make a quantitative estimation of the proportional contribution of this time window to the total (adult) bone mass. Before puberty there is no difference in BMD between boys and girls (Table 3.3.1).

Development of bone density during puberty

Puberty is a relatively short period of 3–5 years in the life of boys and girls. This short period seems to be a very important one for the development of bone mass, if we review the literature. The results of six cross-sectional studies[16–21] report increases of BMD in girls that vary between 17 and 70% and in boys between 11 and 75% of total adult values. Table 3.3.2 summarizes the percentage increase in BMD found in the lumbar spine and in the radial region during the pubertal years of boys and girls.

The high variation in the results can be attributed to several factors:

(1) differences in the classification of puberty;

(2) confounding factors such as nutritional and/or activity patterns that are different for the populations studied;

(3) the possible influence of early or late maturation: early maturation coincides with a relatively longer exposure to sex specific hormones than late maturation; oestrogen levels in girls and testosterone levels in boys seem to be related to bone mass development.

The cross-sectional data shown in Table 3.3.2 suggest that in boys and girls the pubertal years add sometimes 50–75% to total bone mass of the lumbar spine, and for the radial bone mass in boys the increase

Table 3.3.1 Estimation of bone mineral density reported in six cross-sectional studies (C) and one longitudinal study (Lo) in prepubertal children in total body (T), lumbar (L), femoral (F) and radial (R) regions of the body

Study	Design	Increase	Sex difference
Gilsanz et al.[18]	C	L	=
Glastre et al.[19]	C	L	=
Gordon et al.[20]	C	L	=
Southard et al.[21]	C	L	=
Bonjour et al.[16]	C	LF	=
Geusens et al.[17]	C	LRT	=
Theintz et al.[23]	Lo	LF	=

L = lumbar; R = radial; F = femoral; T = total body.

Table 3.3.2 Estimation of bone mineral density reported in six cross-sectional studies in boys and girls during their pubertal years

Study	Percentage increase	
	Girls	Boys
Lumbar spine		
Gilsanz et al.[18]	17%	—
Glastre et al.[19]	41%	—
Geusens et al.[17]	70%	75%
Gordon et al.[20]	38%	11%
Bonjour et al.[16]	51%	53%
Grimston et al.[22]	48%	48%
Radial		
Riis et al.[24]	–	31%

is 31%.[24] However, Bailey et al.[25] reported that BMD changes should be interpreted with caution because of the methods used. Determination of BMD by projectional methods like dual X-ray absorptiometry (DEXA) provide areal densities (g cm^{-2}) which are confounded by the earlier mentioned size changes accompanying growth. Consequently calculated volumetric BMD percentage increases are substantially less than the corresponding area BMD value increases. This dimensional consideration explains why Gilsanz et al.[18] showed the lowest increase (15%), since they were the only ones that used the quantified computerized tomography (QCT) method to measure BMD and this method provides real volumetric BMD values.

The BMD changes during the growth period that are reported in the literature, indicating that around puberty 50% of BMD is accrued, are measured with DEXA and must therefore be doubted. The only study with QCT methodology reports a 15% volume BMD increase in pubertal girls, which seems to be a more realistic value.

Age at which maximal bone mass is reached (peak bone mineral density, PBMD)

Most of the anatomical structures and physiological functions, such as muscle mass, cardiorespiratory functions, immune system and central nervous system, show a typical pattern over time. This is characterized by a steep increase during the growth period till the age of 20 years, and thereafter a much slower decrease and gradually a decline during ageing.[22] This pattern implies that there is a point or period in time where the human functions reach their maximal capacities. The question is, if there is a similar pattern observable in the development of bone mass, and if so, at what point in time of life peak bone mineral density (PBMD) occurs.

Twelve cross-sectional studies have been published since 1981; seven were performed on girls and five on both boys and girls. In principle, a cross-sectional design is not adequate to indicate individual changes over time. It also has methodological constraints (such as cohort effects, secular trend etc.). With these flaws in mind the results of six cross-sectional studies, with acceptable methodology and with sufficient information from the publication, are taken into account.[16–19,26,27] They report an age period of reaching PBMD in girls between 16 and 23 and in boys between 16 and 25 years. In Table 3.3.3 the results of estimated age of peak bone mineral density (PBMD) of each of the six valid studies are given separately for boys and girls.

Eight longitudinal studies investigated the development of BMD and PBMD. All of them used female subjects. From a methodological point of view the quality of three studies can be questioned seriously. These studies tend to confirm the cross-sectional results that PBMD occurs before the age of 20 years. However, the two high quality studies from Davies et al.[28] with a follow up of 4 years and from Recker et al.[29] with a follow up of 5 years, show very clearly that, at least in females, the age of PBMD is reached much later than 20 years: both lumbar, radial and total BMD reach the highest values around the age of 30 years. In Table 3.3.4 the estimated age at PBMD found in three low quality[30–32] and two high quality[28,29] longitudinal studies is summarized. Because no data are available for males it remains still unknown at what age PBMD is reached in males.

The discrepancies between the results of cross-sectional and longitudinal studies should be attributed to confounding factors. In general, high quality cross-sectional studies tend to establish PBMD in females between 16 and 25 years of age and the high quality longitudinal investigations much later, around the age of 30. Because longitudinal data are more valid in detecting age changes, it is more likely that PBMD in females occurs not in their late teens but in their late twenties.

Recently Bailey[33] investigated bone mineral accretion in growing children from the Saskatchewan Pediatric Bone Mineral Accrual Study. To investigate how bone mineral at clinically important sites

Table 3.3.4 Estimated age at peak bone mineral density (PBMD) reported in three low quality and two high quality longitudinal studies in females*

Longitudinal studies	Age at PBMD (years)
Invalid studies	
Riggs et al.[31]	17
Moen et al.[30]	17–18
Slemenda et al.[32]	< 20
Valid studies	
Davies et al.[28]	> 26
Recker et al.[29]	29

*Eight studies found with females.

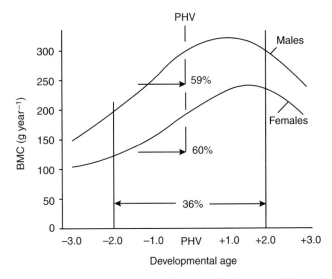

Fig. 3.3.4 Total body bone mineral content velocity curves of boys and girls aligned on age at PHV (after Bailey[33]).

proceeds in relation to maturation, distance and velocity curves for body height and bone mineral content (BMC) were made in both boys and girls, measured every six months for six years. Figure 3.3.4 shows the results: in both boys and girls over 35% of total body BMC was laid down during the four-year circumpubertal period and peak BMC was reached about 1–1.5 years after peak height velocity (PHV).

Effects of physical activity and physical fitness on bone mass

Physical fitness (including neuro-motor and cardiorespiratory fitness) is often used as a proxy measure of physical activity. In theory, however, physical fitness is the result of both genetic and environmental influences. For most of the physical fitness parameters, the genetic component is responsible for about 80% of the variance (e.g. maximal aerobic power, maximal muscle force, flexibility). Physical activity is only one of the several other environmental factors that can modify physical fitness. Therefore in this section the relationship between bone health and physical fitness is not taken into consideration.

Table 3.3.3 Estimated age at peak bone mineral density (PBMD) reported in six cross-sectional studies*

Cross-sectional study	Age at PBMD (years)	
	Females	**Males**
Gilsanz et al.[18]	16–17	—
Buchanan et al.[26]	15–23	—
Glastre et al.[19]	> 15	> 15
Geusens et al.[17]	16–20	21–25
Bonjour et al.[16]	14–15	17–18
Rico et al.[27]	15–19	—

*Twelve studies found between 1981 and 1992, six valid studies are considered.

Longitudinal studies that include interventions with extra physical activity are indispensable to prove that bone mass can be influenced by the daily activity pattern of the subjects involved. The majority of these studies, so called randomized controlled trials (RCTs), are done in females older than 45 years in order to prevent postmenarchal bone loss osteoporosis.

In a recent meta-analysis the effects of exercise training programmes in pre- and post-menopausal women on BMD of the lumbar spine (LS) and the femoral neck (FN) were studied.[34] The study treatment effect was defined as the difference between percentage change in BMD per year in the training and the control group. Seventeen articles were included. The summary treatment effects were in premenopausal women 0.9% (95% CI: 0.4–1.4) in LS and 0.9% (0.3–1.5) in FN, and in postmenopausal women 0.9% (0.4–1.3) in LS and 1.0% (0.4–1.5) in FN. It showed that exercise prevents almost 1% BMD loss per year in both pre- and post-menopausal women. The separate analysis for endurance and strength training type did not reveal large differences. The main reasons for this are: (1) the small number of studies with specific strength training and (2) the endurance programmes also might have included exercises with high strains.

The number of studies in young subjects is scarce: three studies in girls[35–37] and two in boys[38,39] are valid for review. The boys' study of Margulies[39] with 268 military recruits, age 18–21 (intensive training 8 hours per day per week) however, had no control group and the period of follow-up was relatively short (14 weeks), but more importantly about 40% of the subjects could not comply because of stress fractures.

In 1998, Bradney et al.[38] published a study in prepubertal boys comparing an eight month, three times per week 30 minutes programme consisting of weight bearing exercise with a control group matched for age, height, weight and BMD. The increase in BMD was site specific and twice that of controls in lumbar spine, legs and total body.

Gleeson et al.[36] performed a one year three times per week weight-training programme of 30 minutes duration, with an intensity of 60% of the one repetition maximum, in 34 women (24–46 year). They compared the bone density in lumbar spine and calcaneus with 38 controls. No changes in BMD could be found in both groups. Blimkie et al.[35] also found non-significant changes in younger girls (14–18 years) on a weight-training programme over a shorter period of 26 weeks.

A ten month intervention in premenarchal girls by Morris et al.[37] with high impact strength-building exercise showed a significant increase at all four bone sites of interest (proximal femur, neck of femur, lumbar spine and total body). This increase was accompanied by a decrease in fat mass, gain in lean mass, shoulder, knee and grip strength.

Non-true-experimental results are available from the Amsterdam Growth and Health Longitudinal Study.[40] About 200 males and females were measured longitudinally from age 13 to age 27. In this follow-up, measurements were taken six times of habitual physical activity and nutritional intake. At age 27 the BMD of the lumbar region was measured by DEXA.[41] The longitudinal information on weight bearing activity and calcium intake were considered over three periods: the adolescent period from 13–18 years, the period between 13 and 22 years and the total period between the age of 13 till 27 years. Results of multiple regression analysis showed that in both sexes weight bearing activity and body mass were significant positive contributors in the prediction of BMD at age 27. Calcium intake never

appeared to be a significant predictor of BMD in the three periods. From these results it can be concluded that BMD in the lumbar spine at age 27 may be influenced by body mass and a high level of weight bearing physical activity carried out during youth.

In the same study, to answer the question what the most important factor is for bone mass development during youth, the physical activity data were scored in two different ways:

(1) by calculating the total weekly energy expenditure of all weight bearing activities (expressed as the number of weight bearing METS week^{-1}; and

(2) by calculating a score that takes into account the ground reaction forces at weight bearing activities as multiples of body weight, irrespective of the frequency and the duration of the activity, i.e. giving a weighted peak strain score.

The two different habitual physical activity scores were again calculated for each subject over three time periods: the adolescent period (four annual measurements between 13 and 17 years of age), the young adult period (two measurements between 17 and 22 years of age), and the adult period (two measurements between 22 and 27 years of age).

Linear regression analyses were performed to analyse the relation between BMD at age 27 and the physical activity scores over three foregoing periods. The physical activity scores were entered in the regression model as independent variables, and gender was added to the model as a covariate. In Fig. 3.3.5, the standard regression coefficients of lumbar BMD and femoral neck BMD, respectively, are given for the MET score and the peak strain scores, and for the three different periods. The results show that as the time period over which the physical activity scores were taken came closer to the BMD measurement at age 27 years, the more important became the peak strain score of physical activity. For this biomechanical component of physical activity, the explained variance of BMD increased from 2% during adolescence to 13% in adulthood. For the energetic score of physical activity the explained variance decreased from 6% during adolescence to 1% in adulthood for both sexes.[42] This strongly supports the validity of the results of animal studies in human subjects. The preventive effect of peak strain, however, has to be confirmed in youth in true experimental design, since the significant differences in BMD can still be explained by self-selection of activity levels during the growing years.

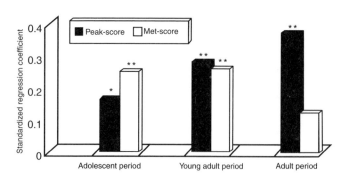

Fig. 3.3.5 The relationship of BMD in the lumbar spine at age 28 years with energetic physical activity (MET-score) and peak strain physical activity (Peak-score) during three different preceding periods in 182 males and females from the Amsterdam Growth and Health Study. (*p < 0.05; **p < 0.01)

Recent results from Mirwald et al.,[43] presented at the first international conference on Children's Bone Health in Maastricht, comparing active subjects (top quartile) with inactive subjects (bottom quartile) suggests that a modifiable lifestyle factor, like physical activity, plays a role in the optimalization of bone mineral acquisition at the lumbar spine in boys and girls during the adolescent growth spurt. A cross-sectional study in tennis and squash female players[44] showed that training started in puberty is maximally beneficial for mineralization of the bone of the playing arm. This training effect on BMD remained also in adult age (age 21–30 years) after four years of cessation of the training.[45]

Summary

Bone mass increases rapidly during growth and development. The mechanism seems to be dependent on three factors: centrally regulated hormonal factors, locally determined mechanical factors and interaction between the hormonal and mechanical factors. Measurement of the quantitative increase of BMD during growth by energy absorption methods, such as DPA, SPA and DEXA, probably gives an overestimation, because these measures do not take into consideration differences in dimensional growth of the bones in question.

Before the age of puberty (around 12 in girls and 13 in boys) no significant differences in BMD between boys and girls are demonstrated. During the pubertal growth spurt it is now clear that the increase in BMC on the average is 35% of total BMC increase. The clinical significance of this high percentage is that as much BMC is laid down during the four adolescent growing years as most people will loose during all adult life.

Investigations that measured BMD longitudinally indicate that boys and girls reach their peak BMD in their late twenties and not in their late teens. In both sexes the greatest change in BMC per year occurs one or two years after PHV.

There are at least two exercise-related strategies to prevent osteoporosis (Fig. 3.3.6). One preventive strategy is to increase bone accrual during youth by increasing the amount of exercise in order to achieve a greater peak bone mass. A second strategy is to ensure that adults maintain a physically active lifestyle until old age, thus minimizing bone loss during ageing. In this way, exercise increases the age at which the osteoporotic fracture limit is reached.

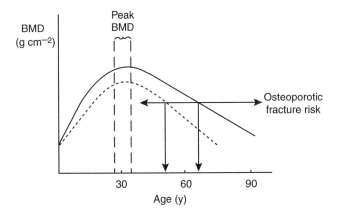

Fig. 3.3.6 The possible effects of lifetime exercise on the developmental curve of BMD: the average curve of inactive people (interrupted line) is shifted to the top-right (solid line) resulting in a higher BMD at any age and crossing the osteoporotic limit at a later age.

In young males and females, studies showing the effects of exercise intervention on BMD are scarce. Recent experimental studies show significant effects of weight bearing activity and high impact strength training programmes on the side specific BMD in both boys and girls. The earlier a child starts with physical activity the more bone is accumulated.

A preventive effect of weight bearing activities on the PBMD is also shown in the Amsterdam Growth and Health Longitudinal study: Both 27 year old males and females, with relative high levels of peak strain weight-bearing physical activity patterns during the foregoing 15 years, show significantly higher PBMD in their lumbar spine than their inactive counter parts.

Further research is needed to establish the most effective type of exercise for increasing bone mass, and also true-experimental studies that are aimed at the possibility of increasing PBMD in both sexes in order to attain optimal maximal bone mass at young adult age.

References

1. **Tanner, J. M.** *Growth at adolescence.* Oxford, Blackwell, 1955.
2. **Tanner, J. M.** *A history of the study of human growth.* Cambridge University Press, London, 1981.
3. **Weiner, J. S.** and **Lourie, J. A.** *Human biology, a guide to field methods IBP Handbook no.9.* Blackwell, Oxford, 1969.
4. **Falkner, F.** and **Tanner, J. M.** *Human growth, part 1, 2 and 3.* Plenum Press, New York, 1978.
5. **Snow-Harter, C.** and **Marcus, R.** Exercise, bone mineral density and osteoporosis. *Exercise and Sport Sciences Reviews* 1991; **19**: 351–88.
6. **Döbeln, W. von.** Anthropometric determination of fat-free body weight. *Acta Medica Scandinavica* 1959; **165**: 37–42.
7. **Roche, A. F., Chumlea, W. C.** and **Thissen, D.** *Assessing the skeletal maturity of the hand-wrist: Fels Method.* C. C. Thomas, Springfield Ill, 1988.
8. **Roche, A. F., Wainer, H.** and **Thissen, D.** *Skeletal maturity: the knee joint as a biological indicator.* Plenum, New York, 1975.
9. **Tanner, J. M., Whitehouse, R. H., Marshall, W. A., Healy, M. J. R.** and **Goldstein, H.** *Assessment of skeletal maturity and prediction of adult height (TW2 method).* Academic Press, London, 1975.
10. **Sievänen, H., Kannus, P., Nieminen, V., Heinonen, A., Oja, P.** and **Vuori, I.** Estimation of various mechanical characteristics of human bones using DEXA: methodology and precision. *Bone* 1996; **18**: 173–275.
11. **Smith, E. L.** and **Raab, D. M.** Osteoporosis and physical activity. *Acta Medica Scandinavica* 1986; (suppl) **711**: 149–56.
12. **Burger, E. H.** and **Klein-Nulend, J.** Mechanotransduction in bone-role of the lacunocanalicular network. *Federation of American Societies for Experimental Biology Journal* 1999; **13** (suppl): S101–S12.
13. **Lanyon, L. E.** Using functional loading to influence bone mass and architecture: objectives, mechanism, and relationship with estrogen of the mechanically adaptive process in bone. *Bone* 1996; **18**: 37S–43S.
14. **Rubin, C. T.** and **Lanyon, L. E.** Regulation of bone formation by applied dynamic loads. *Journal of Bone and Joint Surgery* 1984; **66A**: 397–402.
15. **Kemper, H. C. G.** *Exercise to fight osteoporosis. A guide for the health care professional.* Medical Forum International Zeist, 1998.
16. **Bonjour, J. F., Theintz, G., Buchs, B., Slosman, D.** and **Rizzoli, R.** Critical years and stages of puberty for spinal and femoral bone mass accumulation during adolescence. *Journal of Clinical Endocrinology and Metabolism* 1991; **73**: 555–63.
17. **Geusens, P., Cantatore, F., Nijs, J., Proesmans, W., Emma, F.** and **Dequeker, J.** Heterogeneity of growth of bone in children at the spine, radius and total skeleton. *Growth, Development and Aging* 1991; **55**: 249–56.
18. **Gilsanz, V., Gibbons, D. T., Roe, T. F.** and **Carlson, M.** Vertebral bone density in children: effect of puberty. *Radiology* 1988; **166**: 847–50.

19. Glastre, C., Braillon, P., David, L., Cochat, P., Meunier, P. J. and Delmas, P. D. Measurement of bone mineral content of the lumbar spine by dual energy X-ray absorptiometry in normal children: correlations with growth parameters. *Journal of Clinical Endocrinology and Metabolism* 1990; **70**: 1330–3.

20. Gordon, C. L., Halton, J. M., Atkinson, S. A. and Webber, C. E. The contributions of growth and puberty to peak bone mass. *Growth, Development and Aging* 1991; **55**: 257–62.

21. Southard, R. N., Morris, J. D., Hayes, J. R., Torch, M. A. and Sommer, A. Bone mass in healthy children: measurement with quantitative DXA. *Radiology* 1991; **179**: 735–8.

22. Grimston, S. K., Morrison, K., Harder, J. A. and Hanley, D. A. Bone mineral density during puberty in Western Canadian children. *Journal of Bone and Mineral Research* 1992; **19**: 85–96.

23. Theintz, G., Buchs, B., Rizolli, R., Slosman, D., Clavien, H., Sizonenko, P. C. and Bonjour, J. P. H. Longitudinal monitoring of bone mass accumulation in healthy adolescents: evidence for a marked reduction after 16 years of age at the levels of lumbar spine and femoral neck in female subjects. *Journal of Clinical Endocrinology and Metabolism* 1992; **75**: 1060–6.

24. Riis, B. J., Krabbe, S., Christiansen, C., Catherwood, B. D. and Deftos, L. J. Bone turnover in male puberty: a longitudinal study. *Calcified Tissue International* 1985; **37**: 213–7.

25. Bailey, D. A., Drinkwater, D., Faulkner, R. and McKay, H. Proximal femur bone mineral changes in growing children: dimensional considerations. *Pediatric Exercise Science* 1993; **5**: 388.

26. Buchanan, J. R., Meyers, C., Lloyd, T. and Greer, R. B. III. Early vertebral trabecular bone loss in normalpremenopausal women. *Journal of Bone and Mineral Research* 1988; **3**: 445–9.

27. Rico, H., Revilla, M., Hernandez, E. R., Villa, L. F. and Alvarez del Buergo, L. Sex differences in the acquisition of total bone mineral mass peak assessed through dual energy X-ray absorptiometry. *Calcified Tissue International* 1992; **51**: 251–4.

28. Davies, K. M., Recker, R. R., Stegman, M. R., Heaney, R. P., Kimmel, D. B. and Leist, J. Third decade bone gain in women. In *Calcium regulation and bone metabolism* (ed. D. V. Cohn, F. H. Glorieux and T. J. Martin). Elsevier Sciences, Amsterdam, 1990; 497–500.

29. Recker, R. R., Davies, K. M., Hinders, S. M., Heaney, R. P., Stegman, R. P. and Kimmel, D. B. Bone gain in young adult women. *Journal of the American Medical Association* 1992; **268**: 2403–8.

30. Moen, S., Sanborn, C., Bonnick, S., Keizer, H., Gench, B. and DiMarco, N. Longitudinal lumbar bone mineral density changes in adolescent female runners. *Medicine and Science in Sports and Exercise* 1992; **5**: S12–24.

31. Riggs, B. L. and Melton, L. J. Involutional osteoporosis. *New England Journal of Medicine* 986; **413**: 1676–86.

32. Slemenda, C. W., Miller, J. Z., Hui, L. S., Reister, T. K. and Johnston, C. C. Role of physical activity in the development of skeletal mass in children. *Journal of Bone Mineral Research* 1991; **6**: 1227–33.

33. Bailey, D. A. The Saskatchewan Pediatric Bone Mineral Accrual Study: bone mineral acquisition during the growing years. *International Journal of Sports Medicine* 1997; **18**, S191–5.

34. Wolff, I., Croonenberg, I. I., Kemper, H. C. G., Kostense, P. J. and Twisk, J. W. R. The effect of exercise training programs on the bone mass: a meta-analysis of published controlled trials in pre- and postmenopausal women. *Osteoporosis International* 1999; **9**: 1–12.

35. Blimkie, C. J., Rice, S., Webber, J., Martin, J., Levy, D. and Parker, D. Bone density, physical activity, fitness, antropometry, gynaecologic, endocrine and nutrition status in adolescent girls. In *Pediatric Work Physiology* (ed. J. Coudert and E. Van Praagh). Masson, Paris, 1993; 201–4.

36. Gleeson, P. B., Protas, E. J., LeBlanc, A. D., Schneider, V. S. and Evans, H. J. Effects of weight lifting on bone mineral density in premopausal women. *Journal of Bone and Mineral Research* 1990; **5**: 153–8.

37. Morris, F. L., Naughton, G. A., Gibbs, J. L., Carlson, J. S. and Wark, J. D. Positive effects on bone and lean mass. *Journal of Bone and Mineral Research* 1997; **12**: 1453–62.

38. Bradney, M., Pearce, G., Naughton, G., Sullivan, C., Bass, S., Beck, T., Carlson, J. and Seeman, E. Moderate exercise during growth in prepubertal boys: changes in bone mass, size, volumetric density and bone strength: a controlled prospective study. *Journal of Bone and Mineral Research* 1998; **13**: 1814–21.

39. Margulies, J. Y., Simkin, A., Leichter, I., Bivas, A., Steinberg, R., Giladi, M., Stein, M., Kashtan, H. and Milgrom, C. Effect of intensive physical activity on the bone mineral density content in power limbs of young adults. *Journal of Bone Joint Surgery* 1986; **68a**: 1090–3.

40. Kemper, H. C. G. *The Amsterdam growth and health study, health, fitness and lifestyle in longitudinal perspective; a follow-up of males and females from 13 to 27 years of age.* Human Kinetics, Champaign, Il., 1995.

41. Welten, D. C., Kemper, H. C. G., Post, G. B., Mechelen, W.v., Twist, J., Lips, P. and Teule, G. J. Weight bearing activity during youth is a more important factor for peak bone mass than calcium intake. *Journal of Bone and Mineral Research* 1994; **9**: 1029–96.

42. Groothausen, J., Siemer, H., Kemper, H. C. G., Twisk, J. W. R. and Welten, D. C. Influence of peak strain on lumbar bone mineral density: an analysis physical activity in young males and females. *Pediatric Exercise Science* 1997; **9**: 159–73.

43. Mirwald, R. L., Bailey, D. A., McKay, H. and Crocker, P. E. Physical activity and bone mineral acquisition at the lumbar spine during the adolescent growth spurt. Abstract at: *First International Conference on Children's Bone Health*, Maastricht. Program and Abstract Book, 1999; 57.

44. Kannus, P., Haapasalo, H., Sankelo, M., Sievanen, H., Pasanen, M., Heinonen, A., Oja, P. and Vuori, I. Effect of starting age of physical activity on bone mass in the dominant arm of tennis and squash players. *Annals of Internal Medicine* 1995; **123**: 27–31.

45. Kontulainen, S., Kannus, P., Haapsalo, H., Heinonen, A., Sievänen, H., Oja, P. and Vuori, I. Changes in bone mineral content with decreased training in competitive young adult tennis players and controls: a prospective 4-year follow-up. *Medicine and Science in Sports and Exercise.* 1999; **31**: 640–52.

3.4 Physical activity, physical fitness and social, psychological and emotional health

Susan R. Tortolero, Wendell C. Taylor and Nancy G. Murray

Introduction

Given the full acceptance of the World Health Organization's definition of health as a positive state of physical, mental and social well being, the mental and social effects of physical activity merit careful and extensive study. Although findings have been summarized among the general population[1–4] and specifically among adults,[5–7] the reviews among children[8–10] have been primarily on selected topics such as self-esteem. Two general reviews[1,12] describe the effects of physical activity on psychological variables, mental health and sense of well-being in paediatric populations. In one review[12] among youth (ages 11–21 years old), self-esteem, self-concept, depressive symptoms and anxiety/stress were related consistently to physical activity, whereas, the evidence for hostility/anger and academic achievement was inconclusive. In an earlier review,[11] the relationship between physical activity and psychological functioning varied depending upon age, sex, state of health, intelligence, past success or failure, appropriateness of activity and subculture values.

Given the importance of psychological, emotional, social and mental health for children and adolescents, we review the literature, identify important gaps in knowledge, and recommend future research. This chapter extends and updates previous reviews by including measures of fitness and expanding the age range and domain of variables, as well as including recent literature.

Method of review

Published articles in English language literature from 1983 through 1998 were reviewed that included:
(1) subjects in the age range of 3–18 years old;
(2) measures of physical activity and/or fitness; and
(3) measures of social, psychological, emotional and/or personality variables.

The focus of our review was on the mental health effects of activity and/or fitness rather than predictors and determinants of activity.

The search techniques were computerized and manual. The computerized search included the following databases: CINAHL, MEDLINE, MEDSCAPE, PsycINFO, Sociological Abstracts, SPORTSDiscus, ProQuest, and publications from the Centers for Disease Control and Prevention. The key words for the computerized searches included children, adolescents, activity, exercise and fitness combined with terms such as social, psychological, emotional, well-being, self-esteem, self-concept, anxiety, affect, depression, cognition, intelligence, hostility, mood states, stress, optimism, psychiatric disorders, substance use, relationships, coping, self-efficacy and body image.

The manual search included consulting experts, reviewing proceedings of recent conferences, identifying references from previous review articles (e.g. Calfas and Taylor[12]) and personal retrieval searches. Unpublished studies, dissertations, case reports and expert opinion were excluded.

This review includes 48 articles published 1983–1998. The tables are organized by self-perceptions, psychosocial and academic functioning, internal emotional and psychological conditions, and risk behaviours. Studies assessing the effects of physical activity and fitness on self perceptions such as self concept, self esteem, self efficacy, perceived physical competence and ability, and body image are presented in Table 3.4.1. Findings related to psychosocial and academic functioning, such as perceived health and well being, academic achievement, social skills, creativity and shyness are described in Table 3.4.2. Results on internal psychological conditions and negative affect such as depression, anxiety, negative affect, emotional distress, stress, loneliness, and hostility are shown in Table 3.4.3. Studies on the effects of physical activity and fitness on risk behaviours such as smoking, alcohol use, aggression, suicide and behavioural problems are shown in Table 3.4.4.

Self perceptions

The related constructs of self-perceptions have been the most extensively studied psychological outcomes of physical activity and fitness. Although many of the constructs of self esteem, self concept, perceived physical competence and ability, self efficacy and body image are highly related, conceptually these constructs are different. Differences and similarities between self-concept, self esteem, and other constructs have been described by several authors (e.g. McAuley[8]). The difficulty in summarizing this literature is that these constructs are used interchangeably, and terms are frequently not defined. Further, the same survey instruments are frequently used to measure different constructs thus making comparisons among studies difficult.

Self concept

Eight studies examined the association between physical activity/fitness and global self-concept among youth.[13–20] Several studies investigated this association using experimental designs;[13,15–17,19–21] however, only one study[13] employed a randomized, controlled trial to examine this association. In a study[13] conducted among 54 boys with learning disabilities, boys participating in an aerobic exercise programme improved self-concept significantly more than boys participating in a less vigorous exercise programme. In a non-randomized, intervention trial,[16] similar results were reported among delinquent boys. Conversely, no improvement in self-concept among boys with behaviour disorders participating in a physical activity intervention was found compared with those not participating in the programme.[17] Although among dance team participants[20] no association between physical fitness and self concept was observed when compared to non-dance team participants, an association between fitness levels and several of the self concept subscales was observed among those participating in dance.

Three studies examined the association between self-concept and physical activity/fitness using cross-sectional designs.[14,18,19] One study found[14] a positive association between parental report of physical activity and positive self concept among elementary children, but did not find an association between physical fitness and self concept. While other studies[18,19] reported a positive association between positive self concept and physical fitness.

Self esteem

Five studies examined the association between physical activity, fitness and self esteem. One study[22] reported significant improvements in self esteem among pregnant adolescent females who participated in a physical activity intervention compared to those who received usual care. Using a pre-test, post-test design without a comparison group,[23] improvements in self esteem among little league baseball players were observed from pre-season to post-season. In a longitudinal study of competitive swim team participants,[24] a significant relationship was observed between improved swim team performance and global self esteem.

A cross-sectional study[25] examining the association between self-esteem and self-reported participation in exercise among 90 youth found no association between self-reported physical activity and self-esteem. Further, no improvements in self-esteem among dance team participants were observed when compared to non-participants.[20]

Body image

Body image or perception of physical appearance is an important construct particularly for adolescents. Both gender and ethnic differences in perceptions of body image have been observed among adolescents.[26] Generally, females are more concerned with physical beauty and maintaining an ideal body image; whereas, boys are more concerned about body size, strength and power.[27] Further, female adolescents generally do not match the perceived ideal body image as determined by society. Also, it has been reported that African American girls are more satisfied with their bodies than European American or Native American girls.[28–35]

A limited number of studies examined the association between body image and physical activity/fitness among youth. We identified three experimental studies; however, results are inconsistent among these studies and methodological problems are apparent. One study[21] found that a physical activity intervention improved positive perceptions of physical appearance among youths aged 9 to 16 years. Among a smaller sample,[15] no association was found between body image after a physical activity intervention among 11 boys and girls aged 9 to 11 years. Similarly, another study[36] reported no association between fitness level and body image among youth attending 4th through 6th grade.

The relationship between physical activity/fitness and body image has not been well studied, and the evidence is inconclusive. Given the importance of body image among youth, and the reported ethnic and gender differences, further research in this area is needed, particularly because adolescents who have an unfavourable body image may engage in physical activity excessively.

Self efficacy/perceived physical competence

According to Bandura, self efficacy is the conviction that one can carry out the desired behaviour to produce the expected outcome.[37] While self efficacy has been shown to be predictive in a variety of health behaviours including physical activity,[38] few studies have determined if engaging in exercise and physical activity increases self efficacy. Three such studies examined this relationship. An exercise intervention study conducted among 27 psychiatrically institutionalized adolescents found that those assigned to the aerobic exercise programme had improved self-efficacy compared with those participating in a regular activity class.[39] Similarly, a reported gain in self efficacy about strength training was observed among 36 girls randomly assigned to a strength training intervention compared to controls.[40] In a longitudinal study,[24] increased swim performance among swim team participants was associated with increased perceived physical competence.

Summary

In general, the conclusions are that physical activity and fitness have positive effects on self perceptions and, in particular, these effects are most evident for self concept, self esteem and self efficacy. However, data are limited about the effects of physical activity on body image because few well-designed studies have been conducted. Many studies have methodological, theoretical and measurement problems such as inadequate study designs, absence of conceptual definitions and theoretical models to guide the research. Horn and Claytor[41] suggested using a unifying theoretical framework of self perceptions such as the multidimensional approach proposed by Fox and Corbin.[26] Given these limitations, there is a need to conduct well-designed, theoretically-based studies to further understand the association between perceptions of self and physical activity and fitness.

Psychosocial and academic functioning

Few studies address the question of whether physical activity improves academic and psychosocial functioning among youth. Findings related to the impact of physical activity and fitness on functioning, such as academic achievement, social skills, creativity, and perceived health and well being, are presented in Table 3.4.2.

Academic functioning

A number of constructs concerning academic functioning and physical activity have been investigated. These include academic performance, intelligence, creativity and confused thinking. Although a number of studies were published between 1950 and 1970 on the association between intellectual ability and sport performance, a limited number of studies have been published more recently.[42] In a review of earlier studies, Kirkendall suggests that while there seems to be a modest relationship between academic and athletic success, little support can be found that physical activity enhances intellectual development.[42] Since 1983, three studies[22,43,44] examined the relationship between physical activity and academic performance among youth. Two experimental

Table 3.4.1 The effects of physical activity/fitness on self perceptions

Study	Related to physical activity/fitness			Unrelated to physical activity/fitness		
	Study design*/pop. characteristics	Psychosocial well-being measures	Physical activity/fitness measures	Study design/pop. characteristics	Psychosocial well-being measures	Physical activity/fitness measures
Self concept						
Overbay and Purath[14]	XSECT Male (n=23) Female (n=38) Age 6–12 y	Martinek-Zaichowsky Self-Concept Scale (MZSCS)	Parental report of exercise	XSECT Male (n=23) Female (n=38) Age 6–12 y	Martinek-Zaichowsky Self-Concept Scale	1-mile walk time, shuttle run time, curl up
Sherrill et al.[18]	XSECT Male/Female (n=393) Grades 4–5	Children's Self Concept Scale	Texas Physical Activity Test			
Hatfield et al.[15]	QEXP Male (n=3) Female (n=11) Age 9–11y	MZSCS Piers-Harris Self-Concept Scale	Physical activity intervention			
MacMahon and Gross[13]	EXP, CLINICAL Male (n=54) Age 7.1–12.8 y M Age 9.7 y	Piers-Harris Self-Concept Scale	Physical activity intervention			
MacMahon and Gross[16]	QEXP, CLINICAL Male (n=98) Age 14–18.3 y M Age 16.3 y	Piers-Harris Self-Concept Scale	Physical activity intervention			
Young[19]	XSECT Female (n=75) Grades 7–10	Tennessee Self-Concept Scale	AAHPER Youth Fitness Test Estimation of Physical Fitness			
Parish-Plass and Lufi[17]				QEXP, CLINICAL Male (n=43) Age 8–13.5 y M Age 10.87 y	Tennessee Self-Concept Scale	Physical activity intervention
Blackman et al.[20]				QEXP Female (n=16) M Age 14.83 y	Tennessee Self-Concept Scale	VO_2 max Fitness tests

276

Table 3.4.1 (Continued)

Study	Related to physical activity/fitness			Unrelated to physical activity/fitness		
	Study design*/pop. characteristics	Psychosocial well-being measures	Physical activity/fitness measures	Study design/pop. characteristics	Psychosocial well-being measures	Physical activity/fitness measures
Self esteem						
Sonstroem et al.[24]	LONG Male (n = 98) High school age	Rosenberg Self-Esteem Scale	Swim performance			
Koniak-Griffin[22]	QEXP, CLINICAL Female (n = 58) Age 14–20 y M Age 16.6 y	Coopersmith Self Esteem Inventory	Physical activity intervention			
Aine and Lester[25]				XSECT Males (n = 28) Female (n = 62) Age 15–24 y	Rosenberg Self-Esteem Scale	Self-report exercise
Boyd and Hrycaiko[21]	QEXP Females (n = 181) Age 9–16 y	Self Description Questionnaire	Physical activity intervention			
Blackman et al.[20]				QEXP Female (n = 16) M Age 14.83 y	Coopersmith Self Esteem Inventory	VO_2 max Fitness tests
Body image						
Boyd and Hrycaiko[21]	QEXP Female (n = 181) Age 9–16 y	Physical Appearance Scale	Physical activity intervention during gym class			

Study	Design & Sample	Measure	Outcome/Intervention
Hatfield et al.[15]			
Tuckman and Hinkle[36]	EXP-No Control Male/Female (n = 11) Age 9–11 y; Devereaux Elementary Male/Female (n = 154) Grades 4–6	Piers-Harris Self Concept Scale; AAHPER Youth School Behaviour Rating Scale; Fitness Test	EXP; Physical activity intervention
Self efficacy/ perceived physical competence			
Sonstroem et al.[24]	LONG, Male (n = 98), High school age	Rosenberg Self-Esteem Scale	Swim performance
Brown et al.[11]	EXP, CLINICAL, Male (n = 16), Female (n = 11), M Age 15.6 y	Self Efficacy Questionnaire	Physical activity intervention
Holloway et al.[40]	QEXP, Female (n = 59), M Age 16 y	Physical Self Efficacy Scale	Strength training intervention
Sonstroem et al.[24]	LONG, Male (n = 98), High school age	Perceived Physical Competence	Swim performance

*XSECT is a cross-sectional study; EXP is an experimental study; QEXP is a quasi-experimental study; CASE is a case-control study; LONG is a longitudinal study; CLINICAL denotes that the study was performed in a clinical setting; M is mean age.

studies examined this association among learning disabled youth and youth with behavioural disturbances.[22,44] These studies reported no differences between treatment groups in academic performance. A third study[43] following 1057 youth concluded that those reporting participation in sports activities had better academic achievement performance than those who did not report participating in sports activities. One study[36] examined the relationship between increased fitness and classroom behaviour among 154 youth and reported that youth who improved physical fitness had increased creativity levels.

Several studies[39,45,46] examined whether increased physical activity levels reduced levels of confused thinking or concentration. In one study, a physical activity intervention decreased levels of confused thinking among females, but not among males.[39] While, among other studies[45,46] physical activity reduced levels of confused thinking and improved concentration levels.

Social skills

While it is generally assumed that involvement in physical activity and fitness can lead to the development of important social skills, few studies have investigated this relationship. An experimental study found that a physical activity intervention improved social skills among youth with a learning disability, but that these gains were no larger in this group than the group that received individualized academic instruction, alone.[44] In a cross-sectional study,[47] those who reported exercising infrequently were more shy than were adolescents who reported exercising frequently. Further, improved emotional development among males with severe perennial asthma was reported after participating in a physical activity intervention.[46]

Perceived health and well-being

Three studies investigated whether physical activity improved perception of physical well being. All three studies[43,48,49] found a significant association between self-reported participation in physical activity and perceived well being. These studies,[43,48,49] however, relied on self-report measures of physical activity and two of the three used cross-sectional designs.[43,49] Although these data support a relationship between physical activity and perceived health and well being, more studies are needed to determine the direction and strength of this relationship while controlling for potential confounding variables.

While it appears that physical activity and fitness may confer some benefit in academic and psychosocial functioning, the lack of well-designed studies limits our ability to form definitive conclusions. Further research is needed to understand if and how physical activity improves psychosocial functioning among youth.

Psychological symptoms and negative affect

A large body of literature has emerged suggesting that physical activity and fitness decreases psychological symptoms and negative affect among adults.[8] Involvement in exercise may be key to enhancing mental health. Since adolescence is characterized as a time of emotional distress, it is particularly useful to understand the benefits of physical activity in decreasing emotional distress and negative affect among youth. The evidence for physical activity and fitness associated with depression, anxiety, negative affect, emotional distress, stress, loneliness and hostility is presented in Table 3.4.3.

Depression

Since 1983, ten studies[16,22,39,48,50–55] have addressed physical activity/fitness and depression among youth. Two quasi-experimental studies[16,22] conducted among high-risk children living in residential facilities found significant decreases in depressive symptoms among youth assigned to the physical activity interventions compared to control conditions. A randomized trial[39] among a small group of psychiatrically institutionalized boys and girls found a significant decrease in depressive symptoms with improved physical fitness among girls but not among boys.

Seven studies used non-clinic, free-living populations. A quasi-experimental study[50] among 47 youth assigned to conditions based on their physical activity history reported long-term exercisers had fewer depressive symptoms than inactive participants. However, these differences were not statistically significant. A longitudinal study[52] among 583 youth found that higher levels of physical activity were related to lower depressive symptoms at follow-up for males, but not for females. Conversely, fitness levels were related to lower depressive symptoms at follow-up for girls, but not for boys.[52] A cross-sectional study[51] among 8 to 12-year olds found that youth who were inactive were about three times more likely to have depressive symptoms than children who were active. Further, they found that youth who were unfit had a four-times greater risk of having depressive symptoms than fit children.[51] Similarly, depressive symptoms were negatively correlated with frequency of sports participation as well as number of hours in sports among a cross-section of 1131 adolescents.[48] In another cross-sectional study,[54] inactive females were more likely to have higher levels of depression than active females.

Two studies found no association between physical activity and depression.[53,55] A randomized, experimental study[53] among 60 youth to examine the effect of participating in a physical activity intervention on depression and other psychological factors found no significant differences in depression levels after a 2-week intervention.[53] Moreover, in a study with cross-sectional and longitudinal data,[55] no association was observed in self-reported physical exercise and depressive symptoms among a sample of 530 adolescents.

In summary, physical activity appears to be associated with decreased depressive symptoms in both free-living and clinic populations. Although much of the research of physical activity and depression has methodological flaws, the evidence points to beneficial effects of physical activity on depressive symptoms. Several possible hypotheses have been proposed to explain how physical activity functions to decrease depressive symptoms, but none has been consistently supported.[56] Some authors have suggested[56] that the beneficial consequences of physical activity may be mediated by several factors (i.e. physiological, chemical and psychosocial).

Anxiety

Five studies assessed the association between physical activity/fitness and anxiety among youth.[39,48,53,55,57] Among a small group of psychiatrically institutionalized adolescents,[39] improving fitness levels decreased tension and anxiety among females but not among males. In a randomized, controlled trial of 60 youth,[53] significant decreases in anxiety levels were observed among those participating in a two-week vigorous exercise intervention compared with youth participating in

Table 3.4.2 The effects of physical activity/fitness on psychosocial and academic functioning

Study	Related to physical activity/fitness			Unrelated to physical activity/fitness		
	Study design/pop. characteristics	Psychosocial well-being measures	Physical activity/fitness measures	Study design/pop. characteristics	Psychosocial well-being measures	Physical activity/fitness measures
Academic achievement						
Mechanic and Hansell[43]	LONG Male/Female (n = 1057) Grades 7–11	Self-report of academic grades	Self-report of sports participation			
MacMahon and Gross[16]				QEXP, CLINICAL Male (n = 98) Age 14–18.3 y M Age 16.3 y	Wide Range Achievement Test	Physical activity intervention
Bluechardt and Shephard[44]				EXP CLINICAL Male (n = 34) Female (n = 11) M Age 9.4 y	Self Perceptions Profile for Learning Disabled Students	Physical activity intervention
Creativity						
Tuckman and Hinkle[36]	EXP Male/Female (n = 154) Grades 4–6	Alternate uses test	AAHPER Youth Fitness Test			
Confused thinking/ concentration						
Brown et al.[39]	EXP, CLINICAL Female (n = 11) M Age 15.6 y	Profile of Mood States	Physical activity intervention	EXP, CLINICAL Male (n = 16) M Age 15.6 y	Profile of Mood States	Physical activity intervention
Aganoff and Boyle[45]	LONG Female (n = 97) Age 14–48 y	Menstrual Distress Questionnaire	Self-report weekly exercise			
Engstrom et al.[46]	QEXP, CLINICAL Male (n = 10) Age 9–12 y	Human figure drawings	Physical activity intervention			

Table 3.4.2   (*Continued*)

Study	Related to physical activity/fitness			Unrelated to physical activity/fitness		
	Study design/pop. characteristics	Psychosocial well-being measures	Physical activity/ fitness measures	Study design/pop. characteristics	Psychosocial well-being measures	Physical activity/ fitness measures
Social skills						
Aganoff and Boyle[45]	LONG) Female (n = 97) Age 14–48 y	Menstrual Distress Questionnaire	Self-report weekly exercise			
Page and Tucker[47]	XSECT Male (n = 654) Female (n = 630) M Age 15.3 y	Cheek Buss Shyness Scale	Self-report exercise			
Bluechardt and Shephard[44]				EXP CLINICAL Male (n = 34) Female (n = 11) M Age 9.4 y	Context-Based Test of Social Skills	Physical activity intervention
Emotional development						
Engstrom et al.[46]	QEXP, CLINICAL Male (n = 10) Age 9–12 y	Human figure drawings	Physical activity intervention			
Perceived health/well being						
Thorlindsson et al.[48]	XSECT Male/Female (n = 1131) Age 15–16 y	Perceived Health) Status (1 item)	Self-report of sports participation			
Leonard[49]	XSECT Male/Female (n = 2560)	Monitoring the Future, well-being scale	Self-report of sports participation			
Mechanic and Hansell[43]	LONG Male/Female (n = 1057) Grades 7–9	Well-being measure	Self-report of sports participation			

280

moderate activity. In a cross-section of Icelandic adolescents,[48] significant correlations between frequency and number of hours spent participating in sports and decreased anxiety levels were reported.

Results on the relationship between physical activity and anxiety are inconclusive. Research is limited, and the available studies are difficult to compare. Researchers used different constructs of anxiety (state versus trait) and many of the measurement instruments were not psychometrically sound.

Stress

Physical activity and in particular physical fitness may have a positive effect on an individual's reactivity to environmental stress. While a number of studies have been performed among adult populations, there is some evidence that children may react to stress differently than adults, which requires research among younger populations.[41] Four studies investigated the relationship between physical activity and stress, whereas no studies examined the relationship between physical fitness and stress. In a well-designed experimental study, those in the high intensity exercise condition had lower perceived stress than those in the moderate intensity, flexibility or control groups.[53] Similarly, long-term exercisers tended to report less overall stress in the prior month than non-exercisers; however, these results were not statistically significant.[50] Two hundred and twelve girls were followed for eight months, and girls who reported higher levels of physical activity were less susceptible to stress-induced illness than inactive girls. Further, among a cross-section of 220 girls,[54] those who reported low levels of exercise had higher stress than those who were more active. Although a limited number of studies have assessed the relationship between physical activity and stress, the conclusion is that physical activity may decrease stress levels among children.

Hostility

Three studies[39,45,53] examined the effect of physical activity on hostility levels among youth; none examined the relationship between physical fitness and hostility levels. While a relationship between improved fitness and decreased hostility was observed among females, this relationship was not found for males.[39] A longitudinal study among 97 women examined the interaction of physical activity levels, hostility and menstrual cycle.[45] Self-reported exercise was predictive of decreased hostility levels, and this relationship was observed after controlling for menstrual cycle.[45] Conversely, in a randomized, controlled trial of 147 youth, Norris and coworkers found no association between participation in a physical activity intervention and hostility levels.[53] Although several studies found that physical activity decreased hostility, in a well-designed controlled trial,[53] no association was observed. Given the dearth of information in this area, future studies are needed.

Psychological well-being

Several studies investigated physical activity and other measures of psychological well-being including loneliness, hopelessness, emotional distress, sadness/happiness and negative affect. Those who reported exercising infrequently had more loneliness, shyness and hopelessness than adolescents who reported exercising frequently.[47] These associations were observed among a cross-section of 1297 adolescents even after statistically controlling for potential confounding effects of gender, grade level, perceived attractiveness, body mass and weight satisfaction.[47]

Among 2223 males and females enrolled in the British Cohort Study, participation in vigorous sports was reported to decrease emotional distress.[58] For participants in non-vigorous sports, no effect was found.[64] Among a cohort of 97 females aged 15 to 24 years, regular exercise decreased sadness and negative affect.[45] Similarly, long-term exercisers reported significantly higher positive affect as a result of thoughts and daily experiences than non-exercisers.[50]

In a cross-sectional sample of 28 males and 62 females,[25] no association between self-reported exercise participation and happiness was found. Similarly, no association in the type of swim training session and mood states among 25 female swimmers was reported in another study.[59]

Although few studies have investigated each construct in depth, it appears that physical activity is associated with decreased negative affect, decreased hopelessness and emotional distress, decreased loneliness and increased happiness. Further studies are needed to examine each construct in more detail and to investigate the mechanisms underlying these relationships.

Risk behaviours

A small number of risk behaviours contribute to adverse health and social consequences for adolescents. These behaviours include tobacco use, drug and alcohol use, sexual behaviours, intentional injury and suicide. In order to examine fully the effect of physical activity on psychosocial health, relationships between physical activity and tobacco use, alcohol and drug use, aggression and delinquency, suicide and sexual behaviours were reviewed (see Table 3.4.4).

Tobacco use

Ten studies investigated the relationship between physical activity and tobacco use among youth.[30,31,33,34,48,60–64] Higher levels of leisure time physical activity and aerobic fitness were protective of initiation of smoking at three-year follow-up for females, but not for males.[60] In cross-sectional designs, an inverse relationship between physical activity or sports participation and smoking for males and females was found.[31,33,48,57,61–64] Findings were inconsistent for males when ethnic background was controlled in the studies. The relationship between leisure-time physical activity and smoking initiation was no longer significant for males after adjusting for age and ethnic background, with European American males more likely to smoke than African American males.[60] The relationship between sports participation and smoking also was non-significant for males after adjusting for ethnic background and grade point average.[33] Perhaps physical activity or sport participation may have a stronger protective effect for females, than for males, but to date the evidence is unclear.

For the relationship between smokeless tobacco use and physical activity, several cross-sectional studies provided conflicting evidence. For male athletes, smokeless tobacco use was significantly higher, even after adjusting for ethnic background and grade point average.[33] However, after adjusting for age, race and gender, two other studies[30,31] found no significant increase in smokeless tobacco use for athletes as compared to non-athletes. For European American males, physical activity level had a protective effect for smokeless tobacco use.[64] These findings may be explained by the low prevalence of smokeless tobacco use among females and African American males but do account for smokeless tobacco use among European American male athletes.

Table 3.4.3 The effects of physical activity/fitness on psychological symptoms

Study	Related to physical activity/fitness			Unrelated to physical activity/fitness		
	Study design/pop. characteristics	Psychosocial well-being measures	Physical activity/fitness measures	Study design/pop. characteristics	Psychosocial well-being measures	Physical activity/fitness measures
Depression						
Brown et al.[39]	EXP, CLINICAL Female (n=11) M Age 15.6 y	Beck's Depression Inventory	Physical activity intervention	EXP, CLINICAL Male (n=16) M Age 15.6 y	Beck's Depression Inventory	Physical activity intervention
Koniak-Griffin[22]	QEXP, CLINICAL Female (n=58) Age 14–20 y M Age 16.6 y	Center for Epidemiologic Studies—Depression (CES_D)	Physical activity intervention			
Thorlindsson, et al.[48]	XSECT Male/Female (n=1131) Age 15–16 y	Three-item depression scale	Self-report of sports participation			
MacMahon and Gross[16]	QEXP, CLINICAL Male (n=98) Age 14–18.3 y M Age 16.3 y	Beck's Depression Inventory	Physical activity intervention			
Michaud-Tomson[51]	XSECT Male/Female (n=933) Age 8–12 y	Dimensions of Depression Profile	Parent and teacher report of physical activity			
Brown and Lawton[54]	XSECT Female (n=220) Age 11–17 y	Multiple Affect Checklist-Depressed	Self-report of sports and physical activity participation			
Dua and Hargreaves[50]				QEXP Male (n=13) Female (n=37) Age 16-48 y	Beck's Depression Inventory	Physical activity intervention
Glyshaw et al.[55]				LONG & XSECT Male/Female (n=530) Grades 7–11	Children's Depression Inventory	Self-report physical exercise
Norris et al.[53]				EXP Male (n=31) Female (n=29) M Age=16.7 y	Multiple Affect Checklist-Depressed	Physical activity intervention

Study	Sample/Design	Measure	PA measure	Sample/Design	Measure	PA measure
Milligan et al.[52]	LONG Male (n=301) M Age 18 y LONG Females (n=282) M Age 18 y	Zung Depression Scale Zung Depression Scale	Self-report physical activity Submax fitness test	LONG Female (n=301) M Age=18 y LONG Males (n=282) M Age=18 y	Zung Depression Scale Zung Depression Scale	Self-report physical activity Submax fitness test
Anxiety						
Brown et al.[39]	EXP, CLINICAL Female (n=11) M Age 15.6 y	Profile of Mood States	Physical activity intervention	EXP, CLINICAL Male (n=16) M Age 15.6 y	Profile of Mood States	Physical activity intervention
Thorlindsson et al.[48]	XSECT Male/Female (n=1131) Age 15–16 y	Three-item anxiety scale	Self-report of sports participation			
Norris et al.[53]	EXP Male (n=31) Female (n=29) M Age 16.7 y	Multiple Affect Checklist-Anxiety	Physical activity intervention			
Bahrke and Smith[57]				EXP Male/Female (n=65) Grades 4–6	STAIC State-Trait Anxiety Inventory for Children	Physical activity intervention
Glyshaw et al.[55]				LONG & XSECT Male/Female (n=530) Grades 7–11	STAIC State-Trait Anxiety Inventory for Children	Self-report physical exercise
Stress						
Brown and Siegel[71]	LONG Female (n=212) M Age 13.10 y	Life Event Survey	Self-report of physical activity			
Brown and Lawton[54]	XSECT Female (n=220) Age 11–17 y	Schedule of Recent Events	Self-report of sports and physical activity participation			

Table 3.4.3 (*Continued*)

Study	Related to physical activity/fitness			Unrelated to physical activity/fitness		
	Study design/pop. characteristics	Psychosocial well-being measures	Physical activity/fitness measures	Study design/pop. characteristics	Psychosocial well-being measures	Physical activity/fitness measures
Norris et al.[53]	EXP Male (n = 31) Female (n = 29) M Age = 16.7 y	Perceived Stress Scale	Physical activity intervention			
Dua and Hargreaves[50]	QEXP Male (n = 13) Female (n = 37) M Age 21.8 y		QEXP	Stress-Arousal Male (n = 13) Female (n = 37) M Age = 21.8y	Physical activity Adjective Checklist Perceived Stress	intervention
Negative affect						
Aganoff and Boyle[45]	LONG Female (n = 97) Age 14–48 y	Menstrual Distress Questionnaire	Self-report weekly exercise			
Dua and Hargreaves[50]	QEXP Male (n = 13) Female (n = 37) M Age 21.8 y	Thoughts and Real Life Experiences Scale	Physical activity intervention			
Berger et al.[59]				LONG Male (n = 23) Female (n = 25) Age 12–20 y	Profile of Mood States	Physical activity intervention
Sadness/happiness						
Aganoff and Boyle[45]	LONG Female (n = 97) Age 14–48 y	Menstrual Distress Questionnaire	Self-report weekly exercise			
Aine and Lester[25]				XSECT Males (n = 28) Female (n = 62) Age 15–24 y	Sadness/Happiness Scale	Self-report exercise

	Design / Sample	Outcome measure	Activity measure	Design / Sample	Outcome measure	Activity measure
Hopelessness						
Page and Tucker[47]	XSECT Male (n = 654) Female (n = 630) M Age 15.3 y	Beck Hopelessness Scale	Self-report exercise			
Loneliness						
Page and Tucker[47]	XSECT Male (n = 654) Female (n = 630) M Age 15.3 y	UCLA Loneliness Scale	Self-report exercise			
Emotional distress						
Steptoe and Butler[58]	LONG Male (n = 2223) Female (n = 2838) M Age 16.3 y	General Health Questionnaire Malaise Inventory	Self-report sports and Vigorous Recreational Activity Index			
Hostility						
Brown et al.[39]	EXP, CLINICAL Female (n = 11) M Age 15.6 y	Profile of Mood States	Physical activity intervention	EXP, CLINICAL Male (n = 16) M Age 15.6 y	Profile of Mood States	Physical activity intervention
Aganoff and Boyle[45]	LONG Female (n = 97) Age 14–48 y	Menstrual Distress Questionnaire	Self-report weekly exercise			
Norris et al.[53]				EXP Male (n = 31) Female (n = 29) M Age 16.7 y	Menstrual Distress Questionnaire	Physical activity intervention

Physical activity may not be a protective factor for smokeless tobacco use among European American male athletes.

Alcohol use

For adolescent males, there is conflicting evidence for the relationship between physical activity, especially participation on sports teams, and alcohol use, particularly binge drinking. In a longitudinal study, males who participated in competitive athletics were significantly more likely to initiate alcohol consumption than non-athletic males.[60] Of four cross-sectional studies,[30,50,67,70] three found a positive relationship between sports participation and binge drinking or frequency of alcohol use.[29,48,62] Despite the use of similar measures in a similar sample, Baumert, et al.[31] did not find a significant relationship between athletic participation and binge drinking after adjusting for age, ethnic background and gender. These authors attribute their differential findings to controlling for confounding factors such as gender. Moreover, in an analysis of national Youth Risk Behaviour Study (YRBS) data, physical activity was not related to alcohol consumption in males, but was negatively related to alcohol consumption in females.[34]

Aggression

For the influence of physical activity on risk behaviours such as aggression or violence, studies do not provide clear evidence. Based on changes in self-reported delinquency and aggressive behaviours from ages 15 to 18 years, males and females who were highly active in physical activity and individual sports were more likely to report delinquent and aggressive behaviours than those who reported lower levels of physical activity.[65] Participation in team sports, however, was not related to delinquency, and sporting behaviours were not related to aggressive behaviour. In another cross-sectional study, physical activity levels were not related to injuries in a physical fight.[34] In two experimental studies, physical activity and/or fitness and psychological well-being in delinquent youth were studied.[16,66] The fitness programmes did improve mood in both studies,[16,66] and a decrease in anger and state anxiety was reported in one study with no significant improvement in self-concept or depression.

Suicide

In one case study of suicidal youth employing retrospective self-reports, no relationship between physical activity and risk of suicide was found.[67] In a cross-sectional study, no relationship between suicidal ideation or suicide attempts and self-reported participation in organized sports was reported.[31] However, a significant inverse relationship between feelings of hopelessness and participation in organized sports was reported.[31] For adolescent males, competitive athletics was unrelated to suicidal behaviours but was related inversely to suicidal ideation, while for females competitive athletics was inversely related to behaviours and ideation.[30] The inconclusive evidence from these studies does, however, suggest further investigation into the relationship between physical activity and suicide is needed.

Drug use

A quasi-experimental study of adolescents in school, hospital or community programmes for substance abuse, found that among adolescents who improved their fitness, significantly fewer used multiple drugs, and significantly more abstained from any drug use.[68] Several cross-sectional studies found marijuana use to be inversely related to physical activity in a population-based high school sample,[30,34,64] while another study found cocaine use to be unrelated to activity.[30]

Sexual activity

In several cross-sectional studies, competitive athletics and sexual activity in adolescents were investigated.[28,32,34,69] For males, two of the studies reported earlier initiation of sexual activity for athletes compared to non-athletes,[28,69] while another study reported no significant differences in initiation rates in sexual activity between athletes and non-athletes.[32] For females, the results are more equivocal. While differences in sexual initiation rates were found for male athletes, female athletes were less likely to have initiated sexual activity compared to female non-athletes.[32] In contrast, higher rates of initiation among female athletes were reported in a different study.[28] In a nationally representative sample, no relationship was found between level of physical activity and number of sex partners in the last three months.[34]

Summary

The relationship between physical activity and risk behaviours is equivocal. While children and adolescents who participate in physical activity may be less likely to use tobacco, marijuana and cocaine, they may be more likely to use alcohol and initiate sexual activity at an earlier age. However, few longitudinal studies have been conducted and many existing studies have methodological weaknesses including inadequate control of confounding factors. Longitudinal studies are needed to determine if there is a risk-taking propensity among some youth that encourages competitive sports and risk-taking behaviours, such as alcohol use, aggression and sexual activity. Research designs that employ randomized, controlled trials implementing physical activities as a preventive intervention for risk behaviours among youth may help to answer some of the questions raised by the current research in this area.

Summary and future directions

Based on our review of 48 articles concerning youth, we found strong and moderate support for several variables and weak support and inconsistent findings for other variables. The variables that were most strongly related to activity and fitness in youth were improved self efficacy, greater perceived physical competence, greater perceived health and well being and decreases in depression and stress. The variables with moderate support were positive self concept, positive self esteem, lower levels of hopelessness and loneliness and greater alcohol use. The variables with inconclusive results were body image, academic functioning, social skills, anxiety, hostility, aggression, suicide, sexual activity and tobacco use.

Our findings are consistent with previous reviews among youth and psychosocial health[5,12] which concluded that physical training is associated with increased self esteem whereas increased fitness is not related to self-esteem. In a review of 20 articles, Calfas and Taylor,[12] reported that activity among youth improves self esteem and decreases depressive symptoms, anxiety and stress. We reviewed 48 articles and report similar results to previous reviews. Additionally, we extended the domains of previous reviews to include a section on risk behaviours.

Table 3.4.4 The effects of physical activity/fitness on risk behaviours

Study	Related to physical activity/fitness			Unrelated to physical activity/fitness		
	Study design*/pop. characteristics	Psychosocial well-being measures	Physical activity/fitness measures	Study design/pop. characteristics	Psychosocial well-being measures	Physical activity/fitness measures
Tobacco use						
Thorlindsson et al.[48]	XSECT Male/Female (n=1131) Age 15–16 y	Self-report smoking behaviour	Self-report of sports participation			
Baumert et al.[31]	XSECT Male/Female (n=6849) Grades 9–12	YRBS Self-report cigarette smoking	Self-report participation in organized sports	XSECT Male/Female (n=6849) Grades 9–12	YRBS self-report smokeless tobacco use	Self-report participation in organized sports
Aaron et al.[60]	LONG Female (n=604) Age 12–16 y	YRBS Self-report cigarette smoking	Self-report leisure time	LONG Male (n=641) Age 12–16 y	YRBS Self report smoking behaviour- (n.s after controlling for age, race and gender)	Self-report leisure time
Coulson et al.[61]	XSECT Male/Female (n=932) M Age 13.5 y	Self-report smoking behaviours	Self-report sports participation			
Oler et al.[30]	XSECT Male (n=409) Female (n=409) Grades 9–12	Self-report smoking	Self-report competitive athletics		Self-report smokeless tobacco	Self-report competitive athletics
Pate et al.[34]	XSECT Male (n=2304) Female (n=1989) Age 12–18 y	YRBS Self-report smoking behaviour	YRBS physical activity items coded as low-high activity			
Rainey et al.[62]	XSECT Male/Female (n=7846) Grades 9–12	YRBS Self-report smoking behaviour	YRBS sports team participation at school			
Escobedo et al.[63]	XSECT Male/Female (n=11248) Grades 8–12	YRBS Self-report smoking behaviour	Self-report sport participation			
Davis et al.[33]	XSECT Male (n=1,200) M Age 15.8 y	Self-report use of smokeless tobacco	Self-report sport participation	XSECT Male (n=1,200) M Age 15.8 y	Self-report smoking (n.s. after controlling for race and GPA)	Self-report sport participation

Table 3.4.4 (*Continued*)

Study	Related to physical activity/fitness			Unrelated to physical activity/fitness		
	Study design*/pop. characteristics	Psychosocial well-being measures	Physical activity/ fitness measures	Study design/pop. characteristics	Psychosocial well-being measures	Physical activity/ fitness measures
Winnail et al.[64]	XSECT Male (n = 1607) Female (n = 1830) Grades 9–12	YRBS Self-report smoking and smokeless tobacco	YRBS number of days sweat/breathe hard			
Suicide						
Baumert et al.[31]	XSECT Male/Female (n = 6849) Grades 9–12	Feelings of hopelessness (− relationship)	Self-report participation in organized sports	XSECT Male/Female (n = 6849) Grades 9–12	Suicide ideation or a attempts	Self-report participation in organized sports
Oler et al.[30]	XSECT Female (n = 409) Grades 9–12	Index of potential suicide Suicide behaviour questionnaire (female only).	Self-report competitive athletics	XSECT Male (n = 409) Grades 9–12	Suicide behaviour questionnaire (male only)	Self-report competitive athletics
DeWilde et al.[67]		Children's Depression Inventory		CASE Male (n = 33) Female (n = 124)	Interviewed in year following suicide attempt	Self-report physical activity
Alcohol						
Thorlindsson et al.[48]	XSECT Male/Female (n = 1131) Age 15–16 y	Self-report alcohol use (binge drinking)	Self-report of sports participation			
Aaron et al.[60]	LONG Male (n = 641) Age 12–16 y	YRBS Self-report alcohol use	Self-report competitive athletics	LONG Female (n = 604) Age 12–16 y	YRBS Self-report alcohol use	Self-report leisure time
Baumert et al.[31]	XSECT Male/Female (n = 6849) Grades 9–12	YRBS Self-report alcohol use		XSECT Male/Female (n = 6849) Grades 9–12	YRBS Self-report alcohol use (binge drinking)	Self-report participation in organized sports
Carr et al.[29]	XSECT Male/Female (n = 1713) Grades 10–12	Self-report alcohol use (frequency) (male only) Abstention (− relationship)	Self-identification as athletic team member			

Study	Design, sample	Substance use measure	Physical activity measure	Design, sample	Substance use measure	Physical activity measure
Pate et al.[34]	XSECT Female (n = 1989) Age 12–18 y	YRBS Self-report alcohol use	YRBS physical activity items coded as low-high activity	XSECT Male (n = 2304) Age 12–18 y	Self-report alcohol use (YRBS)	YRBS physical activity items coded as low–high activity
Oler et al.[30]				XSECT Male (n = 409) Female (n = 409) Grades 9–12 y	Self-report alcohol use	Self-report competitive athletics
Rainey et al.[62]	XSECT Male/Female (n = 7846) Grades 9–12	YRBS self-report alcohol use and binge drinking	Self-report athletic teams and physical activity (+ relationship)			
Drug use						
Winnall et al.[64]	XSECT Male (n = 1607) Female (n = 1830)	YRBS self-report marijuana use	YRBS number of days sweat/breathe hard			
Oler et al.[30]	XSECT Male (n = 409) Female (n = 409) Grades 9–12	Self-report marijuana use	Self-report competitive athletics	XSECT Male (n = 409) Female (n = 409) Grades 9–12	Self-report cocaine use	Self-report competitive athletics
Pate et al.[34]	XSECT Male (n = 2304) Female (n = 1989) Age 12–18 y	YRBS Self-report marijuana and cocaine use	YRBS physical activity items coded as low-high activity			
Collingwood et al.[68]	QEXP, CLINICAL Male (n = 46) Female (n = 28) M Age 16.8 y	Self-report substance use	Fitness test			

Table 3.4.4 (Continued)

Study	Related to physical activity/fitness			Unrelated to physical activity/fitness		
	Study design*/pop. characteristics	Psychosocial well-being measures	Physical activity/ fitness measures	Study design/pop. characteristics	Psychosocial well-being measures	Physical activity/ fitness measures
Aggression						
Pate et al.[34]				XSECT Male (n = 2304) Female (n = 1989) Age 12–18 y	Injured in a physical fight (past 30 d)	YRBS physical activity items coded as low-high activity
Begg et al.[65]	LONG Male/Female (n = 1037) Age 15–18 y	Self-reported delinquency, aggressive behaviours, social competence index	Self-report leisure time physical activity	LONG Male/Female (n = 1037) Age 15–18 y	Self-reported delinquency, aggressive behaviours, social competence index	Sports participation
Sexual behaviours						
Smith and Caldwell[28]	XSECT Male/Female (n = 1071) Grades 9 to 11	Self-report of participation in sexual intercourse	Self-report of high school interscholastic sports (participants more likely to have had sex)			
Miller et al.[32]	XSECT Female (n = 335) Age 15–18 y	Self-report participation in sexual activities	Self-report athletic participation (– relation for girls)	XSECT Male (n = 276) Age 15–18 y	Self-report participation in sexual activities	Self-report athletic participation
Pate et al.[34]				XSECT Male (n = 2304) Female (n = 1989) Age 12–18 y	No. of sex partners in past 3 months	YRBS physical activity items coded as low-high activity
Forman et al.[64]	XSECT Male (n = 1112) Age 13–19 y	Self-report participation in sexual intercourse	Self-report of high school interscholastic sports			

YRBS = Youth Risk Behaviour Survey.

The challenges are many for future research studies on the effects of physical activity and fitness on the social, psychological and emotional health of children and adolescents. One challenge is to improve the reliability and validity of the activity and fitness and psychosocial measures. Many studies did not present evidence for reliability and validity of the measures. Further, the developmental appropriateness of the measures should be documented. Another challenge is conducting more studies with longitudinal and experimental designs. Many of the findings are based on cross-sectional studies or studies without control groups. In these cases, caution is required in interpreting results and confidence in findings is limited. A third challenge is generalizability. More studies are needed with girls, diverse racial and ethnic groups, diverse social classes, varied age groups and diverse health statuses (e.g. obese youth, hypertensive youth, etc.). By including a broader range of youth, the confidence in the robustness of the findings increases.

A fourth challenge is to understand the processes or mediators underlying the relationship and the context of the activity. Three potential mediating factors are:

(1) 'time out' theory;
(2) self significance; and
(3) biochemical changes.[70]

The 'time out' theory is that physical activity diverts attention away from environmental stressors and thus positive benefits are achieved. The self-significance mechanism is that regular physical activity provides a sense of self-mastery, competence and control. The biochemical mechanism is that as a result of physical activity alterations in central neurotransmitters, cortisol levels, body temperature, cerebral blood flow and endogenous opiates influence psychological states.[70] Potential biological changes are endorphins and plasma catecholamine and monoamine levels.[8] These factors as well as other potential factors should be explored in greater depth.

To better understand mediating factors, distinctions should be reported between fitness versus activity effects. Also, extra programme influences (e.g. attention and social support) should be carefully moni-tored and evaluated. These influences can affect results and may be unrelated to the activity. Another important consideration is the context of the activity. The context can be competition, self-appraisal, individual versus group activities, or structured activities to lose weight or improve strength and endurance. The context and the perceptions of youth should be described to better understand the meaning of results.

In summary, future research should demonstrate consistency in methods and measurement techniques. More reliable, valid, and developmentally appropriate measures, longer time periods, repeated assessments, and more youth from more diverse income levels, ages, cultural settings and ethnic backgrounds are needed. More data on the stability and permanence of effects (long term follow-up) can improve the research in this area. Finally, findings from scientifically grounded research will result in more definitive conclusions. Then, the effects of activity and fitness on the social, psychological and emotional health of children and adolescents will be better understood.

Acknowledgements

We gratefully acknowledge the assistance of Ms Regina Jones Johnson and Ms Sandra De la Garza in identifying relevant literature.

References

1. Biddle, S. Exercise and psychosocial health. *Research Quarterly for Exercise and Sport* 1995; 66: 292–7.
2. Dishman, R. K. Medical psychology in exercise and sport. *Medical Clinics of North America* 1985; 69: 123–43.
3. Folkins, C. H. and Sime, W. E. Physical fitness training and mental health. *American Psychologist* 1981; 36: 373–89.
4. Shephard, R. J. Physical activity, health, and well-being at different life stages. *Research Quarterly for Exercise and Sport* 1995; 66: 298–302.
5. Byrne, A. and Byrne, D. G. The effect of exercise on depression, anxiety and other mood states: a review. *Journal of Psychosomatic Research* 1993; 37: 565–74.
6. LaFontaine, T. P., DiLorenzo, T. M., Frensch, P. A., Stucky-Ropp, R. C., Bargman, E.P. and McDonald, D. G. Aerobic exercise and mood: a brief review, 1985–1990. *Sports Medicine* 1992; 13: 160–70.
7. Taylor, C. B., Sallis, J. F. and Needle, R. The relation of physical activity and exercise to mental health. *Public Health Reports* 1985; 100: 195–202.
8. McAuley, E. Physical activity and psychosocial outcomes. In *Physical activity, fitness, and health: international proceedings and consensus statement* (ed. C. Bouchard, R. J. Shephard and T. Stephens). Human Kinetics, Champaign, IL, 1994; 551–68.
9. Sonstroem, R. J. Exercise and self esteem. *Exercise and Sport Sciences Reviews* 1984; 12: 123–55.
10. Weiss, M. R. Self-esteem and achievement in children's sport and physical activity. *Advances in Pediatric Sport Sciences* 1987; 2: 87–119.
11. Brown, R. S. Exercise and mental health in the pediatric population. *Clinics in Sports Medicine* 1982; 1: 515–27.
12. Calfas, K. J. and Taylor, W. C. Effects of physical activity on psychological variables in adolescents. *Pediatric Exercise Science* 1994; 6: 406–23.
13. MacMahon, J. R. and Gross, R. T. Physical and psychological effects of aerobic exercise in boys with learning disabilities. *Journal of Developmental and Behavioral Pediatrics* 1987; 8: 274–7.
14. Overbay, J. D. and Purath, J. Self-concept and health status in elementary-school-aged children. *Issues in Comprehensive Pediatric Nursing* 1997; 20: 89–101.
15. Hatfield, B. D, Vaccaro, P. and Benedict, G. J. Self-concept responses of children to participation in an eight-week precision jump-rope program. *Perceptual and Motor Skills* 1985; 61: 1275–9.
16. MacMahon, J. R. and Gross, R. T. Physical and psychological effects of aerobic exercise in delinquent adolescent males. *American Journal of Diseases of Children* 1988; 142: 1361–6.
17. Parish-Plass, J. and Lufi, D. Combining physical activity with a behavioral approach in the treatment of young boys with behavior disorders. *Small Group Research* 1997; 28: 357–69.
18. Sherrill, C., Holguin, O. and Caywood, A. J. Fitness, attitude toward physical education, and self-concept of elementary school children. *Perceptual and Motor Skills* 1989; 69: 411–4.
19. Young, M. L. Estimation of fitness and physical ability, physical performance, and self-concept among adolescent females. *Journal of Sports Medicine and Physical Fitness* 1985; 25: 144–50.
20. Blackman, L., Hunter, G., Hilyer, J. and Harrison, P. The effects of dance team participation on female adolescent physical fitness and self-concept. *Adolescence* 1988; 23: 437–48.
21. Boyd, K. R. and Hrycaiko, D. W. The effect of a physical activity intervention package on the self-esteem of pre-adolescent and adolescent females. *Adolescence* 1997; 32: 693–708.
22. Koniak-Grifin, D. Aerobic exercise, psychological well-being, and physical discomforts during adolescent pregnancy. *Research in Nursing and Health* 1994; 17: 253–63.
23. Hawkins, D. B. and Gruber, J. J. Little League baseball and players' self-esteem. *Perceptual and Motor Skills* 1982; 55: 1335–40.
24. Sonstroem, R. J., Harlow, L. L. and Salsbury, K. S. Path analysis of a self-esteem model across a competitive swim season. *Research Quarterly for Exercise and Sport* 1993; 64: 335–42.
25. Aine, D. and Lester, D. Exercise, depression, and self-esteem [comment]. *Perceptual and Motor Skills* 1995; 81: 890.

26. Fox, K. R. and Corbin, C. C. The Physical Self-perception Profile: development and preliminary validation. *Journal of Sport and Exercise Psychology.* 1989; **11**: 408–430.

27. Gill, D. Gender issues: a social-educational perspective. In *Sport psychology interventions* (ed. S. M. Murphy). Human Kinetics, Champaign, IL, 1995: 205–34.

28. Smith, E. A. and Caldwell, L. L. Participation in high school sports and adolescent sexual activity. *Pediatric Exercise Science* 1994; **6**: 69–74.

29. Carr, C. N., Kennedy, S. R. and Dimick, K. M. Alcohol use among high school athletes: a comparison of alcohol use and intoxication of male and female high school athletes and non-athletes. *Journal of Alcohol and Drug Education* 1990; **36**: 39–43.

30. Oler, M. J., Mainous, A. G. 3d, Martin C. A., Richardson, E., Haney, A., Wilson, D. and Adams, T. Depression, suicidal ideation, and substance use among adolescents: Are athletes at less risk? *Archives of Family Medicine* 1994; **3**: 781–5.

31. Baumert, P. W. Jr., Henderson, J. M. and Thompson, N. J. Health risk behaviors of adolescent participants in organized sports. *Journal of Adolescent Health* 1998; **22**: 460–5.

32. Miller, K. E., Sabo, D. F., Farrell, M. P., Barnes, G. M. and Melnick, M. J. Athletic participation and sexual behavior in adolescents: the different worlds of boys and girls. *Journal of Health and Social Behavior* 1998; **39**: 108–23.

33. Davis, T. C., Arnold, C., Nandy, I., Bocchini, J. A., Gottlieb, A., George, R. B. and Berkel, H. Tobacco use among male high school athletes. *Journal of Adolescent Health* 1997; **21**: 97–101.

34. Pate, R. R., Heath, G. W., Dowda, M. and Trost, S. G. Associations between physical activity and other health behaviors in a representative sample of US adolescents. *American Journal of Public Health* 1996; **86**: 1577–81.

35. Jaffe L. Adolescent girls: factors influencing low and high body image. *Melpomen: A Journal for Women's Health Research* 1995; **14**: 14–22.

36. Tuckman, B. W. and Hinkle, J. S. An experimental study of the physical and psychological effects of aerobic exercise on school children. *Health Psychology* 1986; **5**: 197–207.

37. Bandura, A. Self-efficacy: toward a unifying theory of behavioral change. *Psychological Review* 1977; **84**: 191–215.

38. Brawley L. R. and Rodgers, W. M. Social-psychological aspects of fitness promotion. In *Exercise psychology: the influence of physical exercise on psychological processes* (ed. P. Seraganian). J. W. Wiley, New York, 1993; 254–98.

39. Brown, S. W., Welsh, M. C., Labbe, E. E, Vitulli, W. F. and Kulkarni, P. Aerobic exercise in the psychological treatment of adolescents. *Perceptual and Motor Skills* 1992; **74**: 555–60.

40. Holloway, J. B., Beuter, A. and Duda, J. L. Self–efficacy and training for strength in adolescent girls. *Journal of Applied Social Psychology* 1988; **18**: 699–719.

41. Horn, T. S. and Claytor, R. P. Developmental aspects of exercise psychology. In *Exercise psychology: the influence of physical exercise on psychological processes* (ed. P. Seraganian). J. W. Wiley, New York, 1993; 299–338.

42. Kirkendall, D. R. Effects of physical activity on intellectual development and academic performance. *American Academy of Physical Education Papers* 1985; **19**: 49–63.

43. Mechanic, D. and Hansell, S. Adolescent competence, psychological well-being, and self-assessed physical health. *Journal of Health and Social Behavior* 1987; **28**: 364–74.

44. Bluechardt, M. H. and Shephard, R. J. Using an extracurricular physical activity program to enhance social skills. *Journal of Learning Disabilities* 1995; **28**: 160–9.

45. Aganoff, J. A. and Boyle, G. J. Aerobic exercise, mood states and menstrual cycle symptoms. *Journal of Psychosomatic Research* 1994; **38**: 183–92.

46. Engstrom, I., Fallstrom, K., Karlberg, E., Sten, G. and Bjure, J. Psychological and respiratory physiological effects of a physical exercise programme on boys with severe asthma. *Acta Paediatrica Scandinavica* 1991; **80**: 1058–65.

47. Page, R. M. and Tucker, L. A. Psychosocial discomfort and exercise frequency: an epidemiological study of adolescents. *Adolescence* 1994; **29**: 183–191.

48. Thorlindsson, T., Vilhjalmsson, R. and Valgeirsson, G. Sport participation and perceived health status: a study of adolescents. *Social Science and Medicine* 1990; **31**: 551–6.

49. Leonard, W. M. *Physical activity and psychological well-being among high school seniors.* Paper presented to the North American Society of the Sociology of Sport: November 16, 1996; Birmingham, Alabama.

50. Dua, J. and Hargreaves, L. Effect of aerobic exercise on negative affect, positive affect, stress, and depression. *Perceptual and Motor Skills* 1992; **75**: 335–61.

51. Michaud-Tomson, L. M. *Childhood depressive symptoms, physical activity and health-related fitness.* Unpublished doctoral dissertation, Arizona State University, Columbia, AZ, 1995.

52. Milligan, R. A. K., Burke, V., Beilin, L. J., Richards, J. Dunbar, D., Spencer, M., Balde, E. and Gracey, M. P. Health-related behaviours and psycho-social characteristics of 18-year-old Australians. *Social Science and Medicine* 1997; **45**: 1549–62.

53. Norris, R., Carroll, D. and Cochrane, R. The effects of physical activity and exercise training on psychological stress and well-being in an adolescent population. *Journal of Psychosomatic Research* 1992; **36**: 55–65.

54. Brown, J. D. and Lawton, M. Stress and well-being in adolescence: the moderating role of physical exercise. *Journal of Human Stress* 1986; **12**: 125–31.

55. Glyshaw, K., Cohen, L. H. and Towbes, L. C. Coping strategies and psychological distress: Prospective analyses of early and middle adolescents. *American Journal of Community Psychology* 1989; **17**: 607–23.

56. Johnsgard, K. W. *The exercise prescription for depression and anxiety.* Plenum Press, New York, 1989.

57. Bahrke, M. S. and Smith, R. G. Alterations in anxiety of children after exercise and rest. *American Corrective Therapy* 1995; **39**: 90–4.

58. Steptoe, A. and Butler, N. Sports participation and emotional wellbeing in adolescents. *Lancet* 1996; **347**: 1789–92.

59. Berger B. G., Grove, J. R., Prapavessis, H. and Butki, B. D. Relationship of swimming distance, expectancy, and performance to mood states of competitive athletes. *Perceptual and Motor Skills* 1997; **84**: 1199–210.

60. Aaron, D. J., Dearwater, S. R., Anderson, R., Olsen, T., Kriska, A. M. and Laporte, R. E. Physical activity and the initiation of high-risk health behaviors in adolescents. *Medicine and Science in Sports and Exercise* 1995; **27**: 1639–45.

61. Coulson, N. S., Eiser, C. and Eiser, J. R. Diet, smoking and exercise: Interrelatioships between adolescent health behaviours. *Child: Care, Health and Development* 1997; **23**: 207–16.

62. Rainey, C. J., McKeown, R. E., Sargent, R. G. and Valois, R. F. Patterns of tobacco and alcohol use among sedentary, exercising, nonathletic, and athletic youth. *Journal of School Health* 1996; **66**: 27–32.

63. Escobedo, L. G., Marcus, S. E., Holtzman, D. and Giovino, G. A. Sports participation, age at smoking initiation, and the risks of smoking among US high school students. *Journal of the American Medical Association* 1993; **269**: 1391–5.

64. Winnail, S. D., Valois, R. F., McKeown, R. E., Saunders, R. P. and Pate, R. R. Relationship between physical activity level and cigarette, smokeless tobacco, and marijuana use among public high school adolescents. *Journal of School Health* 1995; **65**: 438–42.

65. Begg, D. J., Langley, J. D., Moffitt, T. and Marshall, S. W. Sport and delinquency: an examination of the deterrence hypothesis in a longitudinal study. *British Journal of Sports Medicine* 1996; **30**: 335–41.

66. Hilyer, J. C., Wilson, D. G., Dillon, C., Caro, L., Jenkins, C., Spenser, W. A., Meadows, M. E. and Booker, W. Physical fitness training and counseling as treatment for youth offenders. *Journal of Counseling Psychology* 1982; **29**: 292–303.

67. DeWilde, E. J., Kienhorst, C. W. M., Diekstra, R. F. W. and Wolters, W. H. G. Social support, life events, and behavioral characteristics of psychologically distressed adolescents at high risk for attempting suicide. *Adolescence* 1994; **29**: 49–60.

68. Collingwood, T. R., Reynolds, R., Kohl, H. W., Smith, W. and Sloan, S. Physical fitness effects on substance abuse risk factors and use patterns. *Journal of Drug Education* 1991; **21**: 73–84.

69. Forman, E., Dekker, A. H., Javors, J. R. and Davidson, D. T. High-risk behaviors in teenage male athletes. *Clinical Journal of Sports Medicine* 1995; **5**: 36–42.

70. Rowland, T. W. *Exercise and children's health*. Human Kinetics Books, Champaign, IL., 1990.

71. Brown, J. D. and Seigel, J. M. Exercise as a buffer of life stress: a prospective study of adolescent health. *Health Psychology* 1998; **7**: 341–535.

3.5 Sport, physical activity and other health behaviours in children and adolescents

Stewart G. Trost, Sarah Levin and Russell R. Pate

Introduction

Millions of children worldwide are involved in organized sports. In the United States alone, an estimated 22 million children between the ages of 5 and 17 years are involved in agency-sponsored sports programmes, such as Little League Baseball and Pop Warner football, with another 24 million involved in club sports, recreational sports programmes, intramural sports programmes and interscholastic sports.[1] Recent data from the US Centers for Disease Control and Prevention (CDC) indicates that approximately 60% of US high school students participate on at least one school or community-based sports team.[2]

Participation in sports has long been thought to promote proper social and moral development in youth.[2] Indeed, when delivered in a responsible, age-appropriate manner, youth sports programmes seemingly provide excellent opportunities for children to increase their self-confidence and learn important lessons about fair play, teamwork and achievement. Besides these outcomes, there is some evidence to suggest that youth sports programmes can deter negative behaviour such as juvenile delinquency, gang membership, and alcohol and drug use.[3] Most youth sports programmes are offered during 'at-risk' times (after-school and on weekends), thus limiting participants' opportunities to engage in negative behaviours. Furthermore, participation in sports is often made contingent upon following rules and regulations that overtly discourage negative behaviours such as skipping school and experimenting with drugs and alcohol. Related to this area of research are the on-going efforts to determine whether health-related behaviours such as physical activity 'cluster' with other health behaviours in youth.[4,5,6] The existence of such clustering implies that positive change in one behaviour (e.g. physical activity) may produce favourable changes in others (e.g. diet, smoking and alcohol use).

The purpose of this review is to summarize the research literature pertaining to the relationships between sports participation and selected health behaviours in children and adolescents. Furthermore, given that sports participation provides substantial amounts of physical activity, we overview the results of studies evaluating the association between physical activity and other health behaviours in youth. The following health behaviours were considered: use of tobacco (cigarettes and smokeless tobacco), alcohol, illegal drugs, anabolic steroids, dietary intake (fruit and vegetable consumption, and high-fat food consumption), weight control practices, sexual activity and violence. The prevalence rates of these health behaviours, as estimated from the 1997 US Youth Risk Behavior Survey (YRBS), are presented in Table 3.5.1.

Method

A search of the scientific literature was conducted using several electronic databases, including MEDLINE, SOCIAL SCIENCES INDEX, ERIC and READER'S GUIDE TO PERIODICAL LITERATURE. Searches were supplemented by direct examination of reference lists of recovered articles. The key words used for the computer searches were: youth, adolescent, physical activity, sports, physical education, health behaviours, tobacco, smoking, alcohol, steroids, drugs, sexual behaviour, violence, weight loss and diet. No limitations were imposed as to publication date or country of origin, except that the article had to be published in the English language. Studies were included if they included children and/or adolescents and provided a measure of association between sports or physical activity participation and a specific health behaviour (e.g. odds ratio, prevalence contrast, correlation coefficient, beta coefficient). The studies included subjects primarily 18 years and younger, although studies including college-aged athletes were cited if they contributed breadth to the topic. In each of the following sections, we first summarize the literature addressing associations between sports participation and the selected health behaviour. Second, associations between physical activity and that behaviour are addressed.

Cigarette smoking

Sports participation

Relative to other health behaviours, the relationship between youth sports participation and cigarette smoking has been studied quite extensively. Escobedo *et al.*[7] examined the relationship between school sport participation and cigarette smoking in a nationally representative sample of US high school students. After adjustments for age, sex, race/ethnicity and academic performance, students reporting participation in three or more scholastic sports teams in the previous 12 months were 2.5 times less likely than non-participants to be classified as regular smokers (smoked on 5 to 15 of the last 30 days). Moreover, when the analyses were restricted to current smokers, students participating in three or more sports in the previous 12 months were 2.5 times less likely than non-participants to be classified as heavy smokers (⩾ 5 cigarettes/day).

Utilizing data from the 1993 YRBS, Pate and colleagues[2] examined the relationship between sports participation and cigarette smoking in US high school students. In contrast to the earlier Escobedo study,[7] the authors examined participation in both school and community-based sports teams. Furthermore, to assess the relationship between sports

Table 3.5.1 Estimated prevalence rates of selected risk behaviours among US high school students

Risk behaviour	Prevalence (%)
Tobacco use	
Smoked cigarettes in the past 30 days	36.4
Used smokeless tobacco	9.3
Alcohol use	
Drank alcohol in the past 30 days	50.8
Had five or more drinks per occasion (at least one time)	33.4
Drug use	
Ever used marijuana	47.1
Ever used cocaine	8.2
Ever used other illegal drugs	17.0
Steroid use	
Ever used steroids	3.1
Dietary habits	
Ate less than 5 servings of fruits & vegetables yesterday	70.7
Ate more than 2 servings of foods high in fat	27.7
Sexual behaviour	
Had sex in the past 3 months	34.8
Had sex with 4 or more partners	16.0
Violence	
Had physical fight in the past year	36.6
Carried a weapon in the past month	18.3
Attempted suicide in the past year	7.7
Weight loss practices	
Dieting to lose weight	30.4
Used laxatives or vomited to lose weight	4.5
Used diet pills to lose weight	4.9

Source: 1997 Centers for Disease Control and Prevention Youth Risk Behavior Survey.

participation *per se* and cigarette smoking, the authors controlled for weekly participation in vigorous physical activity. After further adjustments for age and race/ethnicity, students reporting participation in one or more sports teams during the previous 12 months were 1.2 to 1.3 times less likely than non-participants to report smoking in the past 30 days. This trend was observed in both genders but was only statistically significant among females.

Thorlindsson and colleagues[8–10] examined the association between sports participation and cigarette smoking in several population-representative samples of Icelandic youth. In two random samples of youth aged 12 to 15 years, sports participation was inversely associated with cigarette smoking. Depending on the definition of sports participation (structured versus non-structured), the correlation ranged from -0.21 to -0.28. Among 15 to 16 year olds, both the frequency ($r = -0.22$) and duration of sports participation ($r = -0.24$) were inversely associated with cigarette smoking.

In a secondary analysis of the 1991 and 1993 South Carolina YRBS data, Rainey *et al.*[11] assessed the relationship between sports participation and cigarette smoking in a sample of 7846 high school students.

After controlling for race/ethnicity, sex and participation in school physical education, non-athletes were significantly more likely to report cigarette smoking in the past 30 days than athletes. When the analyses were restricted to current smokers, sedentary non-athletes were found to be the heaviest smokers, smoking approximately 11 packs during the past 30 days. In a further analysis of the 1993 YRBS data, Winnail and colleagues[12] reported sports participation to be inversely related to cigarette smoking among white males and females. However, among African-American students, athletes were approximately twice as likely as non-athletes to report cigarette smoking in the past 30 days.

Baumert *et al.*[13] compared the prevalence of smoking among athletes ($n = 4036$) and non-athletes ($n = 2813$) from a single school district in southern Georgia. After controlling for age, race/ethnicity and gender, athletes were significantly less likely than non-athletes to report smoking one or more cigarettes in the past 30 days. Oler *et al.*[14] compared cigarette smoking rates in high school athletes ($n = 243$) and non-athletes ($n = 575$) from Kentucky. After controlling for age, sex, race/ethnicity and academic performance, non-athletes were four times more likely than athletes to smoke cigarettes. Davis et al.[15] examined the relationship between sports participation and cigarette smoking in 1200 high school males from northwest Louisiana. Medium- and high-intensity athletes were significantly less likely to be heavy smokers than athletes participating in low-intensity sports and non-athletes. However, when these relationships were adjusted for race/ethnicity and academic performance, the association between sports participation was no longer significant. Lastly, Forman et al.[16] compared the smoking rates of 1117 male high school athletes from northwest Indiana with the prevalence estimates obtained from the 1989 National Survey of American High School Seniors. Relative to the survey participants (65.7%), athletes (27.9%) were significantly less likely to experiment with cigarettes.

Physical activity

Results from population-based studies conducted in the United States and Finland provide consistent evidence of a significant inverse association between physical activity and cigarette smoking among adolescent youth. Pate et al.[17] assessed the relationship between physical activity and cigarette smoking in a nationally representative sample of US high school students ($n = 11 631$). After controlling for age, sex and race/ethnicity, low active youth were found to be 1.42 times more likely than active students to have smoked one or more cigarettes in the past 30 days. As part of the Cardiovascular Risk in Young Finns study, Raitakari et al.[18] prospectively examined the association between physical activity and cigarette smoking in a nationally representative sample of Finnish youth aged 12 to 18 years. Male adolescents who remained sedentary over the six-year follow-up period were significantly more likely than their active counterparts to either begin smoking (33.3% versus 0%) or smoke on a daily basis (46.9% versus 9.3%). Similarly, females who remained sedentary over the six-year follow-up period were significantly more likely than active females to either begin smoking (25.9% versus 4.6%) or smoke on a daily basis (45.5% versus 8.7%).

Smaller scale studies involving less broadly representative samples of youth also provide evidence of an inverse relationship between physical activity and cigarette smoking. Winnail and coworkers[19] assessed the relationship between physical activity level and cigarette use among high school students from a single state in the southern United States. Among white males, low-activity students were almost twice as likely as high-activity students to report cigarette use in the past 30 days. However, no association was observed in black males or females. Aaron et al.[20] prospectively examined the relationship of leisure-time physical activity and cigarette smoking in high school students from a single city in the northeastern United States. After controlling for gender, race/ethnicity and academic performance, a significant inverse association was observed among females but not males. The percentage of females reporting cigarette smoking among the highest tertile for physical activity (10%) was significantly lower than the percentage observed for the moderate (23%) and low physical activity tertiles (22%). Kelder and colleagues[21] noted a similar trend among students participating in the Minnesota Class of 1989 Study. The prevalence of cigarette smoking among low-active students was at least 14% higher than students in the highest physical activity tertile.

A small number of studies have investigated the relationship between physical activity and cigarette smoking in preadolescent youth. Valois et al.[22] investigated the relationship between physical

activity and cigarette smoking in 374 fifth grade students from rural South Carolina. The authors found no relationship between physical activity and experimentation with cigarette smoking. D'Elio et al.[23] studied the relationship between physical activity level and experimentation with cigarette smoking in 303 urban African-American fourth grade students. Unexpectedly, students with moderate to very high levels of physical activity were 3.7 to 8 times more likely than low active students to try cigarette smoking. However, the number of students experimenting with cigarettes was small, and none of the reported associations were significant at the 0.05 level. The negative findings of this study of preadolescents are likely attributable to the relatively low prevalence of cigarette smoking in this population.

Conclusion

Studies examining the relationship between cigarette smoking and sports participation or physical activity are numerous and generally consistent in identifying an inverse association. For sports participation, it appears that athletes are about 1.2 to 4 times less likely than non-athletes to smoke cigarettes. For physical activity, it appears that active adolescents are about 1.4 to 5 times less likely to smoke cigarettes than their low-active counterparts. Only two of the identified studies did not report an inverse association, and both of these studies focused on elementary aged school children among whom the prevalence of cigarette smoking is low.

Smokeless tobacco
Sports participation

Pate et al.[2] assessed the relationship between sports participation and smokeless tobacco use in a nationally-representative sample of US high school students. After controlling for age, race/ethnicity and participation in vigorous physical activity, sports participants were significantly more likely than their non-sporting counterparts to report smokeless tobacco use in the previous 30 days; however, this association reached statistical significance among the males only. Karvonen et al.[24] assessed the relationship between sports participation and smokeless tobacco use in three population-representative samples of Finnish adolescents aged 16 and 18 years. After controlling for socioeconomic status, participation in organized sports was significantly associated with smokeless tobacco use, but only among boys living in urban areas. For boys living in less urbanized areas, the prevalence of smokeless tobacco use was low and unrelated to physical activity or sports participation.

Smaller studies involving less representative samples of children and adolescents have produced equivocal findings. While some studies report a positive relationship between sports participation and smokeless tobacco use, others have found no association whatsoever. Rainey et al.[11] evaluated the relationship between sports participation and smokeless tobacco use among respondents to the 1991 and 1993 South Carolina Youth Risk Behavior Survey. After controlling for race/ethnicity, sex and participation in school physical education, high school sports participation was positively associated with smokeless tobacco use in the 30 days preceding the survey; however, this trend failed to reach statistical significance. In a separate analysis of the 1993 South Carolina YRBS data set, Winnail and colleagues[12] reported no association between high school sports participation and smokeless tobacco use. Oler et al.[14] contrasted smokeless tobacco use in 243 athletes and 575 non-athletes attending a suburban high school in Kentucky. Consistent with the findings of Rainey and Winnail, the prevalence of chewing tobacco and snuff use was found to be similar in athletes and non-athletes (~10%). Davis et al.[15] examined the association between sports participation and smokeless tobacco use in 1200 high school males from northwest Louisiana. After controlling for race, grade point average and sport intensity, athletes were significantly more likely than non-athletes to use chewing tobacco or snuff. On average, the rate of smokeless tobacco use was approximately 1.5 times higher among athletes than non-athletes.

Sussman et al.[25] examined the predictors of smokeless tobacco use in two successive cohorts of seventh grade students residing in the Los Angeles metropolitan area. Cross-sectional analyses of data collected during the participants' seventh and eighth grade years showed sports participation to be unrelated to experimentation with smokeless tobacco. However, among girls in the second cohort, sports participation in the seventh grade was significantly associated with smokeless tobacco use in the eighth grade. Seventeen per cent of the girls who reported participation in four or more competitive sports reported having tried smokeless tobacco, compared with 8.5% of girls who reported participation in three or less competitive sports over the same period. Sports participation in the seventh grade was not associated with smokeless tobacco use in the eighth grade among boys from either cohort or girls from cohort one.

Physical activity

Winnail and coworkers[18] assessed the relationship between physical activity level and smokeless tobacco use among high school students from a single state in the southern United States ($n = 4800$). Among white males and African-American females, students with low and moderate levels of physical activity were significantly more likely than those with high levels of physical activity to report smokeless tobacco use in the previous 30 days. Among white females and African-American males, low and moderate levels of physical activity were associated with decreased risk of smokeless tobacco use compared to those with high levels of physical activity; however, none of these associations reached statistical significance.

Conclusion

The question of whether youth sports participants are at greater risk for smokeless tobacco use has received a moderate amount of research attention. Results from population-based studies suggest that sports participation is positively associated with smokeless tobacco use, but only in specific population groups (i.e. males). Smaller studies involving less broadly representative samples of adolescent youth have produced mixed results. While some studies report a positive association between sports participation and smokeless tobacco use, others have found no association. To date only one study has assessed the association between physical activity and smokeless tobacco use in youth. Consistent with the results of sports participation studies, the relationship between physical activity and smokeless tobacco use varies considerably with sex and race/ethnicity. More studies related to youth physical activity and smokeless tobacco use are needed.

Alcohol use

Sports participation

Buhrman[26] examined the relationship between sport participation and alcohol use in 857 high school females from rural Iowa. After controlling for parental occupation, mother's education, cumulative grade point average, membership in out-of-school organizations and social status, a significant inverse correlation of -0.40 was observed between sports participation and alcohol use. Thorlindsson[8] examined the relationship between sports participation and alcohol use in two large samples of rural Icelandic youth age 12 to 15 years old. The correlation between sports participation and use of alcohol ranged from -0.04 to 0.12, indicating a weak to non-existent association between sports participation and alcohol use. In a further study of Icelandic youth, Thorlindsson et al.[10] examined the relationship between sports participation and alcohol consumption in a nationally representative sample of 1200 15 to 16-year-olds. Both the frequency of sports participation and the hours engaged in sport were inversely associated with alcohol consumption ($r = -0.19$ and -0.17, respectively).

Donato et al.[27] compared the drinking habits of 330 elite male athletes to those of 366 male high school students residing in the same area of northern Italy. After controlling for social class, parental education, parental alcohol use, peer alcohol use, smoking status and judgement of alcohol as harmful, sports participation was found to have a significant inverse relationship with total alcohol intake, frequency of wine drinking and amount of spirits consumed. Nativ and Puffer[28] contrasted the drinking practices of 109 intercollegiate athletes and 110 non-athletic controls. After controlling for age, sex, race and campus living status, athletes were significantly more likely than non-athletes to report drinking three or more alcohol beverages per sitting. Athletes and non-athletes did not differ significantly with respect to the frequency of alcohol consumption.

Physical activity

Aarnio et al.[29] examined the association between leisure time physical activity and alcohol consumption among 1097 boys and 1014 girls from Finland. Participants were categorized into one of five physical activity levels ranging from sedentary (no leisure time physical activity in the previous month) to very active (vigorous physical activity 4–5 times/week). An inverse relationship was observed between physical activity and the frequency of alcohol use; however, this association reached statistical significance only among the girls. Faulkner and Slattery[30] (1990) investigated the relationship between physical activity and alcohol use among 257 Canadian high school students. After placing students into gender specific activity tertiles, a significant positive association between physical activity level and alcohol consumption was observed in males but not females. Rainey and colleagues[11] studied the relationship between physical activity level, participation in school sports and alcohol use in a random sample of high school students from South Carolina. After controlling for race/ethnicity, gender and physical education status, sports participants with moderate and high levels of physical activity were found to be significantly more likely to report drinking on 6 to 19 of the 30 days preceding the survey. Physically active sports participants also reported drinking more frequently than non-sports participants, and were more likely than sedentary non-sports participants to have engaged in episodes of binge drinking in the previous month ($\geqslant 5$ drinks at a sitting).

Utilizing data from the 1990 Youth Risk Behavior Survey, Pate et al.[17] examined the association between physical activity and alcohol consumption in a nationally representative sample of US high school students. After controlling for age group, gender and race/ethnicity, females classified as physically active were significantly less likely than their low active counterparts to report alcohol use in the 30 days preceding the survey. No association was found between physical activity and alcohol use among male high school students.

A small number of studies have investigated the association between physical activity and experimentation with alcohol in children. In a study of 381 sixth grade students, Hastad et al.[31] reported experimentation with alcohol or tobacco to be approximately 10% lower among sports participants (24.1% versus 34.0%). This difference remained intact when participants were stratified into low and high socioeconomic groups. In conflict with this finding, Felton et al.[32] reported no association between participation in moderate to vigorous physical activity and alcohol experimentation in rural fifth grade children from South Carolina. D'Elio et al.[23] evaluated the association between exercise level and alcohol experimentation in 303 African-American fourth and fifth grade students. Students reporting moderate and high levels of physical activity were more likely than their low-active counterparts to report alcohol use; however, this association was not statistically significant when adjusted for gender, socioeconomic status, use of other abusable substances, friends' use, self-esteem and academic performance.

Aaron et al.[20] prospectively examined the relationships between leisure time physical activity, participation in competitive sports and alcohol consumption in high school students from Pittsburgh. After controlling for gender, race/ethnicity and age, a significant positive association between leisure time physical activity and alcohol consumption was observed for male students. Furthermore, males who reported participation in competitive sports were significantly more likely than their non-sporting counterparts to report alcohol use in the month preceding the survey. No associations were found between physical activity, sports participation and alcohol use among female students.

Conclusion

The results of studies related to alcohol consumption and participation in sports and physical activity participation are inconsistent. Among adolescents under the age of 18, sports participation appears to be inversely associated with alcohol use. However, among older adolescents (i.e. college athletes), sports participation may be positively associated with alcohol use. The relationship between physical activity and alcohol consumption is even less clear. Among high school aged males, physical activity appears to be weakly associated with greater alcohol consumption. Among high school aged females, however, physical activity appears to be weakly associated with lower alcohol consumption.

Illegal drugs
Sports participation

Baumert et al.[13] compared the prevalence of marijuana use among athletes (n = 4036) and non-athletes (n = 2813) residing in a large city in the southern United States. After controlling for age, race and gender, athletes were significantly less likely than non-athletes to report marijuana use. Oler et al.[14] compared illicit drug use in high school athletes

(n = 243) and non-athletes (n = 575) from a single suburban high school in Kentucky. After controlling for age, sex, race and academic performance, non-athletes were found to be twice as likely as athletes to report marijuana use. No association was found between athletic participation and cocaine use. Winnail et al.[12] examined the relationship between sports participation and illicit drug use in 4800 public high school students from South Carolina. After adjusting for race and gender, sports participants were significantly less likely than non-participants to report using marijuana, cocaine and other illicit drugs, such as LSD, PCP and heroin. Forman et al.[16] compared the prevalence rates of drug use of 1117 male high school sport participants from the Chicago area with those reported in the 1989 National Survey of American High School Seniors. Relative to the survey participants, athletes were less likely to report use of marijuana, cocaine, amphetamines, barbiturates, heroin, PCP and LSD.

Physical activity

Using data from the South Carolina YRBS, Winnail et al.[19] contrasted marijuana use in high school students reporting low, moderate and high levels of physical activity. After stratifying the sample by gender and race, moderate and high levels of physical activity were found to be negatively associated with marijuana use among white males. No association was observed among African-American males and females. Robinson et al.[33] examined the predictors of substance use in 1447 tenth grade students. Self-reported participation in aerobic activity did not correlate significantly with use of illegal substances. Pate et al.[17] examined the relationship between physical activity status and illicit drug use in a population-representative sample of US high school students. After controlling for grade level, sex and race, students classified as physically active were significantly less likely to report using cocaine and marijuana in the 30 days preceding the survey.

Conclusion

A relatively small number of studies have examined the relationship between physical activity or sports participation and use of illegal drugs such as marijuana, cocaine, amphetamines and LSD. Most studies have focused on the potential of organized sports to prevent drug use and abuse among young people. Collectively, the results of these studies suggest an inverse relationship between sport participation and illicit drug use.

Anabolic steroids
Sports participation

Buckley et al.[34] were the first to comprehensively examine the prevalence of steroid use among high school athletes. They drew a sample of 12th grade male students from 150 high schools across the nation. Of those eligible, only 50.3% voluntarily participated. Eleven questions were used to establish current or previous use of steroids. Steroid users were more likely to participate in school sports programmes than non-users. When examined on a sports specific basis, steroid users were more likely to participate in football and wrestling than other school sports. Of interest, it was noted that 35.2% of users did not intend to participate in school-sponsored athletics. The largest percentage of users (47%) reported their main reason for using steroids was to improve athletic performance. Using the 1993 national YRBS data, Pate and colleagues[2] found that sports participation was associated with increased steroid use, but only among African-American males. These analyses were adjusted for age and participation in regular, vigorous physical activity.

DuRant et al.[35] used the 1991 national YRBS data set ($n = 12\,267$) to assess the relationship between steroid use and sports participation, and steroid use and strength training. After controlling for age, sex, academic performance, other drug use and region of the country, students who engaged in strength training were found to be significantly more likely to report lifetime steroid use than students who did not engage in strength training. Students who participated on a sports team were more likely than non-participants to report steroid use; however, this association did not reach statistical significance. In the midwest, both strength training and sports participation were significantly associated with increased likelihood of using anabolic steroids; while in the northeast, only strength training was significantly associated with steroid use. In the southern and western states, neither strength training nor sports participation was significantly associated with steroid use.

The 1993 South Carolina YRBS ($n = 3437$) revealed that non-athletes were slightly more likely to report steroid (non-significant) use in their lifetime compared to athletes (OR = 1.17 95% CI: 0.71–1.94).[12] When stratified by race and gender, it was found that white male and female non-athletes were significantly more likely to use other drugs including steroids than their athletic counterparts. In a study conducted in seven high schools in Georgia ($n = 6849$), no significant difference in steroid use (ever or current) between athletes and non-athletes was found after controlling for age, race and gender.[13]

Several studies conducted with non-representative samples of adolescent youth have observed a positive association between sports participation and steroid use among youth. Windsor and Dumitru[36] surveyed 901 high school students from one relatively affluent school district and one relatively lower socioeconomic status (SES) school district regarding their steroid use. Five per cent of males and 1.4% of females reported they had used steroids. In comparison, more than six per cent (6.7%) of male athletes, and 1.8% of male non-athletes took steroids. The males athletes from the higher SES schools reported significantly more steroid use than the male athletes from the lower SES schools (10.2% versus 2.8%). Tanner and colleagues[37] conducted a confidential survey questionnaire to assess anabolic steroid use among 6930 students from 10 high schools in Denver, Colorado. The overall prevalence of anabolic steroid use was 2.7% (4.0% for boys and 1.3% for girls). Use was slightly higher among sports participants (2.9%) than non-participants (2.2%).

Conclusion

The literature examining the relationship between youth sports participation and steroids use is inconsistent with the strength and direction of the association varying by race/ethnicity and by region of the country. A positive association may exist, but this may be limited to athletes such as football players and wrestlers. No studies were identified that examined physical activity and steroid use.

Dietary practices

Sports participation

French et al.[38] surveyed students in grades seven through ten (708 males and 786 females) in a mostly white, upper-middle class school district in Minnesota. Sports participation was assessed with a 28-item checklist representing activities of light to vigorous-intensity. Students were asked to check the activities that they performed for 20 minutes or more and indicate one of five choices as to when the activity was last performed (e.g. today, rarely or never). Dietary constructs were assessed with a 25-item questionnaire for preference (1 through 5) and recency of consumption (1 through 5) of various foods representing sweets, salty snacks, fruits and vegetables, and protein entrees. Factor analysis was used to group the activities into leisure sports, conditioning sports and atypical sports (sports played less frequently). Factor analysis was also used to group the foods into junk food or empty calories, salty snacks, healthy foods (e.g. fruits and vegetables, yoghurt) and protein entree (e.g. hamburger). Among both males and females, participation in leisure sports and conditioning sports was found to be correlated with recent healthy food choices ($r = 0.26$ to 0.36), and healthy food preferences ($r = 0.13$ to 0.20). Among females, conditioning sports ($r = -0.10$) and atypical sports ($r = -0.09$) were inversely correlated with salty snack preference, while conditioning sports were inversely associated with junk food preference ($r = -0.10$). Among males, conditioning sports was associated with protein entree preference ($r = 0.11$).

Baumert et al.[13] examined the relationship between sports participation and dietary intake in 7179 high school students from a single county in the southern United States. Compared to non-athletes, athletes were significantly more likely to report consuming breakfast, fruits and vegetables, and one serving from the dairy food group on a daily basis. They were also less likely to add salt to their foods. No differences were found in reported consumption of red meats, fried foods and snack foods.

Among the 14 747 US high school students who completed the 1993 YRBS, sports participants were more likely to report recent consumption of fruits and vegetables than non-participants. In addition, female sports participants were less likely to report recent consumption of high fat foods than non-participants.[2]

Physical activity

Pate et al.[17] analysed data from the national YRBS to determine if physically active adolescents were more likely than their low-active counterparts to report consumption of fruit or vegetables on the previous day. After adjustment for age group, sex and race, students who did not eat vegetables on the previous day were almost twice as likely to be low active than students who reported eating at least one serving of vegetables. Among the Hispanic and White subgroups, students who ate no fruit on the previous day were 2.3 and 3.1 times, respectively, more likely to be low active than those who ate one or more serving of fruit on the previous day.

Aarnio et al.[29] surveyed 1097 girls and 1014 boys in Finland from 1991–1993. Physical activity behaviour was classified into one of five categories from very active to inactive based on reported frequency and intensity of physical activity performed outside of school.

Saturated fat intake was estimated with a single item regarding use of spread on bread. Response choices included: (1) usually nothing; (2) mostly margarine; (3) mostly butter; (4) butter/margarine mixtures; (5) light spread; and (6) other.

Results indicated that the highest activity group was significantly more likely to use no spread on their bread than the inactive group. For example, in the very active group, 15.4% of girls and 5.2% of boys reported using no spread; whereas among the inactive, only 1.6% of girls and none of the boys reported using no spread.

Raitakari et al.[18] tracked the health-related behaviours of 961 Finnish adolescents, aged 12 to 18 years. Leisure time physical activity was assessed by questionnaire. A physical activity index, ranging from 1 to 225, was calculated from the product of intensity, duration and frequency. Participants with a score greater than or equal to 85 in three examinations, three years apart (i.e. 1980, 1983, 1986) were considered constantly active. Those with an index value less than 15 over the three examinations were considered constantly sedentary. Diet was assessed by a trained nutritionist using a 48-hour recall at the baseline examination in 1980 and again in 1986. Comparing the constantly active to the constantly sedentary, it was found that the sedentary young males consumed significantly more saturated fat and had a lower polyunsaturated to saturated fat ratio than the active males.

Lytle et al.[39] examined cross-sectional data from grades 6 though 12 of the Class of 1989 Study which was part of the Minnesota Heart Health Project. Subjects from the intervention communities were examined separately from the comparison communities. Frequency and intensity of physical activity was used to create an exercise score ranging from zero to nine. Dietary behaviour was summarized on a scale of zero to 18 with each point on the scale representing a healthier food choice. In both the intervention and control communities, students in the highest two quintiles for healthy food choices exhibited significantly higher levels of physical activity than students in lowest two quintiles. This difference was most evident among females in the intervention communities.

Terre et al.[6] studied the interrelationships among health-related behaviours in 1092 children between the ages 11 to 18 years. To examine potential developmental differences in these relationships, participants were grouped into four groups: Grade 6 (age 11), Grades 7–8 (ages 12–13), Grades 9–10 (ages 14 –15) and Grades 11–12 (ages 16–18). Students completed a 35-item self-reported questionnaire designed to assess five health-related behaviours including diet and exercise. Exploratory factor analyses performed within each group revealed sedentary behaviour to be related to poor eating habits in all grade level groups with the exception of students in Grades 11 and 12.

Conclusion

Based on three studies of sports participation and five studies of physical activity, there appears to be a positive association between physical activity and healthy dietary practices. However, it is important to note that this association may not be consistent for all dietary behaviours. Given the scarcity of information available and the difficulty of assessing both physical activity and dietary behaviour in this population, caution should be used when making conclusions about the relationship between physical activity and dietary behaviour in youth.

Weight control practices

Sports participation

There is evidence to suggest that those who participate in sports in which leanness is emphasized, such as ballet or gymnastics, are more likely to diet inappropriately or have eating disorders such as bulimia and anorexia nervosa.[40,41] Leon[40] suggests that with the increasing participation of females in sports activities, a greater number of adolescent females may be at risk for the development of eating disorders. Others have recognized that owing to the rules of their sport, certain athletes are subject to a particular pressure to maintain a low body weight.[42]

A study of 955 competitive male and female swimmers aged 9–18 years showed that girls, irrespective of actual weight, were more likely to engage in weight loss efforts, while boys were more likely to try to gain weight.[43] Girls were more likely than boys to use unhealthy weight loss methods such as fasting (27.0% versus 16.4%), self-induced vomiting (12.7% versus 2.7%) and diet pills (10.7% versus 6.8%). Boys used laxatives and diuretics more than girls (4.1% versus 2.5%, 2.8 versus 1.5%, respectively). At least one unhealthy method of weight control was used by 15.4% of the girls (24.8% among postmenarcheal girls) and 3.6% of the boys.[43]

In a sample of high school females in a midwestern US city, the eating disorder inventory (EDI) was used to assess psychological traits known to be associated with eating disorders. Female athletes were significantly more likely than non-athletes to be perfectionistic and to engage in bulimic behaviour, such as uncontrollable overeating and self-induced vomiting. Yet, no significant differences were found on current dieting practices (28% of athletes versus 25% of non-athletes were on a diet to lose weight.[44]

Among 64 female university students, athletes involved in sports that provide an advantage to those with a slim body (e.g. gymnastics, synchronized swimming, diving, figure skating, long-distance running and ballet) had greater weight concerns and diet concerns, and were more emotionally liable and dissatisfied than female athletes participating in hockey, basketball, sprinting, downhill skiing and volleyball.[45] Analyses of the 1993 national YRBS found no association between high school sports participation and weight loss behaviour including use of vomiting or diet pills to lose weight. In fact, young girls (less than 16 years) involved in sports were less likely to report trying to lose weight than non-athletes.[2]

Physical activity

Few studies have examined the association between physical activity and weight loss practices or eating disorders. Those that have been conducted have utilized very limited samples. French et al.[38] collected data from 708 males and 786 females in grades 7 through 10 from a suburban school district in the mid-western United States. A 21-item eating disorder checklist was developed for the study, based on previous research and DSM-III-R criteria for eating disorders. The number of affirmative responses constituted a risk score for eating disorders. Physical activity was measured using a 28-item checklist of activities. Principal components analysis resulted in three categories of activities: leisure or outdoor sports, conditioning sports and atypical sports. Among males, atypical sports participation (e.g. bowling, aerobics, softball) was a significant predictor of the risk score for eating disorders. Among females, all three categories of physical activity (conditioning sports, leisure sports and atypical sports) were significant predictors of the risk score for eating disorders. In the Massachusetts YRBS data-set, vigorous exercise, stretching and toning were associated with trying to lose weight among females and trying to gain weight among males.[46]

Conclusion

Relatively few studies have examined the relationship between sports and physical activity participation and weight loss practices in adolescent youth. The majority of these studies have been conducted with small samples that may not be representative of the general population of youth. The available evidence, although limited, suggests that participation in sports which emphasize leanness and artistic ability is associated with an increased risk for inappropriate weight control methods and eating disorders, especially among female athletes.

Sexual activity

Sports participation

Smith and Caldwell[47] examined the prevalence of sexual activity in 1071 high school students from a large city in the southern United States. Students classified as sports participants were significantly more likely than non-participants to report having sexual intercourse on at least one occasion (60.6% versus 41.8%). Miller *et al.*[48] examined the effects of sports participation on sexual behaviour in a sample of 611 Western New York adolescents. The authors found the relationship between sports participation and sexual behaviour to be highly gender-specific. Whereas male athletes were more likely than non-athletes to report sexual activity, female athletes were significantly less likely than their non-athletic counterparts to report sexual activity. These findings remained intact after controlling for race, age, socioeconomic status, quality of family relations and participation in other extracurricular activities.

Physical activity

Pate *et al.*[17] examined the relationship between physical activity status and sexual activity in a national sample of US high school students. In unadjusted analyses, students classified as low active were significantly more likely than active students to report having one or more sexual partners in the previous three months. However, no association was observed between physical activity and sexual activity after controlling for age group, gender and race/ethnicity.

Conclusion

There is a very limited literature on which to base a conclusion regarding the potential association between sports participation/physical activity and sexual behaviour in youth. There is some evidence to suggest that sports participation may be associated with increased sexual behaviour among males but not females. In fact, female athletes may be less likely than their non-sporting counterparts to engage in sexual activity. More research is warranted in this area.

Violence

Sports participation

Levin *et al.*[49] examined the relationship between violent behaviours and sports participation in 2436 high school students from a single county in the southeastern United States. The violent behaviours examined included assault, trouble at school, stealing, trouble with police, damaging property, carrying a weapon to get something, and carrying a weapon for protection. Among males, sports participation was not significantly associated with any of the violent behaviours; however, when male athletes were divided into contact and non-contact sports, athletes in contact sports were significantly more likely than their non-contact counterparts to assault others, get into trouble at school and carry a weapon for protection. Among females, athletes from any sport were significantly less likely than non-athletes to get into trouble at school. Similar to the males, females involved into contact sports were significantly more likely than their non-contact counterparts to engage in assault and carry a weapon for protection.

Physical activity

Pate and colleagues[17] examined physical activity participation and the relative odds of being injured in a physical fight in a nationally-representative sample of US high school students. After controlling for age, sex and race/ethnicity, no association was found between physical activity level and injury from physical fighting (OR = 0.90, 95% C.I. 0.71–1.15). Aaron *et al.*[20] contrasted the prevalence of weapon carrying in high school students reporting low, medium and high levels of leisure time physical activity. Boys were significantly more likely than girls to report carrying a weapon in the previous 30 days; however, within gender groups, the prevalence of weapon carrying was similar across the three physical activity groups. When students were classified on the basis of participation in competitive sports, no association was found in either boys or girls; however, it is notable that the prevalence of weapon carrying among female athletes (8%) was almost half of that observed among female non-athletes (15%).

Conclusion

A small number of studies have examined the relationship between sports and/or physical activity participation and violent behaviour in youth. Collectively, the results of these studies indicate that sports participation is not related to violent behaviour in adolescents. However; when athletes from different types of sports are compared, there is some evidence that athletes in 'contact sports' exhibit a higher prevalence of violent behaviours than athletes in 'non-contact' sports.

Summary

This review examined the relationship between sport, physical activity and nine health behaviours associated with significant morbidity and mortality in children and adolescents. These relationships are summarized in Table 3.5.2. The available evidence, although limited, suggests that sports participation and/or physical activity may be associated with other health behaviours. However, the strength and direction of these associations vary markedly with the health behaviour under examination and the population under study. Depending on one's age, gender and race/ethnicity, sports and physical activity participation may be

Table 3.5.2 Overview of the associations between specific health behaviours and participation in sport and physical activity

Health behaviour*	Sports participation	Physical activity
Cigarette smoking	− −	− −
Smokeless tobacco	−	↔
Alcohol use	−	− +
Illegal drugs	−	−
Anabolic steroids	+	?
Improper dietary practices	−	
Improper weight control practices	+	+
Sexual activity	+	↔
Violence	↔	↔

*Each health behaviour is presented as a health compromising behaviour. Thus, a negative association indicates that athletes and/or physically active youth are less likely to engage in that behaviour.

− − = repeatedly documented inverse association; − = weak or mixed evidence of an inverse association; ↔ = consistent evidence of no association; + = weak or mixed evidence of a positive association; + + = repeatedly documented positive association; ? = no data available.

somewhat of a double-edged sword. On the positive side, sport and physical activity participation may reduce the risk for cigarette smoking, alcohol consumption and illicit drug use. However, on the negative side, sport and physical activity may marginally increase the risk for sexual activity, smokeless tobacco use and inappropriate weight loss practices. Considerable caution should be exercised in interpreting such relationships as the literature is, at best, inconsistent and almost entirely comprised of cross-sectional studies. Clearly, more longitudinal studies are needed to establish causal relations between sports, physical activity and other health behaviours in youth.

References

1. Seefeld, V. D. and Ewing, M. E. Youth sports in America: an overview. *Physical Activity and Fitness Research Digest* 1997; **2**: 1–2.
2. Pate, R. R., Trost, S. G., Levin, S. and Dowda, M. Sports participation and health-related behaviors among US high-school students. *Medicine and Science in Sports and Exercise* 1999; **31**(Suppl): S85.
3. Poinsett, A. *Carnegie meeting papers: the role of sports in youth development*. Carnegie Corporation, New York, 1996.
4. Burke, V., Milligan, R. A. K., Beilin, L. J., Dunbar, D., Spencer, M., Balde, E. and Gracey, M. P. Clustering of health-related behaviors among 18-year-old Australians. *Preventive Medicine* 1997; **26**: 724–33.
5. Johnson, M. F., Nichols, J. F., Sallis, J. F., Calfas, K. J. and Hovell, M.F. Interrelationships between physical activity and other health behaviors among university women and men. *Preventive Medicine* 1998; **27**: 536–44.
6. Terre, L., Drabman, R. S. and Meydrech, E. F. Relationships among children's health-related behaviors: multivariate, developmental perspective. *Preventive Medicine* 1990; **19**: 134–6.
7. Escobedo, L. G., Marcus, S. E., Holtzman, D. and Giovano, G. A. Sports participation, age of smoking initiation, and the risk of smoking among US high school students. *Journal of the American Medical Association* 1993; **269**: 1391–5.
8. Thorlindsson, T. Sports participation, smoking, and drug and alcohol use among Icelandic youth. *Society and Sport Journal* 1989; **6**: 136–43.
9. Thorlindsson, T. and Vilhjalmsson, R. Factors related to cigarette smoking and alcohol use among adolescents. *Adolescence* 1991; **26**: 399–417.

10. Thorlindsson, T., Vilhjalmsson, R. and Valgeirsson, G. Sports participation and perceived health status: a study of adolescence. *Social Science in Medicine* 1990; **31**: 551–6.
11. Rainey, C. J., McKeown, R. E., Sargent, R. G. and Valois, R. F. Patterns of tobacco and alcohol use among sedentary, exercising, non-athletic, and athletic youth. *Journal of School Health* 1996; **66**: 27–32.
12. Winnail, S. D., Valois, R. F., Dowda, M., McKeown, R. E., Saunders, R. P. and Pate, R. R. Athletics and substance abuse among public high school students in a southern state. *American Journal of Health Studies* 1997; **13**: 187–94.
13. Baumert, P. W. Jr., Henderson, J. M., and Thompson, N. J. Health risk behaviors of adolescent participants in organized sports. *Journal of Adolescent Health* 1998; **22**: 460–5.
14. Oler, M. J., Mainous, A. G. 3rd, Martin, C. A., Richardson, E., Haney, A., Wilson, D. and Adams, T. Depression, suicide ideation, and substance abuse among adolescents. Are athletes at less risk? *Archives of Family Medicine* 1994; **3**: 781–5.
15. Davis, T. C., Arnold, C., Nandy, I., Bocchini, J. A., Gottlieb, A., George, R. B. and Berkel, H. Tobacco use among high school athletes. *Journal of Adolescent Health* 1997; **21**: 97–101.
16. Forman, E. S., Dekker, A. H., Javors, J. R. and Davison, D. T. High-risk behaviors in teenage male athletes. *Clinical Journal of Sports Medicine* 1995; **5**: 36–42.
17. Pate, R. R., Heath, G. W., Dowda, M. and Trost, S. G. Associations between physical activity and other health behaviors in a representative sample of US adolescents. *American Journal of Public Health* 1996; **86**: 1577–81.
18. Raitakari, O. T., Porkka, K. V., Taimela, S., Telama, R., Rasanen, L. and Viikari, J. S. Effects of persistent physical activity and inactivity on coronary risk factors in children and young adults. The Cardiovascular Risk in Young Finns Study. *American Journal of Epidemiology* 1994; **140**: 195–205.
19. Winnail, S. D., Valois, R. F., McKeown, R. E., Saunders, R. P. and Pate, R. R. Relationship between physical activity level and cigarette, smokeless tobacco use, and marijuana use among public high school adolescents. *Journal of School Health* 1995; **65**: 438–42.
20. Aaron, D. J., Dearwater, S. R., Anderson, R., Olsen, T., Kriska A. M. and LaPorte R. E. Physical activity and the initiation of high-risk health behaviors in adolescents. *Medicine and Science in Sport and Exercise* 1995; **27**: 1639–45.

21. Kelder, S. H., Perry, C. L., Klepp, K. I. and Lytle, L.L. Longitudinal tracking of adolescent smoking, physical activity, and food choices. *American Journal of Public Health* 1994; **84**: 1121–6.
22. Valois, R., Dowda, M., Trost, S. G, Weinrich, M., Felton, G. and Pate, R. R. Cigarette smoking experimentation among rural fifth grade students. *American Journal of Health Behavior* 1998; **22**: 101–7.
23. D'Elio, M. A., Mundt, D. J., Bush, P. J. and Iannotti, R. J. Healthful behaviors: do they protect African-American, urban preadolescents from abusable substance use. *American Journal of Public Health* 1993; **7**: 354–63.
24. Karvonen, J. S., Rimpela, A. H., and Rimpela, M. Do sports clubs promote snuff use? Trends among Finnish boys between 1981 and 1991. *Health Education Research* 1995; **10**: 147–54.
25. Sussman, S., Holt, L., Dent, C. W., Flay, B. R., Graham, J. W., Hansen, W. B. and Johnson, C. A. Activity involvement, risk-taking, demographic variables, and other drug use: prediction of trying smokeless tobacco. *National Cancer Institute Monograph*, 1989; **8**: 57–62.
26. Buhrman, H. G. Athletics and deviance: an examination of the relationship between athletic participation and deviant behavior of high school girls. *Review of Sport and Leisure* 1977; **2**: 17–35.
27. Donato, F., Assanelli, D., Marconi, M., Corsini, C., Rosa, G. and Monarca, S. Alcohol consumption among high school students and young athletes in north Italy. *Revue Epidemiology de la Sante Publique* 1994; **42**: 198–206.
28. Nativ, A. and Puffer, J. C. Lifestyle and health risk of collegiate athletes. *Journal of Family Practice* 1991; **33**: 585–90.
29. Aarnio, M., Kujala, U. M. and Kaprio, J. Associations of health-related behaviors, school type and health status to physical activity patterns in 16 year old boys and girls. *Scandinavian Journal of Social Medicine* 1997; **25**: 156–67.
30. Faulkner, R. A. and Slattery, C. M. The relationship of physical activity to alcohol consumption in youth, 15–16 years of age. *Canadian Journal of Public Health* 1990; **81**: 168–9.
31. Hastad, D. N., Segrave, J. O., Pangrazi, R. and Peterson, G. Youth sport participation and deviant behavior. *Sociology of Sport Journal* 1984; **1**: 366–73.
32. Felton,G. M., Parsons, M. A., Pate, R. R., Ward, D., Saunders, R. P., Valois, R. F., Dowda, M. and Trost, S. G. Predictors of alcohol use among rural adolescents. *Journal of Rural Health* 1996; **12**: 378–85.
33. Robinson, T. N., Killen, J. D., Taylor, C. B., Telch, M. J., Bryson, S. W., Saylor, K. E., Maron, D. J., Maccoby, N. and Farquhar, J. W. Perspectives on adolescent substance use. A defined population study. *Journal of the American Medical Association*, 1987; **258**: 2072–6.
34. Buckley, W. E., Yesalis, C. E. III., Friedl, K. E., Anderson, W. A., Streit, A. L. and Wright, J. E. Estimated prevalence of anabolic steroid use among male high school students. *Journal of the American Medical Association* 1988; **260**: 3441–5.
35. DuRant, R. H., Escobedo, L. G. and Heath, G. W. Anabolic-steroid use, strength training and multiple drug use among adolescents in the United States. *Pediatrics*, 1995; **96**: 23–8.
36. Windsor, R. and Dumitru, D. Prevalence of anabolic steroid use by male and female adolescents. *Medicine and Science in Sports and Exercise* 1989; **21**: 494–7.
37. Tanner, S. M., Miller, D. W. and Alongi, C. Anabolic steroid use by adolescents: prevalence, motives, and knowledge of risks. *Clinical Journal of Sports Medicine*, 1995; **5**: 108–15.
38. French, S. A., Perry, C. L., Leon, G. R. and Fulkerson, J. A. Food preferences, eating patterns, and physical activity among adolescents: correlates of eating disorders symptoms. *Journal of Adolescent Health* 1994; **15**: 286–94.
39. Lytle, L. A., Kelder, S. H., Perry, C. L. and Klepp, K-I. Covariance of adolescent health behaviors: the Class of 1989 study. *Health Education Research* 1995; **10**: 133–46.
40. Leon, G. R. Eating disorders in female athletes. *Sports Medicine* 1991; **12**: 219–27.
41. Ponton, L. E. A review of eating disorders in adolescents. *Adolescent Psychiatry* 1995; **20**: 267–85.
42. Thiel, A., Gottfried, H. and Hesse, F. W. Subclinical eating disorders in male athletes. A study of the low weight categories in rowers and wrestlers. *Acta Psychiatrica Scandanavia* 1993; **88**: 259–65.
43. Drummer, G. M., Rosen, L. W., Heusner, W. W., Roberts, P. J. and Counsilman, J. E. Pathogenic weight control behaviors of young competitive swimmers. *The Physician and Sports Medicine* 1987; **15**: 75–84.
44. Taub, D. E. and Blinde, E. M. Eating disorders among adolescent female athletes: influence of athletic participation and sport team membership. *Adolescence* 1992; **27**: 833–48.
45. Davis, C. and Cowles, M. A comparison of weight and diet concerns and personality factors among female athletes and non-athletes. *Journal of Psychosomatic Research* 1989; **33**: 527–36.
46. Middleman, A. B., Vazquez, I. and Durant, R. H. Eating patterns, physical activity, and attempts to change weight among adolescents. *Journal of Adolescent Health* 1998; **22**: 37–42.
47. Smith, E. A. and Caldwell, L. L. Participation in high school sports and adolescent sexual activity. *Pediatric Exercise Science* 1994; **6**: 69–74.
48. Miller, K. E., Sabo, D. F., Farrel, M. P., Barnes, G. M. and Melnick, M. J. Athletic participation and sexual behavior in adolescents: the different worlds of boys and girls. *Journal of Health and Social Behavior* 1998; **39**: 108–23.
49. Levin, D. S., Smith, E. A., Caldwell, L. L. and Kimbrough, J. Violence and high school sports participation. *Pediatric Exercise Science*, 1995; **7**: 379–88.

3.6 Health education and the promotion of physical activity

Herman Schaalma, Ree Meertens, Willem van Mechelen and Gerjo Kok

Introduction

Nowadays it is widely acknowledged that physical activity has a positive impact on the physiological and psychological health of adults, and that the same observation may hold for teenagers. If young people indeed do benefit from a physically active lifestyle, this leads us to consider the question how we can promote such a lifestyle. In this chapter a general approach will be presented for the theory and data-based development of health education interventions. This approach will be illustrated with examples concerning the promotion of physical activity amongst young people.

Health education and health promotion: concepts

Although *health education* has been defined in many ways, a generally accepted definition is:

> any planned combination of learning experiences designed to predispose, enable, and reinforce voluntary behaviour conducive to health in individuals, groups, or communities.[1]

Health education needs to be distinguished from the concept of *health promotion*, defined as

> any planned combination of educational, political, regulatory, and organisational supports for actions and conditions of living conducive to the health of individuals, groups, or communities.[1]

Health promotion objectives are:

(1) primary prevention;

(2) early detection and treatment (secondary prevention); and

(3) patient care and support (tertiary prevention).

Health promotion strategies include:

(1) legislation and regulations designed to enforce behaviour change;

(2) the provision of non-compulsory services; and

(3) education that focuses on encouraging and helping people to change their behaviour of their own accord.

As such, health education is one of the instruments or strategies of achieving the goals of health promotion. Generally, health promotion is most effective when it involves several mutually reinforcing strategies, and when it affects different levels of society.[2,3]

Evidence-based health education

When developing health education programmes various decisions have to be made with regard to programme objectives, the target population, educational methods and strategies, useful media, etc. Unfortunately, these decisions cannot be made without careful analysis of the health problem, the behavioural and environmental factors affecting this problem, and the options for corrective action. Figure 3.6.1 depicts a planning and evaluation model for the development of health education interventions.[1,4]

The first phase in the planning process addresses the social and epidemiological diagnosis of the health problem. This phase should make clear whether the health problem is linked to individual and social perceptions of the quality of life, whether the assumed problem has serious individual and social consequences, and whether it relates to other health problems. This phase should also reveal which people or institutions are involved.

The second planning phase includes the diagnosis of the behavioural, social and environmental factors that are linked to the health problem of interest. This phase should reveal whether the health problem is linked to specific behaviours, and if it is, to whose behaviours. This phase should also make clear whether reduction of the health problem needs an environmental change, and if so, the decision-makers that are responsible for environmental change should be identified.

The third phase of the model, needs assessment, examines the determinants of the behavioural and environmental conditions that are linked to health status or quality-of-life concerns. It also identifies the factors that must be changed to initiate and sustain the process of behavioural and environmental change. According to Green and Kreuter[1] any given behaviour can be explained as a function of three categories of factors. *Predisposing factors* are those cognitive antecedents that provide a rationale or motivation for behaviour (e.g. knowledge, attitudes, values and goal priorities). *Enabling factors* are

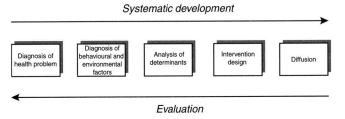

Fig. 3.6.1 Evidence-based development of health education.

the cognitive antecedents that enable the enactment of intentions (e.g. availability and accessibility of health resources, government laws, as well as individual competencies). *Reinforcing factors* are the factors that, following a behaviour, determine its persistence or repetition (e.g. social support, physical consequences, feedback provided by health-care providers).

The fourth phase, intervention development, addresses the analysis of the possible usefulness of (components of) health education and other potential interventions (resources, regulations). This phase may include:

(1) the assessment of the usefulness of current health education interventions;
(2) the development and small-scale evaluation of new interventions or intervention components; and
(3) a diagnosis of the political, regulatory and organizational factors that may facilitate or hinder the development and widespread implementation of a health education intervention.

The fifth planning phase addresses the diffusion of an intervention programme. This phase includes the diagnosis of the factors that are linked to the adoption, actual implementation and institutionalization of a health promotion programme, and the launching of activities to enhance widespread programme diffusion. Awareness of the outcomes of this phase is necessary before starting the design of a practical health education programme.

Subsequent phases of the model all refer to the evaluation of the process, impact and outcomes of the health promotion programme, resulting in feedback and adjustment. The core evaluation question—whether a programme results in a reduction of the health problem—often cannot be answered because of a delay between behaviour change and observable effects on the health problem. Generally, a change of behaviour is the best possible indication of the effectiveness of health promotion programmes.[5]

Health promotion and physical activity

Problems and problem-causing factors

Nowadays in Western society premature death is strongly related to chronic diseases like heart disease, cancers, stroke and diabetes. Lifestyle factors, such as smoking, alcohol abuse, improper diet and physical inactivity, play an important role in the aetiology of these chronic diseases. Epidemiological studies have demonstrated that, together with smoking, physical inactivity is the most important independent risk factor for the leading causes of death in Western society.[6] Consequently, it is generally accepted that a physically active lifestyle has enormous direct and indirect health advantages for both adults and adolescents.[7–10] Not only the health of individuals, but also a nation's public health status will benefit from a physically active lifestyle. Estimates by Powell and Blair[11] showed that in the USA 35% of the coronary heart disease deaths, 32% of the colon cancer deaths and 35% of the diabetes mellitus deaths could, theoretically, be prevented if everyone was vigorously active.

Whereas it is generally recognized that adult populations in Western society are rather inactive, young people seem to have a fairly active lifestyle. Small children play, jump, bike and run throughout the day. When they grow older, most of them participate in school-based physical education, organized sports and leisure time activities in which they are physically active. For example, a nation-wide survey among Dutch teenagers[12] showed that almost all participated in school-based physical education with a mean of about two hours per week, and that about two out of three participated in organized sports for about three hours per week. In addition, most of them used a bicycle as a means of transportation with a mean of at least two hours per week, and many enjoyed leisure time activities in which they were physically active for another four hours per week (such as street soccer, mountain biking, dancing).

Although young people seem to be fairly physically active, many young people in Western society gradually develop an inactive lifestyle during secondary school years, at least partly because of competing daily activities such as homework, watching television, playing computer games, part-time jobs and going out.[13–17] For instance, Schaalma and colleagues found a decline in physical activity with growing age for physical education, organized sports and unorganized leisure time activities, as well as for the use of a bicycle as a means of transportation. Van Mechelen and Kemper[15] found that young people who had an average of four hours per week of moderate physical activity at age 13, only had one hour of comparable activity at age 27.

These results suggest that most young people are physically active. Therefore, health promotion activities aimed at a physically active lifestyle amongst young people should focus on the maintenance of regular physical activity.

Predisposing antecedents of participation in physical activity

Theory

Consideration of social and cognitive determinants of behaviour can highlight differences between young people's preparedness to exercise. Various social-psychological models predicting goal-oriented behaviour can be applied to health-related behaviours. Although these models include a broad range of variables, basically five general categories of core cognitive antecedents of health behaviours can be distinguished.[18]

1. *Attitude.* This category refers to what someone himself feels and thinks with regard to the behaviour in question. It includes affects, beliefs and personal assessments of the advantages and disadvantages (e.g. health risks) of behaviour, resulting in an overall evaluation of a health behaviour. Health considerations may be secondary in forming attitudes towards behaviours such as exercise.
2. *Social influences.* This category includes injunctive social norms (i.e. subjective beliefs about what important others, such as parents, partners and friends, think ought to be thought or done), descriptive social norms (i.e. perceptions of what others generally do), and perceived social pressures (i.e. perceptions of direct social sanctions and rewards for behaviour).
3. *Self-efficacy.* This category refers to perceptions of one's own capability to successfully perform a particular behaviour, also referred to as perceived behavioural control.
4. *Identity concerns.* This type of determinant refers to the extent to which a behaviour allows expression of, or contradicts, a valued social or personal construction of the self.
5. *Action Control.* This category concerns the extent to which, having decided to act, people are able to, or are prompted to, plan on how to enact their intentions amidst competing everyday priorities.

Whereas attitudes, perceived social influences, self-efficacy and identity concerns generally are reliable predictors of people's intentions to act, action control refers to the cognitive factors that distinguish between those who intend to act and succeed, and those who fail to act despite their intentions.[18]

Figure 3.6.2 presents a general model for these social cognitive determinants of behaviour. Distal factors, such as gender, socio-economic status and educational degree, are not included in the model because these factors affect behaviour via cognitions. However, such cognitive models operate in social contexts and culture; laws and the availability of resources and facilities critically curtail an individual's construction of health-related behaviour, including exercise.

An example: determinants of physical activity in young people

Many researchers have focused on determinants of young people's exercise behaviour or their physical activity.[12,19,20] These studies suggest that cognitive factors (attitudes and self-efficacy expectations) and social factors (the influence of peers and family) strongly relate to the frequency of physical activity.

Recent research among Dutch young people revealed that they, generally, had positive attitudes with regard to being physically active in their leisure time.[12] In their view, leisure time physical activity was pleasurable, healthy, sociable and relaxing. The most important psychological barriers were lack of interest and lack of time. Students who intended to maintain being physically active generally had more positive attitudes than students with ambivalent intentions did; they attached more value to the advantages of physical activity and less importance to the disadvantages. Students who intended to continue being physically active also perceived a supportive and stimulating social environment. The role of parents seemed to be important, although most of the students indicated that their parents did not exert direct pressure on them to participate in sports. Important barriers to exercise were 'feeling tired', 'a good movie on TV' and 'a lot of homework'.

This analysis suggests that, since lack of time appears to be an important barrier to maintaining a physically active lifestyle amongst young people, health promotion activities should focus on increasing the number of hours that young people have available to participate in school-based physical education programmes. A second objective could be the reinforcement of young people's attitudes, for instance by emphasizing the social advantages of participation in sports. In addition, sports clubs could focus more on the social aspects of sports instead of competition.

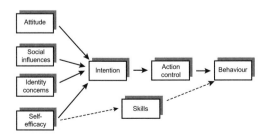

Fig. 3.6.2 Determinants of health behaviour.

Health education interventions

Theory

The phase following the need assessment addresses the development of a health education programme. In this stage, insights from theory and research have to be translated into educational methods and strategies. A shift must be made from *explaining* behaviour to *changing* behaviour. There is no such thing as a *magic bullet*: no intervention method is universally effective.[21] Intervention programmes have to be tailored very carefully to the behaviour, behavioural determinants and target population. The process of intervention design includes several steps.[22] First, general intervention objectives and specific learning outcomes must be specified. Second, theoretical methods that may be useful for the accomplishment of these learning objectives have to be selected. Third, useful theoretical methods have to be translated into feasible educational strategies and materials, while anticipating implementation barriers. Fourth, at different development stages the process and effects of the intervention should be monitored and evaluated. Systematically going through these 'intervention mapping' steps more or less guarantees the explicit link between programme objectives, theoretical methods and the final educational strategies and materials.[22,23]

Current social psychological theoretical frameworks for behaviour change through communication distinguish steps, phases or stages of behaviour change. One of these general frameworks is McGuire's *Persuasion-Communication* model.[24] This model describes the various steps that people take, from the initial response to an educational message to, hopefully, a continuous change of behaviour in the desired direction. This framework was simplified and extended into seven phases:[25] successful communication ((1) *attention* and (2) *comprehension*); changes in social cognitive determinants of behaviour ((3) *attitude*, (4) *social influence*, (5) *self-efficacy*); and (6) *change of behaviour* and (7) *maintenance* of behaviour change. The essence of this framework is that interventions or intervention components may be different for each of these phases. For instance, an intervention method that is useful for attracting the attention of a target group may be unsuitable for changing self-belief in skills, or a messenger that is useful for the transfer of facts about health risks (e.g. a medical doctor), may be useless for the accomplishment of attitude change.

Another framework for behaviour change that has become very popular in the field of health education is the *Stages of Change Model*.[26] This model describes behaviour change as a process that takes time to develop: people go through a series of stages before they internalize a new behaviour. In the first stage, *precontemplation*, people do not think about changing a particular behaviour; they have a low motivation towards change. In the second stage, *contemplation*, people consider behavioural change and make decisions as to that. In the third stage, *action*, people actually change their behaviour. In the last stage, *maintenance*, people have internalized the new behaviour and they have integrated the new behaviour in their daily routines. An important implication of the Stages of Change model is that people in different stages of change may need different educational interventions. Educational interventions tailored to different stages of change may be very different with respect to educational methods and strategies.

Within these general frameworks, various specific theories can be applied to guide the development of specific components of health education programmes.[27,28] For example, theories about fear-arousal and persuasive communication can guide the design of educational strategies to improve people's attitudes towards health behaviours.[29]

Other theories, such as Goal Setting[30] and Relapse Prevention[31] can be helpful in developing interventions that focus on particular aspects of change. Although these theories often cover only specific phases in the process of behaviour change, they can be helpful in the design of specific intervention components.

An example: goal setting and feedback

Although many programme developers claim that their intervention is theoretically and empirically based, descriptions of the way in which data and theories were actually applied in health education interventions are rare. Consequently, we have little knowledge about the efficacy of specific teaching methods or approaches with regard to the promotion of healthy behaviours.[22] As Almond and Harris[33] concluded:

> current research does little to promote our understanding of what kind of programmes bring about health gains or outcomes that we value.

Recent reviews do provide some insight into the effectiveness of programmes promoting physical exercise. Physical education programmes appear to have short-term positive physiological, clinical and behavioural outcomes. The value of school-based physical education in stimulating further participation in physical exercise, however, is unclear.[32,33] Evaluations of interventions aimed at the enhancement of participation in organized exercise programmes showed that social support, commitment enhancing techniques (e.g. making a contract to complete the programme) and drop-out prevention training based on Relapse Prevention theory[31] can be useful in motivating young people to maintain their participation in organized sports. Motivation oriented programmes, mostly based on social cognitive and social influence techniques, are least effective at this point.[32,34]

The analyses of behaviour and determinants showed that the maintenance of a physically active lifestyle is one of the main problems with physical activity amongst young people. One of the theoretical methods that can be useful for the development of intervention components with beneficial effects on the maintenance of a physically active lifestyle is Relapse Prevention theory.[31] A study by King and Frederiksen[35] that evaluated a drop-out prevention training that was based upon Relapse Prevention theory resulted in a higher attendance to a five week jogging programme. This drop-out training included (1) the identification of so-called high risk situations, that is situations in which it would be difficult to maintain participation in the programme, and (2) the development and practice of adequate coping responses to deal with these high risk situations.

Diffusion of health education

Theory

The diffusion of a prevention programme is an essential part of the health promotion planning process. Underestimating diffusion barriers is one of the major causes of ineffectiveness in health promotion. While the need for information about the determinants of individual behaviour is commonly accepted, the need for information about the antecedents of institutional 'behaviour' (such as the adoption of a prevention programme by organizations) is not widely recognized. Consequently, many expensive programmes are never adequately applied in the contexts where they are most likely to be effective.

The diffusion of a health promotion programme can be described as a process consisting of four phases: dissemination, adoption, implementation and maintenance.[36] Dissemination concerns the transfer of information about the programme to potential users. This phase involves the selection of communication channels and systems that facilitate the diffusion of the programme to a target population. Adoption refers to potential users' intention to use the programme. This phase includes a diagnosis of the target population with regard to their needs, values and attitudes, and their perception of programme attributes and adoption of barriers, such as the relative advantage of the programme, its fit with the target population, its complexity and the observability of programme outcomes. This phase also includes the diagnosis of the ways target adopters can be motivated to adopt the programme, and the ways to overcome barriers. Implementation refers to the actual use of the programme. The major focus in this phase is on the enhancement of the adopters' self-efficacy and skills, and on encouraging trial programme implementation. Maintenance or continuation succeeds initial implementation. This phase refers to the stage in which the programme has become current practice and in which the allocation of resources are routinely made.[37]

According to Orlandi and colleagues[38] many health promotion innovations have failed because of 'the gap that is frequently left unfilled between the point where innovation-development ends and diffusion planning begins', as if innovation-development barriers and diffusion barriers were aspects of unrelated problems. To bridge this gap, Orlandi and colleagues stressed the need for a *linkage system* between the resource system that develops and promotes the intervention (e.g. a Health Education Authority), and the user system that is supposed to adopt the intervention (e.g. sports organizations, schools). Such a liaison group should include representatives of the user system, representatives of the resource system and a change agent facilitating the collaboration. Diffusion of the innovation may be carried out by any of the members of this liaison group. The essential point is that the innovation-development process and the diffusion planning process have been developed through cooperation, to improve the fit between innovation and user, to attune intervention innovations to practical possibilities and constraints, and to facilitate widespread implementation.

The development of a diffusion strategy can be based on a planning process that is similar to the planning of health education programmes. A diffusion strategy should be based on insights in the determinants of potential users' decisions regarding the adoption, implementation and continuation of a health promotion programme. These determinants can be measured with the same kind of protocol as is used in the determinants of behaviour analyses, using the same kind of theories.[23] A diffusion strategy should further be based on useful theoretical methods and theory-based strategies.

An example: school-based programmes to promote physical activity

Social Cognitive Theory[39] provides a valuable framework for the development of interventions aimed at improving the diffusion of school-based health education programmes.[40,41] A strategy for the diffusion of a school-based programme to promote physical activity may include the following objectives and methods. The objectives of a dissemination strategy could be that teachers and administrators are aware of the programme, view the programme favourably and communicate with colleagues about the programme. Useful methods to reach these objectives are personal communication by opinion leaders, and the use of modelling, showing teachers successfully using the programme, for example, through a video or role-model stories in newsletters. An adoption strategy could focus on the advantages of the exercise programme in terms of outcomes, expectancies and social reinforcements. Useful methods to reach these objectives are modelling (e.g. peer model stories in written material), incentives and social contracting, for instance through a newsletter. An implementation strategy could focus on the reinforcement of teachers' skills and their self-efficacy to use the exercise programme with acceptable completeness, fidelity and proficiency. Data from other implementation studies showed the importance of in-service training.[42] Methods to reach these objectives are direct modelling and guided enactment through a live workshop training, and symbolic modelling through video training. The objectives of a continuation strategy could be that teachers and administrators will have experienced positive feedback and reinforcement on the use of the exercise programme after one year and will continue to use it. These objectives may be accomplished by means of various kinds of incentives (social, monetary, status and self-evaluative incentives).

Summary

From a public health perspective the promotion of physical activity has many benefits. Inactivity is a risk factor for multicausal chronic disease, and a physically active lifestyle helps to maintain body weight, and leads to favourable health habits, such as non-smoking and a healthy diet. In our view, the promotion of physical activity should be evidence-based. Physical activity promoting programmes should be based on a design approach combining empirical findings, theoretical insights and practical considerations.

Of course, the same observation also holds for the prevention of sports injuries, the other side of the exercise picture. Just as for exercise promoting programmes, injury prevention programmes should be based on a careful epidemiological and medical diagnosis of the injuries in question, on a careful identification of injury-causing behavioural and environmental factors and related determinants, and on a thorough analysis of the possibilities for corrective action. The greater the extent to which programmes are designed systematically along these lines, the more likely it will be that they effectively affect behaviour.

In the past many researchers have addressed the determin-ants of physical activity behaviour of various target groups.[20,43] Others have addressed the effectiveness of physical education programmes[33] or programmes promoting physical activity.[16,32,34] The scientific literature, however, hardly provides any insight into the ways in which social science theory and empirical findings are applied in the design of physical activity promoting interventions, or in the effectiveness of attempts to facilitate large-scale implementation of such interventions. Future research on physical activity behaviour should fill this gap.

It took a while before health decision-makers acknowledged that stimulating a physically active lifestyle may be one of public health's best buys. It may take more time before decision-makers acknowledge that the development of programmes promoting such a lifestyle does need an evidence-based development and evaluation approach, but as with physical activity, it will be rewarding to hold out.

Acknowledgement

The authors thank Charles Abraham (University of Sussex, UK) for his helpful comments on an earlier draft of this paper.

References

1. Green, L. W. and Kreuter, M. W. *Health promotion planning: an educational and environmental approach.* Mountain View, Mayfield, 1991.
2. De Leeuw, E. D. *The sane revolution. Health promotion: backgrounds, scope, prospects.* Van Gorcum, Assen, 1989.
3. Milio, N. Strategies for health promoting policy: a study of four national case studies. *Health Promotion International* 1988; 3: 307–11.
4. Kok, G. J. Quality of planning as decisive determinant of health education *Hygie* 1992; 11: 5–8.
5. Tones, K., Tilford, S. and Robinson, Y. K. *Health education: effectiveness and efficiency.* Chapman, London, 1990.
6. Pate, R. R., Pratt, M., Blair, S. N., Haskell, W. L., Macera, C. A., Bouchard, C., Buchner, D., Ettinger, W., Heath, G. W. and King, A. C. Physical activity and public health. A recommendation from the Centers for Disease Control and Prevention and the American College of Sports Medicine. *Journal of the American Medical Association* 1995; 273: 402–7.
7. Tell, G. S. and Vellar, O. D. Physical fitness, physical activity, and cardiovascular disease risk factors in adolescents: the Oslo study. *Preventive Medicine* 1988; 17: 12–24.
8. US Department of Health and Human Services. *US physical activity and health; a report of the Surgeon General.* US Department of Health and Human services, National Center for Disease Control and Prevention, Atalanta, GA, 1996.
9. NIH Consensus Development Panel and Physical Activity and Cardiovascular Health. Physical activity and cardiovascular health. *Journal of the American Medical Association* 1996; 276: 241–6.
10. Suter, E. and Hawes, M. R. Relationship of physical activity, body fat, diet, and blood lipid profile in youth 10–15 yr. *Medicine and Science in Sports and Exercise* 1993; 25: 748–54.
11. Powell, K. E. and Blair, S. N. The public health burden of sedentary living habits: theoretical but realistic estimates. *Medicine and Science in Sports and Exercise* 1994; 26: 851–6.
12. Schaalma, H.P., Bolman, C., Nooijer, J. de, Vries, H. de, Paulussen, Th., Aarts, H. and Willemse, G. Jangeren en de preventie van hart- en vaatziekten. Een leefstijl—en determinanten-analyse. Den Haag, Nederlandse Hartstichting, 1997. Foundation, The Hague, 1997.
13. Schaalma, H., Bolman, C., Nooijer, J. de, Aarts, H., Paulussen, Th., Vries, H. de, Willemse, G. and Kolner, C. Preventie van hart- en vaatziekten: een leefstijlanalyse onder jongeren. *Tijdschrift voor Gezondheidswetenschappen* 1998; 76: 458–65.
14. Robinson, T. N., Hammer, L. D., Killen, L. D., Kraemer, H. C., Wilson, D. M. Hayward, C. and Taylor, C. B. Does television viewing increase obesity and reduce physical activity in adolescents? *Preventive Medicine* 1993; 19: 541–51.
15. Van Mechelen, W. and Kemper, H. Habitual physical activity in longitudinal perspective. In *The Amsterdam Growth Study: a longitudinal analysis of health, fitness, and lifestyle, HK Sport Science Monographs Series, Vol. 6,* (ed. H. Kemper), Human Kinetics, Champaign, Il. 1995; 135–59.
16. Kelder, S. H., Perry, C. L. and Klepp, K.-I. Community-wide youth exercise promotion: long term outcomes of the Minnesota Heart Health Program and the Class of 1989 study. *Journal of School Health* 1993; 63: 218–23.
17. Gortmaker, S. L., Dietz, W. H. and Cheung, L.W.Y. Inactivity, diet and the fattening of America. *Journal of American Diet Association* 1990; 90: 1247–55.
18. Abraham, C., Sheeran, P., and Johnston, M. From health beliefs to self-regulation: theoretical advances in the psychology of action control. *Psychology and Health* 1998; 13: 569–91.

19. **Bourdeauhuij, I. de.** Behavioural factors associated with physical activity in young people. In *Young and active?* (ed. S. Biddle, J. Sallis and N. Cavill), Health Education Authority, London, 1998; 98–118.

20. **Dishman R. K.** and **Sallis, J. F.** Determinants and interventions for physical activity and exercise. In Physical activity, fitness and health: international proceedings and consensus statement, (eds C. Bouchard, R. J. Shephard, and T. Stephens). Human Kinetics, Champaign, Il. 1994; 214–38.

21. **Mullen, P. D., Green, L. W.** and **Persinger, G.** Clinical trails for patient education for chronic conditions: a comparative meta-analysis of intervention types. *Preventive Medicine* 1985; **14**: 753–81.

22. **Bartholomew, K., Parcel, G.** and **Kok, G.** Intervention mapping: a process for developing theory- and data-based health education programs. *Health Education and Behavior* 1998; **25**: 545–63.

23. **Kok, G., Schaalma, H., De Vries, H., Parcel, G.** and **Paulussen, Th.** Social psychology and health education. In *European Review of Social Psychology*, Vol. 7 (eds W. Stroebe and M. Hewstone), John Wiley & Sons, Chichester, 1996; 210–40.

24. **McGuire, W. J.** Attitudes and attitude change. The handbook of social psychology, Vol. 2 (ed. M. Lindsay and E. Aronson), Random House, New York, 1985; 233–346.

25. **Kok, G.** Health education theories and research for Aids prevention. *Hygie* 1991; **10**: 32–9.

26. **Prochaska, J. O.** and **DiClemente, C. C.** *The transtheoretical approach: crossing traditional boundaries of therapy.* Dow Jones-Irwin, Homewood, 1984.

27. **Zimbardo, P. G.** and **Leippe, M. R.** The psychology of attitude change and social influence. McGraw-Hill, Philadelphia, 1991.

28. **Glanz, K., Lewis, F. M.** and **Rimer, B. K.** Linking theory, research, and practice. In *Health behavior and health education: theory, research and practice*, 2nd edn (eds K. Glanz, F. M. Lewis and B.K. Rimer). Jossey-Bass, San Francisco, 1997; 19–35.

29. **Maibach, E.** and **Parrott, R. L.** (eds) *Designing health messages: approaches from communication theory and public health practice.* Sage Publications Ltd, London, 1995.

30. **Strecher, V. J., Seijts, G. H., Kok, G. J., Latham, G. P., Glasgow, R., DeVellis, B., Meertens, R. M.** and **Bulger, D. W.** Goal setting as a strategy for health behaviour change. *Health Education Quarterly* 1995; **22**: 190–200.

31. **Marlatt, G. A.** and **Gordon, J.** *Relapse prevention.* Guilford Press, New York, 1985.

32. **Aarts, H., Paulussen, Th., Willemse, G., Schaalma, H., Bolman, C.** and **De Nooijer, J.** *Prevention of cardiovascular disease: an analysis of international effect research on the promotion of physical exercise among young people.* Netherlands Heart Foundation, The Hague, 1997.

33. **Almond, L.** and **Harris, J.** Interventions to promote health-related physical education. In *Young and active?* (ed. S. Biddle, J. Sallis, and N. Cavill), Health Education Authority, London, 1998; 133–49.

34. **Sallis, J.** Family and community interventions to promote physical activity in young people. In *Young and active?* (eds S. Biddle, J. Sallis, and N. Cavill), Health Education Authority, London, 1998; 150–61.

35. **King, A. C.** and **Frederiksen, L. W.** Low-cost strategies for increasing exercise behavior. *Behavior Modification* 1984; **8**: 3–21.

36. **Oldenburg, B., Hardcastle, D.** and **Kok, G.** Diffusion of innovations. In *Health behavior and health education: theory, research and practice*, 2nd edn (eds K. Glanz, F. M. Lewis, and B. K. Rimer), Jossey-Bass, San Francisco, 1997; 270–86.

37. **Miles, M. B.** and **Louis, K. S.** Research on institutionalization: a reflective review. In *Lasting school improvement: exploring the process of institutionalization* (ed. M. B. Miles, M. Ekholm, and R. Vandenberghe). ACCO, Amersfoort, 1987; 241–82.

38. **Orlandi, M. A., Landers, C., Weston, R.** and **Haley, N.** Diffusion of health promotion innovations. In *Health behavior and health education: theory, research and practice*, 1st edn. (eds K. Glanz, F. M. Lewis., and B. K. Rimer), Jossey-Bass, San Francisco, 1990; 288–313.

39. **Bandura, A.** *Social foundation of thought and action: a social cognitive theory.* Prentice-Hall, New Jersey, 1986.

40. **Parcel, G., Taylor, W. C., Brink, S. G., Gotlieb, N., Enquist, K., O'Hara, N. M.** and **Erikson, M. P.** Translating theory into practice: intervention strategies for the diffusion of a health promotion innovation. *Family and Community Health* 1989; **12**: 1–13.

41. **Parcel, G., Erikson, M. P., Lovato, C. Y., Gottlieb, N. H., Brink, S. G., Green, L. W.** The diffusion of school-based tobacco-use prevention programmes; project description and baseline data. *Health Education Research* 1989; **4**: 111–24.

42. **Joyce, B.** and **Showers, B.** *Student achievement through staff development.* Longman, New York, 1988.

43. **Godin, G.** Theories of reasoned action and planned behaviour: usefulness for exercise promotion. *Medicine and Science in Sports and Exercise* 1994; **26**: 81–102.

PART IV

Chronic Health Conditions and Physical Activity

4.1 Exercise testing and daily physical activity in children with congenital heart disease

Tony Reybrouck and Marc Gewillig

Introduction

Exercise testing in adult cardiac patients has mainly focused on ischaemic heart disease. The results of exercise testing with ECG monitoring are often helpful in diagnosing the presence of coronary artery disease. In children with heart disease, the type of pathology is different. Ischaemic heart disease is very rare. The majority of patients will present congenital heart defects which will affect exercise capacity. In patients with congenital heart disease, exercise tests are frequently performed to measure exercise function or to assess abnormalities of cardiac rhythm. The risk of exercise testing is very low in the paediatric age group.[1]

To perform cardiopulmonary exercise testing in children, the same types of ergometers can be used as have been used with adults (bicycle ergometer, treadmill).[2–6] Differences from adult exercise testing procedures[2] include adaptations of the ergometer in order to fit the size of the child, and modifications of the exercise protocols due to cooperation (motivation, anxiety).[3] Since the motivation of young children to sustain incremental exercise testing is lower than in adults, the duration of the exercise testing procedure should be shorter than for adults. Several protocols have been recommended for bicycle exercise, the most commonly used is the James protocol.[3] However, in children, especially younger children, treadmill exercise testing is preferred, since younger children are used to walking rather than to performing bicycle exercise. The most widely used protocol is the Bruce test, where the inclination and speed of the treadmill are simultaneously increased every 3 minutes, until exhaustion.[4] Normal values have been reported for the paediatric age group.[3,6] Other frequently used protocols are the Balke protocol[7] or variants, where the speed is a function of the age of the child ($4.8\,km\,h^{-1}$ for children below 6 years of age and $5.6\,km\,h^{-1}$ for children above that age).[8,9]

Review of commonly used parameters to assess aerobic exercise function in the paediatric age group

In adult exercise physiology, aerobic exercise function is traditionally assessed by determination of the maximal oxygen uptake. This reflects the highest level of oxygen uptake($\dot{V}O_2$), which does not further increase despite an increase in exercise intensity. In paediatric exercise testing the $\dot{V}O_2$ max test is frequently applied, but its use in children is more limited since only a minority (one third) is able to reach a levelling off in $\dot{V}O_2$,[10] which is a prerequisite for objective evidence that a true $\dot{V}O_2$ max is reached (see chapter 1.7). Moreover at maximal exercise, many patients with congenital heart disease reach a lower value for maximal heart rate than normal controls. Furthermore, many children are not motivated to exercise to that point of exhaustion.[11] Other parameters of maximal exercise function are the measurement of the maximal work rate (W),[5] which can be indexed by expressing it to body mass and the maximal endurance time on a treadmill, while performing the Bruce protocol. Although the latter test has been shown to correlate with $\dot{V}O_2$ max (indexed per kg body weight; $r = 0.88$ to 0.92),[6] this measurement is strongly influenced by the motivation of the child and also by the encouragement of the investigator.

Because maximal exercise tests have several drawbacks in the paediatric population, clinical investigators have tried to use submaximal exercise test procedures for application in children. In the past, heart rate response to exercise has frequently been used to assess cardiovascular exercise performance.[12] The advantage of this measurement is its submaximal nature and minimal ergometric equipment. However, in patients with congenital heart disease several drawbacks exists, as many patients may show a relative bradycardia during exercise, which is not associated with a high value for $\dot{V}O_2$ max, as should theoretically be expected. For example, in patients after total surgical repair of tetralogy of Fallot, we found a reduced value for heart rate during graded exercise, which was not associated with a normal value for ventilatory anaerobic threshold.[13] Therefore, the use of heart rate response to exercise in the assessment of cardiovascular exercise performance can be misleading in patients with congenital heart disease, and cannot be considered to be a valid determinant of aerobic fitness.[3]

A more sensitive assessment of aerobic exercise function can be obtained by analysis of gas exchange. Therefore considerable attention has been focused on the determination of the ventilatory anaerobic threshold in children.[14–16] This reflects the highest exercise intensity at which a disproportionate increase in CO_2 elimination ($\dot{V}CO_2$) is found relative to $\dot{V}O_2$.[17,18] Although in adult subjects a concomitant disproportional increase is found between the excessive CO_2 elimination and lactate accumulation or bicarbonate decrease in the blood, a lot of experimental conditions exist where this relationship can be disturbed (e.g. in patients with McArdle's disease who have an inability to produce lactate[19] and after glycogen depletion[20]). However, despite this scientific debate, this exercise level has been shown also to be a very useful and reproducible indicator of aerobic exercise function in the paediatric age group.[16,18] Moreover, the recent development of breath-by-breath analysis of gas exchange, with rapid response gas analysers or mass spectrometers, allows precise and reproducible measurements of this parameter. More specifically in the paediatric age group, no ventilatory anaerobic threshold can be detected in about

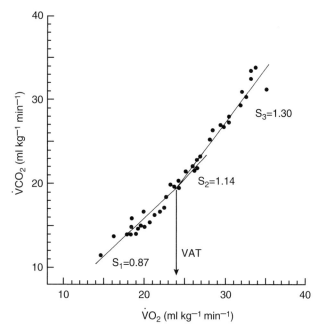

Fig. 4.1.1 Typical response of CO_2 output ($\dot{V}CO_2$) versus oxygen uptake ($\dot{V}O_2$) during graded treadmill exercise in an 11 year old boy after total repair for tetralogy of Fallot. Data represent average value for breath-by-breath measurements of $\dot{V}O_2$ and $\dot{V}CO_2$ in 10 s intervals. Exercise intensity was increased until a heart rate of 170 beats.min[-1] was reached. S_1 is the calculated slope for increase of $\dot{V}CO_2$ versus $\dot{V}O_2$ from onset of exercise to ventilatory anaerobic threshold (VAT). S_2 is the slope between VAT and the respiratory compensation point, and S_3 is the slope between VAT and exercise intensity reached at a heart rate of 170 beats.min[-1]. (Reproduced from Reybrouck et al[18], with permission).

10 % of the children.[15,16] Normal reference values have been reported for European[15,21] and North American children.[14,16]

More recently, newer concepts have been developed to assess dynamic changes of respiratory gas exchange during exercise, in patients with congenital heart disease. The study of the steepness of the slope of $\dot{V}CO_2$ versus $\dot{V}O_2$ above the ventilatory anaerobic threshold, has been found to be a very sensitive and reproducible index for the assessment of cardiovascular exercise function in this patient group (Fig. 4.1.1).

Furthermore, time constants for the assessment of the initial response of $\dot{V}O_2$, $\dot{V}CO_2$ and pulmonary ventilation ($\dot{V}_E$) during constant rate exercise, together with the recovery (half time measurement for $\dot{V}O_2$), have been found to be sensitive indicators for the evaluation of aerobic exercise function.[22] Also the calculation of the normalized oxygen deficit, which reflects the oxygen debt at the onset of exercise, subtracted from the steady state value, reached after 6 minutes of constant work rate exercise and expressed as a percentage of the total oxygen cost of a 6 minutes exercise test, has been found to be a useful parameter for the assessment of cardiovascular exercise function[23] (Fig. 4.1.2).

Parameters of aerobic exercise function, such as the steepness of the slope of $\dot{V}CO_2$, time constants, oxygen deficit and recovery kinetics, have the advantage that they all study the dynamic change of the cardiovascular response during constant work rate exercise. The evaluation of the non-steady state phase of the cardiorespiratory response to exercise is much more relevant to activities during daily life than maximal exercise testing. In particular, paediatric patients and normal children perform a lot of activities during non-steady state exercise.

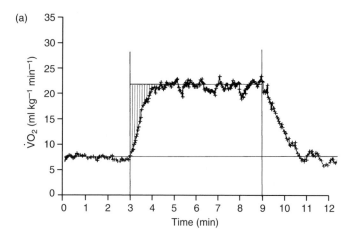

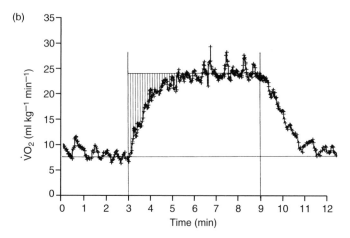

Fig. 4.1.2 Normalized oxygen deficit. Data for oxygen uptake were collected during a 3 min rest period, followed by 6 min treadmill exercise at a speed of 5 km h[-1] and inclination of 4%, and finally a recovery period for 3 minutes. The normalized oxygen deficit was calculated at onset of exercise as the difference between the single breath values and the steady state value. Each point represents a five-breaths moving average value for oxygen uptake, expressed as ml kg[-1]min[-1]. Data were cumulated and expressed as a percentage of the total oxygen cost for 6 min of exercise. A typical example is presented for (a) a normal child with an oxygen deficit of 8% and (b) a patient with Fontan circulation with an oxygen deficit of 14%.

The speed of the response of the cardiovascular system will affect the exercise tolerance and consequently the ability to perform a subsequent bout of exercise.

One should bear in mind that when evaluating exercise tolerance in patients with congenital heart disease, it is recommended that each laboratory determines its own normal values, because geographical differences may influence the results of aerobic exercise performance. For example, in the classical studies of Åstrand[24] on (normal) Swedish children, these subjects (both adults and children) always showed superior values for maximal aerobic power, which may be related to a more active life-style in the Scandinavian countries.[24]

Assessment of the habitual level of physical activity in patients with congenital heart disease

Different methods for assessing the daily level of physical activity in paediatric patients have been applied. These vary from history taking, questionnaires and interviews to more direct observations, measurements of heart rate, $\dot{V}O_2$ and even long-term video recording.[25] More sophisticated methods are pedometers and actometers which record the number of steps and vertical displacements of the body. Each of these methods has its limitations. For recall questionnaires a low reliability and low objectivity has been experienced. The same holds true for a self-keeping log. Even more sophisticated methods do not give a precise estimation of energy expenditure. For example, the measurement of $\dot{V}O_2$ under real life conditions is cumbersome, and video recording is limited to a specific space and is hard to quantify. Holter and ECG recorders are complex devices and require individual calibration. Furthermore, pedometers do not give information about vertical displacement or the nature of the activity (e.g. walking or running). Therefore these devices may give an underestimation at high activity levels. A review of advantages and disadvantages of different systems has been published by Bar-Or[25] (see chapter 1.8).

However, despite these limitations and the lack of accuracy of questionnaires, we found that the use of a standardized questionnaire, with questions about school sport, leisure time physical activity and formal sports participation during leisure time, was reproducible in young children (9–13 years of age; $r=0.98$). Furthermore, these questionnaires were able to show reduced levels of physical activity in patients with congenital heart disease and subnormal exercise tolerance.[26]

In conclusion, although the use of a standardized questionnaire to assess the daily level of physical activity is superior to the classical medical history taking, it cannot replace the objective assessment of aerobic exercise function by performing an exercise test. It should rather be considered as complementary information which is useful in the interpretation of the exercise results.

Cardiorespiratory response to exercise in specific congenital heart defects

Left-to-right shunts

Atrial septal defect

Children with atrial septal defect (ASD) usually have a normal or near normal exercise capacity. These children can attain normal values for $\dot{V}O_2$ max or near normal values. A number of haemodynamic abnormalities to exercise have been documented. The increase of cardiac output during exercise may be smaller than normal, and maximal heart rate response has been found to be lower than normal.[27] In those who underwent surgical closure of the ASD, the age at surgery has been shown to influence exercise performance. In a consecutive series of 50 patients with ASD or ventricular septum defect evaluated in our laboratory, the ventilatory anaerobic threshold (as an estimate of aerobic exercise performance) was at the lower limit of normal (89 $\pm$ 14.4% of normal).[9] When studying the exercise response in children who underwent surgical closure of an ASD, a normal value was found in children who underwent surgery before 5 years of age, whereas a significantly lower value was found in children operated after that age.[28]

In general, abnormalities detected in children either with unoperated or surgically closed ASD are usually minor and do not result in major limitations in exercise performance. Unless arrhythmia is a complication, these children should be encouraged to perform physical exercise and participate in all sports at all levels. Exercise testing is generally indicated if symptoms of arrhythmia or dyspnoea on exercise are reported.

Ventricular septal defect

A small ventricular septal defect (VSD) will transmit only a small amount of blood from the left to the right site of the heart. Also during exercise the shunt will remain small. Haemodynamic studies in this patient group showed that during graded exercise, patients with a VSD had a higher pulmonary circulation than systemic circulation, as could be expected. However, the relative shunt fraction decreased with increasing exercise intensity.[29] Subnormal values for cardiac output were found in this patient group. Exercise performance, assessed by measurement of maximal endurance time, maximal work rate on the bicycle ergometer and also maximal heart rate were slightly reduced, when compared to normal controls (90.8 $\pm$ 1.6%).[30] Studies during submaximal exercise testing, using gas exchange measurements, showed suboptimal values for ventilatory anaerobic threshold in a consecutive series of 43 patients with an unoperated VSD, evaluated in our laboratory. This value averaged 90 $\pm$ 15.3% of normal and was below the lower limit of the 95% confidence interval.[9] In this patient group, the decreased level of exercise capacity was correlated with a decreased level of habitual physical activity. In another series of patients, studied after surgical closure of a VSD, a significantly lower value was found for the ventilatory threshold (86 $\pm$ 12% of the normal value), which remains stable at re-evaluation about 3 years later on the average (see Fig. 4.1.3 below).[26] Finally in a group of 18 patients who underwent surgical closure of a large VSD with pulmonary hypertension before 1 year of life, the value for aerobic exercise performance was at the lower limit of normal (92 $\pm$ 17% of normal).[31] This shows that surgical correction of a congenital heart defect early in life can normalize the child's exercise performance.

Patent ductus arteriosus

Similarly in this group of patients, results of exercise testing will generally be normal if the size of the shunt is moderate or small. These subjects will ordinarily be asymptomatic. In most conditions, these defects will be closed surgically or percutaneously, at an age when exercise testing is not feasible. Exercise testing will add little to the routine clinical evaluation of these patients.[1]

Valvular heart lesions

Aortic stenosis

Exercise testing in patients with aortic stenosis may show ST segment changes on the ECG, reflecting ischaemia, a drop in blood pressure or an inadequate rise in blood pressure with increasing exercise intensity, and eventually arrhythmia during exercise testing. The major haemodynamic determinant of ST segment changes during exercise is the inadequate oxygen delivery to the left ventricle. After surgical relief of the gradient, improvement of ST segment changes on the ECG during exercise has been reported.[11] A critical aortic stenosis can be identified by clinical findings and confirmed by echo-Doppler examination and eventually by cardiac catheterization.

During exercise testing, most of the patients show a reduced aerobic exercise performance.[26] This may be related both to the inability of the cardiac output to increase adequately during exercise and further also to the effect of a medically imposed restriction of heavy physical activity and competitive sports.

Pulmonary valve stenosis

The transvalvular pressure gradient in pulmonary stenosis may increase during graded exercise testing.[1] In mild cases (gradients <30 mmHg), values for ventilatory anaerobic threshold have been found to be at the lower limit of normal.[26] In cases with moderate to severe pulmonary stenosis, right ventricular pressures may rise considerably during exercise, which may limit exercise capacity.[32] In severe cases, balloon valvuloplasty (or surgery) will be performed. However, exercise performance may be limited in cases with severe pulmonary incompetence.[33]

Cyanotic heart disease

Tetralogy of Fallot

Post-operative children who are felt to have good results (no residual VSD and a pressure gradient between right ventricle and pulmonary artery below 20 mm Hg), are generally asymptomatic at rest. However, a variety of abnormalities, may be brought out by intensive exercise.[13,34] These include:

(1) a high right ventricular pressure with values as high as 100 mm Hg during maximal exercise, caused by a pressure gradient between right ventricle and pulmonary artery;

(2) a blunted increase in stroke volume and heart rate; and

(3) the appearance of ventricular arrhythmia.

Despite these abnormalities, children who underwent total surgical repair for tetralogy of Fallot are usually well during daily life. However, formal exercise testing has repeatedly shown subnormal values for maximal oxygen uptake and also for ventilatory anaerobic threshold in this patient group.[13,18,35] Some individuals though may reach normal values (100% normal or even higher than normal values). Furthermore, after training, patients with this type of pathology can increase maximal work capacity by 25%.[36] On the other hand, low values for exercise capacity have also been reported.[1,18] This is mostly attributed to significant residual haemodynamic abnormalities, such as severe pulmonary regurgitation and right ventricular dysfunction.

Post-operative tetralogy of Fallot patients may have ventricular ectopy during exercise (exercise-induced arrhythmia). Patients with important residual haemodynamic abnormalities such as those mentioned above are at risk for cardiovascular events.[33,37]

Transposition of the great arteries

In simple transposition of the great arteries (TGA), the aorta arises from the right ventricle, while the pulmonary artery originates from the left ventricle. This results in severe cyanosis, as desaturated systemic venous blood is pumped in the systemic circulation, while the pulmonary venous return is pumped via left atrium and left ventricle in the lungs. Since this blood is already fully oxygenated, no more oxygen will be added to the blood.

The surgical approach to TGA from the late 1960s to early 1980s involved baffling or rerouting the systemic venous return (from the superior and inferior vena cava) to the mitral valve and left ventricle (Mustard or Senning procedure). The desaturated blood would be pumped from the pulmonary artery (arising from the left ventricle) to the lungs. The interatrial septum was removed and the pulmonary venous return (arterial blood) was drained to the right ventricle, and pumped into the aorta (arising from the right ventricle). In these atrial switch procedures, the right ventricle functions as the systemic ventricle. However, two major problems exist: (1) there have been extensive atrial incisions, and (2) the right ventricle is left as the systemic ventricle. Long-term problems include sinus node dysfunction, slow junctional rhythms, supraventricular tachycardias, depressed right ventricular function, right ventricular failure, and tricuspid valve insufficiency. Furthermore, because of extensive atrial surgery, the reservoir function of the atrium is seriously compromised. During ventricular filling, blood cannot 'just drop' into the ventricle, but has to come along a much longer way. Any tachycardia will shorten diastole and may critically impair ventricular filling, especially if an obstruction of the pathway is present. This may result in sudden death.[38]

Exercise testing following atrial switch procedures has shown a variety of abnormalities, even in patients who were asymptomatic at rest. Decreased endurance times, decreased $\dot{V}O_2$ max, subnormal $\dot{V}O_2$ during submaximal exercise and subnormal values for ventilatory anaerobic threshold have been reported.[11,18,39] Also a variety of arrhythmias have been documented during exercise testing (junctional rhythm, premature atrial contractions, premature ventricular contractions). In addition to these abnormalities, potentially detrimental effects of vigorous training in these patients have been reported. It is unknown, whether the right ventricle can dilate and hypertrophy during endurance training as does the left ventricle in highly trained young athletes.[34] For these reasons, high intensity isometric exercise or high intensity dynamic exercise and competitive sports are discouraged.

Nowadays the arterial switch operation is the current surgical technique for transposition of the great arteries in the majority of cases. Normal values for exercise performance and normal ST on ECG have been reported in this patient group. However, the length of the follow up with this procedure is still limited.[1]

Fontan-circulation

In tricuspid atresia, there is a congenital absence of the tricuspid valve. To survive, a communication is made between the caval veins and the pulmonary artery, bypassing the right ventricle. This means that there is no effective right heart pump. Although the survival and also preoperative exercise performance of these patients improve dramatically, most of these subjects still have a limited exercise tolerance,[40,41,42] which is due to the subnormal value for cardiac output during exercise.[43]

Rhythm disturbances and conduction defects

Congenital complete atrioventricular block

In congenital complete atrioventricular block, the atrial rate increases normally during exercise, but ventricular rate does not accelerate adequately. In some cases, these patients may develop dizziness and syncope.[44] Exercise testing in these patients shows subnormal values for $\dot{V}O_2$ max or ventilatory anaerobic threshold and even for the increase of oxygen uptake versus exercise intensity.[45] This results from the lack of acceleration of heart rate during exercise, one of the major components which increase cardiac output and consequently oxygen delivery to the exercising tissues. In some cases with severe bradycardia and syncope, a pacemaker is inserted. It is obvious that these children should avoid competitive sports and physical activities with a danger of body collision.

In the paediatric population, the frequency and significance of arrhythmia differs from adults.[44] As a general rule, the assessment of cardiac arrhythmia during exercise is useful in the management of these patients. If arrhythmia disappears with increasing exercise intensity, the arrhythmia is usually benign.

A common form of chronotropic impairment is abnormal function of the sinus node. This anatomic structure is vulnerable to damage during cardiac surgery. Damage of the sinus node has frequently been observed after surgical procedures that require extensive manipulations and sutures in the atria. Specific defects include D-transposition of the great arteries, repaired by atrial baffling procedures.[46] However, fortunately, surgically acquired complete atrioventricular block, despite extensive surgery in the atria as for D-transposition of the great arteries, is relatively uncommon. Pacemaker technology, when applied in young patients, has significant limitations, because the upper limit of the pacemaker is often too low for these youngsters to achieve a physiological normal value for heart rate during exercise.[46]

Natural evolution of aerobic exercise performance and daily level of physical activity in patients with congenital heart disease

To study the natural evolution of aerobic exercise performance during medium-term follow-up in patients with congenital heart disease, exercise performance tests were compared in patients who underwent exercise testing at least twice with a time interval of about 3 years. Between 1980 to 1992, at our department of Paediatric Cardiology, 1982 exercise tests were performed. In 79 patients from this database,[26] exercise tests were performed at least twice in the same patient, with satisfactory respiratory gas exchange measurements on a breath-by-breath basis and a time interval of at least two years. These patients were divided into six subgroups. Three groups were studied for a non-operated congenital heart defect. Fourteen patients were followed for a ventricular septal defect (VSD), which did not require surgical closure; 12 patients were followed for a mild pulmonary stenosis (PS), with a gradient of less than 41 mm Hg (average 17 ± 11 mm Hg); and 12 patients were followed with a mild aortic stenosis (AS) with a mean gradient of 36 ± 17 mm Hg. All underwent exercise testing. Furthermore, three groups of patients who underwent surgical repair of a congenital heart defect were also studied twice. Sixteen patients who underwent total correction for tetralogy of Fallot (TF-PO), 13 patients who underwent surgical closure of a VSD (VSD-PO), and 12 patients with a Fontan circulation for tricuspidatresia, 1.9 ± 1.1 years after the Fontan operation, were studied.

The results of this study showed that at the initial evaluation all patients were in class I of the New York Heart Association (NYHA). Aerobic exercise performance, assessed by determination of the ventilatory anaerobic threshold, was at the lower limit of the normal mean

value or below (Fig. 4.1.3). Significant differences for aerobic exercise performance were found between the different pathologies. The lowest values were found in the patients with the Fontan circulation and the highest values in patients with a VSD.

At reassessment, about three years later, all patients remained in NYHA class I, except for two patients with a Fontan circulation, who belonged to class II and III at re-evaluation. For patients in whom no medical restriction of physical activity was imposed (VSD, PS and VSD-PO), no significant change was found for the value of ventilatory anaerobic threshold (expressed as a percentage of the mean value obtained in a pool of normal controls of the same age and gender) (Fig. 4.1.3). At variance, in patients with AS, with a medically imposed restriction of heavy physical exercise and competitive sports, a decrease was found for aerobic exercise performance of about 8%. In patients with surgical repair of tetralogy of Fallot, a decrease in the value of ventilatory anaerobic threshold of about 9% was found over the same time interval, which was related to residual haemodynamic lesions, such as pulmonary valve incompetence.[35] Finally, also in the patients with a Fontan circulation, a significant decrease of aerobic exercise performance was found over this time interval. Similarly, at reassessment the lowest values were found in this patient group. This was related to the fact that these patients were unable to perform intensive physical exercise during daily life activities and also to residual haemodynamic dysfunction.

The daily level of physical activity, assessed by a standardized questionnaire, was significantly lower both at the first and second evaluation, in patients with AS, surgical repair of tetralogy of Fallot and Fontan repair. These subnormal values for daily physical activity level were associated with a significant decrease in aerobic exercise function at reassessment. In the other patient groups (VSD, PS, VSD-PO), no significant change was found for aerobic exercise performance between the two assessments (Fig. 4.1.3).

These data show the combined effect of residual haemodynamic lesions and hypoactivity on the evaluation of aerobic exercise performance in these groups of patients. In children and adolescents with aortic stenosis, significantly lower values for aerobic exercise

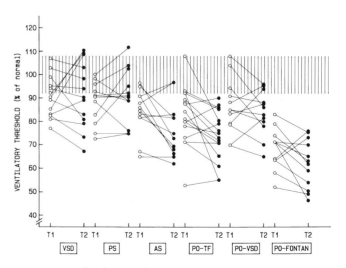

Fig. 4.1.3 Serial evaluation of cardiovascular exercise performance in children with congenital heart disease. (Reproduced from Reybrouck *et al.*,[26] with permission.)

Table 4.1.1   Guidelines for exercise restriction in different types of congenital heart disease

Type of cardiac disorder	Exercise restriction
Atrial septal defect, untreated	
Normal pulmonary artery pressures	No[1]
Pulmonary hypertension	Moderate[3]
Atrial septal defect, closed at operation or by interventional catheterization	
$\geqslant$6 months after operation	No
Pulmonary hypertension, arrhythmia or myocardial dysfunction	Mild[2] to moderate
Ventricular septal defect, untreated	
Normal pulmonary artery pressures	No
Mild to moderate pulmonary hypertension	Moderate
Ventricular septal defect, closed at operation or by interventional catheterization	
$\geqslant$6 months after operation	No
Residual moderate or large defects	Moderate
Persistent pulmonary hypertension	Moderate to severe
Patent ductus arteriosus, closed at operation or by interventional catheterization	
Normal cardiac examination	No
Aortic stenosis, untreated	
Mild (gradient <30 mmHg PIG)	No
Moderate (gradient 30–70 mmHg PIG)	Mild
Severe (gradient >70 mmHg PIG)	Moderate
Aortic stenosis, treated by surgery or balloon valvuloplasty	
If residual stenosis	Same rules as for untreated aortic stenosis
If moderate to severe regurgitation	
– normal ventricular size	No
– with moderate left ventricular enlargement	Moderate, no static exercise
Pulmonary valve stenosis, untreated	
<50 mm Hg PIG, normal right ventricular function	No
>50 mm Hg PIG	Moderate
Pulmonary valve stenosis, treated by surgery or balloon valvuloplasty	
Adequate relief	No
Residual stenosis (PIG >50 mm Hg)	Moderate
Severe pulmonary incompetence	Individual assessment
Repaired tetralogy of Fallot	
Excellent surgical result, no arrhythmia	No
Marked pulmonary regurgitation	Moderate
Transposition of the great arteries	
Venous switch	Mild to moderate
Arterial switch, if excellent surgical outcome	No restriction for dynamic exercise avoidance of static exercise

Adapted from Graham et al.[33]

Exercise restriction: (1) *No restriction*: all sports activities at school, during leisure time and also competitive sports are allowed. (2) *Mild restriction*: exercises of maximal intensity or near maximal intensity should be avoided. (3) *Moderate restriction*: team sports participation is discouraged. (4) *Severe restriction*: patients are advised to perform only activities with low energy expenditure (e.g. bowling, low intensity callisthenics, golf).

   PIG: peak instantaneous gradient.

performance were found both at first and second assessment. Similar data have been reported by Driscoll et al.[30] In this group of patients heavy physical exercise and competitive sports are discouraged because of the risk of ischaemia and arrhythmia. In the other patient groups, residual haemodynamic dysfunction may impede the child in performance of aerobic exercise of heavy intensity, which is necessary for the normal development of the oxidative metabolism. In these patient groups (Fontan and TF-PO), subnormal values for increase in $\dot{V}O_2$ during graded exercise have also been observed.[18,42]

The results of these studies show that the suboptimal aerobic exercise performance in children and adolescents with congenital heart disease is to some extent attributable to residual haemodynamic lesions after corrective surgery of the defect, and also to some degree of hypoactivity, which results from overprotection of the parents and the environment. However, in some patients there may also be an increase of the severity of the disease, which may impede the individual in performing the same amount of physical exercise as healthy peers. Therefore, except for some cases with progression of the severity of the disease and medical imposed restriction of intensive dynamic or static physical exercise, children and adolescents with congenital heart disease and their parents should be strongly encouraged to be more active and to prevent the deleterious effect of physical deconditioning.

Exercise recommendations and rehabilitation of patients with congenital heart disease

Nowadays most children with congenital heart disease are encouraged to be fully active and to participate in all recreational sport activities, also after corrective surgery. These recommendations are based on clinical findings which have shown that physical exercise in children with congenital heart disease has beneficial effects on the physical, psychological and social level, both for the children and also for the parents. In the majority of cases, these children do not need to participate in a formal rehabilitation programme, but they should be encouraged to participate in recreational physical activities in leisure time and at school. Even after corrective surgery a formal rehabilitation programme is mostly restricted to the hospitalization period and consists mainly of chest physiotherapy (breathing exercises) and early mobilization. As soon as the children are discharged from the hospital, they are encouraged to resume their normal physical activities at home.

In the majority of cases of congenital heart disease there are only a few contraindications for physical exercise for the non-operated cardiac defects as for the operated ones.[33] The final decision to allow a child with congenital heart disease to participate in physical exercise should always be based on a full cardiological examination.

A few controlled exercise studies in patients with congenital heart disease have shown that maximal exercise capacity can be improved following a period of physical training.[36,47] However, $\dot{V}O_2$ max was not improved in all subjects. The improvement of maximal exercise performance (expressed in watts, assessed during bicycle ergometry) without an increase in $\dot{V}O_2$ max represents an improved mechanical efficiency during exercise. This may be beneficial for the patients, since the same level of exercise will be perceived as easier to perform and will induce less dyspnoea. Furthermore, especially in young children, the measurement of $\dot{V}O_2$ max is often difficult as it depends on the motivation of the child. In fact, a plateau in $\dot{V}O_2$ with increasing exercise intensity (which is a prerequisite for a true $\dot{V}O_2$ max) is difficult to obtain in young children.[10]

Cumulative medical experience has shown that the potential risk of physical exercise in patients with congenital heart disease is very low.[33] In fact, only a few heart defects have been associated with sudden cardiac death during sports participation. These include mainly: hypertrophic cardiomyopathy, aortic stenosis, congenital anomalies of the coronary arteries, Marfan's syndrome, and myocarditis. Fortunately, these anomalies represent only a small percentage of the total number of congenital heart defects for which sport participation is allowed.

A restriction of heavy physical exercise and competitive sports is imposed in moderate to severe aortic stenosis, in left to right shunts with pulmonary hypertension, hypertrophic cardiomyopathy, pulmonary hypertension and arrhythmia which worsens during exercise. As a general rule, cardiopulmonary exercise testing is advised in children with congenital heart defects, before sport participation is allowed. More detailed guidelines for different types of congenital heart defects have been published jointly by the American College of Sports Medicine and the American College of Cardiology (1994)[48]; see also Table 4.1.1.

Summary

As the majority of patients with congenital heart disease belong to the paediatric age group, exercise testing equipment and exercise protocols have to be adapted for children. Functional performance should be assessed by performing exercise testing with measurement of gas exchange. Nowadays new concepts for exercise testing in the paediatric age group are analysis of gas exchange during the non-steady state of exercise and determination of the kinetics of gas exchange during the recovery phase of exercise. In some groups of patients with congenital heart disease, suboptimal values have been found for aerobic exercise capacity, which can be ascribed to haemodynamic dysfunction or residual haemodynamic lesions after surgery (e.g. in transposition of the great arteries, tetralogy of Fallot, Fontan repair for univentricular heart). In other types of pathologies medical imposed restriction of intensive physical exercise or competitive sports may determine to some extent a subnormal value of exercise performance. Finally in some other types of congenital heart disease without overt haemodynamic dysfunction (e.g. ventricular septal defect or atrial septal defect, with normal pressures in the pulmonary circulation) a suboptimal value for aerobic exercise capacity is often related to overprotection by the parents or environment of the child. Therefore, except for some cases with medically imposed restriction of intensive physical exercise, most patients are encouraged to be fully active during leisure time and to participate in all types of physical exercise at school.

References

1. Gibbons, R. J., Balady, G. J., Beasley, J. W., Bricker, J. T., Duvernoy, W. F. C., Froelicher, V. F., Mark, D. B., Marwich, T. H., McCallister, B. D., Thompson, P. D, Winters, W. L. and Yanowitz, F. G. ACC/AHA Guidelines for Exercise Testing. A Report of the American College of Cardiology/ American Heart Association Task force on Practice Guidelines (Committee on Exercise Testing), *Journal of the American College of Cardiology* 1997; 30: 260–15.

2. Pina, I. L., Balady, G. J., Hanson, M., Labovitz, A. J., Madonna, D. W. and Myers, J. Guidelines for Clinical Exercise Testing Laboratories. A Statement for Healthcare Professionals from the Committee on Exercise and Cardiac Rehabilitation, American Heart Association. *Circulation* 1995; **91**: 912–21.

3. Washington, R. L., Bricker, J. T., Alpert, B. S., Daniels, S. R., Decelbaum, R. J., Fisher, E. A., Gidding, S. S., Isabel-Jones, J., Kavey, R. E. W., Marx, G. R., Strong, B. W., Teske, D. W., Wilmore, J. H. and Winston, M. Guidelines for Exercise Testing in the Pediatric Age Group. *Circulation* 1994; **90**: 2166–79.

4. Cumming, G. R., Everatt, D. and Hastman, L. Bruce treadmill test in children: normal values in a clinic population. *American Journal of Cardiology* 1978; **41**: 69–75.

5. James, F. W., Blomqvist, C. G., Freed, M. D., Miller, W. W., Moller, J. H, Nugent, E. W., Riopel, D. A., Strong, W. B. and Wessel, H. U. Standards for Exercise Testing In the Pediatric Age Group. *Circulation* 1982; **66**: 1377A–97A.

6. Rowland, T. W. Aerobic exercise testing protocols. In *Pediatric laboratory exercise testing. Clinical guidelines* (ed. T. W. Rowland), Human Kinetics Publishers. Champaign, Il. 1993; 19–41.

7. Riopel, D. A., Taylor, A. B. and Hohn, A. R. Blood pressure, heart rate, pressure-rate product and electrocardiographic changes in healthy children during treadmill exercise. *American Journal of Cardiology* 1979; **44**: 697–704.

8. Chandramouli, B., Ehmke, D. A. and Lauer, R. M. Exercise-induced electrocardiographic changes in children with congenital aortic stenosis. *Journal of Pediatrics* 1973; **87**: 725–30.

9. Reybrouck, T., Weymans, M., Stijns, H. and van der Hauwaert, L. G. Ventilatory anaerobic threshold for evaluating exercise performance in children with congenital left-to right intracardiac shunt. *Pediatric Cardiology* 1986; **7**: 19–24.

10. Armstrong, N., Welsman, J. and Winsley, R. Is peak $\dot{V}O_2$ a maximal index of children's aerobic fitness. *International Journal of Sports Medicine* 1996; **17**: 356–59.

11. Driscoll, D. J. Exercise testing. In *Moss' heart disease in infants, children, and adolescents* (ed. F. H. Adams, G. C. Emmanouides and T. A. Riemenschneider), Williams & Wilkins, Baltimore, 1989; 293–310.

12. Adams, F. H., Linde, L. M. and Niyake, H. The physical working capacity of normal school children. *Pediatrics* 1961; **28**: 55–64.

13. Reybrouck, T., Weymans, M., Stijns, H. and van der Hauwaert, L. G. Exercise testing after correction of tetralogy of Fallot: The fallacy of a reduced heart rate response. *American. Heart Journal* 1986; **112**: 998–1003.

14. Cooper, D. M., Weiler-Ravell, D., Whipp, B. J. and Wasserman, K. Aerobic parameters of exercise as a function of body size during growth in children. *Journal of Applied Physiology* 1984; **56**: 628–34.

15. Reybrouck, T., Weymans, M., Stijns, H. and Van der Hauwaert, L. G. Ventilatory anaerobic threshold in healthy children. *European Journal of Applied Physiology* 1985; **54**: 278–84.

16. Washington, R. L., van Gundy, J. C., Cohen, C., Sondheimer, H. M. and Wolfe, R. R. Normal aerobic and anaerobic exercise data for North American school-age children. *Journal of Pediatrics* 1988; **112**; 223–33.

17. Wasserman, K., Beaver, W. L. and Whipp, B. J. Gas exchange threshold and the lactic acidosis (anaerobic) threshold. *Circulation* 1990; **81**, (Suppl) 11: 14–30.

18. Reybrouck, T., Mertens, L., Kalis, N., Weymans, M., Dumoulin, M., Daenen, W. and Gewillig, M. Dynamics of respiratory gas exchange during exercise after correction of congenital heart disease. *Journal of Applied Physiology* 1996; **80**: 458–63.

19. Hagberg, J. M., Coyle, E. F., Carroll, J. E., Miller, J. M., Martin, W. H. and Brooke MH. Exercise hyperventilation in patients with McArdle's disease. *Journal of Applied Physiology* 1982; **52**: 991–4.

20. Heigenhauser, G. J. F., Sutton, J. R. and Jones, N. L. Effect of glycogen depletion on ventilatory response to exercise. *Journal of Applied Physiology* 1983; **54**: 470–4.

21. Schulze-Neick, I., Austenat, I., Wessel, H. U. and Lange, P. Submaximum exercise parameters in normal children. *Pediatric Research* 1985; **38**: 454.

22. Cooper, D. M., Kaplan, M. R., Baumgarten, L., Weiler-Ravell, D., Whipp, B. J. and Wasserman, K. Coupling of ventilation and CO_2 production during exercise in children. *Pediatric Research.* 1987; **21**: 568–72.

23. Mertens, L., Gewillig, M., Eyskens, B., Dumoulin, M., Brown, S., Daenen, W. and Reybrouck, T. Slow kinetics of oxygen uptake at onset of exercise in patients with a Fontan circulation. *Proceedings 2nd World Congress of Paediatric Cardiology and Cardiac Surgery* 1997: 824–26.

24. Åstrand, P. O. (1952). *Experimental studies of physical working capacity in relation to sex and age.* Munsgaard, Copenhagen.

25. Bar-Or, O. Clinical implications of pediatric exercise physiology. *Annals of Clinical Research* 1982; **14**, (Suppl) 34: 97–106.

26. Reybrouck, T., Rogers, R., Weymans, M., Dumoulin, M., Vanhove, M., Daenen, W. and Van der Hauwaert, L. Serial cardiorespiratory exercise testing in patients with congenital heart disease. *European Journal of Pediatrics* 1995; **154**: 801–6.

27. Perrault, H., Drblik, S. P., Montigny, M., Davignon, A., Lamarre, A., Chartrand, C. and Stanley, P. Comparison of cardiovascular adjustments to exercise in adolescents 8 to 15 years of age after correction of tetralogy of Fallot, ventricular septal defect or atrial septal defect. *The American Journal of Cardiology* 1989; **64**: 213–17.

28. Reybrouck, T., Bisschop, A., Dumoulin, M. and Van der Hauwaert, L. G. Cardiorespiratory exercise capacity after surgical closure of atrial septal defect is influenced by the age at surgery. *American Heart Journal* 1991; **122**: 1073–78.

29. Bendien, C., Bossina, K. K., Buurma, A. E., Gerding, A. M., Kuipers, J. R. G., Landsman, M. L. J, Mook, G. A. and Zijlstra, W. G. Hemodynamic effects of dynamic exercise in children and adolescents with moderate-to-small ventricular septal defects. *Circulation* 1984; **70**: 929–34.

30. Driscoll, D. J., Wolfe, R. R., Gersony, W. M., Hayes, C. J., Keane, J. F., Kidd, L., O'Fallon, M., Pieroni, D. R. and Weidman, W. H. Cardiorespiratory responses to exercise of patients with aortic stenosis, pulmonary stenosis, and ventricular septal defect. *Circulation* 1993; **87**, (Suppl): I-102–I-13.

31. Reybrouck, T., Mertens, L., Schulze-Neick, I., Austenat, I., Eyskens, B., Dumoulin, M. and Gewillig, M. Ventilatory inefficiency for carbon dioxide during exercise in patients with pulmonary hypertension. *Clinical Physiology* 1998; **18**: 337–44.

32. Rowland, T. W. Congenital obstructive and valvular heart disease. In *Sports and exercise for children with chronic health conditions* (ed. B. Goldberg), Human Kinetics, Leeds (UK). 1995; 225–36.

33. Graham, T. W. Jr, Bricker, T., James, F. W. and Strong, W. B. Congenital heart disease. *Medicine and Science in Sports and Exercise* 1994; **26** (suppl): S246–S253.

34. Fahey, J. T. Congenital heart disease-shunt lesions and cyanotic heart disease. In *Sports and exercise for children with chronic health conditions* (ed. B. Goldberg), Human Kinetics, Leeds (UK), 1995; 208–24.

35. Rowe, S. A., Zakha, K. G., Manolio, T. A, Hornheffer, P. J. and Kidd, L. Lung function and pulmonary regurgitation limit exercise capacity in postoperative tetralogy of Fallot. *Journal of the American College of Cardiology* 1991; **17**: 461–66.

36. Goldberg, B., Fripp, R. R., Lister, G., Loke, J., Nicholas, J. A. and Talner, N. S. Effect of physical training on exercise performance of children following surgical repair of congenital heart disease. *Pediatrics* 1981; **68**: 691–99.

37. Garson, A. Jr, Gillette, P. C., Gutgesell, H. P., M. C. and Namara, D. G. Stress-induced ventricular arrhythmia after repair of tetralogy of Fallot. *American Journal of Cardiology* 1980; **46**: 1006–12.

38. Gewillig, M., Balaji, S., Mertens, B., Lesaffre, E. and Deanfield, J. Risk factors for arrhythmia and death after Mustard operation for simple transposition of the great arteries. *Circulation* 1991; **84**: 187–92.

39. Reybrouck, T., Gewillig, M., Dumoulin, M. and van der Hauwaert, L. G. Cardiorespiratory exercise performance after Senning operation for transposition of the great arteries. *British Heart Journal* 1993; **70**: 175–79.

40. Driscoll, D. J., Danielson, G. K., Puga, F. J., Schaff, H. F., Heise, C. T. and Staats, B. A. Exercise tolerance and cardiorespiratory response to exercise after Fontan operation for tricuspidatresia or functional single ventricle. *Journal of the American College of Cardiology* 1986; **7**: 1087–94.

41. Gewillig, M. The Fontan Circulation: late functional results. *Seminars in Thoracic and Cardiovascular Surgery* 1994; **6**: 56–63.

42. Mertens, L., Rogers, R., Reybrouck, T., Dumoulin, M. Vanhees, L. and Gewillig, M. Cardiopulmonary response to exercise after the Fontan operation—a cross sectional and longitudinal evaluation. *Cardiology in the Young* 1996; **6**: 136–42.

43. Gewillig, M., Lündstrom, R., Bull, C., Wyse, R. K. H. and Deanfield, J. E. Exercise responses in patients with congenital heart disease after Fontan repair : Patterns and determinants of performance. *Journal of the American College of Cardiology* 1990; **15**: 1424–32.

44. Park, M. K. *Pediatric cardiology for practitioners* (3rd edn). Mosby, St Louis, 1996.

45. Reybrouck, T., Vanden Eynde, B., Dumoulin M. and Van der Hauwaert, L. G. Cardiorespiratory response to exercise in congenital complete atrio ventricular block. *American Journal of Cardiology* 1989; **64**: 896–99.

46. Parridon, S. M. Congenital heart disease : cardiac performance and adaptations to exercise. *Pediatric Exercise Science* 1997; **9**: 308–323.

47. Balfour, I. C., Drimmer, A. M., Nouri, S., Pennington, D. G., Hemkens, C. and Harvey, L. L. Pediatric cardiac rehabilitation. *American Journal of Diseases of Children* 1991; **145**: 627–30.

48. American College of Sports Medicine and American College of Cardiology. Recommendations for determining eligibility for competition in athletes with cardiovascular abnormalities. *Medicine and Science in Sports and Exercise* 1994; **26**(Suppl): 223–76.

4.2 Exercise and physical activity in the child with asthma

Helge Hebestreit

Introduction

Asthma is a lung disease with the following characteristics:[1]

(1) airway obstruction that is reversible (but not completely so in some patients) either spontaneously or with treatment;

(2) airway inflammation; and

(3) increased airway responsiveness to a variety of stimuli.

Information on the prevalence of asthma in children and adolescents is dependent on the diagnostic criteria used. In a recent study in Denmark, the prevalence of asthma in 8–10 year old children, as diagnosed by their general practitioner or during a medical assessment of children who were selected based on a screening interview and monitoring of peak flow, was 6.6%.[2] In a survey on 12 year old children,[3] a history of asthma was reported in 16.8% of children in New Zealand, while other countries showed lower prevalences (South Africa, 11.5%; Sweden, 4.0%; Wales, 12.0%). In another epidemiological study surveying 12–15 year-old children in Australia, England, Germany and New Zealand, 20–27% of the participants experienced wheezing during the past 12 months, and 4–12% reported more than three episodes per year.[4] Thus, the prevalence of asthma in childhood and adolescence varies among countries and can be estimated to be somewhere between 5–20%. Over the last decades, there seems to be an increasing asthma prevalence in the western countries.[5,6]

One of the characteristics of asthma is that the bronchial system is hyper-responsive to a variety of triggers. These stimuli include airway infections, exposure to allergens or air pollutants, inhalation of dry and cold air, and, last but not least, exercise. Thus, exercise-induced asthma (EIA) is a feature of asthma and may affect any patient with asthma, provided that the exercise is of a sufficient intensity and duration.[7] Thus, knowledge about the interrelationships between asthma and exercise is of immense importance when dealing with an active paediatric population.

This chapter reviews the existing data on exercise capacity and physical activity of children with asthma. The mechanisms underlying pathologic responses to exercise in these children are summarized. Most of the information provided in this chapter is valid not only for children but also for adults.

Exercise induced asthma

Children at risk

As stated above, EIA may possibly affect any child diagnosed to suffer from asthma. Furthermore, EIA has been described in patients with a history of bronchopulmonary dysplasia, or with a diagnosis of hay fever or cystic fibrosis.[8,9] There are also children or adolescents suffering from EIA, who do not exhibit any of the above risk factors. It has been suggested that some 10% of adolescent athletes suffer from EIA without it being recognized.[10]

Symptoms of EIA

In most patients, EIA leads to coughing, wheezing and shortness of breath shortly following exercise.[11] However, rather than reporting these typical respiratory symptoms, some patients complain about chest discomfort, nausea or stomach-ache following exercise. In children, symptoms usually resolve within 10 to 90 min after cessation of exercise, although some may experience a progressive worsening of bronchoconstriction.

Pathophysiology of exercise-induced bronchoconstriction

It has long been recognized that children with asthma are less likely to experience an attack when exercising in a warm and humid environment than when inhaling cold and dry air. Based on this observation, it was suggested that either the heat loss from the respiratory epithelium and/or the loss of water might trigger the bronchoconstriction.[12] Based on subsequent studies, the role of airway cooling/drying during exercise and/or rewarming of the bronchi after cessation of exertion is now generally accepted as the major mechanism responsible for EIA.[13] However, even if the respiratory heat loss is controlled for, the likelihood and severity of EIA is influenced by exercise intensity (low versus high) and exercise mode (swimming versus running).[14,15] Whether these latter findings indicate that airway cooling/drying/rewarming are not the exclusive pathogenic triggers responsible for EIA remains a matter of debate. It could be possible that significant local differences in respiratory heat loss occurred under the various conditions in the studies by Bar-Yishay *et al.*[14] and Noviski *et al.*[15] even though the respiratory heat loss at the level of the mouth was identical.[16]

The exact pathway linking airway cooling/rewarming/drying to bronchial obstruction is not yet completely understood.[13] The following mechanisms have been suggested:

1. The cooling of the bronchial wall stimulates the parasympathetic system which then leads to a broncoconstriction.[17]

2. The cooling of the airways, or the increase in bronchial surface osmolality paralleling airway drying, triggers the release of

neutrophil chemotactic factor of anaphylaxis, histamine and/or leukotrienes which then initiate a bronchoconstriction.[18,19]

3. The rewarming of the airways following exercise induces either a contraction of smooth airway muscles, or a hyperaemia and swelling of the bronchial mucosa.[13,20]

Late response

Several studies have suggested that a considerable number of patients suffering from EIA experience a second fall in pulmonary function parameters several hours after the first exercise-induced airway narrowing has resolved.[21,22] These 'late responses' were reported to begin 2–4 hours following the exercise challenge, peak between 4–8 hours and resolve after 12–24 hours. There are, however, some recent studies which could not detect a significant exercise-induced late response compared to a placebo visit.[23,24] The authors attributed the reports of late asthmatic responses following exercise to the increased spontaneous within-day variation of pulmonary mechanics in children with asthma.[23,24]

Refractory period

In patients with EIA, a second bout of exercise 1–2 hours following a first exercise task may induce less bronchial obstruction than a task of similar exercise intensity and duration which is administered without a preceding exercise.[25] This reduced responsiveness is referred to as 'refractory period', and may occur even if the first challenge did not induce a significant bronchial narrowing or was performed with other muscle groups than the subsequent exercise.[26] Refractoriness can be induced by continuous submaximal exercise but also by intermittent sprints.[27,28]

It is important to stress that only about 40–60% of all patients with EIA show a refractory period.[29] In those patients who do exhibit this phenomenon the most effective exercise protocol seems to vary among individuals. Therefore, asthma patients who wish to utilize the refractory period to prevent EIA during training and competition should be counselled to try several exercise procedures and select the most effective routine.

The mechanisms underlying the refractory period are not yet understood. It has been suggested that mast cells might be depleted from mediators, including histamine, with the first exercise challenge and that the replenishment of the stores takes up to 2 hours.[30] Another explanation put forward is that prostaglandins, possibly type E_2, are released with the initial exercise bout and prevent a bronchial obstruction with a subsequent exercise challenge.[31] A third hypothesis is based on the assumption that a second exercise task induces less airway cooling than the first task.[32]

Diagnosing EIA

EIA should be suspected if a patient complains about shortness of breath, wheezing or coughing during or following exercise. In children or adolescents who complain about chest pain with exercise, EIA should also be suspected.[33]

In patients diagnosed to have asthma, a history of exercise-related symptoms typical for EIA justifies a medical treatment (see below) without further evaluation.[13] Only if the improvement with medication is less than expected, is a further evaluation including an exercise challenge necessary.

Children and adolescents who have no established diagnosis of asthma should be tested for impairment of resting pulmonary functions. If this test reveals bronchial obstruction which is markedly improved with inhalation of β-adrenergic drugs, asthma as the cause for the exercise-related symptoms can be assumed. No further testing is necessary to establish the diagnosis if an adequate treatment leads to satisfactory results. In all other cases, a standardized challenge to prove bronchial hyper-responsiveness is recommended.

Physical activity and exercise capacity of children and adolescents with asthma or EIA

Acute asthmatic attacks are often triggered by exercise.[34] It would, therefore, not be surprising if children with asthma were less active than their peers. Astonishingly little information is available on this issue. One survey suggests that children with known asthma are physically as active as their peers,[35] another study found children with asthma to be even more active than healthy children.[36] Thus, nowadays the average child who is known to suffer from asthma probably is as active as healthy children. This is in contrast to findings reported in the 1970s and might be the consequence of improved therapy and counselling towards physical activity. In agreement with this hypothesis, two studies have shown that children who suffer from undiagnosed or poorly controlled asthma are still at risk for hypoactivity.[37,38]

Most[39,40,41] but not all[42] studies have shown that children with asthma have a decreased short-term and endurance exercise capacity compared to healthy controls. The different findings between studies might reflect, in part, differences in disease severity.[40,41] Mechanisms limiting exercise capacity in asthmatic patients could be an increase in end-expiratory lung volume with exercise, which results in increased work for ventilation and limitation of minute ventilation,[43] and a disturbance of the ventilation–perfusion relationship in the lung.[44] However, the latter mechanism should lead to oxygen desaturation with exercise, which is rarely seen in patients with asthma.[20]

Since there is increasing evidence that a reduced level of physical activity in children with asthma is a more important predictor of low fitness than disease severity,[42,45] a reduced fitness in a child with asthma should be primarily 'treated' with education and conditioning. An adjustment of medication might only be necessary in some cases.

Exercise related benefits to children with asthma

Several studies have evaluated the benefits of increased physical activity in children and adolescents with asthma. In general, the effects are more pronounced in patients with severe disease compared to those with moderately severe asthma. Patients with mild asthma may not benefit from specific exercise programmes more than healthy children.

While many studies showed an improvement in fitness or psychological variables in structured and supervised training programmes, some,[46] but not all,[47] observed a beneficial effect from a home-based unsupervised exercise programme. It is therefore advocated to refer those patients with moderate to severe asthma who might benefit from exercise rehabilitation to a structured programme. Possibly, the advantage of a structured exercise programme might be related to the effects of education[48] in addition to a more regular and intense physical training.

Improvement in fitness

Regular exercise training is effective in enhancing cardiovascular fitness and motor coordination in children with asthma.[40,49] The mechanisms underlying this improvement may act via the training effect, but also by helping children with asthma and their parents to feel comfortable when the child engages in physical activities.

Psychological benefits

Children with asthma show disturbances in their psychological development which might be treated with an exercise programme.[50] Specifically, positive effects have been shown for ego structure, body image, social development and concentration capacity.[50]

It should also be kept in mind that children with asthma strongly value the ability to engage in physical activities. For example, when 71 children aged 9–11 years were asked 'How do you know when you are healthy?', 46% of all responses referred to activity or other physical/functional abilities.[51] In contrast, only 9% of the responses related to the absence of asthma specific symptoms. In other words, many children with asthma consider physical activity as an integral part of daily life. To them, being allowed to exercise means to be normal.

Reduction in asthma symptoms and EIA

Even relatively short exercise programmes with a duration of 2–6 months may reduce the frequency of asthma symptoms, hospitalizations, emergency room visits and school absenteeism.[52,53] However, the effects of an exercise programme on EIA are less clear. While Fitch et al.[54] did not see any change in the severity of EIA after a 3-months running training, Svenonius et al.[46] and Henrikson and Nielsen[55] found a significant improvement in EIA following a combined landbased and swimming interval training for 3–4 months and a 6-week training, respectively. At least part of the improvement in hyperresponsiveness observed in the latter two studies might be attributed to the fact that the exercise challenge to determine EIA was not adjusted for the improvements in physical fitness with training. Thus, the relative intensity of the exercise was lower for the post-training tests compared to the pre-training challenge, which might have been paralleled by a lower minute ventilation.

Exercise testing in children with asthma or suspected EIA

Indications

As pointed out above, exercise testing might be helpful to establish the diagnosis of EIA. Furthermore, once a treatment for EIA has been started, the effectiveness of that therapy can be assessed using a follow-up exercise test.

In addition, exercise testing in patients with asthma or EIA can serve several other purposes:

1. According to the guidelines of the US National Asthma Education Program,[1] the diagnosis of asthma is based on the patient's medical history, physical examination, and, last but not least, laboratory tests. Therefore, when asthma is suspected but cannot be proven otherwise, an exercise test may help to establish the diagnosis by demonstrating a hyper-responsive airway system. The same objective can, however, be met with provocation tests using other triggers, such as hyperventilation with room air or cold air or histamine/metacholine provocation. It should be kept in mind that most of these tests including an exercise challenge have a sensitivity to diagnose asthma of about 40–60%.[56–59] The specificity is generally somewhat higher (around 80–90%).

2. Exercise testing has been used as a screening tool for asthma in epidemiological research.[3] A relatively low sensitivity and a poor stability of the bronchial responses over time, however, challenge its value for this purpose.[60,61]

3. Several studies have shown that children who are not known to have asthma, but who show a pathological fall in pulmonary function parameters following an exercise challenge, are at high risk of developing clinically recognizable asthma during the subsequent years.[57] Exercise testing could, therefore, be used to screen for children at risk of developing asthma. To date, however, a pathological airway response to an exercise test without any other signs of respiratory disease would not result in any treatment, so that this indication for an exercise test is hypothetical. In future, cromoglycate sodium might be advocated to prevent the development of asthma.

4. Many children with asthma and their parents are afraid of EIA. The patient and her/his parents might be convinced during an exercise test that exercise can be safe under certain conditions. Furthermore, the appropriate behaviour before, during and after exercise can be practised to prevent EIA.

5. In children with significant asthma, a decreased level of aerobic fitness might be suspected. Exercise testing can provide quantitative measures of fitness and may thereby help to document the deficit and to follow-up changes during an exercise intervention.

Who should not be tested

Exercise testing in asthmatic patients always includes the risk of severe exercise-induced bronchoconstriction. In most exercise tests, this pathological response is actually striven for. Since the decrease in pulmonary function is larger in patients with a bronchial obstruction prior to the test, a patient should not be subjected to an exercise test if the patient's baseline forced expiratory volume in 1 second (FEV_1) is below 60% of predicted or less than 80% of the patient's usual values.[62–64] No exercise testing should be performed during infections and in times of high seasonal allergen exposure. Furthermore, health conditions other than pulmonary impairment, such as cardiovascular or neuromuscular diseases, should also be considered.[65]

Preparation before the test and safety procedures

Based on the purpose of the exercise test, the child should discontinue cromoglycate sodium and short-acting β-adrenergic drugs eight hours prior to testing.

Four hours before the exercise test, the child should refrain from any strenuous activities and should not ingest large amounts of food.

After arrival at the laboratory, the patient should be seen by a physician to obtain a recent medical history and to perform a physical examination. A test of pulmonary function at rest is mandatory to estimate the risks of an exercise test and to reconsider the indication. A resting ECG should also be written unless congenital conduction abnormalities can be excluded from an older ECG. The exercise test should then be explained in detail to the child and parents and, at least, verbal consent should be obtained.

During the exercise challenge, at least power output on the cycle ergometer or slope and speed of the belt on the treadmill, heart rate and breath sounds should be monitored. In patients with unclear respiratory disease or severe asthma, it is recommended to further monitor ECG, blood pressure, oxygen saturation (SaO_2), minute ventilation, end tidal PCO_2 and oxygen uptake.[62] Based on these latter parameters, a list of situations has been compiled in which an exercise test should be terminated (Table 4.2.1).

Conducting the exercise challenge

Mode of exercise

Early studies indicated that the most effective exercise challenge to induce EIA was a run outdoors. However, recent research shows that treadmill running is as effective as free running in triggering EIA if climatic conditions and exercise intensity are controlled for.[66] Since there are concerns with the standardization of an exercise challenge outdoors as well as with monitoring and safety, usually a laboratory based exercise test is used to test for EIA.

Although some studies indicate that cycling is less effective than treadmill running in triggering an EIA,[67] others suggest that the asthmatic response to various land-based exercises might be of equal magnitude, provided that the volume, temperature and humidity of the inspired air is similar among challenges.[68,69] Both treadmill and cycle ergometer are used to test for EIA in laboratories around the world.

Duration and intensity of exercise

It is generally agreed that exercise of 6–10 min duration and at an intensity severe enough to raise heart rate to at least 85% of predicted (about 170 beats min^{-1} in children and adolescents) or oxygen uptake to 60–80% of maximum is best suited to induce EIA.[13] Using a shorter exercise, but supramaximal exercise intensities, might also be effective in inducing EIA.[70] However, an exercise of longer duration (and lower intensity) may result in a false negative test, because the subject may run through the temporary EIA. Although several studies suggest that a higher exercise intensity than stated here would neither affect the sensitivity of the tests to pick up EIA, nor increase the severity of bronchoconstriction EIA, others have shown that a heart rate of about 180 beats min^{-1} during treadmill exercise is more advantageous than a heart rate of 170 beats min^{-1}. The required exercise intensity is usually achieved employing work rates on the cycle ergometer of 2 to 2.5 W kg^{-1} body weight. Due to developmental changes in running economy, the optimal speed and slope during a treadmill challenge are less easy to predict.

Criteria to identify EIA with an exercise challenge

In order to detect an EIA, pulmonary function is assessed before the exercise challenge, immediately afterwards and thereafter in 3–5 min intervals. Brudno et al.[71] suggested continuing collecting data at least until 30 min after exercise.

Post-exercise pulmonary function is expressed as a percentage of pre-exercise values. A fall below a certain percentage is considered indicative of EIA.

Although many different parameters derived from pulmonary function testing have been used to diagnose EIA, forced expiratory volume in one second (FEV_1) is most commonly employed. The forced expiratory flow between 25 and 75% of forced vital capacity (FEF_{25-75}) and the peak expiratory flow rate (PEFR) might also be used, although sensitivity and specificity of the exercise test seems to be less with these variables compared with FEV_1.[72] Custovic et al.[72] suggested using a combination of two criteria. They felt that a fall either in FEV_1 or in FEF_{25-75} below the 95%-confidence limits of normal values was most sensitive to diagnose EIA. No increase in false positive tests was observed using this approach.

Most recent reviews on exercise testing in asthma refer to the criteria published by Cropp[62] to diagnose EIA and to determine the severity of bronchoconstriction (see Table 4.2.2). However, the cut-off for FEV_1 and PEFR as suggested by Cropp,[62] 80% and 75% respectively, might be to conservative. For example, based on the data of Custovic et al.,[72] the lower borders of the 95%-confidence interval for FEV_1 and PEFR in 48 healthy children can be calculated to be roughly 90% and 83%. Indeed, many authors have used a fall in FEV_1 of more than 10%[73] or 15%[74] as a criterion for EIA. In our laboratory, we assume EIA if the fall in FEV_1 exceeds 15%.

Table 4.2.1 Reasons to terminate an exercise test in children (based on Cropp[62] and Washington et al.[65])

- Patient request
- Diagnostic findings have been established
- Failure of monitoring equipment
- Cardiac arrhythmias precipitated or aggravated by the exercise test
- Myocardial ischaemia on ECG (ST segment depression or elevation >0.3 mV)
- Progressive decrease in systolic blood pressure
- Significant respiratory distress
- Rise in end tidal PCO_2 of more than 10 torr or exceeding 55 torr
- Drop in SaO_2 of more than 10% or below 85%

Table 4.2.2 Criteria for assessing the severity of EIA. Values are post-exercise pulmonary function measurements as a percentage of pre-exercise determinations (based on Cropp[62])

Parameter	Mild EIA	Moderate EIA	Severe EIA
FVC	81–90%	70–80%	<70%
FEV_1	66–80%	50–65%	<50%
FEF_{25-75}	61–75%	40–60%	<40%
PEFR	61–75%	40–60%	<40%

Reliability of bronchial responsiveness to a standardized exercise challenge

Intraclass correlation coefficients for the fall in FEV_1 with treadmill exercise while breathing dry air were reported to be 0.57.[75] The reliability, as described by coefficient of variation, is higher in subjects with a fall in FEV_1 >20% (CV 26%) than in subjects with a fall in FEV_1 <20% (CV 81%).[76] This moderate reliability limits the information gained from repeated testing of one individual in order to assess the effectiveness of medication in preventing EIA.

Prevention of EIA and exercise counselling

Based on the reported benefits of exercise and physical activity for patients suffering from asthma or EIA (see above), every physician should try to enable a child with asthma to engage in as much physical activity as possible. The following section will summarize different approaches and principles which might be adopted to minimize exercise-related risks for the child with asthma (see also Table 4.2.3). The average daily doses of various drugs used to control asthma are summarized in Table 4.2.4.

Control of asthma

During periods of airway inflammation, patients with asthma respond to an exercise challenge with a larger than usual fall in pulmonary function parameters. Long-term treatment of asthmatic patients with inhaled steroids such as budesonide or fluticasone propionate may decrease the hyper-responsiveness of the bronchi to a variety of stimuli, including exercise,[77,78] thereby lowering the frequency or severity of EIA. Long acting β2-adrenoceptor agonists, such as salmeterol or formoterol, may help to reduce the risk of EIA in patients who are not symptom free with inhaled steroids alone.[79–81] Leucotriene antagonists are also effective in reducing EIA.[82]

Table 4.2.3 Recommendations to reduce the risk of EIA in patients with asthma

- Control asthma (use anti-inflammatory drugs whenever bronchodilators are necessary on several days per week)
- Prefer swimming over running or cycling
- Do not exercise during a period of severely reduced airway patency
- Be especially careful if you exercise after inhalation of allergens
- Do not exercise at high ozone levels (above 180 ppm) or in an environment with a high concentration of allergens
- Warm-up before exercise
- Inhale β2-adrenergic agonists or cromolyn nebulizers 10–20 min before exercise
- Wear a face mask in cold weather (prevents heat/water loss from bronchial system)
- In case of EIA, use β2-adrenergic agonists

Table 4.2.4 Recommended average daily dose for long-term nebulizer therapy in children with asthma (adapted from Reinhardt[93] and Berdel et al.[94])

Drug	Age 2–5 years	Age ≥6 years
Budenoside	2×50–$200\ \mu g$	1–3×200–$400\ \mu g$
Cromoglycate sodium	3–4×2–$4\ mg$	3–4×2–$4\ mg$
Fluticasone	2×25–$100\ \mu g$	1–4×125–$250\ \mu g$
Formoterol		$2 \times 6\ \mu g$
Nedocromil sodium	3–4×2–$4\ mg$	3–$4 \times 4\ mg$
Salbutamol	4–$6 \times 100\ \mu g$	4–6×100–$200\ \mu g$
Salmeterol		2×25–$50\ \mu g$

Select the least asthmogenic activity

As pointed out above, inhaling cold and dry air while exercising increases the risk for a severe broncho-obstruction. Therefore, children with asthma are sometimes advised not to participate in winter sport activities. Using the precautions outlined in this section, such as wearing a face mask, properly administered medications and monitoring of peak flow, exercise in cold-weather can be safe for children with asthma.[83] However, if the physician is asked to provide an activity recommendation, he should emphasize swimming since EIA is less common during swimming than during land based activities.

Select the right time to exercise

In patients with EIA, pulmonary function at rest is positively related to the exercise-induced fall in pulmonary function.[84] Therefore, exercise should be avoided in times of bronchial obstruction. Although monitoring PEFR is not the best method to detect airway narrowing, it is recommended to measure PEFR before engaging in physical activity. If PEFR is below 80% of the child's average PEFR, short-acting β-mimetic drugs should be administered (see below) and exercise should be postponed until PEFR has improved.

The exercise-induced bronchial response is enhanced for several days after inhalation of allergens.[85] Avoiding allergens for one month has been shown to reduce the risk for EIA.[86] For practical reasons, however, this recommendation can rarely be implemented. It should, however, be emphasized that exercising in an environment with a high allergen concentration may trigger EIA. Likewise, a high level of dust or ozone in the air has been linked to an increase in EIA.

Prevention of EIA shortly before and during exercise

As outlined above, a specific warm-up might be effective in some patients to lower the risk for EIA during the subsequent 2 hours.[27–29] However, the optimal pattern and efficacy of a warm-up protocol should be determined individually.

Several substances, such as sodium cromoglycate sodium 20 mg, nedocromil sodium 4 mg, ipatropium bromide 80 g and salbutamol 0.2–0.4 mg, administered 10–20 min prior to exercise have been shown to offer protection against EIA.[87–89] β-Adrenergic agonists seem to be more effective compared to cromoglycate or ipatropium bromide.[37,90] Using the same absolute dose, spacers do not improve the effect of cromoglycate or nedocromil.[91]

Based on the finding that an asthmatic attack with exercise most likely results from cooling and/or fluid loss of the bronchial system, the use of face masks has been recommended in cold or dry air.

Treatment of EIA

Once EIA has developed, it can be treated successfully with nebulized short-acting β-adrenoceptor agonists such as terbutaline sulphate or salbutamol.[92]

Summary

Provided that the child with asthma and her or his parents are well educated and trained in the management of EIA, that the disease is treated adequately, and that the methods to prevent bronchoconstriction with exercise are consequently employed, exercise can be safe. Under these conditions, nearly every patient with asthma can engage in all types of physical activities[95] and may even be successful at the very elite level of competitive athletics, like the Olympic Games.[96]

References

1. **National Asthma Education Program** I. Definition and diagnosis. *Journal of Allergy and Clinical Immunology* 1991; **88**: 427–38.
2. **Prahl, P., Christiansen, P., Hjuler, I. and Kaae, H. H.** Prevalence of asthma in Danish children aged 8–10 years. *Acta Paediatrica* 1997; **86**: 1110–3.
3. **Burr, M. L., Limb, E. S., Andrae, S., Barry, D. M. and Nagel, F.** Childhood asthma in four countries: a comparative survey. *International Journal of Epidemiology* 1994; **23**: 341–7.
4. **Pearce, N., Weiland, S., Keic, U., Longridge, P., Anderson, H. R., Strachow, D.** *et al.* Self-reported prevalence of asthma in children in Australia, England, Germany and New Zealand: An international comparison using the JAAC protocol. *European Respiratory Journal* 1993; **6**: 1455–61.
5. **Robertson, C. F., Heycock, E., Bishop, J., Nolan, T., Olinsky, A. and Phelan, P. D.** Prevalence of asthma in Melbourne schoolchildren: Changes over 26 years. *British Medical Journal* 1991; **302**: 1116–8.
6. **Skjonsberg, O. H., Clench-Aas, J., Leegaard, J., Skarpaas, I. J., Giaever, P., Bartonova, A. and Moseng, J.** Prevalence of bronchial asthma in schoolchildren in Oslo, Norway. Comparison of data obtained in 1993 and 1981. *Allergy* 1995; **50**: 806–10.
7. **McFadden, E. R.** Exercise induced asthma. Assessment of current etiologic concepts. *Chest* 1987; **91**: 151S–7S.
8. **Badger, D., Ramos, A. D., Lew, C. D., Platzker, A. C. G., Stabile, M. W. and Keens, T. G.** Childhood sequelae of infant lung disease: Exercise and pulmonary function abnormalities after bronchopulmonary dysplasia. *Journal of Pediatrics* 1987; **110**: 693–9.
9. **Silverman, M., Hobbs, F. Gordon, I. and Carswell, F.** Cystic fibrosis, atopy and airways lability. *Archives of Diseases in Children* 1978; **47**: 882–9.
10. **Rupp, N., Guill, M. and Brudno, D.** Unrecognized exercise-induced bronchospasm in adolescent athletes. *American Journal of Diseases of Children* 1992; **146**: 941–4.
11. **Storms, W. W.** Exercise-induced asthma: diagnosis and treatment for the recreational or elite athlete. *Medicine and Science in Sports and Exercise* 1999; **31** (Suppl 1): S33–S38.
12. **Chen, W. Y. and Horton, D. J.** Heat and water loss from the airways and exercise-induced asthma. *Respiration* 1977; **34**: 305–10.
13. **McFadden, E. R. and Gilbert, I. A.** Exercise induced asthma. *New England Journal of Medicine* 1994; **330**: 1362–7.
14. **Bar-Yishay, E., Gur, I., Inbar, O., Neuman, I., Dlin, R. A. and Godfrey, S.** Differences between swimming and running as stimuli for exercise-induced asthma. *European Journal of Applied Physiology* 1982; **48**: 387–97.
15. **Noviski, N., Bar-Yishay, E., Gur, I. and Godfrey, S.** Exercise intensity determines and climatic conditions modify the severity of exercise-induced asthma. *American Review of Respiratory Disease* 1987; **136**: 592–4.
16. **Sheppard, D.** What does exercise have to do with 'exercise-induced' asthma? *American Review of Respiratory Disease* 1987; **136**: 547–9.
17. **McNally, J. F., Enright, P., Hirsch, J. E. and Souhrada, J. F.** The attenuation of exercise-induced bronchoconstriction by oro-pharyngeal anaesthesia. *American Review of Respiratory Disease* 1984; **118**: 247–52.
18. **Anderson, S. D.** Is there a unifying hypothesis for exercise induced asthma? *Journal of Allergy and Clinical Immunology* 1984; **73**: 660–5.
19. **Kikawa, Y., Hosoi, S., Inoue, Y., Saito, M., Nakai, A., Shigematsu, Y., Hirao, T. and Sudo, M.** Exercise-induced urinary excretion of leukotriene E4 in children with atopic asthma. *Pediatric Research* 1991; **29**: 455–9.
20. **Lemanske, R. F. and Henke, K. G.** Exercise-induced asthma. In *Youth, exercise, and sport. Perspectives in exercise science and sports medicine*, Vol. 2 (ed. C. V. Gisolfi and D. R. Lamb). Benchmark Press, Indianapolis, IN, 1989; 465–511.
21. **Koh, Y. Y., Lim, H. S. and Min, K. U.** Airway responsiveness to allergen is increased 24 hours after exercise challenge. *Journal of Allergy and Clinical Immunology* 1994; **94**: 507–16.
22. **Speelberg, B., Panis, E. A., Bijl, D., van Herwaarden, C. L. and Bruynzeel, P. L.** Late asthmatic responses after exercise challenge are reproducible. *Journal of Allergy and Clinical Immunology* 1991; **87**: 1128–37.
23. **Boner, A. L., Vallone, G., Chiesa, M., Spezia, E., Fambri, L. and Sette, L.** Reproducibility of late phase pulmonary response to exercise and its relationship to bronchial hyperreactivity in children with chronic asthma. *Pediatric Pulmonology* 1992; **14**: 156–9.
24. **Hofstra, W. B., Sterk, P. J., Neijens, H. J., Kouwenberg, J. M., Mulder, P. G. and Duiverman, E. J.** Occurrence of a late response to exercise in asthmatic children: multiple regression approach using time-matched baseline and histamine control days. *European Respiratory Journal* 1996; **9**: 1348–55.
25. **Hamielec, C. M., Manning, P. J. and O'Byrne, P. M.** Exercise refractoriness after histamine inhalation in asthmatic subjects. *American Review of Respiratory Disease* 1988; **138**: 794–8.
26. **Wilson, B., Bar-Or, O. and Seed, L.** Effects of humid air breathing during arm or treadmill exercise on exercise-induced bronchoconstriction and refractoriness. *American Reviews of Respiratory Diseases* 1990; **142**: 349–52.
27. **Reiff, D. B., Choudry, N. B., Pride, N. B. and Ind, P. W.** The effect of prolonged submaximal warm-up exercise on exercise-induced asthma. *American Review of Respiratory Disease* 1989; **139**: 479–84.
28. **Schnall, R. P. and Landau, R. I.** Protective effects of repeated short sprints in exercise-induced asthma. *Thorax* 1980; **35**: 828–32.
29. **Lin, C. C., Wu, J. L., Huang, W. C. and Lin, C. Y.** A bronchial response comparison of exercise and methacholine in asthmatic subjects. *Journal of Asthma* 1991; **28**: 31–40.
30. **Ben-Dov, I., Bar-Yishay, E. and Godfrey, S.** Refractory period after exercise-induced asthma unexplained by respiratory heat loss. *American Review of Respiratory Disease* 1982; **125**: 530–4.
31. **Wilson, B., Bar-Or, O. and O'Byrne, P. M.** The effects of indomethacin on refractoriness following exercise both with and without a bronchoconstrictor response. *European Respiratory Journal* 1994; **7**: 2174–8.
32. **Gilbert, I. A., Fouke, J. M. and McFadden, E. R.** The effect of repetitive exercise on airway temperatures. *American Review of Respiratory Disease*, 1990; **142**: 826–31.
33. **Wiens, L., Sabath, R., Ewing, L., Gowdamarajan, R., Portnoy, J. and Scagliotti, D.** Chest pain in otherwise healthy children and adolescents is frequently caused by exercise-induced asthma. *Pediatrics* 1992; **90**: 350–3.

34. Sarafino, E. P., Paterson, M. E. and Murphy, E. L. Age and the impacts of triggers in childhood asthma. *Journal of Asthma* 1998; **35**: 213–7.

35. Nystad, W. The physical activity level in children with asthma based on a survey among 7–16 year old school children. *Scandinavian Journal of Medical Science in Sports* 1997; **7**: 331–5.

36. Weston, A. R., Macfarlane, D. J. and Hopkins, W. G. Physical activity of asthmatic and nonasthmatic children. *Journal of Asthma* 1989; **26**: 279–86.

37. Hussein, A., Forderer, A., Abelitis, M. and Koch, I. Der Einfluss von Diagnose und Prophylaxe der anstrengungsinduzierten Bronchialobstruktion auf die sportlich Aktivitat asthmatischer Schulkinder. [Effect of the diagnosis and prevention of exercise-induced bronchial obstruction on sports participation by asthmatic school children]. *Monatsschrift Kinderheilkunde* 1988; **136**: 819–23.

38. Siersted, H. C., Boldsen, J., Hansen, H. S., Mostgaard, G. and Hyldebrandt, N. Population based study of risk factors for underdiagnosis of asthma in adolescence: Odense schoolchild study. *British Medical Journal* 1998; **316**: 651–5.

39. Counil, F. P., Varray, A., Karila, C., Hayot, M., Voisin, M. and Prefaut, C. Wingate test performance in children with asthma: aerobic or anaerobic limitation? *Medicine and Science in Sports and Exercise* 1997; **29**: 430–5.

40. Ludwick, S. K., Jones, J. W., Jones, T. K., Fukuhara, J. T. and Strunk, R. C. Normalization of cardiopulmonary endurance in severely asthmatic children after bicycle ergometry therapy. *Journal of Pediatrics* 1986; **109**: 446–51.

41. Strunk, R. C., Mrazek, D. A., Fukuhara, J. T., Masterson, J., Ludwick, S. K. and LaBreque, J. F. Cardiovascular fitness in children with asthma correlates with psychologic functioning of the child. *Pediatrics* 1989; **84**: 460–4.

42. Santuz, P., Baraldi, E., Filippone, M. and Zacchello, F. Exercise performance in children with asthma: is it different from that of healthy controls? *European Respiratory Journal* 1997; **10**: 1254–60.

43. Kiers, A., van der Mark, T. W., Woldring, M. G. and Peset, R. Determination of the functional residual capacity during exercise. *Ergonomics* 1980; **23**: 955–9.

44. Freyschuss, U. G., Hedlin, G. and Hedenstierna, G. Ventilation-perfusion relationships during exercise-induced asthma in children. *American Review of Respiratory Disease*, 130, 888–94.

45. Garfinkel, S., Kesten, S., Chapman, K. and Rebuck, A. Physiologic and nonphysiologic determinants of aerobic fitness in mild to moderate asthma. *American Review of Respiratory Disease* 1992; **145**: 741–5.

46. Svenonius, E., Kautto, R. and Arborelius, M. Improvement after training of children with exercise-induced asthma. *Acta Paediatrica Scandinavia* 1983; **72**: 23–30.

47. Holzer, F. J., Schnall, R. and Landau, L. I. The effect of a home exercise programme in children with cystic fibrosis and asthma. *Australian Paediatric Journal* 1984; **20**: 297–301.

48. Perrin, J. M., MacLean, W. E., Gortmaker, S. L. and Asher, K. N. Improving the psychological status of children with asthma: a randomized controlled trial. *Journal of Developmental and Behavioral Pediatrics* 1992; **13**: 241–7.

49. Schmidt, S. M., Ballke, E. H., Nuske, F., Leistikow, G. and Wiersbitzky, S. K. Der Einfluß einer ambulanten Sporttherapie auf das Asthma bronchiale bei Kindern. [Effect of ambulatory sports therapy on bronchial asthma in children]. *Pneumologie* 1997; **51**: 835–41.

50. Engstrom, I., Fallstrom, K., Karlberg, E., Sten, G. and Bjure, J. Psychological and respiratory physiological effects of a physical exercise programme on boys with severe asthma. *Acta Paediatrica Scandinavia* 1991; **80**: 1058–65.

51. Kieckhefer, G. M. The meaning of health to 9-, 10-, and 11-year-old children with asthma. *Journal of Asthma* 1988; **25**: 325–33.

52. Huang, S. W., Veiga, R., Sila, U., Reed, E. and Hines, S. The effect of swimming in asthmatic children—participants in a swimming program in the city of Baltimore. *Journal of Asthma* 1989; **26**: 117–21.

53. Szentagothai, K., Gyene, I., Szocska, M. and Osvath, P. Physical exercise program for children with bronchial asthma. *Pediatric Pulmonology* 1987; **3**: 166–72.

54. Fitch, K. D., Blitvich, J. D. and Morton, A. R. The effect of running training on exercise-induced asthma. *Annals of Allergy* 1986; **57**: 90–4.

55. Henriksen, J. M. and Nielsen, T. T. Effect of physical training on exercise-induced bronchoconstriction. *Acta Paediatrica Scandinavia* 1983; **72**: 31–6.

56. Foresi, A., Corbo, G. M. and Valente, S. Airway responsiveness to exercise and ultrasonically nebulized distilled water in children: relationship to clinical and functional characteristics. *Respiration* 1988; **53**: 205–13.

57. Jones, A. and Bowen, M. Screening for childhood asthma using an exercise test. *British Journal for the General Practitioner* 1994; **44**: 127–31.

58. Ponsonby, A. L., Couper, D., Dwyer, T., Carmichael, A. and Wood-Baker, R. Exercise-induced bronchial hyperresponsiveness and parental ISAAC questionnaire responses. *European Respiratory Journal* 1996; **9**: 1356–62.

59. Riedler, J., Reade, T., Dalton, M., Holst, D. and Robertson, C. Hypertonic saline challenge in an epidemiologic survey of asthma in children. *American Journal of Respiratory and Critical Care Medicine* 1994; **150**: 1632–9.

60. Powell, C. V., White, R. D. and Primhak, R. A. Longitudinal study of free running exercise challenge: reproducibility. *Archives of Diseases in Children* 1996; **74**: 108–14.

61. West, J. V., Robertson, C. F., Roberts, R. and Olinsky, A. Evaluation of bronchial responsiveness to exercise in children as an objective measure of asthma in epidemiological surveys. *Thorax* 1996; **51**: 590–5.

62. Cropp, G. The exercise bronchoprovocation test: standardization of procedures and evaluation of response. *Journal of Allergy and Clinical Immunology* 1979; **64**: 627–33.

63. Eggleston, P. A., Rosenthal, R. R., Anderson, S. A., Anderton, R., Bierman, C. W., Bleecker, E. R., et al. Guidelines for the methodology of exercise challenge testing of asthmatics. *Journal of Allergy and Clinical Immunology* 1979; **64**: 642–5.

64. Russo, G. H., Bellia, C. A. and Bodas, A. W. Exercise-induced asthma (EIA): its prevention with the combined use of ipratropium bromide and fenoterol. *Respiration* 1986; **50** (Suppl. 2): 258–61.

65. Washington, R. L., Bricker, J. T., Alpert, B. S., Daniels, S. R., Deckelbaum, R. J., Fisher, E. A., et al. Guidelines for exercise testing in the pediatric age group. *Circulation* 1994; **90**: 2166–79.

66. Garcia de la Rubia, S., Pajaron Fernandez, M. J., Sanchez-Solis, M., Martinez-Gonzalez-Moro, I., Perez-Flores, D. and Pajaron-Ahumada, M. Exercise-induced asthma in children: a comparative study of free and treadmill running. *Annals of Allergy, Asthma and Immunology* 1998; **80**: 232–6.

67. Fitch, K. Comparative aspects of available exercise systems. *Pediatrics* 1975; (Suppl.), **56**: 904–7.

68. Bundgaard, A., Ingemann-Hansen, T., Schmidt, A. and Halkjaer-Kristensen, J. Exercise-induced asthma after walking, running and cycling. *Scandinavian Journal of Clinical Laboratory Investigations* 1982; **42**: 15–8.

69. Kilham, H., Tooley, M. and Silverman, M. Running, walking, and hyper-ventilation causing asthma in children. *Thorax* 1979; **34**: 582–6.

70. Inbar, O., Alvarez, D. and Lyons, H. Exercise-induced asthma—a comparison between two modes of exercise stress. *European Journal of Respiratory Disease* 1981; **62**: 160–7.

71. Brudno, D. S., Wagner, J. M. and Rupp, N. T. Length of postexercise assessment in the determination of exercise-induced bronchospasm. *Annals of Allergy* 1994; **73**: 227–31.

72. Custovic, A., Arifhodzic, N., Robinson, A. and Woodcock, A. Exercise testing revisited. The response to exercise in normal and atopic children. *Chest* 1994; **105**: 1127–32.

73. Tan, R. A and Spector, S. L. Exercise-induced asthma. *Sports Medicine* 1998; **25**: 1–6.

74. Shapiro, G. G., Pierson, W. E., Furukawa, C. T. and Bierman, C. W. A comparison of the effectiveness of free-running and treadmill exercise for assessing exercise-induced bronchospasm in clinical practice. *Journal of Allergy and Clinical Immunology* 1979; **64**: 609–11.

75. Hofstra, W. B., Sont, J. K., Sterk, P. J., Neijens, H. J., Kuethe, M. C. and Duiverman, E. J. Sample size estimation in studies monitoring

exercise-induced bronchoconstriction in asthmatic children. *Thorax* 1997; **52**: 739–41.

76. **Eggleston, P. A.** and **Guerrant, J. L.** A standardized method of evaluating exercise-induced asthma. *Journal of Allergy and Clinical Immunology* 1976; **58**: 414–25.

77. **Vathenen, A. S., Knox, A. J., Wisniewski, A.** and **Tattersfield, A. E.** Effect of inhaled budesonide on bronchial reactivity to histamine, exercise, and eucapnic dry air hyperventilation in patients with asthma. *Thorax* 1991; **46**: 811–6.

78. **Pedersen, S.** and **Hansen, O. R.** Budesonide treatment of moderate and severe asthma in children: a dose-response study. *Journal of Allergy and Clinical Immunology* 1995; **95**: 29–33.

79. **Adkins, J. C.** and **McTavish, D.** Salmeterol. A review of its pharmacological properties and clinical efficacy in the management of children with asthma. *Drugs* 1997; **54**: 331–54.

80. **De Benedictis, F. M., Tuteri, G., Pazzelli, P., Niccoli, A., Mezzetti, D.** and **Vaccaro, R.** Salmeterol in exercise-induced bronchoconstriction in asthmatic children: comparison of two doses. *European Respiratory Journal* 1996; **9**: 2099–103.

81. **Daugbjerg, P., Nielsen, K. G., Skov, M.** and **Bisgaard, H.** Duration of action of formoterol and salbutamol dry-powder inhalation in prevention of exercise-induced asthma in children. *Acta Paediatrica* 1996; **85**: 684–7.

82. **Leff, J. A., Busse, W. W., Pearlman, D., Bronsky, E. A., Kemp, J., Hendeles, L.,** *et al.* Montelukast, a leucotriene receptor antagonist, for the treatment of mild asthma and exercise induced bronchoconstriction. *New England Journal of Medicine* 1998; **339**: 147–52.

83. **Silvers, W., Morrison, M.** and **Wiener, M.** Asthma ski day: cold air sports safe with peak flow monitoring. *Annals of Allergy* 1994; **73**: 105–8.

84. **Nolan, P.** Clinical features predictive of exercise-induced asthma in children. *Respirology* 1996; **1**: 201–5.

85. **Mussaffi, H., Springer, C.** and **Godfrey, S.** Increased bronchial responsiveness to exercise and histamine after allergen challenge in children with asthma. *Journal of Allergy and Clinical Immunology* 1986; **77**: 48–52.

86. **Benckhuijsen, J., van den Bos, J. W., van Velzen, E., de Bruijn, R.** and **Aalbers, R.** Differences in the effect of allergen avoidance on bronchial hyperresponsiveness as measured by methacholine, adenosine 5'-monophosphate, and exercise in asthmatic children. *Pediatric Pulmonology* 1996; **22**: 147–53.

87. **Ben-Dov, I., Bar-Yishay, E.** and **Godfrey, S.** Heterogeneity in the response of asthmatic patients to pre-exercise treatment with cromolyn sodium. *American Review Respiratory Disease*, 1983; **127**: 113–6.

88. **Boner, A. L., Antolini, I., Andreoli, A., de Stefano, G.** and **Sette, L.** Comparison of the effects of inhaled calcium antagonist verapamil, sodium cromoglycate and ipratropium bromide on exercise-induced bronchoconstriction in children with asthma. *European Journal of Pediatrics* 1987; **146**: 408–11.

89. **Novembre, E., Frongia, G. F., Veneruso, G.** and **Vierucci, A.** (1994). Inhibition of exercise-induced-asthma (EIA) by nedocromil sodium and sodium cromoglycate in children. *Pediatric Allergy and Immunology*, 5, 107–10.

90. **Svenonius, E., Arborelius, M., Wiberg, R.** and **Ekberg, P.** Prevention of exercise-induced asthma by drugs inhaled from metered aerosols. *Allergy* 1988; **43**: 252–7.

91. **Comis, A., Valletta, E. A., Sette, L., Andreoli, A.** and **Boner, A. L.** Comparison of nedocromil sodium and sodium cromoglycate administered by pressurized aerosol, with and without a spacer device in exercise-induced asthma in children. *European Respiratory Journal* 1993; **6**: 523–6.

92. **Dos Santos, J. M., Costa, H., Stahl, E.** and **Wiren, J. E.** Bricanyl Turbuhaler and Ventolin Rotahaler in exercise-induced asthma in children. *Allergy* 1991; **46**: 203–5.

93. **Reinhardt, D.** *Asthma bronchiale im Kindesalter.* [Bronchial asthma in childhood]. Springer Verlag, Berlin, 1996.

94. **Berdel, D., Reinhardt, D., Hofmann, D., Leupold, W.** and **Lindemann, H.** Therapie-Empfehlungen der Gesellschaft für Pädiatrische Pneumologie zur Behandlung des Asthma bronchiale bei Kindern und Jugendlichen. [The German Society of Paediatric Pulmonology: Guidelines for asthma therapy in children] *Monatsschrift Kinderheilkunde* 1998; **146**: 492–7.

95. **Bundgaard, A.** Exercise and the asthmatic. *Sports Medicine* 1985; **2**: 254–66.

96. **Voy, R. O.** The U. S. Olympic Committee experience with exercise-induced bronchospasm, 1984. *Medicine and Science in Sports and Exercise* 1986; **18**: 328–30.

4.3   Exercise capacity and daily physical activity in children with cystic fibrosis

Susi Kriemler

Cystic fibrosis and decreased exercise performance

Cystic fibrosis (CF) is the most common genetic autosomal recessive disease of the Caucasian race, generally leading to death in early adulthood. The frequency of the gene carrier (heterocygot) is 1 : 20–25 in Caucasian populations, 1 : 2000 in African-Americans, and practically non-existent in Asian populations. The disease occurs in about one in every 2500 live births of the white population. The genetic defect causes a pathological electrolyte transport through the cell membranes by a defective chloride channel membrane transport protein (Cystic Fibrosis Transmembrane Conductance Regulator or CFTR). Functionally, this affects mainly the exocrine glands of the human body leading to a highly viscous, water depleted secretion. The secretion cannot leave the glands and in consequence causes local inflammation and destruction of various organs. The main symptoms include chronic inflammatory pulmonary disease with a progressive loss of lung function, exocrine and sometimes endocrine pancreas insufficiency, and an excessive salt loss through the sweat glands.[1] A brief summary of the signs and symptoms of CF will be given with a special emphasis on the effect of exercise performance and capacity.

Exercise tolerance in the patient with CF shows a wide variation. Some patients perform marathons or triathlons and others are hardly able to walk for a few minutes. Most CF patients suffer from some limitations in exercise performance with progression of the disease for which several factors can be responsible. In CF patients, aerobic exercise capacity correlates significantly with resting pulmonary function. Increasing the lung function parameters, normally results in an improved exercise capacity.[2] In a normal population, maximal exercise is limited by symptoms of breathlessness or muscle fatigue when the muscles become oxygen depleted and accumulate lactic acid. Patients with pulmonary disease are ventilatorily limited to a degree which is normally correlated to the severity of the underlying lung disease.

Respiratory and cardiac system

The defect of the CFTR protein complex results in an increase of the viscosity of the bronchial secretion and its retention,[3] with the consequence of bronchial obstruction and recurrent or chronic infections in the lungs. A complex inflammatory mechanism, involving protease–antiprotease and the oxidants–antioxidants balance, as well as the excessive de-liberation of DNA from distracted epithelium and neutrophils, which increases the viscosity of the mucus, plays an important role. The recurrent inflammation/infection leads to a progressive destruction of the bronchial mucosa with bronchi-ectasis, and to a

progressive bronchial lability with a tendency to bronchial collapse, which further provokes mucostasis and inflammation. The development of atelectatic, emphysematic and fibrotic areas implies a progressive decline of functional lung tissue, the so called cystic-fibrotic degeneration of the lung. The disease severity varies tremendously among patients, ranging from severe obstructive pulmonary disease in the infant up to a mild cough with normal pulmonary function in a 40-year-old patient. About 10% of adolescent or adult CF patients develop a spontaneous pneumothorax mainly presenting as sharp thoracic pain and consequent tachypnea or dyspnea. Respiratory insufficiency with hypercapnia, chronic hypoxemia and an exhaustion of the respiratory muscles is the cause of death in more than 95% of all CF patients.[4]

The patients normally show an obstruction in their resting pulmonary function, including a decreased forced vital capacity (FVC), forced expiratory flow in 1 sec (FEV_1),[5] forced expiratory flow between 25 and 75% of vital capacity (FEF_{25-75})[6] and peak flow (PEF), and an increased residual volume to total lung capacity (RV/TLC).[7] In other words, the pulmonary function shows hyperinflation and atelectasis which results in an increase of dead space ventilation. Ventilation at exercise is therefore higher for a given work load, and at high work intensities maximal oxygen uptake and peak work capacity will become limited.[8] Likewise, forced vital capacity (FVC) may be limited by progressive airway obstruction, which further prevents a sufficient increase of tidal volumes (V_T) at increasing work loads. Increased dead space ventilation (V_D) occurs. Healthy people show a V_D/V_T of about 30% at rest and a lower percentage at exercise. In patients with moderate or severe CF, V_D/V_T is increased at rest and even more at exercise due to a limited V_T and a poor matching of ventilation and perfusion of the lungs.[9] Other specific patterns of ventilatory limitations of exercise are a low maximal voluntary ventilation (MVV) at rest,[8] a low peak $\dot{V}O_2$,[10,11] as well as high heart rates[10,12,13] and a high respiratory equivalent for oxygen as a consequence of a high dead space ventilation at submaximum exercise.[2,8,10]

With progression of the disease, an increased arterio-alveolar oxygen gradient occurs as a manifestation of a ventilation–perfusion mismatch. The consequence might be an oxygen desaturation, first during exercise and finally also at rest.[14] It has to be mentioned, however, that oxygen saturation at rest does not predict the risk of desaturation at peak exercise.[15] Some patients with severe disease might even increase their oxygen saturation during exercise.[8,15] In general, patients with an FVC or an FEV_1/FVC ratio of >50% predicted are unlikely to desaturate even at high intensity exercise.[15] In early reports, it was speculated that exercise performance in CF might be limited by oxygen availability, as indicated by a positive relationship between oxygen saturation at peak exercise and peak oxygen uptake.[10] The desaturation, if it occurs, does, however, not seem to limit maximal exercise performance.

Nixon et al.[16] could not induce an increase in peak work load despite oxygen supplementation in hypoxemic CF patients. Oxygen supplementation might, however, help to improve exercise performance at submaximal levels by lowering minute ventilation and as such conserving energy of the respiratory muscles. Likewise, it lowers heart rate and pulmonary artery hypertension with the consequence of an improved ventilation–perfusion-time.[16] It also seems to improve aerobic metabolism in the peripheral muscles as shown in calf muscles of patients with COPD.[17]

Maximal voluntary ventilation is usually assessed by a manoeuvre in which the child is coached to 'blow, blow' as hard and fast as possible for 12 or 15 seconds, and thereafter values are extrapolated to litres per minute. While a healthy child uses only about 70% of the maximal voluntary ventilation during maximal exercise, the patient with progressed CF uses 100% or even more.[13] Likewise, the relative ventilation for a given work load is increased resulting in a higher oxygen cost of ventilation.[18] At peak exercise the healthy child is limited by his/her heart minute volume and the peripheral muscle tissue, while the child with CF experiences a ventilatory limitation. This is true despite the fact that children and adults with CF have a higher ventilatory muscle endurance than the healthy population induced by the chronic hyperventilation.[19] While the respiratory muscles during exercise use about 10–15% of the total body oxygen consumption in a healthy population, those with a chronic pulmonary disease may use up to 40%.[20]

Some patients experience a severe cough at exercise. It is important to mention to the patient, family and teacher that this is not dangerous. To our experience and based on scientific evidence[21] coughing is helpful, because it facilitates the clearing of mucus from the bronchial system. Usually, a short break during exercise is sufficient to stop the spells. In some patients, however, the cough is a sign of exercise-induced bronchoconstriction,[22–24] and should then be treated accordingly (see chapter 4.2). The therapy is the same as for EIB in the non-CF population, but some CF patients do not respond to bronchodilators as well as asthmatics. Note that some authors also found the opposite scenario of an improvement of the obstructive pattern with bronchodilation during or after exercise.[25,26] An exercise-induced increase in mucus clearance or the reopening of collapsed bronchi are thought to be reasons for the improvement in lung function. EIB might also be present if the child develops shortness of breath.

The reason for shortness of breath is often not asthma or the impaired pulmonary function, but rather a low habitual physical activity with a low aerobic exercise capacity as seen in children[27] and adults[28] with chronic disease. There is virtually no information available about the habitual physical activity in the CF population. There are some loose statements of a correlation between maximal oxygen uptake during exercise and the level of physical activity.[29] In our own clinical population, the activity level especially among adolescents, and more so in girls, is clearly less than in an age-matched healthy group. Inactivity is correlated with a low aerobic exercise performance capacity independent of the coincident chronic disease. Simple encouragement and the explanation that exercise is beneficial and certainly not harmful might help to make the child more active. Sometimes an exercise test is useful to show the child and the parent that all the physical parameters are normal, and to prove to the child that he/she can perform even at high intensity.[27]

With disease progression, CF patients often show a significant cor pulmonale as a consequence of the pulmonary artery hypertension caused by the lung deterioration. Benson et al.[30] found both right and left ventricular pathology using equilibrium radionuclide cineangiography at rest and exercise. Right as well as left ventricular function were significantly reduced, sometimes at rest and more so during exercise (30% of 31 CF patients). No correlation was found between the degree of right and left ventricular dysfunction and clinical variables such as resting pulmonary function, arterial oxygen saturation or the severity of the disease as expressed by the Shwachman Score (combined score of radiological and clinical picture). This study might explain some of the non-pulmonary induced exercise performance limitations. Chipps et al.[31] could also show an impairment of resting left ventricular function in 19% at rest and in 37% at exercise, but others basically found no abnormalities.[8,32]

Gastrointestinal system

The exocrine pancreas insufficiency with maldigestion and failure to thrive is a hallmark of CF. The impairment of the intraluminal digestion varies widely, from the life-threatening event of a meconium ileus in the newborn, to a subclinical digestive residual function in the adult patient, and the severity seems to be related to the genetic defect.[33,34] It is nowadays well accepted that external factors such as enzyme therapy or nutrition influence the progression and severity of the disease.[35,36] Malnutrition is the factor that mostly influences exercise performance.[37–39] The genetic defect increases energy demands per se, malassimilation causes energy loss, and external factors decrease energy intake. Consequently, there is a net energy deficit which is believed to impair the respiratory muscles, lead to a progressive destruction of the pulmonary parenchyma and decrease immune regulation. This causes a worsening of the pulmonary function and increases the likelihood of pulmonary infections. Those pulmonary infections again provoke a further decrease of the lung function and on the other side may cause anorexia and vomiting which closes the vicious circle.[40]

A better nutritional status is associated with higher aerobic[37] and anaerobic[38,39] exercise capacity. It has to be considered that total daily energy expenditure, in a resting state as well as during exercise, is increased in persons with CF,[41,42] especially in the advanced stage with severe lung disease. It is therefore important, that the energy intake is adjusted to the disease severity and the activity level. Koletzko et al.[43] developed a simple equation to calculate a crude estimate of energy demand, based on the activity level and the pulmonary function (Table 4.3.1).

In order to be able to calculate proper energy requirements, one needs to assess the nutritional status and body composition. While those with a normal weight and body composition can maintain their actual regimen, those who are undernourished have to adjust the energy balance and increase intake accordingly.

In epidemiological surveys of a healthy population, age adjusted percentiles for height and weight or the body mass index (BMI = body weight/height^2) usually provide a good estimate of body composition. Nevertheless, Lohman[44] has shown that it is difficult to interpret BMI values in terms of body composition in children and adolescents. He demonstrated that at the 50th percentile, the BMI ranges from 15.4 for the 6 year old male to 21.5 for the 17 year old male. In the CF population, BMI might be even more variable, because the lean body mass as well as the fat mass are often unproportionally decreased. Table 4.3.2 presents the BMI, skinfold and bioelectrical impedance (BIA) measurements of a 15 to 24 year old CF population assessed during a summer camp (unpublished data). Despite a similar BMI in the male and female population, there is a striking difference in percent body fat (t-test, $p < 0.0001$) between the different genders. The percentage fat mass was not significantly different between the assessment by skinfolds and by BIA (t-test, $p > 0.4$), as also shown by others.[45,46] Note that the girls were underweight based on BMI standards despite a normal percentage of fat mass. In such cases, an increase in physical activity is probably more suitable to improve than increasing the energy intake. We therefore suggest using skinfold measurements or bioelectrical impedance to get information about the percentage of fat and lean body mass. Newer studies propose dual-energy X-ray absorptiometry (DEXA) measurements as a good, but expensive, alternative to the methods mentioned above to evaluate body composition.[47,48]

A poor nutritional status is considered as a risk factor for limited exercise capacity.[32] Age-adjusted body mass was significantly correlated to work performance in 20 children with CF of varying severity.[49] Likewise, anaerobic capacity is significantly correlated to the nutritional status.[38,39] Diaphragmatic muscle strength seems to be significantly decreased with malnutrition,[50] suggesting that general muscle strength might be affected as well. A magnetic resonance spectroscopy study looking at forearm and calf muscles of 12 to 17 year old CF patients during exercise found higher intracellular pH values than in the healthy controls.[51] The authors concluded that oxidative work performance of skeletal muscles might be reduced due to secondary pathophysiological changes of the skeletal muscle, such as decreased mitochondrial function and density. Whether the muscle function deficit is caused by the malnutrition or by the genetic defect itself is not clear.

Table 4.3.1 Daily energy requirements, based on basal metabolic rate, activity level and lung function at rest. Daily energy requirement = BMR × activity factor + lung function factor

Activity factor	
Bedrest	1.3
Moderate activity	1.5
Normal activity	1.7
Lung function factor	
$FEV_1 >/= 80\%$	0.1
FEV_1 40–79%	0.2
$FEV_1 < 40\%$	0.3
BMR for 10–18 year old children (WHO guidelines)	
12.2 × body weight + 746 (girls)	17.5 × body weight + 651 (boys)

BMR = basal metabolic rate in kcal day^{-1}.

An increase in body weight through an adequate nutrition has been shown to improve exercise capacity[52] and muscle strength.[53] When the increase in energy intake was combined with exercise training, an improved exercise capacity and lean tissue gain was attained in some[54] but not all studies.[53,55]

Diabetes

About 10% of the total CF population, and 30% of patients over 35 years, develop a CF related diabetes mellitus (CFRDM).[56] Most of the patients are treated the same way as type I diabetics. CFRDM can be associated with exercise intolerance, is almost always non-ketotic and has a slow, insidious onset. The disease is usually mild because there is some insulin production left. Physical activity should be specially promoted because it is able to smooth the glucose peaks in the blood. As in type I diabetes, the physically active child should be motivated to eat and drink before and during physical activity, especially when it is prolonged and intense, in order to avoid hypoglycaemia. Patients with CFRDM tend to be more prone to hypoglycaemia than type I diabetics, because glucagon deficiency frequently accompanies the insulin deficiency[57] and because of a tendency towards increased peripheral insulin sensitivity.[58] Based on the better and better long-term prognosis in CF it is more important than ever to provide good management of the diabetes in order to prevent microangiopathy. One way is to promote physical activity.

Osteopenia

Children as well as adults with CF demonstrate low bone mass which may lead to osteoporosis with the potential of atraumatic bone fractures. CF patients show a reduced bone density in dual energy X-ray absorptiometry (DEXA) mass[59–63] and peripheral computer tomography (qCT).[64] The more ill patients tend to have the least bone mass, showing a decrease in bone formation and an increase in bone resorption.[65] As in a healthy population, risk factors such as nutrition, physical inactivity, delayed puberty and steroid therapy are major causes of osteopenia. There is a consistent correlation between body mass and bone density, with underweight patients showing the lowest bone mass.[59,60,62–64] This pattern might be caused by a reduced mechanical loading of the bone as well as by inadequate quantitative and qualitative nutrition. However, most studies have failed to show a correlation between calcium or vitamin D intake and bone mass.[60,62,63] Weight-bearing physical activity has been found to correlate with bone mass in a healthy population, but this pattern was found in only one study.[61] Nevertheless, treatment goals should emphasize general weight-bearing activity, beside an optimal nutrition with adequate calorie, protein, calcium and vitamin D intake. Hormonal replacement

Table 4.3.2 Body composition of 22 15–24 yearold CF patients

n = 22	Age (y)	BW (kg)	HT (cm)	BMI (kg cm^{-2})	SFI (% FM)	SF2 (% FM)	BIA (% FM)
All	17.8	48.6	165.7	17.6	16.5	16.7	15.1
Male	18.4	49.9	169.7	17.3	7.7	10.2	7.9
Female	17.3	47.6	163.0	17.8	22.5	21.2	19.6

Comparison of various approaches to assess body composition in 22 14–25-year-old CF patients, collected during a summer camp.
SF1 = Slaughter equation with triceps and subscapular skinfolds, SF2 = Slaughter equation with subscapular and calf skinfolds,
BIA = bioelectrical impedance (Valhalla Inc., California, USA).

should take place in adolescents with delayed puberty and women with low oestrogen levels when a low bone mass exists.

Dehydration

CF patients have a low tolerance to climatic heat stress which has been shown to increase morbidity and mortality among CF patients.[66,67] Dehydration might decrease strength[68] and aerobic exercise performance.[69]

The thermoregulatory ability among children with CF, who exercised 1.5 to 3 hours in a hot climate, nevertheless, seems to be normal. However, unlike healthy people who usually increase their extracellular osmolality as a result of sweating, CF patients had a decline in serum NaCl and osmolality during exposures to the heat.[70,71] This resulted from the much higher loss of NaCl in the sweat of exercising CF patients, compared to healthy controls. One of the triggers for thirst is an increase in extracellular osmolality which, in turn, stimulates hypothalamic osmoreceptors.[72–74] It is thus possible that patients with CF, whose sweating does not induce a normal increase in extracellular osmolality, would be deprived of this trigger for thirst. Indeed, children with CF, when allowed to drink water *ad libitum* during exposure to a hot climate, drank half as much and dehydrated almost three times as much as healthy controls.[71] Children and adolescents with CF must therefore be encouraged to drink above and beyond thirst, especially when they exercise in warm or humid climates. In addition, they should be encouraged to ingest electrolyte solutions with a high NaCl content (preferably 50 mmol litre^{-1} or more) rather than water alone. It is possible that improvement in palatability of a high-sodium beverage would induce an even greater voluntary fluid intake.

Beneficial effects of exercise and physical activity

There is little knowledge about the long-term effects of exercise on pulmonary function, because the performed studies generally included too-short intervention periods. Zach et al.[75,76] in their two studies over 2.5 and 7 weeks of intense exercise could show an improvement of FEV$_1$ and FVC during the intervention, but the values were back to normal within 8 weeks. Cerny et al. confirmed this increase in pulmonary function over a two-week hospital treatment, including exercise.[2] Likewise Andréasson et al.[77] found a decrease in residual volume (RV) over an unsupervised home exercise training for 30 months. Most of the other exercise studies did not elucidate any changes in pulmonary function during and after the intervention.[13,78,79] One reason might be that the natural course of the disease normally induces a constant decline of pulmonary parameters, and no change might thus mean a relative improvement.

Mucus clearance is difficult to measure, because patients normally do not pay attention to the clearance and have a poor documentation ability. However, some authors described improved mucus clearance with various exercise programmes including swimming[76] and cycling.[80] The improved pulmonary function described above might be an indirect hint that the exercising patients manage to clear mucus from the bronchial tree.

One of the most important studies in the field of exercise in CF has been written by Nixon et al.[81] They found a significant positive correlation between the fitness level and survival in a population of more than 100 CF patients. Eight year survival was significantly higher when peak oxygen consumption was over 80% of predicted than when it was less than 60% of predicted. Colonization with *Pseudomonas cepacea* was also an important factor, but surprisingly resting pulmonary function was a weaker predictor of mortality than exercise performance. Exercise might not only improve survival, but it also acts positively on the patients quality of life as shown by Orenstein et al.[82]

By looking at the exercise training studies, there is indeed evidence of a beneficial effect of an exercise programme on various physiological parameters, and no harmful effects of exercise have been reported. Exercise studies over the last 30 years can be divided up into:

(1) ventilatory muscle exercise;
(2) aerobic training with running, walking, biking and swimming;
(3) strength training; and
(4) various sports combined.

Keens et al.[19] and Asher et al.[83] focused on ventilatory muscle training. Both could document an increased endurance of these muscles over a four-week training period. There was no effect on the exercise performance. The endurance returned to baseline after cessation of the programme.[19]

Zach et al.[76] described improved expiratory flow rates after a seven-week swim training (two to three times a week). The sputum production was improved on training days compared to the non-training days. Exercise performance was not measured. The pulmonary function tests were back to baseline 10 weeks after the programme. The opposite scenario was reported in another swimming programme of 10 weeks duration,[84] with unchanged pulmonary function but an improved treadmill endurance. Salh et al.[80] implemented cycling training for two months on five days of the weeks. There was no change in FVC and FEV$_1$, a non-significant increase in sputum production but a significant increase in peak oxygen consumption (from 25.9 up to 30.3 ml kg^{-1} min^{-1}) in 65% of the patients who finished the programme. Orenstein et al.[13] could improve ventilatory muscle endurance (but not pulmonary function), exercise tolerance and peak $\dot{V}O_2$ with a progressive walking–jogging programme for three months on three days a week. Braggion et al.[79] performed a similar jogging programme over three months but was unable to show any significant changes in either exercise endurance, cardiorespiratory fitness or pulmonary function.

There is only one study in an adult CF population which has looked at the effect of strength training over the time of six months.[85] A significant increase in upper body strength was documented together with a decrease in hyperinflation of the lungs possibly due to stronger expiratory muscle strength.

Zach et al.[75] performed a strenuous combined exercise programme with 12 CF children over a period of 17 days during a summer camp. Sports for several hours a day included swimming, hiking, cycling, jogging, gymnastics, skipping and table tennis. No chest physiotherapy nor inhalation was done. The children showed a significant increase in peak flow but the values were back to normal 8 weeks after the programme. Andréasson et al.[77] let seven CF patients perform a daily unsupervised exercise programme of 30 min duration over 30 months. Activities included jogging, swimming, ball games and sit-ups. After 12 months, the usual chest physiotherapy was withdrawn. At the end pulmonary function testing as well as exercise tolerance were unaltered. The authors concluded that conventional physiotherapy can be replaced by an efficient exercise programme. Another daily programme over three months including various activities did not find any effect of training on performance and pulmonary function.[78] However, this programme was performed at home without supervision.

In summary, there seems to be a beneficial effect of different exercise and physical activity regimens on exercise capacity and pulmonary function in youth with CF. Many of these studies have to be interpreted with caution. Factors such as small sample sizes,[19,77] the lack of an adequate control group,[75,76,78–80,86] short intervention periods of less than two months,[19,75,76] or unsupervised training[77,78,80,86] are some of the possible limitations to be considered.

Harmful effects of exercise and physical activity

Exercise might cause arterial oxygen desaturation, especially in the more severely affected CF population.[87,88] Nevertheless, most patients with CF tolerate even maximal exercise without desaturation and some even improve it during exercise.[13,89] It has been recommended[13] that patients with an $FEV_1 < 50\%$ are at higher risk and should undergo a supervised exercise testing with oximetric measurements before and during an exercise programme. Prolonged desaturation levels of below 90% might contribute to the development or worsening of the pulmonary artery hypertension and cor pulmonale as well as to an encephalopathy.[10,30,90]

While some patients experience bronchodilation at and following exercise,[25,26] some might show the opposite scenario and develop exercise-induced bronchoconstriction (EIB). The reported proportion of reactive airways ranges from as high as 65%[91] down to 2%,[26] but averages around 40%.[22,24,25] It is noteworthy that airway reactivity cannot be defined by improvement in pulmonary function with brochodilator administration due to the pathology of the CF lung. It must be assessed by response of provocation, such as metacholine, histamine, exercise or inhalation of cold air. Typical complaints include shortness of breath, tightness or cough, and these symptoms are more often simply related to the CF lung disease without an asthmatic component. An inhalation therapy with physiologic NaCl solution before exercise is often helpful to prevent especially the coughing spells, but usually a short break helps.

Especially when exercise is prolonged and takes place in a warm environment, dehydration and salt depletion might occur.[70,71] With the proper supply of a salt and carbohydrate containing beverage before and during exercise, this adverse effect can easily be prevented.[92] In rare circumstances, exercise induced hypoglycaemia might occur in those with a manifest CFRDM.

Oxygen desaturation in patients with CF might not only occur during exercise but also at altitude or in airplanes[93] due to the lower oxygen tension of the ambient air. Flying aircrafts usually keep an oxygen tension comparable to 2000 m of altitude, which is equivalent to breathing an air mixture containing 15% oxygen at sea level. Oades et al.[94] suggested an easy approach of a laboratory-based hypoxic challenge to predict desaturation during flights and at altitude. The patient in question simply breathes an air mixture of 15% oxygen while the O_2 saturation is measured transcutaneously. If the patient desaturates to O_2 saturations below 90%, s/he should refrain from high altitudes and use additional oxygen during flights. Resting pulmonary function and oxygen saturation at rest by breathing room air are imprecise predictors of the saturation at low oxygen tensions, and might underestimate individual hypoxic responses. Taking into consideration that children who wish to spend some time at altitude are usually active, it might be advisable to perform the hypoxic laboratory test not only at rest, but also during exercise.

Exercise testing

An exercise test in a child or adolescent with CF can cause early fatigue of respiratory and other muscles, ventilation–perfusion abnormalities with arterial desaturation, alveolar hypoventilation and EIB. These limitations seem to occur more often in patients with advanced disease than those with an early stage [10] and are only moderately correlated to the pulmonary function at rest.[10,11,89] If a child or adolescent with CF performs an aerobic exercise test, there are some differences compared to an age-matched healthy youngster.

Heart rate is elevated at rest only in the most severely affected patients,[10] and maximal heart rate is usually lower than in a comparable healthy population, mainly due to the ventilatory limited maximal exercise capacity. For a given work load, CF patients require a higher minute ventilation than a healthy population due to a higher dead space ventilation.[95] The milder the disease, the higher the minute ventilation at maximal exercise. Exercise in the moderately to severely affected patient is mainly limited by respiratory muscle exhaustion. CF patients use maximal ventilations which reach or even exceed MVV.[95] Maximal ventilation might not be sufficient to provide an adequate gas exchange. In consequence, CO_2 retention and O_2 desaturation might occur, leading to an oxygen deficit and lactic acid accumulation. This is especially true for those with an $FEV_1 < 50\%$.[95]

Anaerobic exercise capacity is limited in youth with CF.[38,39] Because the anaerobic performance is only marginally dependent on oxygen, one has to search for other contributing factors. One important factor seems to be the nutritional status,[38,39] which influences substrate supply and utilization in the muscle cell.

Exercise testing is suggested in all patients who:

(1) experience some sort of symptoms at exercise, such as cough, dyspnea, cyanosis;

(2) those with an FEV_1 and/or $FVC < 50\%$;

(3) those who fear having any harmful effect from any type of physical activity; and

(4) those who want to start a training programme.

Some laboratories advocate a yearly exercise test in all individuals with CF in order to monitor the disease progress. It makes sense to choose an exercise test which is the most similar to the activity the child or adolescent wants to perform on a regular basis. Most studies looking at exercise performance cross-sectionally or longitudinally have used a progressive bicycle or a treadmill test. The Godfrey protocol[96] (Table 4.3.3) has been used most frequently. In our experience, this is an easy protocol which is not too strenuous and takes the body size and low levels of physical fitness into consideration. Likewise, simple walking tests have been suggested which can easily be performed.[97,98] Patients walk in a hospital corridor over a distance of 8 m[97] and 40 m[98] back and forth while the walking distance over a 6 min period is measured. The test has been validated by the same authors with an incremental bicycle test. The walking distance significantly correlated with the maximal work load ($r = 0.76$ and 0.64, respectively) and the maximal oxygen uptake ($r = 0.76$ and 0.7, respectively).

Table 4.3.3 Protocol to assess aerobic exercise capacity

Rate (rpm)	Load (watt)	Increment (watt)	Height (cm)	Stage duration (min)
60	10	10	<120	1
60	15	15	120–150	1
60	20	20	>150	1

If more than three levels of exercise are necessary, add 16–33 W until exhaustion from Godfrey.[96]

Whatever test is performed, it should identify the patients whose oxygen levels fall during exercise. It is recommended that patients with CF should exercise at an intensity level which allows the oxygen saturation to stay above 90%. The heart rate at which desaturation below 90% occurs can be noted and the patient can make sure that his exercise intensity does not exceed this level. If desaturation occurs at a very low intensity level, oxygen supplementation during exercise can be discussed. Another aim of the test is to evaluate each patient's own maximal heart rate, to be able to prescribe an optimal training intensity. Generally, 70–80% of maximal heart rate is considered to be beneficial for efficient aerobic training in health and disease. Retesting will reinforce the benefits to the patient and allow the physician to evaluate the progression of the disease. We recommend doing an exercise test every 3–6 months; however, one should always consider a change in body composition when comparing the data longitudinally. We recommend, that the performance should at least be related to body weight, but better to lean body mass.

Each training recommendation should include information about the frequency, intensity and duration or time of the sport programme. As for healthy persons it should be performed at least three times, better five times per week, at an intensity level of 70–80% of maximal capacity and for a duration of 30 min. Most beginners are not capable of performing such a programme initially and should be allowed to reach this level within 2 or 3 months. A good rule of increase is 10% per week, either in intensity or duration. Very often, an intermittent training programme with a lot of breaks helps at the beginning. Based on the information from training programmes with CF patients, the youngsters should be informed that a clear training effect is not expected before 2–3 months. Strength training can be applied as in the healthy population.

Exercise recommendations

There are two specific sports which should be prohibited for the young patient with CF, especially in an advanced stage of disease. One is scuba diving, the other is sports at high altitude. In both types of activities, detrimental situations can occur in which oxygen becomes limited and severe desaturation can occur over longer periods. For all other sports there is no contraindication.

We always recommend that the young CF patient performs various sports in combination. Team sports are extremely important for the self-esteem and social integration of any child with a chronic disease. When they are well integrated in a team, they feel healthy and 'normal' and even forget about their disease. It is helpful to inform the team and coach about the child's disease and allow him/her to take breaks or run slower whenever needed. An individual sport has the advantage that it can be performed at an individual pace without interfering with any-

body else. This type is specially important if the disease becomes advanced, in order to keep the young person active but without constantly showing him/her the progression of the disease. In those progressed stages, it can be very helpful to search for sports where skills like reactivity, coordination and flexibility are more important than aerobic capacity or strength: goal keeping, tennis, table tennis, rock climbing, dance and golf are some examples.

In general, the child should be allowed to perform any sport beside the two exceptions mentioned above. As long as the motivation and fun aspect is apparent, the best possible adherence and compliance is reached. Again, the orientation of the coach and team members about the child's health condition seems to be the best way to allow an optimal tolerance and integration of the young patient with CF into the sports world.

References

1. Davis, P. B. *Cystic fibrosis.* Marcel Dekker Inc., New York, 1993.
2. Cerny, F. J., Cropp, G. J. A. and Bye, M. R. Hospital therapy improves exercise tolerance and lung function in cystic fibrosis. *American Journal of Diseases of Children* 1984; **138**: 261–65.
3. Sturgess, J. M. Morphological characteristics of the bronchial mucosal in cystic fibrosis. In *Fluid and electrolyte abnormalities in exocrine glands in cystic fibrosis* (ed P. M. Quinton, J. R. Martinez and U. Hopfer). San Francisco Press, San Francisco, 1982; 254–70.
4. Davis, P. B. Pathophysiology of the lung disease in cystic fibrosis. In *Cystic fibrosis* (ed. P. B. Davis). Marcel Dekker Inc., New York, 1993; 193–218.
5. Wagener, J. S., Taussig, L. M. and Burrows, B. Comparison of lung function and survival patterns between cystic fibrosis and emphysema or chronic bronchitis patients. In *Proceedings of the Candian Fibrosis Foundation* (ed. J. Sturgess). 1980; 236.
6. Landau, L. I. and Phelan, P. D. The spectrum of cystic fibrosis. *American Review of Respiratory Disease* 1973; **108**: 593–602.
7. Zapletal, A., Motoyama, E. K., Gibson, L. E. and Bouhuys, A. Pulmonary mechanics in asthma and cystic fibrosis. *Pediatrics* 1971; **48**: 64.
8. Godfrey, S. and Mearns, M. Pulmonary function and responses to exercise in cystic fibrosis. *Archives of Disease in Childhood* 1971; **46**: 144–51.
9. Webb, A. K., Dodd, M. E. and Moorcroft, J. Exercise in cystic fibrosis. *Journal of Royal Society in Medicine* 1995; **88** (Suppl): 30–6.
10. Cropp, G. J A, Pullano, T. P. and Cerny, F. J. and Nathannson, I. T. Exercise tolerance and cardiorespiratory adjustments at peak work capacity in cystic fibrosis. *American Review of Respiratory Disease* 1982; **126**: 211–16.
11. Cerny, F. J., Pullano, T. and Cropp, G. J. A. Cardiorespiratory adaptations to exercise in cystic fibrosis. *American Review of Respiratory Disease* 1982; **126**: 217–20.
12. Moss, A. J. The cardiovascular system in cystic fibrosis. *Pediatrics* 1982; **70**: 728–41.
13. Orenstein, D. M., Franklin, B. A., Doershuk, C. F., Hellerstein, H. K., Germann, K. J., Horowitz, J. G. and Stern, R. C. Exercise conditioning and cardiopulmonary fitness in cystic fibrosis. The effects of a three-month supervised running program. *Chest* 1981; **80**: 392–98.
14. Marcus, C. L., Bader, D., Stabile, M. W., Wang, C-I., Osher, A. B. and Keens, T. G. Supplemental oxygen and exercise performance in patients with cystic fibrosis with severe pulmonary disease. *Chest* 1992; **101**: 52–7.
15. Henke, K. G. and Orenstein, D. M. Oxygen saturation during exercise in cystic fibrosis. *American Review of Respiratory Disease* 1984; **129**: 708–11.
16. Nixon, P. A., Orenstein, D. M., Curtis, S. E. and Ross, E. A. Oxygen supplementation during exercise in cystic fibrosis. *American Review of Respiratory Disease* 1990; **142**: 807–11.
17. Payen, J. F., Wuyam, B. and Levy, P. Muscular metabolism during oxygen supplementation in patients with chronic hypoxemia. *American Review of Respiratory Disease* 1993; **147**: 592–8.

18. Mador, M. J. Respiratory muscle fatigue and breathing pattern. *Chest* 1991; **100**: 1430–5.

19. Keens, T. G., Krastins, I. R., Wannamaker, E. M., Levison, H., Crozier, O. N. and Bryan, C. Ventilatory muscle endurance training in normal subjects and patients with cystic fibrosis. *American Review of Respiratory Disease* 1977; **116**: 853–60.

20. Levison, H. and Cherniack, R. M. Ventilatory cost of exercise in chronic obstructive pulmonary disease. *Journal of Applied Physiology* 1968; **25**: 21–7.

21. King, M., Brock, G. and Lundell, C. Clearance of mucus by simulated cough. *Journal of Applied Physiology* 1985; **58**: 1776–82.

22. Holzer, F. J., Olinsky, A. and Phelan, P. D. Variability of airways hyper-reactivity and allergy in cystic fibrosis. *Archives of Diseases in Childhood* 1981; **56**: 455–9.

23. Mellis, C. M. and Levison, H. Bronchial reactivity in cystic fibrosis. *Pediatrics* 1978; **61**: 446–50.

24. Silverman, M., Hobbs, F. D. and Gordon, I. R. Cystic fibrosis, atopy and airways lability. *Archives of Diseases in Childhood* 1978; **53**: 873–8.

25. Price, J. F., Weller, P. H., Harper, S. A. and Metthew, D. J. Response to bronchial provocation and exercise in children with cystic fibrosis. *Clinical Allergy* 1979; **9**: 563–70.

26. Skorecki, K., Levison, H. and Crozier, D. N. Bronchial lability in cystic fibrosis. *Acta Pediatrica Scandinavia* 1976; **65**: 39–42.

27. Bar-Or, O. *Pediatric sports medicine for the practitioner.* Springer Verlag, Berlin, New York, 1983.

28. Préfaut, C., Varray, A. and Vallet, G. Pathophysiological basis of exercise training in patients with chronic obstructive lung disease. *European Respiratory Review* 1995; **5**: 27–32.

29. Stanghelle, J. K., Michalsen, H. and Skyberg, D. Five-year follow-up of pulmonary function and peak oxygen uptake on 16-year-old boys with cystic fibrosis with special regard to the influence of regular physical exercise. *International Journal of Sports Medicine* 1988; **9**: 19–24.

30. Benson, L. N., Newth, C. J., Desouza, M., Lobraico, R., Kartodihardjo, W., Corkey, C., Gilday, D. and Olley, P. M. Radionuclide assessment of right and left ventricular function during bicycle exercise in young patients with cystic fibrosis. *American Review of Respiratory Disease* 1984; **130**: 987–92.

31. Chipps, B. E., Alderson, P. O., Roland, J. M. A., Yang, A. V., Martinez, C. R. and Rosenstein, B. J. Non-invasive evaluation of ventricular function in cystic fibrosis. *Journal of Pediatrics* 1979; **95**: 379–84.

32. Marcotte, J. E., Grisdale, R. K., Levison, H., Coates, A. L. and Canny, C. J. Multiple factors limit exercise in cystic fibrosis. *Pediatric Pulmonology* 1986; **2**: 274–81.

33. Borgo, G., Astella, G., Gasparini, P., Zorzanella, A., Doro R. and Pignatti, P. F. Pancreatic function and gene deletion F508 in cystic fibrosis. *Journal of Medicine and Genetics* 1990; **27**: 665–9.

34. Kerem, E., Corey, M., Kerem, B-S., Rommens, J., Markiewicz, D., Levison, H., Tsui, L-C. and Durie, P. The relation between genotype and phenotype in cystic fibrosis. *New England Journal of Medicine* 1990; **323**: 1517–22.

35. Levy, L. D., Durie, P. R., Pencharz, P. B. and Corey, M. L. Effects of long-term nutritional rehabilitation on body composition and clinical status in malnourished children and adolescents with cystic fibrosis. *Journal of Pediatrics* 1985; **107**: 225–30.

36. Shepherd, R. W., Holt, T. L. and Thomas, B. J. Nutritional rehabilitation in cystic fibrosis: controlled studies of effects on nutritional growth retardation, body protein turnover, and course of pulmonary disease. *Journal of Pediatrics* 1986; **109**: 788–94.

37. Coates, A. L., Boyce, P., Muller, D., Mearns, M. and Godfrey, S. The role of nutritional status, airway constriction, hypoxia and abnormalities in serum lipid composition in limiting exercise tolerance in children with cystic fibrosis. *Bulletin of European Physiopathology in Respiration* 1979; **15**: 341–2(Abstract).

38. Cabrera, M. E., Lough, M. D., Doershuk, C. F. and DeRivera, G. A. Anaerobic performance—assessed by the Wingate Test—in patients with Cystic Fibrosis. *Pediatric Exercise Science* 1993; **5**: 78–87.

39. Boas, S. R., Joswiak, M. L., Nixon, A. P. A., Fulton, J. A. and Orenstien, D. M. Factors limiting anaerobic performance in adolescent males with cystic fibrosis. *Medicine and Science in Sports and Exercise* 1996; **28**: 291–8.

40. Durie, P. R. and Forstner, G. G. Pathophysiology of the exocrine pancreas in cystic fibrosis. *Journal of Royal Society of Medicine* 1989; **16**: 1–20.

41. Vaisman, N., Penchanrz, P. B., Corey, M. and Canny, G. J. Energy expenditure of patients with cystic fibrosis. *Journal of Pediatrics* 1987; **111**: 496–500.

42. Fried, M. D. The cystic fibrosis gene and resting energy expenditure. *Journal of Pediatrics* 1991; **119**: 913–6.

43. Koletzko, S. and Koletzko, B. Zystische Fibrose—Normalernaehrung oder Ernaehrungstherapiezn. In *Ernaehrung chronisch kranker Kinder und Jugendlicher* (ed. B. Koletzko). Springer, Berlin, 1983.

44. Lohman, T. G. *Advances in body composition assessment: current issues in exercise science.* Human Kinetics, Champaign, Il, 1992.

45. Holt, T. L., Cui, C., Thomas, B. J., Ward, L. C., Quirk, P. C., Crawford, D. and Shepherd, R. W. Clinical applicability of bioelectrical impedance to measure body composition in health and disease. *Nutrition* 1994; **10**: 221–4.

46. Spicher, V., Roulet, M. and Schutz, Y. Assessment of total energy expenditure in free-living patients with cystic fibrosis. *Journal of Pediatrics* 1991; **118**: 865–72.

47. Rochat, T., Slosman, D. O., Pichard, C. and Belli, D. C. Body composition analysis by dual-energy x-ray absorptiometry in adults with cystic fibrosis. *Chest* 1994; **106**: 800–5.

48. Lands, L. C., Gordon, C, Bar-Or, O. Blimkie, C. J., Hanning, R. M., Jones, N. J., Moss, L. A., Webber, C. E., Wilson, W. M. and Heigenhauser, G. J. F. Comparison of three techniques for body composition analysis in cystic fibrosis. *Journal of Applied Physiology* 1993; **75**: 162–6.

49. Coates, A. L., Boyce, P., Muller, D. Mearns, M. and Godfrey, S. The role of nutritional status, airway obstruction, hypoxia, and abnormalities in serum lipid composition in limiting exercise tolerance in children with cystic fibrosis. *Acta Paediatrica Scandinavia* 1980; **69**: 353–8.

50. Pradal, U., Polese, G., Braggion, C., Poggi, R., Zanolla L., Mastella, G. and Rossi, A. Determinants of maximal transdiaphragmatic pressure in adults with cystic fibrosis. *American Journal of Respiratory and Critical Care Medicine* 1994; **150**: 167–73.

51. de Meer, K., Jeneson, J. A., Gulmans, V. A., van der Laag, J. and Berger, R. Efficiency of oxidative work performance of skeletal muscle in patients with cystic fibrosis. *Thorax* 1995; **50**: 980–3.

52. Skeie, B., Askanazi, J., Rothkopf, M. M., Rosenbaum, S. H., Kvetan, V. and Rose, E. Improved exercise tolerance with long-term parenteral nutrition in cystic fibrosis. *Critical Care Medicine* 1987; **15**: 960–2.

53. Hanning, R. M., Blimkie, C. J. R., Bar-Or, O., Lands, L. C., Moss, L. A. and Wilson, W. M. Relationships among nutritional status and skeletal and respiratory muscle function in cystic fibrosis: does early dietary supplementation make a difference? *American Journal of Clinical Nutrition* 1993; **57**: 580–7.

54. Heijerman, H. G. M., Bakker, W., Sterk, P. J., and Dijkman, J. H. Long-term effects of exercise training and hyperalimentation in adult cystic fibrosis patients with severe pulmonary dysfunction. *International Journal of Rehabilitation Research* 1992; **15**: 252–7.

55. Bertrand, J. M., Morin, C. L., Lasalle, R., Patrick, J. and Coates, A. L. Short-term clinical, nutritional, and functional effects of continuous elemental enteral alimentation in children with cystic fibrosis. *Journal of Pediatrics* 1984; **104**: 41–6.

56. Lanng, S., Thorsteinsson, B., Erichsen, G., Nerup, J. and Koch, C. Glucose tolerance in cystic fibrosis. *Archives of Diseases in Childhood* 1991; **66**: 612–16.

57. Moran, A., Pyzdrowski, K. L., Weinreb, J., Kahn, B. B., Smith, S. A., Adams, K. S. and Seaquist, E. R. Insulin sensitivity in cystic fibrosis. *Diabetes* 1994; **43**: 1020–6.

58. Cucinotta, D., Nibali, S. C., Arrigo, T., Di Benedetto, A., Magazzu, G., Di Cesare, E., Costantino, A., Pezzino, V. and De Luca, F. Beta cell function, peripheral sensitivity to insulin and islet cell autoimmunity in cystic

fibrosis patients with normal glucose tolerance. *Hormones in Research* 1990; **34**: 33–8.

59. Henderson, R. C. and Madsen, C. D. Bone density in children and adolescents with cystic fibrosis. *Journal of Pediatrics* 1996; **128**: 28–34.

60. Bhudhikanok, G. S., Lim, J., Marcus, R., Hawkins, A. and Moss, R. B. and Bachrach, L. K. Correlates of osteopenia in patients with cystic fibrosis. *Pediatrics* 1996; **97**: 103–11.

61. Bhudhikanok, G. S., Wang, M-C., Marcus, R., Hawkins, A., Moss, R. B. and Bachrach, L. K. Bone acquisition and loss in children and adults with cystic fibrosis: a longitudinal study. *Journal of Pediatrics* 1998; **133**: 18–27.

62. Grey, A. B., Ames, R. W., Matthews, R. D. and Reid, I. R. Bone mineral density and body composition in adult patients with cystic fibrosis. *Thorax* 1993; **48**: 589–93.

63. Bachrach, L. K., Loutit, C. W. and Moss, R. B. Osteopenia in adults with cystic fibrosis. *American Journal of Medicine* 1994; **96**: 27–34.

64. Gibbens, D. T., Gilsanz, V., Boechat, M. I., Dufer, D., Carlson, M. E. and Wang, C.-I. Osteoporosis in cystic fibrosis. *Journal of Pediatrics* 1988; **113**: 295–300.

65. Baroncelli, G. I., De Luca, F., Magazzu, G., Arrigo, T., Sferlazzas, C., Catena, C., Bertelloni, S. and Saggese, G. Bone demineralization in cystic fibrosis: evidence of imbalance between bone formation and degradation. *Pediatrics in Research* 1997; **41**: 397–403.

66. Kessler, W. R. and Andersen, D. H. Heat prostration in fibrocystic disease of the pancreas and other conditions. *Pediatrics* 1951; **8**: 648–56.

67. Williams, A. J., McKiernan, J. and Harris, F. Heat prostration in children with cystic fibrosis. *British Medical Journal* 1976; **2**: 297.

68. Bosco, J. S., Terjung, R. L. and Greenleaf, J. E. Effects of progressive hypohydration on maximal isometric muscular strength. *Journal of Sports Medicine and Physical Fitness* 1968; **8**: 81–6.

69. Saltin, B. Aerobic and anaerobic work capacity after dehydration. *Journal of Applied Physiology* 1964; **19**: 1114–18.

70. Orenstein, D. M. Exercise in the heat in cystic fibrosis patients. *Medicine and Science in Sports and Exercise* 1981; **13**: 91(Abstract).

71. Bar-Or, O., Blimkie, C. J., Hay, J. D., Macdougall, J. D., Ward, D. S. and Wilson, W. M. Voluntary dehydration and heat intolerance in cystic fibrosis. *Lancet* 1992; **339**: 696–9.

72. Nose, H., Yawata, T. and Morimoto, T. Osmotic factors in restitution from thermal dehydration in rats. *American Journal of Physiology* 1985; **249**: R166–71.

73. Morimoto, T., Slabochova, Z., Naman, R. K. and Sargent, F. Sex differences in physiological reactions to thermal stress. *Journal of Applied Physiology* 1967; **22**: 526–32.

74. Nose, H., Mack, G. W., Shi, X. and Nadel, E. R. The role of plasma osmolality and plasma volume during rehydration in humans. *Journal of Applied Physiology* 1988; **65**: 1–7.

75. Zach, M., Oberwaldner, B. and Hauslen, F. Cystic Fibrosis: physical exercise vs. chest physiotherapy. *Archives of Diseases in Childhood* 1982; **57**: 587–9.

76. Zach, M., Purrer, B. and Oberwalder, B. Effect of swimming on forced expiration and sputum clearance in cystic fibrosis. *Lancet* 1981; **2**: 1201–3.

77. Andréasson, B., Jonson, B. and Kornfält, R., Nordmark, E. and Sandström, S. Long-term effects of physical exercise on working capacity and pulmonary function in cystic fibrosis. *Acta Paediatrica Scandinavia* 1987; **76**: 70–5.

78. Holzer, F. J., Schnall, R. and Landau, L. I. The effect of a home exercise program in children with cystic fibrosis and asthma. *Australian Paediatric Journal* 1984; **20**: 297–302.

79. Braggion, C., Cornacchia, M., Miano, A., Schena, F., Verlato, G. and Mastella, G. Exercise tolerance and effects of training in young patients with cystic fibrosis and mild airway obstruction. *Pediatric Pulmonology* 1989; **7**: 145–52.

80. Salh, W., Bilton, D., Dodd, M. and Webb, A. K. Effect of exercise and physiotherapy in aiding sputum expectoration in adults with cystic fibrosis. *Thorax* 1989; **44**: 1006–8.

81. Nixon, P. A., Orenstein, D. M., Kelsey, Sf. and Doershuk, C. F. The prognostic value of exercise testing in patients with cystic fibrosis. *New England Journal of Medicine* 1992; **327**: 1785–8.

82. Orenstein, D. M., Nixon, P. A., Ross, E. A. and Kaplan, R. M. The quality of well-being in cystic fibrosis. *Chest* 1989; **95**: 344–7.

83. Asher, M. I., Pardy, R. L., Coates, A. L. Thomas, E. and Macklem, P. T. The effects of inspiratory muscle training in patients with cystic fibrosis. *American Review of Respiratory Disease* 1982; **126**: 855–9.

84. Edlund, L. D., French, R. W., Herbst, J. J., Ruttenberg, H. D., Ruhling, R. O. and Adams, T. D. Effects of a swimming program on children with cystic fibrosis. *American Journal of Diseases of Children* 1986; **140**: 80–3.

85. Strauss, G. D., Osher, A. and Wang, C.-I., Goodrich, E., Gold, F., Colman, W., Stabile, M., Dobrenchuck, A. and Keens, T. G. Variable weight training in cystic fibrosis. *Chest* 1987; **92**: 273–6.

86. O'Neill, P., Dodds, M. and Phillips, B., Poole, J. and Webb, A. Regular exercise and reduction of breathlessness in patients with cystic fibrosis. *British Journal of Disease in the Chest* 1987; **81**: 62–9.

87. Goldring, R., Fishman, A. P., Turino, G. M., Cohen, H. I., Denning, C. R. and Andersen, D. H. Pulmonary hypertension and cor pulmonale in cystic fibrosis of the pancreas. *Journal of Pediatrics* 1964; **65**: 501–24.

88. Cerny, F. J., Pullano, T. and Cropp, G. J. A. Adaptation to exercise in children with cystic fibrosis. In *Exercise in health and disease* (eds F. J. Nagle and H. J. Montoye). Thomas, Springfield, Il, 1982; 36–42.

89. Godfrey, S. and Mearns, M. Pulmonary function and response to exercise in cystic fibrosis. *Archives of Diseases in Childhood* 1971; **46**: 144–51.

90. Hortop, J., Desmond, K. J. and Coates, A. L. The mechanical effects of xpiratory airflow limitation on cardiac performance in cystic fibrosis. *American Review of Respiratory Disease* 1988; **137**: 132–7.

91. Day, G. and Mearn, H. B. Bronchial lability in cystic fibrosis. *Archives of Diseases in Childhood* 1973; **48**: 355–9.

92. Kriemler, S., Wilk, B., Schurer, W., Wilson, W. M. and Bar-Or, O. Preventing dehydration in children with cystic fibrosis who exercise in the heat. *Medicine and Science in Sports and Exercise* 1999; **31**: 774–9.

93. Speechly-Dick, M. E., Rimmer, S. J. and Hodson, M. E. Exacerbations of cystic fibrosis after holiday at high altitude-a cautionary tale. *Respiratory Medicine* 1992; **86**: 55–6.

94. Oades, P. J., Buchdahl, R. M. and Bush, A. Prediction of hypoxaemia at high altitude in children with cystic fibrosis. *British Medical Journal* 1994; **308**: 15–18.

95. Orenstein, D. M., Franklin, B. A., Doershuk, C. F., Hellerstein, H. K., Germann, K. J., Horowitz, J. G. and Stern, R. C. Exercise conditioning and cardiopulmonary fitness in cystic fibrosis. *Chest* 1981; **80**: 392–8.

96. Godfrey, S. *Exercise testing in children: applications in health and disease.* W. B. Saunders Co. Ltd., London, 1974.

97. Upton, C. J., Tyrrell, J. C. and Hillser, E. J. Two minute walking distance in cystic fibrosis. *Archives of Diseases in Childhood* 1988; **63**: 1444–8.

98. Nixon, P. A., Joswiak, M. L. and Fricker, F. J. A six-minute walking test for assessing exercise tolerance in severely ill children. *Journal of Pediatrics* 1996; **129**: 362–6.

4.4 Exercise, daily physical activity, eating and weight disorders in children

Andrew P. Hills and Nuala M. Byrne

Introduction

In most industrialized countries, the combination of poor dietary habits and sedentary lifestyle behaviours has led to an increased incidence of paediatric obesity. However, obesity is not the only eating and weight-related problem facing many societies.

In recent years there has been an increasing preoccupation by many adults with body size, shape, weight and fatness.[1,2] Diet and exercise are cited as the primary strategies used in attempts to alter body size and shape.[3] Unfortunately, diet and exercise are commonly abused, and cosmetic benefits are often the primary motivation for change rather than the enhancement of health.

A low level of body fat is recognized as a 'desirable' physical characteristic for most sports performances, particularly where body weight needs to be lifted or where aesthetics are important.[4] Consequently, many athletes work hard to attain a lean and perceived 'ideal' body size and shape for their sport. Concerns about eating and weight usually relate to optimal eating habits and body weight (or body composition) in relation to athletic performance. Unfortunately, drastic adjustments to body composition to meet an imposed size or shape can be problematic.[5,6]

As obesity in adulthood is increasing, reducing body fat is a relevant issue for the wider community.[7] Unfortunately, a proportion of the population who are 'normal' weight or underweight perceive themselves as fat and desire to be thinner. To what extent are similar physical characteristics and concerns relevant to the growing individual? What do we know of the eating, exercise and weight-related behaviours of children and adolescents? What is the role of the medical practitioner and other health professionals in this area?

Consistent with the trends displayed in adults, the weight-control practices employed by children and adolescents appear to reflect a heightened concern with body image.[1,8–12] The potential long-term consequences of inappropriate weight-control practices are serious. They include the adoption of disordered eating practices,[13,14] growth retardation, delayed menarche, amenorrhoea, osteoporosis and psychological disturbances.[4,15–17] The commonly employed weight-control practices, dietary modification and exercise, are pervasive, whether for health or aesthetic reasons.[2] There is also evidence to suggest that these practices are not limited to the female population but are of concern for both genders. As medical practitioners are widely consulted and held in high esteem by members of the public, they are in a good position to identify potential problems in children and adolescents in their care.

The central problem: fear of fatness?

A societal preference for leanness stigmatizes body fatness, which in turn places a social and psychological burden on many people.[18] Paradoxically, the preference for leanness coexists with an increased prevalence of obesity in childhood, adolescence and adulthood.

Too often, physical activity and dietary restriction are taken to extremes in attempts to attain unrealistic physical characteristics such as low levels of body fatness. The net result has been a proliferation of poor diets, extreme behaviours to reduce body fat, including exercise,[7] body image disturbances, including weight dissatisfaction[19] and an apparent increase in eating disorders.

Dieting could play a role in the development of eating and weight disorders, including obesity.[20] The practice of adolescent girls, and to a lesser extent boys, attempting to lose weight is widespread, commonly through self-imposed dieting.[21,22] Whilst the practice of dieting is commonplace in youngsters who are overweight, it is practised by children as young as 9 years of age[23] and those who are normal weight or underweight.[21,24] As many dieters regain weight it may be reasonable to suggest that periods of dietary restraint may lead to episodes of excessive eating.[25] There may also be associated adverse psychological effects including the emergence of clinical eating disorders.[26]

Rodin *et al.*[27] have suggested that for a large number of women in society, being a woman means feeling too fat and wishing to weigh less. Perhaps the perception of fatness and fear of overweight in girls are more powerful determinants of the eating behaviours and related attitudes than is weight *per se*. If fear of fatness is a central concern for adolescent girls or boys, they must be protected from additional pressures to lose weight.[22] This is a key area in which health professionals must be vigilant. The encouragement of a sensible approach to nutrition and exercise, along with an appreciation of individual differences in body size and shape is critical.

The 'eating and weight disorders'

The term 'eating disorder' has traditionally been reserved for the conditions of anorexia nervosa and bulimia nervosa and, more recently, binge eating disorder. Each condition has a significant psychological component and consequent implications for health and body weight. Whilst not commonly cited as an eating disorder, obesity, at least in some individuals,[28] has some similarities with other conditions. For example, obesity is often an allied issue for a number of bulimics and binge eaters. Each of these complex conditions appears to be more prevalent in individuals who lack self esteem and a sense of effectiveness, and they are often related to the cultural obsession with an unrealistically 'thin' body image.[7] Like many chronic diseases each condition can have its genesis in the paediatric years.

There are conflicting reports of the extent of the eating and weight disorders in different populations,[1] the predisposing genetic and environmental factors, and the level of associated psychological ill-health.[29] Some of the confusion stems from the use of different approaches to define these conditions. Stanton[6] has suggested that the inability to clearly define the boundaries between normality and abnormality in terms of body weight and eating behaviour in athletes is difficult. This may well be true of the wider population.

Given the level of community interest in anorexia and bulimia nervosa, one would expect the prevalence of these conditions to be high. However, the number of individuals who meet DSM-IV[30] criteria is relatively low. There are many more individuals who display sub-clinical behaviours such as a preoccupation with weight and food, crash diets, fasting, binge eating and purging behaviours. The impact these behaviours may have on health status should not be underestimated. Stanton[6] contends that in athletes it may be difficult to distinguish eating disorders from a conscientious desire to follow guidelines for eating and exercise.

This chapter addresses some of the major issues relevant to the continuum from obesity to anorexia nervosa. These include eating, weight and exercise behaviours of children and adolescents. Wherever possible, implications for health professionals and practical suggestions are provided.

Contrasting scenarios: over-nutrition and physical inactivity, under-nutrition and excessive physical activity

Over-nutrition and under-nutrition may lead to impaired health. When over-nutrition is combined with physical inactivity, or under-nutrition is combined with excessive physical activity, there is an increased risk of an eating or weight disorder. The former scenario is the classic prescription for increased body fatness and a perpetuation of low levels of physical fitness. Conversely, the latter scenario is relevant to individuals who attempt to modify their body weight (generally level of body fatness), whilst participating in heavy physical training. Consequently, there is concern for the health status of gymnasts, dancers, swimmers and endurance athletes, predominantly females, who engage in heavy training over an extended period, often with an inappropriate energy intake.[1]

Obesity

Obesity is a complex, multi-factorial condition that often consists of psychosocial, anatomical and metabolic adaptations. There are a number of interrelated causes of the condition that may include over-nutrition, physical inactivity, genetic predisposition, psychologically determined eating disorders and social factors.[31–33] A number of

studies[28,34] have claimed that the recent increase in obesity has occurred alongside a population decrease in energy intake. Therefore, the decrease in energy expenditure has resulted primarily from lower levels of physical activity.

Participation in regular physical activity and exercise may provide a protective effect against the accumulation of excess body fat and assist in long-term weight control.[35–37] There are numerous examples of a higher prevalence of obesity in groups whose spontaneous habitual and occupational activity has decreased. In contrast, there is a low incidence of obesity in athletic populations.

Appropriate levels of body weight and adiposity are related to good health, and excess body fatness is associated with cardiorespiratory, articular, metabolic, locomotor, social and psychological complications.[38–41] Unfortunately, the prevalence of obesity in childhood and adolescence has increased in recent years.[42–44]

Assessment of body fatness and criteria for obesity

A range of indirect and doubly indirect methods has been used to assess body fatness, and include skinfold thickness, bioelectrical impedance (BIA), densitometry (underwater weighing), dual energy X-ray absorptiometry (DEXA) and others. In turn, criteria employed to categorize obesity range from simplistic to more complex measures. Criteria include 120 per cent of ideal body weight, the Body Mass Index (BMI), weight-for-age percentiles and skinfold thickness. Using weight-for-age, the 85th percentile is commonly used to classify those 'at risk' of overweight,[45,46] whilst the 95th percentile weight-for-age is used as a cut-off for obesity.[45,47–49] Bar-Or and Baranowski[50] suggest that when criteria used are based on excess body mass, such as mass per age, height or height squared (BMI), the term overweight should be used rather than obesity.

An alternative approach was proposed in a recent study by Dwyer and Blizzard.[51] These researchers suggested that the biomedical status and sum of skinfold measurements of individual children can be used to define obesity. Suggested cut-offs for obesity are 30% of body mass as fat for girls and 20% for boys.[51]

The BMI has been used extensively as an indicator of overweight and obesity in epidemiological studies of adults and in some studies of children and adolescents.[2,46,52] The major shortcoming of this index is its inability to distinguish weight from fatness, and the instability of the index in the growing individual. According to Lazarus et al.,[46] the BMI percentiles for moderate obesity are between 85 and 94 and for marked obesity, over 94. Tell et al.[53] have suggested age-based cut-offs for obesity using BMI: 14 years of age and less, a BMI of 19–20; 15 years of age, a BMI of 25; and 16 years and older, a BMI of 28. These cut-offs may be considered arbitrary as they consider chronological age and not developmental age.

Treatment and management

The treatment and management of obesity in adulthood is a major challenge. This is particularly the case for individuals who have been over-fat for an extended period and experienced multiple failures in weight loss. The key to the treatment and management of obesity in children and adolescents, and eventually its prevention, is to modify body composition whilst promoting regular physical activity and sound nutritional practices.[54–56]

Individual assessment is highly recommended as the child and family can be provided with an insight into the basis for the child's obesity, and be helped to make appropriate changes in the lifestyle of the family. Further, the process may also help parents to remove guilt and modulate blame which is common in families with an obese child.[32]

Exercise, diet and behavioural interventions

The three traditional components of obesity intervention programmes are diet, exercise and behaviour modification. Court[32] and Nuutinen and Knip[57] have suggested that the active involvement of parents and family members be an additional element. An intervention with a single component is relatively limited. For example, weight loss through dietary intervention is easy to achieve in the short term but is far more difficult to sustain for an extended period.[58] Whilst diet and behavioural interventions have been widely utilized their value and efficacy has been challenged. Body composition improvement, on the basis of a reduction in body fat and a maintenance or enhancement of fat-free mass, should be considered important rather than the commonly held view or measure of success, a decrease in body mass.[41]

Severe dietary restriction, particularly in young children, is contraindicated as this may jeopardize the process of normal growth and development.[54] For most children and adolescents who are carrying excess body fat, the maintenance of a stable body weight may be more important as they increase in height during the growing years, rather than attempts to drastically reduce body weight.

Whilst exercise alone does not usually result in successful weight loss it should be the major component of obesity treatment.[41,59] The enhancement of health, motor skills and psychosocial benefits should be stressed. Moore and Burrows[60] indicate that because exercise is active, unrestricted and positive, whereas dieting is passive, restrictive and negative, it is healthier to promote the benefits of a positive and rewarding activity.

Readers are referred to a number of recent reviews on the use of exercise in treating childhood and adolescent obesity.[50,54,61,62] Although not specific to a single age group, the paper by Foreyt and Goodrick[58] is also recommended.

The work of Epstein[36] in the area of family-based behavioural weight control provides an excellent approach to the use of diet and exercise and the incorporation of behaviour change techniques. Techniques include self-monitoring, social reinforcement, modelling and social skills. Using this approach, children can make changes in eating and exercise behaviours that result in long-term improvements in relative body weight.[63]

Whilst greater shifts in negative energy balance are possible through reductions in energy intake than increases in physical activity,[62] a combined approach will be more efficacious in terms of body weight and composition. Further, to increase the likelihood of maintenance of weight loss, numerous researchers have stressed the importance of an active lifestyle.[58,64,65]

It is difficult to identify definitive criteria that may be used by a clinician to determine whether or not an obese individual should be actively involved in an intervention. The process of treatment and management of obesity in children and adolescents is often emotionally charged and challenging. Whilst guidelines for management are consistent for all individuals the process must be individualized and personalized with a strong commitment and involvement of the

family in this process. Key questions that may help a clinician in decision-making include the following:

1. How long has the individual been overweight or obese?
2. What is the nature of the family environment, for example physical characteristics of parents and siblings?
3. Is the child or adolescent's willingness to participate in physical activity limited by a lack of self-confidence and/or low self-esteem which may have resulted from their weight status?
4. Has the individual's behaviour been influenced by repeated teasing and ridicule by peers as a function of his or her size and shape?
5. Is the individual concerned about their physical size and do they desire to improve their body composition status? Any intervention work that is driven by parents, without a commitment from the individual child, is unlikely to succeed.
6. Has the individual been relatively inactive for an extended time period?
7. Is the young person willing to make a commitment to changes in eating and physical activity behaviours?
8. What is the individual's current health status and estimated risk should he or she continue to carry excess fatness?

From treatment and management to prevention

The prevention and management of obesity in children should be a high priority.[66–69] Prevention strategies during childhood should include the initiation of prevention through primary care, family-based programmes and school-based programmes.[66]

For some young people, an increase in energy expenditure through an increased participation in physical activity may be sufficient to prevent obesity.[54] Physical activity should be a non-negotiable component of one's lifestyle from birth. Epstein *et al.*[54] have proposed that a change in activity status may be simpler for non-obese youngsters than to encourage older individuals to be active once obese. Parents, teachers, coaches, medical practitioners and other adults have a collective responsibility to provide every opportunity for young people to be physically active.

All children, irrespective of age, size and shape, love to move. Unfortunately, an increasing number of children are not given sufficient opportunity and encouragement. Physical activity can take many forms, from spontaneous play and incidental activity through to more structured activity in the form of physical education and sport. It is reasonable to suggest that quality experiences during childhood and adolescence may set the scene for a more active adulthood.

Amongst the key elements in the maintenance of activity behaviours from childhood through to adulthood are the success, fun and enjoyment one experiences in the activities undertaken during the younger years.[50] Activity should never be a chore, but rather should be relevant and personally challenging for the individual. The recent review by Epstein *et al.*[54] summarized the work to date on the use of exercise programmes with obese children. Activity programmes using lifestyle activities were more effective than programmed aerobic exercise across a two year period.[70,71]

Differences in body size and shape play a large role in determining physical ability in activity tasks. An appreciation of individual differences and an empathy for all individuals, irrespective of their size, shape and body composition, particularly level of fatness, is extremely important. The predisposition for some individuals to gain weight more readily than others, and to have more difficulty in losing weight, may be biologically determined in the same way size and shape is genetically mediated.[33,72,73] It is very important that medical and other health professionals responsible for obesity interventions are conscious of the possibility of precipitating the development of eating disorders associated with a fear of fatness.[68]

The school setting could also be better utilized to foster active behaviours,[33] with physical education programmes in infant, primary and secondary schools and the harnessing of available professionals and equipment a high priority.[74,75] Such programmes should cater for all individuals, not just those who are physically capable.

The major risk factors for childhood obesity include parental obesity[33,36] and parental exercise.[33] Parents may facilitate and contribute to the maintenance of sedentary lifestyle behaviours.[76] Parental exercise is related to lower levels of fatness in children, irrespective of whether the parent exercises with the child. For many children there is often a lack of adult supervision at home before and after school. Therefore, the opportunity for young people to make poor food choices and choose inactive behaviours, such as television viewing, may be heightened. Under such circumstances the potential time for active pursuits is reduced.[62]

Klesges et al.[77] claim that children's food choices are likely to be less healthy than their parents' choices, if left to their own resources. Even when parents are present, inactive pursuits such as passive television viewing may be chosen as a convenient child-minding tool. Consequently, television has been postulated as a cause of increasing obesity among children,[78] and may also enhance the energy intake of snacks low in nutritional value.[79] Further, television advertising usually promotes less healthy food options,[80] the types of food that parents may wish to limit.[81]

Young people determine activity patterns, for example choices between sedentary and more vigorous activities, on the basis of access to alternatives and the relative reinforcing value of the choices.[82] Generally, research has indicated that obese children choose to be sedentary rather than active.[82,83]

There is considerable merit in further research to consider the effects of reinforcing obese children for being more active and less sedentary.[71,84,85] Epstein et al.[85] found that reducing access to preferred sedentary behaviours was superior to reinforcing active behaviour choices for weight control and fitness improvement at one year. Saelens and Epstein[86] found that highly valued sedentary activities can reinforce physical activities. By making television activities available only while children were physically active, activity time increased from 5 minutes during baseline free choice to greater than twenty minutes when the contingency was in effect. Parents should be encouraged to praise children who are active and refrain from eating foods that are energy-dense and low in nutritional value.

Direct involvement of at least one parent as an active participant in the weight management process with a child improves short- and long-term weight regulation.[36] All family members can benefit from encouragement and support needed in the adoption of new eating and exercise habits. As active role models, parents can encourage the whole family to participate in physical activity. Examples may include walking to and from school, taking the dog and children for a walk rather than sitting or pursuing other inactive behaviours, walking to the shops, parking the car further away from the shopping centre entrance, taking the stairs rather than lifts or escalators and so on.

Social and community efforts to encourage more physical activity should include changes to the physical environment and the provision of greater opportunity and inducement to exercise.[66] Some of the better options in terms of prevention and support of obese children and adolescents are to:

- educate and inform them
- discourage dieting to promote dramatic weight loss
- re-educate to correct poor eating and exercise habits whilst encouraging an improvement in overall health and well-being
- increase self-esteem and body image including a positive mental attitude
- encourage a positive 'can do' mentality—everyone, irrespective of size and shape, has the ability to improve their health status
- encourage acceptance of individual variability in body size and shape
- focus on health status not on weight *per se*
- foster an enjoyment in regular, low to moderate intensity physical activity
- downplay the 'shame and blame' mentality about weight and fatness
- eat well (following recommended guidelines)

Bar-Or and Baranowski[50] provide a succinct summary of the challenges facing the research community with respect to exercise and weight control. It is difficult to assess the association between adiposity and enhanced physical activity (training) because there is a lack of standardized assessment of adiposity, physical activity and energy expenditure. The authors contend that there are too few data to recommend a dose–response or minimal dose of exercise to maintain a desirable body composition. Epstein et al.[54] similarly contend that a major challenge is to identify the ideal type of exercise programme that promotes weight loss beyond that of diet alone, and which promotes long-term changes in physical activity.

As a function of growth and maturation, differential approaches to exercise prescription are logical. Therefore, intervention programmes should respect age-related changes in activity levels and spontaneity along with activity preferences.[54] These sentiments parallel the findings of Taylor et al.[87] who have suggested that the active participation of children in decision making related to physical activity and sports participation may be important. The relationship between activity experiences in the growing years and likelihood of the maintenance of physical activity in adult life is an important area of study. A generalized approach would contend that level of enjoyment of activity in early years may be a key determinant of continued participation. A recent study by Trudeau et al.[88] suggested that daily physical education in primary school (even without a health orientation) had a long-term positive effect on exercise habits in women.

Body satisfaction during the growing years: implications for eating and weight disorders

The physical and psychosocial development of children proceeds at variable rates according to maturational status. The nature of external influences on size and shape, and aspects of psychological health, are relatively poorly understood. For example, whilst there is a strong association between increased body fatness and levels of body dissatisfaction, it is unclear when dissatisfaction commences and/or at what age indicators of body image, like dissatisfaction with one's body, is important enough to influence the global construct of self-esteem. Are some of the key psychological indicators of health status linked, and do they track with physical growth changes? Is the pubertal barrier important in distinguishing particular traits in this area? What is the role of physical activity participation in relation to the psychological constructs?

Relatively few studies have considered the interrelationships between body composition and body satisfaction during childhood and adolescence.[2] Nevertheless, as with adults, preoccupation with body weight appears to be commonplace in childhood and adolescent populations.[2,9,38,90–94] However, the strength of the association between body satisfaction and weight-related behaviours is unclear. A recent study with 9 year old children[95] found that overweight and obese girls had significantly lower physical appearance and athletic competence self-esteem than their normal-weight peers, but body weight had no impact on girls' rated importance of self-esteem domains. Heavier girls were less likely to be peer nominated as pretty, but did not differ in their popularity. The stereotypes of thinness as attractive and desirable, and fatness as neither, are well established by 9 years of age.[96]

One of the key factors in this area is the suitability of the methodology employed. In studies concerning the body image and weight-control practices of children and adolescents, the utilization of measures designed for adults can be problematic.[90] To investigate whether ratings of body image were affected by the scale employed, the authors[92] tested a group of adolescents using both adult and adolescent body-figure silhouette scales. Significant between-scale differences were found, with adolescents displaying consistently lower body-image ratings when viewing adult as opposed to adolescent scales. The results confirm the need for population-specific measurement scales and the implementation of standardized assessment procedures.

Further, differences exist among the measures used to assess body satisfaction, particularly with reference to the body composition of subjects. Hills and Byrne[93] investigated the effect of body composition on the association among three indices of body satisfaction in a group of adolescents. For individuals with a higher weight-for-height, Pearson correlation coefficients for body satisfaction were stronger than those for normal weight individuals. The magnitude of association was similarly influenced by body fat levels with stronger correlations between indices for individuals having more body fat.

Hills and Byrne[2] also assessed appearance and weight-control attitudes and behaviours in a group of adolescents. As for previous work with this population,[90–93] males were significantly more satisfied than females with their physical appearance in general, and with weight-related aspects in particular. Although both male and female adolescents were less satisfied with a fatter physique, males wished to be more muscular, while females desired to be thinner. That is, more males perceived themselves as too thin and more females felt they were too fat.

Research by Smolak et al.[38] documented an association between puberty and an increase in body dissatisfaction in females. Koff et al.[89] suggested that the relationship between body image and self-concept is much higher for females at this age, coincidental with the onset of

puberty for females at approximately 12 years of age. Earlier work by an Australian group[98] found that between nine and ten years of age, males and females do not differ significantly in their level of body satisfaction.

Hills and Byrne[2] also agree that the onset of puberty may influence body satisfaction, but for both sexes. A significant gender difference in this study was found at 12 years of age. Females displayed a marked level of body dissatisfaction while males were satisfied with their physical appearance. At 14 years of age males displayed a level of dissatisfaction with their physical appearance comparable with that displayed by females two years younger. This change for males dovetailed with the average age of puberty for males. Gender differences resumed by 16 years of age with males as a group more satisfied as they moved towards their mature adult physique, whilst females remained dissatisfied with their appearance.

It appears that current body size influences body satisfaction to some extent. A higher weight-for-height ratio and higher adiposity levels were associated with lower body satisfaction for both male and female adolescents. Those with a higher level of adiposity thought and felt they were larger than their peers who displayed less adiposity.

The gender differences in body and weight satisfaction noted above, were not evident when adolescent males and females with lower levels of adiposity were compared. In addition, when categorized according to weight-for-height, females were no more likely than males to perceive themselves as overweight. These results suggest that due to their centrality to physical appearance, body weight and level of adiposity are fundamental elements of physical attractiveness standards for both sexes.

The influence of body composition on disordered eating tendencies of adolescents

Given the increasing prevalence of obesity in childhood, and because being above average weight is a major predictor of dieting in adolescence,[8] it may be hypothesized that the number of adolescents who employ restrictive dietary practices has increased.

More research in this area has focused on girls rather than boys with the majority of studies reporting dieting behaviours as a predominantly female characteristic. Some researchers have suggested that concerns about weight and physical appearance, and the use of dieting to address these preoccupations, have become so pervasive among females in recent years that they may be considered normal behaviour.[13,14,99,100] Wertheim et al.[9] and Maude et al.[10] noted that a substantial proportion of adolescent girls used extreme weight-loss behaviours at least occasionally. However, many studies of weight-control practices have not made reference to the actual physical size of individuals studied.

Work by Hills and Byrne[2] assessed weight concerns and dieting activities in a group of adolescent boys and girls. Consistent with previous work with a similar population[3,100,101] females were significantly more likely than males to diet and fast for weight-control. Similarly, females employed more pathogenic weight-control practices and counted the energy content of foods they consumed. It is very difficult to assess the normalcy of these results given the range of reported prevalence in adults and adolescents.

The gender differences found by Hills and Byrne[2] may be due to the greater number of females perceiving themselves as overweight. Streigel-Moore et al.[99] proposed that the concerns of adolescent females with body weight are due to them equating 'normal' weight with 'underweight.' Another explanation[13] may be that females are aware of appropriate weight norms, but deliberately try to violate them, reflecting dissatisfaction with body weight.

Both relative weight-for-height (BMI) and body fat levels influenced both body satisfaction and drive-for-thinness in males and females. In both sexes, individuals who were bigger and fatter according to these measures, were more dissatisfied with their physique, and displayed a greater concern with dieting, preoccupation with weight and pursuit of thinness. These results suggest that body composition does influence the prevalence of restrictive dietary practices. However, despite these findings, gender differences were still evident within each body composition categorization.

Exercise motivations of adolescents

In order to minimize distorted attitudes about body size and weight-control there is a need to determine what motivates these attitudes, when they begin, how they evolve over time and which individuals are most vulnerable.[92,103] Hills and Byrne[94] investigated whether gender differences in exercise motivations exist during adolescence and the extent to which any differences could be attributed to body composition status. Males in this study displayed significantly greater body satisfaction than females, while females reported a significantly greater concern and preoccupation with weight and thinness. While a similar proportion of males and females were overweight, nearly twice as many females perceived themselves to be overweight.

Significantly more females than males reported exercising for weight-control and to improve body tone. While individuals motivated to exercise for fitness, health and enjoyment reported less disturbances in body image, those motivated to exercise for weight-control, tone and attractiveness displayed greater body dissatisfaction. This finding is consistent with other studies.[101,104]

Accounting for body composition, however, there were no significant gender differences in exercise motivation for individuals with higher body fat levels. Thus, while gender differences cited in studies of adults are evident by adolescence, differences in exercise motivation may be attributed both to level of body dissatisfaction and to body composition. As suggested by McDonald and Thompson,[104] there is cause for concern for individuals, particularly females, whose motivation for exercise is primarily cosmetic. From the available research, it appears that body composition, weight-control behaviours and health status are associated from an early age. There is a need for all health professionals to promote exercise as a means of achieving health and wellness, rather than the restrictive approach of using exercise merely as an avenue for weight-control.[90]

Anorexia nervosa, bulimia nervosa and binge eating disorder

Anorexia nervosa and bulimia are complex, closely related alterations in eating behaviour.[105] Crisp[106] suggests that both are pubertally driven disorders, the common element being the underlying 'dyslipophobia' (or distressing fear of 'fatness'). Anorexia is characterized by weight loss, poor body image, an intense fear of weight gain and obesity, particularly the 'fatness' of the normal mature female body which is instigated at puberty.[106,107] Excessive physical activity also figures prominently as a symptom.[108,109]

Mainstream bulimia, by contrast, occurs at or above normal adult weight. The condition is also characterized by an intense fear of fatness and the belief that other people consider this as a loss of control.[106] Bulimia is characterized by eating large quantities of food at one time (bingeing) which is purged from the body by vomiting, using laxatives or diuretics, fasting and/or excessive exercise. Bulimia is frequently related to weight reduction diets.[105] Early attention to binge eating focused on bulimia in which binge eating was accompanied by strict dieting, self-induced vomiting and low body weight.[110] Obese girls who diet may be at particular risk of developing an eating disorder.

Numerous diagnostic criteria have been employed to define each condition. The following is adapted from the DSM-IV[30] criteria.

Diagnostic criteria for anorexia nervosa

1. Refusal to maintain body weight at or above a minimally normal weight for age and height (for example, weight loss leading to maintenance of body weight less than 85% of that expected; or failure to make expected weight gain during a period of growth, leading to body weight less that 85% of that expected).
2. Intense fear of gaining weight or becoming fat, even though underweight.
3. Disturbance in the way in which one's body weight or shape is experienced, undue influence of body weight or shape on self-evaluation, or denial of the seriousness of the current low body weight.
4. In postmenarcheal females, amenorrhea, that is, the absence of at least three consecutive menstrual cycles.

Diagnostic criteria for bulimia nervosa

1. Recurrent episodes of binge eating. An episode of binge eating is characterized by both of the following:
   (a) eating, in a discrete period of time (for example, within any 2-hour period), an amount of food that is definitely larger than most people would eat during a similar period of time and under similar circumstances; and
   (b) a sense of lack of control over eating during the episode (for example, a feeling that one cannot stop eating or control what or how much one is eating).
2. Recurrent inappropriate compensatory behaviour in order to prevent weight gain, such as self-induced vomiting; misuse of laxatives, diuretics, enemas or other medications; fasting; excessive exercise.
3. The binge eating and inappropriate compensatory behaviours both occur, on average, at least twice a week for three months.
4. Self-evaluation is unduly influenced by body shape and weight.
5. The disturbance does not occur exclusively during episodes of anorexia nervosa.

Criteria for binge eating disorder

1. Recurrent episodes of binge eating. An episode of binge eating is characterized by both of the following:

(a) eating, in a discrete period of time (for example, within any 2-hour period), an amount of food that is definitely larger than most people would eat in a similar period of time under similar circumstances; and

(b) a sense of lack of control over eating during the episode (for example, a feeling that one cannot stop eating or control what or how much one is eating).

2. The binge-eating episodes are associated with three (or more) of the following:
   (a) eating much more rapidly than normal;
   (b) eating until feeling uncomfortably full;
   (c) eating large amounts of food when not feeling physically hungry;
   (d) eating alone because of being embarrassed by how much one is eating;
   (e) feeling disgusted with oneself, depressed, or very guilty after overeating.

3. Marked distress regarding binge eating is present.

4. The binge eating occurs, on average, at least two days a week for six months.

5. The binge eating is not associated with the regular use of inappropriate compensatory behaviours (for example, purging, fasting, excessive exercise) and does not occur exclusively during the course of anorexia nervosa or bulimia nervosa.

Aetiology of anorexia and bulimia

Whilst the specific aetiology of the eating disorders and the normal development of eating behaviour is yet to be established,[111] literature supports the recognition of certain critical elements that may be responsible for the development and maintenance of these disorders.[112] The risk factors identified include familial influences and genetic predisposition,[113,114] biological mechanisms such as a serotonin deficiency,[115,116] and personality and individual psychopathology.[117–119]

Casper[120] has outlined two categories of precipitating event in relation to the onset of anorexia nervosa, psychological or physical. Examples of psychological events include extreme disappointment in relation to an important relationship, the birth of a sibling, moving house, the loss of a friend or a death in the family. Physical events may include early physical maturation and anxiety about puberty.

A number of researchers[1,121] have stated that participation in sport increases the risk for eating and weight problems. The biological risk for eating disorders relates to the common trend in many athletes to restrict energy intake. The dietary restraint needed to control intake may influence attitudes, such as a preoccupation with eating and weight, and behaviours such as binge eating.[1]

The transition from childhood to adolescence is a time of substantial biological change. In females, body fat stores increase as one changes from a child to a mature young woman. As organized sport and competition in the physical activity setting are commonplace, many individuals are faced with a dilemma, a biological change in physical characteristics and a desire to control eating and weight for both appearance and performance reasons.[1]

Crisp[106] indicates that anorexia has physical, social and psychological handicaps, many of which the anorectic recognizes. At the same time the individual denies the presence of illness and weight concerns. The individual will often be secretive and manipulative in an attempt to defend her bio-psychological avoidant stance. The individual with bulimia nervosa may also be secretive, commonly experiencing guilt, low self-esteem and anger at her incapacity to control food intake.[106]

The dieting–eating disorder continuum

There is considerable support for a continuum of risks for eating disorders.[9,38,123] Eating disturbances are reported to lie on a continuum ranging from normative concerns about body weight and shape, to rigid dieting, to sub-clinical, and to diagnosable eating disorders.[99,112] In addition, Nylander[124] proposed that dieting behaviour lies on a continuum with no dieting behaviour and eating disorder at the extremes, and increasing levels of dieting severity between.

Although not all individuals who diet develop eating disorders, dieting has been recognized as a prelude to anorexia and bulimia nervosa.[3,99,114,125] Smolak et al.[38] suggested that dieting should be viewed as problematic behaviour, as it may lead to health threatening weight cycling and binge-eating. Dieting during adolescence is of particular concern, due to anorexia nervosa having its highest incidence at the beginning of adolescence and bulimia nervosa at the end.[99,126]

Prevalence of eating disorders

A number of issues need to be addressed when discussing the prevalence of disordered eating behaviours. Brownell et al.[1] noted that to deal only with the 'clinical' entities of anorexia and bulimia nervosa would miss many 'sub-clinical' problems, such as preoccupation with food, obsessive thinking about weight and disturbed body image. While the prevalence of anorexia nervosa in the general population is approximately 1% and bulimia between 1% and 3%,[127] the number of people who suffer with eating and weight problems but do not meet strict diagnostic criteria is much greater.[125,128,129] In adolescent girls, only 3–5% suffer from clinically diagnosable eating disorders,[114] but the majority report dieting behaviours.[19]

Many individuals may have eating patterns considered unusual, but do not meet established diagnostic criteria.[131] Thus, it is important that the terminology for clinically disordered eating practices is used only where appropriate. Misuse of such terminology may be a reason for the diversity in the reported figures regarding the prevalence of eating disorders.

Binge eating disorder (BED)

A recognized sub-population of the obese, estimated to approximate 25 per cent of those seeking treatment for obesity,[132] undertake periodic bouts of binge eating. Obese binge eaters have been described as a group that may have experienced multiple weight loss failures followed by an abandonment of dietary restraint.[28] Wilson et al.[132] have reported that obese binge eaters are more dissatisfied with their weight and have more preoccupation with their weight and food than other obese individuals.

Binges are often precipitated by negative emotions and individuals report feeling out of control.[133] When binge eaters experience guilt, binges can be followed by increased dietary restraint which perpetuates an unbalanced relationship with food.[58]

Prevention, treatment and management

Treatment for each condition is largely experiential and behavioural.[106] Goals for the anorectic individual include weight gain, whilst weight maintenance may be more important for the bulimic or obese individual with binge eating disorder. Robin et al.[134] have stressed the differential expression of anorexia and bulimia in children and adolescents compared to adults. Further, they suggest that multidisciplinary treatments should be tailored to the unique developmental, medical, nutritional and psychological needs of young people. The use of exercise in the treatment and management of these conditions appears to have considerable merit. For example, anorexic adolescents who are constantly looking for opportunities to participate in aerobic-based activities may benefit from individualized resistance training sessions to help preserve and strengthen skeletal muscle tissue.

The reader is referred to a number of other excellent sources for comprehensive details of prevention, treatment and management.[29,108,120,130,135–141]

References

1. Brownell, K. D., Rodin, J. and Wilmore, J.H. Eating, body weight and performance in athletes: an introduction. In *Eating, body weight and performance* (ed. K. D. Brownell, J. Rodin and J. H. Wilmore). Lea and Febiger, Philadelphia, 1992.

2. Hills, A.P. and Byrne, N.M. Body composition, body satisfaction, eating and exercise behaviour of Australian adolescents. In *Physical fitness and nutrition during growth* (ed. J. Parizkova and A. P. Hills). Karger, Basel, 1998.

3. Emmons, L. Dieting and purging behaviour in black and white high school students. *Journal of the American Dietetic Association* 1992; **92**: 306–12.

4. Treble, G.F., and Morton, A.R. A recipe for success or tragedy? Selection for Australian Rhythmic Gymnastic Representation. *Sport Health* 1994; **12**: 5–10.

5. Davis, C. Body image, dieting behaviours and personality factors: a study of high performance athletes. *International Journal of Sport Psychology* 1992; **23**: 179–92.

6. Stanton, R. Dietary extremism and eating disorders in athletes. In *Clinical sports nutrition* (ed. L. Burke and V. Deakin). McGraw-Hill, Sydney, 1994; 285–306.

7. Brownell, K. D. Dieting and the search for the perfect body: where physiology and culture collide. *Behavior Therapy* 1991; **22**: 1–12.

8. Paxton, S. J., Wertheim, E. H., Gibbons, K., Szmukler, G. I., Hillier, L. and Petrovich, J. Body image satisfaction, dieting belief and weight-loss behaviours in adolescent girls and boys. *Journal of Youth and Adolescence* 1991; **20**: 361–79.

9. Wertheim, E. H., Paxton, S. J., Maude D, Szmukler GI, Gibbons K. and Hillier L. Psychosocial predictors of weight loss behaviors and binge eating in adolescent girls and boys. *International Journal of Eating Disorders* 1992; **12**: 15–160.

10. Maude, D., Wertheim, E. H., Paxton, S., Gibbons, K. and Szmukler, G. Body dissatisfaction, weight loss behaviours and bulimic tendencies in Australian adolescents with an estimate of female data representativeness. *Australian Psychologist* 1993; **28**: 128–32.

11. O'Dea, J. Food habits, body image and self-esteem of adolescent girls from disadvantaged and non-disadvantaged backgrounds. *Australian Journal of Nutrition and Dietetics* 1994; **51**: 74–8.

12. Nowak, M., Speare, R. and Crawford, D. Gender differences in adolescent weight and shape related beliefs and behaviours. *Journal of Paediatrics and Child Health* 1996; **32**: 148–52.

13. Koff, E. and Rierdan, J. Perceptions of weight and attitudes toward eating in early adolescent girls. *Journal of Adolescent Health* 1991; **12**: 307–12.

14. Mellin, L. M., Irwin, C. E. and Scully, S. Prevalence of disordered eating in girls: a survey of middle-class children. *Journal of the American Dietetic Association* 1992; **92**: 851–3.

15. Greenfeld, D., Quinlan, D., Harding, M., Glass, E. and Bliss, A. Eating behaviour in an adolescent population. *International Journal of Eating Disorders* 1987; **6**: 99–111.

16. Carbon, R. J. Exercise, amenorrhoea and the skeleton. *British Medical Journal* 1992; **48**: 546–60.

17. Davis, C. and Fox, J. Excessive exercise and weight preoccupation in women. *Addictive Behaviors* 1993; **18**: 201–11.

18. Spring, B., Pingitore, R., Bruckner, E. and Penava, S. Obesity: idealized or stigmatized? Sociocultural influences on the meaning and prevalence of obesity. In *Exercise and obesity* (ed. A. P. Hills and M. L. Wahlqvist). Smith-Gordon, London, 1994; 49–60.

19. Rosen, J., Gross, J. and Vara, L. Psychological adjustment of adolescents attempting to lose or gain weight. *Journal of Consulting and Clinical Psychology* 1987; **55**: 742–7.

20. Polivy, J. and Herman, P. Dieting and bingeing: a causal analysis. *American Psychologist* 1985; **40**: 193–7.

21. Wadden, T. A., Foster, G. D., Stunkard, A. J. and Linowitz, J. R. Dissatisfaction with weight and figure in obese girls: discontent but not depression. *International Journal of Obesity* 1989; **13**: 89–97.

22. Flynn, M. A. T. Fear of fatness and adolescent girls: implications for obesity prevention. *Proceedings of the Nutrition Society* 1997; **56**: 305–17.

23. Hill, A. J., Draper, E. and Stack, J. A weight on children's minds: body shape dissatisfaction at 9 years old. *International Journal of Obesity* 1994; **18**: 383–9.

24. Whitaker, A., Davies, M., Shaffer, D, Johnson, J., Abrams, S., Walsh, B. T. and Kalikow, K. The struggle to be thin: a survey of anorexic and bulimic symptoms in a non-referred adolescent population. *Psychological Medicine* 1989; **19**: 143–63.

25. Hill, A. J. Pre-adolescent dieting: implications for eating disorders. *International Review of Psychiatry* 1993; **5**: 87–100.

26. Hill, A. J. Causes and consequences of dieting and anorexia. *Proceedings of the Nutrition Society* 1993; **52**: 211–18.

27. Rodin, J., Silberstein, L. and Striegel-Moore, R. Women and weight: a normative discontent. In *Psychology and gender* (ed. T. B. Sonderegger). University of Nebraska Press, Lincoln, 1985; 267–307.

28. Jebb, S. A. and Prentice, A. M. Is obesity an eating disorder? *Proceedings of the Nutrition Society* 1995; **54**: 721–8.

29. Garfinkel, P. E. and Dorian, B. J. Factors that may influence future approaches to the eating disorders. *Eating and Weight Disorders* 1997; **2**: 1–16.

30. American Psychiatric Association. *Diagnostic and statistical manual of the American Psychiatric Association.* American Psychiatric Association, Washington, DC, 1994.

31. Gortmaker, S. L., Must, A., Perrin, J. M., Sobol, A. M.and Dietz, W. H. Social and economic consequences of overweight in adolescence and young adulthood. *New England Journal of Medicine* 1993; **329**: 1008–12.

32. Court, J. M. Strategies for management of obesity in children and adolescents. In *Exercise and obesity* (ed. A. P. Hills and M. L. Wahlqvist). Smith-Gordon, London, 1994; 181–93.

33. Dietz, W. H. Childhood obesity. In *Child health, nutrition and physical activity* (ed. L. W. Y. Cheung and J. B. Richmond). Human Kinetics, Champaign, 1995; 155–70.

34. Andersen, R. E., Wadden, T. A., Bartlett, S. J., Zemel, B. Verde, T. J. and Franckowiak, S. C. Effects of lifestyle activity vs structured aerobic exercise in obese women. *Journal of the American Medical Association* 1999; **281**: 335–40.

35. Parizkova, J., Hainer, V., Stich, V., Kunesova, M. and Ksantini, M. Physiological capabilities of obese individuals and implications for exercise. In *Exercise and obesity* (ed. A. P. Hills and M. L. Wahlqvist). Smith-Gordon, London, 1994; 131–40.

36. Epstein, L. H. Family-based behavioural intervention for obese children. *International Journal of Obesity* 1996; **20** (Suppl 1): S14–S21.

37. Wilmore, J. H. Increasing physical activity. *American Journal of Clinical Nutrition* 1996; **63**: 456S–60S.

38. Smolak, L., Levine, M. P. and Gralen, S. The impact of puberty and dating on eating problems among middle school girls. *Journal of Youth and Adolescence* 1993; **22**: 355–69.

39. Hills, A. P. Locomotor characteristics of obese children. In *Exercise and obesity* (ed. A. P. Hills and M. L. Wahlqvist). Smith-Gordon, London, 1994; 141–50.

40. **Milligan, R. A., Thompson, C., Vandongen, R., Beilin, L. J.** and **Burke, V.** Clustering of cardiovascular risk factors in Australian adolescents: association with dietary excesses and deficiencies. *Journal of Cardiovascular Risk* 1996; **2**: 515–23.

41. **Hills, A. P.** and **Byrne, N. M.** Exercise prescription for weight management. *Proceedings of the Nutrition Society* 1998; **57**: 93–103.

42. **Gortmaker, S. L., Dietz, W. H., Sobol, A. M.** and **Wehler, C. A.** Increasing paediatric obesity in the United States. *American Journal of Diseases of Children* 1987; **141**: 535–40.

43. **Chinn, S.** and **Rona, R. J.** Trends in weight-for-height and triceps skinfold thickness for English and Scottish children, 1972–82 and 1982–90. *Paediatric and Perinatal Epidemiology* 1994; **8**: 90–106.

44. **Barth, N., Ziegler, A., Himmelmann, G. W., Coners, H., Wabitsch, M., Hennighausen, K., Mayer, H., Remschmidt, H., Schafer, H.** and **Hebebrand, J.** Significant weight gains in a clinical sample of obese children and adolescents between 1985 and 1995. *International Journal of Obesity* 1997; **21**: 122–6.

45. **Himes, J. H.** and **Dietz, W. H.** Guidelines for overweight in adolescent preventive services: recommendations from an expert committee. *American Journal of Clinical Nutrition* 1994; **59**: 307–16.

46. **Lazarus, R., Baur, L., Webb, K., Blyth, F.** and **Gliksman, M.** Recommended body mass index cut-off values for overweight screening programmes in Australian children and adolescents: comparisons with North American values. *Journal of Paediatric and Child Health* 1995; **31**: 143–7.

47. **Hills, A. P.** and **Parker, A. W.** Obesity management via diet and exercise intervention. *Child: Care, Health and Development* 1988; **14**: 409–16.

48. **Hills, A. P.** and **Parker, A. W.** Anthropometric and body composition assessment of obese children. *Journal of Sports Sciences* 1990; **8**: 175–6.

49. **Hills, A. P.** Effects of diet and exercise on body composition of pre-pubertal children. *Journal of Physical Education and Sports Science* 1991; **3**: 22–6.

50. **Bar-Or, O.** and **Baranowski, T.** Physical activity, adiposity, and obesity among adolescents. *Pediatric Exercise Science* 1994; **6**: 348–60.

51. **Dwyer, T.** and **Blizzard, C. L.** Defining obesity in children by biological endpoint rather than population distribution. *International Journal of Obesity* 1996; **20**: 472–80.

52. **O'Callaghan, M. J., Williams, G. M., Andersen, M. J., Bor, W.** and **Najman, J. M.** Prediction of obesity in children at 5 years: a cohort study. *Journal of Paediatric Child Health* 1997; **33**: 311–16.

53. **Tell, G. S., Tuomilehto, J., Epstein, F. H.** and **Strasser, T.** Studies of atherosclerosis determinants and precursors during childhood and adolescence. *Bulletin of the World Health Organization* 1986; **64**: 595–605.

54. **Epstein, L. H., Coleman, K. J.** and **Myers, M. D.** Exercise in treating obesity in children and adolescents. *Medicine and Science in Sports and Exercise* 1996; **28**: 428–35.

55. **Must, A.** Morbidity and mortality associated with elevated body weight in children and adolescents. *American Journal of Clinical Nutrition* 1996; **63**: 445S–447S.

56. **Barlow, S. E.** and **Dietz, W. H.** Obesity evaluation and treatment: Expert Committee recommendations. The Maternal and Child Health Bureau, Health Resources and Services Administration and the Department of Health and Human Services. *Pediatrics* 1998; **102**: E29.

57. **Nuutinen, O.** and **Knip, M.** Predictors of weight reduction in obese children. *European Journal of Clinical Nutrition* 1996; **46**: 785–94.

58. **Foreyt, J. P.** and **Goodrick, G. K.** Living without dieting: motivating the obese to exercise and to eat prudently. *Quest* 1997; **47**: 264–73.

59. **Schiffman, S.** Biological and psychological benefits of exercise in obesity. In *Exercise and obesity* (ed. A. P. Hills and M. L. Wahlqvist). Smith-Gordon, London, 1994; 103–13.

60. **Moore, K. A.** and **Burrows, G. D.** Behavioural management of obesity in an exercise context. In *Exercise and obesity* (ed. A. P. Hills and M. L. Wahlqvist). Smith-Gordon, London, 1994; 207–16.

61. **Epstein, L. H.** Exercise and obesity in children. *Journal of Applied Sports Psychology* 1992; **4**: 120–33.

62. **Epstein, L. H.** Exercise in the treatment of childhood obesity. *International Journal of Obesity* 1995; **19**(Suppl. 4): S117–21.

63. **Epstein, L. H., Saelens, B. E.** and **O'Brien, J. G.** Effects of reinforcing increases in active behavior versus decreases in sedentary behavior for obese children. *International Journal of Behavioral Medicine* 1995; **2**: 41–50.

64. **Brownell, K. D.** and **Wadden, T. A.** The heterogeneity of obesity: fitting treatments to individuals. *Behavior Therapy* 1991; **22**: 153–77.

65. **Saris, WHM.** and **van Baak, M. A.** Consequences of exercise on energy expenditure. In *Exercise and obesity* (ed. A. P. Hills and M. L. Wahlqvist). Smith-Gordon, London, 1994; 85–102.

66. **Gill, T. P.** Key issues in the prevention of obesity. *British Medical Bulletin* 1997; **53**: 359–88.

67. **National Health and Medical Research Council.** *Acting on Australia's weight.* Australian Government Publishing Service, Canberra, 1997.

68. WHO (World Health Organization) *Obesity: Preventing and managing the global epidemic.* World Health Organization, Geneva, 1997.

69. **Wilmore, J. H.** Weight gain, weight loss, and weight control: what is the role of physical activity. *Nutrition* 1997; **9**: 820–1.

70. **Epstein, L. H., Wing, R. R., Koeske, R., Ossip, D.** and **Beck, S.** A comparison of lifestyle change and programmed aerobic exercise on weight and fitness changes in obese children. *Behaviour Therapy* 1982; **13**: 651–65.

71. **Epstein, L. H., Wing, R. R., Koeske, R.** and **Valoski, A.** A comparison of lifestyle exercise, aerobic exercise, and calisthenics on weight loss in obese children. *Behaviour Therapy* 1985; **16**: 345–56.

72. **Bouchard, C., Tremblay, A., Despres, J. P., Nadeau, A., Lupien, P. J., Theriault, G., Dussault, J., Moorjania, S., Pineault, S.** and **Fournier, G.** The response to long-term overfeeding in identical twins. *New England Journal of Medicine* 1990; **322**: 1477–82.

73. **Stunkard, A. J., Harris, H. R., Pedersen, N. L.** and **McClearn, G. E.** The body mass index of twins who have been reared apart. *New England Journal of Medicine* 1990; **322**: 1483–7.

74. **Ward, D.** and **Bar-Or, O.** Role of the physician and physical education teacher in the treatment of obesity at school. *Pediatrician* 1986; **13**: 44–51.

75. **Sallis, J. F., Chen, A. H.** and **Castro, C. M.** School-based interventions for childhood obesity. In *Child health, nutrition and physical activity* (ed. L. W. Y. Cheung and J. B. Richmond). Human Kinetics, Champaign, 1995; 179–203.

76. **Dietz, W. H.** The role of lifestyle in health: the epidemiology and consequences of inactivity. *Proceedings of the Nutrition Society* 1996; **55**: 829–40.

77. **Klesges, R. C., Stein, R. J., Eck, L. H., Isbell, T. R.** and **Klesges, L. M.** Parental influence on food selection in young children and its relationship to childhood obesity. *American Journal of Clinical Nutrition* 1991; **53**: 859–64.

78. **Gortmaker, S. L., Must, A., Sobol, A. M., Peterson, K., Colditz, G. A.** and **Dietz, W. H.** Television viewing as a cause of increasing obesity among children in the United States, 1986–90. *Archives of Pediatric and Adolescent Medicine* 1996; **150**: 356–62.

79. **Dietz, W. H.** and **Gortmaker, S. L.** Do we fatten our children at the television set? Obesity and television viewing in children and adolescents. *Pediatrics* 1985; **75**: 807–12.

80. **Lewis, M. K.** and **Hill, A. J.** Food advertising on British children's television: a content analysis and experimental study with nine-year olds. *International Journal of Obesity* 1998; **22**: 206–14.

81. **Wardle, J.** Parental influences on children's diets. *Proceedings of the Nutrition Society* 1995; **54**: 47–58.

82. **Epstein, L. H., Smith, J. A., Vara, L. S.** and **Rodefer, J. S.** Behavioral economic analysis of activity choice in obese children. *Health Psychologist* 1991; **10**: 311–16.

83. **Epstein, L. H., Valoski, A.** and **McCurley, J.** Effect of weight loss by obese children on long-term growth. *American Journal of Diseases of Children* 1993; **147**: 1076–80.

84. **Epstein, L. H., Wing, R. R., Penner, B. C.** and **Kress, M. J.** The effect of diet and controlled exercise on weight loss in obese children. *Journal of Pediatrics* 1985; **107**: 358–61.

85. **Epstein, L. H., Valoski, A., Vara, S., McCurley, J., Wisniewski, L., Kalarchian, M. A., Klein, K. R.** and **Shrager, L. R.** Effects of decreasing

sedentary behaviour and increasing activity on weight change in obese children. *Health Psychologist* 1995; **14**: 109–15.

86. Saelens, B. E. and Epstein, L. H. Behavioral engineering of activity choice in obese children. *International Journal of Obesity* 1998; **22**: 275–7.

87. Taylor, W. C., Blair, S. N., Cummings, S. S., Wun, C. C. and Malina, R. M. Childhood and adolescent physical activity patterns and adult physical activity. *Medicine and Science in Sports and Exercise* 1999; **31**: 118–23.

88. Trudeau, F., Laurencelle, L., Tremblay, J., Rajic, M. and Shephard, R. Daily primary physical education: effects on physical activity during adult life. *Medicine and Science in Sports and Exercise* 1999; **31**: 111–17.

89. Koff, E., Rierdan, J. and Stubbs, M. Gender, body image, and self-concept in early adolescence 1990; **10**: 56–68.

90. Hills, A. P. and Byrne, N. M. Relationships between body dissatisfaction, disordered eating and exercise motivations. *International Journal of Obesity* 1994; **18** (Suppl 2): S31.

91. Byrne, N. M. and Hills, A. P. Assessment of eating practices in adolescence. *Proceedings of the Nutrition Society (Australia)* 1995; **19**: 106.

92. Byrne, N. M. and Hills, A. P: Should body-image scales designed for adults be used with adolescents? *Perceptual and Motor Skills* 1996; **82**: 747–53.

93. Hills, A. P. and Byrne, N. M. Body composition and body image: implications for weight-control practices in adolescents. *International Journal of Obesity* 1997; **21** (Suppl 2): S115.

94. Hills, A. P. and Byrne, N. M. Body composition, body satisfaction and exercise motivation of girls and boys. *Medicine and Science in Sports and Exercise* 1998; **30**: S120.

95. Phillips, R. G. and Hill, A. J. Fat, plain, but not friendless: self-esteem and peer acceptance of obese pre-adolescent girls. *International Journal of Obesity* 1998; **22**: 287–93.

96. Hill, A. J. and Silver, E. K. Fat, friendless and unhealthy: 9 year-old children's perception of body shape stereotypes. *International Journal of Obesity* 1995; **19**: 423–30.

97. Byrne, N. M. and Hills, A. P. Correlations of body composition and body-image assessments of adolescents. *Perceptual and Motor Skills* 1997; **84**: 1330.

98. Tiggemann, M. and Pennington, B. The development of gender differences in body-size satisfaction. *Australian Psychologist* 1990; **25**: 306–13.

99. Striegel-Moore, R. H., Silberstein, L. R. and Rodin, J. Toward an understanding of risk factors for bulimia. *American Psychologist* 1986; **41**: 246–63.

100. Moses, N., Banilivy, M. M. and Lifshitz, F. Fear of obesity among adolescent girls. *Pediatrics* 1989; **118**: 215–19.

101. Silberstein, L., Striegel-Moore, R. H., Timko, C. and Rodin, J. Behavioural and psychological implications of body dissatisfaction: do men and women differ? *Sex Roles* 1988; **19**: 219–32.

102. Krowchuk, D. P., Kreiter, S. R., Woods, C. R., Sinal, S. H. and Du Rant, R. H. Problem dieting behaviours among young adolescents. *Archives of Pediatric and Adolescent Medicine* 1998; **152**: 884–8.

103. Killen, J. D., Taylor, C. B., Hammer, L. D., Litt, I., Wilson, D. M., Rich, T., Haywood, C., Simmonds, B., Kraemer, H. and Varady, A. An attempt to modify unhealthful eating attitudes and weight regulation practices of young adolescent girls. *International Journal of Eating Disorders* 1993; **13**: 369–84.

104. McDonald, K. and Thompson, J. K. Eating disturbance, body image dissatisfaction, and reasons for exercising: gender differences and correlational findings. *International Journal of Eating Disorders* 1992; **11**: 289–92.

105. Westerterp, K. R. and Saris, W. H. M. Limits of energy turnover in relation to physical performance, achievement of energy balance on a daily basis. In *Food, nutrition and performance* (ed. C. Williams and J. T. Devlin). E. & F. N. Spon, London, 1992; 1–18.

106. Crisp, A. H. The dyslipophobias: a view of the psychopathologies involved and the hazards of construing anorexia nervosa and bulimia nervosa as 'eating disorders'. *Proceedings of the Nutrition Society* 1995; **54**: 701–9.

107. Herzog, D. and Copeland, P. Eating disorders. *New England Journal of Medicine* 1985; **318**: 295.

108. Beumont, P. J., Arthur, B., Russell, J. D. and Touyz, S. W. Excessive physical activity in dieting disorder patients: proposals for a supervised exercise program. *International Journal of Eating Disorders* 1994; **15**: 21–36.

109. Davis, C. Eating disorders and hyperactivity: A psychobiological perspective. *Canadian Journal of Psychiatry* 1997; **42**: 168–75.

110. Russell, G. F. M. Bulimia nervosa: An ominous variant of anorexia nervosa. *Psychological Medicine* 1979; 429–48.

111. Sokol, M. S., Steinberg, D. and Zerbe, K. J. 1998 Childhood eating disorders. *Current Opinion in Pediatrics* 1998; **10**: 369–77.

112. Wilson, G. T. and Eldredge, I. I. Pathology and development of eating disorders: implications for athletes. In *Eating, body weight, and performance in athletes* (ed. K. D. Brownell, J. Rodin and J. H. Wilmore). Lea and Febiger, Philadelphia, 1992; 128–45.

113. Fitcher, M. M. and Noegel, R. Concordance for bulimia nervosa in twins. *International Journal of Eating Disorders* 1990; **9**: 255–63.

114. Hsu, L. K. G., Chestler, B. E. and Santhourse, R. Bulimia nervosa in eleven sets of twins: a clinical report. *International Journal of Eating Disorders* 1990; **9**: 275–82.

115. Goodwin, G. M., Fairburn, C. G. and Cowen, P. J. Dieting changes serotonergic function in women, not men: Implications for the aetiology of anorexia nervosa? *Psychological Medicine* 1987; **17**: 839–42.

116. Kay, W. H., Balenger, J. C. and Lydiard, R. B. CSF monoamine levels in normal weight bulimia: evidence for abnormal noradrenergic activity. *American Journal of Psychiatry* 1990; **147**: 225–9.

117. Laeesle, R., Wittchen, H., Fichter, M. and Pirke, K. The significance of sub-groups of bulimia and anorexia nervosa: Lifetime frequency of psychiatric disorders. *International Journal of Eating Disorders* 1989; **8**: 569–74.

118. Garner, D. M., Olmstead, M. P., Davis, R., Rockert, W., Goldbloom, D. and Eagle, M. The association between bulimic symptoms and reported psychopathology. *International Journal of Eating Disorders* 1990; **9**: 1–15.

119. Laberg, J. C., Wilson, G. T., Eldredge, K. and Nordby, H. Effects of mood on heart rate reactivity in bulimia nervosa. *International Journal of Eating Disorders* 1991; **10**: 169–78.

120. Casper, R. C. Fear of fatness and anorexia nervosa in children. In *Child health, nutrition and physical activity* (ed. L. W. Y. Cheung and J. B. Richmond). Human Kinetics, Champaign, 1995; 211–34.

121. Davis, C., Kennedy, S. H., Ravelski, E. and Dionne, M. The role of physical activity in the development and maintenance of eating disorders. *Psychological Medicine* 1994; **24**: 957–67.

122. Kishchuk, N., Gagnon, G., Belisle, D. and Laurendeau, M. Sociodemographic and psychological correlates of actual and desired weight insufficiency in the general population. *International Journal of Eating Disorders* 1992; **12**: 73–81.

123. Garfinkel, P. E., Kennedy, S. H. and Kaplan, A. S. Views on classification and diagnosis of eating disorders. *Canadian Journal of Psychiatry* 1995; **40**: 445–56.

124. Nylander, I. The feeling of being fat and dieting in a school population. Epidemiological interview investigation. *Acta Sociomedicine Scandinavia* 1971; **1**: 17–26.

125. King, A. C., Taylor, C. B., Haskell, W. L. and DeBusk, R. F. Influence of regular aerobic exercise on psychological health: a randomized controlled trial of healthy middle-aged men. *Health Psychologist* 1989; **8**: 305–24.

126. Attie, I. and Brooks-Gunn, J. The development of eating problems in adolescent girls: a longitudinal study. *Developmental Psychology* 1989; **25**: 70–9.

127. Fairburn, C. G., Phil, M. and Beglin, S. J. Studies of the epidemiology of bulimia nervosa. *American Journal of Psychiatry* 1990; **147**: 401–8.

128. Bunnell, D. W., Shenker, I. R., Nussbaum, M. P., Jackobson, M. S. and Cooper, P. Subclinical vs formal eating disorders: differentiating psychological features. *International Journal of Eating Disorders* 1990; **9**: 345–55.

129. **Brownell, K. D.** and **Fairburn, C. G.** (eds). *Eating disorders and obesity.* Guilford Press, New York, 1995.
130. **Fairburn, C. G., Jones, R., Peveler, R. C., Carr, S. J., Solomon, R. A., O'Connor, M. E., Burton, J.** and **Hope, R. A.** Three psychological treatments of bulimia nervosa. *Archives of General Psychiatry* 1991; **48**: 463–9.
131. **Wilmore, J. H.** Eating and weight disorders in the female athlete. *International Journal of Sport Nutrition* 1991; **1**: 104–17.
132. **Wilson, G. T., Nonas, C. A.** and **Rosenblum, G. D.** Assessment of binge eating in obese patients. *International Journal of Eating Disorders* 1993; **13**: 25–34.
133. **Spitzer, R. C., Devlin, M., Walsh, B. J., Hasin, D., Wing, R. R., Marcus, M. D., Stunkard, A., Wadden, T., Yanovski, S., Agras, S., Mitchell, J.** and **Nonas, C.** Binge eating disorder: a multisite field trial of the diagnostic criteria. *International Journal of Eating Disorders* 1992; **11**: 191–203.
134. **Robin, A. L., Gilroy, M.** and **Dennis, A. B.** Treatment of eating disorders in children and adolescents. *Clinical Psychology Reviews* 1998; **18**: 421–46.
135. **Lacey, J. H.** An out-patient treatment for bulimia nervosa. *International Journal of Eating Disorders* 1983; **2**: 209–14.
136. **Crisp, A. H.** Some possible approaches to prevention of eating and body weight/shape disorders, with particular reference to anorexia nervosa. *International Journal of Eating Disorders* 1988; **7**: 1–17.
137. **Beumont, P. J., Russell, J. D.** and **Touyz, S. W.** Treatment of anorexia nervosa. *Lancet* 1993; **341**: 1635–40.
138. **Crisp, A. H., Norton, K., Gowers, S., Halek, C., Bowyer, C., Yeldham, D., Levett, G.** and **Bhat, A.** A controlled study of the effect of therapies aimed at adolescent and family psychotherapy in anorexia nervosa. *British Journal of Psychiatry* 1991; **159**: 325–33.
139. **Doyle, M. M.** Practical management of eating disorders. *Proceedings of the Nutrition Society* 1995; **54**: 711–9.
140. **Halmi, K. A.** Prevention strategies for eating disorders. In *Child health, nutrition and physical activity* (ed. L. W. Y. Cheung and J. B. Richmond). Human Kinetics, Champaign, 1995; 243–6.
141. **Friedman, S. S.** Girls in the 90s: a gender-based model for eating disorder prevention. *Patient Education and Counselling* 1998; **33**: 217–24.

4.5 Exercise capacity, physical activity, cerebral palsy and other neuromuscular diseases

Jost Schnyder, Susan Rochat-Griffith and Carlos Rodriguez

Introduction

In cases of neuromuscular diseases, exercise can be helpful in the assessment of physiological functions, but also as a therapeutic tool and as a means for sociocultural integration. It offers the handicapped patient better self-esteem and gives a feeling of self-responsibility. Children with cerebral palsy (CP) and other neuromuscular diseases (NMD), such as progressive muscular dystrophy (PMD), spinal cord impairments (SCI), traumatic brain injury (TBI), myelomeningocele and poliomyelitis, were at one time restricted from physical activity. Therefore, we find little information in the literature about their ability to perform, the state of their physiological parameters or their response to exercise. We know even less about the kind, intensity, duration or frequency of the physical activity they may be able to perform.

This chapter intends to give an understanding of the principal neuromuscular diseases, the present knowledge of the role of exercise in the functional assessment of such patients, like energy-cost and mechanical efficiency, aerobic and anaerobic capacity, muscle strength, endurance and explosive power, as well as the clinical management. Doctors, educators, physical therapists, schoolteachers, parents and, of course, the children should get helpful practical advise and suggestions on how to build up and how to execute an adapted programme for physical activity, sports and exercise. Among the large variety of paediatric NMD, the most frequent are CP, PMD and SCI. Data will be summarized to recognize the possibilities as well as the limits of exercise, and also to permit a regular evaluation and a constant adaptation of a programme. The results of a multidisciplinary programme from the author's laboratory (Center for Exercise Medicine, SSJ, Geneva, CH) may contribute to a better understanding of the necessity of a regular physical activity programme for these children. It also shows the effects of an interruption or cessation of being physically active in these children. Finally, the chapter emphasizes the physical, psychological and sociocultural benefits of exercise and encourages more research in this difficult field.

Cerebral palsy

CP is certainly the most common condition encountered in the large field of neuromuscular diseases. It can be defined as a disorder of movement and posture that is due to non-progressive damage to the immature brain. Depending on the location and the amount of damage, symptoms may vary, ranging from severe (total inability to control movements) to very mild (only a light clumsiness). Although the brain continues to grow into early adulthood, essential events in its development occur during intrauterine life and early childhood. Events or conditions that disturb the usual unfolding of this process can result in CP and also produce several other associated disabilities (mental retardation, seizures, visual and auditory impairments, learning difficulties, behaviour problems and obesity),[1] which aggravate the neuromotor behaviour and development.

CP may result from numerous conditions (genetic abnormalities, intrauterine infections, prematurity, problematic labour or delivery, traumatic brain injury). In each case, normal developmental processes are disturbed or actual brain damage occurs, resulting in different motor abnormalities and functional impairments called CP. Damage to the brain contributes to abnormal reflex development and muscle response. Abnormal muscle tone and agonist–antagonist imbalance lead to contractures and deformities. This results in difficulty coordinating and integrating basic movement patterns. Therefore physical activity results in a high energy cost for qualitative changes in the muscle (constant hypertonia, involuntary movements and stabilizing movements during exercise),[2–4] and explains the general low mechanical efficiency compared with healthy children.[5] A significant correlation between mechanical efficiency and nature of the handicap was found.[6] A high energy cost of locomotion causes the patient to exert at a high percentage of his maximal aerobic power and thus to fatigue easily.[7,8] Associated disabilities and lower mechanical efficiency influence the acquisition and the application of new motor skills and eventually limit the exercise performances.

Classification

Individuals with CP typically present a variety of observable symptoms depending on the degree and location of brain damage. Over the years, classification has evolved that categorizes CP according to topographical (anatomical) site, neuromotor (medical) and functional (most recent) perspectives. The topographical classification is based on the body segments involved (mono-, di-, hemi-, tri-, quadri- or tetra- and paraplegia). The neuromotor classification describes the medical aspects such as spasticity, athetosis, ataxia, rigidity, tremor and mixed forms. Finally, the functional classification,[9] commonly used in education and sports, is based on an eight ability group list (from severe to minimal impairment), which allows integration of the patients in an adequate programme and equalizes competition among the participants.

Physiological parameters

The assessment of CP patients may be difficult. A precise knowledge of the neuromotor definitions is necessary and it often seems impossible to relate the state of the disease to the degree of possible exercise performances. Thus, an overview of the classical parameters can be helpful to evaluate a patient, to establish a series of reliable and easy to perform laboratory or field tests,[10] and to set up an adequate exercise or physical activity programme.

Mechanical efficiency and aerobic capacity

As shown by Lundberg,[3] mechanical efficiency is low in CP patients, particularly among the spastic ones. Assuming that ATP/mol is no different from that of healthy children,[5] the low efficiency must be due to the wasteful movements caused by mobility problems (contractures and deformities).[11] Dresen et al.[6] and Jones[12] showed a significant reduction in mechanical efficiency at maximum stable workload, as there were no differences in resting energy expenditure between nine CP and non-disabled gender-matched children. As the measurement of $\dot{V}O_2$ is sometimes difficult to perform, Rose et al.[13] suggested, following a study with CP patients and healthy children, that there is a good linear relationship between oxygen uptake and heart rate. They also proposed an Energy Expenditure Index (EEI) based on oxygen uptake and heart rate to compare the economy of walking at various speeds between normal and cerebral palsied children. Mean EEI values for normal children were significantly lower and occurred at faster walking speeds than those for children with CP.[14] Training, however, seemed to have a beneficial effect on handicapped children. A ten-week training programme was followed by six handicapped and five healthy children. Intensity was measured by heart rate recording (attempts were made to achieve HR higher than 160 beats min^{-1} as long as possible). The relationship $\dot{V}O_2$/HR/workload was determined before and after the end of the training programme by submaximal ergometer bicycle tests. The results showed a significant decrease of $\dot{V}O_2$ at different workloads, but no effect on the relationship of oxygen uptake and heart rate was found. So Dresen et al.[15] concluded that these children can perform the same amount of work after training as before, but with a lower aerobic energy expenditure. This has been confirmed by Fernandez and Pitetti[16] who showed a significant effect on the physical work capacity after an eight-week training, suggesting that CP patients could benefit from a training programme.

In CP patients, it is muscle function rather than cardiorespiratory function and consequently aerobic power that is usually affected.[17] Bar Or[2] reported a decreased mechanical efficiency in both trained and untrained children with CP, despite improvements in aerobic capacity in a training group. Nevertheless, a lower aerobic power has been documented by several authors.[2,4,5,7,12,18] Lundberg[19] showed in a longitudinal study that absolute values for aerobic capacity and physical working capacity increased in children with spastic diplegia during adolescence, whereas mechanical efficiency decreased. Therefore, the conclusion is that CP patients present a lower, but trainable, aerobic capacity compared with healthy children, but the effect of an improvement by training is annulled by the lower mechanical efficiency due to the high energy cost.

Anaerobic capacity

As seen above, the lower mechanical efficiency influences the aerobic and consequently also the anaerobic power. The degree of the disability, the muscle tone and contracture, as well as the importance of associated handicaps, are limiting factors and explain the lower anaerobic power. Bar Or,[8] Parker et al.[20] and Emons et al.[21] showed, using the Wingate Anaerobic Test (WAnT), a lower peak and mean power output in young spastic CP patients than in healthy children. Bar Or[22] reviewed several possible explanations mentioned in the literature: it could be due to the low functional muscle mass, an insufficient stretch in the spastic muscle caused by an exaggerated tonic reflex or a preferential reduction in type II fibres that may take place in CP as well as in other NMDs. This would reduce performance in high intensity tasks such as the WAnT.[23] The deficient synchronization between the agonist and antagonist muscle groups[24] is also a reason for the higher energy cost of locomotion, and could therefore explain an underestimation of the mechanical power as measured by anaerobic tests based on performance.

Today it is still difficult to say if anaerobic power can be trained in children. Some collected but not yet published data from The Children's Exercise and Nutrition Center at MacMaster (personal communication Oded Bar Or) and from the Center for Exercise Medicine in Geneva, seem to corroborate the results published in 1992 by O'Connell et al.[25] They had trained three CP patients and three patients with spina bifida and noted an increase in muscle endurance. In contrast, Emons and van Baak[26] could not confirm an improvement in anaerobic power after a nine-month training programme with 6–12 year old children with spastic CP. More investigation has to be done to see whether and how exercise can influence the anaerobic capacity.

Muscle strength and muscle endurance

In CP, muscle mass is low,[7] and muscle strength is reduced. Bar Or[8] showed, as assessed by the Wingate anaerobic test, that local muscle endurance is particularly deficient in some neuromuscular diseases like spastic CP. Chretien et al.[27] mentioned that further impairment in strength is likely due to a peripheral nerve degeneration. Asymmetry of muscle deterioration leads to contractures and deformities leading to hypoactivity, which increases atrophy and therefore a loss of mechanical efficiency due to less economical movements. Low strength probably also reflects alterations in muscle fibre characteristics towards a higher rate of fast-twitch fibres.[28] Winnick and Short[29] documented a lower handgrip strength in 141 paraplegic children and adolescents. Muscle endurance is also reduced in children with CP as in other NMDs, and this reduction may reflect the high energy cost of ambulation and resultant hypoactivity.[11] Anaerobic power and endurance in children is significantly reduced. Parker et al.[20] showed that, in the Wingate test, when corrected for body mass, peak and mean power output in children aged 6 to 14 was 3–4 SD below normal in moderate to severe CP.

The following question arises: if muscle strength and endurance are trainable, is there a positive effect on the spasticity and mechanical efficiency? The use of strength training in cerebral palsied children is still controversial. Bar Or[8] mentioned the studies from Spira[30] and Rotzinger and Stoboy[31] which could not give a clear answer about a beneficial effect. Recent results shown by Damiano et al.[32,33] encourage a strengthening programme to obtain an improvement in walking and crouch gait. Quadriceps strength had significantly improved after a six-week muscle strengthening programme, three times weekly, at 30°, 60° and 90° of knee flexion. The maximal voluntary contraction of the quadriceps muscle did not differ statistically from normal at the end of the programme. Gait analysis resulted in an improvement in crouch gait. Quadriceps weakness was shown to be a factor in crouch gait. Restoring strength through resistance exercise therefore may be a useful adjunct in the treatment of CP. MacPhail and Kramer[34] observed, after an eight-week isokinetic strength training programme, a significant increase in gross motor ability and strength gains of 21 to 25%, similar to those previously reported for healthy individuals. O'Connell and Barnhart[35] also reported an improvement in strength after a progressive resistance exercise training programme.

Aerobic, anaerobic and muscle strength as well as endurance can be trained. The limiting factor will still remain the high energy cost and the lower mechanical efficiency, even if an improvement in walking velocity has been demonstrated.

Associated handicaps

One point has to be remembered also: many CP patients suffer from hypoactivity or inactivity resulting in some degree of obesity. Therefore, precise follow-up and counselling by a nutritionist, should be part of the therapeutic approach. Preventing obesity may significantly delay the decline in functional status of the patient. This point is even more important as the patient grows into adolescence. Impaired vision and hearing aggravates the often observed learning difficulties. It is necessary to take any concentration problem into consideration.

Summary concerning CP

One can state that all exercise physiological parameters are important and can be trained. The most important aspect is certainly the low mechanical efficiency, and a training programme should therefore be oriented towards an improvement of the spasticity and imbalance between muscle groups. Training aerobic and anaerobic power may help to improve the basis for a strengthening programme and also contribute to a better muscle endurance.

Neuromuscular dystrophy (Duchenne, Becker) and myopathy

Defined as a progressive degeneration of muscle cells, diseases of skeletal muscles (myopathies) produce two major patterns of exercise intolerance. In disorders of muscle energy metabolism, muscle bulk and resting strength are preserved, but an imbalance in muscle energy production and utilization in exercise leads to exertional muscle pain, cramps, weakness or fatigue. It may be caused by an impaired anaerobic glycolysis in isometric exercise, a disorder of oxidative metabolism in dynamic exercise, or a reduced maximal oxygen uptake as in case of mitochondrial myopathies.[36] In muscular dystrophy, there is a progressive loss of muscle fibres which results in increasing muscle weakness and reduced $\dot{V}O_2$ max, due to a progressive loss of functional muscle mass.

Muscular dystrophy is considered as a group of inherited diseases. Muscle cells degenerate and are replaced by adipose and connective tissues. The dystrophy itself is not fatal, but these patients suffer progressively from cardiovascular and respiratory complications due to the weakness of the muscles. There are different types of dystrophies like myotonic (Steinert), fascio-scapulo-humeral, limb-girdle and Duchenne, as well as Becker's dystrophy. Duchenne muscular dystrophy is the most frequent and severe form of the disease in childhood. It affects more boys than girls and usually starts between ages two and six years. The patients present a pseudohypertrophic appearance,

especially of the calves and forearms, due to an excessive accumulation of adipose and connective tissues within the interstitial spaces between degenerated muscle cells. The genetic origin has now been proved and a specific protein, called dystrophin, is linked to the gene. In Duchenne disease, this protein is absent. In animals, muscle cells transplantation has shown positive results,[37] but much more research is necessary before this kind of treatment can be applied to humans. The disease shows itself in atrophy and weakness of the thigh, hip, back, shoulder-girdle and respiratory muscles. The progression is rapid and results in walking inability within about ten years of onset. Difficulty in rising from a recumbent position, tendency to fall down and pain in climbing stairs are typical symptoms. Blood creatine phosphokinase (CPK) is high. As the disease progresses, patients become confined to wheelchairs and develop obesity. Contractures may also result from asymmetrical atrophy.[37] Three deficient fitness components characterize the physical working capacity of a patient with neuromuscular dystrophy: muscle strength, muscle endurance and maximal aerobic power.

Muscle strength

This factor is essential to the child's ability to accomplish daily activities like standing, rising or walking. Many authors have assessed muscle strength in NMD, especially in PMD. Lewis and Haller[38] reviewed skeletal muscle disorders and associated factors that limit exercise performance, and noted a low muscle strength in all types of NMD, such as Duchenne, Becker's or Steinert dystrophy, where exercise is severely impaired due to muscle wasting and weakness in spite of largely normal pathways for muscle ATP resynthesis. McDonald et al.[39] studied 162 patients with DMD to provide a profile of impairment and disability. The normal growth was markedly reduced after age of ten. Younger boys gained more weight, whereas older individuals actually showed a weight loss. Manual muscle test (MMT) measurements showed loss of strength in a fairly linear fashion from age 5 to 13 years, −0.25 MMT units per year. Isometrically measured strength was 40–50% below normal values.

Joint contractures were rare before age nine, but increased in frequency and severity with age. The prevalence of scoliosis increased between age 11 and 16 years, corresponding with the onset of the adolescent growth spurt. Percent predicted forced vital capacity (FVC) declined at different yearly rates. There was a direct relationship between per cent predicted FVC and MMT scores. Thirty per cent of DMD boys had a history of respiratory complications. There was a high occurrence (79%) of abnormal ECGs, but only 30% had cardiovascular complications. One point is important: while healthy children have a constant increase in muscle strength, either measurement approach shows a continuous decline in muscle strength in DMD.[5] Bar Or also comments on the fact that these children grow, and as their strength does not progress, such a non-progression in absolute muscle strength during growth is equivalent to a marked drop in function.

Concerning the question of trainability of muscle strength in DMD, Florence and Hagberg[40] reported the result of a 12-week programme to develop cardiovascular training adaptation. Resting CPK and myoglobin did not change with training. $\dot{V}O_2$ max and heart rate increased at the same levels as in healthy children. They concluded that training improves adaptation, but each disease has to be considered separately. McCartney et al.[41] reported the results of a dynamic nine-week weight training programme, three times a week, in a group of five patients with different types of dystrophy. They observed a strength gain from 19–50% in the trained limb. Different measures showed that the gains in strength were apparently due to a neural adaptation, rather than muscle hypertrophy. Milner-Brown and Miller[42] quantified muscle performance in 16 patients with gradually progressive neuromuscular disorders. They concluded that a high resistance weight training programme can significantly increase muscle performance of patients with neuromuscular disorders, if the disease progression is slow and initial muscle strength is greater than 15% of normal. Bar Or,[17] in his review, also finds evidence to suggest that muscle strength is trainable in NMD.

Muscle endurance and peak anaerobic power

Clinical observations show that children with PMD have a low muscle endurance and peak anaerobic power. This can be judged from their easy fatigability in daily activities. Different attempts have been made to assess muscle endurance objectively. Two tests, however, are useful. Sargeant[43] and van Praagh[44] have shown the feasibility and reliability of the force velocity test (FVT). In 1990, Tirosh et al.[45] found a highly reliable correlation for the Wingate test (WAnT) in PMD (test–retest: $r = 0.99$ for mean and peak power). The advantage of the WAnT is the fact that one can carry out the measures by pedalling and arm cranking. According to the anatomical distribution of the disease, this point is important. The anaerobic tests are also easier to perform in NMD than longer lasting aerobic protocols, this being due to the muscle weakness and the resulting fatigue limiting the duration of the test. Children with PMD always show lower scores. As the disease progresses, it is difficult to give norms for anaerobic performance for children with PMD.

Maximal aerobic power

Children with PMD progressively undergo a reduction of functional motor units in the muscles and, to a lesser extent, present lower respiratory functions. This explains the long-time observed low peak power output and maximal oxygen uptake.[46,47] PMD patients cannot reach a very high peak HR and therefore have to terminate an aerobic test whereas the cardiovascular system is not fully in demand. One can assume that the main limiting factor in these children is not the oxygen transport system but rather their reduced muscle strength, endurance and anaerobic power.

Muscle endurance and peak anaerobic power are trainable. Several studies showed that strength and endurance can be improved as long as they remain within residual functional motor units. The result will be reflected in a prolongation of walking, standing and rising ability. The type of exercise seems to be important. Recently, Wright et al.[48] suggested that moderate intensity aerobic exercise training is well tolerated and may provide modest improvement of aerobic capacity in slowly progressive NMD. Kilmer et al.[49] found no advantage of a high resistance exercise programme in slowing PMD, whereas in an earlier study,[50] the same group noted significant increases in most strength measures after a 12-week moderate resistance exercise programme.

Concerning muscular fatigue in PMD, Sharma et al.[51] studied a group of 11 boys (age five to ten years) with DMD. They found that, after a four minute sustained maximum voluntary contraction of the tibialis anterior muscle, the patients with DMD and controls had similar intramuscular fatigability and excitation–contraction coupling. Central activation in patients was also functioning as well as, or

better than, that in healthy controls. These findings corroborate the fact that muscle strength, muscle endurance, anaerobic power and aerobic power are trainable in this group of children. A progressive loss of strength can be slowed down and, at least for a while, reversed, which is one of the goals of any exercise programme.

Respiratory muscles

In PMD, as mentioned above, there is also a deterioration of lung functions. The changes are of a restrictive type, reflecting a weakness and a decrease of the lung compliance. Rothman[52] has shown an increase in respiratory functions after a breathing exercise programme. More recently, to study the usefulness of a specific inspiratory muscle training in DMD, Wanke et al.[53] found an improvement of inspiratory muscle function, even six months after a training programme, in 10 of 15 patients. In the other five there was no training effect, but all had vital capacity values of less than 25% predicted. They concluded that specific inspiratory muscle training is useful in the early stage of DMD.

Associated handicaps

Obesity is an important problem in PMD. Muscle cells are replaced by adipose and connective tissues. The body weight increases. Diet is controversial as its influence on the residual muscle mass is still unclear. Immobilization is probably the worst handicap accompanying PMD. As shown by Bar-Or,[5] bedrest must be avoided imperatively. Some patients never recover from a prolonged intercurrent illness or surgery, after having been bed-ridden for several weeks. Exercise is therefore an important therapeutic tool for PMD patients, and no study can scientifically prove a damaging effect of exercise.

The group of myopathies has to be distinguished from muscle dystrophies. Genetic, metabolic or infectious origins generate the pathology of mitochondrial myopathy, neurofibromatosis, myasthenia gravis, McArdle's disease, Prader Wili syndrome, Friedreich's ataxia or others. The genetic origin of several diseases is known, but still remains unclear for some others. Many recent studies have shown an improvement of muscle strength in different myopathies through exercise.[54–58] As far as exercise is concerned, these diseases can be assimilated to the group of progressive neuromuscular disorders. The questions are: what kind of activity, what intensity and what frequency of exercise are indicated?

Spinal cord impairments (SCI) and traumatic brain injuries (TBI)

Three categories of SCI have to be distinguished. In the first group, there are inherited diseases like spina bifida, myelomeningocele or spinal myatrophy. The second group consists of acquired diseases like poliomyelitis, Guillain-Barré syndrome or other infectious conditions affecting the brain or the vertebral column and spinal cord. The third group concerns traumatic brain and spinal cord injuries. All these conditions restrict patients from experiencing normal movement patterns that are essential to normal motor development.

An important factor is the onset of the disease or injury. The psychological impact is therefore evident. For a child who has lived under normal conditions before, the re-apprenticeship of all the motor skills he used to perform is very often difficult. Patients have to learn to live with a different body, they must adapt a different approach of learning and develop a new personality. They have to know their new limits to prevent training stress and overuse, but also their new capabilities. This is even more important if sports play a crucial part of life, especially in an adolescent's life. Strong psychological and pedagogical support has to be offered to help the patient recover a healthy self-esteem and body-image.

Physical fitness and the ability to exercise depend on the severity and the localization of the lesion, the associated lesions or handicaps, the age, the sociocultural environment and the disease itself. Some conditions can be improved, some cannot. Muscular strength, endurance and maximal aerobic power are secondarily reduced. Winnick and Short[29] have shown decreased muscle endurance in children and adolescents with paraplegia due to SCI, as indicated by flexed arm-hang and pull-ups scores. Bar-Or[8] demonstrated a reduced muscle strength, even if some compensation through the valid part of the body may exist. Aerobic and anaerobic power can be normal if there is no associated pathology. Important intrinsic factors play a role too. The adolescent growth spurt and its influence on the child's ability to perform, can exert positive and negative effects. Obesity has to be expected if a regular programme of physical activity is not set up. This is important as several studies have shown a positive effect of muscle strength and muscle endurance training. Einarsson,[59] Gordon and Mao,[60] Spector et al.[61] and recently Hutzler et al.[62] have demonstrated strength gains in patients with post-polio muscular atrophy without serological or histological evidence of muscular damage. Many studies show the trainability of all the physiological parameters in SCI, but the paucity of data for children requires deductions from observation in adults. As more and more children are involved in TBI and SCI, research has to be done in this area to help set up adapted facilities and programmes for these patients.

Fitness assessment in NMD

Children respond in a different way to chronic or acute exercise stress than adults.[63] This point is even more important for patients with NMD. As tests often represent a strong demand on physical resources and may fatigue excessively, one has to decide whether they are necessary, useful and safe for the patient, and which type of tests is best indicated. One has to consider their feasibility, reproducibility and reliability. A certain number of protocols exists for laboratory tests. Tomassoni[64] provides information about paediatric laboratory exercise testing, and Rowland[65] gives an overview of aerobic exercise tests. A review of evaluation by exercise testing of the child with CP published by Unnitham et al.[66] gives a clear understanding of the actual state of research. In view of the fact that expensive computer-linked equipment is not commonly available, a battery of field tests can be used. Children will anyway prefer to perform tests in a group and under familiar conditions. To set up a protocol for field tests, some points have to be considered: the tests have to be carried out under the same conditions and with the same testing person; and learning effects must be eliminated from initial measurements by repeated testing. In order to evaluate a patient with NMD, a series of easy to perform field tests can be used. In relation to a multidisciplinary programme at the CME in Geneva, a study comparing the reliability between laboratory tests and these tests is close to completion, and the initial results indicate a probable correlation.

Table 4.5.1 Field tests to assess physical fitness in disabled children (neuromuscular diseases, CP, poliomyelitis, myopathy, PMD, SCI, TBI)

	Endurance, Aerobic power	Resistance, Anaerobic power	Explosive power, Muscle endurance	Coordination
Laboratory	Léger shuttle run	Wingate anaerobic test	Bosco vertical jump	Fitronic agility
Field	Léger shuttle run 15 min swim 3 min water run	Obstacle race	Standing long jump	Obstacle race Eurofit Juggling

References for the tests
Léger test: see Table 4.5.2. Wingate test: Bar-Or, O.[63] Bosco vertical jump test: Bosco et al.[67] Agility test, Fitronic: Hamar, D. University Bratislava, Slovakia. Obstacle race: see Table 4.5.2. Standing long jump: see Table 4.5.2.

Table 4.5.1 shows a series of field tests. In Table 4.5.2 a short description of the tests is given. The tests provide information about the child's development of fitness and about the quality of the programme, but they can serve as a motivational tool as well.

What kind of physical activity is suitable for young patients with NMD?

As seen above, children with NMD can and should exercise. The question is: what kind of physical activity is indicated for them? Since 1992, a multidisciplinary programme for children with NMD has been set up at the CME in Geneva. Twice a week, children take part in organized activities: one in the pool (45 minutes) and one in the gymnasium (90 minutes). They are followed by a physician, a nutritionist and a psychologist. A medical and a physiological evaluation (see Tables 4.5.1 and 4.5.2) are done twice a year. Before integrating children with NMD in an adapted physical activity programme, one has to specify the physiological and psychological status of each candidate. A medical history and a general clinical examination are necessary to provide information about possible general health problems, which may have an influence on the disease itself. Any underlying pathology independent from the NMD should be clarified to prevent damaging interactions. Associated handicaps, such as hearing disorders, troubles of vision and obesity must be taken into account particularly.

A nutritional evaluation also has to be part of this multidisciplinary approach. It is known that sociocultural factors can strongly influence the evolution of obesity in healthy children, and they become even more important in disabled patients. A questionnaire concerning eating habits and measurements of body mass, stature and body composition are performed, and constitute a starting basis. The results allow the evolution of the patient to be followed, and for the introduction or adaptation of the programme to each case individually. The role of the nutritionist is to give advice and information to the children

Table 4.5.2   Description of the field tests carried out at the CME

15 min swimming Test elaborated after a five year test period by the physiotherapist and physical education teacher of the CME Geneva.	Endurance test: the child must swim (front crawl) the longest possible distance in 15 min. The test is performed in shallow water (approx. 55 cm) in order not to penalize participants due to their swimming technique, the endurance being the only parameter measured. The children touch the bottom of the pool with their hands at each stroke.
Léger test Léger, L., Cloutier, J., Rowan, C.: University of Montreal, April 1985.	Determines the maximal aerobic power ($\dot{V}O_2$ max) expressed in METS or ml kg^{-1} min^{-1}. Progressive maximal indirect shuttle run test, that can be used in the field as well as in the laboratory. The children have to run a distance of 20 m at a given speed, which is accelerated every minute.
Obstacle race Devised by the physiotherapist and physical education teacher at the CME Geneva, this test aims at integrating notions of coordination, speed and anticipation of the forthcoming obstacle.	This test is comprised of different exercises which have to be performed in a minimum time. The race includes a slalom between flags, jumping feet together from one hoop to the other, crawling under a horse, crossing a landing mattress and climbing over a box.
Standing long jump Eurofit. Handbook for the EUROFIT Tests of Physical Fitness. Committee of experts on sports research. Rome, 1988.	The tested exercise consists of a standing long jump from an upright position. At the reception of the jump, a balanced position must be held.

and the parents for their specific needs. Occasionally, the nutritionist also participates in the physical activity lessons to be able to understand better the problems the child may encounter.

A psychological evaluation is of major importance to assess the patients' motivations to adhere to the programme and to reveal disfunctioning thoughts and self-perceptions which might aggravate their condition. The evaluation thus serves as a basis to set realistic goals for each patient in the group concerning his/her progress, and also to provide topics on which to work, such as self-acceptance, self body image, social integration and unrealistic expectations about the programme. The model used for the psychological intervention is cognitive-behavioural. It allows work to be done on specific situations, the emotions and thoughts arising in the patient, and their consequences on his/her behaviour. What has proved to be critical in the therapeutic approach is the notion of physical activity. By encouraging the children to find activities which are suited to their actual capabilities, the psychologist is able to create some sense of perceived competence and trust. This psychological aspect helps the patients to cope better with their impairment and becomes the basis for self-acceptance in many of them. It is stressed that they have the right to do things their own way, compared to their peers. This approach is highly beneficial to the children, it fosters group cohesion and helps give them a new significance to their life. The psychologist, like the nutritionist, sometimes takes part in the physical activity lessons.

The multidisciplinary approach of such a programme has numerous advantages. Lifestyle, self-esteem and integration are often problematic concerns in these patients. Obesity represents an important issue and a regular follow-up is beneficial in controlling obesity. The physical activity programme is established by a therapist specialized in

NMD (e.g. Bobath) and a specially trained physical educator. According to the severity of the handicaps, one instructor is necessary for a group of three to six children.

Aims of the course

Increased autonomy

Autonomy is increased through carefully planned lessons, which include exercises aimed at improving physical resistance, endurance, strength, balance, coordination, speed of reaction and reasoning, flexibility and swiftness of execution. In as many different situations as possible, one aims at helping children with NMD to become more autonomous in everyday life. Developing body awareness and acceptance of a handicap with its limitations and emphasizing the possibilities—which must be used to a maximum—also helps towards independence. Notions such as reinforcing antagonist muscle groups for those suffering from CP to increase range of motion (ROM), strength and speed in spastic limbs are applied whenever possible.[36,68,69] The necessity of exercising and maintaining maximum muscle power without fatigue in children with any form of muscular dystrophy is also taken into consideration.[70] It is thought that active stimulation of muscles, either by volition or impulse from intact muscle groups, can reactivate some fibres that may have remained innervated amongst muscles weakened by poliomyelitis.[71] Controlled physical activity for people with motor deficiencies following poliomyelitis can help prevent overuse syndromes in cardiac deconditioning later in life.[72] Joining a group for specialized physical education can be a means of reducing medical support and physiotherapy sessions and be a help in becoming more independent. It can also be a way of stimulating someone who refuses to continue therapy when it is still considered necessary, e.g. during the growth spurt of adolescence.

Well-being

Being able to participate in activities adapted to each patient's special needs and level of abilities, without the fear of failure or the need to compete against non-handicapped peers, is often a novel experience. Success motivates further effort resulting in feeling fitter and getting an improved self-image. Psychological support in a group or individual situation should be available to help the children overcome unpleasant reminiscences.

Enjoyment and fun

These are important factors in stimulating effort and participation in new, and possibly at first frightening, experiences. Learning to climb and to jump from a height can be encouraged if the descent is fun (slide, big mattress, etc.). Games can make the hard work necessary to improve endurance enjoyable.

Creating a team spirit

Among individuals generally isolated by their handicap, this notion is as important as the physiological benefits derived from sport. Children with NMD often show great solidarity and help each other, without adults having to artificially create an atmosphere. Of course, as in any other mini-society, there can be conflicts.

Integration

The activities proposed are designed to bring the youngsters up to a sufficient standard, physically and psychologically, so that they are able to join a local club, group or school lesson for some kind of sport.

Different activities within a course

Physical activities for children with NMD should not differ too much from those for healthy children. The problem for the animators of such a course is to choose the correct degree of difficulty, intensity, frequency and duration. One must show the child what he is able to do. Success in varied situations is the key to all functioning programmes.

In the pool

Water is a fantastic medium in which a handicapped person can move more freely (effect of buoyancy). Special attention is given to ensure that the temperature is adequate (29–30°C). Sufficient time is spent in ensuring there is an adaptation to water with little or no fear. Basic swimming techniques are taught in varying depths of water and different positions. Increased physical resistance and endurance can be trained in various ways: running, walking or hopping, depending on the handicap, in different levels of water; swimming in shallow water—with hands touching the bottom of the pool for non or poor swimmers—and, of course, swimming in medium to deep water for the good ones. Circuit training on, in and under water are great fun and improve balance. Jumping in and out of hoops or air rings and over submerged ropes, climbing into floating objects, rowing rafts, doing tasks forwards and backwards, are means to exercise coordination in an entertaining way. All these activities increase cardiorespiratory demand and optimize the adaptation to water.

Individual work, where participants are grouped according to their handicap, allows for specific needs to be catered for: relaxation and floating for the spastic or anxious, the use of floats as resistance to increase the work of hemiplegic limbs, and many other possibilities. Games play an important part in all courses, fun and motivation being excellent stimuli.

A typical lesson in the pool

Warm-up and making contact can be achieved with games such as 'catch', either running through shallow water or crawling in a lizard fashion. The main part of the course can be based on teaching swimming techniques in different depths of water. Towards the end, the children could be allowed to take it in turns to demonstrate and choose the style for the whole class to swim. Jumping, diving or relaxation on floating mats are fun ways to end a lesson.

In the gymnasium

Varied relay games have many advantages, such as memorizing instructions and planning oneself for action. Speed is an important factor which provokes an increase in heart rate. Care must be taken when selecting teams so that each group has a similar variety of handicaps, and therefore equal chances of success. Although the aim of each relay race is the same for all, the way in which it is performed can be varied according to individual possibilities. Trampolining is wonderful exercise, climbing onto the apparatus can be a challenge in itself. The proprioceptive input and rhythmic bouncing balance out muscle tone, stimulate back extension, righting and parachute reactions, and decrease asymmetry. There are many ways of using the trampoline: lying, long sitting, prone kneeling, high kneeling or standing. Balance, climbing and swinging can be combined in a lot of different activities and circuits. Children and adolescents often enjoy the challenge of big apparatus and moving surfaces; all senses (tactile, vestibular and proprioceptive) are stimulated and motor response is often maximal. Adapted team games, such as uni hockey, volley ball, net ball, etc., need breaking down into small elements and careful teaching over weeks or months in order to build up an activity where all members of the team can function and enjoy a group situation. Stretching should be a part of all lessons and adapted to the activity of the day and the individual needs of the participants.

A typical lesson in the gymnasium

Force, endurance and physical resistance are elements included in all lessons in many different ways. Typically, one would start with a warm-up comprised of a team game, for example, 'cat catches the mice tails' (physiological warm-up plus physical resistance). The main part of the lesson could be a circuit using large apparatus. Strength, dexterity, balance and possibly speed and endurance can be included depending on the aims and the instructions given. A calm game or stretching can be done at the end (physiological cool-down and flexibility).

Precautions to be taken when organizing specialized physical activities

A certain selection of candidates must be made in order to obtain a smoothly running group. One should check that future participants and their families are aware of the handicap, already have some degree of acceptance, and are also prepared to tolerate other children's disabilities. The purpose of the course should be carefully explained so that the children know that the difficulties will be adapted to their individual possibilities, and that regular participation is needed in order to gain benefit from the programme. Each participant must find a level of activity within the course which corresponds to his/her abilities. If an exercise is too easy, boredom can set in; on the contrary, too high a level of difficulty can lead to frustration and negative feed-back. Constant stimulation through fun learning situations, attainable aims and encouraging course leaders (teachers, physiotherapists, educators) must result in regular effort and performance from the children. Any notion of competition on an individual basis must be avoided in a heterogeneous group to prevent detriment to the self-image of the more severely handicapped. One must be vigilant so that the children do not avoid using their handicapped limbs, nor that they refrain from trying difficult activities. As a long-term aim is reintegration into non-specialized physical activities, the participants must not be overprotected within the group and should gain in independence progressively.

Care must be taken with children with CP so that excitement and effort do not excessively increase associated reactions and spastic patterns. Relaxation, stretching and correct postures at the end of a lesson help in the recovery of a more normal muscle tone and body position. Children with PMD must be carefully monitored to ensure that they do not go over their fatigue level and increase CPK, which may initiate accelerated degradation of residual muscle.[73,74] Children with polio must be vigilant not to damage their skin whilst swinging or dragging

their flaccid limbs. Other problems linked to handicaps can arise during a programme. Caution must be used when asking for speed of execution to ensure that not too much quality of movement is lost. Correction of trick movements must be systematic to avoid abnormal postures and eventual overuse syndromes. Hand holds in climbing and swinging must be closely supervised: a spastic hand can slip during motion, and children with PMD are known to let go suddenly when their muscles tire. Foot and hand deformities can make running, jumping and climbing very difficult and even contraindicated. All course leaders must ensure that the activity has the desired effect and not a detrimental one, may it be physical or psychological.

During the programme, continuous information must be given, especially to those suffering from progressive diseases (PMD, Recklinghausen), so that poor results are correctly interpreted and that disappointment and unreasonable expectations are avoided.

Evaluation

In order to determine if the aims of the course have been attained, a series of useful tests can be chosen. These should be performed twice a year and clear information has to be given to the parents, the child and his doctor. The tests serve also as a motivation for the children and their parents, and show the doctors the possible therapeutic utility of exercise. Some results from the author's laboratory where seven children followed the multidisciplinary programme including one session in the gymnasium and one in the pool per week show the importance of physical activity and the necessity of its continuity (Table 4.5.3 and Figs 4.5.1–4.5.3).

Table 4.5.3 Results of laboratory and field tests after a nine month training programme and after a three month summer vacation in seven children with NMD

	Aerobic power						Anaerobic power						Explosive Power					
	Laboratory			Field			Laboratory			Field			Laboratory			Field		
	Léger, shuttle run			15 min. swimming			Wingate			Obstacle race			Bosco			Standing long jump		
Subject	R 97	F 98	R 98	R 97	F 98	R 98	R 97	F 98	R 98	R 97	F 98	R 98	R 97	F 98	R 98	R 97	F 98	R 98
C.Z.	2.5	3	3	283.2	341.5	312.4	5.7	6	6	28.5	29.6	24.9	19	20.5	19	130	120	135
F.M.	1.5	1	1.5	362.4	399.8	410.8	3	3.9	3	28.5	22.7	26.8	12.5	13.1	12.5	90	95	100
H.J.	0.5	1	3.5	254.1	258.2	372	1.8	1.8	2.3	34.8	33.1	33.9	9.3	9.8	10.3	65	80	75
T.C.	0.5	0.5	0.5	145.8	125	174.9	3.1	3.7	2.2	62.7	61.3	59.2	10.3	10.9	10.3	30	65	50
W.S.	4.5	5.5	4.5	533.1	558.1	641.4	6.9	7.7	7.7	23.6	20.8	19.7	19.78	21.3	22	150	160	160
D.A.	1	1.5	–	337.4	288.7	333.2	3.7	3.7	4.7	38.1	30.7	33.1	8.3	12	12.2	85	100	–
H.D.	0.5	0.5	0.5	241.6	299.9	266.6	3.1	2.9	2.3	40.1	34.9	33.2	9.7	9.8	9.8	85	90	95

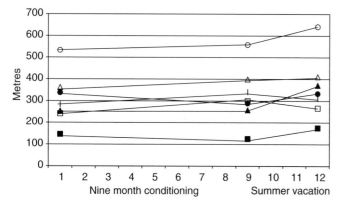

Fig. 4.5.1 Results of the 15 minutes swimming testing aerobic power in 7 children with NMD after a 9 month training programme and 3 month summer vacation.

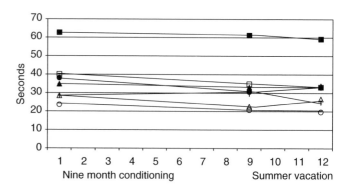

Fig. 4.5.2 Results of the obstacle race testing anaerobic power and coordination in 7 children with NMD after a 9 month training programme and 3 month summer vacation.

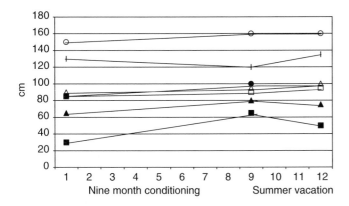

Fig. 4.5.3 Results of the standing long jump testing explosive power in 7 children with NMD after a 9 month training programme and 3 month summer vacation.

Several interesting points have to be taken into consideration:

1. One cannot expect extraordinary progression in children with NMD.

2. The course is very positive if no deterioration has occurred (PMD) or if only little improvement of the physical parameters has been observed, as its initial goal is to slow down the progression of the physical deterioration, and secondarily to improve the performance.

3. The regularity of physical activity seems to be an important determinant. Intercurrent illness or surgery immediately provoke a stop or regression of any previously achieved acquisition.

4. Continuity and the possibility of following a physical activity programme during the long period of the summer vacation is imperative to prevent a regression, as already mentioned by Berg in 1970.[75]

5. The improvement of self-esteem and well being and the possibility of integration within a group are of greatest value, not only for the patient, but also for his family.

6. Children also seem to overcome possible associated handicaps more effectively. Learning difficulties, problems of vision and hearing, and prevention of obesity can be improved through an individual and group approach.

7. A multidisciplinary approach is certainly advantageous and stimulating for patients, parents and therapists.

Summary

Physical activity is beneficial for most of the children with NMD. Even if the disease is progressive like PMD or myopathies, the fact of being able to delay the negative evolution and to help the patient to walk as long as possible and to achieve most common daily activities should encourage all the people involved in the approach of these diseases to motivate the patients and their families to invest in physical activity.

A lot of research is still needed to progress, but many positive results are already available. A better knowledge of the innocuity of sports, if correctly practised, as well as a precise appreciation of the clinical and physiological parameters, should also help to decrease fear and overprotection and, finally, to delay as long as possible the course towards wheelchair status.

References

1. **Pellegrino, L.** Cerebral palsy. In *Children with disabilities* (4th edn) (ed. M. L. Batshaw). Paul. H. Brookes Publishing Company, Baltimore, 1997; 499–510 and 516–21.

2. **Bar-Or, O.** Physiological effects of a sports rehabilitation program on cerebral palsied or postmyelitic adolescents. *Medicine and Science in Sports and Exercise* 1976; **8**: 157–61.

3. **Lundberg, A.** Mechanical efficiency in bicycle ergometer work of young adults with cerebral palsy. *Developmental Medicine and Child Neurology* 1975; **17**: 434–9.

4. **Lundberg, A.** Oxygen consumption in relation to work load in students with cerebral palsy. *Journal of Applied Physiology* 1976; **40**: 873–5.

5. **Bar-Or, O.** *Pediatric sports medicine for the practitioner.* Springer Verlag, New York, 1983; 227.

6. **Dresen, M. H., de Groot, G., Corstius, J. J., Krediet, G. H., and Meijer, M. G.** Physical work capacity and daily physical activities of handicapped and non-handicapped children. *European Journal of Applied Physiology* 1982; **48**: 241–51.

7. **Lundberg, A.** Maximal aerobic capacity of young people with spastic cerebral palsy. *Developmental Medicine and Child Neurology* 1978; **20**: 205–10.

8. **Bar–Or, O.** Pathophysiological factors which limit the exercise capacity of the sick child. *Medicine and Science in Sports and Exercise* 1986; **18**: 276–82.

9. **Peacock, G.** Classification for competition. In *A training guide for CP sports* (ed. J.A. Jones). Human Kinetics, Champaign, Il., 1988; 27–39.

10. **van den Berg-Emons, R. J., van Baak, M. A., de Barbanson, D. C., Speth, L., and Saris, W. H.** Reliability of tests to determine peak aerobic power, anaerobic power and isokinetic muscle strength in children with spastic cerebral palsy. *Developmental Medicine and Child Neurology* 1996; **38**: 1117–25.

11. **Steadward, R. D. and Wheeler, G. D.** The young athlete with a motor disability. In *The encyclopaedia of sports medicine, VI: the child and adolescent athlete* (ed. O. Bar-Or). Blackwell Science, Oxford, 1996; 493–520.

12. **Jones, J.** Mechanical efficiency of children with spastic cerebral palsy. *Developmental Medicine and Child Neurology* 1993; **35**: 614–20.

13. **Rose, J., Gamble, J. G., Medeiros, J., Burgos, A. and Haskell, W. L.** Energy cost of walking in normal children and in those with cerebral palsy: comparison of heart rate and oxygen uptake. *Journal of Pediatric Orthopaedics* 1989; **9**: 276–9.

14. **Rose, J., Gamble, J. G., Burgos, A., Medeiros, J. and Haskell, W. L.** Energy expenditure index of walking for normal children and for children with cerebral palsy. *Developmental Medicine and Child Neurology* 1990; **32**: 333–40.

15. **Dresen, M. H., de Groot, G., Mesa Menor, J. R. and Bouman, L. N.** Aerobic energy expenditure of handicapped children after training. *Archives of Physical Medicine and Rehabilitation* 1985; **66**: 302–6.

16. **Fernandez, J. and Pitetti K.H.** Training of ambulatory individuals with cerebral palsy. *Archives of Physical Medicine and Rehabilitation* 1993; **74**: 468–72.

17. **Bar-Or, O.** Role of exercise in the assessment and management of neuromuscular disease in children. *Medicine and Science in Sports and Exercise* 1996; **28**: 421–7.

18. **Lundberg, A.** Effect of physical training in school children with cerebral palsy. *Acta Paediatrica Scandinavica* 1967; **56**: 182–8.

19. **Lundberg, A.** Longitudinal study of physical working capacity of young people with spastic cerebral palsy. *Developmental Medicine and Child Neurology* 1984; **26**: 328–34.

20. **Parker, D. F., Carrière, L., Hebestreit, H. and Bar-Or, O.** Anaerobic endurance and peak muscle power in children with spastic cerebral palsy. *American Journal of Diseases of Children* 1992; **146**: 1069–73.

21. **Emons, H. J. G., Groenenboom, D. C., Burggraaff, Y. I., Janssen, T. L. E., and Van Baak, M. A.** Wingate anaerobic test in children with cerebral palsy. In *Children and exercise XVI* (ed. J. Coudert and E. Van Praagh). Masson, Paris, 1992; 187–9.

22. **Bar-Or, O.** Neuromuscular disease and anaerobic performance during childhood. In *Pediatric anaerobic performance* (ed. E. Van Praagh). Human Kinetics, Champaign, Il., 1998; 291–303.

23. **Bar-Or, O.** Anaerobic capacity and muscle fiber type distribution in man. *International Journal of Sports Medicine* 1980; **1**: 89–92.

24. **Berbrayer, D.** Reciprocal inhibition in cerebral palsy. *Neurology* 1990; **40**: 653–6.

25. **O'Connell, D. G., Barnhart, R.** and **Parks, L.** Muscular endurance and wheelchair propulsion in children with cerebral palsy or meningomyelocele. *Archives of Physical Medicine and Rehabilitation* 1992; **73**: 709–11.

26. **Emons, H. J. G.,** and **Van Baak, M. A.** Effect of training on aerobic and anaerobic power and mechanical efficiency in spastic cerebral palsied children. *Pediatric Exercise Science* 1993; **5**: 412.

27. **Chretien, R., Simard, C. P.** and **Dorion, A.** *International perspectives on adapted physical activity* (ed. M. Berridge and C. Ward). Human Kinetics, Champaign, Il., 1987; 65–72.

28. **Castle, M. E., Reyman, T. A.** and **Schneider, M.** Pathology of spastic muscle in cerebral palsy. *Clinical Orthopaedics and Related Research* 1979; **142**: 223–33.

29. **Winnick, J. P.** and **Short, F. X.** The physical fitness of youngsters with spinal neuromuscular conditions. *Adapted Physical Activity Quarterly* 1984; **1**: 37–41.

30. **Spira, R.** Contribution of the H-reflex to the study of spasticity in adolescents. *Developmental Medicine and Child Neurology* 1974; **16**: 150–7.

31. **Rotzinger, G.** and **Stoboy, H.** Comparison between clinical judgement and electromyographic investigations of the effect of a special training program. *Acta Paediatrica Belgica* 1974; **28**: 121–8.

32. **Damiano, D. L., Vaughan, C. L.** and **Abel, M. F.** Muscle response to heavy resistance exercise in children with spastic cerebral palsy. *Developmental Medicine and Child Neurology* 1995; **37**: 731–9.

33. **Damiano, D. L., Kelly, L. E.** and **Vaughan, C. L.** Effects of quadriceps femoris muscle strengthening on crouch gait in children with spastic diplegia. *Physical Therapy* 1995; **75**: 731–9.

34. **MacPhail, H. E.** and **Kramer, J. F.** Effect of isokinetic strength-training on functional ability and walking efficiency in adolescents with cerebral palsy. *Developmental Medicine and Child Neurology* 1995; **37**: 763–75.

35. **O'Connell, D. G.** and **Barnhart, R.** Improvement in wheelchair propulsion in pediatric wheelchair users through resistance training: a pilot study. *Archives of Physical Medicine and Rehabilitation* 1995; **76**: 368–72.

36. **Haller, R. G.** and **Lewis, S.F.** Pathophysiology of exercise performance in muscle disease. *Medicine and Science in Sports and Exercise* 1984; **16**: 456–9.

37. **Poretta, D. L.** CP, TBI, stroke, amputations, dwarfism and other orthopedic impairments. In *Disability and sport* (ed. K. P. De Pauw and S. J. Gavron). Human Kinetics, Champaign, Il., 1995; 167–91.

38. **Lewis, F. S.** and **Haller, R. G.** Skeletal muscle disorders and associated factors that limit exercise performance. *Exercise and Sport Sciences Reviews* 1989; **17**: 67–113.

39. **McDonald, C. M., Abrech, R. T., Carter, G. T., Fowler, W. M. Jr., Johnson, E. R., Kilmer, D. D.** and **Sigford, B. J.** Profiles of neuromuscular diseases, Duchenne muscular dystrophy. *American Journal of Physical Medicine Rehabilitation* 1995; **74**: 870–92.

40. **Florence, J. M.** and **Hagberg, J. M.** Effect of training on the exercise response of neuromuscular disease patients. *Medicine and Science in Sports and Exercise* 1984; **16**: 460–5.

41. **McCartney, N., Moroz, D., Garner, S. H.** and **McComas, A.** The effects of strength training in patients with selected neuromuscular disorders. *Medicine and Science in Sports and Exercise* 1988; **20**: 362–8.

42. **Milner-Brown, H. S.** and **Miller, R. G.** Muscle strengthening through high resistance weight training in patients with neuromuscular disorders. *Archives of Physical Medicine and Rehabilitation* 1988; **69**: 14–9.

43. **Sargeant, A.** Short term muscle power in children and adolescents. In *Advances in pediatric sports sciences* (ed. O. Bar-Or). Human Kinetics, Champaign, Il., 1989; 42–65.

44. **Van Praagh, E.** Testing anaerobic performance. In *The encyclopaedia of sports medicine VI: the child and adolescent athlete* (ed. O. Bar-Or). Blackwell Science, Oxford, 1996; 603–16.

45. **Tirosh, E., Bar-Or, O.** and **Rosenbaum, P.** New muscle power test in neuromuscular disease. Feasibility and reliability. *American Journal of Diseases of Children* 1990; **144**: 1083–7.

46. **Sockolov, R., Irwin, B., Dresseuderfer, R. H.** and **Bernauer, E. M.** Exercise performance in 6–11 year old boys with Duchenne muscular dystrophy. *Archives of Physical Medicine and Rehabilitation* 1977; **58**: 195–201.

47. **Carroll, J. E., Hagberg, J. M., Brooke, M. H.** and **Shumate, J. B.** Bicycle ergometry and gas exchange. Measurements in NMD. *Archives of Neurology* 1979; **36**: 457–61.

48. **Wright, N. C., Kilmer, D. D., McCrory, M. A., Aitkens, S. G., Holcomb, B. J.** and **Bernauer, E. M.** Aerobic walking in slowly progressive neuromuscular disease : effect of a 12-week program. *Archives of Physical Medicine and Rehabilitation* 1996; **77**: 64–9.

49. **Kilmer, D. D., McCrory, M. A., Wright, N. C., Aitkens, S. G.** and **Bernauer, E. M.** The effect of a high resistance exercise program in slowly progressive neuromuscular disease. *Archives of Physical Medicine and Rehabilitation* 1994; **75**: 560–3.

50. **Aitkens, S. G., McCrory, M. A., Kilmer, D. D.** and **Bernauer, E. M.** Moderate resistance exercise program : its effect in slowly progressive neuromuscular disease. *Archives of Physical Medicine and Rehabilitation* 1993; **74**: 711–5.

51. **Sharma, K. R., Mynhier, M. A.** and **Miller, R. G.** Muscular fatigue in DMD. *Neurology* 1995; **45**: 306–10.

52. **Rothman, J. G.** Effects of respiratory exercises on the vital capacity and forced expiratory volume in children with cerebral palsy. *Physical Therapy* 1978; **58**: 421–5.

53. **Wanke, T., Toifl, K., Merkle M., Formanek, D., Lahrmann, H.** and **Zwick, H.** Inspiratory muscle training in patients with Duchenne muscular dystrophy. *Chest* 1994; **105**: 475–82.

54. **Erwin, J. H., Keller, C., Anderson, S.** and **Costa, J.** Hand and wrist strengthening exercises during rehabilitation of a patient with hereditary distal myopathy. *Archives of Physical Medicine and Rehabilitation* 1991; **72**: 701–2.

55. **Koch, B. M.** and **Simenson, R. L.** Upper extremity strength and function in children with spinal muscular atrophy type II. *Archives of Physical Medicine and Rehabilitation* 1992; **73**: 241–5.

56. **Chaussain, M., Camus, F., Defuolihny, C., Eymard, B.** and **Fardeau, M.** Exercise intolerance in patients with McArdle's disease or mito-chondrial myopathies. E*uropean Journal of Medicine* 1992; **1**: 457–63.

57. **Lohi, E. L., Linberg, C.** and **Andersen, O.** Physical training effects in myasthenia gravis. *Archives of Physical Medicine and Rehabilitation* 1993; **74**: 1178–80.

58. **Taivassalo, T., De Stefano, N, Argov, Z., Matthews, P. M., Chen, J., Genge, A., Karpati, G.** and **Arnold, D. L.** Effects of aerobic training in patients with myochondrial myopathies. *Neurology* 1998; **50**: 1055–60.

59. **Einarsson, G.** Muscle conditioning in late poliomyelitis. *Archives of Physical Medicine and Rehabilitation* 1991; **72**: 11–4.

60. **Gordon, T.** and **Mao, J.** Muscle atrophy and procedures for training after SCI. *Physical Therapy* 1994; **74**: 50–60.

61. **Spector, S. A., Gordon, P. L., Feuerstein, I. M., Sivakumar, K., Hurley, B. F.** and **Dalakas, M. C.** Strength gains without muscle injury after strength training in patients with postpolio muscular atrophy. *Muscle Nerve* 1996; **19**: 1282–90.

62. **Hutzler, Y., Ochana, S., Bolotin, R.** and **Kalina, E.** Aerobic and anaerobic arm-cranking power outputs of males with lower limb impairments: relationship with sport participation: intensity, age, impairment and functional classification. *Spinal Cord* 1998; **36**: 205–12.

63. **Bar-Or, O.** Non-cardiopulmonary pediatric exercise tests. In *Pediatric laboratory exercise testing* (ed. T. W. Rowland). Human Kinetics, Champaign, Il., 1993; 165–85.

64. **Tomassoni, T. L.** Conducting the pediatric exercise test. In *Pediatric laboratory exercise testing* (ed.T. W. Rowland). Human Kinetics, Champaign. Il., 1993; 1–17.

65. **Rowland, T. W.** Aerobic exercise testing protocols. In *Pediatric laboratory exercise testing* (ed. T.W. Rowland). Human Kinetics, Champaign, Il., 1993; 19–41.

66. **Unnitham, V. B., Clifford, C.** and **Bar-Or, O.** Evaluation by exercise testing of the child with cerebral palsy. *Sports Medicine* 1998; **26**: 239–51.

67. **Bosco, C., Luhtanen, P.** and **Komi, P. V.** A simple method for measurement of mechanical power in jumping. *European Journal of Applied Physiology* 1983; **50**: 273–82.

68. **Surburg, P. R.** New perspectives for developing range of motion and flexibility for special populations. *Adapted Physical Activity Quarterly* 1996; **3**: 227–35.

69. **Damiano, D. L.** and **Abel, A. F.** Functional outcomes of strength training in spastic cerebral palsy. *Archives of Physical Medicine and Rehabilitation* 1998; **79**: 119–25.

70. **Siegel, M.** Update on Duchenne muscular dystrophy. *Comprehensive Therapy* 1989; **15**: 45–52.

71. **Birk, T. J.** Poliomyelitis and the post-polio syndrome: exercise capacities and adaptation ; current research, future directions, and widespread applicability. *Medicine and Science in Sports and Exercise* 1993; **25**: 466–72.

72. **Dean, E., Agboatwalla, M., Dallimore, M., Habib, Z.** and **Akram D. S.** Poliomyelitis: an old problem revisited. *Physiotherapy* 1995; **81**: 17–28.

73. **Agre, J. C.** The role of exercise in the patient with post-polio syndrome. *Annals of the New York Academy of Sciences* 1995; **25**: 321–34.

74. **Siegel, I.** *The clinical management of muscle disease.* William Heinemann Medical Books Ltd., London, 1977; 112.

75. **Berg, K.** Effect of physical training of school children with cerebral palsy. *Acta Paediatrica Scandinavica* 1970; **204**: 27–33.

4.6 Exercise, sport and diabetes mellitus

Keith D. Buchanan

What is diabetes mellitus?

The *American Diabetes Association* (ADA) during its annual meeting in 1997 approved new diagnostic criteria for diabetes mellitus.[1] The revised criteria are symptoms of diabetes mellitus and a casual plasma glucose $\geqslant 11.1$ mmol litre^{-1} or a fasting plasma glucose $\geqslant 7.0$ mmol litre^{-1} or a 2 hour plasma glucose $\geqslant 11.1$ mmol litre^{-1} during a standard 75 g oral glucose tolerance test. Therefore, the criteria rest solely on the estimation of glucose levels in the blood.

Classification of diabetes mellitus

There are two main types:
(1) Type 1 diabetes mellitus or insulin dependent diabetes mellitus (IDDM), and
(2) Type 2 diabetes mellitus or non-insulin dependent diabetes mellitus (NIDDM).

A number of other conditions are associated with diabetes mellitus, i.e.

- gestational diabetes
- maturity onset diabetes of the young (MODY)
- pancreatic disease
- endocrinopathies
- chemical-induced
- infection-related
- immune-mediated forms
- genetic syndromes

Of these the most important related to children and exercise and sport is Type 1 diabetes mellitus. The impact of other types in childhood is negligible.

The aetiology of Type 1 diabetes mellitus

Type 1 diabetes mellitus is associated with deficient insulin secretion. The beta cells of the pancreas are largely destroyed. Insulin secretory responses to standard glucose tolerance tests are markedly reduced or absent. C-peptide responses are used instead of insulin to check beta cell capacity when the diabetic is already receiving exogenous insulin. Type lA diabetes mellitus refers to immune-mediated diabetes mellitus which results in destruction of the beta cells of the pancreas, and features anti-islet autoantibodies.[2] Genetic factors are involved. The risk for type 1 diabetes mellitus in first degree relatives of patients is about 15-fold higher than the disease prevalence of about 0.004 in Caucasian populations. The HLA (human leukocyte antigen) region, also known as the human major histocompatibility complex (MHC), influences type 1 diabetes mellitus susceptibility.[3]

Type 1 diabetes mellitus is also associated with other autoimmune disorders. This includes coeliac disease, Addison's disease, thyroid disease and atrophic gastritis. Environmental influences are incriminated in the aetiology of type 1 diabetes mellitus. A study showed correlation between the decline in breast feeding and an increased incidence of diabetes mellitus suggesting milk proteins may be involved.[4] There have been substantial studies on the relationship of viral illnesses to Type 1 diabetes mellitus, but conclusive evidence has not yet been found.

The incidence of Type 1 diabetes mellitus

Type 1 diabetes mellitus is one of the commonest chronic diseases of childhood with prevalence rates for US Caucasians of approximately 3 per 1000. Incidence figures appear to be rising in a number of countries around the World. In a study from N. Ireland a standardized rate of 19.6 per 1 000 000 persons of diabetes mellitus was obtained for children under the age of 15 years.[5] Interestingly, these authors found the incidence to be lower in socially deprived areas with overcrowding.

The clinical spectrum of Type 1 diabetes mellitus

The presentation

The presentation is usually abrupt with a short preceding illness. The patient feels tired, loses weight and has a dramatic thirst and polyuria. This may lead to a critical illness with diabetic ketoacidosis. Patients suffering from diabetic ketoacidosis may be drowsy, even comatose, are markedly dehydrated and have a severe metabolic acidosis due to the accumulation of ketone bodies because of insulin lack. The condition is a grave emergency and necessitates hospital admission. The diagnosis is made by finding an elevated blood glucose and a biochemical profile of metabolic acidosis. Treatment consists of rehydration and insulin administration.

The management of Type 1 diabetes mellitus

The aims

The main aim is to render as normal a lifestyle as possible to the diabetic, although certain differences are inevitable. The main differences are that the patient must receive insulin by injection and there must be attention given to dietary factors.

The young person with diabetes also faces a number of hurdles mainly in the form of complications. Complications can be divided into acute and chronic. The acute complications include hypoglycaemia and diabetic ketoacidosis. The chronic complications are the triopathy of retinopathy, nephropathy and neuropathy. Although the chronic complications may not affect the young person with diabetes, nevertheless the control of the diabetes during this time may have impact on the development of such complications in later life. The Diabetes Control and Complications Trial (DCCT)[6] established criteria to be achieved which will lead to the prevention, at least in part, of the triopathy of complications. In an excellently controlled study, the research group concluded that intensive therapy effectively delays the onset and slows the progression of diabetic retinopathy, nephropathy and neuropathy. Intensive therapy included delivery of insulin by an external pump or three or more daily insulin injections. This resulted in maintaining blood glucose concentrations close to the normal range in addition to glycosylated haemoglobin. The major side-effect was a two- to three-fold increase in severe hypoglycaemia. In a thoughtful article, Watkins[7] considers the advantages and disadvantages of conclusions of DCCT. The price of achieving excellent control will almost certainly result in more frequent insulin injections and a greater risk of hypoglycaemia. The choice for the patient and the physician is a difficult one, especially in the case of a child with diabetes. Such intensive regimes are even more daunting when the child is faced with exercise and sport. The major problems in the management of Type 1 diabetes is that no matter how intensive the regime, it is impossible to mimic the physiological state and the second-to-second control of blood glucose by the normal pancreas.

The main aims in the management of a child or teenager with diabetes are as follows:

Diet (a)   The diet should have sufficient calories balanced among protein, fat and carbohydrate to result in normal growth and body weight.

Diet (b)   The diet has to be regimented in that the patient must eat on a regular basis including snacking between meals, in order to prevent hypoglycaemia.

The insulin regime should be such that it achieves the goals of DCCT within the tolerance of the young person and/or the parents.

The practical aspects

To achieve such aims requires a considerable amount of education of the young patient and the parents. What can be achieved will be dependent on the age of the patient, and the younger the patient the more management will fall on the parents. The patient should be taught the core concepts of diabetes mellitus, the self-monitoring of blood glucose levels and their interpretation, and the practicalities of self-injection of insulin. The patient should fully understand the warning symptoms of hypoglycaemia, how to prevent this, and how to take action should symptoms occur. Hypoglycaemia will be covered more extensively when exercise and sport are considered. The patient (and parents) should also be aware of possible situations which may lead to ketoacidosis, and know what regimes to employ when the patient becomes ill for other reasons (most often an infective illness).

The psychological aspects of diabetes are not to be ignored. The impact of diabetes can lead to emotional reactions including anger, grief, depression, anxiety and denial.[8]

The adolescent with diabetes presents special problems. The secretion of sex hormones and an increased secretion of growth hormone in a pulsatile fashion leads to growth spurts and the development of secondary sex characteristics. The impact of new social interests will lead to changes in lifestyle, and feelings of independence sometimes amounting to rebelliousness. Eating disorders may occur at this age.[9] This will result in increased dosage of insulin, but may also lead to deterioration in control due to all the quoted factors. So-called 'brittle diabetes' is common at this age group, where the diabetic experiences wild swings in blood sugar with frequent hypoglycaemic attacks and ketoacidosis. The period of adolescence with all its physiological and psychological changes may be responsible, although behavioural disturbances are often behind the 'brittleness'.[10]

The insulin regime in childhood diabetes offers two major choices. In the younger child, a two dose insulin regime is common. This will usually consist of a mixture of soluble insulin and intermediate acting insulin before breakfast, and this is repeated in the evening prior to the main evening meal. This is conveniently given in cartridges by the pen system in a 'pre-mix' of insulin, where the ratio of the soluble and intermediate insulin can be varied. Parents and patient will be instructed to vary the dose dependent on a number of factors including the prevailing blood glucose, and other factors such as intercurrent illness, exercise etc. The alternative regime is to administer three soluble injections prior to meals and an intermediate acting insulin injection usually around supper time. Again this can be given conveniently in a cartridge and pen system. This might not offer better control but more mimics the physiological situation. It also confers greater flexibility and is very suited to a busy adolescent especially one involved in sport.

Hypoglycaemia

As this is a significant problem in the exercising diabetic, it will be covered in more detail. It is also the most feared acute complication in the insulin dependent diabetic creating havoc with lifestyle. As previously stated insulin injections, no matter how sophisticated the regime, cannot mimic the physiological state. If the blood glucose runs high to avoid hypoglycaemia, then the feared chronic complications are an ever-present worry.

In the normal subject hypoglycaemia (blood glucose $<2.5\,mmol$ $litre^{-1}$) is prevented by inhibition of insulin secretion, secretion of counter regulatory hormones, in particular adrenaline and glucagon, and by neural influences.[11]

The main symptoms of hypoglycaemia are a combination of the effects on the brain and catecholamines. Palpitations (tachycardia), sweating, hunger and shaking are early warning symptoms. In mild hypoglycaemia, double vision, difficulty in concentration and slurring of the speech occur. In moderate cases, there is confusion and behavioural changes. In severe cases, the patient can become unconscious with fits and neurological deficits such as hemiplegia.[12] The major precipitating factors are insufficient carbohydrate at meals, delayed meals, over dosage with insulin and exercise, especially severe.

There are other problems the diabetic has to contend with. Loss of awareness of hypoglycaemia is a worrying development, probably due to loss of neurohumoral responses to hypoglycaemia in the diabetic.[13] There is, however, evidence that hypoglycaemic awareness can be restored by scrupulous hypoglycaemic avoidance.[14]

Transferring patients from animal insulin to human insulin can result in increased attacks of hypoglycaemia. Patients transferring should take less insulin (approximately 30%) to avoid hypoglycaemia, but animal insulins should be continued if the patient prefers it.[15] Hypoglycaemic avoidance is covered by Amiel.[16] Preventative actions include frequent snacking, and reduced bedtime intermediate insulin after vigorous or sustained exercise on the evening after. Excess alcohol should be avoided. Both patient and doctor should be educated.

Exercise

The normal subject

In order to understand the problems facing the insulin dependent diabetic a knowledge of glucose homeostasis during exercise in the normal subject is required. During exercise insulin falls and the counter regulatory hormones glucagon and catecholamines rise. The glucagon: insulin molar ratio appears critical to glucose output from the liver, and a very small amount of insulin is all that is necessary to control glucose uptake.[17] Carbohydrate is stored as glycogen in muscle and liver, and fatty acids are stored, mainly as triglycerides, in adipose tissue. Protein may also be used as a fuel but to a lesser extent.[18] Exercise in the normal subject is usually accompanied by eugly-caemia.[19] Therefore, in exercising man the glucose output from the liver matches the glucose uptake by muscle.

At relatively low energy levels, up to 50% $\dot{V}O_2$ max, fat is the main source of fuel. However, as exercise intensity increases carbohydrate becomes the main source of fuel. Depletion of carbohydrate stores in muscle are the main causes of fatigue in athletes. The liver has only 2–3 hours of storage glycogen to meet the needs of a person exercising at high intensity.[20] Feeding on a high carbohydrate diet (70% of energy intake as carbohydrate) enabled runners who were training for 2 hours per day to maintain muscle glycogen levels.[21] A dietary carbohydrate intake of 500–600 g may be necessary to ensure adequate glycogen resynthesis.[22]

The conclusion must be that in athletes who are competing in prolonged events at a high energy level, increased dietary intake of carbohydrate is essential. The athlete who is also training frequently and for prolonged times must ensure that sufficient carbohydrate is ingested between training times to ensure adequate stores of glycogen in muscle and liver, otherwise fatigue will result.

Carbohydrate feeding during prolonged exercise has been shown to enhance performance.[23] This probably works to spare muscle glycogen thus delaying fatigue.[24] Alternatively, it may improve performance by maintaining blood glucose at a critical point in endurance exercise, when liver and glycogen levels are low and the uptake of glucose by skeletal muscle is increased.[25]

Physical training enhances insulin-stimulated glucose disposal in proportion to the improvement in physical fitness.[26] This appears to be mediated through increases in blood flow, muscle glucose transport protein (Glut-4 concentration) and glycogen synthase activity.[27] The increased insulin sensitivity is seen in aerobic events but not in subjects in anaerobic events.[28]

Exercise can influence intestinal absorption of fluids and glucose. Gastric emptying may be affected by exercise, the process being inhibited.[29] In post-absorptive humans, splanchnic blood flow decreases during supine[30] and upright exercise.[31] Hypoxia to mucosal cells affects sugar absorption, leading to the conclusion that intense exercise will also have this effect due to diminished blood flow.[32]

The diabetic subject

The insulin dependent diabetic must therefore face exercise with disordered or indeed absent insulin secretion, and possibly with other problems relating to complications including disordered autonomic function.

Exercise may be divided into two categories:

1. Random and recreational exercise. This will certainly be the category the young child with diabetes will inevitably be involved in. This will include the normal activity of the young child but on occasion will involve somewhat more extensive exercise, e.g. an outing, a sports day etc.

2. Sport and training. Children from about eight years old begin to become involved in organized sport such as running, gymnastics, football, hockey, swimming etc. This will include some training but usually not involving more than 2–3 hours per week.

When the subject reaches 11 or 12 years, training will increase and intensify and will continue into adolescence and teenage years.

Philosophy of involvement of diabetics in sport

It may be argued that because of potential risks, children and teenagers with diabetes should not be involved in sport. Certainly life without sport and training will be a more sedate and less complicated existence.

Michael Hall, Chairman of the Board of Trustees, British Diabetic Association, writes[33] that diabetics should not be sheltered from the normal activities of mankind, and should be able to undertake a full range of sporting activities. He quotes outstanding athletes in many sports who are diabetic and reach the highest levels. He finds it regrettable that some sports bodies treat diabetics as disabled, and that they have been refused entry to some events. There is an International Diabetes Athletes' Association which caters for diabetics in sport.

Safety, however, must be the watchword, and a complete understanding by the patient as to how to control his/her diabetes is essential. Most sports have safety standards so that training is supervised and it is vital that a coach or attendant is informed that the athlete is a diabetic.

The effect of exercise in diabetes

Regular exercise will improve the health of the insulin dependent diabetic in the following ways:

- Increased cardiorespiratory fitness
- Increased insulin sensitivity
- Maintenance of ideal body weight
- Reduction in serum lipids
- Improvement in hypertension
- Improved quality of life

However, diabetics will respond to exercise differently from normal subjects, particularly with respect to glucose homeostasis. The key problem is that the insulin-dependent diabetic does not have the normal insulin response to exercise. As previously stated plasma insulin levels fall to low levels in normal subjects during exercise. The diabetic has a very significant problem in mimicking this, and indeed injected insulin often rises in the blood during exercise in the diabetic.[34] This is caused by more rapid absorption of the injected insulin particularly if the insulin is injected into the exercising part of the body.[35] This rapid absorption is more marked when the insulin is given shortly before the exercise, than if given 60–90 mins before the exercise.

The inappropriately elevated insulin levels during exercise will have undesirable effects by inhibiting hepatic glucose output and by enhancing peripheral glucose uptake and stimulating glucose oxidation by exercising muscle.[36] Gluconeogenesis is also inhibited. Counter-regulatory responses, such as glucagon, can be deficient in the diabetic. These changes inevitably lead to hypoglycaemia during exercise.

Post-exercise hypoglycaemia can also be encountered up to several hours after exercise and even the following day.[37] This is probably due to increased glucose uptake and glycogen synthesis in the previously exercised muscle groups.

Should exercise be undertaken during a state of severe insulin deficiency exercise induced ketoacidosis can occur. During exercise under such circumstances, peripheral glucose utilization is impaired, hepatic glucose output enhanced as is lipolysis.[38]

The type of exercise will make differences. Low to moderate intensity exercise especially for longish spells increases the risk of hypoglycaemia.[39] In very high intensity exercise (>85% $\dot{V}O_2$ max), blood glucose levels rise. Therefore hypoglycaemia will be encountered in aerobic exercise especially if prolonged.

The insulin dependent diabetic may also have gastrointestinal motor dysfunction. This can include gastric motor dysfunction, known as gastroparesis, with significant delay in stomach emptying.[40] This can result in delay of emptying of meals and enhancing the possibility of hypoglycaemia during exercise.

Practical considerations for the exercising diabetic

An exact prescription for the exercising young diabetic cannot be made. However, if major precautions and preparations are taken, then the acute problems of severe hypoglycaemia can be largely prevented. Probably the childhood diabetic athlete who undertakes regular training and competition is more likely to be well educated in actions than the child who undertakes occasional and variable exercise, and will, therefore, be safer. There is extensive literature in this field.[41–46] In addition there are publications which specifically cover the diabetic child athlete.[47–51] The author will attempt to summarize the points made in these articles introducing discussion as required.

Pre-exercise assessment

Education of the patient and, if very young, the parents is essential. No young diabetic should embark on sport and exercise without having substantial awareness of the problems and how to overcome these problems. This can be appropriately undertaken by a doctor experienced in diabetes management, a specialist diabetic nurse, a dietitian and possibly also an exercise physiologist who can advise on the energy requirements of the type of exercise.

The patient should have the following training:

(1) self-monitoring of blood glucose levels;
(2) monitoring of ketone levels in urine;
(3) knowledge of dietary factors; and

(4) awareness of the symptoms of hypoglycaemia, methods of prevention and how to treat it.

The patient should preferably be receiving the pen injection system of three or four soluble insulin injections per day and one longer acting bolus injection. Although possibly not introducing better control, the flexibility afforded is a major advantage.

Should the child be undertaking regular physical training for a sport, the club, coach or teacher must be informed. Often a doctor may be involved in this sport.[52] The diabetic should wear identity indicating that he/she is a diabetic. Those supervising the training should be aware of the symptoms of hypoglycaemia and the treatment required.

It is generally recommended that the patient should have a full medical assessment prior to undertaking exercise, in order to identify complicating factors such as vascular disease, microangiopathy, nephropathy and neuropathy. Significant disease may preclude some sports, or require a modified approach to exercise. It is, however, unlikely that a young diabetic will have such significant disease. The so-called 'brittle' diabetic, or someone with psychological problems should be cautious about involvement in highly demanding sports.

Prior to the exercise

The type of exercise should be assessed. This may be regularly recurring, for example, training 1–2 hours of swimming, football, athletics etc. The diabetic may, therefore, have a standard regime. Alternatively, the exercise may be unusual, e.g. a sports day with several intermittent events. If the exercise is prolonged and aerobic, there is probably greater danger of hypoglycaemia than if the exercise is short and anaerobic.

The patient should already be well and repleted in carbohydrate stores. A meal should be taken 1–3 hours before the exercise. The meal should have a large carbohydrate component with mainly complex 'slowly absorbable' carbohydrates.

Short acting insulin should preferably be used. The dose should be taken prior to a meal and a reduction in dosage is essential. This reduction varies by 30–50%, but will depend on the type of exercise, and the previous experience of the patient concerning insulin dosage. The insulin should not be injected into an exercising extremity, thus an abdominal site is usually preferable. This will prevent rapid absorption of insulin.

Metabolic control should be assessed. If the blood glucose is <5 mmol litre^{-1} extra calories prior to exercise will be required. If blood glucose is >15 mmol litre^{-1}, measure urinary ketones, and if positive, take more insulin, and delay exercise until blood glucose is satisfactory and urinary ketones are negative.

During exercise

If the exercise is prolonged, then further monitoring of blood glucose may be required. This will obviously be awkward and will lose time in a prolonged marathon type event, but in a training situation should be possible. Again, if the exercise is prolonged >30 minutes, supplemental rapidly absorbable carbohydrate (15–40 g) should be taken every 30 minutes. This can be made up in drinks, as fluid replacement is also essential. Should the subject experience symptoms of hypoglycaemia he/she should inform someone else, and take rapidly absorbable carbohydrate. Exercise can then be continued when the subject has recovered. Should severe hypoglycaemia occur and if oral administration is impossible, then intravenous glucose and/or intramuscular 1 mg glucagon will be required.

After exercise

The main problem is delayed hypoglycaemia and a reduction in insulin dosage may be required, and possibly increased calorie intake for 12–14 hours after the activity.

Other points

It should be emphasized that exact prescriptions are impossible. Campaigne et al.[53] concluded that general recommendations on how to adjust insulin or diet before exercise are difficult to give. Individualized recommendations for treatment modification appear most appropriate.

Short acting insulin analogues

Tuominen et al.[54] found that a short acting insulin analogue [Lys (B28) Pro (B29)] peaked earlier than human insulin and post-prandial blood glucose was lower. Exercise induced hypoglycaemia was also 2.2-fold greater during early exercise, but less by 46% during late exercise. They concluded that as exercise is usually not performed until 2–3 h after a meal, short acting insulin analogues may be more feasible than soluble human insulin.

References

1. World Health Organisation Study Group. *Diabetic mellitus*. WHO Technical Report Series 1985; **727**: 1–104.
2. Atkinson, M. A. and Maclaren, N. K. The pathogenesis of insulin-dependent diabetes mellitus. *New England Journal of Medicine* 1994; **331**: 1428–36.
3. Erlich, H. A., Zeidler, A., Chang, J., Shaw, S., Raffel, L. J., Klitz, W., Beshkov, Y., Costing, G., Pressman, S. and Bugawan, T. HLA class II alleles and susceptibility and resistance to insulin dependant diabetes mellitus in Mexican-American families. *Nature Genetics* 1993; **3**: 358–64.
4. Martin, J. M., Trink, B., Daneman, D., Dosch, H. M. and Robinson, B. Milk proteins in the aetiology of insulin-dependant diabetes mellitus (IDDM). *Annals of Medicine* 1991; **23**: 447–52.
5. Patterson, C. C., Carson, D. J. and Hadden, D. R. Epidemiology of childhood IDDM in Northern Ireland 1989–1994: Low incidence in areas with highest population density and most household crowding. *Diabetologia* 1996; **39**: 1063–9.
6. Diabetes Control and Complications Trial Research Group. The effect of intensive treatment on the development and progression of long-term complications in insulin dependent diabetes mellitus. *New England Journal of Medicine* 1993; **329**: 977–86.
7. Watkins, P. J. DCCT: The ecstasy and the agony. *Quarterly Journal of Medicine* 1994; **87**: 315–6.
8. Bradley, C. (ed). *Handbook of psychology and diabetes: A guide to psychological management measurement in diabetes research and practice.* Harwood Academic Press, Chur, Switzerland, 1994.
9. Steel, J. M., Young, R. J., Lloyd, G. G. and Macintyre, C. C. Abnormal eating attitudes in young insulin-dependant diabetics. *British Journal of Psychiatry* 1989; **155**: 515–21.
10. Thompson, C. J., Cummings, F., Chalmers, J. and Newtown, R. W. Abnormal insulin treatment behaviour: a major cause of ketoacidosis in young adults with type 1 diabetes. *Diabetic Medicine* 1986; **12**: 429–32.
11. Frier, B. M. Hypoglycaemia and diabetes. *Diabetic Medicine* 1986; **3**: 513–25.
12. Watkins, P. J. ABC of diabetes. *British Medical Journal* 1982; **285**: 278–9.
13. Ryder, R. J., Owens, D. R., Hayes, H. M., Ghatei, M. A. and Bloom, S. R. Unawareness of hypoglycaemia and inadequate hypoglycaemic counter-regulation. *British Medical Journal* 1980; **301**: 783–7.
14. Cranston, I., Lomas, J., Maran, A., Macdonald, I. and Amiel, S. A. Restoration of hypoglycaemia awareness in patients with long-duration insulin-dependent diabetes. *Lancet* 1994; **344**: 287–7.
15. Transferring diabetic patients to human insulin. *Lancet Editorial* 1989; 762–3.
16. Amiel, S. A. Hypoglycaemic avoidance—technology and knowledge. *Lancet* 1998: **352**: 502–3.
17. Wasserman, O. H. and Vranic, M. Interaction between insulin and counter regulation hormones in control of substance utilisation in health and diabetes during exercise. *Diabetes and Metabolism Reviews* 1986; **1**: 359–84.
18. Cahill, G. F. Starvation in man. *New England Journal of Medicine* 1970; **282**: 668–75.
19. Dill, D. B., Edwards, H. T. and Mead, S. Blood sugar regulation in exercise. *American Journal of Physiology* 1935; **111**: 21–30.
20. Maughan, R. J. Nutritional aspects of endurance exercise in humans. *Proceedings of the Nutrition Society* 1994; **53**: 181–8.
21. Costill, D. L. Carbohydrate for exercise: dietary demands for optimal performance. *International Journal of Sports Medicine* 1988; **9**: 1–18.
22. Coyle, E. Timing and method of increased carbohydrate intake to cope with heavy training, competition and recovery. *Journal of Sports Science* 1991; **9**: 29–52.
23. Wilker, R. L. and Moffatt, R. J. Influence of carbohydrate ingestion on blood glucose and performance in runners. *International Journal of Sport Nutrition* 1992; **2**: 317–27.
24. Hargreaves, M., Costill, D. L., Coggan, A., Fink, W. J. and Nishibata, I. Effect of carbohydrate feeding on muscle glycogen utilisation and exercise performance. *Medicine and Science in Sports and Exercise* 1984; **16**: 219–22.
25. Coyle, E. F., Hagberg, J. M., Hurley, B. F., Martin, W. H., Ehsani, A. A. and Holloszy, J. O. Carbohydrate feeding during prolonged strenuous exercise can delay fatigue. *Journal of Applied Physiology* 1983; **55**: 230–5.
26. Soman, V. R., Koivisto, V. A., Deibert, D., Felig, P., and DeFronzo, R.A. Increased insulin sensitivity and insulin binding to monocytes after physical training. *New England Journal of Medicine* 1979; **301**: 1200–4.
27. Ebeling, P., Bourey, R., Koranyi, L., Touminen, J. A., Groop, L.C. Henriksson, J., Mueckler, M., Sovijarvi, A. and Koivisto, V. A. Mechanisms of enhanced insulin sensitivity in athletes. Increased blood flow, muscle glucose transport protein (GLUT-4) concentration, and glycogen synthase activity. *Journal of Clinical Investigation* 1993; **92**: 1623–31.
28. Yki-Järvihen, H. and Koivisto, V. A. Effect of body composition on insulin sensitivity. *Diabetes* 1983; **32**: 965–9.
29. Costill, D. L. and Saltin, B. Factors limiting gastric emptying during rest and exercise. *Journal of Applied Physiology* 1974; **37**: 679–83.
30. Wade, O. L., Combes, B., Childs, A. W., Wheeler, H. O., Cournand, A. and Bradley, S. E. Effects of exercise on the splanchnic blood flow and splanchnic blood volume in normal man. *Clinical Science* 1956; **15**: 457–63.
31. Rowell, L. B., Blackmon, J. R. and Bruce, R. A. Indocyanine green clearance and estimated hepatic blood flow during mild to maximum exercise in upright man. *Journal of Clinical Investigation* 1964; **43**: 1677–90.
32. Darlington, W. and Quastel, J. Absorption of sugars from isolated surviving intestine. *Archives of Biochemistry* 1953; **43**: 194–207.
33. Hall, M. Sport and diabetes. *British Journal of Sports Medicine* 1997; **3**: 3.
34. Berger, M., Halban, Pa., Assal, J. P., Offord, R. E., Vranic, M. and Renold, A.E. Pharmacokinetics of subcutaneously injected titiated insulin: effects of exercise. *Diabetes* 1979; **28** 53–7.
35. Koivisto, V. and Felig, P. Effect of leg exercise on insulin absorption in diabetic patients. *New England Journal of Medicine* 1978; **298**: 77–8.
36. Zinman, B., Murray, F. T., Vranic, M., Albisser, A. M., Leibel, B. S., McClean, P. A. and Marliss, E. B. Glucoregulation during moderate exercise in insulin-treated diabetes. *Journal of Clinical Endocrinology and Metabolism* 1977; **45**: 641–52.

37. **McDonald, M. J.** Post exercise late-onset hypoglycaemia in insulin-dependent diabetic patients. *Diabetes Care* 1987; **10**: 584–8.

38. **Horton, E. S.** Exercise and diabetes mellitus. *Medical Clinics of North America* 1988; **72**: 1301–21.

39. **Ruegemer, J. J., Squires, R. W., Marsh, H. M., Haymond, M. W., Cryer, P. E., Rizza, R. A.** and **Miles, J. M.** Difference between prebreakfast and late afternoon glycaemic responses to exercise in IDDM patients. *Diabetes Care* 1990; **13**: 104–10.

40. **Horowitz, M.** and **Dent, J.** Disordered gastric emptying: mechanical basis, assessment and treatment. *Baillere's Clinical Gastroenterology* 1991; **5**: 371–407.

41. **Tsuei, E. Y. L.** and **Zinman, B.** Exercise and diabetes—new insights and therapeutic goals. *The Endocrinologist* 1995; **5**: 263–71.

42. **Choi, K. I.** and **Chisholm, D. J.** Exercise and insulin-dependent diabetes mellitus (IDDM): benefits and pitfalls. *Australian and New Zealand Journal of Medicine* 1996; **26**: 827–33.

43. **Landry, G. L.** and **Allen, D. B.** Diabetes mellitus and exercise. *Clinics in Sports Medicine* 1992; **11**: 403–17.

44. **Horton, E. S.** Exercise and diabetes mellitus. *Medical Clinics of North America* 1998; **72**: 1301–21.

45. **Fahey, P. J., Stallkamp, E. T.** and **Kwartra, S.** The athlete with Type 1 diabetes: managing insulin, diet and exercise. *American Family Physician* 1996; **55**: 1611–22.

46. **American College of Sports Medicine** and **American Diabetes Association** Joint Position Statement. Diabetes mellitus and exercise. *Medicine and Science in Sports and Exercise* 1996; **28**: 1675–80.

47. **Byrne, G.** Children, diabetes and sport—yes, they do mix. *Aussie Sport Action (Canberra, Aust)* 1993; **4**: 10–11.

48. **Bar-Or, O.** Effects of training on the child with a chronic disease: Beauty and the beast? (Editorial) *Clinical Journal of Sport Medicine* 1993; **3**: 2–5.

49. **Lording, D.** The diabetic athlete today. *Sports Training, Medicine and Rehabilitation* 1991; **2**: 197–201.

50. **Dorchy, H.** and **Poortmans, J.** Sport and the diabetic child. *Sports Medicine* 1989; **7**: 246–62.

51. **Horton, E. S.** Exercise and diabetes in youth. In *Youth, exercise and sport* (ed. C. V. Gisolfi and D. R. Lamb). Benchmark, Indianapolis Ind., 1980: 539–74.

52. **Jimenez, C. C.** Diabetes and exercise: the role of the athletic trainer. *Journal of Athletic Training* 1997; **32**: 339–43.

53. **Campaigne, B. N., Wallberg-Henriksson, H.** and **Gunnarsson, R.** Glucose and insulin responses in relation to insulin dose and calorie intake 12 h after acute physical exercise in men with IDDM. *Diabetes Care* 1987; **10**: 716–21.

54. **Tuominen, J. A., Karonen, S. L., Melamies, L., Bolli, G.** and **Koivisto, V. A.** Exercise-induced hypoglycaemia in IDDM patients treated with a short acting insulin analogue. *Diabetologia* 1995; **38**: 106–11.

4.7 Young athletes with a physical or mental disability

Merrilee Zetaruk

Introduction

Children with disabilities, whether mental or physical, have a right to the same respect and dignity afforded to able-bodied children. Although sports participation may present more of a challenge for many with disabilities, the rewards of such activities are immeasurable. The physical and psychological benefits can have a lasting effect throughout the life of the child. Physical benefits include decreased obesity, lower lifetime risk of cardiovascular disease, improved physical skills, improved functional ability, maintenance or improvement in range of motion of joints and increased independence.[1-4] Those with physical disabilities may have a low self-esteem,[5] and children with mental disabilities often are affected more by social stigma than by their own limitations. Through sports, these children develop confidence in themselves and learn important social skills as they work together with their peers. At the same time, able-bodied children observe that despite an apparent 'handicap', disabled children can excel in many sports. They learn that it is ability rather than disability which makes each child unique.

Deaf athletes became involved in organized sports in the United States in the 1870s when the Ohio School for the Deaf began to offer baseball for its students.[6] Soon after, football and basketball were introduced in a number of schools for the deaf. Because there were no neuromuscular deficits in this population, deaf athletes often played against hearing athletes. Today, we see many deaf athletes who are successful in both the deaf and hearing worlds of sport.

Despite the early progress made in deaf sports, it was not until the Second World War that it was recognized that children and adults with visible disabilities, such as amputations, spinal cord injuries or cerebral palsy, could benefit from sports participation. The first wheelchair sports began at the Stoke Mandeville Hospital in England. Since that time, national and international organizations representing a variety of disabled athletes have flourished and international, elite level competitions have been established. Today, spectators watch in awe as these athletes reach new heights, at times rivalling their able-bodied counterparts.

Many disabled athletes have demonstrated great achievements beyond the competitive field. Two athletes who deserve special mention are Terry Fox and Rick Hansen. Terry Fox lost his right leg to cancer in 1977. Three years later, with the aid of a lower limb prosthesis, he began a run across Canada to raise money for cancer research. Although his journey was terminated early due to a recurrence of the disease, he was able to raise $24 million for his cause. He received the prestigious Order of Canada award in 1980, one year before his death. Rick Hansen became paraplegic following a motor vehicle accident in 1973. In order to raise money and awareness about spinal cord injuries, this elite athlete began a world tour which took him to 34 different countries over a two-year period. He completed over 40 000 km by wheelchair and raised millions of dollars for spinal cord research. These men have served not only as role models for young athletes with disabilities, but have become national heroes.

Athletes with sensory impairments

The deaf athlete

Permanent, moderate to severe bilateral sensorineural hearing loss affects 0.5–1/1000 live births. Such hearing loss can also occur at any time during childhood, resulting in a prevalence of 1.5–2/1000 children under 6 years of age.[7] Speech and language development can be impaired by hearing loss at a very young age, as can social and emotional development, behaviour, attention and academic achievement.[7] Sports participation for children, regardless of the status of their hearing, helps foster a healthy, active lifestyle and promotes positive attitudes toward competition and fair play.[8] There is also an opportunity for social development and increased confidence through sports participation.

Hearing loss does not predispose the young athlete to any specific patterns of injury. Coexisting dysfunction of the vestibular apparatus affects equilibrium; therefore, sports which require balance are more challenging. Activities which require climbing to heights, jumping on a trampoline or diving into a pool should only be permitted if adequate safeguards are in place to prevent injury if the athlete loses balance and falls. Tumbling activities which require rotation should be attempted only if close supervision and spotting is available.[9] In the absence of concomitant vestibular dysfunction, the performance of deaf athletes compares favourably with that of able-bodied athletes since their muscle function, strength, sensation and coordination do not differ significantly.[10] The greatest problem for the hard-of-hearing or deaf athlete is communication with other athletes, making participation in team sports more difficult.[11] Deaf children often participate in sports with hearing athletes but are unable to hear verbal instructions or auditory cues from coaches and other athletes. Hearing aids may be helpful for some children. Coexisting speech impairments make communication even more difficult; however, many deaf athletes facilitate communication through sign language, lip reading and other methods of visual cueing.[12] These skills, along with maximizing powers of observation and peripheral vision, allow athletes with hearing losses to participate in almost any sport; however, individual activities which require minimal communication (e.g. running or skiing) allow for the greatest success.

The World Games for the Deaf take place every four years. Winter events include Alpine and Nordic skiing, ice hockey and speed skating. Summer events include badminton, basketball, cycling, men's wrestling, shooting, soccer, swimming, table tennis, team handball, tennis, track and field, volleyball and water polo. The rules are essentially the same as those used in hearing competitions, with minor modifications such as visual cues to replace or supplement auditory cues.

The blind athlete

Visual impairment in children presents a challenge for sports participation. Approximately three in every thousand people are blind; as a result, a number of programmes have been developed in order to allow blind athletes to participate in various sports. According to the International Blind Sports Association (IBSA), any person with less than 10% of useful vision is eligible to compete as a blind athlete. The IBSA uses the following classification of athletes, based on testing of the better, corrected eye:[12]

1. B1: No light perception or light perception with inability to recognize the shape of a hand at any distance or in any direction.
2. B2: Ability to recognize the shape of a hand, up to a visual acuity of 2/60 and/or a field of vision less than 5 degrees.
3. B3: Visual acuity greater than 2/60 up to 6/60 and/or a field of vision greater than 5 degrees but less than 20 degrees.

Although visual impairment itself does not affect neuromuscular function, a fear of falling or colliding with objects results in a different pattern of movement than is observed in sighted children. Blind children have a stiffer posture, shorter stride, slower pace and a shuffling gait. There is often hyperlordosis with a protruding abdomen.[13] Because of their restricted free movement in space, without early intervention through physical activity, blind children are apt to lead a sedentary lifestyle. Sedentary children become sedentary adults; therefore, it is important to encourage physical activity in all children, especially those with visual impairments.

There are many aspects of sports participation that are of particular benefit to visually impaired children. Physical activity helps develop a sense of orientation in space and improved mobility through enhancement of sense of touch, proprioception, balance, posture and body control.[9,13] Early physical activity enhances coordinated associated movements of the hands. Sports participation also provides psychosocial benefits such as increased self-confidence, improved social skills and a competitive spirit.[13]

Auditory and tactile cues can be substituted for visual cues in a number of sports, thereby facilitating participation of blind athletes. Through voice and touch, a guide can communicate with blind athletes to teach downhill skiing. The ski bra, invented in 1974, can be used initially to help with balance. This is a rigid device which keeps the ski tips about 7.5–10 cm apart, preventing crossing of the skis. Blind skiers, instructors and guides wear a distinctive jacket or bib to allow easy identification by sighted skiers on the slopes.[14]

In addition to skiing, blind athletes compete in many different types of sports that athletes without visual impairment participate in, including competitive swimming, skating, baseball, track and field, and judo. Goal ball is a game uniquely designed for blind athletes. The ball has a bell inside it, allowing athletes to identify the trajectory of the ball and prevent it from crossing their goal line or entering the net. Like hearing loss, visual impairment alone does not affect the general fitness of individuals;[13] therefore, with modifications of rules and equipment, children with visual impairment can not only become physically active, but can attain a high level of performance in many sports.

Wheelchair athletes

Athletes who have a disability which impairs their mobility and necessitates the use of a wheelchair for sports participation may compete in wheelchair sports. Most commonly, wheelchair sports include athletes with cerebral palsy, myelomeningocoeles, spinal cord injuries or lower-extremity amputations. Not all athletes with these conditions require wheelchairs; therefore, this section will include discussion of a range of disabilities from ambulatory to wheelchair athletes.

The athlete with cerebral palsy

Cerebral palsy (CP) is a non-progressive disorder of posture and movement resulting from a defect or lesion of the developing brain. CP affects 4/1000 live births, with an estimated prevalence of 2/1000 in the general population.[15] Injuries to the cerebral cortex result in spasticity in one or more of the extremities, whereas injuries to the cerebellum or basal ganglia produce ataxia or athetosis, respectively. The most common patterns of spasticity as well as physiological parameters of exercise in CP are described below:

1. Monoplegia: one extremity, usually a lower extremity.
2. Hemiplegia: involvement of the extremities on one side of the body; associated seizure disorder in one-third of affected children and cognitive impairments in one-quarter.
3. Paraplegia: spasticity affects both lower extremities.
4. Diplegia: spasticity noted in all four extremities, with the upper extremities being involved to a much lesser extent; likely to have normal intellectual development with a low incidence of seizure disorders.
5. Triplegia: three extremities involved, with sparing of one upper extremity.
6. Quadriplegia: involvement of all four limbs; high rate of mental retardation and seizures.

Athetoid CP is the least common form of this disorder. It is characterized by hypotonia, athetoid movements and slurring of speech. Seizures and intellectual impairment are uncommon in this group.

There are a number of benefits to sports participation for the child with CP. A carefully designed and monitored programme of strength and flexibility training will improve flexibility, range of motion and strength in these children.[4] Early physical activity helps maximize compensatory mechanisms of the central nervous system in order to decrease abnormal patterns of movement or posture.[16] The psychological benefits of sports are equally important to the young athlete with CP. Many forms of CP are accompanied by intellectual impairments or emotional disorders which often cause social difficulties among peers. Children with CP experience greater self-esteem and confidence through sports participation.

Although risk factors for injury are not unique to the athlete with CP, many risk factors are magnified in this population. Richter *et al.*[17] found an injury rate of 60% among athletes with CP at the 1988

Paralympic Games in South Korea. Imbalances in strength between agonist and antagonist muscle groups are a risk factor for injury in children.[18] These imbalances are even greater in CP due to the predilection of spasticity to affect primarily agonist muscle groups. A good example of the effect of spasticity on muscle balance can be observed in the ankles. Spasticity of the gastrocnemius and soleus muscles results in tight heel cords and excessive plantar flexion of the foot.[21] Children with CP tend to be less active than their able-bodied peers, leaving them little opportunity to stretch their muscles on a regular basis.[11] Joint contractures occur frequently in this population, adding to imbalances about the joints.

Patellofemoral dysfunction occurs with increased frequency as growth and spasticity lead to tightening of the quadriceps and hamstring muscles. Gait disturbances predispose children with CP to joint malalignments.[20] The result is increased stress across the patellofemoral joint, which leads to overuse injuries of the extensor mechanism. Patellofemoral syndrome, while similar to that seen in able-bodied athletes, tends to be more severe in the CP population. In addition, there is increased risk of fragmentation of the distal patellar pole, such as is seen in Sinding–Larsen–Johansson syndrome. Athletes with this condition will present with pain and tenderness of the lower pole of the patella.

Spasticity not only causes an imbalance of muscles of the hip, but also can result in abnormal development of the hip joint itself. These abnormalities range from acetabular dysplasia and progressive arthritis to frank dislocation of the joint. These athletes present clinically with increasing hip pain associated with physical activity such as running. Marked adductor spasticity (scissor gait) contributes to the malalignments observed in the lower extremities.[11,16]

Athletes with athetoid CP exhibit slow, writhing, involuntary movements of the extremities, head and neck. Activities which require accuracy, such as kicking a soccer ball, may be difficult in the more severely affected children. Sports which require balance will pose the greatest challenge, and perhaps the greatest risk, to children with the ataxic or atonic forms of CP. Their unsteady gait and lack of coordination make basic skills such as running and jumping quite difficult, and may lead to injury from falls.

The diverse presentations and range of severity of CP have necessitated the development of classification systems for athletic competition. The Functional Classification System (FCS) used in the Paralympic Games assesses trunk control, gross motor control and strength of the extremities, as well as balance and fine motor control, with or without assistive devices.[12,21] Such a classification system is designed to permit more equitable competition among CP athletes with a wide range of disabilities. Athletes with CP compete in many different sports, including cycling, power lifting, shooting, track, archery, bowling, table-tennis, snooker, football, basketball, volleyball and swimming. The latter is a very good sport for children with CP, as swimming improves coordination and may relax spasticity.[16] Due to the high prevalence of epilepsy in CP, drowning is a real risk in this group; therefore, very close observation must be provided for all athletes with a seizure disorder. Regardless of the sport, children with CP can benefit from physical activity and experience success in the competitive arena.

Athletes with myelomeningoceles

Myelomeningocele is the most common congenital anomaly of the nervous system. It results from a failure of the neural tube to close and affects approximately 1/1000 live births. Three-quarters of myelomeningoceles occur in the lumbosacral region.[15] They produce motor and sensory deficits as well as impairments in bowel and bladder function. Lesions in the lower sacral region have sparing of motor function. Eighty per cent of affected children have an associated hydrocephalus which can affect cognitive function and can further impair motor function.

Children with myelomeningoceles are classified according to their functional level, which corresponds to the most caudal nerve root which is functioning. Lower lesions may simply require bracing of the foot and ankle to permit sports participation, while athletes with higher lesions may perform best in a wheelchair. Swimming is a popular sport for many athletes with myelomeningoceles since the upper extremities are often unaffected (Fig. 4.7.1). Sports participation depends not only on the functional level, but on the presence of mental retardation and degree of spasticity that result from associated hydrocephalus. These factors make this group of athletes extremely heterogeneous in abilities.

Skin, bone and muscle–tendon units are all at increased risk of injury in athletes with myelomeningoceles. The lack of sensation below the level of the lesion leads to bruising, pressure sores and skin breakdown from braces or wheelchair seats. The risk of skin breakdown can be minimized by teaching children and their parents to inspect the skin regularly and to shift weight frequently. Children who

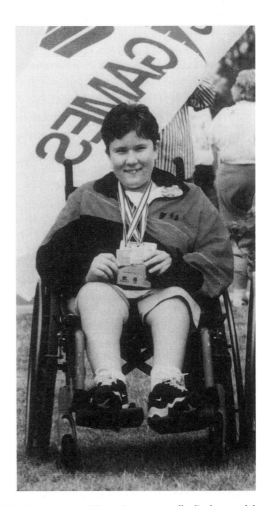

Fig. 4.7.1 Young competitive swimmer proudly displays medals.

use braces should ensure that they are correctly positioned after each fall to reduce the likelihood of skin irritation from the brace.

Limited weight-bearing results in osteopenia and increased risk of fractures. Fractures are particularly problematic in this group because of the sensory deficits which often result in delayed diagnosis. The incidence of fractures can be reduced by encouraging weight-bearing where possible and by limiting the period of immobilization following a fracture.

Soft-tissue injuries such as muscle strains occur with greater frequency in this population. This is due to muscle weaknesses just above the level of the lesion and muscle imbalances resulting from spasticity. These athletes frequently have joint contractures which can significantly limit their range of motion. Special emphasis should be placed on range of motion and flexibility in the affected limbs, particularly if joint contractures are present.

Athletes with spinal cord injuries

Between 13% and 15% of all spinal cord injuries occur in children.[11] Such injuries result in variable degrees of paralysis and sensory loss, along with dysfunction in other areas such as thermoregulation, circulation, and bowel and bladder control. The extent of the disability depends on the level of the spinal cord lesion and whether or not it is complete. Incomplete injuries allow some communication with areas distal to the injured cord. This results in some residual motor or sensory function below the level of the injury. Classification of spinal cord injury is based upon the lowest level of motor function;[21] however, the Functional Classification System used in the Paralympic Games categorizes athletes according to their functional abilities.[12]

There are many benefits associated with participation in wheelchair sports. These include an improvement in maximal oxygen uptake by an average of 20%, reduced risk of cardiovascular disease and respiratory infection, and improved self-image. Sedentary individuals with paraplegia are at a threefold increased risk of hospitalizations compared with paraplegic athletes.[22]

The most common injuries reported in young wheelchair athletes are blisters, wheel burns, bruises and abrasions. These result from contact with the wheelchair seat back, brakes, push rims and wheels.[22] Lacerations can occur from collisions with other wheelchairs. Spinal-cord-injured athletes experience many of the same problems as athletes with myelomeningoceles, due to sensory and motor deficits. Contractures and muscle imbalances place the athletes at increased risk, with the shoulder being the most common site of injury to muscle–tendon units. The anterior shoulder is prone to excessive tightness due to poor posture and wheelchair pushing.[21] The latter can also result in muscle imbalances, with the shoulder flexor muscles being stronger than the extensors. Wheelchair athletes are at increased risk of shoulder injuries such as impingement syndromes and rotator cuff tendinitis. The elbow and wrist are also frequent sites of overuse injuries, with medial and lateral epicondylitis as well as de Quervain's tenosynovitis being among the more common injuries at these sites.[22] Those who present with shoulder pain often have a relative weakness of the adductor muscles. Careful attention to stretching and to achieving balanced strength can reduce the likelihood of overuse injuries in the upper extremities. Skin breakdown and osteopenia also occur in the spinal-cord-injured athlete. The principles of management are the same as for athletes with myelomeningoceles.

Nerve entrapment syndromes in the upper extremities are a problem for many wheelchair athletes. The numbness and weakness associated with carpal tunnel syndrome result from repetitive pressure of the heel of the hand on the push rim. Compression of the median or ulnar nerves can occur at the elbow as well. Radial tunnel syndrome should be considered in the differential diagnosis of lateral epicondylitis.[22]

Of particular concern for the spinal cord injured athlete is impairment of thermoregulation. Able-bodied children are less efficient than adults at compensating for changes in ambient temperature. Children with lesions above T8 cannot maintain normal body temperature in the face of extreme environmental stresses.[11] Autonomic dysfunction impedes heat production mechanisms, such as shivering, as well as heat dissipation mechanisms, such as sweating below the level of the spinal cord injury. While this problem also occurs in athletes with myelomeningoceles, as mentioned earlier, most of these neural tube defects occur in the lumbosacral region. The higher the lesion, the greater the impairment of thermoregulation; therefore, spinal-cord-injured athletes with thoracic lesions are at greatest risk. Careful observation of both groups during events that take place in either high or low ambient temperatures will prevent hyperthermia or hypothermia, respectively. Physicians who provide medical coverage at wheelchair athletic events must be prepared to deal with either outcome.

Autonomic dysreflexia occurs most frequently in quadriplegics and paraplegics with lesions above T6.[21] Noxious stimuli such as a full bladder or a fracture below the lesion cause mass activation of the sympathetic nervous system. Blood pressure rises dramatically as peripheral and splanchnic blood vessels vasoconstrict.[20] Due to sympathetic activation distal to the lesion, skin will be pale, cool and clammy below the injury. Above the lesion, parasympathetic activation from the stimulation of carotid and aortic baroreceptors leads to marked vasodilation as well as facial flushing, sweating, nasal stuffiness and bradycardia. This condition has been considered a medical emergency for years because of the potential for stroke. It also appears to enhance performance in wheelchair racing, which has prompted athletes to intentionally induce the condition by drinking excessively prior to a race or by clamping urinary catheters. This practice is extremely dangerous and is to be condemned. In the event that a wheelchair athlete presents with signs of autonomic dysreflexia, the urinary catheter should be inspected for a clamp or kink, and tight clothing or strapping of the lower extremities should be loosened. As it is difficult to place controls on the intentional induction of autonomic dysreflexia, athlete education may be the best defence against the potentially catastrophic outcome of this condition.

Amputee athletes

Amputation refers to a partial or complete loss of one or more limbs and may be either congenital or acquired. Acquired amputations may be the result of trauma, tumour, infection or vascular insufficiency.[23] Because the number of limbs affected and the level of the amputation varies considerably among amputee athletes, classification systems based on these variables have been established. The classification systems take into account whether the amputation is confined to a single arm or leg, or whether there are multiple amputations present. Athletes with amputations above the knee are distinguished from those with below knee amputations. Similarly, athletes with above elbow amputations compete in separate categories from those with below elbow deficiencies. These systems provide a more equitable playing field for athletes whose disabilities vary greatly.[12]

Many amputee athletes participate in sports with the use of a prosthesis. The prosthetic device is designed to compensate for any loss of function associated with the specific amputation. In the case of acquired amputations, early use of the prosthetic device facilitates its incorporation into the child's normal body actions.[19] It is very important that the prosthesis fit the child well; any discomfort may result in posture or gait disturbances. A good prosthesis alone is not enough to replace the deficient limb. The amputee athlete must learn how to use the prosthesis, with some devices requiring more extensive training. The higher the arm or leg amputation, the greater the time and effort needed to master use of the prosthetic device.[19,24]

A number of highly specialized terminal prosthetic devices have been developed in order to allow children with amputations to participate in a wide variety of activities. Upper-limb prostheses have been used very successfully for swimming, baseball (Fig. 4.7.2), golf, basketball, skiing and ice hockey. A device developed at the Rehabilitation Centre for Children in Winnipeg, Canada (Fig. 4.7.3) has allowed many young amputees to participate in hockey on a level equal to their able-bodied peers up to the Bantam division (ages 14 and 15 years) (personal communication, Doug Paulsen, Rehabilitation Centre for Children, Winnipeg, Canada). Refinements in prosthetic design are ongoing, allowing improved performance in many different sports. New lower-limb prosthetic devices provide athletes with near normal foot function. These carbon graphite prostheses store and release energy, which allows for an active push-off during running or jumping.[19] These advances in material and design of prostheses facilitate involvement in sports such as volleyball, basketball and track (Fig. 4.7.4).

Special mention should be made of snow skiing for amputee athletes. In the early 1940s, Franz Wendel of Germany became the first person to compete as a handicapped skier after sustaining a leg injury which required amputation. Short ski tips were attached to the bottoms of crutches to aid in balance while skiing.[14] Since that time, significant improvements have been made to equipment design. *Three-track skiing* is used by athletes with a single leg amputation with or without one upper-extremity prosthesis. One full-length ski is attached to the sound leg, while two short outrigger skis on forearm crutches are manoeuvred by the upper extremities. Children tend to ski without their lower limb prosthesis for improved balance and agility, while those with below-knee amputations who begin to ski

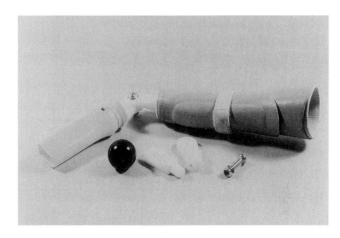

Fig. 4.7.3a   Upper limb prosthesis for participation in ice hockey.

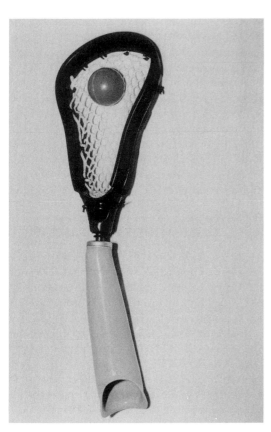

Fig. 4.7.2   Terminal prosthesis to facilitate participation in baseball by children with upper limb amputations.

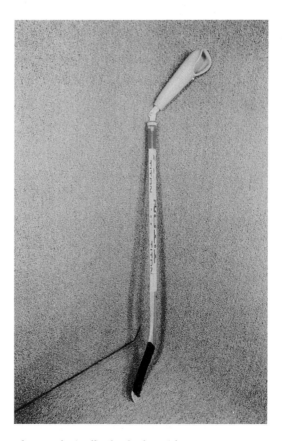

Fig. 4.7.3b   Prosthesis affixed to hockey stick.

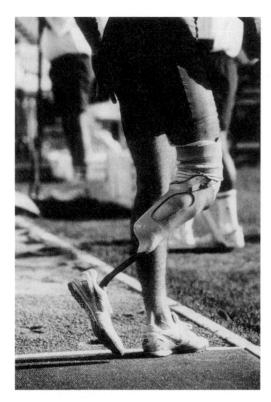

Fig. 4.7.4 Specialized prosthesis worn by an athlete at the Paralympic Games, Barcelona, 1992.

during late adolescence tend to ski with the prosthesis, primarily for cosmetic reasons. Athletes with above-knee amputations usually ski without their prosthesis.

Children and adolescents with amputations may have a decreased range of motion due to tight musculature or contractures. For example, a below-knee amputee who spends more time sitting than ambulating may develop tight hip and knee flexors. These athletes need to emphasize range of motion exercises in their training in order to reduce the risk of injuries to the muscle–tendon units. Balance is also adversely affected in athletes with amputations. For those with lower-limb amputations, this is due to the loss of proprioceptive feedback from the extremity. For those with acquired upper-limb amputations, the change in weight across the shoulder girdle affects balance. This is particularly hazardous in a sport such as figure skating, where balance is critical in preventing serious injuries from falls.[24]

In children, stump overgrowth is a frequent problem.[11,25] The bone begins to grow through the soft tissue left at the end of the stump, resulting in skin breakdown during physical activities. Young athletes should be instructed to inspect the stump for erythema or skin breakdown, particularly if the stump begins to lose the cushioned feeling of the soft tissues. Surgical revision of the stump will prevent severe overgrowth and will facilitate continued pain free participation in sports.[11] For those who wear their prosthesis during skiing, padding of the stump end can help prevent pressure sores and keep the stump warm.

An additional concern is for the integrity of the prosthesis. The stresses on the prosthesis during sports participation can be quite substantial, resulting in minor or major breakdowns of the device. Amputee athletes should be instructed to inspect the prosthetic device regularly in order to detect problems before they develop into major breakdowns.

Finally, children with limb deficiencies are at risk for psychological and social adjustment problems. Prejudices toward cosmetic handicaps, such as amputations, are greater than those toward functional handicaps, such as needing a wheelchair. Self-esteem can be adversely affected by these attitudes from peers; however, athletic competence in these individuals has been shown to correlate with higher self-esteem.[5]

Wheelchair sports

The concept of sports participation for individuals with spinal cord injuries was introduced by Sir Ludwig Guttman during the Second World War, at a time when the prevailing feeling was that very little could be done for paraplegics and quadriplegics. His revolutionary approach to the spinal-cord-injured patient included the introduction of the first competitive team sport for paraplegics, namely wheelchair polo. Soon after, wheelchair basketball and badminton were added to the list of sports for patients with spinal cord injuries, followed by archery and table tennis. On 28 July 1948, the Stoke Mandeville Games for the Paralysed were founded. They are held annually in Aylesbury, England, except every fourth year, when they are held in the country hosting the Olympic Games. The first city to host the International Stoke Mandeville Games outside of England was Rome in 1960, when 400 athletes from 23 countries competed in the Olympic Stadium following the Olympic Games. These Games became known as the Paraplegic Olympic Games, or Paralympics, and have grown dramatically since their inception. In 1992, more than one-million spectators attended the Paralympics in Barcelona. In 1996, 3350 athletes from 120 countries participated in the Atlanta Paralympics (Fig. 4.7.5).

Wheelchair basketball was the first organized sport for paraplegics in the United States, with athletes achieving high skill levels. Certain modifications to the rules have been made for wheelchair basketball. For example, a travelling violation occurs when an athlete performs three or more pushes of the wheelchair without bouncing the ball. Other popular wheelchair sports include tennis, volleyball, archery, bowling, track-and-field, marathon road racing and quad rugby. The latter is played on a regulation basketball court with four quadriplegic players on each team. Players attempt to bring the ball across the goal line, while opposing players impede the advancement of the ball. Thanks to the initiative of Sir Ludwig Guttman and others around the world, spinal-cord-injured individuals who were thought of as 'hopeless cripples'[3] 50 years ago now participate in sports at an elite level and achieve things unimaginable to many able-bodied athletes.

Athletes with mental retardation

Mental retardation (IQ less than 70), which affects approximately 3% of the population, is characterized by impairments in measured intelligence and adaptive behaviour.[26] The severity of mental retardation is based upon level of IQ. Children with borderline mental retardation (IQ 68–83) do not all meet the criteria for mental retardation; however, they are all likely to have difficulties in school. The vast majority of children classified as mentally retarded fall into the category of mild mental retardation (IQ 52–67). These children may require special class placement at school, but those with higher adaptive skills can become independent adults. Moderate mental retardation (IQ 36–51) limits academic achievements to a second grade level. As adults, those who are in this category require supervision of daily activities. Children with severe mental retardation (IQ 20–35) may learn minimal self-care

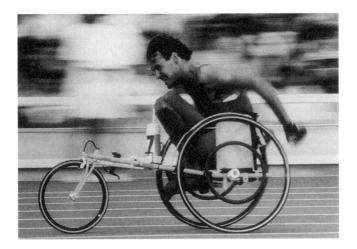

Fig. 4.7.5 Paralympic athlete displays speed in highly specialized wheelchair.

skills, but require extensive supervision. Profound mental retardation (IQ less than 20) affects only 1% of children with cognitive impairment. These children require total supervision for all aspects of daily life.

For children with borderline or high functioning mild mental retardation, the social stigma attached to the impairment can be more handicapping than the condition itself. Sports participation can provide a means of social interaction for children with mental retardation, while improving their fitness and self-concept.[27] Exercise and activity in this population may delay the need for institutionalization as well.[28]

Adults with mild to moderate mental retardation have a higher prevalence of obesity than do their peers without mental handicaps; however, there appears to be no difference in obesity between mentally retarded children and children without cognitive impairments.[28] Physical activity reduces the likelihood of obesity in adults with mental retardation, so the trend to obesity with age in this population is most likely the result of lifestyle. Perhaps by encouraging mentally retarded children to participate in sports or other physical activities, as adults they may be more active and therefore at lower risk of obesity and all its health implications.

Cardiovascular fitness is important in the prevention of coronary artery disease. Cardiovascular disease is the most common medical problem in adults with mental retardation.[29] Maximal oxygen uptake as a measurement of cardiovascular fitness appears to be similar among children with and without mental retardation.[28] As adolescents, those with mental retardation have a substantially lower maximal oxygen uptake than their unaffected peers.[28] This trend continues into adulthood and is particularly true for adults with Down Syndrome.[28] It appears that training can improve cardiovascular fitness in all individuals with mental retardation.[28] In order to reduce the risk of premature death due to coronary artery disease, children and adults with mental retardation should be encouraged to participate in activities that improve cardiovascular fitness.

Muscular strength and endurance appear to be lower in individuals of all ages with mental retardation compared to those with normal cognitive function.[28] Like obesity, this difference is thought to be primarily due to lifestyle. Through training programmes aimed at increasing muscular endurance, this problem can be largely rectified.[28] By improving muscular strength, work performance and level of independence also improve.

Down Syndrome

Down Syndrome, or Trisomy-21, is the most frequent human chromosomal syndrome, occurring in 1.5/1000 live births.[30,31] It occurs when an extra No. 21 chromosome is present through non-disjunction or translocation. If non-disjunction occurs after the first cell division following conception, only some of the cell lines will have trisomy 21, while others will have a normal chromosomal complement. An individual affected by this mosaicism may have a nearly normal phenotype or may have all the characteristics of Down Syndrome.[32] The craniofacial features, including oblique palpebral fissures, epicanthic folds, brushfield spots, protruding tongue, prominent malformed ears, flat nasal bridge and flat occiput, make Down Syndrome the best recognized of the chromosomal syndromes. Of particular interest to the sport medicine physician are the musculoskeletal and cardiovascular anomalies, as well as the cognitive impairment associated with this syndrome. Through proper screening prior to sports participation, many children with Down Syndrome can become active in a wide variety of sports and leisure activities.

Most of the musculoskeletal abnormalities result from a defect in collagen synthesis which leads to generalized hypotonia and ligamentous laxity. As a result, children with Down Syndrome are at increased risk of problems associated with hyperflexibility, such as pes planus and joint instability. Atlantoaxial instability subluxation (AAI) is potentially the most serious musculoskeletal problem associated with Down Syndrome. It is also the most controversial area in the management of these athletes. The incidence of AAI in children under 21 years of age with Down Syndrome is approximately 15%[33] and 1–2% of individuals with Down Syndrome have symptomatic AAI.[34] The subluxation is due to laxity of the annular ligament of C1 as well as the generalized hypotonia in Down Syndrome. Bony abnormalities, such as odontoid hypoplasia, odontoid dysplasia and the presence of os odontoideum, occur in 6% of those with Down Syndrome and increase the risk of atlantoaxial dislocation.

Because of the potential for permanent neurologic disability resulting from AAI, the Special Olympics issued a bulletin in 1983 restricting athletes with Down Syndrome from participating in any activities that might cause injury to the neck and upper spine until they had been examined for AAI. Individuals who were found to have asymptomatic AAI were permanently restricted from participation in certain Special Olympics activities that placed them at increased risk of injury. These activities include gymnastics, diving, pentathlon, butterfly stroke in swimming, diving starts in swimming, high jump and warm-up activities that place undue stress on the head and neck muscles.[35] The following year, the American Academy of Pediatrics (AAP) issued a policy statement recommending that all children with Down Syndrome who wished to participate in sports that involve possible trauma to the head and neck have lateral cervical spine radiographs in neutral, flexion and extension prior to beginning training or competition. This recommendation applied only to those who had not previously had normal radiologic findings. The AAP recommended restriction from high risk sports when the distance between the odontoid process of the axis and the anterior arch of the atlas exceeded 4.5 mm or the odontoid was abnormal. Repeated radiographs were not indicated for those with previously normal findings. The AAP policy stated that persons with atlantoaxial subluxation or dislocation and neurologic signs or symptoms should be restricted from all strenuous activities and operative stabilization of the cervical spine be considered.

The statement concluded that persons with Down Syndrome who did not have evidence of AAI could participate in all sports with no further follow-up unless neurologic signs or symptoms developed.[36]

The AAP retired the 1984 policy statement following a subject review in 1995. The AAP reviewed the data on which their earlier recommmendation was made and decided that there was uncertainty regarding the value of cervical spine radiographs in screening for possible catastrophic neck injury in athletes with Down Syndrome. The AAP felt that radiologic screening for AAI failed to meet the criteria of Sackett et al.,[37] stating that:

1. Symptomatic AAI is rare in the paediatric age range.
2. One study has shown poor reproducibility of the radiologic tests for AAI.[38] Other studies have shown changes in radiologic status over time.[39,40]
3. Asymptomatic AAI, which is common, has not been proven to be a significant risk factor for symptomatic AAI, which is rare.
4. The AAP feels that the intervention to prevent symptomatic AAI has never been tested.
5. Screening is expensive.
6. Undue anxiety may result from labelling a child as having AAI.
7. Many patients with symptomatic AAI have symptoms and signs of cervical spinal cord compression for weeks to years before they are recognized as having neurologic disease.

Although not a frequent finding, symptomatic AAI may be present in as many as 5000 individuals with Down Syndrome in the United States. It is argued by some experts that the associated high morbidity and mortality of symptomatic AAI should justify a screening programme.[34] O'Connor et al.[41] suggest that a single lateral radiograph at 1.85 m in active flexion is adequate to detect any potential AAI, since flexion views are unlikely to demonstrate a lesser gap than neutral or extension views. By eliminating the neutral and extension views, the cost of screening would be reduced significantly. Standardized interpretation is essential in improving reproducibility. It may also be argued that the lack of sports-related symptomatic AAI may be the result of the preventative measures in place since the 1983 bulletin by the Special Olympics restricting participation of Down Syndrome athletes with AAI. Seventeen per cent of Down Syndrome patients with symptomatic AAI have a history of cervical spine injury which either caused or contributed to the onset of symptoms.[42] Avoiding sports which have a high risk of injury to the cervical spine could reduce the risk of symptomatic AAI in Down Syndrome athletes significantly. Regarding the potential for anxiety among parents of athletes with Down Syndrome and given that Special Olympics still require assessments for AAI, a screening programme would be more likely to allay fears than to create undue anxiety, since the vast majority of radiographic examinations would be negative. Identification of neurologic abnormalities in Down Syndrome children may be more predictive of impending progression to a more serious symptomatic AAI; however, reliance on history and physical examination alone would fail to identify any children with asymptomatic AAI who may be at risk of progression to symptomatic AAI. In addition, assessing children with Down Syndrome for neurologic signs and symptoms can be extremely challenging.[43] Their ability to verbalize regarding neuromotor difficulties or neck discomfort is often limited and they may not be cooperative during physical examinations.[39] Taking all of the aforementioned issues into account, the author recommends a single lateral radiograph of the cervical spine in flexion to screen for AAI.

White et al.[44] have found a significant relationship between neural canal width and subarachnoid space width, but not with atlanto-dens interval. Narrow neural canal width appears to be a predictor of potential spinal cord compression.[44] As such, it is recommended that lateral radiographs be done with careful positioning of the neck in flexion with the chin tucked. Abnormal atlanto-dens interval should be correlated with neural canal width, and any patients with narrowing of the canal or evidence of AAI should be evaluated with MRI before imposing restrictions on activities or considering surgery. White suggests that those patients with a marginally widened atlanto-dens interval but normal neural canal width may be followed up with serial radiographs; however, more research needs to be done in this area.

Cervical spine abnormalities occur in 40% of Down Syndrome persons.[45] Although AAI is by far the most common, other cervical spine abnormalities exist, such as abnormal vertebral bodies (especially C-2), multiple vertebral fusions, hypoplastic posterior arch of C-1, odontoid abnormalities, and spondylolysis and spondylolisthesis of the midcervical vertebrae.[46] Instability may also occur between the atlas and the occiput, increasing the risk of neurologic injury particularly if the neck is extended. Although radiographic evaluation and normative values for Down Syndrome have not been well defined for the atlanto-occipital region,[11] instability may be detected on lateral radiographs.[34,35] If lateral views are performed for the purposes of screening prior to sports participation, not only should AAI be evaluated, but other craniocervical abnormalities should be ruled out.

Patellofemoral instability is a concern for many Down Syndrome athletes. In 32%[32] of patients with Down Syndrome, the patella subluxes or dislocates, resulting in significant impairment in sports and activities of daily living. This instability results from ligamentous laxity in conjunction with anatomic abnormalities such as genu valgus, patella alta or hypoplastic medial femoral condyle. Pes planus, also due to severe, generalized ligamentous laxity, is seen frequently in Down Syndrome children; therefore, use of orthotics may be necessary both in the management of patellofemoral symptoms and in the treatment of foot pain.

Excessive joint laxity may affect the hips and often presents as a loud clunking or popping sound. This condition causes gradual degeneration of the hip joint, the extent of which is not certain. These individuals have a poor gait and limited ambulation.[32] Prevention of hip damage is difficult but may be attempted using casting or abduction bracing. Even with surgical correction, hip instability may recur.

Special Olympics

Special Olympics International began serving mentally handicapped children and adults in 1968. Participation in Special Olympics helps develop better socialization and physical skills among children and adults with mental retardation. It increases the athletes' self-confidence and independence. Today, over 150 countries around the world offer this programme for children and adults with mental disabilities. Athletes, who are grouped according to age and ability, compete in summer sports such as track-and-field, swimming, powerlifting, rhythmic gymnastics, soccer, softball and bowling (Fig. 4.7.6). Official winter sports include Alpine and Nordic skiing, figure skating, speed skating, snowshoeing and floor hockey. Over 20 000 athletes participate in the programme in Canada, and many more are involved throughout the world. Athletes begin with local level competitions and, like their peers without mental retardation, can progress to international competitions which are held every four years and are analogous to the Olympic Games.[47,48] The spirit of Special Olympics is encompassed in the Special Olympics athlete oath: 'Let me win but if I cannot win, let me be brave in the attempt' (Fig. 4.7.7).

Summary

The twentieth century has witnessed a dramatic change in the public's perception of individuals with disabilities. New opportunities have allowed these young athletes to experience the many benefits of sports

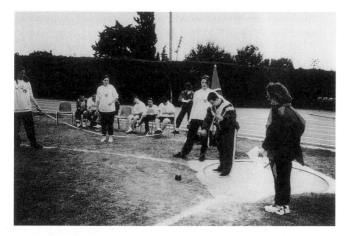

Fig. 4.7.6   Track and field athlete competing in the Special Olympics.

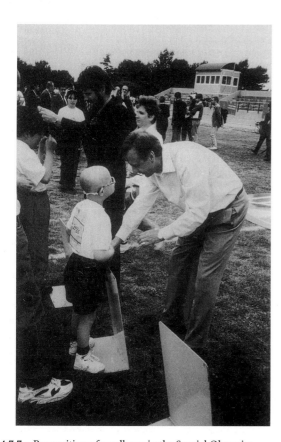

Fig. 4.7.7   Recognition of excellence in the Special Olympics.

participation once reserved exclusively for the able-bodied child. With this new participation, the field of sport medicine has had to expand in order to allow a greater understanding of the issues unique to each athlete with a disability. From the late 1800s, when baseball was first introduced at the Ohio School for the Deaf, to the World Games for the Deaf, and from labels such as 'hopeless cripples' of 50 years ago to the world-class Paralympic Games of today, athletes with disabilities have reached heights many of us will never achieve.

You are the living demonstration of the marvels of the virtue of energy. You have given a great example, which We would like to emphasize, it can be a lead to all: you have shown what an energetic soul can achieve, in spite of apparently insurmountable obstacles imposed by the body. (Pope John XXIII, at the International Stoke Mandeville Games in Rome, 1960.[49])

References

1. **Rimmer, J. H., Braddock, D.** and **Fujiura, G.** Prevalence of obesity in adults with mental retardation: implications for health promotion and disease prevention. *Mental Retardation* 1993; **31**: 105–10.
2. **Lockette, K. F.** and **Keyes, A. M.** Strength training. In *Conditioning with physical disabilities* (ed. M. E. Fowler). Human Kinetics, Windsor, Ontario, 1994: 15–38.
3. **Guttman, L.** Wheelchair sports for spinal para- and tetraplegics. In *Textbook of sport for the disabled* (ed. L. Guttman). H. M. & M. Publishers, Aylesbury, 1976: 21–46.
4. **Richter, K. J., Gaebler-Spira, D.** and **Mushett, C. A.** Sport and the person with spasticity of cerebral origin. *Developmental Medicine and Child Neurology* 1996; **38**: 867–70.
5. **Varni, J. W.** and **Setoguchi, Y.** Correlates of perceived physical appearance in children with congenital/acquired limb deficiencies. *Journal of Developmental and Behavioral Pediatrics* 1991; **12**: 171–6.
6. **Winnick, J. P.** An introduction to adapted physical education and sport. In *Adapted physical education and sport* (ed. J. P. Winnick). Human Kinetics, Windsor, Ontario, 1995: 3–16.
7. **Arnold, J. E.** The Ear. In *Nelson textbook of pediatrics* (15th edn) (ed. W. E. Nelson). W. B. Saunders, Philadelphia, 1996: 1804–26.
8. **Hyndman, J. C.** The Growing Athlete. In *Oxford textbook of sports medicine* (2nd edn) (ed. M. Harries, C. Williams, W. D. Stanish and L. J. Micheli). Oxford University Press, Oxford, 1998: 727–41.
9. **Craft, D. H.** Visual impairments and hearing losses. In *Adapted physical education and sport* (ed. J. P. Winnick). Human Kinetics, Windsor, Ontario, 1995: 143–66.
10. **Guttman, L.** Sports for the deaf. In *Textbook of sport for the disabled* (ed. L. Guttman). H. M. & M. Publishers, Aylesbury, 1976: 170–3.
11. **Chang, F. M.** The disabled athlete. In *Pediatric and adolescent sports medicine*, Vol. 3 (ed. C. L. Stanitski, J. C. DeLee and D. Drez). W. B. Saunders, Philadelphia, 1994: 48–76.
12. **Booth, D. W.** and **Grogono, B. J.** Athletes with a disability. In *Oxford textbook of sports medicine* (2nd edn) (ed. M. Harries, C. Williams, W. D. Stanish and L. J. Micheli). Oxford University Press, Oxford, 1998: 815–31.
13. **Guttman, L.** Sports for the blind and partially sighted. In *Textbook of sport for the disabled* (ed. L. Guttman). H. M. & M. Publishers, Aylesbury, 1976: 150–61.
14. **Laskowski, E. R.** Snow skiing for the physically disabled. *Mayo Clinic Proceedings* 1991; **66**: 160–72.
15. **Haslam, R. H. A.** The nervous system. In *Nelson textbook of pediatrics* (15th edn) (ed. W. E. Nelson). W. B. Saunders, Philadelphia, 1996: 1667–738.
16. **Guttman L.** Sports for sufferers from cerebral palsy. In *Textbook of sport for the disabled* (ed. L. Guttman). H. M. & M. Publishers, Aylesbury, 1976: 162–69.

17. **Richter K. E., Hyman, S. C.** and **Mushett-Adams, C. A.** Injuries in world-class cerebral palsy athletes at the 1988 South Korea Paralympics. *Journal of Osteopathic Sports Medicine* 1991; **5**: 15–18.

18. **O'Neill, D. B.** and **Micheli, L. J.** Overuse injuries in the young athlete. *Clinics in Sports Medicine* 1988; **7**: 591–610.

19. **Poretta, D. L.** Cerebral palsy, traumatic brain injury, stroke, amputations, dwarfism, and other orthopedic impairments. In *Adapted physical education and sport* (ed. J. P. Winnick). Human Kinetics, Windsor, Ontario, 1995: 167–91.

20. **Steadward, R. D.** and **Wheeler, G. D.** The young athlete with a motor disability. In *The child and adolescent athlete* (ed. O. Bar-Or). Blackwell Science, Oxford, 1996: 493–520.

21. **Lockette, K. F.** and **Keyes, A. M.** Conditioning with spinal cord injuries, spina bifida, and poliomyelitis. In *Conditioning with physical disabilities* (ed. M. E. Fowler). Human Kinetics, Windsor, Ontario, 1994: 91–116.

22. **Schutz, L. K.** The wheelchair athlete. In *Sports medicine and rehabilitation: a sport-specific approach* (ed. R. M. Buschbacher and R. L. Braddom). Hanley & Belfus, Philadelphia, 1994: 267–74.

23. **Lockette, K. F.** and **Keyes, A. M.** Conditioning with Amputations. In *Conditioning with physical disabilities* (ed. M. E. Fowler). Human Kinetics, Windsor, Ontario, 1994: 117–34.

24. **Guttman, L.** Sports for amputees. In *Textbook of sport for the disabled* (ed. L. Guttman). H. M. & M. Publishers, Aylesbury, 1976: 119–49.

25. **Marquardt, E, Correll, J.** Amputations and Prostheses for the lower limb. *International Orthopedics (SICOT)* 1984; **8**: 139–46.

26. **Shonkoff, J. P.** Mental retardation. In *Nelson textbook of pediatrics* (15th edn) (ed. W. E. Nelson). W. B. Saunders, Philadelphia, 1996: 128–31.

27. **Compton, D. M., Eisenman, P. A.** and **Henderson, H. L.** Exercise and fitness for persons with disabilities. *Sports Medicine* 1989; **7**: 150–62.

28. **Fernhall, B.** Physical fitness and exercise training of individuals with mental retardation. *Medicine and Science in Sports and Exercise* 1993; **25**: 442–50.

29. **Pitetti, K. H.** and **Campbell, K. D.** Mentally retarded individuals—a population at risk? *Medicine and Science in Sports and Exercise* 1991; **23**: 586–93.

30. **Harley, E. H.** and **Collins, M. D.** Neurologic sequelae secondary to atlantoaxial instability in down syndrome: Implications in Otolaryngologic Surgery. *Archives of Otolaryngology Head and Neck Surgery* 1994; **120**: 159–65.

31. **Hall, J. G.** Chromosomal clinical abnormalities. In *Nelson textbook of pediatrics* (15th edn) (ed. W. E. Nelson). W. B. Saunders, Philadelphia, 1996: 312–21.

32. **Diamond, L. S., Lynne, D.** and **Sigman. B.** Orthopedic disorders in patients with down's syndrome. *Orthopedic Clinics of North America* 1981; **12**: 57–71.

33. American Academy of Pediatrics. Atlantoaxial instability in down syndrome: subject review. *Pediatrics* 1995; **96**: 151–54.

34. **Pueschel, S. M.** Should children with Down syndrome be screened for atlantoaxial instability? *Archives of Pediatric and Adolescent Medicine* 1998; **152**: 123–25.

35. **Cohen, W. I.** Atlantoaxial instability: what's next? *Archives of Pediatric and Adolescent Medicine* 1998; **152**: 119–12.

36. Committee on Sports Medicine. Atlantoaxial instability in Down syndrome. *Pediatrics* 1984; **74**: 152–54.

37. **Sackett, D. L., Haynes, R. B., Guyatt, G. H.** and **Tugwell, P.** *Clinical epidemiology: a basic science for clinical medicine* (2nd edn). Little, Brown, Boston, 1991: 153–70.

38. **Selby, K. A., Newton, R. W., Gupta, S.** and **Hunt, L.** Clinical predictors and radiologic reliability in atlantoaxial subluxation in Down's Syndrome. *Archives of Disease in Childhood* 1991; **66**: 876–878.

39. **Peuschel, S. M., Scola. F. H.** and **Pezzullo, J. C.** A longitudinal study of atlanto-dens relationships in asymptomatic individuals with Down Syndrome. *Pediatrics* 1992; **89**: 1194–8.

40. **Peuschel, S. M.** and **Scola, F. H.** Atlantoaxial instability in individuals with Down Syndrome: epidemiologic, radiographic, and clinical studies. *Pediatrics* 1987; **80**: 555–60.

41. **O'Connor, J. F., Cranley, W. R., McCarten, K. M.** and **Feingold, M.** Commentary: atlantoaxial instability in down syndrome: reassessment by the committee on sports medicine and fitness of the American Academy of Pediatrics. *Pediatric Radiology* 1996; **26**: 748–9.

42. **Peuschel, S. M., Herndon, J. H., Gelch, M. M., Senft, K. E., Scola, F. H.** and **Goldberg, M. J.** Symptomatic atlantoaxial subluxation in persons with Down Syndrome. *Journal of Pediatric Orthopedics* 1984; **4**: 682–8.

43. **Msall, M. E., Reese, M. E., DiGaugdio, K., Granger, C. V.** and **Cooke, R. E.** Symptomatic Atlantoaxial instability associated with medical and rehabilitative procedures in children with Down Syndrome. *Pediatrics* 1990; **85**: 447–9.

44. **White, K. S., Ball, W. S., Prenger, E. C., Patterson, B. J.** and **Kirks, D. R.** Evaluation of the craniocervical junction in Down Syndrome: correlation of measurements obtained by radiography and MR imaging. *Radiology* 1993; **186**: 377–82.

45. **Cope, R.** and **Olson, S.** Abnormalities of the cervical spine in Down's Syndrome: Diagnosis, risks, and review of the literature, with particular Reference to the Special Olympics. *Southern Medical Journal* 1987; **80**: 33–6.

46. **Goldberg, M. J.** Spine instability and the Special Olympics. *Clinics in Sports Medicine* 1993; **12**: 507–15.

47. Manitoba Special Olympics. *Volunteer orientation handbook.* Pamphlet, obtainable from: Manitoba Special Olympics, 200 Main Street, Winnipeg, Manitoba R3C 4M2.

48. Canadian Special Olympics. *Canadian Special Olympics.* Pamphlet, obtainable from Canadian Special Olympics, 40 St. Clair Avenue W., Suite 209, Toronto, Ontario M4V 1M2.

49. **Guttman, L.** In *Textbook of sport for the disabled* (ed. L. Guttman). H. M. & M. Publishers, Aylesbury, 1976.

PART V
Sports and Exercise Injuries

5.1 Current concepts on the aetiology and prevention of sports injuries

Willem van Mechelen

Introduction

A physically active lifestyle and active participation in sports is important, both for adults as well as for children. Reasons to participate in sports and physical activity are many; pleasure and relaxation, competition, socialization, maintenance and improvement of fitness and health, etc. In general, when compared to adults, in children the risk for sports injury resulting from participation in sports and free play is low.[1] Despite this relatively low risk, sports injuries in children are a fact of life, which calls for preventive action. In order to set out effective prevention programmes, epidemiological studies need to be done on incidence, severity and aetiology of sports injuries. Also the effect of preventive measures needs to be evaluated. In the following chapters various authors will describe these aspects of sports injuries in children, regarding specific sports. This chapter describes briefly some current concepts regarding the epidemiology and prevention of sports injuries as a means of introduction to these chapters.

The sequence of prevention

Measures to prevent sports injuries do not stand by themselves. They form part of what might be called a sequence of prevention[2] (Fig. 5.1.1). First, the problem must be identified and described in terms of incidence and severity of sports injuries. Then the factors and mechanisms that play a part in the occurrence of sports injuries have to be identified. The third step is to introduce measures that are likely to reduce the future risk and/or severity of sports injuries. Such measures should be based on the aetiologic factors and the mechanisms as identified in the second step. Finally, the effect of the measures must be evaluated by repeating the first step, which will lead to so-called time-trend analysis of injury patterns. However, from an epidemiological standpoint it is preferable to evaluate the effect of preventive measures by means of a randomized controlled trial (RCT). Unfortunately RCTs have only very rarely been conducted in sports injury prevention studies, and most of the RCTs that have been conducted so far in this area of research were carried out in adults.

When conducting (and also when interpreting the outcomes of) epidemiological sports injuries studies one is confronted with a number of methodological issues. The first issue of importance here is the definition of sports injury. In general, sports injury is a collective name for all types of damage that can occur in relation to sporting activities. Various studies of incidence define the term sports injury in different ways. In some studies, a sports injury is defined as any injury sustained during sporting activities for which an insurance claim is submitted; in other studies the definition is confined to injuries treated at a hospital

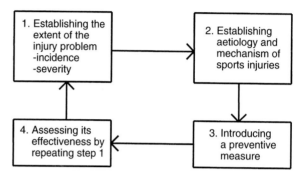

Fig. 5.1.1 The sequence of prevention of sports injuries. From van Mechelen et al.[2]

casualty or other medical department.[2] Different definitions partly explain the differing incidences found in the literature. The results of various sports injury incidence surveys are therefore not comparable. If sports injuries are recorded through medical channels (for instance through hospital emergency rooms), a fairly large percentage of serious, predominantly acute injuries will be observed and less serious and/or overuse injuries will not be recorded. If such a 'limited' definition is used, only part of the total sports injury problem is revealed. This 'tip-of-the-iceberg' phenomenon is commonly described in epidemiological research.[3] This problem is to a large extent found in sports injury epidemiology in youth, where many overuse injuries are thought to be found, as well as 'minor' acute injuries.

To make sports injury surveys comparable and to avoid the 'tip-of-the-iceberg' phenomenon as far as possible, an unambiguous, universally applicable definition of sports injury is the first prerequisite. This definition should be based on a concept of health other than that customary in standard medicine, and should, for instance, take incapacitation for sports or school into account. Even if one single uniform definition of sports injury is applied, the need remains for uniform agreement on other issues. These concern, for instance, the way in which sports injury incidence is expressed and the ways in which reliable estimates are made of both the number of people engaging in sports and the number of injured sports persons.

Sports injury incidence

One way of getting an impression of the extent of the sports injury problem is by counting the absolute number of injuries. When these absolute numbers are compared with, for instance, the number of traffic accidents or the number of injuries sustained during leisure time activities, the relative extent of the sports injury problem can be revealed. However, such data do not give estimates of injury risk and are inferior from an epidemiological perspective.

The most appropriate indication of the spread of disease in the population or in a section of the population is incidence. If one substitutes 'sports injury or sports accident' for 'disease', incidence can be defined as 'the number of new sports injuries or accidents sustained during a particular period, divided by the total number of sports persons at the start of the period (i.e. the population-at-risk)'. Incidence thus defined also gives an estimate of risk. If one multiplies the obtained figure by 100, one gets the incidence percentage rate.[4] Expressed in this way, sports injury incidence figures give insight into the extent of the sports injury problem in a particular population-at-risk. It is clear from this definition of incidence that incidence can only be assessed properly if both a clear definition of sports injury, as well as of the population-at-risk are present.

In many studies the incidence rate of sports injuries is usually defined as the number of new sports injuries during a particular period (e.g. 1 year) divided by the total number of sports persons at the start of that period (population-at-risk). When interpreting and comparing incidence rates found in different studies it is important to know what definition of sports injury was used. One should also have information on the comparability of the populations-at-risk. It is clear that the methods used to count injuries and to count the population-at-risk will also influence sports injury incidence figures. Finally, the length of the observation period has to be taken into account, since different lengths of observation periods will have a distinct influence on the incidences calculated.

In terms of risk assessment, another problem lies in the way incidence rates are expressed. In most cases, the number of injuries in a particular category of sports persons per season or per year is taken, or the number of injuries per player per match. In both examples no allowance is made for any differences in the actual exposure to injury risk (i.e. the number of hours of active play during which the sports person actually runs the risk of being injured). This is peculiar because this factor certainly has great influence on the risk of sustaining a sports injury. Incidence figures that take no account of exposure are therefore not a good indication of the 'true' risk one runs, nor can such incidence rates be used for a comparison of risk between different sports or between age and sex groups participating in the same sport. It would therefore be better to calculate the incidence of sports injuries in relation to exposure time (hours).

The equation of Chambers,[5] adapted by De Loës and Goldi,[6] can be used to calculate injury incidence (ii) taking exposure into account:

$$ii = \frac{(\text{no. of sports injuries/yr}) \times 10^4}{(\text{no. of participants}) \times (\text{hrs of sports participation/wk}) \times (\text{wks of season/yr})}$$

Research design

The extent to which sports injury incidence and sports injury risk can be assessed depends on the definition of sports injury, the way in which incidence is expressed, the method used to count injuries, the method to establish the population at risk and the representativeness of the sample. Here, clearly, research design also comes into play.

Injuries as well as time-at-risk can be assessed retrospectively or prospectively, using questionnaires or person-to-person interviews. However, prospective studies can, by closely monitoring exposure time and injury outcome, more accurately estimate the risk and incidence of sports injury according to the level of sports participation and type of exposure of an athlete. They are therefore superior to retrospective studies. One of the main problems of retrospective studies is the inherent recall bias of the subjects participating in such a study.

A word should be said here about case studies. In sports medical journals, clinical case studies are often described. Conclusions are drawn from these case studies regarding the incidence and the risk of sustaining sports injuries. However, case studies have the drawback that no information on the population-at-risk is available. Consequently, no valid conclusions can be drawn from case studies; either with respect to sports injury incidence, or with respect to injury risks.[3]

Depending on the methods used the researcher will be confronted to a greater or lesser extent with phenomena such as recall bias, overestimation of the hours of sport participation,[7] incomplete responses, non-response, drop-out, invalid injury description and problems related to the duration and cost of research. These factors will clearly affect the internal validity of a study.

Special attention has to be paid to the method of assessing the population-at-risk and to the representativeness of the sample. If the population-at-risk is not clearly identified, it is not possible to calculate reliable incidence data. With regard to the representativeness of the sample, it has to be taken into consideration that the performance of athletes in sports, and therefore the incidence of sports injuries, is highly determined by selection. Bol et al.[8] recognized four different kinds of selection:

(1) self-selection (personal preferences) and/or selection by social environment (parents, friends, school, etc.);

(2) selection by the sports environment (trainer, coach, etc.);

(3) selection by sports organizations (organization of competition by age and gender, the setting of participation standards, etc.); and

(4) selection by social, medical and biological factors (socio-economic background, mortality, age, ageing, gender, etc.).

For example, within a certain sport, competing at a high level increases sports injury risk; more injuries are sustained during matches than during training; in contact sports more injuries are sustained as compared with non-contact sports; during and shortly after the growth spurt boys sustain more injuries than during other periods of growth; etc.

The severity of sports injuries

A description of the severity of sports injuries is important in making a decision about whether or not preventive measures are needed, since the need to prevent serious injuries in a particular sport need not coincide with a high overall incidence of injuries in that sport. According to the literature the severity of sports injuries can be described on the basis of six criteria.[9] These criteria are briefly described below.

Nature of sports injuries

The nature of sports injuries can be described in terms of medical diagnosis: sprain (of joint capsule and ligaments), strain (of muscle or tendon), contusion (bruising), dislocation or subluxation, fracture (of bone), etc. It is the nature of the sports injury that determines whether assistance (medical or otherwise) is sought. Recording of the nature of sports injuries enables those sports with relatively serious injuries to be identified. The nature of sports injuries can also be described according to the part of the body injured.

Duration and nature of treatment

Data on the duration and nature of treatment can be used to determine the severity of an injury more precisely, especially if it is a question of what medical bodies are involved in the treatment and what therapies used.

Sports time lost

It is important for a sports person to be able to take up his or her sport again as soon as possible after an injury. Sport and exercise play an essential part in people's free time and thus influence their mental well-being. The loss of sporting time is an important psychosocial factor. The length of sporting time lost gives the most precise indication of the consequences of an injury to a sports person.

Working or school time lost

Like the cost of medical treatment, the length of working or school time lost gives an indication of the consequences of sports injuries at a societal level. Data of working or school time lost are used to compare the cost to society of sports injuries with that of other situations involving risks, such as traffic accidents.

Permanent damage

The vast majority of sports injuries heal without permanent disability. Serious injuries, such as fractures, ligament, tendon and intra-articular injuries, spinal injuries and eye injuries, can leave permanent damage (residual symptoms). Excessive delay between the occurrence of an injury and medical assistance can aggravate the injury. If the residual symptoms are slight, they may cause the individual to modify his or her level of sporting activity. In some cases, however, the sports person may have to choose another sport or give up sport altogether. Serious physical damage can cause permanent disability or death, thus reducing or eliminating the individual's capacity for work or school. When taking precautions, then, priority should be given to measures in sports where such serious injuries are common, even though the particular sport itself is characterized by a low incidence of sports injuries and/or a low absolute number of participants.

Costs of sports injuries

The calculation of the costs of sports injuries essentially involves the expression of the above mentioned five categories of seriousness of sports injuries in economic terms. The economic costs can be divided into:

(1) direct costs, i.e. the cost of medical treatment (diagnostic expenses such as X-rays, doctor's fee, cost of medicines, admission costs, etc.); and

(2) indirect costs, i.e. expenditure incurred in connection with the loss of productivity due to increased morbidity and mortality levels (loss of school or working time and loss of expertise due to death or handicap).

Conceptual models for the aetiology and prevention of sports injuries

Risk indicators for sports injuries can be divided into two main categories: internal personal risk indicators and external, environmental risk indicators.[2] This division is based on partly proven and partly supposed causal relationships between risk factors and sports injuries. However, merely to establish the causes of sports injuries, i.e. the internal and external factors, is not enough; the mechanism by which they occur must also be identified.

As can be seen in Fig. 5.1.2, sports injuries result from a complex interaction of multiple risk factors, of which only a fraction have been identified. Despite this multicausality, many epidemiological studies have concentrated on identifying single internal and external risk indicators from a medical, monocausal point of view, rather than from a multicausal point of view. However, studies on the aetiology of sports injuries require a dynamic model that accounts for this multifactorial nature of sports injuries, and that also takes the sequence of events eventually leading to an injury into account. One such dynamic model is the model described by Meeuwisse.[10] This model describes how multiple factors interact to produce injury (see Fig. 5.1.3).

In studies on the aetiology of sports injuries, this model can be used to explore the inter-relationships between risk factors and their contribution to the occurrence of injury. Meeuwisse[10] classifies the intrinsic or athlete-related factors as predisposing factors that are necessary, but seldom sufficient, to produce injury. In his theoretical model, extrinsic risk factors act on the predisposed athlete from without, and are

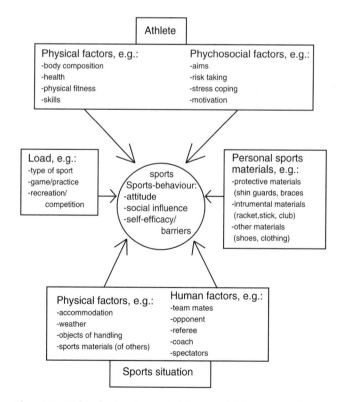

Fig. 5.1.2 Risk indicators for sports injuries and determinants of sports and preventive behaviour. From van Mechelen *et al.*[2]

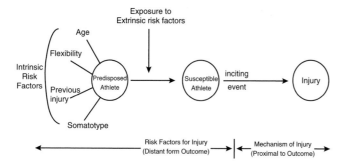

Fig. 5.1.3   A dynamic, multifactorial model of sports injury aetiology. Reprinted with permission from Meeuwisse.[10]

classified as enabling factors in that they facilitate the manifestation of injury. It is the presence of both intrinsic and extrinsic risk factors that render the athlete susceptible to injury, but the mere presence of these risk factors is usually not sufficient to produce injury. It is the sum of these risk factors and the interaction between them that 'prepare' the athlete for an injury to happen at a given place, in a given sports situation. Meeuwisse describes an inciting event to be the final link in the chain of causation to sports injury, and states that such an inciting event is usually directly associated with the onset of injury. Such events are regarded as necessary causes. Studies on the aetiology of sports injuries tend to focus on factors proximal to the injury event (i.e. the inciting events) and tend to neglect factors more distant from the injury event (i.e. the intrinsic and extrinsic risk factors), thereby revealing only a small fraction of the factors and events that lead to sports injury. Although understandable, focusing on inciting events may lead to overweighing the importance of such events in the aetiology and prevention of sports injuries. If in aetiological studies distant factors are studied, they usually concern intrinsic, person-related risk factors. These factors are relatively easier to measure than extrinsic risk factors. It is a multifactorial model, like the model of Meeuwisse,[10] that should be used to study the aetiology of sports injuries.

Finally, a word should be said here about the determinants of sports behaviour. When trying to prevent sports injuries one should realize that participation in sports is a form of behaviour. Usually the introduction of preventive measures implies a change or modification of behaviour of the athlete. It may very well be that the desired preventive behaviour conflicts with the actual sport behaviour, for instance because it is believed by the athlete that the preventive behaviour will affect sports performance negatively. When introducing preventive measures and when evaluating the effect of such measures, it is therefore necessary to have knowledge of the determinants of both sports and preventive behaviour. Many models are used to explain preventive behaviour. In general, these models include three sets of determinants: (1) knowledge and attitude, (2) social influence and (3) barriers and self-efficacy[11] (see Fig. 5.1.2). These determinants are described as follows:

1. 'Attitude refers to the knowledge and beliefs of a person concerning the specific consequences of a certain form of behaviour. An attitude is the weighing of all consequences of the performance of the behaviour, as seen by the individual. Health is only seen as one of the considerations, and is often an unimportant one. When health is part of attitude one may suppose that healthy motivation is a combination of the perceived severity of the health risk, the perceived susceptibility to the health risk, and the effectiveness of the preventive behaviour.'

2. 'Social influence is the influence by others; directly by what others expect, indirectly by what others do (modelling).' 'Social influence is often underestimated as a determinant of behaviour. It can lead to behaviour that conflicts with previous attitudes. Most sports situations are social situations.'

3. 'Self-efficacy-cum-barriers stands for the determinant whether one is able to perform the (desired) behaviour. It involves an estimation of ability, taking into account possible internal (e.g. insufficient skill, knowledge, endurance) or external barriers (e.g. resistance from others, time and money not available, etc.). Self-efficacy is the people's perception of their ability to perform the behaviour, and barriers are the real problems they face in actually performing the behaviour.'

It is these determinants that should be accounted for when trying to prevent sports injuries.

Summary

The outcome of research on the extent of the sports injury problem is highly dependent on the definitions of 'sports injury', 'sports injury incidence' and 'sports participation'. The outcome of sports epidemiological research also depends on the research design and methodology, the representativeness of the sample, and on whether or not exposure time was considered when calculating incidence. The severity of sports injuries can be expressed by taking six indices into consideration. The aetiology of sports injuries is highly multicausal. This fact, as well as the sequence of events leading to a sports injury, should be accounted for when studying the aetiology of sports injuries and when trying to prevent them. Finally, one should take determinants of sports and preventive behaviour into account in attempts to solve the sports injury problem.

References

1. **van Mechelen, W.** Etiology and prevention of sports injuries in youth. In *Exercise and fitness—Children and exercise XVIII* (ed. K. Froberg, P. Pedersen, H. Steen Hansen and C. J. R. Blimkie), Odense University Press, Odense, 1997; 209–28.
2. **van Mechelen. W., Hlobil, H.** and **Kemper, H. C. G.** Incidence, severity, aetiology and prevention of sports injuries. *Sports Medicine* 1992; **14:** 82–99.
3. **Walter, S. D., Sutton, J. R., McIntosh, J. M.** and **Connolly, C.** The aetiology of sports injuries. A review of methodologies. *Sports Medicine* 1985; **2:** 47–58.
4. **Sturmans, F.** *Epidemiologie.* Dekker & van de Vegt, Nijmegen, 1984.
5. **Chambers, R. B.** Orthopedic injuries in athletes (ages 6 to 17), comparison of injuries occurring in six sports. *American Journal of Sports Medicine* 1979; **7:** 195–7.
6. **de Loës,** and **Goldi, M. K.** Incidence rate of injuries during sport activity, and physical exercise in a rural Swedish municipality: incidence rates in 17 sports. *International Journal of Sports Medicine* 1988; **9:** 461–7.
7. **Klesges, R. C., Eck, L. H., Mellon, M. W., Fulliton, W., Somes, G. W.** and **Hanson, C. L.** The accuracy of self-reports of physical activity. *Medicine and Science in Sports and Exercise* 1990; **22:** 690–7.
8. **Bol E, Schmickli, S. L., Backx, F. J. G.** and **van Mechelen, W.** *Sportblessures onder de knie;* NISGZ publication 38, Papendal, 1991.
9. **van Mechelen W.** The severity of sports injuries. *Sports Medicine* 1997; **24:** 176–180.
10. **Meeuwisse, W.** Assessing causation in sport injury: a multifactorial model. *Clinical Journal of Sports Medicine* 1994; **4:** 166–170.
11. **Kok, G.J.** and **Bouter, L.M.** On the importance of planned health education: prevention of ski injury as an example. *American Journal of Sports Medicine* 1990; **18:** 600–605.

5.2 Aetiology and prevention of injuries in physical education classes

Frank J. G. Backx

Introduction

In most western countries, school-aged children get one or two hours of physical education classes (PE classes) a week. Although it is questionable if this number of PE classes contribute substantially to the physical development and health of a young individual, it is presumed to be beneficial in the short and long term.[1]

In most countries in Europe, sports activities are not explicitly incorporated into the school system as much as in the USA. On the one hand, this has resulted in PE classes being less competitive. On the other hand, club sports activities in Europe have increased. The latter has been accompanied by an increase in sports injuries.[2]

Physical education at school, in which all school-aged children participate, is aimed at an all-round physical conditioning by a diversity of movements. However, the participation in PE classes diminishes as one grows older.[3] Nowadays, for instance in the Netherlands, not all secondary schools offer obligatory physical education classes at every grade level anymore. Remarkably this trend seems to be independent of the increased number of injuries during PE classes. Data concerning injuries in PE classes are mostly obtained from large epidemiological studies that do not specifically address the issue. Consequently, there are only limited specific data on this theme.

This chapter summarizes the available specific information on the epidemiology and prevention of injuries sustained in physical education.

Incidence rates

In general, sports participation and consequently the number of sports injuries in young people have increased considerably in the last three decades. Nowadays, it is evident that despite the fact that the number of school children is declining in most European countries, there still is a general increase in sports accidents.[4] Unfortunately, data concerning injuries specifically incurred in PE lessons are scarce at present. Only a few studies on sports injuries in children and adolescents have outlined the incidence and types of injuries in PE lessons. Analogous to studies performed outside the school system, these studies suffer from a lack of comparability because of:[5]

(1) a lack of uniform definitions of sports injury;

(2) limited reliability of collected data;

(3) insufficient information on the population at risk; and

(4) insufficient information on the sports exposure time.

Furthermore, these investigations vary enormously in extent and depth. The scope of data gathered depends strongly on the methods of data acquisition, particularly on the locus of measurement.

Overall in the literature, studies on children and adolescents have rarely been population-based. Some were registrations in out-patient clinics or in casualty departments,[6,7] and other registrations were based on reports of PE teachers.[2,8] Probably the number of injuries that actually occur in PE classes is much higher than found in these studies, because many schools do not maintain good injury records.[2,3] Another problem arises when pupils themselves have to fill in a registration form. In addition, retrospective study designs introduce recall-bias resulting in under- or over-recording.

As a result of several differences in definitions of injury, the locus of measurement and the contents of the PE classes, it is not surprising that incidence rates of injuries sustained in PE classes vary between 0.75[9] and 11.7 per 100 school children per year.[10]

Obviously, diagnosis by medical staff or assessment by PE teachers and school-aged children themselves will affect results of studies on the incidence of injuries in PE classes considerably. It is clear that the medical system is aware of only a small and distorted segment of the total injury problem. In this context, reference is made to the well-known 'iceberg' phenomenon, discussed in Chapter 5.1. Therefore, the population approach to injury is preferable, as it allows considerable insight into the rate of occurrence, the causes of injury and the identification of high-risk groups.[11] The disadvantage of this approach is the registration of a large number of less severe injuries.

The very wide variety of activities during PE classes is another point of concern. If, despite these problems, one still attempts to compare injuries sustained in physical education, because each kind of sports activity has its own characteristics, one has to deal with important differences in sports specific risk factors. This will also affect the number of injuries sustained during PE classes.

Risk of injury

First of all, it is interesting to compare the risk of getting injured during PE classes with the risk during organized and non-organized sports. Tursz and Crost[5] stated that the frequency of accidents in out-of-school sports in France was much higher than for those in PE classes. This is in line with data from a population-based study in the Netherlands,[2] where sports injuries were also more likely to occur during the competition games of sports clubs rather than during PE classes or non-organized sports activities (Table 5.2.1; risk ratio = 1.75). Especially, the injuries sustained in organized sports matches led to more absence from physical education classes and to more medical consultation (risk ratios for both, 1.50). A comparison of year incidence rates per 1000 young athletes in organized sports and physical education is given in Table 5.2.2.

Table 5.2.1 Observed versus expected numbers[a] of injuries (risk ratios) according to the nature of sports participation[2]

Nature of sport	No. of school children	Risk ratio			
		All injuries	Injuries followed by non-attendance of		Injuries with medical consultation
			PE[b] classes	School	
PE	7468	0.63	0.97	1.05	0.66
Club training[c]	6458	1.04	0.99	0.76	1.05
Club match[c]	4439	1.75	1.50	1.11	1.50
Non-organized sports	4762	0.81	0.95	1.14	1.01
Total	23127	1	1	1	1

[a] Expected numbers are based on the injury rate: i.e. all injuries occurred in the total study population.
[b] Physical education.
[c] Pupils with 2, 3 memberships respectively are counted as 2, 3 persons, respectively. From Backx et al.[2]

The finding that the risk of injury in PE classes and non-organized sports is low relative to the number of exposure hours is explained mainly by the lower intensity of the physical exertion involved. Additionally, activities during PE lessons are mostly adapted to the abilities of the pupils,[4] which is in contrast to the common practice when participating in team sports.

PE lessons containing activities like gymnastic activities (specifically trampolining) and ball games (especially basketball) provoke most damage.[6,12] Rümmele[4] registered nationwide sports accidents in German schools. He found that three areas (ball games; apparatus gymnastics; athletics) accounted for 88% of all sports accidents registered in schools. In comparison with the preceding two decades, accidents from ball games had increased tremendously, while accidents arising from gymnastics and track-and-field had remained relatively constant. This trend has also been seen in other countries.[10]

Location of injury

Comparison of medically treated home, school and road accidents reveals that medically treated sports accidents have the highest proportion (43%) of upper limb injuries.[5] Naturally, the distribution of injuries relative to body area depends substantially on the activities programmed and instructed by the PE teachers. Figure 5.2.1 summarizes reported injuries by body area found in the study of Backx et al.[10] The distribution of injuries relative to body area and to category of sports activity revealed that PE classes gave rise to relatively more upper extremity injuries.

Based on the popularity of ball games in school, the ball is considered to be an important factor in sustaining a finger injury. Finger injuries are dominant with younger children, while ankle joint injuries occur more in older pupils.[4] This is in accordance with an injury registration in an Austrian hospital in which hand and finger injuries were most frequently treated.

Type of injury

The distribution of injury type in relation to PE classes shows no uniform pattern, which primarily is caused by the difference in injury definition, the locus of measurement and the type of activity.

Table 5.2.2 Incidence rates in organized sports with more than 15 participants

Sport	Incidence per 1000 hours practice	Sport	Incidence per 1000 hours games
Volleyball	6.7	Basketball	23
Handball	4.3	Handball	14
Martial arts	3.8	Korfball	12
Club gymnastics	3.6	Soccer	8
Korfball	3.4	Field hockey	7
Baseball	3.0	Baseball	3
Horseback riding	1.7	Ballet[a]	
Soccer	1.6	Track and field[a]	
Tennis	1.5	Martial arts[a]	
Swimming	1.2	Volleyball[a]	
Field hockey	1.2	Badminton[a]	
Track and field	1.0	Tennis[a]	
Basketball[a]		Swimming[a]	
Table tennis[a]		Table tennis[a]	
Badminton[a]		Horseback riding[a]	
Ice skating[a]		Ice skating[a]	
Ballet[a]		Club gymnastics[a]	
Dance[a]		Dance[a]	

[a] The incidence rate was not calculated for types of sport in which fewer than five sports injuries were registered in practice or games. From Backx et al.[10]

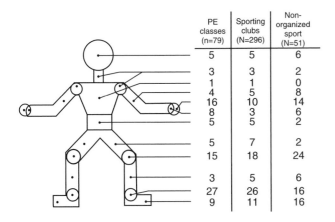

	PE classes (n=79)	Sporting clubs (N=296)	Non-organized sport (N=51)
	5	5	6
	3	3	2
	1	1	0
	4	5	8
	16	10	14
	8	3	6
	5	5	2
	5	7	2
	15	18	24
	3	5	6
	27	26	16
	9	11	16

Fig. 5.2.1 Distribution of 399 sports injuries involving 426 body areas (%) in school children (aged 8–17) related to sports activity category. From Backx et al.[2]

In studies using a broad injury definition, the fracture rate is low and most injuries are light contusions and sprains.[2] Measurements in hospitals have shown a different picture. Depending on the type of sport, the number of fractures varies between 15 and 60% of the total number of sports traumata.[7]

In the study of Backx et al.,[2] significantly more fractures or dislocations occurred in PE classes in comparison with out-of-school sports. Nearly all of these fractures were located at the upper limb. Also sprains, especially involving the ankle, did often occur, although less frequently than during organized sports.[2]

Besides acute macrotrauma, the importance of microtrauma and overuse injuries in children are still growing. The latter type of injury will not be described in the context of this chapter because the direct influence of PE classes on the origin of overuse injuries is unknown. Furthermore, it is important to realize that registrations of acute and chronic injuries sustained during PE classes in school will also include injuries that should primarily be attributed to biological growth. The magnitude of growth as an independent risk factor has yet to be confirmed.

Severity of injuries

It is obvious that a high incidence rate of sports injuries is no indicator of injury severity. Therefore, van Mechelen et al.[13] have distinguished six factors of importance to describe the severity of injuries in an efficient and practical manner. Using these factors, the following can be concluded concerning young athletes.

1. The nature of the sports injury

Very serious sports accidents in youth, e.g. brain or spinal cord damage, or lesions of the heart or submersion, leading to permanent handicap or death, are exceptional.[5] This is in correspondence with a Swedish study[14] in which only a few such injuries were registered, ranging from life-threatening to fatal, according to the Abbreviated Injury Scale (AIS severity codes 4, 5, 6). The AIS is commonly used to classify the severity of traffic accidents. Most of the injuries sustained in PE classes have to be coded as AIS 1 and 2. Sprains are considered the most common type of injury and the ankle the most frequently injured body area.

2. Nature and duration of treatment

From an epidemiological point of view, one may assume, according to the Backx et al. study,[10] that only 25% of all injuries registered call for medical attention from a general practitioner or a medical specialist. In that particular study, pupils who were injured in PE classes had to consult a medical doctor more frequently compared with those injured in other sports activities.

Watson[16] observed that 13% of injured Irish school children spent one or more days in a hospital. In two other studies concerning macro-trauma requiring medical care, the proportion of hospitalization was 10–11%. There is no consensus on the influence of age and gender on hospital admission.[5,12]

The type and duration of treatment in the case of sports injuries in school-aged children has not been analysed well, although there are indications that the claim on the health care system seems to be less than in adults.

3. Time lost from sport

The actual number of days elapsed until the athlete returns to sports activity is often reported as a measure of injury severity. Although van Mechelen et al.[13] stated that the length of sports absenteeism gives the most precise indication of the consequences of a sports injury to an athlete, this is questionable with regard to school-aged children. Bias can easily be introduced, caused by factors such as an individual's tolerance to pain, type of treatment, parents and coach. A time-loss definition of a sports injury is therefore not useful in studies that focus on non-organized sports and PE classes.

4. Work absenteeism

In the case of youngsters, injury severity in terms of work absenteeism must be transformed into school absenteeism. Similar to days off work, defining the severity of an injury by the amount of time lost in school is highly subjective, as it is with time lost from sports. Those estimates of injury severity are more practical rather than valid parameters.

This parameter was studied only in a Dutch study.[10] In general, most sports injuries found in this study were neither severe nor long-lasting and resulted in little loss of time from PE classes or school. Pupils who were injured in PE classes had more time loss of physical education and total school days in comparison with those whose injuries were sustained during club sports.

5. Permanent damage

Up to this moment there are no solid data available assessing the residual and long-term effects of injuries sustained in PE lessons. Zaricznyj et al.[12] recorded in school children participating in sports and physical education that 1.2% of the injured ones got a more severe injury, such as a compression fracture of the spine or a ruptured spleen, resulting in more or less permanent damage. Actually, it is rather difficult to predict correctly whether or not such injuries will be permanent.

6. Costs

Severity in terms of costs have to include the direct costs resulting from (para)medical treatment and also the indirect social costs (i.e. sick leave) to the injured pupil, his family and school.[13,14] The financial costs stemming from sports injuries in youth are not explored as a single category. Only rough calculations are known, being derived from figures concerning adults.

Aetiology

Usually the most important factors affecting sports injuries are divided in two main categories named internal and external factors (see Fig. 5.2.2). It is clear that injuries are mostly caused by a combination of factors.[2,12] Generally, it seems that internal factors, such as physical build, physical fitness, skills and joint stability are much more important than external factors such as the referee, the opponent or sports material.

It is noticeable that specific information on the aetiology and, consequently, on the prevention of sports injuries in school-aged children is minimal. Most of the investigations according to this target group do mention causes, but this information is primarily retrieved from the subject himself or is reconstructed by the coach or physician. For example, retrospective data from a population-based study revealed that most reported causes of sports injuries were falling/stumbling (24%), misstep/twist (22%) and kick/push (18%) induced by the child himself instead of by other pupils.[10] In the near future, more prospective data from observational studies have to be gathered in order to get more valid information, which can than be transferred into preventive measures.

Prevention

Injury prevention is a must, when everybody is proclaiming 'sports, a life-long activity', based on the potential benefits on health. One of the strategies in the battle against sports injuries is aimed at behaviour modification of the participants in sports.[15] Health education as a tool in realizing behavioural change can be implemented in the school's curriculum and, consequently, should be given by well educated teachers in physical education or biology.[18]

The need for the physical educator to become involved in the field of sports injury prevention may vary from one country to another, depending on the number of other groups of professionals working in the same area. In Table 5.2.3, some conditions are listed which determine the need for involvement in case of the PE teacher. The primary tasks of the physical educator must not be limited to a stimulating role in the development of skills and to applying preventive measures for safety in PE classes. The PE teacher should be, at a minimum, a message mediator, by educating school-aged children in practical and theoretical aspects of injury prevention. This kind of information will also be valuable for out-of-school sports activities. Although in this specific area the effects of health education still have to be proven, there are strong indications that in the short term it can be beneficial in reducing the number of sports injuries. The effects in the long run are only speculative.

In Holland a controlled experimental study, focused on students of a secondary school (12–18 years old), has been performed. In this study, 24 PE lessons and six biology lessons were given in injury prevention.[18] The practical topics instructed in PE classes included warming up, stretching exercises, cooling down, exercises for ankle stabilization and general coordination, and techniques to fall correctly. Those practical items were supported by theoretical information, instructed by teachers in biology. Additional education took place

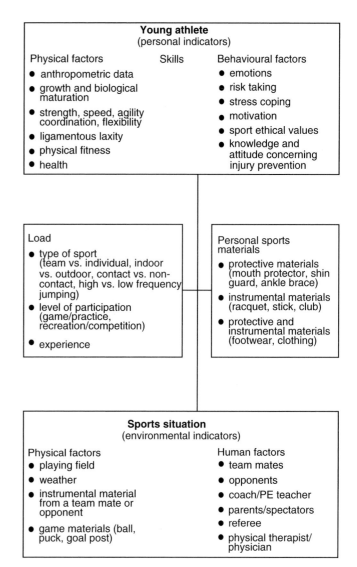

Fig. 5.2.2 Schematic expression of the most important risk indicators affecting sports injuries in youth. From Backx.[20]

Table 5.2.3 Aspects upon which the role of the PE teacher depends

- Creating an environment for safe and fair play[19]
- Checking appropriate equipment and good condition of the playing sites
- Screening of physical defects
- Qualification in sports medicine and injury prevention
- Public awareness

concerning adequate sporting shoes, protective materials and first aid in sports. In this study, success was achieved by clearly improving knowledge about injury prevention. This increase in knowledge led to an increase in attitude. Although the attitude change over the one-year period of follow-up was small, it nevertheless had a favourable influence on injury incidence, even though the explained variance was minimal. No reduction in the severity of sports injuries was seen. It can be speculated that if the intervention had been executed more frequently and for a longer period of time, the effectiveness of the educational programme would have been greater. Based on this study it was also recommended that the effects on the incidence should be monitored for a period longer than one year, because in health education, effects are particularly expected in the long term. Because the results of this health educational programme were very encouraging, it seems worthwhile to implement this kind of health educational intervention into the school's curriculum on a more regular basis. To do so, it is, however, necessary to compose a post-academic course for the teachers concerned, in order to optimize their role in the prevention of sports injuries.

References

1. Jüngst, B. K. Schulsport; Traume und Wirklichkeit. *Deutsche Zeitschrift fur Sportmedizin* 1991; **42**: 87.
2. Backx, F. J. G., Erich, W. B. M., Kemper, A. B. A. and Verbeek, A. L. M. Sports injuries in school-aged children; an epidemiologic study. *American Journal of Sports Medicine* 1989; **17**: 234–40.
3. Calvert, R. Jr. *Athletic injuries and deaths in secondary schools and Colleges, 1975–76.* National Center for Education Statistics, Washington, 1979.
4. Rümmele, E. Sports injuries in the Federal Republic of Germany. Part two. In *Council of Europe: Sport for all; Sports injuries and their prevention. Proceedings of the 2nd meeting* (ed. C. R. van der Togt, A. B. A. Kemper and M. Koornneef). National Institute for Sports Health Care, Oosterbeek, The Netherlands, 1987; 37–49.
5. Tursz, A. and Crost, M. Sports-related injuries in children. A study of their characteristics, frequency and severity, with comparison to other types of accidental injuries. *American Journal of Sports Medicine* 1986; **14**: 294–9.
6. Hammer, A., Schwartzbach, A. L. and Paulev, P. E. Children injured during physical education lessons. *Journal of Sports Medicine* 1981; **21**: 423–31.
7. Sahlin, Y. Sport accidents in childhood. *British Journal of Sports Medicine* 1990; **24**: 40–4.
8. Medved, R. and Pavisic-Medved, V. Causes of injuries during the practical classes on physical education in schools. *Journal of Sports Medicine and Physical Fitness* 1973; **13**: 32–41.
9. Pospiech, R. Analyse von 1.000 Unfällen beim Schulsport. *Medicine Sport* 1981; **21**: 78–82.
10. Backx, F. J. G., Beijer, H. J. M., Bol, E. and Erich, W. B. M. Injuries in high-risk persons and high-risk sports. A longitudinal study of 1,818 school children. *American Journal of Sports Medicine* 1991; **19**: 124–30.
11. Walter, S. D., Sutton, J. R., and McIntosh, J. M., *et al.* The aetiology of sports injuries: A review of methodologies. *Sports Medicine* 1985; **2**: 47–58.
12. Zaricznyj, B., Shattuck, L. J. M., Mast, T. A., Robertson, R. V. and D'Elia, G. Sports-related injuries in school-aged children. *American Journal of Sports Medicine* 1980; **8**: 318–24.
13. Mechelen, W. van, Hlobil, H. and Kemper, H. C. G. *How can sports injuries be prevented?* National Institute for Sports Health Care, Oosterbeek, The Netherlands, 1987.
14. Nathorst Westfelt, J. A. R. Environmental factors in childhood accidents. A prospective study in Götenborg, Sweden. *Acta Paediatrica Scandinavica* 1982; **291** (suppl): 6–61.
15. Kok, G. J. and Bouter, L. M. On the importance of planned health education. Prevention of ski injury as an example. *American Journal of Sports Medicine* 1990; **18**: 600–605.
16. Watson, A. W. S. *Sports injuries in Irish second-level schools during the school year 1984–85.* Department of Education, Dublin, 1986.
17. Watson, A. W. S. The role of the physical educator in the prevention of sports injuries. In *Council of Europe: Sport for all; Sports injuries and their prevention. Proceedings of the 2nd meeting* (ed. C. R. van der Togt, A. B. A. Kemper and M. Koornneef). National Institute for Sports Health Care, Oosterbeek, The Netherlands, 1987.
18. Backx, F. J. G. *Sports injuries in youth; Etiology and prevention (thesis).* Janus Jongbloed Research Center on Sports and Health, Utrecht, The Netherlands, 1991.
19. Stanitski, C. L. Pediatric and adolescent sports injuries athletes. *Clinics in Sports Medicine* 1997; **16**: 613–33.
20. Backx, F. J. G. Epidemiology of paediatric sports-related injuries. In *The Olympic book of sports medicine. Part 6. The child and adolescent athlete* (ed. O. Bar-Or). Blackwell Science, London, 1996; 163–72.

5.3 Aetiology and prevention of injuries in youth competition: contact sports

Evert A. L. M. Verhagen, Willem van Mechelen, Adam D. G. Baxter-Jones and Nicola Maffulli

Introduction

Chapters 5.1 and 5.4 have covered the theoretical framework regarding the aetiology and prevention of sports injuries, and the aetiology and prevention of injuries in non-contact youth competition sports has been addressed in chapter 5.4. This chapter will focus on sport specific injuries in contact sports. A number of sports where contact with the opponent is intentional or common have therefore been selected. Each sport is covered in a systematic way by describing some practical information concerning the particular sport, as well as the epidemiology and aetiology of sport specific injuries, and by giving facts about preventive strategies related to the latter.

In general, sports injuries in contact sports are more frequent than in non-contact sports.[1–4] One should, however, bear in mind that a large proportion of sports pathology is common to both contact and non-contact sports where similar movements are involved that potentially can lead to injury; e.g. running and cutting.

It should also be noted that for certain contact sports little information is available on children, and that, therefore, extrapolation from adult data has been used when appropriate. Taking this into consideration, the following chapter summarizes certain trends that can be drawn from the literature and that give a reasonable basis on which to develop and promote prevention strategies.

American football

American football, a violent collision and contact sport, has been one of the most popular sports in the United States within the past century, and has recently received support and increased participation from European nations. Given that football is a collision sport, it would be expected that most football injuries are acute, as opposed to overuse or gradual onset injuries.

To reflect the incidence and aetiology of American football injuries in youth athletes, most literature used describes high school football.

Epidemiology of American football injuries

With an increased number of athletes playing American football an increased number of football related injuries has been documented.[5] The US National Athletic Trainers Association (NATA)[7] found incidence rates of 8.2 injuries per 1000 athlete exposures for high school football. Another study shows that at high school level, injury incidence rates range from 11.8 to 81.1 per 100 players.[6] When keeping the same definition for injury, similar incidence rates are found in college football. A note of caution in interpreting such results is needed. Although rates of injuries per 100 players are frequently cited in the literature, they do not take into account the varying numbers of games and practice sessions taking place. The rate of re-injury has not been extensively studied, but a study in 1989 by the NATA[7] found that 10% of high school players' injuries were re-injuries to a previously hurt area.

Different studies regarding high school football[7–11] found that the three most commonly occurring types of injuries are sprains (ligaments), strains (muscles) and contusions. This result was fairly consistent across all the studies.

The head is particularly susceptible to injury (approximately 10% of all reported injuries),[12–15] with cerebral concussions (5%) as the most frequently occurring type of head injury.[12,16,17] Injuries to the upper extremities commonly occur in the game of American football (approximately 30% of all reported injuries). Of those, the most commonly reported cases concern the shoulders (9%) and the hands/fingers (10%).[7–11] From the lower extremities (approximately 50% of all reported injuries), the knee (18%) and ankle (12%) are particularly vulnerable to injury.[7–11]

Aetiology of American football injuries

Concussions may occur when the skull is put into motion before the contained brain. This occurs when a moving object strikes the head in a resting state, or when the head collides with a non-moving object.[13] Injuries to the cervical spine traditionally have been attributed to hyperflexion and/or hyperextension mechanisms.[18,19]

The shoulder is often the initial contact point in tackling and blocking.[6] The hand is vulnerable to injury because it is often used in direct contact against the facemask, the opponents' body, headgear and the shoulder pads.[6] Injuries to the fingers may occur as players grasp the opponent's pads, belts and jerseys while blocking and tackling.[6]

Normally knee motion is limited to internal and external rotation when the leg is in extension and flexion. Therefore injury to the knee may occur when the joint is stressed into unusual positions as the result of direct contact from other players. Non-contact injuries to the knee often involve unnatural twisting motions that prevent the natural rotation of the knee joint.

Intrinsic and extrinsic risk factors of football injuries described in the literature are listed in Table 5.3.1.

Table 5.3.1   Intrinsic and extrinsic risk factors for football injuries, with their respective references

Intrinsic risk factors	Extrinsic risk factors
Leg deficiencies[20–25]	Players position[30–33]
Body dimensions[24,26,27]	Lack of well-rounded full year conditioning[21,34]
Previous injuries[16,28,29]	Cleats[8]
	Playing surface[37,38]
	Equipment[39–41]

Leg deficiencies

There is evidence in the literature that lower extremity injuries may be the result of lower body strength imbalances and other leg deficiencies.[22] It is also believed that athletes with tight heel cords may be more susceptible to lower extremity injury.[23] Other researchers, however, have found contradicting evidence.[24,25] The role of leg deficiencies as a risk factor in injuries therefore is not totally clear.

Height, weight

There is a lack of statistical evidence with regards to the relationship between size, age, weight and height and football injuries.[24,26] It is also often debated that with children of the same calendar age, the less mature player has a greater risk of sustaining an injury due to the inequality in body dimensions. Lindner et al.,[27] however, found contradicting results, which they ascribed to more aggressive play by the more mature boys due to the advanced growth.

Previous injuries

Especially previous head injuries lead to a higher risk for future injuries to this body area.[16,28] There is also strong evidence that ankle sprains lead to chronic instability of the ankle, which will result in a higher risk of sustaining ankle sprains.[29]

Players' position

Research showed that defensive and offensive line players have the highest injury incidence,[33] possibly due to the fact that these players are involved in physical contact in every play. However, it is also stated that this high incidence in defensive and offensive line players is due to the fact that there are more line players on the field than other players.[32] When adjusting for exposure, running backs seem to be at the highest risk.[32]

Lack of well-rounded full year conditioning

Cahill and Griffith[34] found in an 8-year prospective study that pre-season conditioning of the total body decreased the incidence and severity of knee injuries throughout the season.

Cleats

Fixation of the foot through rigid cleating has been shown to be a primary factor in the production of lower extremity injuries, particularly of the knee/ankle.[8,35,36]

Playing surface

Grass and artificial surfaces produce similar injury rates; however, the most serious injuries occur on artificial turf.[37,38]

Equipment

Longitudinal research has shown that different helmets bring different concussion rates.[39] On the effectiveness of knee braces in the prevention of knee injuries, there is little agreement among researchers.[40,41] However, most of the contradiction between results stems from the variety in study designs and methodologies, which does not allow a proper comparison between study results.

Prevention of American football injuries

Blyth and Mueller[8] found that 1.7% of all football injuries were caused by defective, broken or ill-fitting equipment. It is also shown that the use of improper cleats is a primary factor in lower extremity injuries.[8,35,36] The use of proven protective equipment therefore needs to be an integral part of all football training programmes. For instance, facial and head injuries may be prevented through the use of properly fitting helmets and padded chin straps, which eliminate helmet rotation.[39] Additional padding and/or taping for ribs, arms, ankles and knees might help prevent some injuries. This additional protection can be individually applied depending on the athlete's position;[6] e.g. defensive and offensive linemen, who have continuously rough physical contact during play, require other additional protection than a wide receiver who sporadically gets extremely hard hits, but needs light protection to maintain speed and agility. Which additional protection should be used for which players' position is not known from the literature. Furthermore the use of additional protective equipment also relies on each player's individual preferences.

Blyth and Mueller[8] found that 3.8% of all injuries were caused by illegal acts. This enforces the belief that stricter enforcement of rules and proper rule awareness might go a long way towards prevention of injuries in general.

Year-round mandatory football-specific conditioning and training programmes should be aimed at improving muscular and ligament imbalances and weaknesses; coordination and timing; flexibility, mobility and agility. Cahill and Griffith[34] have already shown an effect of pre-season conditioning on an incidence reduction of knee injuries. It is maybe reasonable to assume an effect of this measure on other injuries.

Furthermore, a qualified sports medicine team needs to be an integral part of all football training programmes. According to Blyth and Mueller,[8] 2.4% of all injuries could have been prevented if adequate medical supervision covered games and practices. This should lead to early and effective diagnosis, evaluation and treatment of injuries. Proper medical supervision should also lead to better rehabilitation from an injury before returning to the game, resulting in fewer reinjuries.[6]

Boxing

Unlike any other sport, boxing is associated with the intentional affliction of traumatic brain injury; i.e. a concussion or knockout. Epidemiological investigations of boxing injuries have been limited both in quality and quantity. Especially with regard to youth in boxing, very little literature can be found. Therefore it is necessary to extrapolate the limited information there is about boxing injuries from adult boxers to youth boxers. When looking at boxing a problem also arises because of differences between professional and amateur boxing. Professional boxing is associated with a higher injury rate than amateur boxing. Youth boxers are predominantly amateur boxers, who often do not even participate in matches, but only participate in training sessions.

Epidemiology of boxing injuries

In Irish competition amateur boxing an injury incidence of 0.92 per man-hour of competition was reported.[46] In the literature, head injuries are described as the most common boxing injury, ranging from 27% to 93% of all injuries.[42–45] The great difference between studies is caused by the relatively flexible definition of head injury. Looking at cerebral injury, due to severe blows to the head, and facial injuries separately gives a clearer view. In Irish competition amateur boxing an incidence of 0.47 per man-hour of competition for cerebral injury was reported, followed by hand/wrist injuries (0.19 per man-hour of competition) and face/head injuries (0.19 per man-hour of competition).[46]

As mentioned youth boxers often only participate in practice sessions. Cerebral and facial injuries are less common during training bouts, where the emphasis lies on training of technique rather than on knocking down the opponent.[46] Therefore the incidence of chronic cerebral injury might be lower and less severe in youth boxers. However, acute cerebral damage might still be a common injury in youth boxers, but unfortunately there are no data on acute cerebral damage in youth boxers.

Facial injuries most often involve facial laceration[42,44] and the nose.[43] Injuries to ears and eyes are uncommon. Injuries to lips and teeth are also rare due to the compulsory wearing of mouth guards. Injury to the spine/trunk are less frequent in boxing and comprise only 2% to 16% of all boxing injuries.[42–45]

Aetiology of boxing injuries

A bout finishing with a knock-out is much rarer in amateur boxing, where the emphasis is on technical superiority and not on power, than in professional boxing.[47] Furthermore, in amateur boxing, the boxer is protected by strict rules which should prevent him from getting serious chronic cerebral injury. Acute cerebral injuries result from intracranial bleeding, caused by a blow to the head. A blow to the head accelerates the head, but there is a delay in the brain following the head movement, which can rupture blood vessels on the surface of the brain.[48]

The incidence of hand injuries in amateur boxing is high. Most hand injuries are related to the execution of blows and/or the vulnerability of the thumb. The thumb is isolated from the other fingers in the glove, which makes it prone to forced abduction on impact.[46] The amateur boxer is only allowed to use a single encircling piece of tape and soft surgical bandages to protect the hands in competition. Shoulder injuries are the result of repetitive and forceful delivery of punches.[49]

Facial abrasions and cuts are relatively common in adult boxing despite the use of headgear. This is because the goal of boxing is the intentional affliction of traumatic brain injury, which is achieved by giving blows to the opponents' head. Lower extremity injuries occur more frequently during training and are likely to include overuse injuries associated with jogging and jumping rope.[49]

The intrinsic and extrinsic risk factors of boxing injuries described in the literature are listed in Table 5.3.2.

Table 5.3.2 Intrinsic and extrinsic risk factors for boxing injuries, with their respective references

Intrinsic risk factors	Extrinsic risk factors
Boxing skills[50,51]	Sparring[43,52]
	Exposure[52,53]

Boxing skills

Intuitively one would expect that more experienced boxers are able to protect themselves better against hard and repetitive blows due to better defensive skills. Research has also shown that there is a positive correlation between lost bouts and chronic brain damage.[50,51] This is only proven for professional boxers but can most likely be extrapolated to youth boxers.

Sparring (i.e. non-competitive boxing)

The absolute number of injuries is higher during sparring, but the incidence is higher for competitive boxing.[43] This reflects the longer duration of time spent on sparring compared to active competition. The hypothesis that an increased exposure to head blows during sparring increases the risk for brain injury has not been confirmed in epidemiological studies.[52] Since no information on total sparring time for youth boxers was found in the literature, nothing can be said about the influence of this risk factor on injuries in youth boxing.

Exposure

This applies more to older boxers instead of youth boxers, as it seems there is a only a correlation between injury and longer periods of boxing, e.g. 10 years or 150 fights. It is proven that the total number of boxing contests, both amateur and professional, are associated with impaired neuropsychological test performance.[52,53]

Prevention of boxing injuries

It is believed that the only way to prevent cerebral injuries, acute as well as chronic injuries, is to change the rules such that they prohibit blows to the head.[54,55] This, however, conflicts with the nature of the game. Preventive strategies more in accordance with the game, might be a well-trained ringside physician, whose duties include pre-fight medical and neurological examinations, injury surveillance during boxing competitions, and post-fight evaluations of suspected injuries.[49]

The monitoring and rehabilitation of injuries is important. A physician should allow injuries to be fully rehabilitated before the boxer re-enters the boxing ring. Length of suspensions following injury or knockout as proposed by the New York State Athletic Commission go some way towards solving this problem. Physicians should be encouraged to apply these suspensions.[49]

It is also suggested that the floor of the ring should be sufficiently shock absorbent to reduce the risk of cerebral damage from head contact in a fall.[48] The floor should, however, not be too soft, since this hastens fatigue, which for instance results in a diminished concentration and a decreased defence.

Soccer

Soccer is considered by many as the most popular game all over the world and is played by at least 40 million people. Many studies have been done to determine the injury pattern in soccer, but only few have been taken prospectively in young players. Several factors combine to make studies of injury in young soccer players important and necessary. The first is the extent of participation in youth soccer, in 1990 it was estimated that more than 6 million youth players under 12 played on a team in the US,[56] while soccer is even more popular in Europe. Second, there is an increased intensity of participation of youth players; some youth players nowadays play whole year round by combining outdoor and indoor soccer. These two factors combine to give a dramatic increase in exposure to injury risk in young soccer players.

Epidemiology of soccer injuries

A four-year prospective study of youth soccer injuries has shown rates of 23.8 per 10 000 player hours.[56] More specifically, 3.4 injuries per player per 1000 hours were found for 12–13 year old players; 3.8 injuries per player per 1000 hours were found for 14–15 year old players; and 4.0 injuries per player per 1000 hours were found for 16–17 year old players.[57] Indoor soccer showed similar injury rates.[58] Sullivan and Gross[59] found player injury rates of 1/100 players in outdoor soccer for under-10 year old players, whereas for under-19 year old players this rate was 7.7 per 100 players.

The same study by Sullivan and Gross[59] concluded that goalies accounted for 17.6% of all injuries, while only comprising 6% of the study population; and females, comprising 27% of the study population, accounted for 44% of all injuries. This difference in injury risk relative to sex and position, is supported by another study of outdoor soccer by Nilsson and Roas.[60] In contrast to outdoor soccer the injury rates of male and female players seem to be similar in indoor soccer.[58]

The lower extremity is the most prevalent site of injury in traumatic injuries; with the thigh and hip area as the most common sites of injury (approximately 45% of all injuries), followed by the ankle (approximately 19% of all injuries) and knee (approximately 16% of all injuries).[56,61] Injuries to arm, groin, lower leg and back are also commonly seen in youth players.[59] Relatively low-grade injuries such as strains and sprains (approximately 50% of all injuries) are the most common injuries, while more serious injuries such as fractures (approximately 7% of all injuries) and meniscal injuries (approximately 4% of all injuries) are less frequent.[56,61] Similar percentages of types of injuries are also found in indoor soccer.[58]

Aetiology of soccer injuries

As would be expected in a contact sport, most of the injuries result from direct contact with other players.[56] Hip and thigh contact is frequent during play, in an attempt to push the opponent away from the ball.

The nature of the game of soccer, in which players make hard cuts, sharp turns off a planted foot, and intense contact with the ball and other players, makes players specifically vulnerable to lower extremity injury.[62] Normally knee motion is limited to internal and external rotation when the leg is in extension and flexion. Therefore injury to the knee may occur when the joint is stressed into unusual positions as the result of direct contact from other players. Non-contact injuries to the knee often involve unnatural twisting motions that prevent the

natural rotation of the knee joint, e.g. kicking the ball which forces rotation in the foot that is planted to the ground. Contact with the ground accounts for the highest number of ankle injuries, mostly ankle inversion sprains.[56] In youth players more upper extremity injuries are found than in adult players. This may be explained by the fact that younger players are not very well coordinated when they try to keep their balance, and thus fall, trying to seek support from the upper extremity.[57]

Head injuries are usually caused when a player heads the ball, when a forcefully striked ball strikes the head, or when two players attempt to head the ball simultaneously and collide head-to-head.[62] Common soccer head injuries resulting from these mechanics include lacerations and concussions.

The higher incidence in outdoor youth female soccer players is attributed to the females' unfamiliarity and inferior technical skills when compared with males of the same age.[63,64]

The intrinsic and extrinsic risk factors of soccer injuries described in the literature are listed in Table 5.3.3.

Age

In younger age groups, Keller et al.[66] documented a higher incidence of upper extremity, head and face injuries. It is believed this higher incidence is due to more frequent falls on outstretched hands, increased fragility of the upper extremity epiphyses, insufficient expertise in heading the ball, mechanical weaknesses of growing dental tissue, increased ball-weight to head-weight ratio, and illegal ball contact. Adolescents who lag behind in skeletal maturity are also at greater risk than 'normal' competitors.[65]

Previous injury

Players with a history of ankle sprains are at 2.3 times greater risk for ankle injuries.[67] The same trend in ankle injuries was found by Nielsen and Yde,[68] who found that 56% of all ankle injuries occurred in players with a history of ankle sprains. In general, it can be concluded that sprains of the lower extremity and overuse injuries are the most common injuries, and persistent symptoms are commonly seen after those injuries.[29]

Gender

It is believed that the females' unfamiliarity and inferior technical skills, compared with males of the same age, in youth soccer leads to the found higher injury rate in females.[63,64,66]

Exposure

Teams with a higher practice-to-game ratio have fewer injuries, likely due to superior physical conditioning.[69] There seems to be no difference between injury occurrence and level of play.[70]

Table 5.3.3 Intrinsic and extrinsic risk factors for soccer injuries, with their respective references

Intrinsic risk factors	Extrinsic risk factors
Age[65,66]	Exposure[69,70]
Previous injury[29,67,68]	Players' position[66,71]
Gender[63,64,66]	Playing surface[72–74]

Players' position

A prospective study by Keller et al.[66] reported no significant differences between injury rates of players in different positions. In contrast to these results, Jörgensen[71] found, in a retrospective study, a significant difference in injury incidence between players' positions. Goalkeepers and defenders sustained more injuries than attackers.

Playing surface

The rate of injury on artificial surfaces is higher than on natural surfaces.[73,74] There is also a difference in injury patterns between playing on natural surfaces and artificial surfaces.[72] More injuries affecting midfielders, injuries in tackling and sliding, and more abrasions occur on artificial surfaces.

Prevention of soccer injuries

Watson[75] found a relation between body mechanics defects and the incidence of certain kinds of sports injuries in senior Irish soccer. Teams with a higher practice-to-game ratio have fewer injuries, likely due to superior physical conditioning.[69] Youth specific conditioning and training programmes aimed at improving muscular and ligament imbalances and weaknesses, coordination and timing, flexibility, mobility and agility, therefore are likely able to reduce the incidence of injuries in youth soccer players who regularly compete at a high level.

An important role in injury prevention lies with the referee. Interviewed players in a study by Cattermole et al.[76] believed that their injury could have been prevented if there had been tighter referee control of the game. Many injuries in soccer occur during tackling and contact with an opposing player.[77] A good referee needs to keep the game under tight control, and must not allow dangerous behaviour on the field.[56] An important role in reducing on-field aggressiveness also lies with the coaches. Coaching within the spirit as well as the letter of soccer laws, so that jersey pulling, deliberate 'take downs' and tackling from behind are not condoned, should be emphasized, since these actions often lead to injuries in youth soccer.[56]

Since females seem to be at more risk of injury, adjustment in playing conditions may need to be explored.[56] Possibilities for adjustments might be ball size, closeness of refereeing and physical conditioning. From studies on brain injury in soccer,[79–81] it is suggested that the ball weight is constant and related to body weight. This implies the use of lighter balls in youth female soccer. Furthermore, it is suggested that soccer players should be advised not to head a ball that is travelling at 'high' velocity; and balls that are too hard or have become heavy with rain-water should be banned.

Proper field policing, including elimination of holes and sharp objects and removal of bags and chairs from the perimeter of the field, should be routine. Protective padding of the goal posts has also been shown to be effective in reducing injuries.[78] The use of shin guards is effective as protection against abrasions, contusions and lacerations. It is believed that further development in shin guard technology could also prevent low impact energy injuries.[76]

Martial arts

Oriental martial sports have become increasingly popular in the west. Tournaments are not only organized for adult participants, but also for young athletes. Despite this interest in martial sports, research on the epidemiology of martial sports injuries is scarce and in some cases even non-existent.

In this section epidemiology, aetiology and prevention of judo, karate and taekwondo injuries will be discussed. These three forms of martial sports offer the majority of injury data.

In non-contact karate competitions, which is the most performed form of karate in youth, rough and uncontrolled contact with the trunk and all contacts to face, head and neck are completely forbidden. In contrast to karate, taekwondo is mostly performed as a full contact sport by youth. At tournaments competitors wear protective equipment: head gear, a chest and abdomen protector, a groin guard, and shin and forearm guards. As in boxing a fight can be won by knockout or on points. Judo involves no punching or kicking; judo techniques have their goal in working the opponent to the ground. This also involves physical contact but in another way than in karate and taekwondo. Competitors of all three forms of martial sports compete in divisions according to age, gender, experience and weight.

Epidemiology of martial arts injuries

In Switzerland an injury incidence of 2.3 injuries per 10 000 hours of exposure was found for both male and female youth judo athletes.[82] Another study involving judo resulted in incidence rates of 122.6 injuries per 1000 athlete exposures for males, and 130.6 injuries per 1000 athlete exposures for females.[83] More detailed information on judo injuries is given by Kujala et al.,[84] unfortunately they used an injury rate that makes their data not comparable with other studies. Overall they found a lower injury rate for athletes under 15 years, than for athletes between the ages of 15 and 19. A higher proportion of injuries occurred in female athletes for both age groups.

In Finland an incidence of 0.28 injuries per bout was found in the national karate competitions.[85] Injuries were most common, however, in bouts between male adults. Buckley[86] found an incidence rate of 46.0 injuries per 1000 athlete exposures in adult karate. No exact injury incidence rates of youth karate in particular were found in the literature. Kujala et al.[84] found overall a lower injury rate for athletes under 15 years, than for athletes between the ages of 15 and 19. A higher proportion of injuries occurred in female athletes for both age groups.

In a prospective study of youth taekwondo, Oler et al.[87] found a rate of 3.4 injuries per 100 athletes in one tournament; this study included both males and females. Another study reported an injury incidence of 58.2 injuries per 1000 athlete exposures in male youth athletes; and an incidence rate of 56.6 injuries per 1000 athlete exposures in female youth athletes.

It is not possible to compare the incidence rates of the different martial sports, due to differences in incidence calculations between studies.

In judo, distortions seem to have the highest incidence in youth male athletes (1.0 per 10 000 hours of exposure), followed by contusions (0.5 per 10 000 hours of exposure), fractures (0.4 per 10 000 hours of exposure) and luxations (0.2 per 10 000 hours of exposure).[82] The same trend was found for youth female athletes. Most injuries involve the upper extremities (45%), followed by the lower extremity (30%) and the head/spine/trunk (25%).[83] Kujala et al.[84] found sprains and strains to be the most frequently occurring type of injury in judo, followed by bruises and wounds; however, they did not mention youth and adult, and male and female athletes separately.

In adult male karate, contusions seem to account for 66% of all injuries, lacerations for 12%, concussions for 10% and epistaxis for 10%.[88] No information on this is available for youth male and female karate, but it seems reasonable to assume that the same trend can be seen there. As in judo, Kujala *et al.*[84] found sprains and strains to be the most frequently occurring type of injury in karate, followed by bruises and wounds.

In taekwondo 82% of all injuries involve sprains, strains or injuries to other soft tissue. The upper or lower leg is the most injured body part (35%), presumably due to the high number of kicks during a match. Injuries to the ankle and foot (16%), head (10%), shoulder (10%) and back (11%) are also commonly seen in taekwondo.[89]

Aetiology of martial arts injuries

Little information on the aetiology of martial arts injuries is available in the literature. Most information comes from case studies. Strangulation, a common occurrence in judo, is a major cause of brain damage; it could lead for instance to subdural haematoma[90] and reduced regional blood flow.[91] Cerebral concussions in karate occur as a result of blows to the head and the neck.[92] Spinning kicks are related to cervical spine injuries.[92] Punches, however, are the lead injury mechanism in karate,[93] accounting for the large amount of contusions. All head and neck injuries in taekwondo are due to kicks.[94]

Fractures in the upper extremity are mostly due to improper falling techniques.[95] Being thrown on the shoulder and poorly executed breakfalls are important mechanisms of injury to the upper extremity.[96,97] In karate, detrimental change and, less often, loss of flexion in the dominant wrist were found.[98]

Since taekwondo has the same goal as boxing it is believed that a majority of taekwondo injuries have the same aetiology as boxing injuries, especially when looking at head injuries.

The intrinsic and extrinsic risk factors of martial arts injuries described in the literature are listed in Table 5.3.4.

Physical characteristics

Age is positively related to the injury prevalence rate.[99] In young males competing at taekwondo, an increased body weight might be a risk factor for injuries, this is not the case for young females.[99]

Skill level

Skill level and flexibility have been implicated in 80% of ruptures and 76% of sprains.[100] In various studies it was found that injury prevalence increases with an increased skill level, while in other studies the contrary was found. Differences in study design, injury definition and populations might account for these contrasting results.

Table 5.3.4 Intrinsic and extrinsic risk factors for martial arts injuries, with their respective references

Intrinsic risk factors	Extrinsic risk factors
Physical characteristics[99]	Exposure[103,104]
Skill level[100]	Equipment[105,106]
Technique[78,101,102]	Opponent[107,108]

Technique

Lack of refined technique may contribute to injury.[87] It is believed that poor fist technique leads to hand fractures in karate and taekwondo.[101,102]

Exposure

The number of bouts fought and repetitive sub-concussive blows to the head could be more related to brain damage than knockouts.[103,104] No data exist, however, that can substantiate this.

Equipment

Although protective equipment may not reduce the chances of brain damage, it will certainly decrease the occurrence of other injuries.[105] No research has been conducted on the protective effect of the helmet and chest protector worn in taekwondo. Some evidence exists that the chest protector may do a better job in absorbing energy from rotational kicks compared with thrust kicks.[106]

Opponent

Receiving a blow is a major injury mechanism in taekwondo.[107] In judo, improper throwing techniques by the opponent are among the major injury mechanisms.[108]

Prevention of martial arts injuries

Referees should have a proper amount of competition experience to better assess the nature of blows being exchanged in the ring and other aspects of the bout.[109] Furthermore, illegal moves should be penalized immediately and bouts interrupted if injuries are imminent.[92]

Athletes and coaches should be made aware of the potential injury risks of martial sports and should be taught not to enter competition prematurely.[87] Athletes should also learn that improper attitude is a risk for injuries; the 'macho' athlete will likely receive and, no less important, deliver avoidable injuries.[110]

Caution by athletes, as well as coach and referee, during strangulation in judo may help prevent injuries and even fatalities.[111] It is recommended that on beginning karate or taekwondo athletes should not be allowed to engage in free exchange of blows.[87] Modification of the rules in karate and taekwondo, which presently allow blows to the head, might help to reduce serious injuries to this body part, e.g. cerebral concussions.

Ice hockey

Ice hockey combines high skating speeds, individual flare for stick handling and accurate puck shooting with team play. It enjoys an enthusiastic worldwide following and is played by all ages. The American Academy of Pediatrics classifies ice hockey as a collision sport with intentional high-energy body contact.[112] The potential for injury is always present in ice hockey, and where intentional collision is allowed, injury rates have increased and the distribution of injury location and frequency has changed.

Epidemiology of ice hockey injuries

Roberts *et al.*[113] studied injury rates in American youth ice hockey tournaments for different age groups. They found incidences of

57.9 injuries per 1000 player hours for 12 to 13 year old males; 42.7 injuries per 1000 player hours for 14 to 15 year old males; 64.8 injuries per 1000 player hours for 15 to 19 year old males in high school; and 44.8 injuries per 1000 player hours for 15 to 19 year old males in the junior gold competition. For females no injuries were found in competition play. Stuart and Smith[114] studied incidence rates for different age groups in ice hockey practice. They found very low incidence rates in practice (from 1.2 injuries per 1000 player-practice hours in 10–11 year old males, to 3.9 injuries per 1000 player-practice hours in 15–19 year old males) compared with injury rates in competition (96.1 injuries per 1000 player-game hours in 15–19 year old males).

From the literature it was impossible to find a single approximation for the incidence rate of ice hockey injuries. This can be related to various factors: some types of soft tissue injuries may not be reported at all times and in all studies; various leagues have different rules regarding protective equipment that might prevent injury; and incidence rates differ between games and practices, while most studies do not stratify for this fact.[115]

Overall contusions are the most frequent type of injury in youth ice hockey, 60% of all injuries according to Roberts et al.,[113] followed by concussions, strains and sprains, and lacerations and fractures. In adult ice hockey, strains and sprains seem to be the most common type of injury.[116] In youth ice hockey, the head and neck appear to be the most frequently injured body parts.[113,114] The leg and arm, however, are also body parts that frequently sustain an injury.

Aetiology of ice hockey injuries

A considerable number of injuries are localized at the face, predominantly lacerations caused by the opponent's stick or less often by the puck.[117] The same mechanism can cause harmless facial wounds, facial fractures, or severe eye injuries resulting in blindness.[118]

The types of head injuries that may occur in ice hockey encompass the entire range, from a mild concussion to a progressive neurosurgical emergency such as an epidural trauma.[118] Most concussions occur from player collisions and rarely from the blow of the puck.

Injuries to the neck, shoulder and arms are regularly caused by collisions with an opponent's stick, the boards, the goalposts or other players by aggressive checking.[119,120] However, most of these injuries are classified as 'minor'.[119,120]

Injuries to the lower extremity predominantly involve soft tissues. The groin is a very common site of muscle strain, because the main thrust of the skating stride involves a forceful contraction of the hip adductor muscles.[118] Contusions of the thigh are common and can occur from direct trauma when a player strikes a goalpost or an opponent's knee. Knee injuries often involve sprains of the collateral ligaments, but disruption of the anterior cruciate ligament also can occur.[118] Ankle sprains are uncommon in ice hockey, due to the stiff protective skate boot. The sharp skate blade, however, can cause tendon and vessel lacerations at the level of the ankle.

The intrinsic and extrinsic risk factors of ice hockey injuries described in the literature are listed in Table 5.3.5.

Physical characteristics

A relation between body weight, height and grip strength with force of impact generated by a body check has been observed.[121,122] Other studies, in youth ice hockey, did not find this relation.[123]

Table 5.3.5 Intrinsic and extrinsic risk factors for ice hockey injuries, with their respective references

Intrinsic risk factors	Extrinsic risk factors
Physical characteristics[121–123]	Aggressive play[121,124,125]
	Equipment[121,122,126,127]

Aggressive play

Over 55% of injuries are attributed to contact with an opponent,[121] these injuries include sprains, strains, contusions, ruptures and fractures. Aggressive play, which involves large amounts of body contact, is seen by many authors as an extrinsic risk factor for ice hockey injuries.[124,125]

Equipment

It has been proven in various studies that proper use of available protective equipment can substantially reduce the incidence of injuries.[121,122,126,127]

Prevention of ice hockey injuries

Brust et al.[128] showed that only half of the 12–15 year old players understood the seriousness of checking another player from behind. The coach has the power to minimize this dangerous attitude by emphasizing the magnitude of the serious injury this move can inflict.

It is also suggested referees are more hesitant to call penalties, because referees share the same stance as players; who might have a feeling of invulnerability due to the protective equipment worn.[129] Some coaches may also share this feeling of invulnerability and may attempt to stretch the rules and instruct players to break them to gain advantage. Most concussions occur from player collisions and referees must be vigilant for checks from behind and checks after more than two strides.[130] The fact that only 8% of injuries are associated with a penalty suggests that referees may presently allow dangerous play.[117]

Mandatory use of visors is presently being introduced into Swedish youth ice hockey, because it is believed to significantly reduce the incidence of facial injuries.[117] The positive effect of mandatory visors on facial injury reduction has already been shown in American junior ice hockey.[114]

Muscle strains involving hip flexor, adductor and lumbar paraspinal muscles correspond to the posture and biomechanics of skating, which places these muscle groups at risk. Stretching programmes that focus on the hip flexor, adductor and lumbar paraspinal musculature may help decrease the incidence of these strains.[114,131]

Basketball

Basketball has long been considered as a non-contact sport, but has nowadays evolved to a game where contact is an inevitable part of the game. Modern basketball is an intense fast-paced game that involves jumping, hard cuts, sharp turns off a planted foot, and intense contact with the ball and other players. Basketball continues to grow in popularity and has participants at all levels of play; and as the number of players increases, so do the number of injuries. Much of the data related to basketball are found in studies comparing various sports.

Epidemiology of basketball injuries

In Swiss youth athletes, an incidence rate of 3.5 injuries per 10 000 hours of exposure was found[82] for males, for females this rate was 4.9 injuries per 10 000 hours of exposure. Since most of the data related to basketball injury incidence are found in studies comparing various sports, not much can be said about the exact incidence rates of males' and females' basketball. Review articles, however, have suggested that males have lower injury rates in basketball than females.[132,133]

In high school male and female basketball, sprains and strains appear to be the most frequent types of injury, accounting for, respectively, 34% and 23% of all injuries.[84,134] Contusions (13% of all injuries) and fracture (10% of all injuries) are also commonly occurring injury types. The lower extremity is the most frequently injured body part (55% of all injuries), followed by the upper extremity (20% of all injuries) and the head (10% of all injuries).[84,135]

From the lower extremity the ankle is the body part most susceptible to injury (31% of all injuries).[84,135] Presumably accounting for the high rate of sprains. The fingers are the most vulnerable part of the upper extremity (11% of all injuries).[84,135] However, injuries to knee, wrist, teeth and back are also not uncommon in basketball.

Aetiology of basketball injuries

Ankle sprains are the most common injuries in basketball. This is due to the high jumping frequency and sharp turns needed to play the game. When jumping there is a great chance of landing on an opponent's foot causing an ankle inversion sprain.[84]

The fingers and wrist are the most commonly injured upper extremity body parts. The proximal interphalangeal joint is the most frequently sprained and dislocated joint in the hand.[136] These result from hyperextension and are usually associated with volar rupture and sparring of the collateral ligaments.[136] This can easily be associated with the inherent nature of the game of constant and aggressive contact with the ball. The majority of ocular injuries sustained in basketball are due to blunt trauma from fingers and elbows of other players.[137]

The intrinsic and extrinsic risk factors of basketball injuries are difficult to assess and are not well presented in the literature.[137] Identifying risk factors in basketball is an extremely complicated problem requiring a large amount of data. There are some small studies in youth that showed some insight into injury risk factors. These studies, however, presented insufficient data to give substantial evidence that any parameter is a clear injury risk factor.

Prevention of basketball injuries

As with any sport, a pre-season conditioning programme is thought to be indicated in preventing a certain number of injuries.[137] Throughout the season a continued condition maintenance programme should lead to less fatigue during the game and intuitively to less abnormal stresses on the lower extremity joints. Therefore a continued conditioning programme might be able to prevent overuse syndromes and injuries.

Since the majority of ocular injuries sustained in basketball are due to blunt trauma from fingers and elbows of other players, protective eyewear is believed to help prevent ocular injury.[137]

Evidence about the effectiveness of braces and/or tape on reduction of the risk for ankle and knee injury exists.[20,22,23] The use of these preventive methods, however, is not well tolerated by the athletes, who believes it restricts their movement and therefore reduces their impact on the game.

Wrestling

Wrestling is a popular sport at both the youth and high school level. Most of its popularity is ascribed to the fact that athletes of all sizes and ages can compete in the sport, although the majority of wrestlers are male. There are three different styles of wrestling and each style requires similar training techniques despite the differences in competition. The competitive season is long and practices are frequent, long and intense. Furthermore in wrestling there is contact 100% of the time, which increases the effective exposure period. Therefore although wrestlers are at the same risks for injury as other contact sport athletes, the exposure for an individual wrestler is high.

Epidemiology of wrestling injuries

The National Collegiate Athletic Association[138] prospectively studied injury incidence rates in wrestling at college level over a period of 8 months. An injury incidence of 9.41 injuries per 1000 athlete exposures was found. Similar results at the same level of wrestling were found by Powell;[139] 9.5 injuries per 1000 athlete exposures. In high school wrestling, lower incidence rates of 7.6 injuries per 1000 athlete exposures were found.[140] Each of these studies defined injury as requiring that participation was restricted for one or more days. Athlete exposure was defined as each opportunity for an athlete to get hurt. This makes the data of these studies comparable, and makes it reasonable to assume a lower injury incidence in high school wrestling in general compared with college wrestling.

The incidence rate in practice is lower than in competitions. In high school, incidence rates were found of 6.45 injuries per 1000 athlete exposures in practice, versus 11.6 injuries per 1000 athlete exposures in competition.[140] At college mean rates were found of 7.4 injuries per 1000 athlete exposures in practice, versus 29 injuries per 1000 athlete exposures in competition.[138,139]

In general, the most commonly reported injuries in wrestling are strain and sprain injuries, accounting for approximately 15% and 28% of all injuries.[138,140] Infections are also commonly encountered problems in wrestling. Infections, like impetigo, folliculitis or herpes simplex, do not seem like injuries at first sight, but they make the athlete to have to stop wrestling for a period of time. Fractures and contusions are also relatively common.

Aetiology of wrestling injuries

Injuries to the head, mainly concussions, are mainly caused by head–knee or head–head collisions during takedowns; i.e. working the opponent to the ground. Concussions can also be caused by contact with the mat.[141] Sprains and strains in the neck region are frequently encountered in wrestling.[142] This injury can occur when a wrestler drives the opponent with his neck and hyperextends it. Auricular haematoma or cauliflower ear result from direct trauma to the ear. This can occur from impact with an opponent's head or knee, or by abrasive friction-causing forces.[141] Lower back injuries commonly occur during takedowns. During a match wrestlers pull and push with the lumbar spine in mild hyperextension. This extension together with twisting results in injuries.[142] Low-back injury, however, may also

Table 5.3.6 Intrinsic and extrinsic risk factors for wrestling injuries, with their respective references

Intrinsic risk factors	Extrinsic risk factors
Body weight[141,144,145]	Exposure[147,148]
Fatigue[141,146,147]	Environment[141,147,149]
Psychosocial characteristics[147]	Protective equipment[141,150]

result from overuse. Chest injuries can be caused in different ways, from direct trauma during takedowns or when direct pressure is applied (i.e. 'bear hug').[141]

Shoulder injuries can be caused when being thrown on the mat from a standing position. The wrestler may attempt to break his fall with an extended arm, imparting force to the shoulder girdle; if unable to extend the arm, the fall is taken directly on the shoulder.[141,142] Elbow injuries are less frequent than shoulder injuries, but are commonly more severe.[143]

Lower extremity injuries are usually caused by the moves used in different wrestling manoeuvres. When a move is not executed correctly or when the opponent makes a countermove, unnatural twisting and stretching of ligaments might occur, resulting in injuries.[141] For instance, meniscus injuries occur frequently via a twisting injury to a weight bearing extremity, and a varus or valgus force to the weight-bearing extremity is commonly the cause of collateral ligament sprains. The same goes for ankle injuries. When, for instance, a wrestler attempts to throw his opponent he rises onto his toes and twists. Loss of balance will cause the wrestler to invert his ankle.

The intrinsic and extrinsic risk factors of wrestling injuries described in the literature are listed in Table 5.3.6.

Body weight

Wrestlers with higher body weights are injured more often; possibly due to the greater forces exerted by heavier wrestlers.[141] The 'weight class system' reduces the risk of injury by reducing discrepancies in weight, size and strength between athletes. This makes it beneficial for a wrestler to lose weight prior to a match in order to fight a weaker opponent.[144,145] This rapid weight loss can be a risk factor for injury in itself, but also the weaker of the two wrestlers has a greater risk for injury.

Fatigue

The exact role of fatigue on injuries in wrestling is not totally clear, mainly due to variety in injury definition and differences in data collection between studies. Overall, studies have shown a higher rate of injuries in the second period of wrestling matches.[146,147] The injury rates are skewed, however, due to the termination of matches after a fall, resulting in lower exposure in the second and third periods of matches. The higher rate of injury in the second period is possibly the result of the initiation of fatigue together with a relatively high exposure.[141]

Psychosocial characteristics

It has been shown for recurrence of knee injuries that compliance to medical advice by the wrestler has an effect on injury.[147] It is not known if this is also true for other injuries.

Exposure

Injury rates increase with an increase in level of wrestling. Injury rates in matches also are higher than in training, due to the higher intensity of matches. Takedowns appear to be manoeuvres that account for most injuries,[147,148] and are common manoeuvres in matches.

Environment

Most injuries occur early in the season.[147,149] At this time in the season athletes are more motivated to get starting roles and to become a member of the team.[141] Another important factor is the conditioning of the athlete, which has not yet reached an optimum. The environment of the wrestling room is also an important factor for injury; e.g. shock absorbency of the mats, cleanliness of the mats, or obstacles near the mats.

Protective equipment

The effect of headgear on a decrease of injury has been shown in wrestling.[150] The role of other protective equipment, e.g. kneepads, shoes or mouth guards, has not been evaluated.[141] In other sports, however, these measures have been effective in preventing injuries.

Prevention of wrestling injuries

Weight reduction should be limited in wrestling. A discrepancy in strength between two wrestlers increases the risk of injury for the weaker athlete. Furthermore, when losing weight the wrestler loses a lot of water and tends to get dehydrated.

Strength training and conditioning might reduce the risk of fatigue on injury, especially in tournaments where there are high numbers of matches per day. Injuries are also common early in the season, suggesting proper year-round conditioning should be introduced.[147,149]

Most shoulder injuries are caused by poor technique.[141] Training on technique will improve technique and therefore reduce the risk of shoulder injuries. For other injuries the same relationship between technique and injury risk may exist, especially if the technique involves takedowns.[147,148] A proper technique is therefore believed to reduce the number of injuries in general.

Dermatological illnesses and bacterial infections are commonly seen in wrestling. Dermatological illnesses are transmitted by contact with the opponent,[151] and bacteria are commonly found on the mats. Proper hygiene by the wrestler, e.g. daily washing of clothes after training, daily showering after training, should reduce dermatological illnesses. Proper cleaning of the mat should reduce bacterial illnesses.[152]

The effect of headgear on a decrease of injury has been shown in wrestling.[150] The role of other protective equipment, e.g. kneepads, shoes or mouth guards, has not been evaluated.[141] In other sports, however, these measures have been effective in preventing injuries. It is reasonable to assume an effect of other protective equipment on injury reduction.

References

1. **de Loës, M.** and **Goldie, I.** Incidence rate of injuries during sport activity and physical exercise in a rural Swedish municipality: incidence rates in 17 sports. *International Journal of Sports Medicine* 1988; **9**: 461–7.

2. Backx, F. J., Beijer, H. J. M., Bol, E. and Erick, W. B. M. Injuries in high-risk persons and high-risk sports. A longitudinal study of 1818 school children. *American Journal of Sports Medicine* 1991; **19**: 124–30.

3. Kujala, U. M., Taimela, S., Antti Poika, I., Orava, S., Tuominen, R. and Myllynen, P. Acute injuries in soccer, ice hockey, volleyball, basketball, judo and karate: analysis of national registry data. *British Medical Journal* 1995; **311**: 1465–8.

4. Van Mechelen, W., Twisk, J., Molendijk, A., Blom, B., Snel, J. and Kemper, H. C. Subject related risk factors for sports-injuries: a 1-year prospective study in young adults. *Medicine and Science in Sports and Exercise* 1996; **28**: 1171–9.

5. Meeuwisse, W. and Fowler, P. Frequency and predictability of sports injuries in intercollegiate athletics. *Canadian Journal of Sports Medicine and Science* 1988; **13**: 35–42.

6. Mueller, F., Zemper, E. D. and Peters, A. American football. In *Epidemiology of sports injuries* (eds D. J. Caine, C. G. Caine and K. J. Lindner). Human Kinetics, Champaign, IL 1996; 41–62.

7. National Athletic Trainers Association. *National high school injury registry report.* NATA, Greenville, SC, 1987.

8. Blyth, C. and Mueller, F. Where and when players get hurt. *Physician and Sports Medicine* 1974; **2**: 45–52.

9. Culpepper, M and Niemann, K. A comparison of game and practice injuries in high school football. *Physician and Sports Medicine* 1983; **11**: 117–22.

10. Lackland, D., Akers, P. and Hirata, I. High school football injuries in South Carolina: a computerized survey. *Journal of the South Carolina Medical Association* 1982; **78**: 75–8.

11. Olson, O. The Spokane study: high school football injuries. *Physician and Sports Medicine* 1979; **7**: 75–82.

12. Alves, W., Rimel, R. and Nelson, W. University of Virginia prospective study of football induced minor head injury: status report. *Clinical Journal of Sports Medicine* 1987; **6**: 211–18.

13. Cantu, R. Cerebral concussions in sports. *Sports Medicine* 1992; **14**: 302–7.

14. Gerberich, S., Priest, J., Boen, J., Staub, C. and Maxwell, R. Concussion incidences and severity in secondary school varsity football players. *American Journal of Public Health* 1983; **73**: 1370–5.

15. Kelly, J., Nichols, J., Filley, C., Lillhei, K., Rubenstein, D. and Kleinschmidt-DeMasters, B. Concussions in sports. *Journal of the American Medical Association* 1991; **266**: 2867–9.

16. Albright, J., McAuley, E., Martin, R., Crowley, E. and Foster, D. Head and neck injuries in college football: an eight-year analysis. *American Journal of Sports Medicine* 1985; **13**: 147–52.

17. Buckley, W. Concussion injury in college football: an eight-year overview. *Athletic Training* 1986; **21**: 207–11.

18. Carter, D. and Frankel, V. Biomechanics of hyperextension injuries to the cervical spine in football. *American Journal of Sports Medicine* 1980; **8**: 302–7.

19. Rogers, B. The mechanics of head and neck trauma to football players. *Athletic Training* 1981; **16**: 132–5.

20. Tamberelli, A. Prevention and care of the knee injury. *Athletic Journal* 1978; **58**: 103–5.

21. Warren, R. Football knee injuries. *Coaching Clinic* 1982; **20**: 16–21.

22. Darden, E. Prevention of knee injuries. *Audible* 1978; **40**: 30–32.

23. Walsh, W. and Blackburn, T. Prevention of ankle sprains. *American Journal of Sports Medicine* 1977; **5**: 243–5.

24. Grace, T., Sweetser, E., Nelson, M., Ydens, L. and Skipper, B. Isokinetic muscle imbalance and knee-joint injuries. *Journal of Bone and Joint Surgery* 1984; **66-A**: 734–40.

25. Kalenak, A. and Morehouse, C. Knee stability and knee ligament injuries. *Journal of the American Medical Association* 1975; **234**: 1143–5.

26. Kaplan, T. A., Digel, S. L., Scavo, S. A. and Arellana, S. B. Effect of obesity on injury risk in high school football players. *Clinical Journal of Sports Medicine* 1995; **5**: 43–7.

27. Lindner, M. M., Towesend, D. J., Jones, J. C., Balkom, Il. and Anthony, C. R. Incidence of adolescent injuries in junior high school and its relation to sexual maturity. *Clinical Journal of Sports Medicine* 1995; **5**: 167–70.

28. Sherk, A. and Watters, W. Neck injuries in football players. *Journal of the Medical Association of New Jersey* 1981; **78**: 579–83.

29. Brynhildsen, J., Ekstrand, J., Jeppson, A. and Tropp, H. Previous injuries and persisting symptoms in female soccer players. *International Journal of Sports Medicine* 1990; **11**: 489–92.

30. Mueller, F. and Blyth, C. North Carolina high school football injury study: Equipment and prevention. *Journal of Sports Medicine* 1974; **2**: 1–10.

31. Powell, J. Pattern of knee injuries associated with college football 1975–1982. *Athletic Training* 1985; **20**: 104–9.

32. Whiteside, J., Fleagle, S., Kalanek, A. and Weber, H. Manpower loss in football: a 12-year study at the Pennsylvania State University. *Physician and Sports Medicine* 1985; **13**: 103–14.

33. Prager, B., Fitton, W., Cahill, B. and Olson, G. High school football injuries: a prospective study and pitfalls of data collection. *American Journal of Sports Medicine* 1989; **17**: 681–5.

34. Cahill, B. and Griffith, E. Effect of pre-season conditioning on the incidence and severity of high school football knee injuries. *American Journal of Sports Medicine* 1978; **6**: 180–4.

35. Cameron, B. M. and Davis, O. The swivel football shoe: a controlled study. *American Journal of Sports Medicine* 1973; **1**: 16–27.

36. Torg, J., Quedenfeld, T. and Landau, S. Football shoes and playing surfaces: from safe to unsafe. *Physician and Sports Medicine* 1973; **1**: 51–4.

37. Henschen, K., Heil, J., Bean, B. and Crain, S. Football injuries: is grass or astroturf the culprit? *UHPERD Journal* 1989; **21**: 5–7.

38. Skovron, M., Levy, I. and Agel, J. Living with artificial grass: A knowledge update. *American Journal of Sports Medicine* 1990; **18**: 510–13.

39. Zemper, E. Analysis of cerebral concussion frequency with the most commonly used models of football helmets. *Journal of Athletic Training* 1994; **29**: 44–50.

40. Hansen, B., Ward, J. and Diehl, R. The preventive use of the Anderson Knee Stabler in football. *Physician and Sports Medicine* 1985; **13**: 75–7.

41. Teitz, C., Hermanson, B., Kronmal, R. and Diehr, P. Evaluation of the use of braces to prevent injury to the knee in collegiate football players. *Journal of Bone and Joint Surgery* 1987; **69**: 1467–70.

42. Estwanik, J. J., Boitano, M. and Ari, N. Amateur boxing injuries at the 1981 and 1982 USA/ABF national championships. *Physician and Sports Medicine* 1984; **12**: 123–28.

43. Welch, M. J., Sitler, M. and Kroeten, H. Boxing injuries from an instructional program. *Physician and Sports Medicine* 1986; **14**: 81–9.

44. Jordan, B. D. and Campbell, E. Acute boxing injuries among professional boxers in New York State: a two-year survey. *Physician and Sports Medicine* 1988; **16**: 87–91.

45. Jordan, B. D., Voy, R. O. and Stone, J. Amateur boxing injuries at the United States Olympic training center. *Physician and Sports Medicine* 1990; **18**: 80–90.

46. Porter, M. and O'Brien, M. Incidence and severity of injuries resulting from amateur boxing in Ireland. *Clinical Journal of Sports Medicine* 1996; **6**: 97–101.

47. Butler, R. J. Neuropsychological investigation of amateur boxers. *British journal of Sports Medicine* 1994; **28**: 187–90.

48. Hlobil, H., van Mechelen, W. and Kemper, H. C. G. Boxing. In *How can sports injuries be prevented.* National Institute for Sports Health Care, Netherlands, 1987; 87–93.

49. Jordan, B. D. Boxing. In *Epidemiology of sports injuries* (ed. D. J. Caine, C. G. Caine and K. J. Lindner). Human Kinetics, Champaign, IL, 1996; 113–23.

50. Drew, R. H., Templer, D. I., Schuyler, B. A., Newell, T. G. and Cannon, W. G. Neuropsychological deficits in active licensed professional boxers. *Journal of Clinical Psychology* 1986; **42**: 520–5.

51. Jordan, B. D., Jahre, C., Hauser, W. A. Zimmerman, R. D., Zarelli, M., Lipsitz, E. C., Johnson, V., Warren, R. F., Tsains, P. and Folk, F. S. CT of 338 active professional boxers. *Radiology* 1992; **185**: 509–12.

52. Stewart, W. F., Gordon, B., Selnes, O., Bandeen-Roche, K., Zeger, S., Tusa, R. J., Celentano, D. D., Schechter, A., Liberman, J. and Hall, C. Prospective study of central nervous system function in amateur boxers in the United States. *American Journal of Epidemiology* 1994; **139**: 573–88.

53. McLatchie, G., Brooks, N., Galraith, S., Hutchinson, J. S., Wilson, L., Melville, I. and Teasdale, E. Clinical neurological examination, neuropsychology, electroencephalography, and computed tomographic head scanning in active amateur boxers. *Journal of Neurology and Neurosurgery*, **50**, 96–9.

54. Unterharnscheidt, F. Boxing injuries. In *Sports injuries* (eds R. C. Schneider, J. C. Kennedy, M. L. Plant, J. T. Hoff and P. J. Fowler). Williams and Wilkins, Baltimore, 1985; 462–95.

55. Kaste, M., Vilkki, J., Sainio, K. and Kuurne, T. Is chronic brain damage in boxing a hazard of the past? *The Lancet* 1982; **8309**: 1186–9.

56. Kibler, W. B. Injuries in adolescent and preadolescent soccer players. *Medicine and Science in Sports and Exercise* 1993; **25**: 1330–32.

57. Schmidt-Olsen, S., Jørgenson, U., Kaalund, S. and Sørenson, J. Injuries among young soccer players. *American Journal of Sports Medicine* 1991; **19**: 273–5.

58. Lindenfeld, T. N., Schmidt, D. J., Hendy, M. P., Mangine, R. E. and Noyes, F. R. Incidence of injury in indoor soccer. *American Journal of Sports Medicine* 1994; **22**: 364–71.

59. Sullivan, J. A. and Gross, D. H. Evaluation of injuries in youth soccer. *American Journal of Sports Medicine* 1980; **8**: 325.

60. Nilsson, J. and Roass, A. Soccer injuries in adolescents. *American Journal of Sports Medicine* 1978; **6**: 358.

61. Xethalis, J. L. and Boiardo, A. Soccer injuries. In *The lower extremity in sports medicine* (ed. J. Nicholas). C. V. Mosby, New York, 1989; 1580–1667.

62. Larson, M., Pearl, A. J., Jaffet, R. and Rudawsky, A. Soccer. In *Epidemiology of sports injuries* (ed. D. J. Caine, C. G. Caine and K. J. Lindner). Human Kinetics, Champaign, IL, 1996; 387–98.

63. Maehlum, S., Dahl, E. and Daljord, O. A. Frequency of soccer injuries in a youth soccer tournament. *Physician and Sports Medicine* 1986; **14**: 73–9.

64. Schmidt-Olsen, S., Bünemann, L. K. H., Lade, V. and Brassoe, J. O. K. Soccer injuries of youth. *British Journal of Sports Medicine* 1985; **19**: 161–4.

65. Backous, D. D., Friedl, K. E., Schmidt, N. J., Parr, T. J. and Carpine, W. D. Soccer injuries and their relation to physical maturity. *American Journal of Diseases of Children* 1988; **142**: 839–42.

66. Keller, C. S., Noyes, F. R. and Buncher, C. R. The medical aspects of soccer injury epidemiology. *American Journal of Sports Medicine* 1987; **15**: 230–7.

67. Ekstrand, J. and Tropp, H. The incidence of ankle sprains in soccer. *Foot and Ankle* 1990; **11**: 41–4.

68. Nielsen, A. B. and Yde, J. Epidemiology and traumatology of injuries in soccer. *American Journal of Sports Medicine* 1989; **17**: 803–7.

69. Ekstrand, J., Gillquist, J., Möller, M., Öberg, B. and Liljedahl, S. Incidence of soccer injuries and their relation to training and team success. *American Journal of Sports Medicine* 1983; **11**: 63–7.

70. Poulsen, T. D., Freund, K. G., Madsen, F. and Sandvej, K. Injuries in high-skilled and low-skilled soccer: a prospective study. *British Journal of Sports Medicine* 1991; **25**: 151–53.

71. Jörgensen, U. Epidemiology of injuries in typical Scandinavian team sports. *British Journal of Sports Medicine* 1984; **18**: 59–63.

72. Ekstrand, J. and Nigg, B. Surface-related injuries in soccer. *Sports Medicine* 1989; **8**: 56–62.

73. National Collegiate Athletic Association Men's Soccer Injury Surveillance System. Unpublished paper, 1992.

74. National Collegiate Athletic Association Women's Soccer Injury Surveillance System. Unpublished paper, 1992.

75. Watson, A. W. S. Sports injuries in footballers related to defects of posture and body mechanics. *Journal of Sports Medicine and Physical Fitness* 1995; **35**: 289–94.

76. Cattermole, H. R., Hardy, J. R. W. and Gregg, P. J. The footballer's fracture. *British Journal of Sports Medicine* 1996; **30**: 171–5.

77. Yde, J. and Nielsen, A. B. Sports injuries in adolescents' ball games: soccer, handball and basketball. *British Journal of Sports Medicine* 1990; **24**: 51–5.

78. Janda, D. H., Bir, C., Wild, B., Olson, S. and Hensinger, R. N. Goal posts injuries in soccer: a laboratory and field testing analysis of a preventive intervention. *American Journal of Sports Medicine* 1995; **23**: 340–4.

79. Schneider, K. Das Risiko einer Hirnverletzung beim Fußball-Kopfstoß. *Unfallheilkunde* 1984; **87**: 40–2.

80. Tysvaer, A. T. and Storli, O. V. Soccer injuries to the brain: a neurologic and electroencephalographic study of active football players. *American Journal of Sports Medicine* 1989; **17**: 573–8.

81. Tysvaer, A. T. and Løchen, E. A. Soccer injuries to the brain: a neuropsychologic study of former soccer players. *American Journal of Sports Medicine* 1991; **19**: 56–69.

82. de Loës, M. Epidemiology of sports injuries in the Swiss organization 'Youth and Sports' 1987–1989: injuries, exposure and risks of main diagnosis. *International Journal of Sports Medicine* 1995; **16**: 134–8.

83. Barrault, D., Achou, B. and Sorel, R. Accidents et incidents survenus au cours de compétitions de judo. In *Medecine du judo* (ed. D. Barrault, J. C. Brondani and D. Rousseau). Masson, Paris, 1991; 144–52.

84. Kujala, U. M., Taimela, S., Antti-Poik a, I., Orava, S., Tuominen, R. and Myllynen, P. Acute injuries in soccer, ice hockey, volleyball, basketball, judo, and karate: analysis of national registry data. *British Medical Journal* 1995; **311**: 1465–8.

85. Tuominen, R. Injuries in national karate competitions in Finland. *Scandinavian Journal of Medicine and Science in Sports* 1995; **5**: 44–48.

86. Buckley, T. Karate injuries. A compilation of 1000 kumite matches. *Unpublished report.* USA Karate Federation of Washington, Everett, WA, 1990.

87. Oler, M., Tomson, W., Pepe, H., Yoon, D., Branoff, R. and Branch, J. Morbidity and mortality in the martial arts: a warning. *Journal of Trauma* 1991; **31**: 251–3.

88. Johanssen, H. V. and Noerregaard, F. O. H. Prevention of injury in karate. *British Journal of Sports Medicine* 1988; **22**: 113–15.

89. Feehan, M. and Waller, A. E. Precompetition injury and subsequent tournament performance in full-contact taekwondo. *British Journal of Sports Medicine* 1995; **29**: 258–62.

90. Nishimura, K., Fujii, K., Maeyama, R., Saiki, I., Sakata, S. and Kitamura, K. Acute subdural hematoma in judo practitioners. Report of four cases. *Neurologica Medico-Chirurgica* 1988; **28**: 991–3.

91. Rodriguez, G., Francione, S., Gardelaa, M., Marenco, S., Nobili, F., Novellone, G., Reggiani, E. and Rosadini, G. Judo and choking: EEG and regional cerebral blood flow findings. *Journal of Sports Medicine and Physical Fitness* 1991; **31**: 605–10.

92. McLatchie, G. R. Injuries in combat sports. In *Sports fitness and sports injuries* (ed. T. Reilly). Faber & Faber, London, 1981; 168–74.

93. Stricevic, M. V., Patel, M. R., Okazaki, T. and Swain, B. K. Karate: historical perspective and injuries sustained in national and international tournament competitions. *American Journal of Sports Medicine* 1993; **11**: 320–4.

94. Siana, J. E., Borum, P. and Kryger, H. Injuries in taekwondo. *British Journal of Sports Medicine* 1986; **20**: 165–6.

95. McLatchie, G. R., Miller, J. H. and Morris, E. W. Combined force injury of the elbow joint: the mechanism clarified. *British Journal of Sports Medicine* 1979; **13**: 176–9.

96. Jerosch, J., Castro, W. H. M. and Geske, B. Damage of the long thoracic and dorsal scapular nerve after traumatic shoulder dislocation: case report and review of the literature. *Acta Orthopedica Belgica* 1990; **56**: 625–7.

97. Russo, M. T. and Maffulli, N. Dorsal dislocation of the distal end of the ulna in a judo player. *Acta Orthopedica Belgica* 1991; **57**: 442–6.

98. Danek, E. Martial arts: the sound of one hand chopping. *Physician and Sports Medicine* 1979; **7**: 140–4.

99. **Pieter, W., Zemper, E. D.** and **Heijmans, J.** Taekwondo blessures. *Geneeskunde en Sport* 1990; **23**: 222–8.

100. **Zandbergen, A.** (no date). Taekwondo blessures en fysiotherapie. *Unpublished thesis.* Twentse akademie voor fysiotherapie, Enschede.

101. **Larose, J. H.** and **Kim, D. S.** Knuckle fracture. A mechanism of injury. *Journal of the American Medical Association* 1968; **206**: 893–4.

102. **Wirtz, P. D., Vito, G. R.** and **Long, D. H.** Calcaneal apophysitis associated with taekwondo injuries. *Journal of the American Pediatric Medical Association* 1988; **78**: 474–5.

103. **Lampert, P. W.** and **Hardman, J. M.** Morphological changes in brains of boxers. *Journal of the American Medical Association* 1984; **251**: 2676–9.

104. **McCunney, R. J.** and **Russo, P. K.** Brain injuries in boxers. *Physician and Sports Medicine* 1984; **12**: 52–67.

105. **Johanssen, H. V.** and **Noerregaard, F. O. H.** Prevention of injury in karate. *British Journal of Sports Medicine* 1988; **22**: 113–15.

106. **Chuang, T. Y.** and **Lieu, D. K.** A parametric study of the thoracic injury potential of basic taekwondo kicks. In *Taekwondo. USTI instructors handbook* (ed. K. Min). United States Taekwondo Union Instructors (sic) Certification Committee, Berkeley, CA, 1991; 118–26.

107. **Zemper, E. D.** and **Pieter, W.** Injury rates during the 1988 US Olympic Team Trials for taekwondo. *British Journal of Sports Medicine* 1989; **23**: 161–4.

108. **Koiwai, E. K.** Major accidents and injuries in judo. *Journal of the Arizona State Medical Association* 1965; **22**: 957–62.

109. **McLatchie, G. R., Commandre, F. A., Zakarian, H., Vanuxem, P., Lamendin, H., Barrault, D.** and **Chau, P. Q.** Injuries in the martial arts. In *Clinical practice of sports injury prevention and care. Volume V of the encyclopedia of Sports Medicine* (ed. P. A. F. H. Renström). Blackwell Scientific Publications, Oxford, 1992; 609–23.

110. **Birrer, R. B.** Martial arts injuries: their spectrum and management. *Sports Medicine Digest* 1984; **6**: 1–3.

111. **Koiwai, E. K.** Deaths allegedly caused by the use of 'choke holds'. *Journal of Forensic Science* 1987; **32**: 419–32.

112. American Academy of Pediatrics Committee on Sports Medicine and Fitness Medical conditions affecting sports participation. *Pediatrics* 1994; **94**: 757–60.

113. **Roberts, W. O., Brust, J. D.** and **Leonard, B.** Youth ice hockey tournament injuries: rates and patterns compared to season play. *Medicine and Science in Sports and Exercise* 1998; **31**: 46–51.

114. **Stuart, M. J.** and **Smith, A.** Injuries in junior A ice hockey: a three year prospective study. *American Journal of Sports Medicine* 1995; **23**: 458–61.

115. **Montelpare, W. J., Pelletier, R. L.** and **Stark, R. M.** Ice hockey. In *Epidemiology of sports injuries* (ed. D. J. Caine, C. G. Caine and K. J. Lindner). Human Kinetics, Champaign, IL, 1996; 247–67.

116. **Mölsä, J., Airaksinen, O., Näsman, O.** and **Torstila, I.** Ice hockey injuries in Finland: a prospective epidemiologic study. *American Journal of Sports Medicine* 1997; **25**: 495–9.

117. **Tegner, Y.** and **Lorentzen, R.** Ice hockey injuries: incidence, nature and causes. *British Journal of Sports Medicine* 1991; **25**: 87–9.

118. **Daly, P. J., Sim, F. H.** and **Simonet, W. T.** Ice hockey injuries: a review. *Sports Medicine* 1990; **10**: 122–31.

119. **Fox, E., Bowers, R.** and **Foss, M.** *The physiological basis for exercise and sport,* 5th edn. Brown and Benchmark, Madison, WI, 1993.

120. **Rielly, M.** The nature and causes of hockey injuries: a five year study. *Athletic Training* 1982; **17**: 88–90.

121. **Roy, A., Bernard, D., Roy, B.** and **Marcotte, G.** Body checking in pee-wee hockey. *Physician and Sports Medicine* 1989; **17**: 119–26.

122. **Bernard, D., Trudel, P., Marcotte, G.** and **Boileau, R.** The incidence, types and circumstances of injuries to ice hockey players at the bantam level (14 to 15 years old). In *Safety in ice hockey: second volume* (ed. C. Castaldi, P. J. Bishop and E. F. Hoerner). American Society for Testing and Materials, Philadelphia, 1993; 45–55.

123. **Kropp, D., Marchant, L.** and **Warshawski, J.** An analysis of head injuries in hockey and lacrosse. Sport safety research report, fitness and amateur sport branch, Department of National Health and Welfare, 1975.

124. **Daly, P., Foster, T.** and **Zarins, B.** Injuries in ice hockey. In *Clinical practice of sports injury prevention and care* (ed. P. Renstrom). Blackwell Scientific Publications, London, 1994; 375–91.

125. **Tator, C., Edmonds, V.** and **Lapczak, L.** Spinal injuries in ice hockey: review of 182 North American cases and analysis of etiological factors. In *Safety in ice hockey: second volume* (ed. C. Castaldi, P. J. Bishop and E. F. Hoerner). American Society for Testing and Materials, Philadelphia, 1993; 95–102.

126. **Goodwyn-Gerberich, S., Finke, R., Madden, M., Priest, J., Aamoth, G.** and **Murray, K.** An epidemiological study of high-school ice hockey injuries. *Child's Nervous System* 1987; **3**: 59–64.

127. **Dick, R. W.** Injuries in collegiate ice hockey. In *Safety in ice hockey: second volume* (ed. C. Castaldi, P. J. Bishop and E. F. Hoerner). American Society for Testing and Materials, Philadelphia, 1993; 21–30.

128. **Brust, J. D., Leonard, B. J., Pheley, A.** and **Roberts, W. O.** Children's ice hockey injuries. *American Journal of the Disabled Child* 1992; **146**: 741–7.

129. **Tator, H. D., Carson, J. D.** and **Edmonds, V. E.** New spinal injuries in hockey. *Clinical Journal of Sports Medicine* 1996; **7**: 17–21.

130. **Honey, C. R.** Brain injury in ice hockey. *Clinical Journal of Sports Medicin* 1997; **8**: 43–6.

131. **Sim, F. H.** and **Chao, E. Y.** Injury potential in modern ice hockey. *American Journal of Sports Medicine* 1978; **15**: 378–84.

132. **Sickles, R. T.** and **Lombardo, J. A.** The adolescent basketball player. *Clinics in Sports Medicine* 1993; **12**: 207–19.

133. **Emerson, R. J.** Basketball knee injuries and the anterior cruciate ligament. *Clinics in Sports Medicine,* **12**: 317–28.

134. **McClain, L. G.** and **Reynolds, S.** Sports injuries in high school. *Pediatrics* 1989; **84**: 446–50.

135. **Whiteside, J. A., Fleagle, S. B.** and **Kalenak, A.** Fractures and refractures in intercollegiate athletes: an eleven-year experience. *American Journal of Sports Medicine* 1981; **9**: 369–77.

136. **Wilson, R. L.** and **McGinty, L. D.** Common hand and wrist injuries in basketball players. *Clinics in Sports Medicine* 1993; **12**: 265–91.

137. **Zvijac, J.** and **Thompson, W.** Basketball In *Epidemiology of sports injuries* (ed. D. J. Caine, C. G. Caine and K. J. Lindner). Human Kinetics, Champaign, IL, 1996; 86–97.

138. National Collegiate Athletic Association Injury Surveillance System. *Wrestling summary.* Shawnee Mission, Kansas, 1992–3.

139. **Powell, J. W.** National athletic injuries/illness reporting system: Eye injuries in college wrestling. *International Ophthalmology Clinics* 1981; **21**: 47–58.

140. National High School Injury Registry reported in *Athletic Training* 1988; **23**: 383–8. 1989; **24**: 360–73.

141. **Wroble, R. R.** Wrestling. In *Epidemiology of sports injuries* (ed. D. J. Caine, C. G. Caine and K. J. Lindner). Human Kinetics, Champaign, IL, 1996; 417–38.

142. **Wroble, R. R.** and **Albright, J. P.** Neck and low back injuries in wrestling. *Clinic in Sports Medicine* 1986; **5**: 295–325.

143. **Estwanik, J. J.** and **Rovere, G. D.** Wrestling injuries in North Carolina high schools. *Physician and Sports Medicine* 1983; **11**: 100–8.

144. **Horswill, C. A.** Applied physiology of amateur wrestling. *Sports Medicine* 1992; **14**: 114–43.

145. **Horswill, C. A.** When wrestlers slim to win. *Physician and Sports Medicine* 1992; **20**: 91–104.

146. **Hartmann, P. M.** Injuries in preadolescent wrestlers. *Physician and Sports Medicine* 1978; **6**: 79–82.

147. **Wroble, R. R., Mysnyk, C. A., Foster, D. T.** and **Albright, J. P.** Patterns of knee injuries in wrestling: a six-year study. *American Journal of Sports Medicine* 1986; **14**: 55–66.

148. **Estwanik, J. J., Bergfeld, J. A., Collins, H. R.** and **Hall, R.** Injuries in interscholastic wrestling. *Physician and Sports Medicine* 1980; **8**: 111–21.

149. **Clarke, K. S.** A survey of sports-related spinal cord injuries in schools and colleges, 1973–1975. *Journal of Safety Research* 1977; **9**: 140–6.

150. Schuller, D. E., Dankle, S. K., Martin, M. and Strauss, R. H. Auricular injury and the use of headgear in wrestlers. *Archives of Otolaryngology Head and Neck Surgery* 1989; **115**: 714–17.

151. Belongia, E. A., Goodman, J. L., Holland, E. J., Andras, C. W., Homann, S. R., Mahanti, R. L., Mizener, M. W. Erice A. and Osterholm, M. T. An outbreak of herpes gladiatorum at a high-school wrestling camp. *New England Journal of Medicine* 1991; **325**: 906–10.

152. Konrad, I. J. *A study of wrestling injuries in high schools throughout seven midwest states.* Thesis, Michigan State College, 1951.

5.4 Aetiology and prevention of injuries in youth competition: non-contact sports

Per Mahler

Introduction

The global approach to the aetiology and prevention of sports injuries has been covered in previous chapters, so this chapter concentrates on sports specific problems and, in particular, those of non-contact sports.

A number of sports, where no intentional contact with an opponent occurs, have therefore been selected based on their worldwide popularity,[1] and are discussed individually or grouped with similar sports. Certain sports that are less universally practised or that are country specific are beyond the scope of this chapter. Each sport is covered in a systematic way covering information about the practice of the sport, epidemiology and aetiology of sport specific injuries, risk factors (intrinsic and extrinsic) and preventive strategies related to the above.

In general, injuries in non-contact sports are less frequent than in contact sport,[2–5] and more frequently fall in the overuse group. One should, however, keep in mind that a large proportion of sports pathology is common to both contact and non-contact sports where similar biomechanical factors are involved (running, cutting, etc.).

Unfortunately, most studies quoted in the following sections are based on case reports and case series rather than randomized prospective or intervention studies, and therefore give limited significant information about risk factors and the influence of prevention on injury.[6] It is also noteworthy that little information is available on children in certain sports and that adult data has therefore been used to extrapolate when appropriate. Taking this into consideration, the following chapter underlines certain trends that can be drawn from the literature and that give a reasonable basis on which to develop and promote prevention strategies.

Bicycling

Apart from being a popular sport, cycling is an equally popular means of transport and leisure activity. It is therefore difficult to differentiate between sports related and sports independent injuries, a lot of the risk factors being present in both activities.

Special emphasis will be placed on competitive cycling injuries when possible.

Epidemiology of cycling injuries

Two studies concerning competitive cycling in adults cite an injury incidence of about 2–3%[7,8] for punctual competitive events, with a potentially higher incidence in mountain biking.[9]

A large scale study drawn from the National Electronic Injury Surveillance System USA 1987,1989 and 1990[10] shows an age and sex related prevalence of injuries with females age 5–9 years (730 injuries) and males age 10–14 years (1311 injuries) having the highest injury rates per 100 000 population. When expressed per million trips, children age 5–15 years (430.7 injuries) and adults over 50 years (296.2 injuries) have the highest injury rates. Injuries can be divided into accidents and overuse (gradual onset), the second group being more specific to competitive cycling. Injuries resulting from accidents include abrasions, lacer-ations (63%), fractures (16%), closed head injuries and concussions (2%).[10] In the overuse group one finds anterior and lateral knee pain,[11] neck and low back pain,[12] ischial pain and pudendal nerve palsy,[13] ulnar nerve pain[14] and stenotic thickening of the external iliac artery,[15] but these mostly concern adults even though the premises may be laid at a younger age.

Aetiology of cycling injuries

Falls are the most frequent source of accidental injuries followed by hitting a stationary object, hitting or being hit by a motor vehicle, hitting another cyclist, pedestrian or animal, and finally bicycle malfunction.[16] Motor vehicles are involved in the minority of accidents (10–35%) but are responsible for about 90% of fatalities. Accidents also correlate with the type of road (more fatal accidents on high speed-limit roads), damaged roads and the availability of cycle tracks. Intersections are a frequent location for accidents.[10]

The non-use of helmets has been shown to be a major risk factor for head and brain injuries and the use of helmets decreases head injuries by up to 80%.[17]

Overuse injuries seem to be linked to biomechanical and training factors. As in other sports, training volume and progression are important. Bicycle fit (saddle position, foot clips, frame size) should be carefully evaluated and re-evaluated in the case of injury.[12,18,19] Cycling technique (foot and hip position) should also be analysed.[20]

The intrinsic and extrinsic risk factors are listed in Table 5.4.1.

Preventive strategies

Accidents are responsible for the most serious injuries and their prevention should therefore receive special attention. The Haddon Matrix[10] that identifies modifiable risk factors and divides them into three phases (pre-impact, during impact, post-impact) is a valuable model for cycle injury prevention. Important factors like helmet use,

Table 5.4.1 Intrinsic and extrinsic risk factors for cycling injuries, with their respective references

Intrinsic risk factors	Extrinsic risk factors
Age, gender[10]	**Protective equipment (helmets)**[17]
Pronation[12,18,19]	Exposure[12,18,19]
Cycling technique[20]	Training quality (progression, programme)[12,18,19]
	Type of roads, intersections, cycle tracks[10]
	Bicycle fit[12,18,19]
	Mechanical malfunction[16]

Bold factors have been confirmed in prospective studies and/or are supported by a general agreement in literature, whilst the others still lack statistical support.

cyclist education, bicycle design, road/path design, emergency service and rehabilitation are stressed.

As previously mentioned, certain age groups are more at risk for cycle accidents and should therefore receive special attention in prevention campaigns.

Overuse injuries are mostly due to bicycle-rider misfit or training errors, hence bicycle choice (accessories) and adjustment should when possible be carried out by a professional and adapted to growth. Other modalities like muscle stretching and strengthening as well as specific protective equipment can also be useful in preventing injury.[14]

Dance

Dance in its various forms (ballet, jazz, rock and roll, fitness etc.) can be compared with other sports when considering athletic qualities required, methodical training programmes and injuries.[21] Dancing is a popular activity amongst youth and often requires intensive involvement in training at a young age.

Because of the paucity of information and the higher age of participants, 'aerobic' (fitness) dancing is not included in this discussion.

Epidemiology of dance injuries

As for other sports, data are flawed by lack of uniformity in injury definition and severity, exposure rates, sample size and controlled data collection. A prospective study conducted by Reid et al.[22] on a group of young (mean age: 13.5 years) ballet dancers, showed an injury incidence of 0.9 injuries per 1000 hours of exposure or 1159 hours of exposure per injury. This was lower than that found by Rovere et al.[23] in slightly older (15–22 years) and more advanced dancers (2.8/1000 h), underlining the probable effect of more intensive and demanding exercise in the older group. The incidence of reinjury reported in the study by Clanin et al.[24] was 0.02 reinjuries per 100 hours of exposure. Few data relate to the type of activity and injury in children, Bowling's data on professional dancers gives us some insight,[25] with 15.5% of injuries occurring in class, 27.6% in rehearsal and 32.8% in performance.

Injuries mostly fall in the overuse group[24] and are two times more frequent in ballet than in modern dance and five times more frequent in ballet than in jazz. This trend was not found by Wiesler et al.[26] who found nearly twice the number of injuries in modern dance than in ballet. The majority (33–60%) of injuries recorded in the literature are sprains and strains, followed by tendinitis and contusions.[27] Stress fractures are not uncommon and concern mainly girls with irregular or absent menses.[28] Overall, knee injuries are the most frequent (14.5–20.1%) followed by ankle (15.4%), foot and toes (13.1–14.8%) and the spine (10.7–12.2%).[22,23]

A number of injuries found in ballet which have been the subject of case reports or case series are summarized by Caine and Garick.[29]

Aetiology of dance injuries

Exposure, as mentioned earlier, can influence occurrence of injury. Kadel et al.[30] found that the risk of sustaining a stress fracture increased significantly in professional dancers who danced over five hours a day or who had amenohroeic intervals extending beyond six months. Dancers are at increased risk of bone injuries because of their extreme nutritional habits (to minimize body fat) and heavy training loads, which when combined can lead to hormonal perturbations and delayed bone growth.[31] It is noteworthy that dancers are at high risk for nutrient deficiency and anorexia nervosa.[32]

Malalignment of the lower extremity and subtalar pronation resulting in a lack of turnout and a shallow 'demi plie' have been shown to be related to knee injuries.[33] Dancing 'en pointe' has been proposed as a potential mechanism for lower-back stress, potentially leading to spondylolysis, because of the biomechanical loading of the pedicles and the pars interarticularis of the vertebrae.[34]

Dancing on 'pointe' and 'demi-pointe', and pronation[35] have also been incriminated in various injuries of the ankle, resulting in tendinitis of the flexor hallucis longus and Achilles tendon,[36] osteochodral fractures of the talus, sprains and anterior impingement syndromes of the ankle.[37] Overstress of the forefoot has been shown to result in injuries to the hallucis longus tendon, to the metatarsophalangeal joints, to the cuboid (subluxations) and to sesamoid bones. Isolated cases of Iselin's disease of the fifth metatarsal[38] and stress fractures involving the Lisfranc joint in dancers with a hyperflexed forefoot have also been reported.[39]

The intrinsic and extrinsic risk factors are listed in Table 5.4.2.

Preventive strategies

A preventive approach includes proper treatment of injuries (rest), good nutritional counselling and follow up, close monitoring of any menstrual irregularities and the constant re-evaluation of training

Table 5.4.2 Intrinsic and extrinsic risk factors for dance injuries, with their respective references

Intrinsic risk factors	Extrinsic risk factors
Previous injury[26]	Exposure[30]
Low body mass index (nutrition)[31]	Dancing surface[40]
Irregular menstrual cycles[28,30]	Type of shoe[41]
Hypermobility[42]	
Restricted joint mobility[22]	
Flaws in technique[43,44]	
Hyperflexed forefoot[39]	
Pronation[33,35]	

Bold factors have been confirmed in prospective studies and/or are supported by a general agreement in literature, whilst the others still lack statistical support.

load. Reid[45] suggests that young dancers should be allowed at least a six week block of rest once a year.

Joint hyper- and hypo-mobility should be recognized and corrected when possible. Adapted shoes, technique and surface may also contribute to preventing injuries.

Preparticipation examination has been shown to be useful in reducing injuries and should include an orthopaedic examination, the rehabilitation of any previous injury and a thorough nutritional and menstrual assessment.[46,47]

Gymnastics

Gymnastics is an increasingly popular sport in certain countries and requires early involvement (6–9 years of age) in intensive training. Training volume can reach 40 hours or more a week for elite gymnasts and generates significant loads to both the upper and lower extremities which potentially result in injury.

Epidemiology of gymnastics injuries

Injury rates vary considerably between studies depending on competitive level, club or school structure, gender and data processing. Injury rates for girls vary between 3.6/1000 h of exposure at club level[3] to 22.7/1000 h in college gymnastics.[48] For men, no data are available per hour but injury incidences of 3.5 to 5.33 injuries per 1000 athletic exposures[49,50] have been observed in college gymnastics, which is lower than that observed in girls: 9.05/1000 athletic exposures.[50] Reinjury rates, including previous seasons, were 0.53 and 2.19 per 1000 athletic exposures in boys and girls, respectively. Injury rates are higher in training than in competition for both boys and girls. However, when computed per athletic exposure, competition results in an approximately threefold higher injury incidence than training for both sexes.[50]

The majority of injuries are of sudden onset, but the difficulty in distinguishing between an acute injury and an acute injury superimposed on a predisposing overuse injury may bias this conclusion. Injury type also tends to be limb specific, more overuse injuries being observed at the upper extremity than at the lower.[51]

Sprains (15.9–43.6%) and strains (6.4–47.1%) are consistently the most frequently observed injuries[52] in women and men,[50] other injuries like fractures, contusions and inflammation being less consistent depending on the groups studied. The lower limb is the most frequently involved body part (54.1–70.2%), followed by the upper extremity (18.1–25%) and the spine and trunk (0–16.7%). The ankle is most frequently injured in the lower limb followed by the knee, the heel/Achilles tendon and the foot/toes. The wrist, followed by the elbow and hands/fingers are most frequently involved in the upper extremity, and the lower back is most often involved in injuries to the spine.[53]

Nutritional, endocrine and psychiatric disorders have also been observed among gymnasts.[54]

Aetiology of gymnastics injuries

The high impact loads and extreme biomechanics seen in gymnastics certainly contribute to both overuse and accidental injuries. Vault takeoffs have been shown to produce ground reaction forces of up to 5.1 times body weight to the lower limb,[55] whereas forces of 8.8 to 14.4 times body weight were found on landing.[56] These forces are transmitted through the lower limbs to the spine and can result in injury.[57] Extreme biomechanics involving hyperflexion, rotation and

hyperextension of the trunk can also be considered causative factors.[58] The high incidence of spondylolysis among gymnasts (19.2% in girls, 11.5% in boys), compared to 3.3% in the general population, tends to confirm the above hypothesis.[59] The upper limb is also exposed to large loads, ranging from 1.57 times body weight in vaulting[55] to 9.2 times body weight in still rings.[60] This might explain the frequently reported stress injuries involving the distal radial growth plate (1.9/100 participant seasons) and osteochondritis dissecans of the humeral capitellum (1.2 and 2.5/100 participant seasons in girls and boys, respectively), which can lead to long term complications.[51] Some data tend to show a dose–response relation between training intensity and ulna–radial-length difference resulting from distal radial physeal arrest in elite[61] and non-elite gymnasts.[62] Femoral nerve palsy due to iliacus muscle injury or direct compression has also been observed.[63] Few catastrophic injuries have been reported in gymnastics and relate mainly to trampoline (trampette) exercises.[64]

Numerous factors have been shown to relate to gymnastics injuries and are summarized below. Anthropometric factors like size, weight and puberty[65–67] are closely related to injury in girls, confirming the advantage of small size, low body weight and retarded puberty to be successful in gymnastics and avoid injuries. Previous injury,[50] which is consistent through most sports, and high lumbar curvature can also be considered intrinsic risk factors.

External factors such as exposure,[68] competitive level[69] and the type of event[48,70] also correlate with injury. The floor exercise has been observed to be the source of most of the acute traumatic injuries in both boys and girls followed by uneven bars in girls and still rings in boys. This was confirmed at the world championships in 1997 where 40% of the injuries occurred during the floor exercise.[72] The first half hour of practice and certain periods of the season (following interruptions, intensive preparation, pre-competition, during competition) have also been shown to be risk factors.[69] Safe equipment is certainly of importance but can lead to more risky behaviour during training. However, due to the high injury incidence during competitions, supplementary protective equipment could prove to be beneficial during competition.[71]

The intrinsic and extrinsic risk factors are listed in Table 5.4.3.

Preventive strategies

Prevention should start with education of the gymnast and the coach concerning sport specific preparation, injuries, injury prevention and treatment, nutrition and coach–child–family interaction.[77,78] Continuing education of coaches should be mandatory and alternate loading, quality training, motivation, individualization, growth and interpersonal skills should all be covered. Equipment should be adapted to exercise level and competition.

Medical support becomes important when children reach competition. Pre-season as well as post-injury medical evaluation is important to re-evaluate risk factors (orthopaedic, schooling and family) and guide the gymnast and his or her support 'team'.

'Achievement by proxy' (parents, coaches, physicians), can be considered to be a risk factor that can lead to health disorders and should therefore be recognized as early as possible.[54]

Running

Running is a widespread activity and is common to a multitude of both contact and non-contact sports. Most of the literature concerns adults, and results concerning injury risk, male to female injury ratios and prevention are unfortunately somewhat contradictory depending on the research design.

Epidemiology of running injuries

One prospective and two retrospective studies conducted on relatively small groups of adolescents show an annual injury incidence of 18–40%[79–81] compared with 25–75% in adults.[82] The most common running injuries observed among adolescents were overuse injuries (19.5% medial tibial stress syndrome, 18% apophyseal injuries, 14.8% non-specific knee pain, 7.3% lower back pain), the rest being mainly composed of sprains and strains (3.4% ankle sprain/strain, 2.4% foot sprain/strain).[83] A majority of injuries concerned the knee and lower leg and no clear difference could be made between males and females. Isolated cases of avulsion fractures of the anterior and posterior iliac spine[84] and the distal femoral epiphysis[85] have been reported in children. Stress fractures of the tibia and fibula[86] as well as epiphyseal stress fractures of the calcaneum[87] and first metatarsal[88] have also been observed in children.

Table 5.4.3 Intrinsic and extrinsic risk factors for gymnastics injuries, with their respective references

Intrinsic risk factors	Extrinsic risk factors
Large body size and weight[65-67]	**Competitive level**[69]
Early maturation (high body fat)[65-67]	**Event (floor)**[48,70,71]
Rapid growth[65-67]	**Event (floor > still rings > horizontal bar)**[48,70,71]
High lumbar curvature[50]	Years of competition (exposure)[68,69]
Previous injury[50]	Training errors[76]
Muscle weakness[73]	Early part of practice[69]
Muscle asymmetry[74]	Period of the sports season[69]
Stressful life events[75]	Coach assisted exercise (spotting)[50] 'Achievement by proxy'[54] Protective equipment[72]

Bold factors have been confirmed in prospective studies and/or are supported by a general agreement in literature, whilst the others still lack statistical support.

Aetiology of running injuries

Most authors agree that a majority of running injuries are of gradual onset and linked to repetitive mechanical loading.[89] This load is more or less well tolerated depending on individual stress tolerance, which is linked to a series of intrinsic and extrinsic risk factors. The only child specific reference in the literature concerns calcaneal apophysitis which was shown to be related to genu varum, subtalar varus, and forefoot varus.[87] Certain risk factors have been shown to be related to running injuries in adults and can be considered relevant in children because of the similarities in biomechanics. Exposure[90] and precious injury[91] have both been shown to be significantly correlated with running injuries. Training errors, inadequate shoes and/or running surface, warm up and stretching, certain psychological factors, lower extremity malalignment, muscular imbalance, restricted range of motion, orthotics, time of year and participation in other sports have also been shown to correlate with injuries.[91] However, none of these factors have been proven in properly controlled studies, and it is therefore difficult to draw clear cut conclusions on how to implement them.

The intrinsic and extrinsic risk factors are listed in Table 5.4.4.

Preventive strategies

Adequate information should be given to the participant with respect to injury risk and risk factors. Lower limb malalignment and muscle imbalance (strength, flexibility) should be identified and corrected (compensated) if possible.

It would seem useful to encourage the young runner to increase running volume progressively and or run on alternate days, to practise a proper warm up, to stretch after exercise, to detect and treat any injury properly and to return to running progressively. Understanding one's body is important as well as knowing how to buy adapted equipment. Preparticipation evaluation by a doctor should be encouraged if intensive participation is considered.

Skiing and snowboarding

Skiing and snowboarding have become increasingly popular over the last 20 years because of the facilitated access and increased capacity of ski areas. One estimate states there are about 200 million leisure skiers in the world today.[93] Snowboarding has also contributed to the popularity of alpine sports, adding a 'fun' dimension which has attracted numerous youngsters.

No specific data are available on competitive skiing in children, so the following data include both recreational and competitive skiers.

Table 5.4.4 Intrinsic and extrinsic risk factors for running injuries, with their respective references

Intrinsic risk factors	Extrinsic risk factors
Lower limb (malalignment, muscle imbalance, restricted range of motion)[87,92]	**Running volume (progression)**[90]
Psychological factors[91]	**Previous injury**[91]
	Shoes (adapted to the foot and biomechanics)[92]
	Running surface (hardness, inclination)[92]

Bold factors have been confirmed in prospective studies and/or are supported by a general agreement in literature, whilst the others still lack statistical support.

Epidemiology of skiing injuries

Deibert et al.[94] prospectively collected data over a 12 year period in a ski area and found an average injury incidence of 2.79 injuries per 1000 skier days. Children (1–10 years of age) showed the highest injury incidence: 4.27 injuries/1000 days, followed by adolescents (11–16 years of age): 2.93 injuries/1000 days. Similar results were found by Macnab and Cadman.[95] This can also be expressed as injuries per 10 km of vertical metres skied, and Matter et al.[96] found rates of four injuries per 10 km in 1972 and one per 10 km in 1986 for adults. This underlines the decrease in injuries over the last 15 years observed in other studies. Snowboarding injuries have been found to have a similar[97–99] or higher[100,101] incidence than skiing injuries, but injury type and location vary considerably between the two. This trend may change with the increasing popularity of snowboarding.

Injuries are principally to the lower extremity (40–70%) and the trend over the last 12 years has shown a decrease in tibial fractures (−89%) and ankle injuries and a clear increase in knee sprains (+280%). The most frequent injuries were knee contusions in children, ulnar collateral sprains of the thumb for adolescents and grade III anterior cruciate sprains in adults.[94] On average (including adults) 10–22% of injuries involve the head and spine,[95,102] and skull fractures seem relatively frequent among children.[102] Upper extremity injuries account for 13–36% of injuries, with ulnar collateral sprains of the thumb being the most frequent injury (10–17%) followed by shoulder fractures and dislocations (5–10%).

Snowboarding injuries vary considerably from skiing injuries in that the upper extremities (mainly hand and wrist) are most frequently involved (45.1–58%). Contrary to skiing, ankle injuries have been found to be more frequent than knee injuries.[97,99,100]

Skiing injuries can on the whole be classified as relatively severe and often result in prolonged absences from sport at both the recreational and competitive level.[104]

Aetiology of skiing injuries

The improving trend in lower extremity injuries is partly due to improvement in equipment (safety bindings, ski stoppers, boots) and better information. However, adjustment of the bindings is paramount and Deibert et al.[94] showed that 71% of children presenting with a spiral fracture of the lower leg had badly adjusted bindings.

Injuries to the head and spine were often due to loss of control, collisions with other skiers or trees, incorrect landings after jumps[105] and negligible helmet use among children.[103] Five mechanisms, involving rotational and translation forces in the knee, have been described by Feagin et al. for anterior cruciate tears.[106] This could lead to a better prevention of this injury by, for example, avoiding skiing from packed to deep snow at high speed.

In snowboarding, injuries seem to affect mainly boys and novices. Injuries vary as a function of the activity (head, face and spine injuries in aerial manoeuvres), type of boots (more severe injuries with stiff boots) and snow conditions (66% of injuries on icy, hard slopes).[98,100,103] Snowboarders have been criticized for their risk-taking behaviour (speed, off piste skiing), but this was not confirmed in Berghold and Seidl's study.[98]

The intrinsic and extrinsic risk factors are listed in Table 5.4.5.

Table 5.4.5 Intrinsic and extrinsic risk factors for skiing and snowboarding injuries, with their respective references

Intrinsic risk factors	Extrinsic risk factors
Novice skiers and snowboarders[98,100,103]	**Binding adjustment**[94]
Age (child, adolescent)[107]	**Helmets**[103]
Common sense[101]	**Snow conditions and weather (avalanches)**[98,100,103]
Conditioning	Fatigue (more injuries in mid-late afternoon)[108]
Risky behaviour[98,105]	Skiing fast from packed to deep snow[106]

Bold factors have been confirmed in prospective studies and/or are supported by a general agreement in literature, whilst the others still lack statistical support.

Preventive strategies

Injury awareness programmes assisted by video presentations on risk behaviour, dangerous situations and how to avoid them have had considerable impact on ACL injuries in Vermont,[109] and can serve as a model for injury prevention in skiing and other sports. Children should receive particular attention because of their relatively high injury risk. They should be informed of risk factors and how to avoid them, especially if they are beginners and/or snowboarders.

Some improvement can certainly be made to safety equipment (skis, bindings, pole handles, gloves) by the industry, but equipment should always be checked and adjusted for weight and expertise. The regular use of helmets should be encouraged for children.

Skiers should take particular care in evaluating snow conditions and the risks in skiing off the piste. Some common sense rules as put forward by Chisell[101] can be of use:

(1) quit before 3 o'clock;

(2) go shopping (or something other than skiing) on the third day; and

(3) be wary when skiing at altitudes over 3000 m.

Swimming

Swimming is among the most popular leisure and competitive sports throughout the world. Participants often begin at a young age, and the swimmers who choose to compete quickly progress to heavy training loads which lead to important loads on the upper extremities and, to a lesser extent, the lower extremity.

Epidemiology of swimming injuries

Few data are available on the epidemiology of swimming injuries in children. Swimming is mostly thought of as a 'safe' sport and the available data tend to confirm this. Maffuli et al.[110] found an injury incidence of 0.3 injuries per 1000 h of swimming in a group of highly trained 10–16 year old swimmers. This is similar to the injury incidence found by Schnyder (personal communication) who found an injury incidence of 0.5 injuries per 1000 h in a group of competitive 12–15 year old swimmers, training an average of 11 hours a week. The injury incidence was similar for boys and girls in both groups.

Most injuries are overuse injuries (62%) and concern mainly the shoulder and arm (35%) followed by the trunk (25%) and the lower extremity (20%).[111] The majority of injuries are benign and lead to short absences from sport. In Rowley's study,[111] 65% of injuries were sustained outside the sports activity, 25% during training and about 6% during competitions.

Aetiology of swimming injuries

Most authors agree that the repetitivity and the high training volume, leading to about 2 million strokes per year in elite swimmers, is the main source of injury.[112] Injury incidence has been shown to correlate with exposure[113,114] and performance, with medal winners showing a higher incidence of injury.[115]

Injury type varies between strokes, shoulder injuries being most common in free-style, back-stroke and butterfly swimming,[112] whilst knee injuries are more common in breast stroke.[116] This can be explained by the varying biomechanics of the strokes, stressing different structures. Shoulder problems mainly result from a sub-acromial impingement mechanism linked to repetitive overhead motion, and which may be aggravated by muscle imbalance between internal and external rotators, shoulder instability[117,118] and acromial shape.[119] Shoulder injuries have also been shown to be related to improper technique, premature strength training and the use of devices such as the pull buoy and paddles.[112]

Knee problems are mainly linked to patello-femoral dysfunction during kicking or medial collateral ligament stress which is more specific to breast stroke. Lower extremity malalignment and patellar instability have been suggested as risk factors.[120]

Back pain can be linked to the repeated flexion and twisting during flip turns, torsional strain if the body is not rolled as a whole unit during the stroke or to swimming techniques that lead to lumbo-sacral hyperextension (breast stroke, butterfly).[121]

The intrinsic and extrinsic risk factors are listed in Table 5.4.6.

Preventive strategies

Ciullo and Stevens[112] suggest a series of factors that may contribute to preventing injuries in youth; emphasis should be placed on proper stroke mechanics, little emphasis on performance, stretching should be carried out before and after swimming, sessions should be started very progressively and terminated at the first signs of fatigue (perturbed mechanics). Strength training should begin in skeletally mature swimmers, when proper swimming mechanics have been acquired, and start with high repetition low resistance exercises. Bak,[122] however, suggests that resistance training in prepubescent swimmers could improve muscle balance and prevent injuries. He also suggests that coaches should be informed on preventive strategies.

Tennis and badminton

Because of similarities in injury profile and biomechanics, this section includes both tennis and badminton. For various reasons, these sports have become increasingly popular amongst youths, leading to early specialization and intensification of training programmes. This has resulted in an increase in injuries in the younger population.[123]

Epidemiology of tennis and badminton injuries

Zaricznyj et al.[124] studied a population of school-aged children and found that 0.3% and 0.1% of the 1576 sports related injures were sustained during tennis and badminton, respectively. This gives an injury incidence of 0.01 per 1000 hours for tennis and quasi 0 for badminton. A similar injury incidence (<1%) was found by Watson[125] in Irish School children. During a two year prospective study on high school children, Garrick and Requa[126] found a 3% incidence of injury in girls and 7% in boys for tennis, and 6% for female badminton players. However, for competitive and elite tennis, injury levels seem to be substantially higher, with about 24% of players at the competitive level[127] and 60% at the elite level having sustained an injury in the two previous years.[123] It would also seem that girls are more often injured than boys at the elite level, contrary to what was found at high school level.[128]

The majority of injuries seem to be from overuse and mainly involve the lower extremity (hamstring, knee, ankle). Injuries to the back, neck and groin occur at a similar frequency to the upper extremity (shoulder, elbow, wrist), but half as frequently as injuries to the lower extremity.[128] In badminton, 74% of injuries are from overuse and involve mainly the lower extremity (83%).[129] In tennis the most frequently observed injuries are rotator cuff tendinitis, epicondylitis, chronic muscle strain and stress fractures. Shoulder subluxation, labral tears, 'Osgood–Schlatter disease of the shoulder', slipped capital humeral epiphysis and a stress fracture of the humeral epiphysis have been described in junior tennis and badminton players' shoulders.[130,131] Eye injuries[132] and neurological injuries involving the suprascapular nerve[133] have also been described.

Aetiology of tennis and badminton injuries

Most injuries are due to repetitive microtrauma as shown by the high incidence of overuse injuries in both tennis and badminton, and may be higher if acute injuries secondary to overuse are included. The overuse mechanism involves mainly the upper extremity,[130] and is often due to poor technique, repetitive movements, fatigue and loss of coordination, as well as inappropriate equipment and training programmes.[134,135] Lower extremity injuries are related to the constant pounding, accelerations and decelerations during games,[136] and to the high eccentric loads which can lead to muscle tears and tendinous injuries.[137] In badminton, however, injuries are often sustained when players stumble while trying to play a stroke.[129] Range of motion may

Table 5.4.6 Intrinsic and extrinsic risk factors for swimming injuries, with their respective references

Intrinsic risk factors	Extrinsic risk factors
Shoulder muscle imbalance[117]	Exposure[113,114]
Shoulder instability[118]	Technique[112,121]
Acromial shape[119]	Using a pull buoy or paddles[112]
Lower extremity malalignment or patellar instability[120]	Premature or unadapted strength training[112] Type of stroke[112,116]

Bold factors have been confirmed in prospective studies and/or are supported by a general agreement in literature, whilst the others still lack statistical support.

also influence predisposition to injury, internal rotation having been shown to be limited in the dominant arm of tennis players.[138] Muscle imbalances and shortness observed in the shoulder, the forearm and the trunk may also predispose the athlete to injury.[128] A higher exposure to matches, as shown by Kibler et al.,[123] may contribute to an increase in the number of injuries in tennis, but the inverse seems to be the case in badminton.[139]

The intrinsic and extrinsic risk factors are listed in Table 5.4.7.

Preventive strategies

Prevention should start by informing players and coaches about the risks of injury linked to the sport, injuries themselves, injury treatment and prevention. Even though statistical evidence is poor, a good basic fitness level, specific strengthening, regular stretching exercises (internal rotation of the dominant arm) and adapted equipment[142] should be encouraged. Varying the playing surface or reducing play on hard courts may also reduce lower limb injuries.

Volleyball

Volleyball is progressively becoming one of the more popular sports for both boys and girls with an estimated 150 million players in the world. It has also become more attractive to children with the introduction of mini volleyball (which is more adapted for younger children) and beach volleyball.

Epidemiology of volleyball injuries

In a six week retrospective study of 1818 school children, Backx et al.[3] found a surprisingly high volleyball injury incidence of 6.7/1000 hours, compared with the data of Zaricznyj et al.[124] who found an injury incidence of 0.13/1000 hours. In the study of Backx et al., the injuries were sustained mainly during practice and were recorded at the beginning of a season. A relatively broad injury definition, however, may bias results and gives little information on the severity of the injuries. Injuries during practice seem to be more frequent than during competitive play.[3,4,143] The evolution from being more of a leisure activity to a highly competitive sport, with the subsequent increase in training volume, may contribute to the increase in injuries as seen over the last 10–15 years.[144]

No data are available on the prevalence of injuries in children, but extrapolating from adult data, sprains (principally ankle and knee) followed by strains and overuse injuries seem to comprise the bulk of observed pathologies. According to Zaricznyj et al.,[124] 50% of injuries are to the hands and fingers, 20% to the ankles and 6% to the knees in children. This contrasts with adult data in an amateur volleyball league where 48% of injuries were to the lower extremity, 26% to the upper extremity and 26% to the trunk and head.[145] Case series including adolescents have shown a high frequency of patellofemoral and patellar tendon pathologies.[146] Isolated cases of long thoracic nerve entrapment[147] and a stress fracture of the ulna[148] have also been reported.

Aetiology of volleyball injuries

The jumping action (eccentric loads) during offensive and defensive play and the numerous contacts between the knee and the playing surface during defensive play are said to be responsible for the majority of injuries around the knee.[3,149] Loss of balance during landing has also been incriminated in both knee and ankle injury. Jumping and landing with the knees in a valgus position,[150] landing with a twisting motion of the knee[151] as well as one legged takeoff and landing[152] all seem to contribute to injury risk. Ankle injuries are mostly sustained during collisions between players and often with the opponent under the net.[145] Shoulder injuries, including supraspinatus tendinopathy, impingement and nerve entrapment, are due to the extreme mechanics of spiking and the jump serve.[153] Fingers are mainly at risk during blocking.

Condensing data from adult literature, blocking seems to be responsible for the largest number of injuries followed by spiking and defence manoeuvres.[154] The intrinsic and extrinsic risk factors are listed in Table 5.4.8.

Preventive strategies

Specific attention should be given to children and their growth phases, adapting training loads to the individual. Malalignment and muscle imbalance should be identified and corrected where possible. Jumping and landing techniques have been shown to be important and can have a protective effect on ankle injuries.[159] Wearing protective equipment should be encouraged and the majority of play should, if possible, be done on wooden or linoleum surfaces.

Table 5.4.8 Intrinsic and extrinsic risk factors for volleyball injuries, with their respective references

Intrinsic risk factors	Extrinsic risk factors
Younger age group[155]	**Exposure (frequency > length)**[149,151]
Growth spurt[156]	**Position (offensive > defensive)**[145]
Poor jumping technique[150–152]	Quality of training[157]
Malalignment of the extensor mechanism	Playing surface[158]
Muscle imbalance	Collision with opponent[145]
Males > females (injury specific trends)	

Bold factors have been confirmed in prospective studies and/or are supported by a general agreement in literature, whilst the others still lack statistical support.

Table 5.4.7 Intrinsic and extrinsic risk factors for tennis and badminton injuries, with their respective references

Intrinsic risk factors	Extrinsic risk factors
Sex ($M > F$)[126]	**Exposure**[123]
Elite tennis ($F > M$)[128]	**Exposure to match**[123]
Low fitness level	Playing surface[141]
Low flexibility[123,138]	Equipment (racket, grip, cord tension, balls)[134,135]
Insufficient shoulder strength[140]	
Muscle imbalance[128]	

Bold factors have been confirmed in prospective studies and/or are supported by a general agreement in literature, whilst the others still lack statistical support. *M*: males, *F*: females.

Summary

Based on the data above, no comparison can be made between sports in terms of relative injury risk (per 1000 h), because of the great disparity in sports practice and data collection. Similarities do, however, exist in epidemiological trends, in injury risk factors and in preventive strategies, but it appears that few data are getting to the field and being used.[160] Factors like insufficient time, stress, money, school and ignorance are often put forward as excuses not to implement this knowledge. Therefore, preventive trends like informing coaches and athletes about prevention and risk factors, adapting the training load to growth, doing a good warm-up, stretching after exercise, taking time for recuperation and regeneration, properly treating injuries, using protective equipment, discouraging 'achievement by proxy', and insuring adequate nutrition and hydration should be encouraged and monitored in all sports even though data are not equivocal.

It is the right of all children to benefit from this information so that we can ensure a safe sports practice and a proper application of the 'Children's Rights in Sport'.[161]

Acknowledgements

My warmest thanks go to Dr P. Fricker and Dr F. Mahler for their help in correcting and improving this text.

References

1. **DeKnop, P., Engström, L. M., Skirstad, B.** and **Weiss, M. R.** *World-wide trends in youth sport,* Human Kinetics, Champaign, IL, 1996.

2. **DeLoes, M.** and **Goldie, I.** Incidence rate of injuries during sport activity and physical exercise in a rural Swedish municipality: incidence rates in 17 sports. *International Journal of Sports Medicine* 1988; **9**: 461–7.

3. **Backx, F. J., Beijer, H. J. M., Bol, E.** and **Erick, W. B. M.** Injuries in high-risk persons and high-risk sports. A longitudinal study of 1818 school children. *American Journal of Sports Medicine* 1991; **19**: 124–30.

4. **Kujala, U. M., Taimela, S., Antti-Poika, I., Orava, S., Tuominen, R.** and **Myllynen, P.** Acute injuries in soccer, ice hockey, volleyball, basketball, judo, and karate : analysis of national registry data. *British Medical Journal* 1995; **311**: 1465–8.

5. **Van Mechelen, W., Twisk, J., Molendijk, A., Blom, B., Snel, J.** and **Kemper, H. C.** Subject-related risk factors for sports injuries: a 1-yr prospective study in young adults. *Medicine and Science in Sports and Exercise* 1996; **28**: 1171–79.

6. **Walter, S. D., Sutton, J. R., McIntosh, J. M.** and **Conolly, C.** The aetiology of sport injuries. A review of methodologies. *Sports Medicine* 1985; **2**: 47–58.

7. **Bohlmann, J. T.** Injuries in competitive cycling. *The Physician in Sports Medicine* 1981; **9**: 117–24.

8. **McLennan, J. G., McLennan, J. C.** and **Ungersma, J.** Accident prevention in competitive cycling. *American Journal of Sports Medicine* 1988; **16**: 266–8.

9. **Chow, T. K., Bracker, M. D.** and **Patrick, K.** Acute injuries from mountain biking. *West Journal of Medicine* 1993; **159**: 145–8.

10. **Baker, S. P., Li. G., Fowler, C.** and **Dannenberg, A. L.** *Injuries to bicyclists: a national perspective.* The Johns Hopkins University Injury Prevention Centre, Baltimore, MD, 1993.

11. **Holmes, J. C., Pruitt, A. L.** and **Whalen, N. J.** Lower extremity overuse in bicycling. In *Clinics in sports medicine* (ed. M. B. Mellion and E. R. Burke), W. B. Saunders, Philadelphia, 1994; 187–206.

12. **Mellion, M. B.** Neck and back pain in cycling. In *Clinics in sports medicine* (ed. M. B. Mellion and E. R. Burke), W. B. Saunders, Philadelphia, 1994; 137–64.

13. **Weiss, B. D.** Clinical syndromes associated with bicycle seats. In *Clinics in sports medicine* (ed. M. B. Mellion and E. R. Burke), W. B. Saunders, Philadelphia, 1994; 175–86.

14. **Richmond, D. R.** Handlebar problems in bicycling. In *Clinics in sports medicine* (ed. M. B. Mellion and E. R. Burke), W. B. Saunders, Philadelphia, 1994; 165–74.

15. **Mosimann, R., Walder, J.** and **Van Melle, G.** Stenotic intimal thickening of the external iliac artery: illness of the competition cyclists?. *Vascular Surgery* 1985; **19**: 258–63.

16. **Friede, A. M., Azzara, C. V., Gallagher, S. S.** and **Guyer, B.** The epidemiology of injuries to bicycle riders. *Paediatric Clinics of North America* 1985; **32**: 141–51.

17. **Thompson, D. C.** and **Patterson, M. Q.** Cycle helmets and the prevention of injuries. *Sports Medicine* 1998; **25**: 213–19.

18. **Burke, E. R.** Proper fit of the bicycle. In *Clinics in sports medicine* (ed. M. B. Mellion and E. R. Burke), W. B. Saunders, Philadelphia, 1994; 1–15.

19. **Nichols, C. E.** Injuries in cycling. In clinical practice of sports injury prevention and care. In *Encyclopaedia of sports medicine* (ed. P. Renstrom). Blackwell Scientific Publications, Oxford, 1994; 514–25.

20. **Mondenard, J. P.** *Technopathies du cyclisme,* Ciba Geigy, Paris, 1989; 12–29.

21. **Bejjani, F. J.** Occupational biomechanics of athletes and dancers: a comparative approach. *Clinics in Paediatric Medicine and Surgery* 1987; **4**: 671–711.

22. **Reid, D. C., Burnham, R. S., Saboe, L. A.** and **Kushner, S. F.** Lower extremity flexibility patterns in classical ballet dancers and their correlation to lateral hip and knee injuries. *American Journal of Sports Medicine* 1987; **15**: 347–52.

23. **Rovere, G. D., Webb, L. Z., Gristina, A. G.** and **Vogel, J. M.** Musculoskeletal injuries in theatrical dance students. *American Journal of Sports Medicine* 1983; **11**: 195–8.

24. **Clanin, D. R., Davidson, D. M.** and **Plastino, J. G.** Injury patterns in university dance students. In *The dancer as athlete* (ed. C. G. Shell), Human Kinetics, Champaign, IL, 1986; 195–99.

25. **Bowling, A.** Injuries to dancers: prevalence, treatment, and perceptions of causes. *British Medical Journal* 1989; **298**: 731–734.

26. **Wiesler, R., Monte Hunter, D., Martin, D. F., Curl, W. W.** and **Hoen H.** Ankle flexibility and injury patterns in dancers. *The American Journal of Sports Medicine* 1996; **24**: 754–7.

27. **Caine, C. G.** and **Garrick, J. G.** Dance. In *Epidemiology of sports injuries* (ed. D. J. Caine, C. G. Caine and K. J. Lindner), Human Kinetics, Champaign, IL, 1996; 130–3.

28. **Benson, J. E., Geiger, C. J., Eiserman, P. A.** and **Wardlaw, G. M.** Relationship between nutrient intake, body mass index, menstrual function, and ballet injury. *Journal of the American Dietetic Association* 1989; **89**: 58–63.

29. **Caine, C. G.** and **Garrick, J. G.** Dance. In *Epidemiology of sports injuries* (ed. D. J. Caine, C. G. Caine and K. J. Lindner), Human Kinetics, Champaign, IL, 1996; 137–9.

30. **Kadel, N. J., Teitz, C. C.** and **Kronmal, R. A.** Stress fractures in ballet dancers. *American Journal of Sports Medicine* 1992; **20**: 445–9.

31. **Warren, M. P., Brooks-Gunn, J., Hamilton, L. H., Warren, L. F.** and **Hamilton, W. G.** Scoliosis and fractures in young ballet dancers: relation to delayed menarche and secondary amennohrea. *The New England Journal of Medicine* 1986; **314**: 1348–53.

32. **Brainsted, J. R., Mellin, L., Gong , E. J.** and **Irwin, C. E. Jr.** The adolescent ballet dancer. Nutritional practices and characteristics associated with anorexia nervosa. *Journal of Adolescent Health Care* 1985; **6**: 365–71.

33. **Clippinger-Robertson, K. S., Hutton, R. S., Miller, D. I.** and **Nichols, T. R.** Mechanical and anatomical factors relating to the incidence and aetiology of patello-femoral pain in dancers. In *The dancer as athlete* (ed. C. G. Shell). Human Kinetics, Champaign IL, 1986; 53–72.

34. Ireland, M. L. and Micheli, L. J. Bilateral stress fracture of the lumbar pedicles in a ballet dancer. *Journal of Bone and Joint Surgery* 1987; **69A**: 140–2.

35. Kravitz, S. R. Pronation as a predisposing factor in overuse injuries. In *Preventing dance injuries: An interdisciplinary perspective* (ed. R. Solomon *et al.*), National Dance Association, 1990; 15–20.

36. Scheller, A. D., Kasser, J. R. and Quigley, T. B. Tendon injuries about the ankle. *Clinics in Sports Medicine* 1983; **2**: 6313–41.

37. Stoller, S. M., Hekmat, F. and Kleiger, B. A comparative study of the frequency of anterior impingement exostoses of the ankle in dancers and non dancers. *Foot Ankle* 1984; **4**: 201–3.

38. Lehmann, R. C., Gregg, J. R. and Torg, E. Iselin's disease. *American Journal of Sports Medicine* 1986; **14**: 494–6.

39. Micheli, L. J., Sohn, R. S. and Solomon, R. Stress fractures of the second metatarsal involving Lisfranc's joint in ballet dancers. *Journal of Bone and Joint Surgery* 1985; **67A**: 1372–5.

40. Fernandez-Palazzi, F., Rivas, S. and Mujica, P. Achilles tendinitis in ballet dancers. *Clinical Orthopaedics and Related Rehabilitation* 1990; **257**: 257–61.

41. Skrinar, M., Carlson, K. and Jeglosky, L. Effect of three brands of pointed shoe on pelvic tilt (abstract). *International Journal of Sports Medicine* 1981; **2**: 283.

42. Klemp, P. and Chalton, D. Articular mobility in ballet dancers, a follow-up study after four years. *American Journal of Sports Medicine* 1989; **17**: 72–5.

43. Gans, A. The relationship of heel contact in ascent and decent from jumps to the incidence of shin splints in ballet dancers. *Physical Therapy* 1985; **65**: 1192–6.

44. Solomon, R. and Micheli, L. Concepts in the prevention of dance injuries: a survey and analysis. In *The dancer as athlete* (ed. C. G. Shell), Human Kinetics, Champaign, IL, 1986; 201–12.

45. Reid, D. C. (1987). Preventing injuries to the young ballet dancer. *Physiotherapy, Canada*, **39**, (4), 231–36.

46. Plastino, J. G. Physical screening of the dancer: General methodologies and procedure. In *Preventing dance injuries: An interdisciplinary perspective* (ed. R. Solomon *et al.*), National Dance Association, 1990; 155–75.

47. Lauffenburger, S. K. Bartenieff fundamentals: Early detection of potential dance injuries. In *Preventing dance injuries: An interdisciplinary perspective* (ed. R. Solomon *et al.*), National Dance Association, 1990; 177–90.

48. Sands, W. A., Schultz, B. B. and Newman, A. P. Woman's gymnastics injuries. A 5 year study. *American Journal of Sports Medicine* 1993; **21**: 271–76.

49. Clark, K. S. and Miller, S. J. The national athletic injury/illness system (NAIRS). In *Sports safety II* (ed. C. H. Morehouse). The American Alliance for Health, Physical Education and Recreation, Washington, 1977; 49–53.

50. NCAA, National Collegiate Athletic Association 1993–94 men's and women's gymnastics injury surveillance system, *NCAA Report*, Kansas, 1994.

51. Dixon, M. and Fricker, P. Injuries to elite gymnasts over 10 years. *Medicine and Science in Sports and Exercise* 1993; **25**: 1322–9.

52. Caine, D. J., Lindner, K. J., Mandelbaum, B. R. and Sands, W. A. Gymnastics. In *Epidemiology of sports injuries* (ed. D. J. Caine, C. G. Caine and K. J. Lindner), Human Kinetics, Champaign, IL, 1996; 219

53. Caine, D. J., Lindner, K. J., Mandelbaum, B. R. and Sands, W. A. Gymnastics. In *Epidemiology of sports injuries* (ed. D. J. Caine, C. G. Caine and K. J. Lindner), Human Kinetics, Champaign, IL, 1996; 220–22.

54. Tofler, I. R., Stryer, B. K., Micheli, L. J. and Herman, L. R. Physical and emotional problems of elite female gymnasts. *New England Journal of Medicine*, 1996; **335**: 281–83.

55. Takai, Y. A comparison of techniques used in performing the men's compulsory gymnastic vault at the 1988 Olympics. *International Journal of Sports Biomechanics* 1991; **7**: 54–75.

56. Panzer, V. P., Wood, G. A., Bates, B. T. and Mason, B. R. Lower extremity loads in landings of elite gymnasts. *Biomechanics XI-B* (ed. G. de Groot *et al.*), Free University Press, Amsterdam, 1988.

57. Too, D. and Adrain, M. Relationship of lumbar curvature and landing surface to ground reaction forces during gymnastic landing. In *Biomechanics in sports III and IV* (ed. J. Terauds *et al.*), Academic Publishers, Del Mar, CA, 1987; 29–34.

58. Hall, S. J. Mechanical contribution to lumbar stress injuries in female gymnasts. *Medicine and Science in Sports and Exercise* 1986; **18**: 599–602.

59. Helleström, M., Jacobsson, B., Sward, L. and Peterson, L. Radiological abnormalities of the thoraco-lumbar spine in athletes. *Acta Radiologica* 1990; **31**: 127–32.

60. Sands, W. A. and Cheltham, P. J. Velocity of the vault run: junior elite female gymnasts. *Technique* 1986; **6**: 10–14.

61. Caine, D., Howe, W., Ross, W. and Bergman, G. Does repetitive physical loading inhibit radial growth in female gymnasts? *Clinical Journal of Sports Medicine* 1997; **7**: 302–8.

62. DiFiori, J. P., Puffer, J. C., Mandelbaum, B. R. and Dorey, F. Distal radial growth plate injury and positive ulnar variance in non elite gymnasts. *The American Journal of Sports Medicine* 1997; **25**: 763–8.

63. Hirasawa, Y. and Sakakida, K. Sports and peripheral nerve injury. *American Journal of Sports Medicine* 1983; **11**: 420–6.

64. Torg, J. S. Trampoline-induced quadriplegia. *Clinics in Sports Medicine* 1987; **6**: 73–85.

65. DeSmet, L., Claessens, A., Lefevre, J., DeCorte, F., Beunen, G., Stijnen, V., Maes, H., and Veer, F. M. Gymnast wrist: an epidemiological survey of the ulnar variance in elite female gymnasts. *American Journal of Sports Medicine* 1994; **22**: 846–50.

66. Meeusen, R. and Borms, J. Gymnastics injuries. *Sports Medicine* 1992; **13**: 337–56.

67. Caine, D. *An epidemiological investigation of injuries affecting young competitive female gymnasts.* Doctoral Dissertation. Microform Publications, University of Oregon, 1988.

68. Dzioba, R. B. Irreversible spinal deformity in Olympic gymnasts. *Orthopaedic Transactions* 1984; **8**: 66.

69. Caine, D., Cochrane, B., Caine, C. and Zemper, E. An epidemiologic investigation of injuries affecting young competitive female gymnasts. *American Journal of Sports Medicine* 1989; **17**: 811–20.

70. Lueken, J., Stone, J. and Wallach, B. A. Olympic training centre report men's gymnastics injuries. *Gymnastics Safety Update* 1993; **8**: 4–5.

71. Goldstein, J. D., Berger, P. E., Windler, G. E. and Jackson, D. W. Spine injuries in gymnasts and swimmers: an epidemiological investigation. *American Journal of Sports Medicine* 1991; **19**: 463–8.

72. Gremion, G., Bielinski, R., Vallotton, J., Augros, R., Laréqui, Y. and Leyvraz, P. F. (Gymnastics World Championships at Lausanne: Medical Backup). Schweizerische Zeitschrift fur 'Sportmedizin und Sporttraumatologie', 1998; **46**: 64–6.

73. Micheli, L. J. Low back pain in the adolescent: differential diagnosis. *American Journal of Sports Medicine* 1979; **7**: 362–6.

74. Irvin, R., Major, J. and Sands, W. A. Lower body and torso strength norms for elite female gymnasts. In *1992 USGF Sport Science Congress Proceedings*, (ed. McNitt Gray *et al.*), USGF publications, Indianapolis, 1992; 5–12.

75. Kerr, G. A. Psychological factors related to the occurrence of athletic injuries. *Journal of Sport and Exercise Psychology* 1988; **10**: 167–73.

76. Sands, W. A., Crain, R. S. and Lee, K. M. Gymnastics coaching survey. *Technique* 1990; **10**: 22–7.

77. Sands, W. A. *Coaching women's gymnastics*, Human Kinetics, Champaign, IL, 1984.

78. Smith, A. D., Andrish, J. T. and Micheli, L. J. Current comment: the prevention of sport injuries of children and adolescents. *Medicine and Science in Sports and Exercise* 1993; **25**: 1–7.

79. Orava, S. and Saarela, J. Exertion injuries to young athletes. *American Journal of Sports Medicine* 1978; **6**: 68–74.

80. Nudel, D. B., Hassett, I., Gurian, A., Diamant, S., Weinhouse, E. and Goodman N. Young long distance runners. Physiological and psychological characteristics. *Clinical Pediatrics* 1989; **28**: 500–5.

81. Rowland, T. W. and Walsh, C. A. Characteristics of child distance runners. *The Physician and Sports Medicine* 1985; **13**: 45–8, 52–3.

82. Van Mechelen, W. Running injuries: A review of the epidemiological literature. *Sports Medicine* 1992; **14**: 320–325.

83. Knutzen, K. and Hart, L. Running. In *Epidemiology of spots injuries* (ed. D. J. Caine, C. G. Caine and K. J. Lindner), Human Kinetics, New York, 1996; 364.

84. Clancy, W. G. and Folz, A. S. Iliac apophysitis and stress fractures in adolescent runners. *American Journal of Sports Medicine*, 1976; **4**: 214–18.

85. Godshall, R. W., Hansen, C. A. and Rising, D. C. Stress fractures through the distal femoral apophysis in athletes. *American Journal of Sports Medicine* 1981; **9**: 114–16.

86. Daffner, R. H., Martinez, S., Gehweiler, J. A. and Harrelson, J. M. Stress fractures of the proximal tibia in runners. *Radiology* 1982; **142**: 63–5.

87. McKenzie, D. C., Taunton, J. E., Clement, D. B., Smart, G. W. and McNicol, K. L. Calcaneal apophysitis in adolescent athletes. *Canadian Journal of Applied Sport Sciences* 1981; **6**: 123–5.

88. Cibulka, M. T. Management of a patient with forefoot pain. *Physical Therapy* 1990; **70**: 41–4.

89. Taunton, J. E., Clement, D. B. and Webber, D. Lower extremity fractures in athletes. *The Physician and Sports Medicine* 1981; **9**: 85–6.

90. Brunet, M. E., Cook, S. D., Brinker, M. R. and Dickijnson, J. A. A survey of running injuries in 1505 competitive and recreational runners. *Journal of Sports Medicine and Physical Fitness* 1990; **30**: 307–15.

91. Marti, B. Benefits and risks of running among women: an epidemiological study. *International Journal of Sports Medicine* 1988; **9**: 92–8.

92. Van Mechelen, W. Can Running injuries be effectively prevented?. *Sports Medicine* 1995; **19**: 161–65.

93. Burns, T. P., Steadman, J. R. and Rodkey, W. G. Alpine skiing and the mature athlete. *Clinics in Sports Medicine* 1991; **10**: 327–38.

94. Deibert, M. C., Aronsson, D. D., Johnson, R. J., Ettlinger, C. F. and Shealy, J. E. Skiing injuries in children. *Journal of Bone and Joint Surgery* 1998; **80**: 25–32.

95. Macnab, A. J. and Cadman, R. Demographics of alpine skiing and snow-boarding injury: lessons for prevention programs. *Injury Prevention* 1996; **2**: 286–9.

96. Matter, P., Ziegler, W. J. and Holzach, P. Skiing accidents in the past 15 years. *Journal of Sports Science* 1987; **5**: 319–26.

97. Pigozzi, F., Santori, N., DiSalvo, V., Parisi, A. and Di-Luigi, L. Snowboard traumatology: an epidemiological study. *Orthopaedics* 1997; **20**: 505–9.

98. Berghold, F. and Seidl, A. M. (Snowboarding accidents in the Alps. Assessment of risk, analysis of the accidents and injury profile). *Schweitzer Zeitung fur Sportmeditzin* 1991; **39**: 13–20.

99. Bladin, C. and McCrory, P. Snowboarding injuries. *Sports Medicine* 1995; **19**: 358–64.

100. Chow, T. K., Corbett, S. W. and Farstad, D. J. Spectrum of injuries from snowboarding. *Journal of Traumatology* 1996; **41**: 321–25.

101. Chissell, H. R., Feagin, J. A., Warme, W. J., Lambert, K. L., King, P. and Johnson, L. Trends in ski and snowboard injuries. *Sports Medicine* 1996; **22**: 141–5.

102. Lystad, H. A one year study of alpine ski injuries in Hemsedal, Norway. *Skiing trauma and safety: fifth international symposium. ASTM STP* 1985; **860**: 314–25.

103. Shorter, N. A., Jensen, P. E., Harmon, B. J. and Monney, D. P. Skiing injuries in children and adolescents. *Journal of Traumatology* 1996; **40**: 997–1001.

104. Higgins, R. W. and Steadman, J. R. Anterior cruciate ligament repairs in world class skiers. *American Journal of Sports Medicine* 1987; **15**: 139–47.

105. Reid, D. C. and Saboe, L. Spine fractures in winter sports. *Sports Medicine* 1989; **7**: 393–9.

106. Feagin, J. A., Lambert, K. L., Cunningham, R. R., Anderson, L. M., Riegel, J., King, P. H. and Van Generen, L. Considerations of the anterior cruciate ligament injury in skiing. *Clinics in Orthopaedic Related Research* 1987; **216**: 13–18.

107. Blitzer, C. M., Johnson, R. J. and Ettlinger, C. F. Downhill skiing injuries in children. *American Journal of Sports Medicine* 1984; **8**: 142–7.

108. Young, L. R. The aetiology of ski injuries: an eight year study of the skier and his equipment. *Orthopaedic Clinics of North America* 1976; **7**: 13–29.

109. Ettliger, C. F., Johnson, R. J. and Shealy, J. E. A method to help reduce the risk of serious knee sprains incurred in alpine skiing. *America Journal of Sports Medicine* 1995; **23**: 531–7.

110. Maffulli, N., King, J. B. and Helms, P. Training in elite young athletes (the training of young athletes (TOYA) study): injuries, flexibility and isometric strength. *British Journal of Sports Medicine* 1994; **28**: 123–36.

111. Rowley, S. *Training of young athletes study: Project description*, The Sports Council, 1992; 1–17.

112. Ciullo, V. C., Stevens G. G. The prevention and treatment of injuries to the shoulder in swimming. *Sports Medicine* 1989; **7**: 182–204.

113. Ciullo, V. C. Swimmer's shoulder. *Clinics in Sports Medicine* 1986; **5**: 115–37.

114. Stocker, D., Pink, M. and Jobe, F. W. Comparison of shoulder injury in collegiate and master's-level swimmers. *Clinical Journal of Sports Medicine* 1995; **5**: 4–8.

115. Bak, K., Bue, P. and Olsson, G. (Injury patterns in Danish competitive swimming), *Ugeskraeft for Laeger* 1989; **151**: 2982–4.

116. Costill, D. L., Maglischo, E. W. and Richardson, A. B. Swimming. Blackwell Science, Oxford, 1992; 190–2.

117. McMaster, W. C. Swimming injuries. *Sports Medicine* 1996; **22**: 332–36.

118. Bak, K. and Magnusson, S. P. Shoulder strength and range of motion in symptomatic and pain-free elite swimmers. *American Journal of Sports Medicine* 1997; **25**: 454–9.

119. Fowler, P. J. and Webster-Bogaert, M. S. Swimming. In *Sports medicine, the school-age athlete* (ed. B. Reider), W. B. Saunders, Philadelphia, 1991; 429–46.

120. Fowler, P. J. and Regan, W. D. Swimming injuries of the knee, foot and ankle, elbow, and back. *Clinics in Sports Medicine* 1986; **5**: 1986.

121. Kenal, K. A. and Knapp, L. D. Rehabilitation of injuries in competitive swimmers. *Sports Medicine* 1996; **22**: 337–47.

122. Bak, K. Nontraumatic glenohumeral instability and coracoacromial impingement in swimmers. *Scandinavian Journal of Medicine and Science in Sports* 1996; **6**: 132–44.

123. Kibler, W. B., McQueen, C. and Uhl, T. Fitness evaluation and fitness findings in competitive junior tennis players. *Clinics in Sports Medicine* 1988; **7**: 403–6.

124. Zaricznyj, B., Shattuck, L. J. M., Mast, T. A., Robertson, R. V. and D'Elia, G. Sports-related injuries in school-aged children. *American Journal of Sports Medicine* 1980; **8**: 318–23.

125. Watson, A. W. Sports injuries during one academic year in 6799 Irish school children. *American Journal of Sports Medicine* 1984; **12**: 65–71.

126. Garrick, J. G. and Requa R. K. Injuries in high school sports. *Paediatrics* 1978; **61**: 465–9.

127. Lehmann, R. C. Shoulder pain in the competitive tennis player. *Clinics in Sports Medicine* 1988; 7: 309–27.

128. Bylack, J. and Hutchinson, M. R. Common sports injuries in young tennis players. *Sports Medicine* 1998; **26**: 119–32.

129. Kroner, K., Schmidt, S. A. and Nielsen, A. B. Badminton injuries. *British Journal of Sports Medicine* 1990; **24**: 169–72.

130. Gregg, J. R. and Torg, E. Upper extremity injuries in adolescent tennis players. *Clinics in Sports Medicine* 1988; 7: 371–85.

131. Boyd, K. T. and Batt, M. E. Stress fracture of the proximal humeral epiphysis in an elite junior badminton player. *British Journal of Sports Medicine* 1997; **31**: 252–3.

132. Larrison, W. I., Hersh, P. S., Kunzweiler, T. and Shingleton, B. J. Sports-related occular trauma. *Ophthalmology* 1990; **97**: 1265–9.

133. Black, K. P. and Lombardo, J. A. Suprascapular nerve injuries with isolated paralysis of the infraspinatus. *American Journal of Sports Medicine* 1990; **18**: 225–8.

134. Nirschl, R. and Sobel, J. Tennis. In *Sports medicine, the school-age athlete* (ed. B. Reider), W. B. Saunders, Philadelphia, 1991; 664–72.

135. Beillot, J. and Parier, J. Tennis: Technological factors and epicondylitis. *Journal de Traumatologie du Sport* 1998; **15**: 62–9.

136. Gecha, S. R. and Torg, E. Knee injuries in tennis. *Clinics in Sports Medicine* 1988; 7: 371–85.

137. **Miller, W. A.** Rupture of the musculotendinous junction of the medial head of the gastrocnemius muscle. *American Journal of Sports Medicine* 1977; **5**: 191–93.

138. **Ellenbecker, T. S., Roetert, E. P., Piorkowski, P. A.** and **Schulz, D. A.** Glenohumeral joint internal and external rotation range of motion in elite junior tennis players. *Journal of Orthopaedics and Sports Physical Therapy* 1996; **24**: 336–41.

139. **Jorgensen, U.** and **Winge, S.** Epidemiology of badminton injuries. *International Journal of Sports Medicine* 1987; **8**: 379–82.

140. **Ellenbecker, T. S., Davies, G. J.** and **Rowinski, M. J.,** Concentric versus eccentric isokinetic strengthening of the rotator cuff. *American Journal of Sports Medicine* 1988; **16**: 64–9.

141. **Nigg, B. M.** and **Saegesser, B.** The influence of playing surfaces on the load of the locomotor system and on football and tennis injuries. *Sports Medicine* 1988; **5**: 375–85.

142. **Knudson, D. V.** Factors affecting force loading on the hand in the tennis forehand. *Journal of Sports Medicine and Physical Fitness* 1991; **31**: 527–31.

143. **Ferrari, G. P., Turra, S., Fama, G.** and **Gigante, C.** (Traumatic injury to the hand and wrist in volleyball, and its evolution). *Journal of Sports Traumatology Related Research* 1990; **12**: 95–9.

144. **Aagaard, H.** and **Jorgensen, U.** Injuries in elite volleyball. *Scandinavian Journal of Medicine and Science in Sports* 1996; **6**: 228–32.

145. **Schafle, M. D., Requa, R. K., Patton, W. L.** and **Garrick, J. G.** Injuries in the 1987 national amateur volleyball tournament. *Austrian Journal of Sports Medicine* 1990; **18**: 624–31.

146. **Ferretti, A.** Epidemiology of jumper's knee. *Sports Medicine* 1986; **3**: 289–95.

147. **Distefano, S.** Neuropathy due to entrapment of the long thoracic nerve. A case report. *Italian Journal of Orthopaedics and Traumatology* 1989; **12**: 159–62.

148. **Mutoh, Y., Mori, T., Suzuki, Y.** and **Sugiura, Y.** Stress fractures of the ulna in athletes. *American Journal of Sports Medicine* 1982; **10**: 365–7.

149. **Ferretti, A., Puddu, G., Mariani, P. P.** and **Neri, M.** Jumpers knee: An epidemiological study of volleyball players. *The Physician in Sports Medicine* 1984; **12**: 97–106.

150. **Sommer, H. M.** Patellar chondropathy and apicitis, and muscle imbalances in the lower extremities in competitive sports. *Sports Medicine* 1988; **5**: 386–94.

151. **Ferretti, A., Papandrea, P., Conteduca ,F.** and **Mariani, P. P.** Knee ligament injuries in volleyball players. *American Journal of Sports Medicine* 1992; **20**: 203–7.

152. **Van Soest, A. J., Roebroeck, M. E., Bobbert, M. F., Huijing, P. A.** and **Van Ingen Schenau, G. J.** A comparison of one-legged and two-legged countermovement jumps. *Medicine and Science in Sports and Exercise* 1985; **17**: 635–9.

153. **Sturbois, X.** and **Surowiecki, R.** Biomechanics and instability of the shoulder in volleyball. *Hermes* (Belgium) 1990; **21**: 423–30.

154. **Lindner, K. J.** and **Ferretti, A.** Volleyball. In *Epidemiology of sports injuries* (ed. D. J. Caine, C. G. Caine and K. J. Lindner), Human Kinetics, Champaign, IL, 1996.

155. **DeHaven, K. E.** and **Lintner, D. M.** Athletic injuries: Comparison by age, sport, and gender. *American Journal of Sports Medicine* 1986; **14**: 218–24.

156. **Backx, F. J., Erich, W. B., Kemper, A. B.** and **Verbeek, A. L.** Sports injuries in school-aged children: an epidemiological study. *American Journal of Sports Medicine* 1989; **17**: 234–40.

157. **Bobbert, M. F.** Drop jumping as a training method for jumping ability. *Sports Medicine* 1990; **9**: 7–22.

158. **Giacomelli, E., Grassi, W.** and **Zampa, A. M.** Athletes diseases affecting volleyball players. *Medicine dello Sport* 1986; **39**: 425–34.

159. **Bahr, R., Lian ,O.** and **Bahr, I. A.** A two-fold reduction in the incidence of acute ankle sprains in volleyball after the introduction of an injury prevention program: a prospective cohort study. *Scandinavian Journal of Medicine and Science in Sports* 1997; **7**: 172–7.

160. **Mahler, P. B., Bizzini, L., Batelaan, C., Schnyder, N.** and **Schnyder, J.** Epidemiology of injuries and their relation to preventive means among adolescents practising high level sports. In *Children in sport* (ed. F. J. Ring), Antony Rowe, Chippenham, UK, 1995; 184–8.

161. Un Champion at tout prix (A Champion at all costs). 5th Seminar on Children's Rights, International Institute for Children's Rights, Institut K. Bosch, CP. 4176, CH-1950 Sion 4, Switzerland, 1998.

5.5 Upper extremity and trunk injuries

Mininder S. Kocher and Lyle J. Micheli

Introduction

Injuries to the trunk and upper extremity in child and adolescent athletes are increasingly being seen with expanded participation and higher competitive levels of youth sports. Injury patterns are unique to the growing musculoskeletal system and specific to the demands of the involved sport. Recognition of injury patterns with early activity modification and the initiation of efficacious treatment can prevent deformity/disability and return the youth athlete to sport. This chapter reviews the diagnosis and management of common upper extremity and trunk injuries in the paediatric athlete.

Upper extremity injuries

Shoulder injuries

General

The shoulder complex involves four articulations and multiple ossification centres. The secondary centre of ossification of the proximal humeral epiphysis is usually seen after 6 months of age. Additional ossification centres appear at the greater tuberosity between 7 months and 3 years of age, and at the lesser tuberosity 2 years later. By age 5 to 7 years, these centres coalesce to form the proximal humeral epiphysis. The proximal humeral physis contributes approximately 80% of the longitudinal growth of the humerus and usually fuses between 19–22 years of age. The proximal humeral physis is extra-articular, except medially where the capsule extends beyond the anatomic neck, inserting on the medial metaphysis. The clavicle forms by intramembranous ossification in its central portion by the sixth gestational week. The medial secondary ossification centre appears between 12 and 19 years of age and does not fuse to the shaft until age 22–25 years. The lateral epiphysis is inconstant: appearing, ossifying and fusing over a period of a few months about age 19 years. The scapula appears as a cartilaginous anlage in the first gestational week at the C4–C5 level and gradually descends to its adult-like position overlying the first to fifth ribs. Failure to descend results in persistent elevation of the scapula and limited glenohumeral motion, Sprengel's deformity. The scapula ossifies via intramembranous ossification with multiple remaining secondary ossification centres. The ossification centre of the coracoid process appears at approximately one year, coalescing with the ossification centre of the upper glenoid by age 10 years. The acromion ossifies by multiple (two to five) ossification centres which usually appear about puberty and fuse by age 22 years. Failure of fusion of one of these ossification centres may result in an os acromionale. Various other scapular malformations may occur including bipartite coracoid, acromion duplication, glenoid dysplasia and scapular clefts.

Injury patterns to the paediatric athlete's shoulder tend to be sport specific. In American gridiron football, the shoulder ranks second only to the knee in number of overall injuries.[1–3] Injury patterns in rugby football are similar. These injuries tend to result from macrotrauma and include glenohumeral dislocation, acromioclavicular separation and clavicle fractures. Bicycling is a popular recreational and sporting activity among children and adolescents. Sixty per cent of all bicycle injuries occur in children between the ages of 5 and 14 years and 85% of injuries involve the upper extremity.[4,5] A common injury pattern during bicycling involves lateral clavicle fracture or acromioclavicular separation from landing on the point of the shoulder when thrown from the bicycle. Shoulder injuries during alpine skiing and snowboarding are being seen with increased frequency and account for approximately 40% of upper extremity injuries and 10% of all injuries.[6] Thirty per cent of wrestling injuries occur in the upper extremity with the shoulder being the most commonly involved location.[7] Injury to the acromioclavicular joint is frequent, resulting from a direct blow of the shoulder against the mat.[7,8]

Overuse injuries to the shoulder, resulting from repetitive overhead use, are becoming more common in the paediatric age group. In baseball, injury to the paediatric shoulder from throwing is a result of microtrauma from repetitive motions of large rotational forces.[9–11] The proximal humeral physis is particularly vulnerable to these large, repetitive forces resulting in a chronic physeal stress fracture, 'little league shoulder'.[10–17] The shoulder in tennis is similarly subjected to repetitive overhead motions involving large torques. Impingement and depression of the shoulder, 'tennis shoulder', may result.[18] Repetitive microtrauma also frequently leads to shoulder dysfunction in swimmers.[19] The risk of injury is related to competitive level and event type. Injuries include impingement syndrome and glenohumeral instability. Multidirectional instability is often seen and is related to the underlying ligamentous laxity often seen in swimmers. Similarly, multidirectional instability can be seen in gymnasts who also frequently demonstrate generalized ligamentous laxity. Additional shoulder injuries unique to gymnasts include cortical hypertrophy at the pectoralis major insertion, ringman's shoulder and supraspinatus tendinitis.[20–22]

Sternoclavicular joint injury

True sternoclavicular joint dislocations are rare in the skeletally immature. The characteristic injury involves a physeal fracture of the medial clavicle (Fig. 5.5.1), commonly a Salter–Harris I or II injury as the medial clavicular physis does not fuse until the early twenties.[23,24] The epiphysis stays attached to the sternum via the stout sternoclavicular ligaments and the medial clavicular shaft displaces posteriorly or anteriorly.

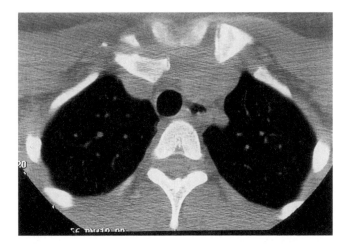

Fig. 5.5.1 Sternoclavicular joint injury. Axial CT scan demonstrating physeal fracture/separation of the medial clavicle with compression of the innominate vein in a 16 year old female.

Medial clavicular injury often results from an indirect force transmitted along the clavicle from a direct blow during contact sports to the lateral shoulder. If the shoulder is driven forward, posterior displacement of the medial clavicle occurs. Conversely, if the shoulder is driven posteriorly, anterior displacement of the medial clavicle occurs. The patient often describes a pop in the region of the sternoclavicular joint and there is tenderness to palpation of the medial clavicle. The direction of displacement may be obscured by marked swelling. Posterior displacement can be a medical emergency as the medial clavicle can impinge on vital mediastinal structures including the innominate great vessels, trachea or oesophagus.[25,26] Venous congestion, diminished pulses, dysphagia or dyspnea should alert the clinician to the possibility of such injury. Standard anteroposterior radiographs of the chest or sternoclavicular joint are often hard to interpret given the overlapping spinal, thoracic and mediastinal structures. A tangential X-ray taken in a 40° cephalad directed manner, the serendipity view, may aid in visualization of the medial clavicle displacement. Definitive delineation of the fracture pattern and direction of displacement is provided by CT scan.[27]

Minimally displaced fractures heal readily. Attempted reduction of anteriorly displaced fractures can be accomplished under local anaesthesia or sedation by placing the patient supine with a bolster between the scapulae. The arm is abducted 90° and then extended with gentle posterior pressure directly over the medial clavicle followed by protraction of the shoulder. After reduction, the shoulder is immobilized in a figure-of-eight dressing or shoulder immobilizer and gentle range of motion exercises are started as pain allows. Most fractures heal in 4–6 weeks and return to sport requires full painless range of motion and strength. Unstable fractures usually heal and remodel rapidly. Posteriorly displaced medial clavicular fractures with impingement of mediastinal structures require emergent reduction with thoracic surgery standby for the rare but potential injury of the major thoracic vessels.[28] Under general anaesthesia with the patient supine, traction is applied to the arm with the shoulder extended, and a towel clip can be used to reduce the medial clavicle. There is occasionally need for open reduction and internal fixation of irreducible medial clavicular physeal fractures. Care should be taken with internal fixation, and pins should

be removed as catastrophic complications of pin migration from hardware about the sternoclavicular joint have been reported.[29] Open reduction with stabilization of the torn periosteum and ligamentous structures with heavy non-absorbable suture should be attempted initially.

Clavicle fracture

The clavicular shaft is vulnerable to injury from direct blows during contact sports. In addition, indirect forces on the outstretched arm may lead to clavicular fracture. The clavicular shaft is mechanically vulnerable as a strut given its S-shaped configuration and the strong ligamentous bindings at either end. With fracture, there is limited shoulder motion, tenderness over the fracture site, and the skin overlying the fracture may be tented and compromised. The proximal fragment may be elevated superiorly due to spasm of the sternocleidomastoid or trapezius muscles. Significant neurovascular injury is rare, but should be assessed clinically given the proximity of the subclavian vessels and the brachial plexus. Plane radiographs are usually sufficient for diagnosis and management. Younger children may exhibit a greenstick fracture or plastic deformation.[30]

The prognosis of clavicular shaft fractures in children is excellent. Immobilization is accomplished by a figure-of-eight bandage or shoulder immobilizer. Slings which exert significant pressure to effect a reduction should be avoided. Even displaced fractures usually heal readily with a bump of healing callus which remodels over a period of 6 to 12 months. Return to sport is allowed when the clavicle is nontender, there is radiographic union, and motion and strength are full. This usually occurs by 4–6 weeks in younger children and 6–10 weeks in the adolescent. Significant malunion which does not remodel and non-union of clavicular shaft fractures in the skeletally immature are rare, but do occur.[31] Open reduction and internal fixation is indicated for open fractures, fractures with significant neurovascular compromise, threatened skin from fracture displacement, and floating shoulder injuries.[32,33]

Acromioclavicular joint injury

A fall on the point of the shoulder usually results in acromioclavicular separation in the adult and older adolescent, but often results in physeal fracture of the lateral clavicle in prepubescents.[28,29,34–37] With lateral clavicle fracture and true acromioclavicular separation in the paediatric patient, displacement of the lateral clavicle occurs superiorly through a tear in the thick periosteal tube surrounding the distal clavicle. The lateral clavicular epiphysis along with the acromioclavicular and coracoclavicular ligaments usually remain continuous with the periosteal tube. The paediatric athlete with lateral clavicle physeal fracture or acromioclavicular injury usually presents after a fall or contact to the point of the shoulder. Pain and deformity are localized to the acromioclavicular joint. Plane radiographs are usually sufficient to evaluate the injury, and stress X-rays with 5–10 pounds of traction may aid in delineating the degree of instability. An axillary lateral demonstrates anteroposterior displacement. Similar to adult acromioclavicular injuries, Rockwood has classified paediatric acromioclavicular injuries based on the position of the lateral clavicle and the accompanying injury to the periosteal tube. Type I injuries involve mild sprain of the acromioclavicular ligaments without disruption of the periosteal tube. Type II injuries involve partial disruption of the dorsal periosteal tube with slight widening of the acromioclavicular joint. Type III injuries involve a large dorsal disruption of the periosteal tube with gross instability of the distal clavicle. Type IV injuries involve disruption of the periosteal tube with posterior displacement of the lateral clavicle (Fig. 5.5.2). Type V injuries involve periosteal tube disruption with >100% superior subcutaneous displacement of the lateral clavicle. Type VI injuries involve an inferior subcoracoid dislocation of the lateral clavicle.

Non-operative management of acromioclavicular injuries in boys under 13 years of age is the mainstay of treatment as these injuries almost always represent a physeal fracture rather than a true acromioclavicular joint dislocation.[34–39] Thus, these injuries exhibit a great potential for healing and remodelling, as the periosteal tube usually remains in continuity with the epiphyseal fragment and acromioclavicular and coracoclavicular ligaments. For type IV, V and VI injuries with large displacement, operative stabilization may be indicated. Repair of the periosteal tube with or without internal fixation is usually performed. As with sternoclavicular injury, hardware should be removed six weeks after repair to avoid complications of pin migration. For late adolescent and adult-type true acromioclavicular joint separations, non-operative management results in good outcomes for type I and II injuries, while operative management is indicated for type IV, V and VI injuries. The management of type III injuries in the athlete remains controversial with many recommending initial non-operative management.[40–42]

Osteolysis of the distal clavicle

Osteolysis of the distal clavicle is an overuse injury resulting from repetitive microtrauma. It is seen most commonly in young adult weightlifters. It has also been described as a sequelae following traumatic injury to the distal clavicle or acromioclavicular joint. In addition, this entity is being identified in other sports, as cross-training has become more popular, and in younger athletes who are weight training year-round for higher level sports. Patients complain of an aching discomfort about the acromioclavicular joint after workouts which progresses to interfere with training and eventually with activities of daily living. There is tenderness to palpation of the distal clavicle and pain with cross-chest adduction. Treatment consists of rest, particularly from weight training, and anti-inflammatory medications. For those who fail conservative treatment or who are unable to refrain from weight training, distal clavicle resection usually results in resolution of pain and return to sport.[43,44] This should be delayed to skeletal maturity, if possible, to lessen the risk of reossification.

Little League shoulder

As a result of repetitive microtrauma from the large rotational torques involved in throwing, chronic stress fracture of the proximal humeral physis can occur. This entity has been termed 'Little League shoulder' and is most commonly seen in high-performance male pitchers between 11 to 13 years old.[10–17,45] In addition to age and the large rotational forces of pitching, poor throwing mechanics may predispose to injury. In an extensive study of Little League pitchers, Albright et al.[12] found that those who had poor pitching skills were more likely to be symptomatic. Patients complain of shoulder pain and there is typically widening of the proximal humeral physis on X-rays. Good results can usually be obtained by enforcing rest from pitching for the remainder of the season, with a vigorous pre-season conditioning programme the subsequent year. Excessive volume of throwing is the most likely risk

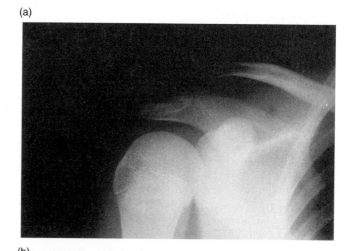
(a)

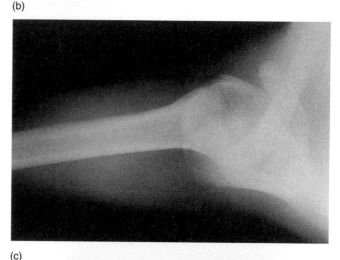
(b)

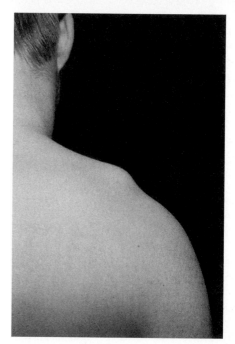
(c)

Fig. 5.5.2 Type IV acromioclavicular injury. (a) AP X-ray, (b) axillary lateral view demonstrating posterior displacement, and (c) photograph showing posterior prominence of lateral clavicle in a 16 year old male.

factor; however, firm evidence-based guidelines concerning throwing volume do not exist. Proper throwing mechanics should be stressed with an emphasis on control instead of speed and intensity.

Proximal humerus fracture

Approximately 20 percent of proximal humeral fractures in the skeletally immature occur in sporting events. The peak age is 10–14 years. Two-thirds involve the proximal humeral metaphysis and one-third involves the proximal humeral physis. Approximately one-fourth of fractures in this region occurs through unicameral bone cysts.[46] Proximal metaphyseal fractures are characteristically more likely in children under 10 years old. The vast majority of physeal fractures in this region are Salter–Harris type I or II lesions, with type II fractures being more common in children over 10 years of age. With physeal fracture, the distal fragment usually displaces anteriorly and laterally through a relatively weaker area of periosteum and the proximal fragment rotates into abduction and forward flexion due to its intact rotator cuff attachments. Patients present with shoulder pain, limited motion and tenderness to palpation. Routine roentgenograms are usually sufficient to demonstrate the fracture pattern, amount of displacement or presence of a unicameral bone cyst.[46–52]

Non-displaced or minimally angulated metaphyseal or physeal fractures can usually be treated adequately with a shoulder immobilizer. Since most of these fractures are intrinsically stable, shoulder motion can be initiated early. There is great potential for remodelling of proximal humerus fractures since the physis is so active. Thus, many moderately displaced, angulated or bayoneted fractures can be accepted in less than anatomic alignment with satisfactory functional outcomes, particularly in younger children. However, in young athletes involved in overhead sports, anatomic reduction must be attained and maintained to prevent loss of abduction and external rotation. Reduction is usually achieved by bringing the distal shaft fragment into flexion, abduction and external rotation to align it with the proximal fragment. If stable after reduction, the fracture can be immobilized next to the chest. If unstable, the reduction must be held immobilized by a shoulder spica cast or shoulder spica brace. These require experience in application and may be poorly tolerated by patients and parents. Percutaneous pinning of the anatomically reduced fracture may allow the arm to be put in a sling after reduction, but maintenance of reduction must be monitored closely with radiographs (Fig. 5.5.3). Open reduction is rarely indicated and often results in poor outcomes.[46–52]

Glenohumeral instability

The glenohumeral joint is the most commonly dislocated large joint in adolescents and adults, but is less commonly involved in children before skeletal maturity. In a large series of patients with glenohumeral instability, the proportion of skeletally immature patients ranges from 1–5%.[53–58] Traumatic anterior dislocation is by far the most common type of instability seen in adolescent athletes; however, multidirectional instability, posterior subluxation and recurrent subluxation are being recognized with increased frequency, particularly in gymnasts, swimmers and throwers. The patient with a traumatic anterior dislocation presents with pain, limited motion and deformity. The humeral head may be palpated anteriorly or in the axilla and the arm is typically held in a slightly abducted, externally rotated position.

(a)

(b)

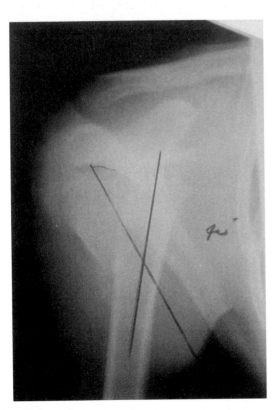
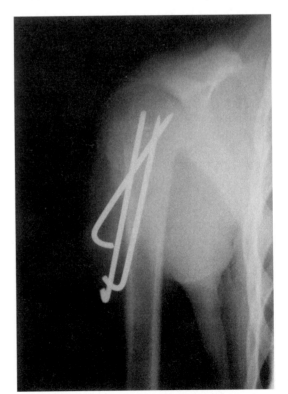

Fig. 5.5.3 Proximal humerus fracture. (a) Oblique view and (b) oblique view after reduction and percutaneous pinning in a 16 year old male.

Careful examination, particularly of the axillary nerve, is essential to rule out neurovascular injury. With posterior dislocation, the coracoid process may be prominent anteriorly and the arm is often held in internal rotation and adduction. Anteroposterior and lateral views of the glenohumeral joint demonstrate the dislocation and identify associated fractures or Hill–Sachs lesions. Posterior dislocations are frequently missed because of inadequate lateral images. Gentle reduction of an anterior dislocation is performed by one of several techniques including traction–countertraction, Stimson manoeuvre or abduction manoeuvres. After a brief period of immobilization, a rehabilitation programme focused on rotator cuff strengthening and avoiding the apprehension position is initiated.

Reported rates of recurrent instability after traumatic dislocation in adolescents and young adults vary between 25–90% in various series.[54,59–61] Rowe reported 100% recurrence in children less than 10 years old and 94% recurrence in patients from 11 to 20 years old.[56,57] Rockwood reported a recurrence rate of 50% in adolescent patients between 14 and 16 years old, and Marans and colleagues reported a 100% recurrence rate in children between 4 and 15 years old with open physes at the time of dislocation.[55] Management of the adolescent patient with significant recurrent instability is usually surgical involving capsulorraphy or a Bankart type repair for capsuloligamentous disruption. Both arthroscopic and open techniques have been utilized, with, in general, higher recurrence rates with arthroscopic repair.

Atraumatic instability can be seen in the paediatric athlete without a clear history of trauma and may occur with throwing, hitting, swimming or overhead serving. There is usually a lack of pain with these episodes of subluxation with spontaneous reduction. Clinical examination often reveals signs of generalized ligamentous laxity including hyper-extensibility of the elbows, knees and metacarpophalangeal joints.[62] Examination may also show signs of multidirectional instability including the sulcus sign and excessive translation with anterior and posterior drawer tests or the load and shift test. A vigorous rehabilitation programme stressing rotator cuff strengthening is successful in most patients.[60] For patients who fail non-operative management, a capsular shift reconstruction is recommended.[63]

Rotator cuff injury

Much less common than in adults, rotator cuff tendinitis and subacromial impingement can occur in the paediatric overhead athlete. Repetitive microtrauma in high level overhead sports, such as swimming, baseball and tennis, can lead to tendinitis, secondary muscle weakness, mechanical imbalance and secondary instability. In the paediatric athlete with joint laxity, true extrinsic impingement with compromise of the subacromial space is uncommon. Rather, impingement secondary to muscle imbalance and anterior instability is seen.[17,64–67] The usual presenting symptom is pain with overhead activities, progressing to constant pain or night pain. As the process continues, range of motion and strength may be diminished with loss of internal rotation, in particular. Hypermobility of the scapula with diminished periscapular strength is common. Impingement may be elicited with forward elevation or secondary to provocative instability tests. MRI may be useful to assess the integrity of the rotator cuff; however, full-thickness tears in the paediatric or adolescent shoulder are uncommon. In competitive swimmers, a variant of impingement syndrome can be seen, 'swimmer's shoulder', involving anterior impingement associated with multidirectional instability and posterior subluxation.

Treatment of rotator cuff impingement consists of rest, non-steroidal anti-inflammatory medications and a rehabilitation programme emphasizing restoration of range of motion, rotator cuff strengthening and scapular stabilization, with the goal of restoring dynamic joint stability. For cases refractory to non-operative management, shoulder arthroscopy may be of benefit to rule out associated intrarticular pathology. Subacromial decompression is rarely indicated in the paediatric athlete.[17,64–67]

Elbow injuries

General

The elbow joint has three major articulations: humeroradial, humeroulnar and proximal radioulnar joints. Delineating injury patterns in children can be challenging given the cartilaginous composition of the distal humerus and the multiple ossification centres. A site-specific clinical exam and radiographs of the contralateral uninjured elbow can prove useful in identifying injury. There are six major secondary centres of ossification, which appear and unite with the epiphysis at characteristic ages (Table 5.5.1). Except for the medial and lateral epicondyles, the remaining ossification centres are intra-articular. The clinical carrying angle of the elbow averages 7° valgus alignment. There are several radiographic lines which are useful in assessing post injury alignment. Bauman's angle, the angle between the capitellar physeal line and a line perpendicular to the humeral shaft, is a guide to the varus attitude of the distal humerus and should be within 5–8° of the contralateral elbow. On the lateral X-ray, the capitellum forms an angle flexed forward 30–40 from the humeral shaft and the anterior humeral line should bisect the capitellum. Elbow stability is provided by congruous articular surfaces and soft tissue constraint via capsular and ligamentous structures.

Elbow injury patterns in the paediatric athlete are dependent on the age-related stage of elbow development and the sport-specific mechanism of injury. Acute macrotraumatic injuries often result in fractures about the elbow. In younger children, supracondylar and lateral condyle fractures predominate. In adolescence and near skeletal maturity, epicondylar and olecranon fractures are more common. In addition, elbow dislocations, ligamentous injuries and muscular avulsions about the elbow can occur.

Repetitive microtraumatic injuries are often sport-specific involving upper extremity overuse. Repetitive throwing places high demands on the vulnerable developing elbow. Tension overload of the medial elbow restraints occurs during late cocking and can lead to medial

Table 5.5.1 Timing of secondary centres of ossification about the elbow

Site	Appearance	Epiphyseal coalescence
Capitellum	18 months	14 years
Radial head	4 years	16 years
Medial epicondyle	5 years	15 years
Trochlea	8 years	14 years
Olecranon	10 years	14 years
Lateral epicondyle	12 years	16 years

epicondyle fragmentation, ulnar collateral ligament strain, flexor muscle strains and traction ulnar neuritis. Compression overload of the lateral articulation also occurs during late cocking and can lead to chondral injuries and growth disturbances of the capitellum or radial head. Posteromedial shear overload of the posterior articular surface occurs during follow-through and can lead to posterior spurs, olecranon apophysistis or avulsion, and traction spurs of the coronoid process.[68] In gymnastics, the elbow becomes a weight-bearing joint often subjected to repetitive large loads. Medial epicondyle traction injuries, partial tears of the flexor origin mass, ulnar collateral ligament strains, subluxation/dislocation often with medial epicondyle avulsion, osteochondral fractures of the capitellum, and posterior elbow spurring have been described.[2,22,69] Osteochondritis dissecans of the capitellum occurs with presentation similar to throwing injuries.

Supracondylar fracture

Supracondylar humerus fractures are the most common elbow fracture in children, accounting for approximately 75% of injuries. The mechanism of injury is usually an acute hyperextension load on the elbow from falling on an outstretched arm. The injury typically occurs in children aged 5 to 10 years, because of thin bony architecture in the supracondylar region and ligamentous laxity. The distal fragment displaces posteriorly in over 95% of cases and the fracture is classified according to displacement: minimally displaced (type I); posterior angulation hinged on an intact posterior cortex (type II); and completely displaced (type III) (Fig. 5.5.4). With complete displacement,

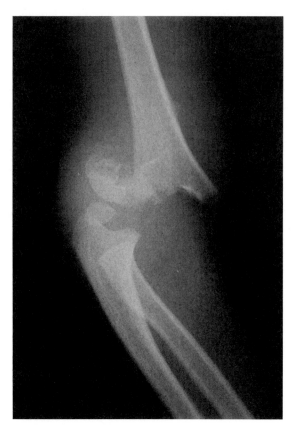

Fig. 5.5.4 Supracondylar humerus fracture. Oblique view of type III displaced fracture in a 6 year old child.

rotational malalignment often occurs and can lead to cubitus varus deformity if unreduced. Injury to the anterior interosseous nerve, radial nerve, median nerve and brachial artery has been reported in 10–18% of displaced fractures.[70,71]

Type I fractures are treated in a long arm cast for three weeks with the elbow flexed 90° to 100°. Type II fractures can be treated with closed reduction and casting alone; however, the elbow should be flexed beyond 90° to maintain reduction, and this position may not be tolerated secondary to vascular insufficiency and swelling. Thus closed reduction and percutaneous pinning with two lateral pins is often the treatment of choice. Closed reduction and percutaneous pinning is the preferred method of treatment for type III fractures, obviating the problems of ischemic contracture (compartment syndrome) and cubitus varus deformity seen with closed treatment. Reduction is accomplished by extension of the elbow, followed by correction of medial–lateral translation, followed by traction and flexion of the elbow with anterior force on the olecranon. For fractures with medial displacement, the forearm is pronated, which tightens the reduction against the intact medial periosteum while closing the lateral column. The most stable pin configuration involves medial and lateral pins crossing above the fracture line. Care must be taken to avoid ulnar nerve injury with the medial pin. Motion is begun after the pins are removed at 3–4 weeks.[70,71] In cases with excessive comminution or other associated extremity injuries, skeletal traction with an olecranon pin may be beneficial.

Lateral condyle fracture

Lateral condyle fractures are the second most common elbow fracture in children and occur typically between 6 and 10 years of age. The mechanism of injury is often a valgus compressive force from the radial head or a varus tensile force on a supinated forearm from the extensor longus and brevis muscles. A significant portion of the fragment is unossified, leaving often only a thin lateral metaphyseal rim of bone to herald the injury. This fracture involves both the physis and the articular surface, making anatomic reduction essential. Displacement and rotation are common due to the lateral extensor muscle mass. Treatment depends on the degree of displacement and fragment stability. Minimally displaced fractures, < 3 mm, which are demonstrated to be stable by clinical examination, are treated with cast immobilization for approximately 3–4 weeks. Follow-up X-rays (particularly the oblique view) are essential one week after injury to rule out further displacement. Any fracture with associated elbow instability should be anatomically reduced and fixed. Fractures with initial displacement of 3–4 mm are at risk of late displacement and non-union, and thus many recommend percutaneous pinning to stabilize these fractures. Fractures with over 4 mm of displacement are often also rotated, necessitating open reduction and internal fixation to restore articular continuity. Complications of lateral condyle fractures include non-union, progressive valgus deformity and tardy ulnar neuritis.[71]

Radial head/neck fracture

Proximal radius injuries in the skeletally immature athlete are either physeal fractures of the radial head or fractures of the radial neck. They occur most commonly in children over the age of 9 years, as the result of valgus stress with longitudinal force on an outstretched arm. Treatment depends on the degree of angulation, amount of displacement, age of child and associated fractures (Fig. 5.5.5). Children less than 10 years old can tolerate up to 40–45° of angulation of the radial neck due to expected remodelling. In older children, less angulation (15–20°) is acceptable due to less remodelling potential. For fractures with acceptable angulation, cast immobilization with early motion in 10 to 14 days is recommended. Closed reduction can be performed by direct pressure over the radial head with a varus stress and rotation. Alternatively, a percutaneous pin can be used to manipulate the proximal fragment. Indications for open reduction include complete displacement of the radial head, irreducible angulation over 45°, or a displaced Salter–Harris IV fracture. Radial head fractures with significant displacement should be anatomically reduced and fixed. Radial head excision is contraindicated, as proximal radial migration, radial deviation of the hand and valgus deviation of the elbow can occur.[71–73]

Medial epicondyle fracture

The medial epicondyle can be avulsed from a valgus load applied to the extended elbow (Fig. 5.5.6). The flexor origin and the ulnar collateral ligament play a role in fracture displacement. These fractures occur typically in children 10 to 14 years old. Almost 50% of these injuries are thought to occur concomitantly with elbow dislocation (Fig. 5.5.7). For the general paediatric population, many advocate closed treatment of this injury, particularly when there is less than 5 mm of displacement. Although non-union may occur, it is often asymptomatic or can be treated with fragment excision when symptomatic. Relative indications for open reduction and fixation include competitive athletes with >2 mm displacement or valgus instability to restore the integrity of the medial collateral ligament and retension the forearm flexors. An absolute indication for open reduction and internal fixation is medial epicondylar entrapment within the joint associated with elbow dislocation (Fig. 5.5.7). A common complication of medial epicondyle fracture is joint stiffness. Internal fixation allows for early post-operative range of motion at 2–3 weeks.[71, 74–76]

Elbow dislocation

Elbow dislocation is relatively uncommon in the child athlete as the peak incidence is in the second decade. However, elbow dislocation may be encountered in the adolescent athlete in contact sports such as football or wrestling, or in non-contact sports such as gymnastics. The most common pattern of injury is posterolateral displacement without disruption of the proximal radioulnar joint. The injury may also involve disruption of the anterior capsule, tearing of the brachialis muscle, avulsion of the medial epicondyle, injury to the ulnar collateral ligament, brachial artery compromise, or nerve injury to the median or ulnar nerves. Prompt and gentle reduction is performed under sedation. Non-concentric reduction should alert the clinician to the possibility of interposed soft tissue or medial epicondyle (Fig. 5.5.7). For simple elbow dislocations, a posterior splint is used for the acute phase of pain and swelling for 10–14 days, followed by assisted range of motion and physical therapy.[71,77] Immobilization beyond three weeks is contraindicated due to stiffness.

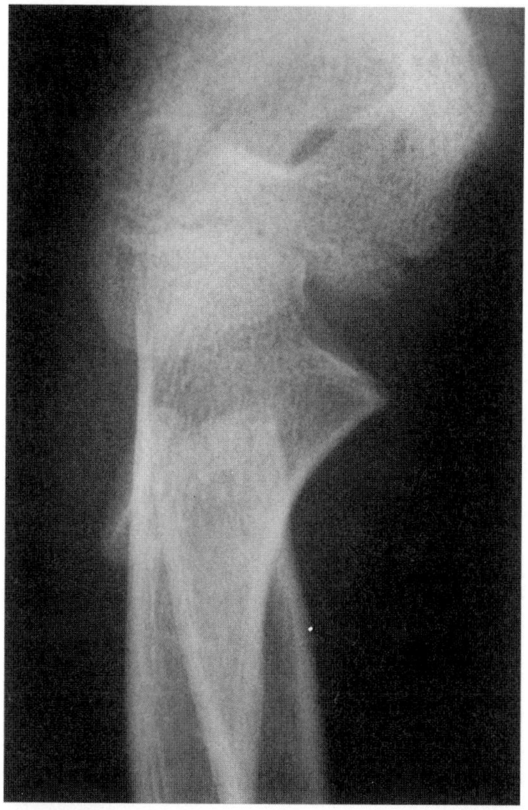

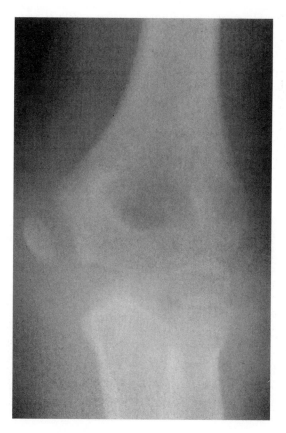

Fig. 5.5.5 Radial head fracture. AP view demonstrating angulation and displacement of proximal radial physeal fracture in a 12 year old boy.

Fig. 5.5.6 Medial epicondyle avulsion. AP view of a displaced medial epicondyle avulsion fracture in a 14 year old male pitcher.

Little League elbow

The term 'Little League elbow' describes a group of pathologic entities about the elbow joint in young throwers. Originally, these findings were noted in baseball pitchers; however, the throwing motion is common to the non-pitcher's throw, the tennis serve, the javelin throw, the cricket bowl and the football pass. The entity includes medial epicondyle fragmentation and avulsion (Fig. 5.5.6), growth alteration of the medial epicondyle, osteochondritis of the capitellum, deformation or osteochondritis of the radial head, hypertrophy of the ulna, and olecranon apophysistis. Osteochondritis of the capitellum may also be seen in high-performance female gymnasts.[54] Most cases

of Little League elbow present with medial elbow complaints: medial pain and decreased throwing effectiveness/distance. Medial tension overload results from repetitive valgus stress and flexor forearm pull. Changes are age dependent. During childhood, irregular appearance of the secondary centres of ossification of the medial epicondyle may be seen. In adolescence with increasing muscle strength, avulsion fracture of the medial epicondyle may occur. After fusion of the medial epicondyle in young adulthood, injuries of the ulnar collateral ligament and flexor muscle origin become more apparent. Laterally, repetitive valgus compression may lead to damage of the radiocapitellar articulation. Osteochondritis dissecans can affect both the capitellum

(a)

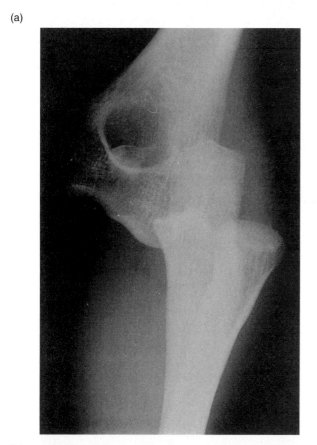

(b)

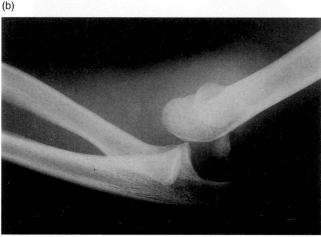

(c)

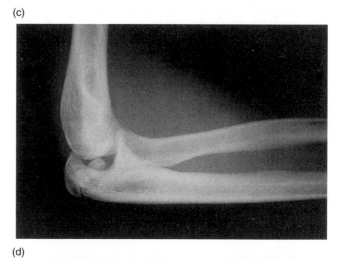

(d)

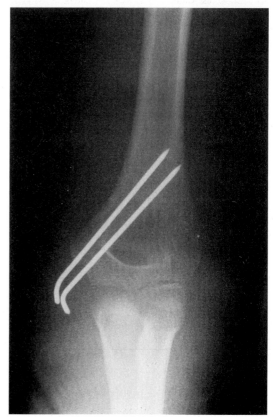

Fig. 5.5.7(a–d)

(e)

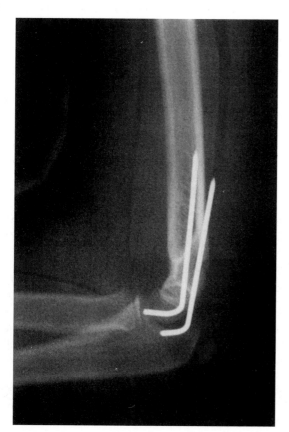

Fig. 5.5.7 Elbow dislocation with medial epicondyle avulsion. AP (a) and lateral (b) views demonstrating elbow dislocation with medial epicondyle avulsion in a 13 year old female gymnast. (c) Entrapped medial epicondyle fragment. AP (d) and lateral (e) views after open reduction and internal fixation.

and the radial head. Changes include chondromalacia with softening and fissuring of the articular surface, subchondral collapse and bony eburnation. Osteochondritis dissecans of the capitellum can present with wide variations in radiographic appearance depending on the extent of osteonecrosis and the presence of loose bodies.

Availability of MRI has given the opportunity for early diagnosis, prior to radiographic changes. Pain, tenderness and contracture dominate the clinical presentation. Additional lateral injuries seen during throwing in the skeletally immature athlete include lateral apophysis avulsion from traction during follow-through and radial physeal injury from repetitive valgus overload. Posterior elbow pain in throwers is frequently due to the powerful contraction of the triceps in the early acceleration phase coupled with the impaction of the olecranon into its humeral fossa in the late follow-through phase. Olecranon apophysistis, avulsion fracture (Fig. 5.5.8), posteromedial osteophytes, and loose bodies may form.[10,12,16,17,68,79–84]

Treatment of Little League elbow is directed at removing the recurrent microtrauma. Cessation of all throwing until the elbow is asymptomatic followed by reassessing throwing mechanics and number of pitches thrown is essential. More than three hundred skilled throws per week may predispose to injury. Range of motion exercises and dynamic splinting may be useful for contractures. Triceps strengthening with stretching of the anterior capsule is helpful for

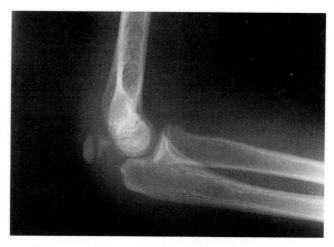

Fig. 5.5.8 Olecranon avulsion. Lateral view demonstrating olecranon apophysis avulsion in a 12 year old male pitcher.

avoidance of contracture. Arthroscopy is useful for assessing chondral injury, removal of loose bodies and management of osteochondritis dissecans through drilling or fragment fixation. Open reduction of displaced medial epicondyle fractures is indicated in the throwing athlete. Results of treatment of Little League elbow are generally favourable when instituted early.[10–12,16,17,68,79–83]

Wrist and hand injuries

General

In most sports, the hand and wrist are exposed and thus are vulnerable to injury. Injury patterns are sport-specific, with macrotraumatic injury or repetitive microtraumatic injury depending upon the demands placed on the upper extremity. Injuries are also age-specific, related to the stage of skeletal development. In several large series of paediatric and adolescent athletic injuries, hand and wrist injury rates vary from 15–65% of all injuries in paediatric and adolescent athletes depending on the sport involved.[85–87] Injuries to the hand are particularly common during basketball, football, boxing, 16-inch softball, skateboarding and alpine skiing. Repetitive stress injuries, particularly of the wrist, are common in gymnasts. Injuries are relatively infrequent during swimming and soccer.[88–90]

Distal radius fractures

Distal radial metaphyseal fracture is the most common fracture of childhood.[91] If treated properly, these fractures usually heal without residual disability. Initial management consists of splinting and careful neurovascular evaluation of the hand. X-Rays are usually sufficient to define the fracture and its angulation/displacement (Fig. 5.5.9). This fracture may occur in association with distal radio–ulnar joint disruption or elbow injury. Torus and greenstick fractures are often fairly stable and may be treated in a short arm cast in older children and a long arm cast in children under 5 years old. The completely displaced distal radial metaphyseal fracture often requires intravenous sedation or general anaesthesia for reduction followed by long arm casting with an appropriate mould. In the young child less than 8 years old, bayonet apposition may be accepted. In the rare irreducible fracture, an

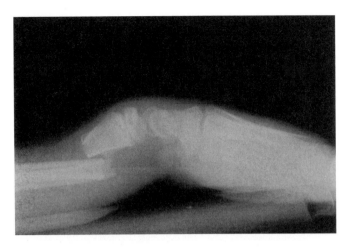

Fig. 5.5.9 Distal radius fracture. Lateral view in a 6 year old boy.

open reduction may be necessary through a volar approach which allows for release of the carpal canal. The position of immobilization of this fracture is controversial, with advocates of pronation, neutral and supination positioning. Approximately 10–30% of distal third radius fractures reangulate to an unacceptable position (> 20°) requiring repeat closed manipulation. For the healing fracture, acceptable limits of angulation are wider. In a child under 8 years, up to 30° may be acceptable due to remodelling potential, with an estimated correction of 1°/month.[92] In the child over 12 years, these fractures become increasingly unstable with less remodelling potential leading to treatment resembling that of an adult.

Physeal fractures of the distal radius occur most commonly in the adolescent. Salter–Harris I and II fracture patterns predominate. The distal fragment is usually dorsally displaced with an intact dorsal peri osteum. This fracture may be associated with acute carpal tunnel syndrome or compartment syndrome. Reduction should be as atraumatic as possible to avoid further injury to the physis. The fracture should be immobilized in the position of stability as determined during reduction. Intraepiphyseal fracture extension, such as in Salter–Harris III or IV injuries is uncommon, but should be treated with anatomical reduction of the articular surface and intraepiphyseal or transphyseal fixation.

Wrist injuries

Wrist pain has become extremely common in young, highly competitive gymnasts related to chronic, repetitive upper extremity weight-bearing during growth and development. Chronic repetitive stress injury to the distal radial and ulnar physes was described by Roy and colleagues in young, highly competitive gymnasts who practised approximately 36 hours/week.[93] The presenting symptoms were stiffness and dorsiflexion pain. Radiographs showed widened physes, cystic changes and distal metaphyseal beaking. Nearly all patients returned to competitive gymnastics without growth arrest after treatment with rest, with or without casting. Subsequently, others have reported acquired Madelung's deformity and increased ulnar variance in young, competitive gymnasts.[94,95] A spectrum of pathologic entities may be found on clinical examination, X-rays, MRI, and arthroscopy, including stress changes of the distal radial/ulnar physes, articular cartilage changes of the wrist/carpal joints, distal radioulnar joint injury, triangular fibrocartilage (TFCC) tears, and ganglion cysts. Management is primarily non-operative with rest, immobilization if necessary, and activity modification.

Distal radioulnar joint injuries in the child and adolescent athlete are rare. Acute dislocations present with pain and deformity of the joint. Acute dislocations are treated with long arm cast immobilization, with the wrist in supination for dorsal dislocations and pronation for volar dislocations. TFCC injuries are increasingly being recognized in patients with repetitive wrist loading, particularly gymnasts. Patients typically present with ulnar wrist pain and injury may be demonstrated on MRI arthrogram or arthroscopy. For patients who fail non-operative management, patients with neutral or negative ulnar variance can be treated by arthroscopic debridement, and patients with positive ulnar variance can be treated by ulnar shortening and/or debridement. In a child or adolescent with significant growth remaining, bony procedures should be delayed until growth ceases.[96]

The scaphoid fracture is the most common carpal fracture in children with a peak incidence between 12 and 15 years of age. In the skeletally immature, the majority of fractures are minimally displaced and involve the distal pole, with fewer waist and proximal pole fractures. However, with increased athletic participation at increasingly intense competitive levels by children and adolescents, more adult-type displaced waist fractures are being seen. Patients present with wrist pain, limited motion and tenderness in the anatomic snuff box. Management of minimally displaced fractures involves a short arm thumb spica cast for six weeks for distal pole fractures, and a long arm thumb spica for four weeks for waist fractures followed by short arm casting until union occurs. Occult fractures can be diagnosed with bone scanning. Acute displaced fractures should be treated with open reduction and internal fixation. Scaphoid non-union usually requires bone grafting with or without fixation (Fig. 5.5.10).[97–99] Scaphoid malunion or non-union can lead to degenerative changes of the wrist in the long term. Stress fracture of the scaphoid waist can be seen, particularly in competitive gymnasts.[100,101] Initial X-rays are often negative, with follow-up X-rays revealing a stress fracture.

Ligamentous injuries of the wrist are unusual in children, but are being seen with increased frequency in the adolescent athlete engaged in high level sports. The volar intercarpal ligaments, particularly the radioscapholunate and radioscaphocapitate ligaments, are important stabilizers of the wrist. Patients present with wrist pain and limited motion. X-Rays may reveal widening of the scapholunate interval or alteration of the scapholunate angle (normal 30–60°). Dorsal intercalated segment instability (DISI) can result from scaphoid fracture or scapholunate dissociation, resulting in an increased scapholunate angle. Volar intercalated segment instability (VISI) can result from disruption of the radiocarpal ligaments on the ulnar side of the wrist, resulting in a decreased scapholunate angle. Wrist arthrography, MRI and arthroscopy can be used to further delineate the extent of ligamentous injury. Partial injuries are treated with immobilization. Acute complete ligamentous injuries are treated with ligament repair and K-wire fixation. Chronic carpal instability is usually treated with limited carpal fusions or proximal row carpectomy, often with unpredictable results.

Hand injuries

The thumb metacarpalphalangeal joint is commonly injured, particularly during skiing. These injuries result from excessive radial deviation during a fall on the outstretched hand with the thumb in abduction.

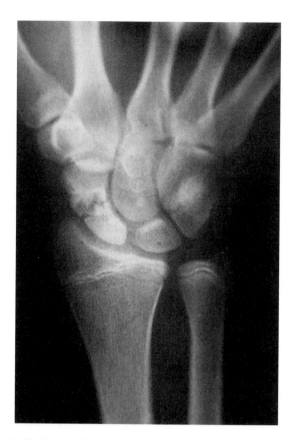

Fig. 5.5.10 Scaphoid non-union.

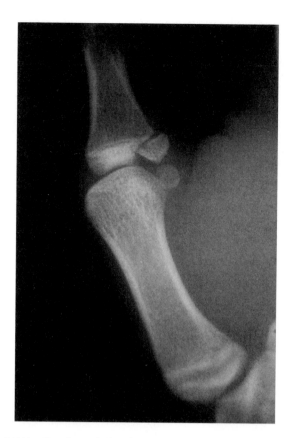

Fig. 5.5.11 Gamekeeper's thumb. Salter–Harris III injury in a 10 year old male.

In adults and older adolescents, injury to the ulnar collateral ligament of the thumb metacarpalphalangeal joint occurs ('gamekeeper's or skier's thumb'). In children and adolescents, physeal fracture at the base of the proximal phalanx is more common. The ulnar collateral ligament inserts onto the proximal phalangeal epiphysis, thus predisposing to a Salter–Harris III fracture, which may involve a large portion of the articular surface (Fig. 5.5.11). Non-displaced fractures and partial ulnar collateral ligament injuries are treated with 4–6 weeks of immobilization in a short arm thumb spica cast. Displaced fractures are treated with open reduction and internal fixation. Complete ligamentous injuries (>35–40° opening in flexion without a firm endpoint) and Stener's lesions (interposition of the adductor aponeurosis) are treated with ligament repair.[102–106]

The 'jammed finger' is the most common joint injury in the paediatric and adolescent athlete's hand. Axial compressive forces applied to the end of the finger can result in proximal interphalangeal joint (PIP) hyperextension with subluxation or dislocation of the joint. This injury is common in ball catching sports such as basketball or football. Reduction of the dislocated joint is accomplished by linear traction. Volar plate injury/avulsion or volar Salter–Harris III fracture may be associated, but rarely requires fixation. Treatment involves a very brief period of immobilization (dorsal alumifoam splint), followed by edema control (elastoplast wrapping) and motion (buddy-taping to adjacent digit) to avoid stiffness and a fixed flexion deformity. Most athletes can return to sports (with buddy-taping) in 1–2 weeks; however, some pain and swelling may persist for months. Axial loading of the finger may also result in boutonniere deformity (PIP flexion, DIP extension) secondary to rupture of the central slip or a dorsally

displaced Salter–Harris III fracture at the base of the middle phalanx. Acute injuries should be splinted in full extension for 4–5 weeks. Chronic reconstruction results in less reliable outcomes.[102–106]

Mallet finger is the most common injury occurring at the DIP joint, resulting from hyperflexion injury producing either extensor tendon (terminal tendon) rupture or Salter–Harris III avulsion of the distal phalangeal epiphysis (Fig. 5.5.12). The patient is unable to actively extend the DIP joint; however, there is full passive motion. Unless there is significant displacement of a substantial epiphyseal fragment, the DIP should be splinted with a dorsal splint in full extension for approximately six weeks. Terminal tendon repair may be necessary if an extensor lag persists after 10 weeks; however, this is unusual.[102–106] Hyperextension of the DIP joint may result in a dorsal DIP dislocation or avulsion of the flexor digitorum profundus (FDP). FDP avulsion most commonly involves the ring finger and occurs during football or rugby as the finger catches on the opposing player's shirt ('jersey finger'). If identified early, the injury can be successfully treated. Missed diagnosis occurs when the patient does not recognize a significant injury or the care provider believes that the inability to flex the DIP joint is secondary to pain and swelling. Direct repair to the distal phalanx is accomplished if possible. With late diagnosis, direct repair is usually not possible as the tendon retracts and fibrosis occurs. In these cases, tendon grafts may be necessary.[107]

Hand fractures are common athletic injuries in children. Fractures involving the physis are frequent, accounting for approximately 40% of hand fractures in the skeletally immature.[103] Ossific nuclei appear in the metacarpals and phalanges by three years of age and fuse between 14 and 17 years. Remodelling potential exists for fractures near the epiphysis

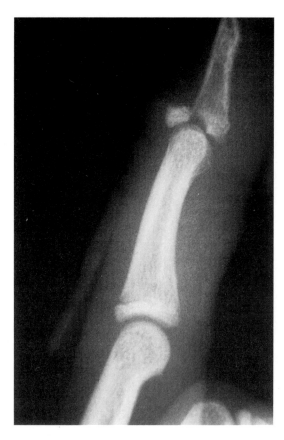

Fig. 5.5.12   Mallet fracture.

in the plane of motion; however, there is minimal remodelling of rotational deformity. The vast majority of hand fractures in children can be managed non-operatively with splinting of non-displaced fractures and closed reduction of angulated or displaced fractures. Fingertip crush injuries occur in tackling and collision sports. These injuries often involve a nailbed laceration and tuft fracture requiring splinting and nailbed repair. Phalangeal neck fractures typically occur between 5 and 10 years of age and involve the proximal phalanx. These fractures may redisplace after reduction and may have substantial rotation not appreciated on X-ray, thus requiring careful clinical examination. Metacarpal fractures in children are less common than adults. Little finger metacarpal neck fractures (boxer's fracture) can usually be managed by closed reduction and cast immobilization for three weeks. Thumb metacarpal fractures often involve a Salter–Harris II fracture through the base of the metacarpal.[102–106]

Trunk injuries

General

Back pain and injuries to the thoracolumbar spine are not infrequent in the school-age athlete. Spine-related complaints constitute almost 10% of athletes' medical problems, and approximately 75% of high-performance athletes have some sort of back pain.[108] Particular sports that require repetitive or high velocity twisting or bending, such as gymnastics, dancing, football and rowing, have a predilection for back injuries.[89,108–117] With the increasing number of young athletes

pursuing rigorous training and intense competition in some of these sports at an early age, the prevalence of back pain in the school-age athlete may be expected to increase.

Effective clinical management of back pain in the child and adolescent athlete requires an accurate diagnosis and a specific treatment plan. Accurate diagnosis necessitates an understanding of the differing aetiologies of back pain in the school-age athlete in contradistinction to back pain in the adult.[118] In the adult, mechanical back pain, degenerative disorders and disc disease predominate, with symptomotology sometimes related to secondary gains including disability and psychologic issues. In the school-age athlete with back pain, a specific diagnosis should be sought, such as spondylolysis, spondylolisthesis, apophysitis, tumour or infection. Macrotrauma and microtrauma must be distinguished. The former involves a single tissue overload while the latter represents cumulative trauma. Macrotrauma is typically seen in high-energy contact sports, such as rugby or football. Microtrauma is typically seen in athletes participating in sports requiring high-energy repetitive bending, twisting or rotation, such as gymnasts, dancers or football lineman. The growing athlete has several unique risk factors relevant to the adolescent spine. The growth cartilage of the vertebral end plates and apophyses are more susceptible to injury. Musculotendinous imbalances are quite common because of periods of rapid longitudinal growth. Eating disorders with irregular menstruation and osteoporosis are not uncommon in adolescent gymnasts and dancers. In addition, extrinsic factors such as poor technique, grouping of children by similar age despite differing abilities and insufficient conditioning may predispose to injury.

Major anatomic differences of the spine in the skeletally immature include an increased cartilage to bone ratio and the presence of secondary centres of ossification at the vertebral end plates, which normally fuse to the vertebral bodies by maturity. Unlike adults who often have asymptomatic pre-existing degenerative changes in the fibrocartilaginous disc, intervertebral discs in the child are generally well hydrated and tightly adhered to the cartilaginous plate. The apophyseal ring is thinner in the middle than the periphery, thus axial compression with forward flexion may force the disc through the end plates into the cancellous bone of the vertebral body as opposed to through the annulus towards the spinal canal as seen in adults. In addition, compressive and bending forces tend to fracture the weaker vertebral end plate rather than producing annulus failure and disc herniation.

A thorough history and discerning physical examination are essential in the assessment of spine injuries in child and adolescent athletes. The athlete's age, sex, pattern of complaints, location and radiation of pain, and chronology of symptoms are essential facts to obtain. Attention should be directed toward the mechanics of the sport producing the pain, such as walkovers in gymnasts, butterfly stroke in swimmers, and hyperextension and loading in linemen. A family history is implicated in scoliosis and spondylolisthesis. Night pain suggests tumour, morning stiffness associated with sacroiliac pain may be the presenting symptoms of juvenile ankylosing spondylitis, and systemic symptoms such as fever and chill suggest infection. Neurologic symptoms such as paresthesias, weakness and bowel/bladder dysfunction require immediate attention. The physical examination should include an assessment of gait and leg lengths. The frontal and sagital contour of the spine should be examined both standing and bending to evaluate any asymmetry or deformity. Range of motion should be measured and localized areas of tenderness elicited. Provocative tests such as hyperextension or straight leg raising should be performed.

Hip range of motion, muscle tightness and generalized laxity should be assessed. Finally, a thorough neurologic examination of muscle strength, sensation and reflexes should be performed. Radiographs and further diagnostic studies such as MRI, CT and radionuclide scanning are individualized depending on the differential diagnosis and symptomatology.

Spondylolysis and spondylolisthesis

Mechanical injury to the pars interarticularis is a common source of discomfort in young athletes involved in competitive sports, and is probably the anatomic lesion diagnosed most frequently in young people with back pain. Spondylolysis refers to a bony defect in the pars interarticularis and spondylolisthesis refers to translation of a vertebral body relative to an adjacent body in the coronal plane. Fracture of the pars interarticularis occurs as a consequence of activity and is usually an overuse injury. Spondylolytic defects are rare in young children, have not been reported in newborns, are absent in other primates and are not seen in patients who have not assumed an upright posture.[119] Nearly 50% of patients with spondylolysis relate the onset of symptoms to competitive sports training.[120] In a series of 177 male high school and college athletes, approximately 21% showed radiographic evidence of spondylolysis.[121] The incidence of spondylolysis is estimated at approximately 4% in the general adolescent population, increasing to 6% in adulthood.[122,123] Many inactive individuals are asymptomatic. The average age of diagnosis in the symptomatic school age athletic population is 15 to 16 years old. LaFond[124] noted that 23% of spondylolysis patients in his series experienced the onset of symptoms before 20 years old; however, only 9% had severe enough symptoms to seek medical attention. Approximately 85% of spondylolysis occurs at the L5 level.

It is postulated that spondylolysis and isthmic spondylolisthesis represent acquired fatigue fractures as a result of repeated microtrauma. Shear stresses of 400 to 600 N due to hyperextension, flexion and torsion are concentrated across the pars interarticularis, an area calculated to be only 0.75 cm^2 at L5.[125,126] Repetitive hyperextension loading sports, such as gymnastics, blocking in football, hurdling, ballet dancing, volleyball spiking, competitive diving, tennis serving, weight lifting and swimming turns, have all been associated with spondylolysis. Pars defects occur four times more frequently in young female gymnasts than the general female population.[113] However, given the same demands within the same sport, it is difficult to determine why one athlete is predisposed to spondylolysis while another avoids injury. Genetic predisposition of spondylolytic defects has been documented.[127,128] Anatomic variations such as transitional vertebrae, spina bifida occulta and an elongated pars may be seen. In addition, poor technique, inadequate supervision, poor conditioning, poor flexibility and hyperlordotic posture may predispose to injury.

It is essential to make the diagnosis and initiate protective treatment as early as possible. The onset of symptoms typically coincides with the adolescent growth spurt and with the onset of strenuous, repetitive training. In athletes, symptoms are usually insidious aching lower back pain without radiation. Initially, the pain is elicited by strenuous activity; however, the pain often becomes progressively more severe and becomes associated with activities of daily living. L5 radicular symptoms may arise from foraminal encroachment, fibrocartilaginous callus at the healing pars or forward displacement of L5 on S1. Physical examination may demonstrate paraspinal tenderness, limited motion, hyperlordosis and hamstring tightness.[129]

Typically, pain can be reproduced with hyperextension and occasionally can be localized with ipsilateral hyperextension. Initial diagnostic work-up includes radiographs of the lumbosacral spine. Slippage through a pars defect may be seen on the standing lateral view, allowing for meas urement of the per cent slippage and slip angle (Figs 5.5.13 and 5.5.14). A 25–45° oblique view may demonstrate the spondylolytic defect (Fig. 5.5.13). Acutely, the defect appears as a narrow gap with irregular edges. Over time, the edges become rounded and smooth. Reactive sclerosis and hypertrophy of the opposite pars or lamina can be seen in unilateral spondylolysis and occasionally confused with osteoid osteoma. If spondylolysis is suspected but not demonstrated on plain films, single photon emission computed tomography (SPECT) scanning is particularly sensitive in detecting pars defects (Fig. 5.5.13).[130] Early diagnosis with SPECT is of great practical significance as fresh pars defects may heal with early effective immobilization.[131] Alternatively, oblique linear tomography or CT scanning may demonstrate the established pars lesion. With radicular symptoms, MRI is useful in demonstrating the aetiology of root compression.

Management must consider the athlete's age, type of sport activity, severity of symptoms and risk of progression. Risk factors for slip progression include slip percentage >50%, high slip angle, spina bifida, convex sacral contour, ligamentous laxity and the adolescent age group.[132–136] The asymptomatic individual should be periodically followed clinically and radiographically if there are risk factors for progression. The symptomatic adolescent athlete can initially be treated with restriction of athletic activity and an abdominal/back strengthening programme. We treat this as a stress fracture with activity modification and immobilization using a rigid polypropylene lumbosacral brace constructed with 0° of lumbar flexion (antilordosis). We advocate full-time brace use for approximately six months. Braced patients are allowed to resume limited activities several weeks after initiation of brace wear, when most have become asymptomatic. Results are promising with this treatment. In our series, 32% of 75 patients achieved bony union and 88% were able to return to previously painful sports even if the pars defect had not healed.[137,138] Bone scans or CT scans may be helpful in following the status of a lesion.[123,139,140] A positive bone scan usually indicates that the defect is healing or has the potential to heal; however, a cold scan should not be taken as a contra indication to bracing.[131] Hamstring tightness is also an indicator of the success of treatment. Patients who fail to improve after an appropriate bracing regimen or who are unable to be weaned from the brace may require surgery. Posterolateral in situ fusion of L5–S1 is usually performed for L5 spondylolysis with post-operative bracing until fusion for up to 6 months. For spondylolysis of L4 or above, direct repair of the pars defect with wiring or osteosynthesis can be attempted, maintaining a motion segment and allowing earlier return to activity.[141–143]

Management of the spondylolisthesis in the adolescent athlete depends on the degree of slippage and the severity of symptoms. Fortunately, it is rare to see progressive listhesis in the adolescent onset stress fracture pars defect seen in young athletes. For patients who remain symptomatic despite bracing, posterolateral in situ fusion of L5–S1 with post-operative bracing is performed.[133,135,144,145] Fusion should be extended to L4 for slips >50%. A slip of over 50% in the immature spine should be stabilized, even in an asymptomatic individual due to the high risk of progression.[135,144,145] The asymptomatic athlete with <25% spondylolisthesis should be allowed to participate

(a)

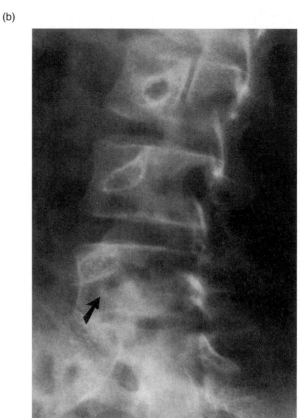

(b)

(c)

Fig. 5.5.13 Spondylolysis. (a) Lateral, (b) oblique and (c) SPECT scans in a 14 year old female gymnast.

in all sports, including contact sports, while being followed periodically for progression (Fig. 5.5.14).[146] Asymptomatic athletes with 25–50% slippage fall into a controversial category. Some advocate observation for progression, some advocate avoidance of contact sports, and some advocate surgical management if the patient wishes to return to competitive sports. The rare individual with high grade slippage and severe lumbosacral kyphosis may benefit from reduction and fusion as opposed to *in situ* fusion; however, this is associated with a higher risk of neurologic complications.[147] Decompression in conjunction with fusion is reserved for a clear neurologic deficit and a readily discernible lesion, such as the hypertrophied fibrocartilaginous mass at the level of the pars defect, irritating the L5 root. With high-grade slips, the sacral dome may stretch the thecal sac and sacral nerve roots.

Discogenic disorders

Although much less common in adolescents than adults, disc herniation and degenerative disc disease can occur in the young adolescent athlete. The true incidence is unknown; however, it is estimated that between 1–4% of all disc herniations occur in the paediatric population, and less than 10% of young athletes' back pain is discogenic.[148–152] The natural history of disc disease in this population is not well understood, although some studies have suggested that these patients continue to have back problems as adults.[153] Acute macrotrauma may result in acute disc herniation as in collision sport athletes and weightlifters, while repetitive microtrauma may result in degenerative disc disease or insidious herniation as in gymnasts. In contrast to adults with pre-existing degenerative disc changes, disc tissue in adolescents is usually noted to be firm, well hydrated and solidly

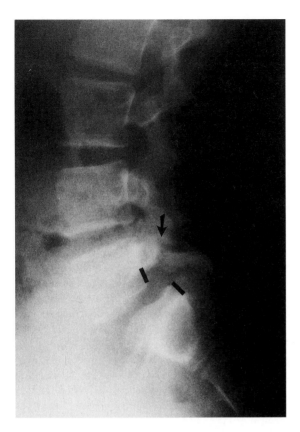

Fig. 5.5.14 Spondylolisthesis. Lateral view in a 17 year old male football lineman.

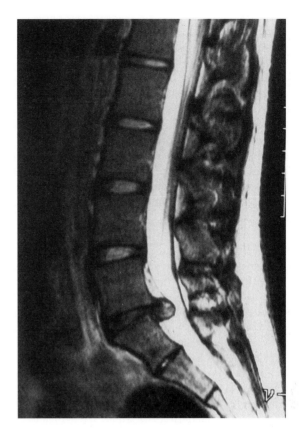

Fig. 5.5.15 Herniated disc. Sagital MRI in a 17 year old gymnast.

attached to the cartilaginous end plate.[152,154–156] These anatomic differences may predispose to disc herniation into the vertebral body or through an endplate fracture, rather than the classic extruded or sequestered disc through the annulus seen in adults. Disc herniations have been associated with sports with repetitive flexion and axial loading of the lumber spine, such as gymnastics, running, football, weight lifting, basketball, soccer and tennis.

The diagnosis can be difficult to determine clinically because the presentation can be quite different from the classic radicular symptom atology of the adult. In the adolescent with a ruptured disc, the most frequent complaint is low back pain with radiation confined to the buttock. There may be a decrease in hamstring flexibility, limited motion, abnormal gait or running pattern, asymmetric paravertebral spasm, or subtle 'sciatic' scoliosis. Neurologic findings of altered reflexes, muscle weakness and atrophy are rare. In cases of severe pain and systemic symptoms, white blood cell count, sedimentation rate and bone scan should be performed to rule out occult disc space infection. Work-up includes lumbosacral spine films which may show end plate fracture. Disc space narrowing is unusual. MRI confirms the presence of a neurocompressive lesion (Fig. 5.5.15). A non-operative approach is the mainstay of management for both disc herniation and discogenic pain. Initial treatment is aimed at resting the back and avoiding sporting activities. Brace treatment with a 15° lumbar lordosis module has been a useful adjunct to the management of adolescent athletes with discogenic pain that does not respond to rest.[137] In our experience, rigid bracing is more effective than use of a soft corset and allows the athlete to return to daily activities and a light training

programme. If the athlete is still symptomatic at 8–12 weeks, epidural corticosteroids are considered.[157] For those who fail non-operative management or have evidence of cauda equina syndrome or severe motor loss, discectomy may be necessary. In general, surgical intervention in this age group has good short-term results; however, return to high level competitive sports may not be possible.[138,148,153,158] In addition, the risk of long-term sequelae, such as degenerative changes at the involved level or herniation at a different level, is not well understood.

A condition that is almost indistinguishable from a herniated lumbar disc is a slipped vertebral apophysis or end plate fracture.[155,159] This condition is often associated with heavy lifting, and typically involves displacement of the posterior inferior apophysis of L4 with its disc attachment into the vertebral canal. Patients present with signs of a herniated disc with neurologic findings. X-Rays reveal the avulsion fragment and MRI reveals an extradural mass. Treatment consists of excision of both the cartilaginous disc and the bony fragment with relief of symptoms.

Scoliosis

Idiopathic scoliosis generally does not cause pain and does not interfere with sports. Scoliotic curves are often detected by asymmetry noted by parents, coaches or screening. Forward bending accentuates the deformity by revealing the rotational deformity associated with coronal plane curvature. After a thorough history and examination to rule out associated abnormalities, full-length standing spine X-rays are obtained and the curve measured. Full time bracing is initiated for progressive curves or, in general, curves over 25° in a child with substantial growth remaining. The braced patient is allowed to participate in sports out of the brace and there is no evidence that sports participation increases the risk of curve progression. On the contrary, physical activity and strengthening are an essential aspect of brace management of scoliosis. After growth is complete, bracing is discontinued and no restrictions are placed on the adolescent with idiopathic scoliosis. Patients with progressive curves despite bracing or curves over 50° have a high incidence of progression after maturity and are treated with spinal instrumentation and fusion. Post-operatively, sports are restricted until the fusion mass heals and matures. Following fusion for scoliosis, contact sports and vigorous gymnastics are restricted due to risks of pseudarthrosis, hardware failure and degenerative changes about the fused levels.[160]

Scheuermann's disease

Scheuermann's disease consists of kyphosis of the thoracic spine with anterior vertebral wedging, Schmorl's nodes and vertebral end-plate deformity. Radiographic criteria include wedging of 5° or more of three consecutive vertebrae.[161] The aetiology is unknown, although repetitive flexion microtrauma and fatigue failure are implicated. Patients typically present due to deformity without pain. On physical examination, patients have a roundback deformity with increased lumbar lordosis in the standing position. Most are unable to correct this deformity with forced hyperextension. Hamstrings are invariably tight. Treatment of Scheuermann's kyphosis consists of posture training, pelvic control, abdominal strengthening, and flexibility exercises to address the tight hamstrings and lumbodorsal fascia. Progressive kyphosis over 50° in an immature child is an indication for bracing, and progression to curves beyond 70° is an indication for spinal fusion. Idiopathic kyphosis without radiographic changes of Scheuermann's disease is seen about the adolescent growth spurt in children with tight lumbodorsal fascia and hamstrings, who subsequently compensate for this pelvic tilt with thoracic kyphosis. In general, this is a flexible kyphosis that can be managed with posture, strength and flexibility training.

Atypical Scheuermann's disease consists of degenerative changes of the disc and vertebral end plates at the thoracolumbar junction. This is seen in adolescent athletes involved in vigorous flexion–extension activity of the spine, such as gymnastics, diving and rowing. Irregularities of the ring apophysis, end-plate wedging and Schmorl's nodes may be seen on radiographs. These changes are often accompanied by pain, and are thought to result from microtrauma with resultant end plate fractures or disc herniation through the anterior ring apophysis with secondary bony deformation of the vertebrae.[151] Typically, the adolescent with atypical Scheuermann's has a flat back with thoracic hypokyphosis and lumbar hypolordosis. Pain is accentuated by forward flexion and relieved with rest. Our treatment utilizes full-time bracing with a moulded thoracolumbar orthosis of 15° extension, advanced to 30° if tolerated. Abdominal strengthening, hamstring stretching and pelvic control are also initiated. The gymnast is often able to slowly return to activity in 3 to 6 months.

Fractures

Fractures of the thoracolumbar spine in child and adolescent athletes are quite rare. Most reports of spinal injuries with neurologic deficits in children involve the cervical spine.[162,163] It takes considerable force

to result in thoracolumbar fracture in the adolescent athlete, and the absence of a major force should prompt a search for a pathologic lesion. The classification and stability of compression fractures can be conceptualized in Denis's three-column model, where the anterior column consists of the anterior longitudinal ligament and the anterior half of the vertebral body, the middle column consists of the posterior half of the vertebral body and the posterior longitudinal ligament, and the posterior column consists of the posterior elements and ligamentous structures. Instability is inferred when two columns are disrupted. Evaluation of these injuries includes a thorough history and physical examination, including neurologic, cardiopulmonary and abdominal assessment. Anteroposterior and lateral X-rays of the spine are obtained and further studies are performed as needed, such as CT to define the extent of bony injury and MRI to evaluate neurologic involvement or disc injury. Stable compression fractures of less than 50% can be treated in a moulded thoracolumbar orthosis or hyperextension brace for 6 to 12 weeks, depending on healing and symptoms (Fig. 5.5.16). Return to sports is allowed when the athlete is pain free and has full strength and flexibility. Unstable fracture-dislocations, fractures with neurologic compromise and fractures with significant deformity may require spinal fusion with possible neurologic decompression.

Apophyseal avulsion injuries resulting from rapid flexion, extension and torsion are specific to the adolescent. Transverse process fractures may occur with contact sports. Associated intra-thoracic, abdominal and retroperitoneal injuries are the initial concerns. Management of these injuries consists of rest, followed by gradually

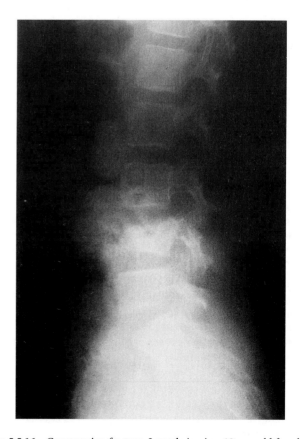

Fig. 5.5.16 Compression fracture, Lateral view in a 10 year old female child.

increased range of motion and strength. Temporary bracing may be helpful. Return to gymnastics and contact sports is allowed when normal flexibility and strength are obtained.

Mechanical back pain

Mechanical back pain secondary to acute or chronic musculoligamentous strains and sprains is rare in the young athlete, and should be a diagnosis of exclusion in children with lower back pain. Such back pain is thought to represent overuse or stretch injuries of the soft tissues including the muscle–tendon unit, ligaments, joint capsules and facets. This is more commonly seen in the older age group and may be related to the adolescent growth spurt. Young athletes with mechanical back pain may be predisposed to injury due to weak abdominal musculature, tight lumbodorsal fascia, tight hamstrings, limited lumbar motion and poor training technique.[164] The pain is often nondescript, exacerbated by activity and relieved by rest. Physical examination reveals paraspinal muscle tenderness, decreased flexibility and limited spinal motion. X-Rays are normal. Acutely, treatment consists of rest. Massage, NSAIDs and phonophoresis may be helpful. Once the acute phase has resolved, a rehabilitation programme consisting of posture control, abdominal strengthening and flexibility is initiated. Return to sport is gradually allowed with resolution of pain and return of strength and flexibility. Proper technique, conditioning and stretching are emphasized.

References

1. Culpepper, M. I. and Niemann, K. M. W. High school football injuries in Birmingham, Alabama. *Southern Medical Journal* 1983; **76**: 873–8.
2. Goldberg, B., Rosenthal, P. P. and Nicholas, J. A. Injuries in youth football. *The Physician and Sports Medicine* 1984; **12**: 122–32.
3. Olson, O. C. The Spokane study: high school football injuries. *The Physician and Sports Medicine* 1979; **7**: 75–82.
4. Consumer Product Safety Commission. Bicycle related injuries: Data from the National Electronic Injury Surveillance System. *Journal of the American Medical Association* 1987; **257**: 3334–7.
5. Kirburz, D., Jacobs, R., Reckling, F. and Mason, J. Bicycle accidents and injuries among adult cyclists. *American Journal of Sports Medicine* 1986; **14**: 416–9.
6. Kocher, M. S. and Feagin, J. A., Jr. Shoulder injuries during alpine skiing. *American Journal of Sports Medicine* 1996; **24**: 665–9.
7. Requa, R. and Garrick, J. G. Injuries in interscholastic wrestling. *The Physician and Sports Medicine* 1981; **9**: 44–51.
8. Snook, G. A. Injuries in intercollegiate wrestling: a 5 year study. *American Journal of Sports Medicine* 1982; **10**: 142–4.
9. Gainor, B. J., Piotrowski, G., Puhl, J., Allen, W. C. and Hagen, R. The throw: biomechanics and acute injury. *American Journal of Sports Medicine* 1980; **8**: 114–8.
10. Tullos, H. S. and Fain, R. H. Little league shoulder: rotational stress fracture of proximal humeral epiphysis. *Journal of Sports Medicine* 1974; **2**: 152–3.
11. Tullos, H. S. and King, J. W. Lesions of the pitching arm in adolescents. *Journal of the American Medical Association* 1972; **220**: 264–71.
12. Albright, J. A., Jokl, P., Shaw, R. and Albright, J. P. Clinical study of baseball pitchers: Correlation of injury to the throwing arm with method of delivery. *American Journal of Sports Medicine* 1978; **6**: 15–21.
13. Barnett, L. S. Little league shoulder syndrome: proximal humeral epiphysis in adolescent baseball pitchers. *Journal of Bone and Joint Surgery* 1985; **67A**: 495–6.
14. Cahill, B. R. and Tullos, H. S. Little league shoulder. *Sports Medicine* 1974; **2**: 150–3.
15. Dotter, W. E. Little leaguer's shoulder: a fracture of the proximal epiphyseal cartilage of the humerus due to baseball pitching. *Guthrie Clinic Bulletin* 1953; **23**: 68–72.
16. Lipscomb, A. B. Baseball injuries in growing athletes. *Journal of Sports Medicine* 1975; **3**: 25–34.
17. Torg, J. S., Pollack, H. and Sweterlitsch, P. The effect of competitive pitching on the shoulders and elbows of preadolescent baseball players. *Pediatrics* 1972; **49**: 267–72.
18. Priest, J. D. and Nagel, D. A. Tennis shoulder. *American Journal of Sports Medicine* 1976; **4**: 28–42.
19. Richardson, A. B., Jobe, F. W. and Collins, H. R. The shoulder in competitive swimming. *American Journal of Sports Medicine* 1980; **8**: 159–63.
20. Fulton, N. N., Albright, J. P. and El-Khoury, G. Y. Cortical desmoid-like lesion of the proximal humerus and its occurrence in gymnasts. *American Journal of Sports Medicine* 1979; **7**: 57–61.
21. Goldberg, M. J. Gymnastic injuries. *Orthopedic Clinics of North America* 1980; **11**: 717–32.
22. Snook, G. A. Injuries in women's gymnastics: a 5 year study. *American Journal of Sports Medicine* 1979; **7**: 242–4.
23. Brooks, A. L. and Henning, G. D. Injury to the proximal clavicular epiphysis. *Journal of Bone and Joint Surgery* 1972; **54A**: 1347–51.
24. Denham, R. H. and Dingley, A. F. Epiphyseal separation of the medial clavicle. *Journal of Bone and Joint Surgery* 1967; **49A**: 1179–83.
25. Lewonowski, K. and Bassett, G. S. Complete posterior sternoclavicular epiphyseal separation: a case report and review of the literature. *Clinical Orthopaedics and Related Research* 1992; **281**: 84–8.
26. Winter, J., Sterner, S., Maurer, D., Varecka, T. and Zarzycki, M. Retrosternal epiphyseal disruption of medial clavicle: case and review in children. *Journal of Emergency Medicine* 1989; **7**: 9–13.
27. Destouet, J. M., Gilula, L. A., Murphy, W. A. and Sagel, S. S. Computed tomography of the sternoclavicular joint and sternum. *Radiology* 1981; **138**: 123–8.
28. Selesnick, F. H., Jablon, M., Frank, C. and Post, M. Retrosternal dislocation of the clavicle. *Journal of Bone and Joint Surgery* 1984; **66A**: 297.
29. Clark, R. L., Milgram, J. W. and Yawn, D. H. Fatal aortic perforation and cardiac tamponade due to Kirschner wire migrating from the right sternoclavicular joint. *Southern Medical Journal* 1974; **67**: 316–8.
30. Bowen, A. Plastic bowing of the clavicle in children: a report of two cases. *Journal of Bone and Joint Surgery* 1983; **65A**: 403–5.
31. Nogi, J., Heckman, J. D., Hakala, M. and Sweet, D. E. Non-union of the clavicle in a child: a case report. *Clinical Orthopaedics and Related Research* 1975; **110**: 19–21.
32. Howard, F. M. and Shafer, S. J. Injury to the clavicle with neurovascular complications: a study of fourteen cases. *Journal of Bone and Joint Surgery* 1965; **47A**: 1335–46.
33. Zenni, E. J., Krieg, J. K. and Rosen, M. J. Open reduction and internal fixation of clavicular fractures. *Journal of Bone and Joint Surgery* 1981; **63A**: 147–51.
34. Black, G. B., McPherson, J. A. and Reed, M. H. Traumatic pseudo-dislocation of the acromioclavicular joint in children. *American Journal of Sports Medicine* 1991; **19**: 644–6.
35. Eidman, D. K., Siff, S. J. and Tullos, H. S. Acromioclavicular lesions in children. *American Journal of Sports Medicine* 1981; **9**: 150–4.
36. Falstie-Jensen, S. and Mikkelsen, P. Pseudodislocation of the acromioclavicular joint. *Journal of Bone and Joint Surgery* 1982; **64B**: 368–9.
37. Havranek, P. Injuries of the distal clavicular physis in children. *Journal of Pediatric Orthopaedics* 1989; **9**: 213–5.
38. Ogden, J. A. Distal clavicular physeal injury. *Clinical Orthopaedics and Related Research* 1984; **188**: 68–73.
39. Rockwood, C. A. Fractures of outer clavicle in children and adults. *Journal of Bone and Joint Surgery* 1982; **64B**: 642–9.
40. Bjerneld, H., Hovelius, L. and Thorling, J. Acromioclavicular separatons treated conservatively. *Acta Orthopaedica Scandinavica* 1983; **54**: 743–5.
41. Galpin, R. D., Hawkins, R. J. and Grainger, R. W. A comparative analysis of operative versus nonoperative management of grade III

acromioclavicular separations. *Clinical Orthopaedics and Related Research* 1985; **193**: 150–5.

42. **Larsen, E., Bjerg-Nielsen, A.** and **Christensen, P.** Conservative or surgical treatment of acromioclavicular dislocation. *Journal of Bone and Joint Surgery* 1986; **68A**: 552–5.

43. **Cahill, B. R.** Atraumatic osteolysis of the distal clavicle: a review. *Sports Medicine* 1992; **13**: 214–22.

44. **Scavenius, M.** and **Iversen, B. F.** Nontraumatic clavicular osteolysis in weight lifters. *American Journal of Sports Medicine* 1992; **20**: 463–7.

45. **Larson, R. L., Singer, K. M., Bergstrom, R.** and **Thomas, S.** Little League survey: the Eugene study. *American Journal of Sports Medicine* 1976; **4**: 201–9.

46. **Kohler, R.** and **Trillaud, J. M.** Fracture and fracture separation of the proximal humerus in children: report of 136 cases. *Journal of Pediatric Orthopaedics* 1983; **3**: 326–32.

47. **Baxter, M. P.** and **Wiley, J.** Fractures of the proximal humeral epiphysis: their influence on humeral growth. *Journal of Bone and Joint Surgery* 1986; **68B**: 570–3.

48. **Dameron, T. B.** and **Reibel, D. B.** Fractures involving the proximal humeral epiphyseal plate. *Journal of Bone and Joint Surgery* 1969; **51A**: 289–97.

49. **Neer, C. S.** and **Horowitz, B. S.** Fractures of the proximal humeral epiphyseal plate. *Clinical Orthopaedics and Related Research* 1965; **41**: 24–31.

50. **Nilsson, S.** and **Svartholm, F.** Fracture of the upper end of the humerus in children: a follow up of 44 cases. *Acta Chirurgica Scandinavica* 1965; **130**: 433–9.

51. **Sherk, H.** and **Probst, C.** Fractures of the proximal humeral epiphysis. *Orthopedic Clinics of North America* 1975; **6**: 401–13.

52. **Williams, D. J.** The mechanisms producing fracture separation of the proximal humeral epiphysis. *Journal of Bone and Joint Surgery* 1981; **63B**: 102–7.

53. **Asher, M. A.** Dislocations of the upper extremity in children. *Orthopedic Clinics of North America* 1976; **7**: 583–91.

54. **Hovelius, L.** Anterior dislocation of the shoulder in teenagers and young adults. *Journal of Bone and Joint Surgery* 1987; **69A**: 393–9.

55. **Marans, H. J., Angel, K. R., Schemitsch, E. H.** and **Wedge, J. H.** The fate of traumatic anterior dislocation of the shoulder in children. *Journal of Bone and Joint Surgery* 1992; **74A**: 1242–4.

56. **Rowe, C. R.** Anterior dislocation of the shoulder: prognosis and treatment. *Surgical Clinics of North America* 1963; **43**: 1609–14.

57. **Rowe, C. R.** Prognosis in dislocation of the shoulder. *Journal of Bone and Joint Surgery* 1956; **38A**: 957–77.

58. **Wagner, K. T.** and **Lyne, E. D.** Adolescent traumatic dislocations of the shoulder with open epiphysis. *Journal of Pediatric Orthopaedics* 1983; **3**: 61–2.

59. **Aronen, J. G.** and **Regan, K.** Decreasing the incidence of recurrence of first time anterior shoulder dislocation with rehabilitation. *American Journal of Sports Medicine* 1984; **12**: 283–91.

60. **Burkhead, W. Z.** and **Rockwood, C. A.** Treatment of instability of the shoulder with an exercise program. *Journal of Bone and Joint Surgery* 1992; **74A**: 890–6.

61. **Simonet, W. T.** and **Cofield, R. H.** Prognosis in anterior shoulder dislocation. *American Journal of Sports Medicine* 1984; **12**: 19–24.

62. **Carter, C.** and **Sweetnam, R.** Recurrent dislocation of the patella and the shoulder: their association with familial joint laxity. *Journal of Bone and Joint Surgery* 1960; **42B**: 721–7.

63. **Neer, C. S.** and **Foster, D. R.** Inferior capsular shift for involuntary inferior and multidirectional instability of the shoulder. *Journal of Bone and Joint Surgery* 1980; **62A**: 897–908.

64. **Bigliani, L. U., D'Alessandro, D. F., Duralde, X. A.** and **McIlveen, S. J.** Anterior acromioplasty for subacromial impingement in patients younger than 40 years of age. *Clinical Orthopaedics and Related Research* 1989; **246**: 111–6.

65. **Hawkins, R. J.** and **Kennedy, J. C.** Impingement syndrome in athletes. *American Journal of Sports Medicine* 1980; **8**: 151–7.

66. **Tibone, J. E.** Shoulder problems of adolescence. *Clinics of Sports Medicine* 1983; **2**: 423–6.

67. **Tibone, J. E., Elrod, B., Jobe, F. W., Kerlan, R. K., Carter, V. S., Shields, L. L., Lombardo, S .J.** and **Yocum, C.** Surgical treatment of tears of the rotator cuff in athletes. *Journal of Bone and Joint Surgery* 1986; **68A**: 887–91.

68. **Pappas, A. M.** Elbow problems associated with baseball during childhood and adolescence. *Clinical Orthopaedics and Related Research* 1982; **164**: 30–41.

69. **Aronem, J. G.** Problems of the upper extremity in gymnastics. *Clinics of Sports Medicine* 1985; **4**: 61–71.

70. **Otsuka, N. Y.** and **Kasser, J. R.** Supracondylar fractures of the humerus in children. *Journal of the American Academy of Orthopaedic Surgeons* 1997; **5**: 19–26.

71. **Skaggs, D. L.** Elbow fractures in children: Diagnosis and Management. *Journal of the American Academy of Orthopaedic Surgeons* 1997; **5**: 303–12.

72. **Bernstein, S. M., McKeever, P.** and **Bernstein, L.** Percutaneous reduction of displaced radial neck fractures in children. *Journal of Pediatric Orthopaedics* 1993; **13**: 85–8.

73. **Gill, T. J.** and **Micheli, L. J.** The immature athlete: common injuries and overuse syndromes of the elbow and wrist. *Clinics of Sports Medicine* 1996; **15**: 401–23.

74. **Dias, J., Johnson, G., Hoskinson, J.** and **Sulaiman, K.** Management of severely displaced medial epicondyle fractures. *Journal of Orthopaedic Trauma* 1987; **1**: 59–62.

75. **Josefsson, P. O.** and **Danielsson, L. G.** Epicondylar elbow fracture in children: 35 year follow-up of 56 unreduced cases. *Acta Orthopaedica Scandinavica* 1986; **57**: 313–5.

76. **Woods, G. W.** and **Tullos, H. S.** Elbow instability and medial epicondyle fractures. *American Journal of Sports Medicine* 1977; **5**: 23–30.

77. **Carlioz, H.** and **Abols, Y.** Posterior dislocation of the elbow in children. *Journal of Pediatric Orthopaedics* 1984; **4**: 8–12.

78. **Jackson, D. W., Silvino, N.** and **Reiman, P.** Osteochondritis in the female gymnast's elbow. *Arthroscopy* 1989; **5**: 129–36.

79. **Brogdon, B. G.** and **Crow, N. E.** Little Leaguer's elbow. *American Journal of Roentgenology* 1960; **83**: 671–5.

80. **Gugenheim, J. J., Stanley, R. F., Wood, G. W.** and **Tullos, H. S.** Little League survey: the Houston study. *American Journal of Sports Medicine* 1976; **4**: 189–200.

81. **Hang, Y. S.** Little League elbow: a clinical and biomechanical study. *International Orthopaedics* 1982; **3**: 70–8.

82. **Slager, R. F.** From Little League to the big league, the weak spot is the arm. *American Journal of Sports Medicine* 1977; **5**: 37–48.

83. **Smith, M. G. H.** Osteochondritis of the humeral capitellum. *Journal of Bone and Joint Surgery* 1964; **46B**: 50–4.

84. **Tiynon, M. C., Anzel, S. H.** and **Waugh, T. R.** Surgical management of osteochondritis dissecans of the capitellum. *American Journal of Sports Medicine* 1976; **4**: 121–8.

85. **Chambers, R. B.** Orthopaedic injuries in athletes (ages 6 to 17). *American Journal of Sports Medicine* 1979; **7**: 195–7.

86. **Watson, A. W.** Sports injuries during one academic year in 6,799 Irish school children. *American Journal of Sports Medicine* 1984; **12**: 65–71.

87. **Zaricznyj, B., Shattuck, L. J., Mast, T. A., Robertson, R. V.** and **D'Elia, G.** Sports-related injuries in school-aged children. *American Journal of Sports Medicine* 1980; **8**: 318–24.

88. **Blitzer, C.M., Johnson, R.J., Ettlinger, C.F.** and **Aggeborn, K.** Downhill skiing injuries in children. *American Journal of Sports Medicine* 1984; **12**: 142–7.

89. **Garrick, J. F.** and **Regua, R. K.** Epidemiology of women's gymnastic injuries. *American Journal of Sports Medicine* 1980; **8**: 261–4.

90. **Sullivan, J. A., Gross, R. H., Grana, W. A.** and **Garcia-Mural, C. A.** Evaluation of injuries in youth soccer. *American Journal of Sports Medicine* 1980; **8**: 325–7.

91. **Mann, D. C.** and **Rajmaira, S.** Distribution of physeal and non-physeal fractures in 2650 long bone fractures in children aged 0–16 years. *Journal of Pediatric Orthopaedics* 1990; **10**: 713–6.

92. Roy, S., Caine, D. and Singer, K. M. Stress changes of the distal radius epiphysis in young gymnasts. *American Journal of Sports Medicine* 1985; **13**: 301–8.

93. Friberg, K. Remodelling after distal forearm fractures. *Acta Orthopaedica Scandinavica* 1970; **50**: 731–50.

94. Mandelbaum, B. R., Bartolozzi, A. R., Davis, C. A., Teurlings, L. and Bragonier, B. Wrist pain syndrome in the gymnast. *American Journal of Sports Medicine* 1989; **17**: 305–17.

95. Vender, M. I. and Watson, H. K. Acquired Madelung-like deformity in a gymnast. *Journal of Hand Surgery* 1988; **13A**: 19–21.

96. Terry, C. L. and Waters, P. M. Triangular fibrocartilage injuries in paediatric and adolescent patients. *Journal of Hand Surgery* 1998; **23A**: 626–34.

97. Mintzer, C. M., Waters, P. M. and Simmons, B. P. Nonunion of the scaphoid in children treated with Herbet screw fixation and bone grafting. A report of five cases. *Journal of Bone and Joint Surgery* 1995; **77B**: 98–100.

98. Riester, J. N., Baker, B. E., Mosher, J. F. and Lowe, D. A review of scaphoid fracture healing in competitive athletes. *American Journal of Sports Medicine* 1985; **13**: 154–61.

99. Southcott, R. and Rosman, M. A. Non-union of carpal scaphoid fractures in children. *Journal of Bone and Joint Surgery* 1977; **59B**: 20–3.

100. Hanks, G. A., Kalenak, A., Bowman, L. S. and Sebastianelli, W. J. Stress fractures of the carpal scaphoid. A report of four cases. *Journal of Bone and Joint Surgery* 1989; **71A**: 938–41.

101. Manzione, M. and Pizzutillo, P. D. Stress fracture of the scaphoid waist. *American Journal of Sports Medicine* 1981; **9**: 268–9.

102. Burton, R. I. and Eaton, R. G. Common hand injuries in the athlete. *Orthopedic Clinics of North America* 1973; **4**: 809–38.

103. Hastings, H. and Simmons, B. P. Hand fractures in children. *Clinical Orthopaedics and Related Research* 1984; **188**: 120–30.

104. McCue, F. C., Baugher, W. H., Kulund, D. N. and Gieck, J. H. Hand and wrist injuries in the athlete. *American Journal of Sports Medicine* 1979; **7**: 275–86.

105. Posner, M. A. Injuries to the hand and wrist in athletes. *Orthopedic Clinics of North America* 1977; **8**: 593–617.

106. Simmons, B. P. and Lovallo, J. L. Hand and wrist injuries in children. *Clinics of Sports Medicine* 1988; **7**: 495–512.

107. Leddy, J. P. and Packer, J. W. Avulsion of the profundus tendon insertion in athletes. *Journal of Hand Surgery* 1977; **2**: 66–9.

108. Ferguson, R. H., McMaster, J. F. and Stanitski, C. L. Low back pain in college football linemen. *American Journal of Sports Medicine* 1974; **2**: 63–9.

109. Ciullo, J. V. and Jackson, D. W. Pars interarticularis stress reaction, spondylolysis, and spondylolisthesis in gymnasts. *Clinics of Sports Medicine* 1985; **4**: 95–110.

110. Hill, S. J. Mechanical contribution to lumbar stress injuries in female gymnasts. *Medicine and Science in Sports and Exercise* 1986; **18**: 599–602.

111. Howell, D. W. Musculoskeletal profile and incidence of musculoskeletal injuries in lightweight women rowers. *American Journal of Sports Medicine* 1984; **12**: 278–81.

112. Ireland, M. L. and Micheli, L. J. Bilateral stress fracture in the lumbar pedicle in a ballet dancer. *Journal of Bone and Joint Surgery* 1987; **69A**: 140–2.

113. Jackson, D. W., Wiltse, L. L. and Cirincione, R. J. Spondylolysis in the female gymnast. *Clinical Orthopaedics and Related Research* 1976; **117**: 68–73.

114. McCarroll, J. R., Miller, J. M. and Ritter, M. A. Lumbar spondylolysis and spondylolisthesis in college football players. *American Journal of Sports Medicine* 1986; **14**: 404–6.

115. Micheli, L. J. Back injuries in dancers. *Clinics of Sports Medicine* 1983; **2**: 473–84.

116. Micheli, L. J. Back injuries in gymnastics. *Clinics of Sports Medicine* 1984; **4**: 85–93.

117. Micheli, L. J. Low back pain in the adolescent: differential diagnosis. *American Journal of Sports Medicine* 1979; **7**: 362–4.

118. Rosenberg, N. J. U., Bargar, W. L. and Friedman, B. The incidence of spondylolysis and spondylolisthesis in nonambulatory patients. *Spine* 1981; **6**: 35–8.

119. Semen, R. L. and Spengler, D. Significance of lumbar spondylolysis in college football players. *Spine* 1981; **6**: 172–4.

120. O'Neill, D. B. and Micheli, L. J. Post-operative radiographic evidence for fatigue fracture as the etiology of spondylolysis. *Spine* 1989; **14**: 1342–55.

121. Hoshina, H. Spondylolysis in athletes. *The Physician and Sports Medicine* 1980; **8**: 75–8.

122. Baker, D. R. and McHolick, W. Spondylolysis and spondylolisthesis in children. *Journal of Bone and Joint Surgery* 1956; **38A**: 933–4.

123. Collier, B. D., Johnson, R. P., Carrera, G. F., Meyer, G. A., Schwab, J. P., Flatley, T. J., Isitman, A. T., Hellman, R. S., Zielonka, J. S. and Knobel, J. Painful spondylolysis or spondylolisthesis studied by radiography or single photon emission computed tomography. *Radiology* 1985; **154**: 207–11.

124. LaFond, G. Surgical treatment of spondylolisthesis. *Clinical Orthopaedics and Related Research* 1962; **22**: 175–9.

125. Hutton, W. C., Stott, J. R. R. and Cyron, B. M. Is spondylolysis a fatigue fracture? *Spine* 1977; **2**: 202–29.

126. Letts, M., Smallman, T., Afanasiev, R. and Gouw, G. Fracture of the pars interarticularis in adolescent athletes: a clinical-biomechanical analysis. *Journal of Pediatric Orthopaedics* 1986; **6**: 40–6.

127. Fredrickson, B. E., Baker, D., McHolick, W. J., Yuan, H. A. and Lubicky, J. P. L. The natural history of spondylolysis and spondylolisthesis. *Journal of Bone and Joint Surgery* 1984; **66A**: 699–707.

128. Winney-Davies, R. and Scott, J. H. S. Inheritance and spondylolisthesis—a radiographic family survey. *Journal of Bone and Joint Surgery* 1979; **61B**: 301–5.

129. Phalen, G. S. and Dickson, J. A. Spondylolisthesis and tight hamstrings. *Journal of Bone and Joint Surgery* 1961; **43A**: 505–12.

130. Bellah, R. D., Summerville, D. A., Treves, S. T. and Micheli, L. J. Low-back pain in adolescent athletes: Detection of stress injury to the pars interarticularis with SPECT. *Radiology* 1991; **180**: 509–12.

131. Morita, T., Ikata, T., Katoh, S. and Miyake, R. Lumbar spondylolysis in children and adolescents. *Journal of Bone and Joint Surgery* 1995; **77B**: 620–5.

132. Saraste, H. Prognostic radiologic aspects of spondylolisthesis. *Acta Radiologica* 1984; **25**: 427–34.

133. Saraste, H. Long-term clinical and radiographic follow-up of spondylolysis and spondylolisthesis. *Journal of Pediatric Orthopaedics* 1987; **7**: 631–8.

134. Turner, R. and Bianco, A. Spondylolysis and spondylolisthesis in children and teenagers. *Journal of Bone and Joint Surgery* 1971; **53A**: 1298–1306.

135. Wiltse, L. L. and Jackson, D. W. Treatment of spondylolisthesis and spondylolysis in children. *Clinical Orthopaedics and Related Research* 1976; **117**: 92–100.

136. Wiltse, L. L., Widell, E. H. and Jackson, D. W. Fatigue fracture: the basic lesion in isthmic spondylolisthesis. *Journal of Bone and Joint Surgery* 1974; **57A**: 17–22.

137. Micheli, L. J., Hall, J. E. and Miller, M. E. Use of modified Boston back brace for back injuries in athletes. *American Journal of Sports Medicine* 1980; **8**: 351–6.

138. Micheli, L. J. and Steiner, M. E. Treatment of symptomatic spondylolysis and spondylolisthesis with the modified Boston brace. *Spine* 1985; **10**: 937–43.

139. Congeni, J., McCulloch, J. and Swanson, K. Lumbar spondylolysis. A study of natural progression in athletes. *American Journal of Sports Medicine* 1997; **25**: 248–53.

140. Papanicolaou, N., Wilkinson, R. H., Emans, J. B., Treves, S. and Micheli, L. J. Bone scintigraphy and radiography in young athletes with low back pain. *American Journal of Roentgenology* 1985; **145**: 1039–44.

141. Bradford, D. S. and Iza, J. Repair of the defect in spondylolysis or minimal degrees of spondylolisthesis by segmental fixation and bone grafting. *Spine* 1985; **10**: 673–9.

142. **Buck, J.** Direct repair of the defect in spondylolisthesis. *Journal of Bone and Joint Surgery* 1970; **52B**: 432–7.

143. **Buring, K.** and **Fredensborg, N.** Osteosynthesis of spondylolysis. *Acta Orthopaedica Scandinavica* 1973; **44**: 91–7.

144. **Boxall, D., Bradford, D., Winter, R.** and **Moe, J. H.** Management of severe spondylolisthesis in children and adolescents. *Journal of Bone and Joint Surgery* 1979; **61A**: 479–95.

145. **Hensinger, R., Lang, J.** and **MacEwen, G.** Surgical management of spondylolisthesis in children and adolescents. *Spine* 1976; **1**: 207–14.

146. **Muschik, M., Hahnel, H., Robinson, P. N., Perka, C.** and **Muschik, C.** Competitive sports and the progression of spondylolisthesis. *Journal of Pediatric Orthopaedics* 1996; **16**: 364–9.

147. **Bradford, D. S.** Treatment of severe spondylolisthesis: a combined approach for reduction and stabilization. *Spine* 1979; **4**: 423–9.

148. **Borgesen, S. E.** and **Vang, P. S.** Herniation of the lumbar interbertebral disk in children and adolescents. *Acta Orthopaedica Scandinavica* 1974; **45**: 540–9.

149. **Epstein, J. A., Epstein, N. E., Marc, J., Rosenthal, A. D.** and **Lavine, L. S.** Lumbar intervertebral disk herniation in teenage children: Recognition and management of associated anomalies. *Spine* 1984; **9**: 427–32.

150. **Garrido, E., Humphreys, R. P., Hendrick, E. B.** and **Hoffman, H. J.** Lumbar disc disease in children. *Neurosurgery* 1978; **2**: 22–6.

151. **Swèrd, L., HellstrÜm, M., Jacobsson, B., Nyman, R.** and **Peterson, L.** Acute injury of the vertebral ring apophysis and intervertebral disc in adolescent gymnasts. *Spine* 1990; **15**: 144–8.

152. **Swèrd, L., HellstrÜm, M., Jacobsson, B., Nyman, R.** and **Peterson, L.** Disc degeneration and associated abnormalities of the spine in elite gymnasts. *Spine* 1991; **16**: 437–43.

153. **DeOrio, J. K.** and **Bianco, A. J.** Lumbar disc excision in children and adolescents. *Journal of Bone and Joint Surgery* 1982; **64A**: 991–5.

154. **Kurihara, A.** and **Kataoka, O.** Lumbar disc herniation in children and adolescents. A review of 70 operated cases and their minimum 5 year follow-up studies. *Spine* 1980; **5**: 443–51.

155. **Lippitt, A. B.** Fracture of a vertebral body end plate and disk protrusion causing subarachnoid block in an adolescent. *Clinical Orthopaedics and Related Research* 1976; **116**: 112–5.

156. **Resnick, D.** and **Niwayama, G.** Intravertebral disk herniation: Cartilaginous (Schmorl's nodes). *Radiology* 1978; **126**: 57–65.

157. **Jackson, D. W., Rettig, A.** and **Wiltse, L. L.** Epidural cortisone injections in the young athletic adult. *American Journal of Sports Medicine* 1980; **8**: 239–43.

158. **Day, A. L., Friedman, W. A.** and **Indelicato, P. A.** Observations on the treatment of lumbar disc disease in college football players. *American Journal of Sports Medicine* 1987; **15**: 72–5.

159. **Techakapuch, S.** Rupture of the lumbar cartilage plate into the spinal canal in an adolescent. A case report. *Journal of Bone and Joint Surgery* 1981; **63A**: 481–2.

160. **Micheli, L. J.** Sports following spinal surgery in the young athlete. *Clinical Orthopaedics and Related Research* 1985; **198**: 152–7.

161. **Sorenson, H. K.** *Scheuermann's juvenile kyphosis.* Munksgaard, Copenhagen, 1964.

162. **Hubbard, D. D.** Injuries of the spine in children and adolescents. *Clinical Orthopaedics and Related Research* 1974; **100**: 56–5.

163. **Kewalramani, M. D.** and **Tori, J. A.** Spinal cord trauma in children: Neurological patterns, radiologic features, and pathomechanics of injury. *Spine* 1980; **5**: 11–8.

164. **Kujala, U. M., Taimela, S., Oksanen, A.** and **Salminen, J. J.** Lumbar mobility and low back pain during adolescence. A longitudinal three-year follow-up study in athletes and controls. *American Journal of Sports Medicine* 1997; **25**: 363–8.

5.6 Lower limb injuries in sporting children

Wolfgang Bruns, Adam D. Baxter-Jones and Nicola Maffulli

Introduction

Sport is an expression of drive for movement, play, activity and competition in humans. Over the past few decades, this has resulted in its great diffusion: 25% of girls and 50% of boys aged 8–16 participate in sport in the US.[1] In the UK, 79% of children aged between 5 and 15 take part in organized sport, 11% of whom are in intensive training.[2] Injuries during sport seem to be unavoidable, and up to 30–40% of all accidents in children and adolescents occur during sports.[3] Nevertheless the rate of injury is lower in children than in mature adolescents.[4] Prevention has been implemented, but, given the large number of participants, healthcare professionals are often confronted by acute and chronic musculoskeletal injuries in young athletes.

Sport injuries depend on the region where the patient is living: for example, a skiing injury would be unusual in a tropical country. The intensity of exercise, the mental and physical readiness for performance, and the type of sports also play a significant role, with swimming having low, ball sports medium, and riding and ice skating high risk. Each sport has a typical pattern of injury: for instance, knee contusions are the most common skiing injuries in children.[5]

The lower extremity is under specific biomechanical demands important in the context of the increasing numbers of athletes in soccer, skiing and running.[6] This chapter will therefore deal with the most common injuries of the lower limb occurring in young athletes.

The musculoskeletal system in childhood

To understand children's injuries, it is important to have an insight into the peculiarities of the growing musculoskeletal system. Tendons and ligaments are relatively stronger than the epiphyseal plate, and considerably more elastic. Therefore, in severe trauma, the epiphyseal plate, being weaker than the ligaments, gives way. Subsequently, growth plate damage is more common than ligamentous injuries.[4,7–10]

In children, bones and muscles show increased elasticity[8] and heal faster.[10–12] Weight bearing is beneficial for the skeleton, but excessive strains may produce serious injuries to joints.[8] Low intensity training can stimulate bone growth, but high intensity can inhibit it.[13,14] There are adaptive changes to sport activity,[15] and up to puberty muscular strength is similar in girls and boys.[16]

Because the skeleton is growing, injuries can result in progressive permanent effects.[8,16–19]

Different metabolic and psychological aspects of childhood sport

Children produce more heat relative to body mass, have a low sweating capacity and also tend not to drink enough compared with adults.[16]

Therefore, heat prostration and exhaustion, especially in hot climates, is more likely than in adults. This may result in an increased number of injuries.[16]

Young competitors may have the same chronological age but not necessarily the same biological age,[10] and children need to be more closely matched with the other competitors not just by chronological age but also by biological age.[22] It is also possible that parents and coaches push children too hard,[10] not appreciating that time is needed to develop high performance abilities.[20] Children may also develop psychological complications following injuries.[21]

Endogenous risk factors

Imbalances in the musculoskeletal system may influence the rate of occurrence of injuries.[10] Common conditions such as pes cavus, pes planus and calcaneus valgus may play a role in the aetiology of some injuries.[10] Anatomical factors have been hypothesized in the aetiology of injuries where overuse is common, such as in patellofemoral stress syndrome, ileotibial band syndrome, medial tibial stress syndrome and plantar fascitis.[23] Compared with adults, children have decreased strength and endurance,[24–26] which has to be taken into account when planning training and competition.

Epidemiology of lower limb injuries

Boys appear to sustain sport injuries approximately twice as often as girls,[3,8,27,28] although Castiglia[16] (1.5:1) and Sahlin[29] (male 53%: female 47%) found a more equal distribution. For some types of sports, such as horse riding, injuries are four times more common in females.[3] Soccer accounts for the majority of injuries,[29,30] but elite athletes have lower injury rates than the general sporting populations.[31]

Schmidt and Höllwarth[3] compared the frequency of sport injuries according to their location. They found that 43.8% of all injuries occur in the upper extremity, 16% in the head, and 34.5% in the lower extremity, with a peak at 12 years of age. Sprains, contusions and lacerations account for the majority (60%) of injuries.[3,32,33]

In the lower extremity, the knee joint is most often involved.[34,35] In adults knee injuries are responsible for 20%[36] of all football (soccer) injuries, and 13%[37,38] of all American football injuries. Ankle injuries are frequent as well, and, in a study of gymnastics[39] and tennis,[40] they were even more common than knee injuries.

Traumatic injuries are often typical of a specific sport: for example, spiral fractures of the tibia are the most common fracture in children with skiing injuries.[41] The pattern of injury has changed over the years, and is related to sporting equipment.[5] Currently, an increased number of overuse injuries are being reported. O'Neill and Micheli[42] relate this to the fact that in highly competitive sports, young athletes tend to train exclusively in their chosen sport. Overuse or chronic injuries as a result of repetitive microtraumata manifest as bursitis, tendinopathy, stress fracture, chondromalacia patellae, osteochondritis dissecans and traction apophysitis,[8,25,26,42–44] and are more common in the lower extremity.[45] Risk factors may include training errors, muscle–tendon imbalance, anatomical alignments, footwear and nutritional factors.[42] However, a prospective study in 136 adult subjects could not prove any influence of flexibility, anthropometric characteristics and malalignment of the lower limb on the total number of injuries.[46]

Ligament, muscle and tendon injuries

Ligaments in youth are considerably more elastic than in adults.[10] Sprains are common, especially in lax individuals,[47] and are normally well tolerated.[26] Ankle sprains are more common in patients with weak and deconditioned peroneal muscles and pes cavus varus deformity.[10] In general, they should be treated conservatively with the use of orthotics if the hindfoot is in varus. The first line management in chronic ankle instability should be strengthening and proprioceptive training.[10,48] The prophylactic effect of external stabilization with strapping remains doubtful, and there appeared to be no effect of high-top shoes in preventing ankle sprains in 622 college basketball players.[49]

Chronic compartment syndrome occurs even in young athletes,[48] and is typical in running.[50] In these patients, compartment pressure monitoring, modification of activity and fasciotomy should be considered.

Tendinopathy

Tendinopathy is a common overuse injury of the lower extremity. Most affected is the site of tendon insertion, the apophysis.[42] In most patients, partial rest and strapping are sufficient. Absolute immobilization leads to musculoskeletal atrophy.[51] Some children will benefit from physiotherapy, especially stretching, and, occasionally, from peritendinous injections. Only rarely is surgery indicated. A brief overview of the most common tendinopathies of the lower limb is given in Table 5.6.1.

Ligament injuries

Injuries of the knee most often result in physeal injuries because ligaments are stronger than growth plates. In 62 young patients with anterior cruciate ligament (ACL) disruptions, Kellenberger and von Laer[53] found avulsions of the tibial spine in 80% of children under 12 years. Over the age of 12 years, 90% of young athletes had intra substance ACL tears. Although ACL tears are considered rare in children, they are becoming increasingly more frequent, and are often associated with medial collateral ligament (MCL) tears.[54]

Operative reconstruction of the ACL can theoretically damage the growth plate, therefore some authors advise conservative management. Although this gives poor results, it allows time for skeletal maturity before reconstructing the ACL.[6,55,56]

Soft tissue grafts seem to have no influence on epiphyseal growth.[57,58] Smith and Tao[6] recommend hamstring tendon grafts using central tibial tunnel placement. In a recent study, no leg-length discrepancy was found in five patients aged 8 to 14 years at surgery. The reconstruction was performed with quadriceps or hamstrings

Table 5.6.1   Common soft tissue injuries of the lower limb[10,42,48,52]

Type	Reason	Remarks	Conservative treatment
Snapping hip	Stenosing tenosynovitis of the ileopsoas tendon	May be subluxation of the hip joint	Exercises to strengthen the hip extensors and abductors
Shin splint syndrome = medial tibial stress syndrome	Overuse of the soleus muscle on its attachment to the tibia	Often in runners	Rest, orthotics to prevent hyperpronation, running on soft surfaces
Posterior tibial tendinopathy	Repetitive excessive traction (with hyperpronation)	Often associated with excessive midfoot pronation	Orthotics to control excessive pronation, cortisone injection, physiotherapy
Achilles tendinopathy	Excessive eccentric loading	Often bilateral and associated with calcaneal apophysitis	Conservative, stretching and eccentric exercises
Peroneal tendinopathy	Impingement in the excessively pronated foot		Orthotics, cortisone injections
Tibialis anterior tendinopathy	Direct pressure in skates or ski boots		Alter footwear, vaseline, pad to reduce friction
Extensor hallucis longus tendinopathy	Tight heel cords with lack of ankle dorsiflexion results in increased activity of the extensor hallucis tendon		Heel lifts and orthotics to support the forefoot
Plantar fasciitis	Predisposition pes cavus or pes planus		Physiotherapy, orthotics, cortisone injections, alteration of activity

grafts.[59] Leg length discrepancies after ACL reconstruction[60,61] may represent normal anatomical variants.

MCL and lateral collateral ligament (LCL) injuries are treated non-operatively, as in adults. Injuries of the posterior cruciate ligament, however, can be treated conservatively or operatively after the growth plates have closed.[6]

Joint injuries

Hip

Direct forces such as dashboard injuries may dislocate the hip and fracture the acetabulum,[62] and such fracture-dislocations are usually posterior.[63] After emergency reduction, patients should be kept in traction for 3 to 6 weeks. A haematoma can be evacuated.[64] MRI is recommended to exclude soft tissue interposition, and later to identify vascular necrosis of the femoral head.

The long-term consequences of hip dislocations can be serious: 50% of patients develop avascular necrosis of the femoral head, and, if the acetabular limbus is torn, the stability of the hip joint can be seriously impaired.[65]

(a)

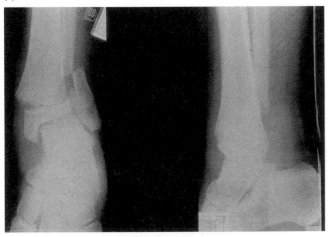

(b)

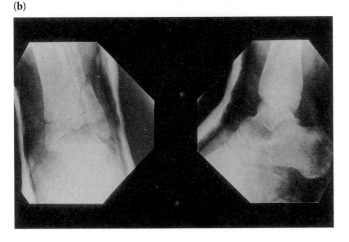

Knee

Patellar subluxation or dislocation occurs in 1 in 1000 children aged between 9 and 15 years.[66] A common cause is a twisting injury, when the femur is twisted medially with the foot planted on the ground, or direct trauma. Patella alta, in which the patella rides high in the femoral groove, predisposes to patellar instability,[8] and may be accompanied by chronic low-grade knee pain due to patellofemoral stress syndrome.[42] Spontaneous reduction is possible, and the patient may present with an effusion at times due to injury of the ACL.[6] Management consists of immediate reduction of the dislocated patella. However, one in six patients will develop recurrent dislocations, and will require realignment surgery. Skyline radiographs are recommended to exclude marginal osteochondral fractures which can result in loose bodies.[8]

In the case of meniscal injuries, repair of torn menisci is recommended because of the extremely poor long-term results following meniscectomy in children.[66,67]

Haemarthrosis of the knee is often accompanied by severe ligamentous or meniscal injury.[68] In 70 young patients with haemarthrosis after acute trauma, Stanitski et al.[69] found that 47% had ACL tears and 47% a meniscal tear. In adolescents (13 to 18 years), the rates were 65% and 45%, respectively. Tightness may be a predisposing factor.[70]

Foot

Pain in the first metatarsal-cuneiform joint is rare, and most often relates to hypermobility of the joint due to hindfoot or subtalar joint pronation.[52] Orthotics limiting such hypermobility may be successful.

Problems of the first metatarso-phalangeal joint in children differ from those in adults due to the lack of arthritic changes.[71] These can occur in children with pes planus and hallux valgus, when a bunion rubs against the shoe. This appears to be a congenital abnormality rather than the results of poorly fitting shoes.[72] Management consists of orthotics and wider fitting shoes, and, if symptoms persist, surgery after the growth plate has closed.[52]

(c)

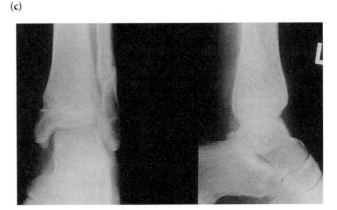

Fig. 5.6.1 Salter–Harris fracture type I of the distal tibia with a fracture of the lower fibula in a 12 year old male horse rider who, while trying to jump an obstacle, fell off the horse and had his ankle trapped in the stirrup (a) at presentation; (b) after manipulation under anaesthesia and application of a lower leg plaster of Paris cast; (c) fracture healing eight weeks after the injury.

Bone injuries

Epiphyseal injuries

Growing bone is characterized by epiphyseal plates which are weaker areas, and therefore predisposed to injury. Such injuries have been classified into five types.[73] A Salter I injury describes epiphysiolysis only (Fig. 5.6.1).

A Salter II injury includes epiphysiolysis, but with the addition of a metaphyseal fragment. After anatomical reduction, the prognosis of both such injuries is very good with conservative management. Salter III and IV injuries consist of fractures of the joint surface limited to the epiphysis (type III) or with a metaphyseal fragment (type IV) (Fig. 5.6.2). In these fractures, open reduction and anatomical reconstruction of the joint surface is generally required.[74] If this is not achieved, growth disturbance is possible.[75]

A Salter V injury describes compression of the epiphyseal plate, and diagnosis is difficult at the time of injury. Growth can be disturbed, and, given the nature of the injury, may only become obvious at a later stage. Physeal injuries can be difficult to diagnose by radiographs. Therefore, if clinically suspected, protection of the limb with a cast and repeat radiographs and examination after two weeks is useful.[76]

Fractures

Pelvis, femur, patella and tibia

Pelvic fractures are mostly found in polytrauma patients, and require careful investigation of internal organs and, in most patients, external fixation. In children, they rarely occur as a result of a sports injury. Similarly, physeal fractures of the proximal femur and acetabulum are seldom associated with sports,[62,77] and are often a result of high energy trauma. Open reduction and internal fixation with pins across the epiphysis is recommended. Patients and their families should be counselled regarding the high risk of avascular necrosis of the femoral head and of premature closure of the epiphysis in such injuries.[62] The risk of avascular necrosis varies with the location of the fracture, and it is possible to identify four categories: transepiphyseal fractures carry a 80–100% risk, proximal femoral neck fractures a 50–80% risk, distal femoral neck fractures a 30–50% risk, and intertrochanteric fractures a 10% risk.[64] Pseudarthrosis, also a result of the limited blood supply to the femoral head, carries a 40% risk. Also common is coxa vara, a complication of early closure of the medial epiphysis, with a 25% risk.[64] Anatomical reduction and internal fixation are necessary to avoid these complications.

Slipped upper femoral epiphysis occurs mainly between the ages of 10 to 16, and may be related to sports.[78] It should be considered in patients with persisting hip and knee pain. Males are more often

(a)

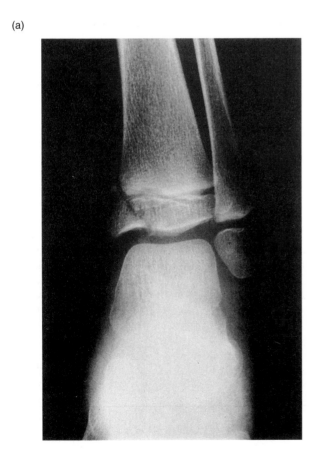

(b)

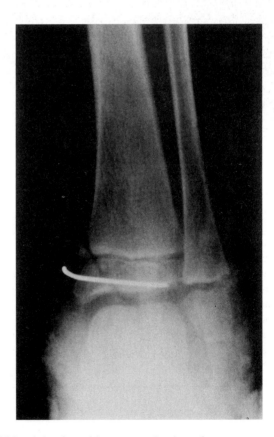

Fig. 5.6.2 Salter–Harris fracture type IV of the distal tibial epiphysis in a 11 year old female ice skater (a) at presentation (note the intra-articular component of the fracture, with a significant step in the articular surface of the lower tibia); (b) after open reduction and fixation with a Kirschner wire.

(a)

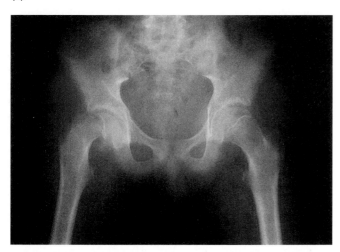

(b)

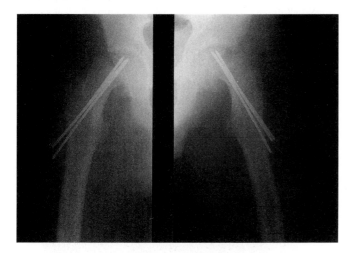

Fig. 5.6.3 Acute slipped upper femoral epiphysis in a 15 year old male gymnast, who sustained this injury on dismounting from the parallel bars (a) at presentation (note the significant slip, with approximately only 50% contact between the head and the neck); (b) after pinning *in situ* with Kirschner wires.

affected, and in up to 25% of patients, both hips are involved. Hypothyroidism and renal osteodystrophy may be associated with epiphysiolysis,[78] and should be excluded. Operative management is generally performed on an emergency basis and pinning *in situ* is recommended[79] (Fig. 5.6.3).

Femoral shaft fractures (Fig. 5.6.4) can often be treated conservatively, especially in younger children, with the application of a spica cast after an initial period of traction,[80,81] because deviation of the femoral axis will correct spontaneously. In older children and adolescents, however, operative treatment with external fixation, plating or intramedullary nailing is indicated.[81] Femoral nailing carries a risk of femoral head necrosis, therefore some authors prefer external fixation or flexible unreamed nails.[64,82,83] In anatomically reduced femoral shaft fractures, leg length discrepancy is also possible because of the increased blood supply to the fracture area,[64] which results in increased growth of the fractured limb.

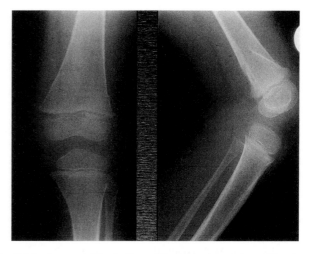

Fig. 5.6.4 Supracondylar fracture of the femur in a six year old male swimmer who slipped on the edge of the swimming pool. The fracture is minimally displaced, and was managed conservatively.

Tibial shaft fractures (Fig. 5.6.5) are the most common fractures in skiing.[5,41] Management should be conservative for closed fractures, while, for open or complicated fractures, anatomical reposition and stable fixation is necessary.[64,84] Osteochondral fractures around the knee are accompanied mostly by severe haemarthrosis.[68]

Table 5.6.2. shows an overview of the different pattern and treatment possibilities of femoral, tibial and patellar fractures.

Ankle

Symptomatic medial malleolar ossifications should be considered in the differential diagnosis of ankle pain in young athletes. On radiographs, spherical ossicles are visible, and conservative treatment is appropriate.[85]

Ankle fractures are caused by major violence and, if undisplaced, they do not need internal fixation. Tillaux–Chaput fractures are Salter–Harris type III fracture of the distal tibia, with an epiphyseal fragment connected to the syndesmosis. This fracture occurs in young athletes close to the end of puberty, and requires internal fixation.[64]

The most common fractures of the ankle after twisting[72] are type I or II Salter injuries with an open distal fibular epiphysis.[8,12,75] These fracture often close up, leaving only tenderness over the epiphysis with normal radiographs. Stress radiographs, however, usually reveal the underlying pathology, and, depending on the age of the patient, internal fixation should be considered.[8,10,81,86] An overview of ankle fractures is given in Table 5.6.3.

Foot

The most common complaint is heel pain due to Severs' disease (see Table 5.6.5). Forefoot problems are common, especially after chronic overload. Osteochondroses typically occur around the tarsal and metatarsal bones of the foot. Freiberg's disease consists of collapse of the articular surface and subchondral bone of the metatarsal head.[72] Most commonly the second metatarsal is affected (68%), but it is also found in the third (27%) or fourth (5%) metatarsal.[87] The collapse is related to reduced blood supply caused by mechanical overload. The main principle of management is to redistribute load, with help from orthotics if necessary.[64,72] Late surgery in adulthood can also be considered for resistant cases.[88,89] Avascular necrosis of the tarsal navicular bone, Köhler's lesion, results in localized pain. It is diagnosed by radiographic increased density of the navicular.[72] Management is usually conservative with orthotics or a period in plaster.[90,91] An overview of the most common bony injuries of the foot is given in Table 5.6.4.

Avulsion fractures and apophysitis

Avulsion fractures are common. They arise because of sudden intense muscular traction exerted on the immature skeleton. Tendons are relatively stronger than bones and avulsion of growth plates is the result of chronic or acute traction. Osgood–Schlatter disease, a traction apophysitis of the tibial tubercle,[92] and Severs' disease, a traction apophysitis of the calcaneal apophysis, are the most common traction apophysites.[25] They are common in boys around the time of growth spurts.[42] The onset of pain is commonly induced by a higher than normal amount of physical activity. Conservative management is normally sufficient.

Severs' disease is often bilateral, and may be due to intensive training and improper shoe wear.[42] A soft heel lift is recommended, and often is all that is required. Table 5.6.5. gives an overview.

Osteochondritis dissecans

Osteochondritis dissecans (OCD) can be due to intense physical activity[94] causing repetitive microtrauma.[42,95] This can be shown by the rate of OCD being three times more prevalent in active boys than girls around puberty, and also in competitive sports involving jumping.[64] OCD usually occurs in the lateral aspect of the medial femoral condyle, femoral head and middle third of the lateral border of the talus.[64,96,97] The radiographic diagnosis can be confirmed by MRI, and, if necessary, definitive treatment can be performed by arthroscopy. In general, management is conservative in stable lesions, and with larger fragments arthroscopic removal of intra-articular loose bodies or fixation is recommended. The long term prognosis associated with excision of the fragment is poor because of an increased risk of osteoarthritis.[98]

Stress fractures

Stress fractures are difficult to diagnose,[42,99,100] and are often associated with training errors.[9,101] Endogenous factors such as body size, sex, diet, hormonal status and anatomical factors are important as well, but difficult to prove.[23,46] Stress fractures occur more often in women, in particular amenorrhoeic athletes with decreased bone density.[102,103] Stress fractures occur more often in organized sports.[104]

Typical locations are the metatarsals, the middle and proximal tibia,[105] the proximal femur and the calcaneus.[42,64] A study of 320 stress fractures reported that 49% of them occur in the tibia, 25% in the tarsal bones and 9% in the metatarsals.[106] Varus alignment seems to play an important role in lower extremity stress fractures. Stress fractures of the

(a)

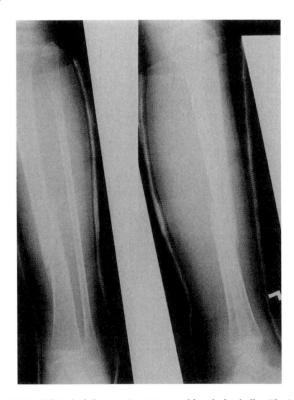

(b)

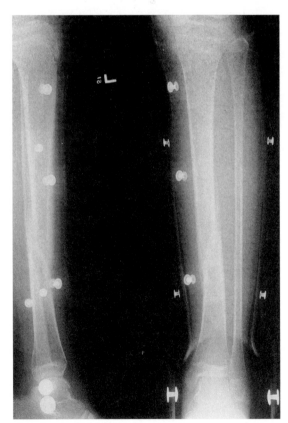

Fig. 5.6.5 Tibia shaft fracture in a 16 year old male footballer. The injury resulted from a tackle by an opponent. The fracture is only minimally displaced, and can be managed conservatively (a) in a plaster of Paris cast; (b) after six weeks, the cast had been removed, and a polypropylene removable brace applied. Note the abundant callus formed at the fracture site, and the periosteal new bone formation.

Table 5.6.2 Common fractures and epiphyseal injuries of femur, patella and tibia[8,68,80]

Type	Cause	Remarks	Treatment
Proximal femur fractures	Direct trauma	High risk of femoral head necrosis, pseudarthrosis and coxa vara	ORIF and non-weight bearing for 3 to 6 months[64]
Femoral stress fractures	Repetitive overload	Rare, crescendo pain, initial radiographs may be normal	Reduction of activity to a pain-free level
Distal femoral physeal fracture	High velocity trauma	Uncommon in sports, often Salter V fractures with disturbance of leg length growth	ORIF for Salter III and IV
Patellar fractures	Direct trauma or avulsion		ORIF in the case of patellar surface disruption
Sleeve fractures of the patella	Periosteum is stripped downwards in continuity with the tendon, results in double patella appearance	Diagnosis usually missed	Early surgery
Proximal tibia fracture	Direct trauma	Often with an avulsion fracture of the patellar tendon, injury to peroneal nerve possible	ORIF if displaced
Tibial shaft fracture	Direct or twisting trauma		Conservative; if displaced or open ORIF
Tibial stress fractures	Repetitive overload	crescendo pain, initial radiographs may be normal	Reduction of activity to a pain-free level for 8 to 12 weeks
Tibial eminence fracture (avulsion of tibial spine)	Direct trauma or forceful hyperextension with rotation	Complication ACL laxity	ORIF for displaced fractures
Tibial tuberosity fracture	Intensive jumping	?Predisposition from Osgood-Schlatter's disease	ORIF in displaced fractures

Table 5.6.3 Ankle fractures and epiphyseal injuries[8,10]

Type	Predisposing factors	Conservative management	Operative management
Epiphyseal fracture	Weak and deconditioned tendons, pes cavus, tarsal coalition	Early motion/taping, casting, Aircast splint	ORIF for Salter III and IV
Osteochondral fractures		Early motion, non-weight bearing	Occasionally but possible, normally undisplaced detached fragment ORIF
Chronic osteochondral fracture (without displacement)		Casting	Failure of non-surgical management dictates surgical debridement, forage, grafting
Isolated fibula fracture	Varus deformity of the hindfoot	Casting or splint	Displaced ORIF
Fibular fracture with medial malleolus fracture		Casting in anatomical position	Unstable fracture needs ORIF
Ankle mortis fracture without displacement			Unstable fracture needs ORIF
Triplane fracture of the distal tibia			ORIF required

Table 5.6.4 Bony foot injuries[8,10,52,68]

Type	Predisposition	Conservative treatment	Operative treatment
Sesamoiditis of the first metatarsal	Pes cavus	Orthotics, metatarsal pad	
Metatarsalgia of the metatarsophalangeal joints	Morton's foot with a short first ray	Modified activity, metatarsal pad	
Freiberg's disease	Long second metatarsal	Modified activity, insert to unload the metatarsal head, rigid soled shoes	Late surgery
Fracture of the metatarsal		Plaster casting	
Stress fracture of 2nd to 4th metatarsals	Pes cavus	Decrease activity, modify footwear	
Navicular stress fracture	Kohler's disease, cricket bowling	Activity reduction, casting for 4-6 weeks	Occasionally screw-fixation
Jones fracture of the fifth metatarsal		Plaster casting	Surgery for non-union
Painful tarsal coalition	Bony or cartilaginous bar in the hindfoot	Physiotherapy, alteration of activity or footwear	Late surgery

Table 5.6.5 Avulsion injuries of the lower extremity[8,12,72,93]

Location		Remarks	Treatment
Pelvis and hip	Anterior inferior iliac spine	Caused by psoas	Conservative non-weight bearing for 3 weeks
	Lesser trochanter	Caused by psoas	
	Iliac crest	Caused by sartorius, abductors and hamstrings	Operative considered when long fragments are displaced
	Whole ischium		
Knee	Osgood Schlatter traction apophysitis of the tibial tubercle		Conservative
			Operative when pain persists with excision of intratendinous ossicles
	Sinding-Larsen-Johannson lower patella pole		Conservative
Ankle and foot	Avulsion of a bony fragment of the anterior tibio-fibular ligament from the distal tibial epiphysis	= Tillaux fracture	Internal fixation
	Iselin's disease apophysitis of the fifth metatarsal	Rare	Conservative
	Severs' disease	Excessive tensile loads Predisposition tight heel cord, often associated with Achilles tendinopathy, Age usually 8 to 13 years	Conservative (shock absorber), avoid barefoot walking physiotherapy, stretching and strengthening, casting if persistent

navicular are associated with a short first metatarsal, metatarsal adductus, and limited ankle dorsiflexion and subtalar motion.[107]

Diagnosis may be difficult on plain radiographs taken at the time of onset of pain, and therefore should be repeated two to three weeks later. At this stage, however, the rapid periosteal response can be confused with infections or tumours. MRI[99] or CT[108,109] may be helpful. If the clinical picture is not typical, a technetium-scan is indicated.[110] Primary management consists of immobilization, with exercise within the limitations of pain.[42]

Legg–Calve–Perthes disease

Legg–Calve–Perthes disease (Fig. 5.6.6), a form of avascular necrosis of the femoral head, occurs mainly between 5 and 10 years of age. The condition is probably due to two or more episodes of raised intra-articular pressure;[111] the influence of sports is doubtful.[8] If in the early stages plain radiographs are normal, isotope bone scanning[112] or MRI scanning[113] can be useful to confirm the diagnosis. Management is either conservative or surgical, depending on various indications and the stage of the disease.[114]

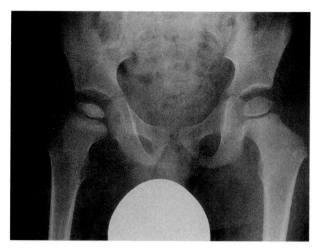

Fig. 5.6.6 Perthes disease in a seven year old male karate player. The boy presented with niggling right knee pain. Physical examination revealed no abnormalities in the right knee, but restriction of motion of the right hip. Note the addensation of the ossific nucleus in the right femoral head and the apparent increase of the joint space in the right hip.

Tarsal coalitions and sinus tarsi problems

Tarsal coalitions can cause pain associated with physical activity and should be suspected after a history of multiple ankle sprains and subtalar stiffness on examination.[72] Most commonly, the subtalar joint is affected, followed by coalition between the calcaneus and navicular.[115] The coalition can be fibrous, cartilaginous or osseous, and is accompanied by loss of supination. Management consists of casting in the painful stage, and surgery for the calcaneal navicular coalition for young children at a later stage.[52]

Sinus tarsi syndrome often occurs after starting a new activity.[52] Patients show tenderness in the sulcus of the sinus tarsi, with, at times, swelling. Management should consist of limiting pronation by orthotics,[52,72] and if the pain persists, surgery is indicated.[116]

Navicular problems

Navicular pain in young athletes is common, and is often accompanied by irritation of the tibialis posterior tendon insertion. It can also be caused by an accessory navicular bone. Excessive pronation can be limited by the use of orthotics.[52]

Summary

We have given an overview on sports related injuries of the lower-limbs in children with emphasis on the management. The special injury-related conditions of childhood, the epidemiology as well as the particular pattern of injuries were reviewed.

The increased participation of children in sports will continue. Permanent damage is a risk, and, as such, prevention should be the most important management in this age group.[117] For instance, stretching exercises should according to some authors be performed with 'warm' muscles.[42,118] Excessive weight training has an unacceptable risk of injury.[119] In endurance sports, the '10 per cent rule', which consists of increasing activity by 10 per cent each week, could probably be applied to prevent overuse injuries.[120] A multifactorial approach may be helpful.[121]

The rationale for high performance competitive sports for children is doubtful.[122] The optimal levels of safe training will remain changeable and not predictable. It should be the responsibility of parents, coaches and healthcare professionals to try and minimize the potential for injury and disability, and allow the children to enjoy the benefits of sports.[8,16,26,123]

References

1. **Metcalfe, J. A.** and **Roberts, S. O.** Strength training and the immature athlete: an overview. *Pediatric Nursing* 1993; **19**: 325–32.
2. **Rowley, S.** *The effect of intensive training on young athletes.* Sports Council, London, 1989; 6–7.
3. **Schmidt, B.** and **Höllwarth, M. E.** Sportunfälle im Kindes- und Jugendalter. *Zeitschrift für Kinderchirurgie* 1989; **44**: 357–62.
4. **Klenerman, L.** Musculoskeletal injuries in child athletes. *British Medical Journal* 1994; **308**: 1556–9.
5. **Deibert, M. C., Aronsson, D. D., Johnson, R. J.** and **Ettlinger, C. F.** Skiing injuries in children, adolescents, and adults. *Journal of Bone and Joint Surgery (American Volume)* 1998; **80**: 25–32.
6. **Smith, A. D.** and **Tao, S. S.** Knee injuries in young athletes. *Clinics in Sports Medicine* 1995; **14** : 629–49.
7. **Kruger-Franke, M., Siebert, C. H.** and **Pfoerringer, W.** Sports-related epiphyseal injuries of the lower extremity. An epidemiologic study. *Journal Sports Medicine and Physical Fitness* 1992; **32**: 106–11.
8. **Maffulli, N., Baxter-Jones, A. D. G.** Common skeletal injuries in young athletes. *Sports Medicine* 1995; **19**: 137–49.
9. **Micheli, L. J.** Overuse injuries in children's sport the growth factor. *Orthopedic Clinics of North America* 1983; **14**: 337–60.
10. **Stanish, W. D.** Lower leg, foot and ankle injuries in young athletes. *Clinics in Sports Medicine* 1995; **14**: 651–67.
11. **Ogden, J. A.** Skeletal injury in the child. Lea & Febinger, Philadelphia, 1982.
12. **Rang, M.** *Children's fracture.* (2nd edn). JB Lippincott, Philadelphia, 1983.
13. **Booth, F. W.** and **Gould, E. W.** Effects of training and disuse on connective tissue. *Exercise and Sports Sciences Review* 1975; **3**: 83–112.
14. **Tipton, C. M., Matthes, R. D.** and **Maynard, J. A.** Influence of chronic exercise on rat bones. *Medical Sciences in Sports* 1972; **4**: 55.
15. **Dalen, N.** and **Olson, K. E.** Bone mineral content and physical activity. *Acta Orthopaedica Scandinavica* 1974; **45**: 170–4.
16. **Castiglia, P. T.** Sports injuries in children. *Journal of Paediatric Health Care* 1995; **9**: 32–3.
17. **Maffulli, N.** The growing child in sport. *British Medical Bulletien* 1992; **48**: 561–8.
18. **Maffulli, N.** and **Helms, P.** Controversies about intensive training in young athletes. *Archives of Diseases in Child* 1988; **63**: 1405–7.
19. **Williams, J. G. P.** Sports injuries in children. *Medisport* 1988; 122–6.
20. **Wojtys, E. M.** Sports injuries in the immature athlete. *Orthopedic Clinics of North America* 1987; **18**: 689–708.
21. **Pillemer, F. G.** and **Micheli, L. J.** Psychological considerations in youth sports. *Clinics in Sports Medicine* 1988; **7**: 679–89.
22. **Baxter-Jones, A. D.** Growth and development of young athletes. Should competition levels be age related? *Sports Medicine* 1995; **20** 59–64.
23. **Krivickas, L.** Anatomical factors associated with overuse sports injuries. *Sports Medicine,* 1997; **24**: 132–146.
24. **Lysens, R., Steverlynck, A., van den.** and **Auweele, Y.,** *et al.:* The accident-prone and overuse-prone profiles of the young athlete. *American Journal of Sports Medicine* 1989; **17**: 612–19.
25. **Maffulli, N.** Intensive training in young athlete. The orthopaedic surgeon's viewpoint. *Sports Medicine,* 1990; **9**: 229–43.

26. **Stanitski, C. L.** Common injuries in preadolescent and adolescent athletes. Recommendations for prevention. *Sports Medicine* 1989; **7**: 32–41.

27. **Crompton, B.** and **Tubbs, N.** A survey of sports injuries in Birmingham. *British Journal of Sports Medicine* 1977; **11**: 12–5.

28. **Zaricznyj, B., Shattuck, L. J. M., Mast, T. A., Robertson, R. V.** and **D'Elia, G.** Sports-related injuries in school aged children. *American Journal of Sports Medicine* 1980; **8**: 3318–24.

29. **Sahlin, Y.** Sport accidents in childhood. *British Journal of Sports Medicine* 1990; **24**: 40–4.

30. **Tursz, A** and **Crost, M.** Sports-related injuries in children a study of their characteristics, frequency, and severity, with comparison to other types of accidental injuries. *American Journal of Sports Medicine* 1986; **14**: 295–9

31. **Baxter-Jones, A., Maffulli, N.** and **Helms, P.** Low injury rates in elite athletics. *Archives of Diseases in Childhood* 1993; **68**: 130–2.

32. **Cotta, H.** and **Steinbrück, K.** *Sportverletzungen und Sportschäden im Breitensport.* Kongreßband Deutscher-Sportärzte-Kongreß Köln 1982; 703–10.

33. **Steinbrück, K.** Analyse einer Sportorthopädischen Ambulanz In *Stellenwert der Sportmedizin in Medizin und Sportwissenschaft* (ed. D. Jeschke). Springer, Berlin, 1984; S 415–20.

34. **Axe, M. J., Newcomb, W. A.** and **Warner, D.** Sports injuries and adolescent athletes. *Delaware Medical Journal* 1991; **63**: 359–63.

35. **DeHaven, K. E.** and **Lintner, D. M.** Athletic injuries Comparison by age, sport and gender. *American Journal of Sports Medicine* 1986; **14**: 218–24

36. **Ekstrand, J.** and **Gillquist, J.** Soccer injuries and their mechanisms a prospective study. *Medicine and Science in Sports and Exercise* 1983; **15**: 267–70

37. **Hale, R. W.** and **Mitchell, W.** Football injuries in Hawaii *Hawaii Medical Journal* 1979, 1981; **40**.

38. **Pritchett, J. W.** A statistical study of knee injuries due to football in high school athletes. *Journal of Bone and Joint Surgery* 1982; **64A**: 240–2.

39. **Lindner, K. J.** and **Caine, D. J.** Injury patterns of female competitive club gymnasts. *Canadian Journal Sport Sciences* 1990; **15**: 254–61.

40. **Hutchinson, M. R., LaPrade, R. F.** and **Burnett, Q. M.,** *et al.*: Injury [surveillance] at the USTA Boy's Tennis Championships a 6 year study. *Medicine and Science in Sports and Exercise* 1995; **27**: 826–30.

41. **Ungerholm, S., Gierup, J., Lindsjo, U.** and **Magnusson, A.** Skiing injuries in children and adults lower leg fractures. *International Journal of Sports Medicine* 1985; **6**: 292–97.

42. **O'Neill, D. B.** and **Micheli, L. J.** Overuse Injuries in the young athlete. *Clinics in Sports Medicine* 1988; **7**(3): 591–610.

43. **Dalton, S. E.** Overuse injuries in adolescent athletes. *Sports Medicine* 1992; **13**: 58–70.

44. **Micheli, L. J.** and **Fehland, A. F. Jr** Overuse injuries to tendons and apophyses in children and adolescents. *Clinics in Sports Medicine* 1992; **11**: 713–26.

45. **Larkins, P. A.** The little athlete. *Australian Family Physician* 1991; **20**: 973–8.

46. **Twellaar, M., Verstappen, F. T. J., Huson, A.** and **van Mechelen, W.** Physical characteristics as risk factors for sport injuries A four year prospective study. *International Journal of Sports Medicine* 1997; **18**: 66–71.

47. **Lysens, R., Steverlynck, A., van den Auweele, Y.,** *et al.* The predictability of sports injuries. *Sports Medicine* 1984; **1**: 6–10.

48. **Bernhardt, D. T.** and **Landry, G. L.** Sport injuries in young athletes. *Advances in Pediatrics* 1995; Mosby-Year Book.

49. **Barrett, J. R., Tanji, J. L., Drake, C., Fuller, D., Kawasaki, R. I.** and **Fenton, R. M.** High- versus low-top shoes for the prevention of ankle sprains in basketball players. A prospective randomized study. *American Journal of Sports Medicine* 1993; **21**: 582–5.

50. **Blue, J. M.** and **Matthews, L. S.** Leg injuries. *Clinics in Sports Medicine* 1997; **16**: 467–78.

51. **Stanish, W. D.** and **Curwin, S.** Tendonitis. Its etiology and treatment. Collamore Press, D.C. Health and Company, Lexington, MA, 1984.

52. **Santopietro, F. J.** Foot and foot-related injuries in the young athlete. *Clinics in Sports Medicine* 1988; **7**: 563–89.

53. **Kellenberger, R.** and **von Laer, L.** Nonosseous lesions of the anterior cruciate ligaments in children and adolescents. *Progresses in Pediatric Surgery* 1990; **25**: 123–132.

54. **Bradley, G. W., Shives, T. C.** and **Samuelson, R. M:** Ligament injuries in the knees of children. *Journal of Bone and Joint Surgery (American Volume)* 1979; **61**: 588–91.

55. **McCarroll, J. R., Shelbourne, K. D., Porter, D. A., Rettig, A. C.** and **Murray, S.** Patellar tendon graft reconstruction for midsubstance anterior cruciate ligament rupture in junior high school athletes. *American Journal of Sports Medicine* 1994; **22**: 478–84.

56. **Nottage, W. M.** and **Matsuura, P. A:** Management of complete traumatic anterior cruciate ligament tears in the skeletally immature patient. Current concepts and review of the literature. *Arthroscopy* 1994; **10**: 569–73.

57. **McCarroll, J. R., Rettig, A. C.** and **Shelbourne, K. D:** Anterior cruciate ligament injuries in the young athlete with open physes. *American Journal of Sports Medicine* 1988; **16**: 44–7.

58. **Parker, A. W., Drez, D.** and **Cooper, J. L:** Anterior cruciate ligament injuries in patients with open physes. *American Journal of Sports Medicine* 1994; **22**: 44–7.

59. **Lo, I. K. Y., Kirkley, A., Fowler, P. J.** and **Miniaci, A:** The outcome of operatively treated anterior cruciate ligament disruptions in the skeletally immature child. *Arthroscopy* 1997; **13**: 627–34.

60. **Lipscomb, A. B.** and **Anderson, A. F:** Tears of the anterior cruciate ligament in adolescents. *Journal of Bone and Joint Surgery (American Volume)* 1986; **68**: 19–28.

61. **Andrews, M., Noyes, F. R.** and **Barber-Westin, S. D:** Anterior cruciate ligament allograft reconstruction in the skeletally immature athlete. *American Journal of Sports Medicine* 1994; **22**: 48–54.

62. **Waters, P. M.** and **Millis, M. B:** Hip and pelvic injuries in the young athlete. *Clinics in Sports Medicine* 1988; **7**: 513–25.

63. **Offrieski, C:** Traumatic dislocations of the hip in children. *Journal of Bone and Joint Surgery (British Volume)* 1981; **63**: 194.

64. **Niethard, F. U.** *Kinderorthopädie.* 1997, Thieme, Stuttgart–New York.

65. **Nietosvaara ,Y., Aalto, K.,** and **Kallio, P. E.** Acute patellar dislocation in children Incidence and associated osteochondral fractures. *Journal of Pediatric Orthopaedics* 1994; **14**: 513–5.

66. **Manzione, M., Pizzutillo, P. D., Peoples, A. B.** and **Schweizer, P. A.** Meniscectomy in children. A long term follow-up study. *American Journal of Sports Medicine* 1983; **11**: 111–5.

67. **Zaman, M.** and **Leonard, M. A.** Meniscectomy in children. A study of 59 knees. *Journal of Bone and Joint Surgery (British Volume)* 1978; **60**: 436–7.

68. **Buckley, S. L.** Sports injuries in children. *Current Opinion in Pediatrics* 1994; **6**: 80–4.

69. **Stanitski, C. L., Harvell, J. C.** and **Fu, F.** Observations on acute knee hemarthrosis in children and adolescents. *Journal of Pediatric Orthopaedics* 1993; **13**: 506–10.

70. **Marshall, J. L.** and **Tischler, H. M.** Screening for sports. *New York Journal of Medicine* 1981; **9**: 68–75.

71. **Coughlin, M.** and **Mann, R.** The pathophysiology of the juvenile bunion. In *Instructional Course Lectures* (ed. P. Griffin) 1987; **26**: 123–36.

72. **Griffin, L. Y.** Common sports injuries of the foot and ankle seen in children and adolescents. *Orthopedic Clinics of North America* 1994; **25**: 83–93.

73. **Salter, R. B.** and **Harris, W. R.** Injuries involving the epiphyseal plate. *Journal of Bone and Joint Surgery (American Volume)* 1963; **45**: 587–622.

74. **Kling, T., Bright, R.** and **Hensinger, R.** Distal tibial physeal fractures in children that may require open reduction. *Journal of Bone and Joint Surgery (American Volume)* 1984; **66**: 647–657.

75. **Ogden, J. A.** *Skeletal injury in the child.* Lea & Febiger, Philadelphia, 1982.

76. **Gregg, J.** and **Das, M.** Foot and ankle problems in the preadolescent and adolescent athlete. *Clinical Sports Medicine* 1982; **1**: 131–47.

77. **Larson, R. L.** Epiphyseal injuries in the adolescent athlete. *Orthopedic Clinics of North America* 1973; **4**: 839–51.

78. **Wolman, R. L., Harries, M. G.** and **Fyfe, I.** Slipped upper femoral epiphysis in an amenorrhoeic athlete. *British Medical Journal* 1989; **299**: 720–721.

79. **Weinstein, S. L., Morrissy, R. T.** and **Crawford, A. H.** Slipped capital femoral epiphysis. In *AAOS Instructional Course Lectures*, 1984; Vol. 33. Mosby, St. Louis.

80. **Albiñana, J.** Pediatric orthopedic problems in lower limbs. *Current Opinion in Orthopedics* 1997; **8**, IV: 10–15.

81. **England, S. P., Sundberg, S.** Management of common pediatric fractures. *Pediatric Clinics of North America* 1996; **43**: 991–1012.

82. **Beaty, J. H., Austin, S. M., Warner, W. C., Canole, S. T.** and **Nichols, L.** Interlocking intramedullary nailing of femoral shaft fractures in adolescents. Preliminary results and complications. *Journal of Pediatric Orthopaedics* 1994; **14**: 178–83.

83. **O'Malley, D. E., Mazur, J. M.** and **Cummings, R. J.** Femoral head avascular necrosis associated with femoral nailing in an adolescent. *Journal of Pediatric Orthopaedics* 1995; **15**: 21–30.

84. **Siegmeth, A., Wruhs, O.** and **Vécsei, V.** External fixation of lower limb fractures in children. *Europaen Journal of Pediatric Surgery* 1998; **8**: 35–41.

85. **Stanitski, C. L.** and **Micheli, L. J.** Observations on symptomatic medial ossification centers. *Journal of Pediatric Orthopaedics* 1993; **13**: 164–8.

86. **Erl, J. P., Barrack, R. L.** and **Alexander, A. H.** Triplane fracture of the distal tibial epiphysis. Long term follow up. *Journal of Bone and Joint Surgery (American Volume)* 1988; **70**: 967–76.

87. **Binek, R., Levisohn, E., Bersani, F.,** *et al.* Freiberg disease complicating unrelated trauma. *Orthopedics* 1988; **11**: 753–7.

88. **Sproul, J., Klaaren, H.** and **Mannarino, F.** Surgical treatment of Freiberg's infarction in athletes. *American Journal of Sports Medicine* 1993; **21**: 381–4.

89. **Gauthier, G.** and **Elbaz, R.** Freiberg's infarction A subchondral bone fatigue fracture. A new surgical treatment. *Clinical Orthopaedics and Related Research* 1979; **142**: 93–5.

90. **Ippolito, E., Ricciari-Pollini, P.** and **Falez, F.** Köhler's disease of the tarsal navicular Long-term follow-up of 12 cases. *Journal of Pediatric Orthopaedics* 1984; **4**: 416–7.

91. **Williams, G.** and **Cowell, H.** Köhler's disease of the tarsal navicular. *Clinical Orthopaedics and Related Research* 1981; **158**: 53–8.

92. **Inoue, G., Kuboyama, K.** and **Shido, T.** Avulsion fractures of the proximal tibial epiphysis. *British Journal of Sports Medicine* 1991; **25**: 52–56.

93. **Lehman, R., Gregg, J.** and **Torg, E.** Iselin's disease. *American Journal of Sports Medicine* 1986; **14**: 494–6.

94. **Aichroth, P.** Osteochondritis dissecans of the knee a clinical study. *Journal of Bone and Joint Surgery (British Volume)* 1971; **53**: 440–7.

95. **Canale, S.** and **Belding, R.** Osteochondral lesions of the talus. *Journal of Bone and Joint Surgery* 1980; **62A**: 97–102.

96. **Twyman, R. S., Desai, K.** and **Aicroth, P. M.** Osteochondritis dissecans of the knee a long term study. *Journal of Bone and Joint Surgery (British Volume)* 1991; **53**: 440–7.

97. **Berndt, A.** and **Harty, M.** Transchondral fractures (osteochondritis dissecans) of the talus. *Journal of Bone and Joint Surgery* 1959; **41A**: 988–1020.

98. **Anderson, A. F.** and **Pagnani, M. J.** Osteochondritis dissecans of the femoral condyles. Long term results of excision of the fragment. *American Journal of Sports Medicine* 1997; **25**: 830–34.

99. **Sallis, R. E.** and **Jones, K.** Stress fractures in athletes. How to spot this under diagnosed injury. *Postgraduate Medicine* 1991; **89**: 185–92.

100. **Riel, K. A.** and **Bernett, P.** Fatigue fractures in sports. Personal experiences and literature review. *Zeitschrift für Orthopädie und ihre Grenzgebiete* 1991; **129**: 471–6.

101. **Martens, R.** *Joy and sadness in children's sports.* Human Kinetics Publishing, Champaign, Illinois, 1978.

102. **Jones, B. H., Bovee, M. W., Harris, J. M.,** *et al.* Intrinsic factors for exercise-related injuries among male and female Army trainees. *American Journal of Sports Medicine* 1993; **21**: 705–10

103. **Barrow, G.** and **Saha, S.** Menstrual irregularities and stress fractures in female collegiate distance runners. *American Journal of Sports Medicine* 1988; **16**: 209–10.

104. **Walker, R. N., Green, N. E.** and **Spindler, K. P.** Stress fractures in skeletally immature patients. *Journal of Pediatric Orthopaedics* 1996; **16**: 578–84.

105. **Beals, R. K.** and **Cook, R. D.** Stress fractures of the anterior tibial diaphysis. Orthopaedic aspects. *Schweizer Zeitschrift für Sportmedizin* 1991; **40**: 869–75.

106. **Matheson, G. O., Clement, D. B., McKenzie, D. C.,** *et al.* Stress fractures in athletes a study of 320 cases. *American Journal of Sports Medicine* 1987; **15**: 46–58.

107. **Torg, J. S., Pavlov, H.** and **Torg, E.** Overuse injuries in sport the foot. *Clinics in Sports Medicine* 1987; **6**: 291–320.

108. **Kiss, Z. S., Khan, K. M.** and **Fuller, P. J.** Stress fractures of the tarsal navicular bone. CT findings in 55 cases. *American Journal of Radiology* 1993; **160**: 111–115.

109. **Khan, K. M., Fuller, P. J.** and **Bruckner, P. D.,** *et al.* Outcome of conservative and surgical management of navicular stress fractures in athletes. Eighty-six cases proven with computerized tomography. *American Journal of Sports Medicine* 1992; **20**: 657–66.

110. **Rosen, P. R., Micheli, L. J.** and **Treves, S.** Early scintigraphic diagnosis of bone stress and fractures in athletic adolescents. *Pediatrics* 1982; **70**: 11–15.

111. **Quain, S.** and **Catterall, A.** Hinge abduction of the hip diagnosis and treatment. *Journal of Bone and Joint Surgery (British Volume)* 1986; **68**: 61–4.

112. **Galasko, C. S. B.** *Imaging techniques in orthopaedics.* Springer-Verlag, London, 1984; 345–362.

113. **Henderson, R. C., Renner, J. B., Sturdivant, M. C.,** *et al.* Evaluation of magnetic resonance imaging in Legg-Perthes disease. A prospective blinded study. *Journal of Pediatric Orthopaedics* 1990; **10**: 289–97.

114. **Evans, I. K., De Luca, P. A.** and **Gage, J. R.** A comparative study of ambulation-abduction bracing and varus derotation osteotomy in the treatment of severe Legg-Calve-Perthes disease in children over 6 years of age. *Journal of Pediatric Orthopaedics* 1986; **6**: 600–4.

115. **Harris, R. I.** and **Beath, T.** Etiology of peroneal spatic flat foot. *Journal of Bone and Joint Surgery (Britsh Volume)* 1948; **30**: 624.

116. **O'Neill, D. B.** and **Micheli, L. J.** Tarsal coalition. *American Journal of Sports Medicine* 1989; **17**(4): 544–9.

117. **Ostrum, G. A.** Sports-related injuries in youth Prevention is the key-and nurses can help! *Pediatric Nursing* 1993; **19**: 333–42.

118. **Bixler, B.** and **Jones, R. L.** High school football injuries Effects of a post-halftime warm-up and stretching routine. *Family Practice in Research Journal* 1992; **12**: 131–9

119. **Brody, T. A.** Weight training related injuries. *American Journal of Sports Medicine* 1982; **10**: 1–5.

120. **Sewall, B. S.** and **Micheli, L. J.** Strength training for children. *Journal of Pediatric Orthopaedics* 1986; **6**: 143–6.

121. **van Mechelen, W., Hlobil, H.** and **Kemper, H. C. G.** Incidence, severity, aetiology and prevention of sports injuries a review of concepts. *Sports Medicine* 1992; **14**: 82–89.

122. **Rowley, S.** Psychological effects of intensive training in young athletes. *Journal of Child Psychology and Psychiatry* 1987; **28**: 371–77.

123. **Mueller, F.** and **Blyth, C.** Epidemiology of sports injuries in children. *Clinics in Sports Medicine* 1982; **1**: 343–52.

5.7 Injuries to the head and cervical spine
Robert C. Cantu

Introduction

The head and cervical spine are unique in that their contents, the brain and spinal cord, are largely incapable of regeneration. Thus, injury to the head and neck takes on a singular importance. Today, many parts of the body can be replaced, either by artificial hardware or transplanted parts; however, the head and spine are not included because their contents cannot be transplanted. Furthermore, injuries to the head and neck are the most frequent catastrophic athletic injury.[1,2]

With these sobering facts in mind the following list contains the most hazardous sports for the head and cervical spine.

1. Auto racing
2. Boxing
3. Cheerleading
4. Cycling
5. Diving
6. Equestrian sports
7. Football
8. Gymnastics
9. Hang gliding
10. Ice hockey
11. Lacrosse
12. Martial arts
13. Motorcycling
14. Parachute
15. Rugby
16. Skating/rollerblading
17. Skiing
18. Sky diving
19. Soccer (goalie)
20. Track (pole vaulting)
21. Trampolining
22. Wrestling

According to statistics from the National Center for Catastrophic Sports Injury Research, the four common school sports with the highest risk of head and cervical spine injury per 100 000 participants are American football, gymnastics, ice hockey and wrestling. There is no statistically significant difference between the four on an incidence per 100 000 participant basis. Because 1 500 000 youths play American football yearly and under 100 000 participate in each of the other sports, the absolute numbers of severe head and spine injuries each year are naturally highest in football. In the USA, the incidence of catastrophic head and spine injury per 100 000 participants is even higher in the activity of cheerleading.

Two other sports have a position or event at high risk of head and spine injury while the overall risks for the sport is low. Soccer goalie is a high-risk position, as is the pole vaulting event in track and field. Additional unsupervised recreational sports, including skiing, skating and equestrian sports, have reports of catastrophic head and neck injuries, but statistics on relative rate of injury are not available.

When considering serious head and spine injury in organized sports, it is important to realize this risk increases with age. American football is an excellent example of this risk. There is virtually no death or quadriplegia at the Pop Warner level, but the risk steadily rises in junior high, then high school, then college, and finally is highest by far at the professional level. This is because at young ages the weight and speed and, thus, the force of impact is low compared with skeletally mature participants.

It is interesting to note that at very young ages (5–14 years of age) the sport of baseball has the highest fatality rate of any youth sport with the least amount of safety equipment mandated. In June 1984, the Consumer Product Safety Commission (CPSC) published a Hazard Analysis on youth baseball injuries and reported that during the years 1973 to 1983 there were 51 baseball-related deaths to children 5 to 14 years of age. In addition the CPSC found that approximately seven out of every 1000 participants in this age group received emergency treatment for injuries. The leading cause of both injury and death is impact with the ball to the chest or head.

Health professionals responsible for the care of athletes who may sustain head and neck trauma should make certain organizational decisions before the season begins. First, a 'captain' of the medical team responsible for supervising on-the-field management of the injured athlete should be designated. Although this will usually be the team physician, in certain localities it may be the athletic trainer or an emergency medical technician. Second, all necessary emergency equipment for the head- or spine-injured athlete should be on the sidelines. At a bare minimum this would include equipment for the initiation and maintenance of cardiopulmonary resuscitation (CPR).

Types of head injury

The differential diagnosis with a head injury includes a cerebral concussion, the second impact syndrome or malignant brain oedema syndrome, intracranial haemorrhage and post-concussion syndrome.

Intracranial haemorrhage

The leading cause of death from athletic head injury is intracranial haemorrhage. There are four types of haemorrhage of which the examining trainer or physician must be aware in every head injury. Because all four types of intracranial haemorrhage may be fatal, rapid and accurate initial assessment as well as appropriate follow-up is mandatory after an athletic head injury.

Epidural haematoma

An epidural or extradural haematoma is usually the most rapidly progressing intracranial haematoma. It is frequently associated with a fracture of the temporal bone and results from a tear of the artery supplying the covering (dura) of the brain. This haematoma accumulates inside the skull but outside the covering of the brain. Arising from a torn artery, it may progress quite rapidly and reach a fatal size in 30 to 60 minutes. Although this does not always occur, the athlete may have a lucid interval. Thus, the athlete may remain conscious initially or regain consciousness after the head trauma and before experiencing an increasing headache and a progressively deteriorating consciousness level. This occurs as the clot accumulates and the intracranial pressure increases. This lesion, if present, will almost always declare itself within an hour or two of the time of injury. Usually the brain substance is free from direct injury; thus, if the clot is promptly removed surgically, full recovery is to be expected. Because this lesion is rapidly and universally fatal if missed, all athletes receiving a major head injury must be very closely and frequently observed during the ensuing several hours, preferably the next 24 hours. This observation should be done at a facility where full neurosurgical services are available immediately.

Subdural haematoma

A subdural haematoma occurs between the brain surface and the dura, and so is located under the dura and directly on the brain. Subdural haematoma often results from a torn vein running from the surface of the brain to the dura. It may also result from a torn venous sinus or even a small artery on the surface of the brain. With this injury, there often is associated injury to the brain tissue. If a subdural haematoma necessitates surgery in the first 24 hours, the mortality rate is high owing not to the clot itself, but to the associated brain damage. With a subdural haematoma that progresses rapidly, the athlete usually does not regain consciousness and the need for immediate neurosurgical evaluation is obvious. This is the most common fatal athletic head injury. Occasionally, the brain itself will not be injured, and a subdural haematoma may develop slowly over a period of days to weeks. This chronic subdural haematoma, although often associated with headache, may initially cause a variety of very mild, almost imperceptible mental, motor or sensory signs and symptoms. Because its recognition and removal will lead to full recovery, it must always be suspected in an athlete who has previously sustained a head injury and who, days or weeks later, is 'not quite right.' A computerized axial tomography (CAT) scan of the head will definitely show such a lesion.

Intracerebral haematoma

An intracerebral haematoma is the third type of intracranial haemorrhage seen after head trauma. In this instance, the bleeding is into the brain substance itself, usually from a torn artery. It also may result from the rupture of a congenital vascular lesion such as an aneurysm or arteriovenous malformation. Intracerebral haematomas are not usually associated with a lucid interval and may be rapidly progressive. Death occasionally occurs before the injured athlete can be moved to a hospital. Because of the intense reaction such a tragic event precipitates among fellow athletes, family, students, and even the community at large, and because of the inevitable rumours that follow, it is imperative to obtain a complete autopsy in such an event to clarify fully the causative factors. Often the autopsy will reveal a congenital lesion, which may indicate that the cause of death was other than presumed and ultimately unavoidable. Only by such full, factual elucidation will appropriate feelings of guilt in fellow athletes, friends and family be assuaged.

Subarachnoid haemorrhage

A fourth type of intracranial haemorrhage is subarachnoid, confined to the surface of the brain. Following head trauma, such bleeding is the result of disruption of the tiny surface brain vessels and is analogous to a bruise. As with the intracerebral haematoma, there is often brain swelling, and such a haemorrhage also can result from a ruptured cerebral aneurysm or arteriovenous malformation. Because bleeding is superficial, surgery is not usually required unless a congenital vascular anomaly is present.

Such a contusion of the brain usually causes headache and, not infrequently, an associated neurologic deficit, depending on the area of the brain involved. The irritative properties of the blood may also precipitate a seizure. If a seizure occurs in a head-injured athlete, it is important to logroll the patient onto his side. By this manoeuvre, any blood or saliva will roll out of the mouth or nose and the tongue cannot fall back, obstructing the airway. If one has a padded tongue depressor or oral airway, it can be inserted between the teeth. Under no circumstances should one insert one's fingers into the mouth of an athlete who is having a seizure, as a traumatic amputation can easily result from such an unwise manoeuvre. Usually such a traumatic seizure will last only for a minute or two. The athlete will then relax, and transportation to the nearest medical facility can be effected.

Following any of the four types of intracranial haemorrhage, prophylactic anticonvulsant therapy with phenytoin is usually given for 1 year. Because the chance of post-traumatic epilepsy is less than 10% with a concussion or contusion, anticonvulsant therapy is given in these conditions only if late epilepsy actually occurs.[3]

Concussion

Concussion is derived from the Latin *concussus* which means 'to shake violently'. Initially it was thought to produce only a temporary disturbance of brain function due to neuronal, chemical or neuroelectrical changes without gross structural damage. We now know that structural damage with loss of brain cells does occur with some concussions. The most common athletic head injury is concussion, with one in five high school American football players suffering one annually.[4] Furthermore, the risk of sustaining a concussion in football is four[4] to six[5] times greater for the player who has sustained a previous concussion. It can occur with direct head trauma in collisions or falls, or may occur without a direct blow to the head when sufficient force is applied to the brain, as in a whiplash injury.[6]

The rates of concussion in some popular sports are listed in Tables 5.7.1 and 5.7.2.[7] Earlier estimates of concussion in American football at all levels put the number at 250 000 per year in the US alone.[8] This number was based on a single survey that found that 20% of high school American football players had sustained some form of concussion[4] and 10% of the college football players sustained concussion in another study.[9]

Current estimates of the incidence of concussion in American football at all levels suggest that about 100 000 per year may be more accurate (personal communication, Powell J, Medical Sports Systems, Iowa City, Iowa, conducting ongoing surveillance of concussion incidence

Table 5.7.1 Sports with helmets

Sport	Rate of concussions per 1000 athlete-exposures[7]
Ice hockey	0.27
Football	0.25
Men's lacrosse	0.19
Women's softball	0.11

Table 5.7.2 Sports with helmets

Sport	Rate of concussions per 1000 athlete-exposures[7]
Men's soccer	0.25
Women's soccer	0.24
Field hockey	0.20
Wrestling	0.20

Table 5.7.3 Severity of concussion

Grade	Feature	Duration of feature
Grade 1 (mild)	PTA	<30 minutes
	LOC	None
Grade 2 (moderate)	PTA	>30 minutes, <24 hours
	LOC	<5 minutes
Grade 3 (severe)	PTA	>24 hours
	LOC	>5 minutes

PTA, post-traumatic amnesia; LOC, loss of consciousness.

Table 5.7.4 Dementia pugilistica: areas of brain damage and resultant deficit

Deficit	Area
1. Abnormalities of the septum pellucidum and the adjacent periventricular grey matter	Altered affect and memory
2. Cerebellar scarring and nerve cell loss	Slurred speech, loss of balance and coordination
3. Degeneration of the substantia nigra	Tremor
4. The regional occurrence of neurofibrillary tangles	Loss of intellect

in NCAA football). No matter whose estimates are used, the dimension of this problem warrants more attention than it has received thus far.

It must be realized that universal agreement on the definition and grading of concussion does not exist.[10–12] This renders the evaluation of epidemiological data extremely difficult. As a neurosurgeon and team physician, I have evaluated many football players who suffered concussion. Most of these injuries were mild and were associated with retrograde amnesia, which is helpful in making the diagnosis, especially in mild cases. I have developed a practical scheme for grading the severity of a concussion based on the duration of unconsciousness and/or post-traumatic amnesia (Table 5.7.3).[1]

The most mild concussion (grade 1) occurs without loss of consciousness and the only neurological deficit is a brief period of confusion or post-traumatic amnesia, by definition lasting less than 30 minutes.

With the moderate (grade 2) concussion there is usually a brief period of unconsciousness, by definition not exceeding five minutes. Less commonly, there is no loss of consciousness but only a protracted period of post-traumatic amnesia lasting over 30 minutes but less than 24 hours.

Severe (grade 3) concussion occurs with a more protracted period of unconsciousness lasting over five minutes. Rarely, it may occur with a shorter period of unconsciousness, but with a very protracted period of post-traumatic amnesia lasting over 24 hours.

In 1991, Kelly *et al.*[10] proposed another guideline regarding the severity of concussion in which the most mild concussion (grade 1) had no loss of consciousness and no post-traumatic amnesia, but rather just a brief period of disorientation or confusion. A grade 2 or moderate concussion was one in which there was no loss of consciousness but post-traumatic amnesia was present. In their guidelines all athletes rendered unconscious were placed in the grade 3, or severe, category. While it can be debated that post-traumatic amnesia of over 24 hours may reflect a more severe brain insult than 30 seconds of unconsciousness, both guidelines will prevent the second impact syndrome, as no athlete still symptomatic from a prior head injury is allowed to return to competition.

Today it is recognized that after concussion the ability to process information may be reduced,[13] and the functional impairment may be greater with repeated concussions.[13,14] Furthermore, these studies suggest that the damaging effects of concussion are cumulative. In proportion to the degree to which the motion of the head is accelerated and to which these forces are imparted to the brain, concussion may produce a shearing injury to nerve fibres and neurons.

The late effects of repeated head trauma of concussive or even subconcussive force leads to anatomical patterns of chronic brain injury with correlating signs and symptoms. Martland[15] first introduced the term 'punch drunk' (dementia pugilistica) in 1928. Although first described in boxers, this traumatic encephalopathy may occur in anyone subjected to repeated blows to the head from any cause.

The characteristic symptoms and signs of the punch drunk state (Table 5.7.4) include the gradual appearance of a fatuous or euphoric dementia with emotional lability, the victim displaying little insight into his deterioration. Speech and thought become progressively slower. Memory deteriorates considerably. There may be mood swings, intense irritability, and sometimes truculence leading to uninhibited violent behaviour. Simple fatuous cheerfulness is, however, the most common prevailing mood, though sometime there is depression with paranoia. From the clinical standpoint, the neurologist may encounter almost any combination of pyramidal, extrapyramidal and cerebellar signs. Tremor and dysarthria are two of the most common findings.

Corsellis *et al.*[16] described the necropsy findings in the brains of men who had been boxers. They described a characteristic pattern of cerebral change that appeared not only to be the result of boxing but also to underlie many features of the punch drunk syndrome. They documented changes in the middle of the brain, which may shear into two layers or even be shredded by the distortions that follow blows to the head. They found destruction of the limbic system, a portion of the brain that governs emotion and has a role in memory and learning. There was a characteristic loss of cells from the cerebellum, a part of the brain that governs balance and coordination. Finally, there was an unusual microscopic change widespread throughout the brain resembling changes that occur with Alzheimer disease, which causes progressive loss of intelligence, but sufficiently different (neurofibrillary tangles only and no senile plaques) to be regarded as a distinct entity, unique to subjects suffering from blows to the head.

Postconcussion symptoms

A second late effect of concussion is the postconcussion syndrome. This syndrome—consisting of headache (especially with exertion), dizziness, fatigue, irritability, and especially impaired memory and concentration—has been reported in football players, but its true incidence is not known. In my experience it is uncommon. The persistence of these symptoms reflect altered neurotransmitter function and usually correlate with the duration of post-traumatic amnesia.[17] When these symptoms persist, the athlete should be evaluated with a computed tomography (CT) scan and neuropsychiatric tests. Return to competition should be deferred until all symptoms have abated and the diagnostic studies are normal.

Malignant brain oedema syndrome

This condition is found in athletes in the paediatric age range and consists of rapid neurological deterioration from an alert conscious state to coma and sometimes death, minutes to several hours after the head trauma.[18,19] Although this sequence in adults almost always is due to an intracranial clot, in children, pathology studies show diffuse brain swelling with little or no brain injury.[19] Rather than true cerebral oedema, Langfitt and colleagues[20,21] have shown that the diffuse cerebral swelling is the result of a true hyperaemia or vascular engorgement. Prompt recognition is extremely important because there is little initial brain injury and the serious or fatal neurological outcome is secondary to raised intracranial pressure with herniation. Prompt treatment with intubation, hyperventilation and osmotic agents has helped to reduce mortality.[22,23]

Second impact syndrome

Recognizing the syndrome

What Saunders and Harbaugh called 'the second impact syndrome of catastrophic head injury' in 1984[24] was first described by Schneider in 1973.[25] The syndrome occurs when an athlete who sustains a head injury—often a concussion or worse injury, such as a cerebral contusion—sustains a second head injury before symptoms associated with the first have cleared.[26–28]

Typically, the athlete suffers postconcussional symptoms after the first head injury. These may include visual, motor or sensory changes and difficulty with thought and memory processes. Before these symptoms resolve—which may take days or weeks—the athlete returns to competition and receives a second blow to the head. The second blow may be remarkably minor, perhaps only involving a blow to the chest that jerks the athlete's head and indirectly imparts accelerative forces to the brain. Affected athletes may appear stunned but usually do not lose consciousness and often complete the play. They usually remain on their feet for 15 seconds to a minute or so but seem dazed, like someone suffering from a grade 1 concussion without loss of consciousness. Often, affected athletes remain on the playing field or walk off under their own power.

What happens in the next 15 seconds to several minutes sets this syndrome apart from a concussion or even a subdural haematoma. Usually within seconds to minutes of the second impact, the athlete—conscious yet stunned—quite precipitously collapses to the ground, semicomatose with rapidly dilating pupils, loss of eye movement and evidence of respiratory failure.

The pathophysiology of second impact syndrome is thought to involve a loss of autoregulation of the brain's blood supply. This loss of autoregulation leads to vascular engorgement within the cranium, which in turn markedly increases intracranial pressure and leads to herniation either of the medial surface (uncus) of the temporal lobe or

lobes below the tentorium or of the cerebellar tonsils through the foramen magnum. Animal research has shown that vascular engorgement of the brain after a mild head injury is difficult if not impossible to control.[29,30] The usual time from second impact to brainstem failure is rapid, taking two to five minutes. Once brain herniation and brainstem compromise occur, ocular involvement and respiratory failure precipitously ensue. Demise occurs far more rapidly than usually seen with an epidural haematoma.

Magnetic resonance imaging (MRI) and CT scan are the neuroimaging studies most likely to demonstrate the second impact syndrome. While MRI is the more sensitive to traumatic brain injuries, especially true oedema,[31,32] the CT scan is usually adequate to show bleeding of midline shifts of the brain requiring neurosurgical intervention. This is important because CT scanning is cheaper, more widely available, and more quickly performed than MRI.

Incidence

While the precise incidence per 100 000 participants is not known, because the precise population at risk is unknown, nonetheless, second impact syndrome is more common than previous reports have suggested. Between 1980 and 1993, the National Center for Catastrophic Sports Injury Research in Chapel Hill, North Carolina, identified 35 probable cases among American football players alone. Necropsy or surgery and MRI findings confirmed 17 of these cases. An additional 18 cases, though not conclusively documented with necropsy findings, most probably are cases of second impact syndrome. Careful scrutiny excluded this diagnosis in 22 of 57 cases originally suspected.[26]

Second impact syndrome is not confined to American football players. Head injury reports of athletes in other sports almost certainly represent the syndrome but do not label it as such. Fekete, for example, described a 16 year old high school hockey player who fell during a game, striking the back of his head on the ice.[33] The boy lost consciousness and afterward complained of unsteadiness and headaches. While playing in the next game four days later, he was checked forcibly and again fell striking his left temple on the ice. His pupils rapidly became fixed and dilated, and he died within two hours while in transit to a neurosurgical facility. Necropsy revealed contusion of several days' duration, an oedematous brain with a thin layer of subdural and subarachnoid haemorrhage, and bilateral herniation of the cerebellar tonsils into the foramen magnum. Though Fekete did not use the label 'second impact syndrome', the clinical course and necropsy findings in this case are consistent with the syndrome.

Other cases include an 18 year old male downhill skier described by McQuillen et al.,[28] who remains in a persistent vegetative state, and a 17 year old football player described by Kelly et al. who died.[10] Such cases indicate that the brain is vulnerable to accelerative forces in a variety of contact and collision sports. Therefore, physicians who cover athletic events, especially those in which head trauma is likely, must understand the second impact syndrome and be prepared to initiate emergency treatment.

Prevention is primary

For a catastrophic condition that has a mortality rate approaching 50% and a morbidity rate nearing 100%, prevention takes on the utmost importance. An athlete who is symptomatic from a head injury *must not* participate in contact or collision sports until all cerebral symptoms have subsided, and preferably not for at least one week after.

Whether it takes days, weeks or months to reach the asymptomatic state, the athlete must never be allowed to practice or compete while still suffering postconcussion symptoms.

Players and parents as well as the physician and medical team must understand this. Files of the National Center for Catastrophic Sport Injury Research include cases of young athletes who did not report their cerebral symptoms. Fearing they would not be allowed to compete and not knowing they were jeopardizing their lives, they played with postconcussional symptoms and tragically developed second impact syndrome.

Diffuse axonal injury

This condition results when severe shearing forces are imparted to the brain and axonal connections are literally severed, in the absence of intracranial haematoma. The patient is usually deeply comatose and with a low Glasgow coma scale and a negative head CT. Immediate neurological triage for treatment of increased intracranial pressure is indicated.

Management guidelines

Immediate treatment

With a head injury the ABCs of first aid must be followed. Before a neurological examination is undertaken, the treating physician must determine if the airway is adequate, and that circulation is being maintained. Thereafter attention may be directed to the neurological examination.

Definitive treatment

Definitive treatment of grade 2 and grade 3 concussions, as well as of the second impact syndrome and intracranial haematoma, should take place at a medical facility where neurosurgical and neuroradiological capabilities are present. In the case of the intracranial haematoma, definitive surgical evacuation is indicated, and in cases of closed head injuries and more severe degrees of concussion, observation is appropriate, with careful neurological monitoring.

What tests to order and when

After a grade 1 concussion, observation alone may be all that is indicated. In instances of grade 2 and grade 3 concussion, however, a CT scan or MRI of the brain is recommended. It is recommended that these athletes be removed from the contest and sent to a definitive neurological facility where such imaging can take place upon arrival. In the case of the second impact syndrome and intracranial haemorrhage, urgent scanning with either a CT or MRI is also appropriate.

When to refer

All head injuries other than a grade 1 concussion should be referred for a neurological or neurosurgical evaluation following removal of the athlete from the contest.

When to operate

Closed head injuries such as a concussion and diffuse axonal injury of the brain do not require surgery. However, significant intracranial blood accumulations, whether epidural, subdural or intracerebral, may require prompt surgical evacuation. Congenital vascular anomalies, such as an aneurysm or arterial venous malformation, may require planned deliberate surgical intervention.

Appropriate time course for resolution

Table 5.7.5 provides guidelines for return to competition after a cerebral concussion whether grade 1, grade 2 or grade 3, and whether this was a first, second or third concussion sustained in a given season. I believe it is important to realize that other concussion guidelines exist.[1,10–12] While none are in precise agreement as to the timing of return to sport after the various degrees and numbers of concussions received in a given season, and thus all are truly only guidelines, all do agree on the most salient point—that is, that no athlete still symptomatic from a previous injury should be allowed to risk a second head injury, either by practice or by event participation. Therefore, while the grading and return dates may vary slightly, all the guidelines will prevent the dreaded second impact syndrome. An athlete who has sustained a second impact syndrome and who is in the small minority that survives without significant morbidity would not be allowed to return to a contact or collision sport. So too, an athlete who has undergone surgery for an intracranial haemorrhage would be ill-advised to return to contact or collision sports, as both the surgery and the underlying haemorrhage have caused an alteration of CSF fluid dynamics and the ability of the CSF fluid to protect the brain from subsequent head injury. Other conditions precluding participation in contact sports are in Table 5.7.6.

A final comment on concussions

Following a concussion, a thorough review of the circumstances resulting in the concussion should occur. In my long experience as a team physician, those athletes subjected to repeated concussions were often using their head unwisely, illegally or both. If available, videotapes of the incident should be reviewed by the team physician, trainer, coach and player to see if this was a factor. Equipment should also be checked

Table 5.7.5 Guidelines for return to sports after concussion

Grade	First concussion	Second concussion	Third concussion
Grade 1 (mild)	May return to play if asymptomatic for 1 week.	Return to play in 2 weeks if asymptomatic at that time for 1 week.	Terminate season; may return to play next season if asymptomatic.
Grade 2 (moderate)	Return to play after asymptomatic for 1 week.	Minimum of 1 month; may return to play then if asymptomatic for 1 week; consider terminating season.	Terminate season; may return to play next season if asymptomatic.
Grade 3 (severe)	Minimum of 1 month; may then return to play if asymptomatic.	Terminate season; may return to play next season.	

Table 5.7.6   Conditions that contraindicate competition in contact sports

1. Persistent postconcussion symptoms.
2. Permanent central neurological sequelae from head injury (e.g. organic dementia, hemiplegia, homonymous heminopsia).
3. Hydrocephalus.
4. Spontaneous subarachnoid haemorrhage from any cause.
5. Symptomatic neurological or pain-producing abnormalities about the foramen magnum.

to be certain that it fits precisely, that the athlete is wearing it properly, and that it is being maintained, especially the air pressure in air helmets. Finally, neck strength and development should be assessed.

Types of spine injuries

Fracture, concussion, contusion, haemorrhage

The same traumatic lesions that affect the brain also may occur to the cervical spinal cord, that is, concussion, contusion and the various types of haemorrhage. Unlike the head where subdural haematoma is the most common and lethal haemorrhage, the subdural haematoma is uncommon in the spine. Since I have been associated with the National Center for Catastrophic Sports Injury Research (NCCSIR), there have been no spinal subdural haematomas. Instead the intraspinal (within the cord) is the most common and epidural next most common type of haemorrhage. Also all spinal haemorrhages have been in the cervical region and none have been in the thoracic or lumbar region.

The major concern with a cervical spinal injury is the possibility of an unstable fracture that may produce quadriplegia. In the NCCSIR registry, all cases of quadriplegia in the absence of spinal stenosis resulted from fracture dislocation of the cervical spine. At the time of injury, on the athletic field, there is no way to determine the presence of an unstable fracture. This requires appropriate radiographs to be taken. There also is no way of differentiating between a fully recoverable and a permanent case of quadriplegia. If the patient is fully conscious, a cervical fracture or cervical cord injury is usually accompanied by rigid cervical muscle spasm and pain that immediately alerts the athlete and physician to the presence of such an injury. It is the unconscious athlete, unable to state that his or her neck hurts and that his or her neck muscles are not in protective spasm, who is susceptible to potential cord severance if caregivers are not aware of the possibility of an unstable cervical spine fracture.

With an unconscious or obviously neck-injured athlete, it is imperative that no neck manipulation be carried out on the field. Definitive treatment must await appropriate radiographs at a medical facility. The athlete must be transported with the head and neck immobilized to the medical facility. There a detailed neurologic examination is carried out. If any motor, sensory or reflex abnormalities are noted, the anal sphincter tone and sensation of perineal and sacral areas must be checked. If the neurologic examination is normal, the next step is a lateral cervical spine radiograph. If this is normal, a complete cervical spine series of anterior, posterior, lateral, oblique and flexion–extension views should be obtained. As high as 20% of unstable cervical spine injuries may be missed when the cross table lateral cervical spine radiograph is used alone.[34] In the adolescent, displacement of the second cervical vertebra

over that of the third occurs because of the hypermobility of those segments. Failure to recognize this normal 1 to 2 mm of subluxation variation may lead to unnecessary treatment of this pseudosubluxation.

When there is spinal cord injury documented on the neurologic examination, a lateral cervical spine radiograph is taken on the still neck-immobilized patient. In this instance, oblique and flexion–extension views are not taken for fear of further injuring the spinal cord. Instead, one proceeds to a computed tomography of the cervical spine to define further the extent of the trauma and presence of spinal cord compression by bone, disc or haematoma. A contrast positive cervical computed tomography often is more sensitive in showing spinal cord compression. In those tertiary institutions with an MR scanner, this modality may be used to define especially intraspinal pathology further.

Stingers

Stingers or burners are colloquial terms used by athletes and trainers to describe a set of symptoms that involve pain, burning or tingling down an arm occasionally accompanied by localized weakness. The symptoms typically abate within seconds or minutes, rarely persisting for days or longer. It has been estimated that a stinger will occur at least once during the career of over 50% of athletes.[35]

There are two typical mechanisms by which stingers may occur—traction on the brachial plexus, or nerve root impingement within the cervical neural foramen. The majority of high-school level injuries are of the brachial plexus type, while most at the college level and virtually all in the professional ranks result from a pinch phenomenon within the neural foramen.

The brachial plexus stinger commonly involves a forceful blow to the head from the side but also can result from head extension or shoulder depression while the head and neck are fixed. Nerve root impingement usually occurs when the athlete's head is driven toward his shoulder pad. The dorsal spinal root ganglion lies close to the posterior intervertebral facet joints and is pinched when the neural foramen is compressed.

With either type of stinger the athlete experiences a shock-like sensation of pain and numbness radiating into the arm and hand. The symptoms are typically purely sensory in nature and most commonly involve the C5 and C6 dermatomes. On occasion weakness may also be present. The most common muscles involved include the deltoid, biceps, supraspinatus and infraspinatus.

Stingers are always unilateral and virtually never involve the lower extremities. Thus if symptoms are bilateral or involve the legs, then the burning hands syndrome with all its implications must be considered.

When stingers are not associated with any neck pain or limitation of neck movement and all motor and sensory symptoms clear within seconds to minutes, the athlete may safely return to competition. This is especially true if the athlete has previously experienced similar symptoms. If there are any residual symptoms or complaints of neck pain, return should be deferred pending further work-up.

On rare occasions a stinger may result in prolonged sensory complaints or weakness. In such a situation, an MR imaging of the cervical spine should be considered to look for a herniated disc or other compressive pathology. If symptoms persist for more than two weeks, then electromyography should allow for an accurate assessment of the degree and extent of injury.

Some athletes seem predisposed to develop a series of recurrent stingers. It has been suggested that repeated stinger injuries over many years may lead to a proximal arm weakness and constant pain. Thus if an athlete suffers two or more stingers, particularly in rapid succession, consideration can be given to the use of high shoulder pads supplemented by a soft cervical roll, which should limit lateral neck flexion and extension. Examining or changing the athlete's blocking and tackling techniques or changing the player's position also may be helpful in preventing recurrences. If the stingers repeatedly recur despite these interventions, then cessation of the causative athletic activity may be necessary.

Transient quadriplegia

Transient quadriplegia or bilateral neurologic symptoms after a player takes a hit in a contact sport raises the spectre of spinal cord compromise. In some athletes, spinal stenosis may be a contributing factor. Although radiographic bone measurements can suggest that the problem may be present, physicians are cautioned against making the diagnosis of spinal stenosis with this technique alone. Instead, diagnostic technologies that view the spinal cord itself, especially MR imaging, contrast positive computed tomography or myelography, should be employed. These imaging methods can determine if the spinal cord has a normal functional reserve: the space largely filled with a protective cushion of CSF between the cord and the spinal canal's interior walls lined by bone, disc and ligament. In addition, these techniques also determine whether the nerve tissue is deformed by an abnormality such as disc protrusion, bony osteophyte or posterior buckling of the ligamentum flavum.

Controversy persists as to whether cervical stenosis increases the risk of spinal cord injury. The author believes very strongly that those who have had spinal cord symptoms from sports-related injuries and are shown to have true spinal stenosis on MR imaging should not be allowed to return to contact sports. Although there are no hard data to back up that recommendation, there is a body of literature in the sports medicine, neurology and radiology fields that indicates that spinal stenosis predisposes a patient to spinal cord injury.[30,35–40]

Matsuura and his group,[41] for example, compared the spinal dimensions of 100 controls with those of 42 patients who had spinal cord injuries. They found that the control group had significantly larger sagittal spinal canal diameters than did the patients who had spinal cord injuries. Furthermore, the National Center for Catastrophic Sports Injury Research has no instance of complete neurologic recovery in spinal stenotic athletes with fracture dislocation of the cervical spine, whereas there are a number of such complete recoveries in athletes with normal size spinal canals. There also are several instances of permanent quadriplegia in athletes with tight spinal stenosis without fracture or demonstrated instability. Thus, we are adamant that following spinal cord symptoms, identification of 'functional spinal stenosis' is a contraindication to further participation in contact collision sports.

Increased attention soon may be focused on this question, however, as several professional football teams now require detailed investigations of the cervical and lumbar spine (some including MR imaging) as a prerequisite to the draft process. Presently, there are no good guidelines to help the physician manage an athlete with a narrow asymptomatic cervical spinal canal. When such an abnormality is encountered, management must be individualized according to the patient's symptoms, the degree of canal stenosis and the perceived risk of permanent neurologic injury.

Vascular injury

A final uncommon but very serious neck injury involves the carotid arteries. By either extremes of lateral flexion or extension or a forceful blow by a relatively fixed, narrow object such as a stiffened forearm or a cross-country ski tip impaling one's neck in a forward fall, the inner layer (intima) of the carotid artery may be torn. This can lead to clot formation at the site of injury, resulting in emboli to the brain, or more commonly, a complete occlusion of the artery causing a major stroke. With a fracture dislocation, injury to the vertebral artery may occur leading to a brainstem stroke.

Return to play

It is recommended that an athlete not return to competition after a neck injury until he or she is free of neck or arm pain, has a full range of neck motion without discomfort or spasm, and neck strength in flexion, extension and on each side has returned to pre-injury levels. If a pre-injury profile is unknown, strength should at least be symmetrical. Also lateral neck radiographs should show return of lordotic curvature in the neutral view, and MR imaging should not reveal significant disc disease or functional spinal stenosis.

Because of their participation in the Special Olympics, it is important to realize that as high as 4% of children with Down's syndrome may have abnormalities of the cervical spine.[42] By far the most common abnormality is a subluxation at the atlantoaxial (C1–2) joint followed by atlanto-occipital subluxation.[43] It is recommended that cervical spine stability be assessed in all patients with Down's syndrome who wish to participate in athletic activities, especially those involving the head and neck, such as soccer.

Summary

Injuries to the head and neck are the most frequent catastrophic sports injury, and head injuries are the most common direct athletic cause of death. Although direct compressive forces may injure the brain, neural tissue is particularly susceptible to injury from shearing stresses, which are most likely to occur when rotational forces are applied to the head.

The most common athletic head injury is concussion, which may vary widely in severity. Intracranial haemorrhage is the leading cause of head injury death in sports, making rapid initial assessment and appropriate follow up mandatory after a head injury. Diffuse cerebral swelling is another serious condition that may be found in the child or adolescent athlete, and the second impact syndrome is a major concern in adult athletes.

Many head injuries in athletes are the result of improper playing techniques and can be reduced by teaching proper skills and enforcing safety promoting rules. Improved conditioning (particularly of the neck), protective headgear and careful medical supervision of athletes will also minimize this type of injury.

References

1. **Cantu, R. C.** Guidelines for return to contact sports after a cerebral concussion. *The Physician and Sports Medicine* 1986; **40**: 10–4.

2. **Cantu, R. C.** *The exercising adult, 2nd ed.* McMillan Publishing Co, New York, 1987.

3. **Gruber, R., Bubl, R.** and **Fruttiger, V.** Anticonvulsant prophylaxis after juvenile craniocerebral injuries: a retrospective evaluation. *Zeitschrift fuer Kinderchirurgie* 1985; **40**:199–202.

4. **Gerberich, S. G., Priest, J. D., Boen, J. R., Straub, C. P.** and **Maxwell, R. E.** Concussion incidences and severity in secondary school varsity football players. *American Journal of Public Health* 1983; **73**:1370–5.

5. **Zemper, E.** Analysis of cerebral concussion frequency with the most common models of football helmets. *Journal of Athletic Training* 1994; **29**:44–50.

6. **Lindberg, R.** and **Freytag, E.** Brainstem lesions characteristics of traumatic hyperextension of the head. *Archives of Pathology and Laboratory Medicine* 1970; **90**:509–15.

7. **Dick, R. W.** A summary of head and neck injuries in collegiate athletes using the NCAA injury surveillance system. In *Head and neck injuries in sports* (ed. E. F. Hoerner). American Society for Testing and Materials, Philadelphia, 1994, 13–9.

8. **Cantu, R. C.** When to return to contact sports after a cerebral concussion. *Sports Medicine Digest* 1988; **10**: 1–2.

9. **Barth, J. T., Alves, W. M.** and **Thomas, V. R.** Mild head injury in sports. Neurophysical sequelae and recovery of function. In *Mild head injury* (ed. H. S. Levin, H. M. Eisenberg and A. L. Benton). Oxford University Press, New York, 1989: 257–75.

10. **Kelly, J. P., Nichols, J. S., Filley, C.M., Lillehei, K. O., Rubinstein, D.** and **Kleinschmidt-DeMasters, B. K.** Concussion in sports: guidelines for the prevention of catastrophic outcome. *Journal of the American Medical Association* 1991; **266**: 2867–9.

11. **Nelson, W. E., Jane, J. A.** and **Gieck, J. H.** Minor head injury in sport: a new classification and management. *The Physician and Sports Medicine* 1984; **12**:103–7.

12. **Torg, J. S.** *Athletic injuries to the head, neck and face.* Mosby Yearbook, St Louis, 1991.

13. **Gronwell, D.** and **Wrightson, P.** Delayed recovery of intellectual function after minor head injury. *Lancet* 1974; **ii**: 445–6.

14. **Symonds, C.** Concussion and its sequelae. *Lancet* 1962; **i**:1–5.

15. **Martland, H. S.** Punch drunk. *Journal of the American Medical Association* 1928; **91**:1103–7.

16. **Corsellis, J. A. N, Bruton, C. J.** and **Freeman-Browne, D.** The aftermath of boxing. *Psychological Medicine* 1973; **3**: 270–303.

17. **Guthkelch, A. N.** Post-traumatic amnesia, post-concussional symptoms and accident neurosis. *Acta Neurochirurgica Supplementum* 1979; **28**: 120–3.

18. **Pickles, W.** Acute general edema of the brain in children with head injuries. *New England Journal of Medicine* 1950; **242**: 607–11.

19. **Schnitker, M. T.** Syndrome of cerebral concussion in children. *Journal of Pediatrics* 1949; **35**: 557–60.

20. **Langfitt, T. W.** and **Kassell, N. F.** Cerebral vasodilatation produced by brain-stem stimulation: Neurogenic control vs autoregulation. *American Journal of Physiology* 1968; **215**: 90–7.

21. **Langfitt, T. W., Tannenbaum, H. M.** and **Kassell, N. F.** The etiology of acute brain swelling following experimental head injury. *Journal of Neurosurgery* 1966; **24**:47–56.

22. **Bowers, S. A.** and **Marshall, L. F.** Outcome in 200 consecutive cases of severe head injury treated in San Diego County: a prospective analysis. *Neurosurgery* 1980; **6**:237–42.

23. **Bruce, D. A. Schut, L., Bruno, L.A., Wood, J. H.** and **Sutton, L. N.** Outcome following severe head injuries in children. *Journal of Neurosurgery* 1978; **48**:679–88.

24. **Saunders, R. L.** and **Harbaugh, R. E.** Second impact in catastrophic contact-sports head trauma. *Journal of the American Medical Association* 1984; **252**:538–9.

25. **Schneider, R. C.** *Head and neck injuries in football.* Williams and Wilkins, Baltimore, 1973.

26. **Cantu, R. C.** Second impact syndrome: immediate management. *The Physician and Sports Medicine* 1992; **20**: 55–66.

27. **Cantu, R. C.** and **Voy, R.** Second impact syndrome a risk in any contact sport. *The Physician and Sports Medicine* 1995; **23**: 27–34.

28. **McQuillen, J. B., McQuillen, E. N.** and **Morrow, P.** Trauma, sports, and malignant cerebral edema. *American Journal of Forensic Medicine and Pathology* 1988; **9**:12–15.

29. **Moody, R. A., Raumsuke, S.** and **Mullen, S. F.** An evaluation of decompression in experimental head injury. *Journal of Neurosurgery* 1968; **29**: 586–90.

30. **Langfitt, T. W., Weinstein, J. D.** and **Kassell, N. F.** Cerebral vasomotor paralysis produced by intracranial hypertension. *Neurology* 1965; **15**: 622–41.

31. **Gentry, L. R., Godersky, J. C., Thompson, B.** and **Dunn, V. D.** Prospective comparative study of intermediate field MR and CT in the evaluation of closed head trauma. *American Journal of Neuroradiology* 1988; **150**: 673–82.

32. **Jenkins, A., Teasdale, G., Hadley, D.M., MacPherson, P.** and **Rowan, J. D.** Brain lesions detected by magnetic resonance imaging in mild and sever head injuries. *Lancet* 1986; **ii**: 445–6.

33. **Fekete, J. F.** Severe brain injury and death following rigid hockey accidents. The effectiveness of the "safety helmets" of amateur hockey players. *Canadian Medical Association Journal* 1968; **99**:1234–9.

34. **Herzog, R. J., Wiens, J. J., Dillingham, M. F.** and **Sontag, M. J.**. Normal cervical spine morphometry and cervical spinal stenosis in asymptomatic professional football players: Plain film radiography, multiplanar computed tomography, and magnetic resonance imaging. *Spine* 1991; **116**: S178–86.

35. **Feldick, H. G.** and **Albright, J. P.** Football survey reveals "missed" neck injuries. *The Physician and Sports Medicine* 1976; **4**: 77–81.

36. **Alexander, M. D., Davis, C. H.** and **Field, C. H.** Hyperextension injuries of the cervical spine. *Archives of Neurology and Psychiatry* 1958; **79**: 146–50.

37. **Eismont, F. J., Clifford, S., Goldberg, M.** and **Green, B.** Cervical sagittal spinal canal size in spine injury. *Spine* 1984; **9**: 663–6.

38. **Mayfield, F. H.** Neurosurgical aspects of cervical trauma. *Clinical Neurosurgery* 1955; **2**: 83–99.

39. **Penning, L.** Some aspects of plain radiography of the cervical spine in chronic myelopathy. *Neurology* (Minneapolis) 1962; **12**: 513–9.

40. **Wolfe, B. S., Khilnani, M.** and **Malis, L.** The sagittal diameter of the bony cervical spinal canal and its significance in cervical spondylosis. *Journal of Mt Sinai Hospital* 1956; **23**: 283–92.

41. **Matsuura, P., Waters, R. L., Atkins, R. H., Rothman, S., Gurbani, N.** and **Sie, I.** Comparison of computerized tomography parameters of the cervical spine in normal control subjects and spinal cord-injured patients. *Journal of Bone and Joint Surgery* 1989; **71**: 183–8.

42. **Cope, R.** and **Olson, S.** Abnormalities of the cervical spine in Down's syndrome: Diagnosis, risks, and review of the literature with particular reference to the Special Olympics. *Southern Medical Journal* 1987; **80**: 33–6.

43. **Rosenbaum, D. M., Blumhagen, J. D.** and **King, H. A.** Altantooccipital subluxation in Down's syndrome. *American Journal of Roentgenology* 1986; **146**: 1269–72.

Index